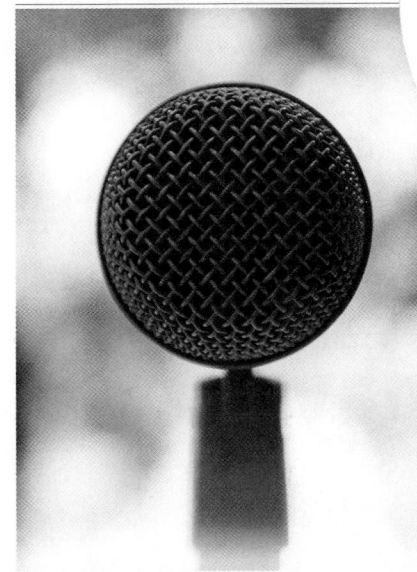

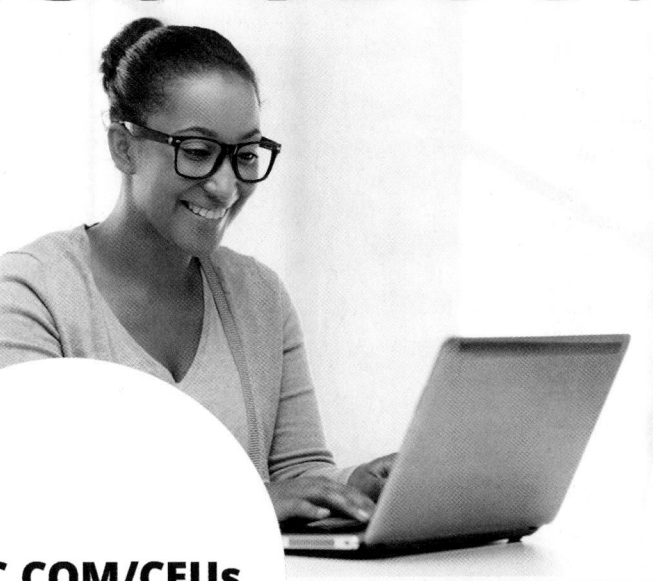

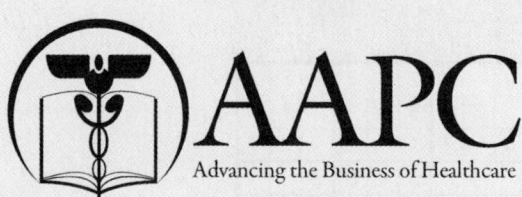

CHOOSING HOSPITAL CODING CREDENTIALS

AAPC now has two certifications representing both inpatient and outpatient hospital coding:

Let's compare to see which one is right for you.

COC

ertified Outpatient Coder (COC)
edicated exclusively
outpatient hospital/facility
ding.

DE SETS TO KNOW
T®, HCPCS Level II, and
D-10-CM

CIC

Certified Inpatient Coder (CIC)
Dedicated exclusively to inpatient hospital/facility coding.

CODE SETS TO KNOW
ICD-10-CM and ICD-10-PCS

LOCATION

COC: ork in a hospital/facility ASC

CIC: Work in a hospital/facility

SALARY

COC: ose who hold e COC™ edential — **Average** 58,822/yr

CIC: Those who hold the CIC™ credential — **Average** 56,544/yr

MEMBER STATS

COC: **11%** — % of AAPC members orking in a hospital tpatient setting.

CIC: **7.6%** — 7.6% of AAPC members working in a hospital inpatient setting

5					8			1
	8	7			1		2	6
		9		3			7	8
			9	4			5	
4	7	8				6		
9				8	6	1	4	7
			2	5				
	5	2	8		4			3
7				6		2	8	5

AAPC

AAPC.com/pcs-puzzle

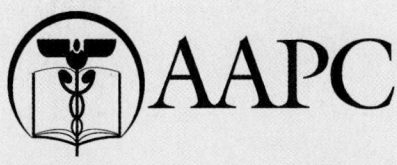

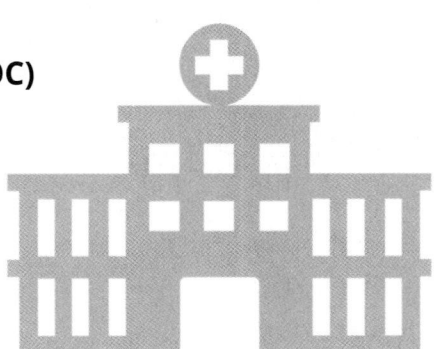

2017

ICD-10-PCS EXPERT

For Hospitals

AAPC
Advancing the Business of Healthcare

PUBLISHER'S NOTICE

AAPC'S COMMITMENT TO ACCURACY

This publisher is committed to providing our members accurate and reliable materials. However, codes and the guidelines by which they are applied change or are reinterpreted through the year. This book contains IPPS FY 2017 proposed rule data for CMS for symbols in the tables which was the latest information available at the time of printing. Visit www.aapc.com periodically for updates. To report corrections and updates, please contact AAPC Customer Service via 1-800-626-2633 or via email to code.books@aapc.com.

Images/Illustrations by the following artists at shutterstock.com:

miucci - 119473492 | ducu59us - 104022683, 125200733 | Alila Medical Media - 228843262, 155445686, 101696095, 96426923, 97755608, 97755611, 147943922, 125899358, 147943910, 155445662, 147943874, 108567068, 106263593, 106263560 | BlueRingMedia - 141162229, 141161560, 141161404 , 149006000, 145028440 | snapgalleria - 142194094 | okili77 - 156466463 | Designua - 180938618, 135935735, 186535475, 165084413 | stockshoppe - 99671552, 180896807, 180896810, 187162247, 187162193, 187162175, 187162163, 187162142, 187162118, 187162106, 187162070, 180896873, 180896855, 180896738, 180896720, 177791516, 177790997 | lotan - 186878060 | sciencepics - 199873508| Blamb - 24129706 | joshya - 226909492, 261971498 | Della_Liner - 324447776 | Marochkina Anastasiia - 414103342 | Alexander_P - 404964388

AAPC
Advancing the Business of Healthcare

ISBN: 978-1-626883-284

Table of Contents

Preface

Thank you for your purchase! We are pleased to offer you the 2017 ICD-10-PCS Complete Code Set.

This manual goes beyond the basics to help you code accurately and efficiently. In addition to including the official Alphabetic Index, Tables, and ICD-10-PCS Official Guidelines, we've crafted a select set of bonus features based on requests from coders in the field as well as the recommendations of our core group of veteran coding educators.

Our goal was to apply our unique approach to focusing on the practical application of the codes to this procedure coding manual. For instance, you will find an overview of the ICD-10-PCS code set as well as step-by-step instructions for assigning ICD-10-PCS codes, numerous examples, and practice exercises.

A few of the other features you'll benefit from page after page include the following:

- Procedures in the Medical and Surgical-related sections, including understanding root operations for various specialties and types of procedures, plenty of examples, and additional coding exercises
- Full illustrations of body systems at the front of the book so you don't have to search the manual for these large color images of body systems
- Medicare Code Edits, including gender edits and edits for limited coverage, noncovered procedures, HAC-associated procedures, combination clusters, and non-OR procedures affecting MS-DRG assignment
- Intuitive color-coded symbols and alerts identify critical coding and reimbursement issues quickly

See the complete List of Features to learn about everything this manual has to offer.

Rely on Our Combination of Official Sources and Experience

This manual includes the official ICD-10-PCS 2017 Alphabetic Index and Tables. We've also included the 2017 ICD-10-PCS Official Guidelines.

Additionally, our dedicated team drew on their years of experience using coding manuals to develop this manual's user friendly symbols, color coding, and tabs, all designed to help you find the information you need quickly.

Let Us Know What You Think

Our goal for this manual is to support those involved in the business side of healthcare, helping them to do their jobs and do them well. We'd appreciate your feedback, including your suggestions for what you'd like to see in an ICD-10-PCS resource, so we can be sure our manuals serve your needs. Thank you.

Changes for 2017

FY 2017 Update Summary

Change Summary Table

2016 Total	New Codes	Revised Titles	Deleted Codes	2017 Total
71,974	3,827	491	12	75,789

ICD-10-PCS Code FY 2017 Totals, By Section

Medical and Surgical	65,676
Obstetrics	300
Placement	861
Administration	1,427
Measurement and Monitoring	342
Extracorporeal Assistance and Performance	41
Extracorporeal Therapies	46
Osteopathic	100
Other Procedures	60
Chiropractic	90
Imaging	2,934
Nuclear Medicine	463
Radiation Oncology	1,939
Rehabilitation and Diagnostic Audiology	1,380
Mental Health	30
Substance Abuse Treatment	59
New Technology	41
Total	**75,789**

ICD-10-PCS Changes Highlights

- In the Medical and Surgical section, root operation definitions for the root operations Control and Creation revised
- In the Extracorporeal Therapies section, new root operation Perfusion created
- ICD-10-PCS guidelines revised in response to public comment and internal review
- Code conversion table, new file available for ICD-10-PCS

The following files provided in preparation for ICD-10 implementation will no longer be updated annually. The last updated versions of these files are posted with the FY 2016 update.

- ICD-10-PCS Reference Manual PDF
- Development of the ICD-10 Procedure Coding System (ICD-10-PCS) PDF
- ICD-10 Procedure Coding System PowerPoint slides

List of FY2017 Files Available from CMS

https://www.cms.gov/Medicare/Coding/ICD10/2017-ICD-10-PCS-and-GEMs.html

2017 Official ICD-10-PCS Coding Guidelines

- Guidelines B2.1a, B3.2, B3.4a, B3.6b, B3.6c, B3.7, B3.9, B4.2 and B4.4 revised in response to public comment and Cooperative Parties review.
- Downloadable PDF, file name **pcs_guidelines_2017.pdf**

2017 ICD-10-PCS Code Tables and Index (Zip file)

- Code tables valid for FY2017, no formatting changes.
- Downloadable PDF, file name **pcs_2017.pdf**
- Downloadable xml files for developers, file names **icd10pcs_tables_2017.xml, icd10pcs_index_2017.xml, icd10pcs_definitions_2017.xml**
- Accompanying schema for developers, file names **icd10pcs_tables_2017.xsd, icd10pcs_index_2017.xsd, icd10pcs_definitions_2017.xsd**

2017 ICD-10-PCS Codes File (Zip file)

- ICD-10-PCS Codes file is a simple format for nontechnical uses, containing the valid FY 2017 ICD-10-PCS codes and their long titles.
- File is in text file format, file name is **icd10pcs_codes_2017.txt**
- Accompanying documentation for codes file, file name is **icd10pcsCodesFile.pdf**
- Codes file addenda in text format, file name is **codes_addenda_2017.txt**

2017 ICD-10-PCS Order File (Long and Abbreviated Titles) (Zip file)

- ICD-10-PCS order file is for developers, provides a unique five-digit "order number" for each ICD-10-PCS table and code, as well as a long and abbreviated code title.
- ICD-10-PCS order file name is **icd10pcs_order_2017.txt**
- Accompanying documentation for tabular order file, file name is **icd10pcsOrderFile.pdf**
- Tabular order file addenda in text format, file name is **order_addenda_2017.txt**

2017 ICD-10-PCS Final Addenda (Zip file)

- Addenda files in downloadable PDF, file names are **tables_addenda_2017.pdf, index_addenda_2017.pdf, definitions_addenda_2017.pdf**
- Addenda files also in machine readable text format for developers, file names **tables_addenda_2017.txt, index_addenda_2017.txt, definitions_addenda_2017.txt**

2017 NEW ICD-10-PCS Conversion Table (Zip file)

- ICD-10-PCS code conversion table is provided to assist users in data retrieval, in downloadable Excel spreadsheet, file name is **icd10pcs_conversion_table_2017.xlsx**
- Accompanying documentation for code conversion table, file name is **icd10pcsConversionTable.pdf**

List of Features

ICD-10-PCS is essential to documenting medical necessity for services rendered, and accurate codes mean better outcomes for the patient, your claims, and your facility.

You can count on this manual to help you choose and report the right ICD-10-PCS code. Unique features, intuitive design, and expert features that coders developed assure this manual will keep your coding on target.

This manual includes the ICD-10-PCS Alphabetic Index and ICD-10-PCS Tables for procedures, effective October 1, 2016 (FY 2017 code set).

To help you make the most of manual, it also includes the following features:

- Introduction to ICD-10-PCS, including the history of ICD-10-PCS, explanations of ICD-10-PCS codes, code structures, design, additional characteristics, and applications
- Procedures in the Medical and Surgical section, including understanding root operations to better help you to choose the right code, along with examples and coding exercises to test your understanding
- Procedures in the Medical and Surgical-related sections, including understanding root operations for various specialties and types of procedures, plenty of examples, and additional coding exercises
- Procedures in the Ancillary sections, including understanding root operations for various ancillary procedures, including imaging, nuclear medicine, radiation therapy, physical rehabilitation, mental health, and substance abuse, many examples, and more practice exercises
- ICD-10-PCS Official Conventions and additional conventions and symbols you'll find in this manual
- ICD-10-PCS Official Guidelines for Coding and Reporting, effective October 1, 2016 (FY 2017)
- Full illustrations of body systems at the front of the book so you don't have to search the manual for these large color images of body systems
- Medicare Code Edits, including gender edits and edits for limited coverage, noncovered procedures, hospital acquired conditions (HAC) associated procedures, combination clusters, and non-OR procedures affecting or not affecting MS-DRG assignment
- Intuitive color-coded symbols and alerts identify critical coding and reimbursement issues quickly
- Appendices for root operations definitions, body part key, device key and aggregation table, character meaning, substance key, and combination clusters
- A user-friendly page design, including dictionary-style headers, colored bleed tabs, and legend keys

Official Conventions and Additional Conventions Specific to this ICD-10-PCS Manual

This manual includes the procedure code set from the International Classification of Diseases, 10th Revision, Procedure Coding System (ICD-10-PCS). Hospitals and third party payers use these codes to classify inpatient procedures.

Official Conventions

Index

Refer to the ICD-10-PCS Index to access the Tables in the manual. The Index mirrors the structure of the Tables, so it follows a consistent pattern of organization and use of hierarchies. The Index is organized as an alphabetic lookup.

Two types of main terms are listed in the Index:

- Based on the value of the third character, such as a root operation (excision, insertion)
- Lists common procedure terms

Main terms

For the Medical and Surgical and related sections, the root operation values are used as main terms in the Index. In other sections, the values representing the general type of procedure performed, such as nuclear medicine or imaging type, are listed as main terms.

For the Medical and Surgical and related sections, values such as Excision, Bypass, and Transplantation are included as main terms in the Index. The applicable body system entries are listed beneath the main term and refer to a specific table. For the ancillary sections, values such as Fluoroscopy and Positron Emission Tomography, are listed as main terms.

To find the code to cross-reference to the Tables, search for the root operation for the procedure in the Index, followed by the subterm for the anatomic site or the subterm that further describes the procedure. Locate the partial code, and cross-reference it to the Table that matches the first three characters of the code.

Tables

The Tables are organized in alphanumeric order in a series by Section, which is the first character of a code. Tables that begin with 0 to 9 are listed first, then tables beginning with B-D, then letters F-X, are listed next.

The same convention is followed within each table for the second through the seventh characters—numeric values in order first, followed by alphabetical values in order.

The Medical and Surgical section (first character 0) is organized by body system values. Each body system subdivision in the Medical and Surgical section contains tables that list the valid root operations for that body system. These are the root operation tables that form the system. These tables provide the valid choices of values available to construct a code.

The root operation tables consist of four columns and a varying number of rows, as in the following example of the root operation Bypass, in the Central Nervous body system.

The values for characters 1 through 3 are provided at the top of each table.

Character 1:	0: MEDICAL AND SURGICAL (Section)
Character 2:	0: CENTRAL NERVOUS (Body system)
Character 3:	1: BYPASS: Altering the route of passage of the contents of a tubular body part (Root operation)

Four columns contain the applicable values for characters 4 through 7, given the values in characters 1 through 3:

Body Part Character 4	Approach Character 5	Device Character 6	Qualifier Character 7
6 Cerebral Ventricle	**0** Open **3** Percutaneous	**7** Autologous Tissue Substitute **J** Synthetic Substitute **K** Nonautologous Tissue Substitute	**0** Nasopharynx **1** Mastoid Sinus **2** Atrium **3** Blood Vessel **4** Pleural Cavity **5** Intestine **6** Peritoneal Cavity **7** Urinary Tract **8** Bone Marrow **B** Cerebral Cisterns
U Spinal Canal	**0** Open **3** Percutaneous	**7** Autologous Tissue Substitute **J** Synthetic Substitute **K** Nonautologous Tissue Substitute	**4** Pleural Cavity **6** Peritoneal Cavity **7** Urinary Tract **9** Fallopian Tube

A table may be separated into rows to specify the valid choices of values in characters 4 through 7. A code built using values from more than one row of a table is not a valid code.

Refer to the ICD-10-PCS Overview section in this manual for detailed guidance on assigning ICD-10-PCS codes.

See Reference

The See reference directs you to go elsewhere in the Index to find the root operation that you need.

Use Reference

The Use reference directs you to a character value selection as an additional reference.

Additional Conventions

Additional conventions that you will find in the Tables in this manual include Medicare Code Edits - Symbols and Brackets.

Medicare Code Edits – Symbols Applied to 4th Characters

LC Limited Coverage

Procedures that are medically complex and serious in nature that incur extraordinary associated costs. Medicare limits coverage to a portion of the cost.

NC Noncovered

Procedures for which Medicare does not typically reimburse.

HAC HAC-associated procedure

Procedures that are associated with hospital-acquired conditions (HAC).

CC Combination Cluster

The procedure is part of a procedure code combination, or cluster, listed in Appendix G of this manual. Medicare does not typically pay for these procedures unless you report them with other specific procedures.

DRG Non-OR-Affecting MS-DRG Assignment

Non-operating room procedures which affect MS-DRG assignment for claims reporting.

⦸ Non-OR-Not Affecting MS-DRG Assignment

Non-operating room procedures which do NOT affect MS-DRG assignment for claims reporting. Codes with this symbol can be from any tables within PCS and are not only limited to medical/surgical or obstetrical procedures.

New/Revised Text in **Orange**

Procedure text was new or revised from the last version of the code set. For new codes, orange text will be shown for all characters in the code. New codes may be shown as their own row in a table and characters 4-7 may be shown in a row that is separate from other characters within that table.

♂ Male

Male procedure only

♀ Female

Female procedure only

Code Lists

Codes that are applicable to each type of symbol in the book are listed after each table.

ICD-10-PCS Overview

The International Classification of Diseases Tenth Revision Procedure Coding System (ICD -10-PCS) was created to accompany the World Health Organization's (WHO) ICD-10 diagnosis classification. The new procedure coding system was developed to replace ICD-9-CM procedure codes for reporting inpatient procedures.

Unlike the ICD-9-CM classification, ICD-10-PCS was designed to enable each code to have a standard structure and be very descriptive, and yet flexible enough to accommodate future needs. Information about the structure, organization, and application of ICD-10-PCS codes, along with reference material for coding with ICD-10-PCS, is provided in this manual.

This overview contains the following parts:

- What is ICD-10-PCS?
  - History of ICD-10-PCS
  - ICD-9-CM Volume 3 Compared with ICD-10-PCS
- ICD-10-PCS Code Structure
- ICD-10-PCS System Organization
- ICD-10-PCS Design
- ICD-10-PCS Additional Characteristics
- ICD-10-PCS Applications

More specific information on coding with ICD-10-PCS is found in other sections of this manual.

What is ICD-10-PCS?

ICD -10-PCS is a procedure coding system that will be used to collect data, determine payment, and support the electronic health record for all inpatient procedures performed in the United States.

History of ICD-10-PCS

The World Health Organization has maintained the International Classification of Diseases (ICD) for recording cause of death since 1893. It has updated the ICD periodically to reflect new discoveries in epidemiology and changes in medical understanding of disease.

The International Classification of Diseases Tenth Revision (ICD-10), published in 1992, is the latest revision of the ICD. The WHO authorized the National Center for Health Statistics (NCHS) to develop a clinical modification of ICD-10 for use in the United States. This version of ICD-10 is called ICD-10-CM. ICD-10-CM is intended to replace the previous U.S. clinical modification, ICD-9-CM, that has been in use since 1979. ICD-9-CM contains a procedure classification; ICD-10-CM does not.

The Centers for Medicare and Medicaid Services, the agency responsible for maintaining the inpatient procedure code set in the U.S., contracted with 3M Health Information Systems in 1993 to design and then develop a procedure classification system to replace Volume 3 of ICD-9-CM. ICD-10-PCS is the result.

ICD-10-PCS was initially released in 1998. It has been updated annually since that time.

ICD-9-CM Volume 3 Compared With ICD-10-PCS

With ICD-10 implementation, the U.S. clinical modification of the ICD will not include a procedure classification based on the same principles of organization as the diagnosis classification. Instead, a separate procedure coding system has been developed to meet the rigorous and varied demands that are made of coded data in the healthcare industry. This represents a significant step toward building a health information infrastructure that functions optimally in the electronic age.

The following information highlights some of the basic differences between ICD-9-CM Volume 3 and ICD-10-PCS:

ICD-9-CM Volume 3

- Follows ICD structure (designed for diagnosis coding)
- Codes available as a fixed/finite set in list form
- Codes are numeric
- Codes are 3 through 4 digits long

ICD-10-PCS

- Designed/developed to meet healthcare needs for a procedure code system
- Codes constructed from flexible code components (values) using tables
- Codes are alphanumeric
- All codes are seven characters long

ICD-10-PCS Code Structure

Undergirding ICD-10-PCS is a logical, consistent structure that informs the system as a whole, down to the level of a single code. This means that the process of constructing codes in ICD-10-PCS is also logical and consistent: individual letters and numbers, called "values," are selected in sequence to occupy the seven spaces of the code, called "characters."

Characters

All codes in ICD-10-PCS are seven characters long. Each character in the seven-character code represents an aspect of the procedure, as shown in the following diagram of characters from the main section of ICD-10-PCS, called Medical and Surgical.

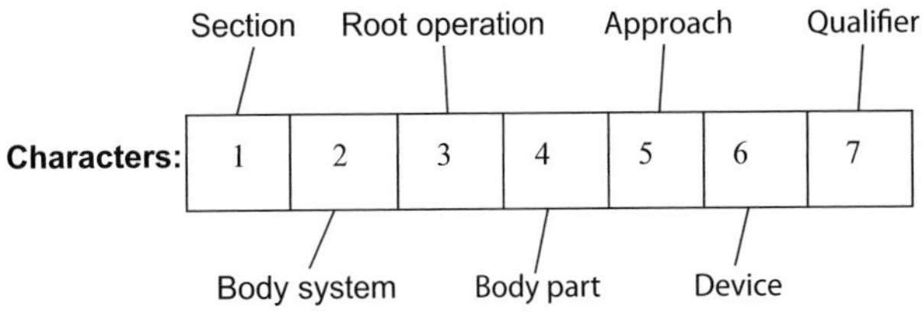

An ICD-10-PCS code is best understood as the result of a process rather than as an isolated, fixed quantity. The process consists of assigning values from among the valid choices for that part of the system, according to the rules governing the construction of codes.

Values

One of 34 possible values can be assigned to each character in a code: the numbers 0 through 9 and the alphabet (except I and O, because they are easily confused with the numbers 1 and 0). A finished code looks like the example below.

```
02103D4
```

This code is derived by choosing a specific value for each of the seven characters. Based on details about the procedure performed, values for each character specifying the section, body system, root operation, body part, approach, device, and qualifier are assigned.

Because the definition of each character is a function of its physical position in the code, the same value placed in a different position in the code means something different. The value 0 in the first character means something different than 0 in the second character, or 0 in the third character, and so on.

Code Structure: Medical and Surgical Section

The following pages define each character using the code 0LB50ZZ, "Excision of right lower arm and wrist tendon, open approach" as an example. This example comes from the Medical and Surgical section of ICD-10-PCS.

Character 1: Section

The first character in the code determines the broad procedure category, or section, where the code is found. In this example, the section is Medical and Surgical. 0 is the value that represents Medical and Surgical in the first character.

For definitions of characters used in the Medical and Surgical section, please refer to the Glossary.

The sample code looks like this so far:

Character 1 Section
Medical and Surgical
0

Character 2: Body System

The second character defines the body system—the general physiological system or anatomical region involved. Examples of body systems include Lower Arteries, Central Nervous System, and Respiratory System. In this example, the body system is Tendons, represented by the value L.

Character 1 Section	Character 2 Body System
Medical and Surgical	Tendons
0	L

Character 3: Root Operation

The third character defines the root operation, or the objective of the procedure. Some examples of root operations are Bypass, Drainage, and Reattachment. In the sample code below, the root operation is Excision. When used in the third character of the code, the value B represents Excision.

Character 1 Section	Character 2 Body System	Character 3 Root Operation
Medical and Surgical	Tendons	Excision
0	L	B

For the complete list of root operations and their definitions, please refer to ICD-10-PCS definitions.

Character 4: Body Part

The fourth character defines the body part, or specific anatomical site where the procedure was performed. The body system (second character) provides only a general indication of the procedure site. The body part and body system values together provide a precise description of the procedure site.

Examples of body parts are Kidney, Tonsils, and Thymus. In this example, the body part value is 5, Lower Arm and Wrist, Right. When the second character is L, the value 5 when used in the fourth character of the code represents the right lower arm and wrist tendon.

Character 1 Section	Character 2 Body System	Character 3 Root Operation	Character 4 Body Part
Medical and Surgical	Tendons	Excision	Lower Arm and Wrist, Right
0	L	B	5

Character 5: Approach

The fifth character defines the approach, or the technique used to reach the procedure site. Seven different approach values are used in the Medical and Surgical section to define the approach. Examples of approaches include Open and Percutaneous Endoscopic.

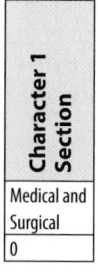

In the sample code below, the approach is Open and is represented by the value 0.

Character 1 Section	Character 2 Body System	Character 3 Root Operation	Character 4 Body Part	Character 5 Approach
Medical and Surgical	Tendons	Excision	Lower Arm and Wrist, Right	Open
0	L	B	5	0

For the complete list of approaches and their definitions, please refer to ICD-10-PCS definitions.

Character 6: Device

Depending on the procedure performed, there may or may not be a device left in place at the end of the procedure. The sixth character defines the device. Device values fall into four basic categories:

- Grafts and Prostheses
- Implants
- Simple or Mechanical Appliances
- Electronic Appliances

In this example, there is no device used in the procedure. The value Z is used to represent No Device, as shown below.

Character 1 Section	Character 2 Body System	Character 3 Root Operation	Character 4 Body Part	Character 5 Approach	Character 6 Device
Medical and Surgical	Tendons	Excision	Lower Arm and Wrist, Right	Open	No Device
0	L	B	5	0	Z

Character 7: Qualifier

The seventh character defines a qualifier for the code. A qualifier specifies an additional attribute of the procedure, if applicable.

Examples of qualifiers include Diagnostic and Stereotactic. Qualifier choices vary depending on the previous values selected. In this example, there is no specific qualifier applicable to this procedure, so the value is No Qualifier, represented by the letter Z.

Character 1 Section	Character 2 Body System	Character 3 Root Operation	Character 4 Body Part	Character 5 Approach	Character 6 Device	Character 7 Qualifier
Medical and Surgical	Tendons	Excision	Lower Arm and Wrist, Right	Open	No Device	No Qualifier
0	L	B	5	0	Z	Z

0LB50ZZ is the complete specification of the procedure "Excision of right lower arm and wrist tendon, open approach."

ICD-10-PCS System Organization

ICD-10-PCS is composed of 16 sections, represented by the numbers 0 through 9 and the letters B through D and F through H. The broad procedure categories contained in these sections range from surgical procedures to substance abuse treatment.

Medical and Surgical section

The first section, Medical and Surgical, contains the great majority of procedures typically reported in an inpatient setting. As shown in the previous section discussing ICD -10-PCS code structure, all procedure codes in the Medical and Surgical section begin with the section value 0.

Character 1 Section	Character 2 Body System	Character 3 Root Operation	Character 4 Body Part	Character 5 Approach	Character 6 Device	Character 7 Qualifier
Medical and Surgical	Tendons	Excision	Lower Arm and Wrist, Right	Open	No Device	No Qualifier
0	L	B	5	0	Z	Z

More complete information on coding procedures in the Medical and Surgical section is found in Procedures in the Medical and Surgical section.

Medical and Surgical-related sections

Sections 1 through 9 of ICD-10-PCS comprise the Medical and Surgical-related sections. These sections include obstetrical procedures, administration of substances, measurement and monitoring of body functions, and extracorporeal therapies, as listed below.

- Section 1: Obstetrics
- Section 2: Placement
- Section 3: Administration
- Section 4: Measurement and Monitoring
- Section 5: Extracorporeal Assistance and Performance
- Section 6: Extracorporeal Therapies
- Section 7: Osteopathic
- Section 8: Other Procedures
- Section 9: Chiropractic

In sections 1 and 2, all seven characters define the same aspects of the procedure as in the Medical and Surgical section.

Codes in sections 3 through 9 are structured for the most part like their counterparts in the Medical and Surgical section, with a few exceptions. For example, in sections 5 and 6, the fifth character is defined as duration instead of approach, as in this code for intra-aortic balloon pump (IABP):

Character 1 Section	Character 2 Body System	Character 3 Root Operation	Character 4 Body Part	Character 5 Approach	Character 6 Device	Character 7 Qualifier
Extracorp. Assist. and Performance	Physiological Systems	Assistance	Cardiac	Continuous	Output	Balloon Pump
5	A	0	2	2	1	0

Additional differences include these uses of the sixth character:

- Section 3 defines the sixth character as substance.
- Sections 4 and 5 define the sixth character as function.
- Sections 7 through 9 define the sixth character as method.

More complete information on coding procedures in the Medical and Surgical-related sections is found in Procedures in the Medical and Surgical-related sections.

Ancillary sections

Sections B through D and F through H comprise the ancillary sections of ICD-10-PCS. These six sections include imaging procedures, nuclear medicine, and substance abuse treatment, as listed in the following table.

- Section B: Imaging
- Section C: Nuclear Medicine
- Section D: Radiation Therapy
- Section F: Physical Rehabilitation and Diagnostic Audiology
- Section G: Mental Health
- Section H: Substance Abuse Treatment

The definitions of some characters in the ancillary sections differs from that seen in previous sections. In the Imaging section, the third character is defined as type, and the fifth and sixth characters define contrast and contrast/qualifier respectively, as in the CT scan example below.

Character 1 Section	Character 2 Body System	Character 3 Type	Character 4 Body Part	Character 5 Contrast	Character 6 Qualifier	Character 7 Qualifier
Imaging	Central Nervous	Computerized Tomography	Brain	High Osmolar	Unenhanced and Enhanced	None
B	0	2	0	0	0	Z

Additional differences include:

- Section C defines the fifth character as radionuclide.
- Section D defines the fifth character as modality qualifier and the sixth character as isotope.
- Section F defines the fifth character as type qualifier and the sixth character as equipment.
- Sections G and H define the third character as a type qualifier.

More complete information on coding procedures in the ancillary sections is found in Procedures in the ancillary sections.

Tables

The complete ICD-10-PCS is presented in three parts: the Tables, the Index, and the Definition.

The Tables are organized in a series, beginning with section 0, Medical and Surgical, and body system 0, Central Nervous, and proceeding in numerical order. Sections 0 through 9 are followed by sections B through D and F through H. The same convention is followed within each table for the second through the seventh characters—numeric values in order first, followed by alphabetical values in order.

The following examples use the Medical and Surgical section to describe the organization and format of the ICD-10-PCS Tables.

The Medical and Surgical section (first character 0) is organized by its 31 body system values. Each body system subdivision in the Medical and Surgical section contains tables that list the valid root operations for that body system. These are the root operation tables that form the system. These tables provide the valid choices of values available to construct a code.

The root operation tables consist of four columns and a varying number of rows, as in the following example of the root operation Bypass, in the Central Nervous body system.

The values for characters 1 through 3 are provided at the top of each table.

0: MEDICAL AND SURGICAL (Section)
0: CENTRAL NERVOUS (Body system)
1: BYPASS: Altering the route of passage of the contents of a tubular body part (Root operation)

Four columns contain the applicable values for characters 4 through 7, given the values in characters 1 through 3.

Body Part Character 4	Approach Character 5	Device Character 6	Qualifier Character 7
6 Cerebral Ventricle	0 Open	7 Autologous Tissue Substitute J Synthetic Substitute K Nonautologous Tissue Substitute	0 Nasopharynx 1 Mastoid Sinus 2 Atrium 3 Blood Vessel 4 Pleural Cavity 5 Intestine 6 Peritoneal Cavity 7 Urinary Tract 8 Bone Marrow B Cerebral Cisterns
U Spinal Canal	0 Open	7 Autologous Tissue Substitute J Synthetic Substitute K Nonautologous Tissue Substitute	4 Pleural Cavity 6 Peritoneal Cavity 7 Urinary Tract 9 Fallopian Tube

A table may be separated into rows to specify the valid choices of values in characters 4 through 7. A code built using values from more than one row of a table is not a valid code.

Index

The ICD-10-PCS Index can be used to access the Tables. The Index mirrors the structure of the Tables, so it follows a consistent pattern of organization and use of hierarchies.

The Index is organized as an alphabetic lookup. Two types of main terms are listed in the Index:

- Based on the value of the third character
- Common procedure terms

Main terms

For the Medical and Surgical and related sections, the root operation values are used as main terms in the Index. In other sections, the values representing the general type of procedure performed, such as nuclear medicine or imaging type, are listed as main terms.

For the Medical and Surgical and related sections, values such as Excision, Bypass, and Transplantation are included as main terms in the Index. The applicable body system entries are listed beneath the main term, and refer to a specific table. For the ancillary sections, values such as Fluoroscopy and Positron Emission Tomography are listed as main terms.

In the example below, the index entry "Bypass" refers to the Medical and Surgical section tables for all applicable body systems, including Anatomical Regions and Central Nervous System.

Bypass

```
by Body System
  Anatomical Regions 0W1....
  Central Nervous System 001....
```

The body system listings may be followed by entries for specific body parts, as in the excerpt below. In the root operations Change, Insertion, Removal, and Revision, the device entries follow the body system listings.

```
by Body Part
  Artery
    Aorta, Abdominal 0410...
    Aorta, Thoracic 021W...
    Axillary 031....
    Brachial 031....
    Common Carotid 031....
```

Common procedure terms

The second type of term listed in the Index uses procedure names, such as "appendectomy" or "fundoplication." These entries are listed as main terms, and refer to a table or tables from which a valid code can be constructed, as shown in the following example.

Cholecystectomy

```
- see Excision, Hepatobiliary System &
Pancreas 0FB....

- see Resection, Hepatobiliary System &
Pancreas 0FT....
```

Definitions

The ICD-10-PCS Definitions contain the official definitions of ICD-10-PCS values in characters 3 through 7 of the seven-character code, and may also provide additional explanation or examples. The definitions are arranged in section order and designate the section and the character within the section being defined.

The Medical and Surgical section body part value definitions refer from the body part value to corresponding anatomical terms. The Medical and Surgical section device definitions refer from the device value to corresponding device terms or manufacturer's names. The Substance value definitions in the Administration section refer from the substance value to a common substance name or manufacturer's substance name. These definitions are also sorted by common term and listed separately as the Body Part Key, Device Key, and Substance Key respectively.

The ICD-10-PCS Device Aggregation Table contains entries that correlate a specific ICD-10-PCS device value with a general device value to be used in tables containing only general device values.

Tabular Order File

The ICD-10-PCS Order file contains a unique "order number" for each valid code or table "header," a flag distinguishing valid codes from headers, and both long and abbreviated title descriptions combined in a single file.

The code descriptions are generated using rules that produce standardized, complete, and easy-to-read code descriptions.

ICD-10-PCS Design

ICD-10-PCS is fundamentally different from ICD-9-CM in its structure, organization, and capabilities. It was designed and developed to adhere to recommendations made by the National Committee on Vital and Health Statistics (NCVHS). It also incorporates input from a wide range of organizations, individual physicians, healthcare professionals, and researchers.

Several structural attributes were recommended for a new procedure coding system. These attributes include

- Multiaxial structure
- Completeness
- Expandability

Multiaxial Structure

The key attribute that provides the framework for all other structural attributes is multiaxial code structure. Multiaxial code structure makes it possible for the ICD-10-PCS to be complete, expandable, and to provide a high degree of flexibility and functionality.

As mentioned earlier, ICD-10-PCS codes are composed of seven characters. Each character represents a category of information that can be specified about the procedure performed. A character defines both the category of information and its physical position in the code.

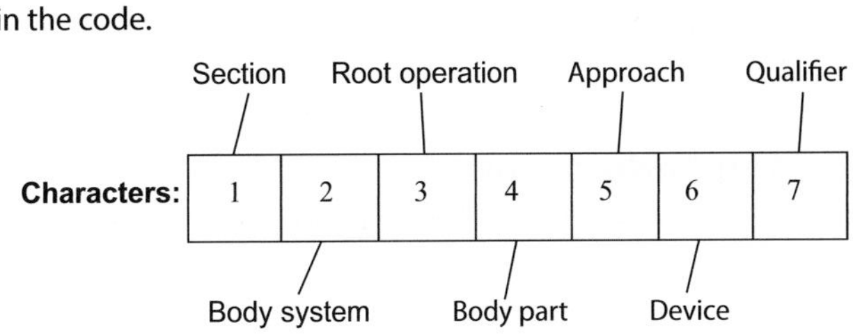

A character's position can be understood as a semi-independent axis of classification that allows different specific values to be inserted into that space, and whose physical position remains stable. Within a defined code range, a character retains the general meaning that it confers on any value in that position. For example, the fifth character retains the general meaning "approach" in sections 0 through 4 and 7 through 9 of the system. Any specific value in the fifth character will define a specific approach, such as Open.

Each group of values for a character contains all of the valid choices in relation to the other characters of the code, giving the system completeness. In the fifth character, for example, each significantly distinct approach is assigned its own approach value and all applicable approach values are included to represent the possible versions of a procedure.

Each group of values for a character can be added to as needed, giving the system expandability. If a significantly distinct approach is used to perform procedures, a new approach value can be added to the system.

Each group of values is confined to its own character, giving ICD -10-PCS a stable, predictable readability across a wide range of codes. In sections 0 through 4 and 7 through 9 of the system, for example, the fifth character always represents the approach.

ICD-10-PCS' multiaxial structure houses its capacity for completeness, expandability, and flexibility, giving it a high degree of functionality for multiple uses.

Completeness

Completeness is considered a key structural attribute for a new procedure coding system. The specific recommendation for completeness includes these characteristics:

- A unique code is available for each significantly different procedure.
- Each code retains its unique definition. Codes are not reused.

In Volume 3 of ICD-9-CM, procedures performed on many different body parts using different approaches or devices may be assigned to the same procedure code. In ICD-10-PCS, a unique code can be constructed for every significantly different procedure.

Within each section, a character defines a consistent component of a code, and contains all applicable values for that character. The values define individual expressions (open, percutaneous) of the character's general meaning (approach) that are then used to construct unique procedure codes.

Because all approaches by which a procedure is performed are assigned a separate approach value in the system, every procedure which uses a different approach will have its own unique code. This is true of the other characters as well. The same procedure performed on a different body part has its own unique code, the same procedure performed using a different device has its own unique code, and so on.

Coronary bypass example

In the case of the coronary artery bypass graft (CABG), ICD-9-CM contains a total of nine codes to describe different versions of the procedure. These codes specify the version based on one aspect of the procedure, and the aspect defined is not consistent for all nine codes. Four of the codes specify the number of coronary arteries bypassed, four specify the source of the new blood flow, and one is an "unspecified" choice.

By contrast, ICD-10-PCS components can be combined to produce 34 unique codes defining all significantly different versions of the comparable CABG procedure. All 34 codes specify the same four aspects of the procedure: the number of coronary artery sites bypassed, the approach to the procedure site, the type of graft if used, and the origin of the bypass (source of the new blood flow). The differences are summarized below.

Table 1. Comparison of CABG procedure codes

ICD-9-CM Volume 3	ICD-10-PCS
36.11	021009W
Aortocoronary Bypass of One Coronary Artery (1 of 4)	Bypass Coronary Artery, One Site to Aorta with Autologous Venous Tissue, Open Approach (1 of 8)
36.15	02100Z8
Single Internal Mammary- Coronary Artery Bypass (1 of 2)	Bypass Coronary Artery, One Site to Right Internal Mammary, Open Approach (1 of 16)
ICD-9-CM Volume 3	**ICD-10-PCS**
36.17	02100AF
Abdominal-Coronary Artery Bypass (1 of 2)	Bypass Coronary Artery, One Site to Abdominal Artery with Autologous Arterial Tissue, Open Approach (1 of 10)
36.10	No Equivalent
Aortocoronary Bypass for Heart Revascularization, Not Otherwise Specified (1 of 1)	ICD-10-PCS codes all contain a minimum level of specificity

Unique definitions

Because ICD-10-PCS codes are constructed of individual values rather than lists of fixed codes and text descriptions, the unique, stable definition of a code in the system is retained. New values may be added to the system to represent a specific new approach or device or qualifier, but whole codes by design cannot be given new meanings and reused.

Expandability

Expandability was also recommended as a key structural attribute. The specific recommendation for expandability includes these characteristics:

- Accommodate new procedures and technologies
- Add new codes without disrupting the existing structure

ICD- 10-PCS is designed to be easily updated as new codes are required for new procedures and new techniques. Changes to ICD-10-PCS can all be made within the existing structure, because whole codes are not added. Instead, one of two possible changes is made to the system:

- A new value for a character is added as needed to the system.
- An existing value for a character is added to a table(s) in the system.

ICD-10-PCS update: PICVA

An example of how the updating of ICD-10-PCS works can be seen in the coronary artery bypass procedure called Percutaneous in-situ coronary venous arterialization (PICVA). This procedure is no more invasive than a percutaneous coronary angioplasty, but achieves the benefits of a bypass procedure by placing a specialized stent into the diseased coronary artery, through its wall into the adjacent coronary vein, and diverting blood flow through the stent into the artery past the blockage.

ICD-10-PCS was updated in 2004 to include an appropriate range of codes for the PICVA procedure (16 possible codes). This was accomplished simply by adding another row to the relevant table (as shown in the example below) containing two approach values for the non-invasive approach, two device values for the possible types of stent, and a single qualifier defining the coronary vein as the source of the new blood flow, as in the example below.

The values for characters 1 through 3 at the top of each table are

0: MEDICAL AND SURGICAL (Section)
2: HEART AND GREAT VESSELS (Body system)
1: BYPASS: Altering the route of passage of the contents of a tubular body part

Body Part Character 4	Approach Character 5	Device Character 6	Qualifier Character 7
0 Coronary Artery, One Artery 1 Coronary Artery, Two Arteries 2 Coronary Artery, Three Arteries 3 Coronary Artery, Four or More Arteries	3 Percutaneous 4 Percutaneous Endoscopic	4 Drug-eluting Intraluminal Device D Intraluminal Device	D Coronary Vein

Structural integrity

As shown in the previous example, ICD-10-PCS can be easily expanded without disrupting the structure of the system.

In the PICVA example, one new value—the qualifier value Coronary Vein—was added to the system to effect this change. All other values in the new row are existing values used to create unique, new codes.

This type of updating can be replicated anywhere in the system when a change is required. ICD-10-PCS allows unique new codes to be added to the system because values for the seven characters that make up a code can be combined as needed. The system can evolve as medical technology and clinical practice evolve, without disrupting the ICD-10-PCS structure.

ICD-10-PCS Additional Characteristics

ICD-10-PCS possesses several additional characteristics in response to government and industry recommendations. These characteristics are

- Standardized terminology within the coding system
- Standardized level of specificity
- No diagnostic information
- No explicit "not otherwise specified" (NOS) code options
- Limited use of "not elsewhere classified" (NEC) code options

Standardized Terminology

Words commonly used in clinical vocabularies may have multiple meanings. This can cause confusion and result in inaccurate data. ICD-10-PCS is standardized and self-contained. Characters and values used in the system are defined in the system.

For example, the word "excision" is used to describe a wide variety of surgical procedures. In ICD-10-PCS, the word "excision" describes a single, precise surgical objective, defined as "Cutting out or off, without replacement, a portion of a body part."

For the complete list of root operations and their definitions, please refer to ICD-10-PCS definitions.

No eponyms or common procedure names

The terminology used in ICD-10-PCS is standardized to provide precise and stable definitions of all procedures performed. This standardized terminology is used in all ICD-10-PCS code descriptions.

As a result, ICD-10-PCS code descriptions do not include eponyms or common procedure names. Two examples from ICD-9-CM are 22.61, "Excision of lesion of maxillary sinus with Caldwell-Luc approach," and 51.10, "Endoscopic retrograde cholangiopancreatography [ERCP]." In ICD-10-PCS, physicians' names are not included in a code description, nor are procedures identified by common terms or acronyms such as appendectomy or CABG. Instead, such procedures are coded to the root operation that accurately identifies the objective of the procedure.

The procedures described in the preceding paragraph by ICD-9-CM codes are coded in ICD-10-PCS according to the root operation that matches the objective of the procedure. Here the ICD - 10-PCS equivalents would be Excision and Inspection respectively. By relying on the universal objectives defined in root operations rather than eponyms or specific procedure titles that change or become obsolete, ICD-10-PCS preserves the capacity to define past, present, and future procedures accurately using stable terminology in the form of characters and values.

No combination codes

With rare exceptions, ICD-10-PCS does not define multiple procedures with one code. This is to preserve standardized terminology and consistency across the system. Procedures that are typically performed together but are distinct procedures

may be defined by a single "combination code" in ICD-9-CM. An example of a combination code in ICD-9-CM is 28.3, "Tonsillectomy with adenoidectomy."

A procedure that meets the reporting criteria for a separate procedure is coded separately in ICD-10-PCS. This allows the system to respond to changes in technology and medical practice with the maximum degree of stability and flexibility.

Standardized Level of Specificity

In ICD-9-CM, one code with its description and includes notes may encompass a vast number of procedure variations while another code defines a single specific procedure. ICD-10-PCS provides a standardized level of specificity for each code, so that each code represents a single procedure variation.

The ICD-9-CM code 39.31, "Suture of artery," does not specify the artery, whereas the code range 38.40 through 38.49, "Resection of artery with replacement," provides a fourth-digit subclassification for specifying the artery by anatomical region (thoracic, abdominal, etc.).

In ICD-10-PCS, the codes identifying all artery suture and artery replacement procedures possess the same degree of specificity. The ICD-9-CM examples above coded to their ICD- 10-PCS equivalents would use the same artery body part values in all codes identifying the respective procedures.

In general, ICD-10-PCS code descriptions are much more specific than their ICD-9-CM counterparts, but sometimes an ICD -10-PCS code description is actually less specific. In most cases this is because the ICD-9-CM code contains diagnosis information. The standardized level of code specificity in ICD-10-PCS cannot always take account of these fluctuations in ICD-9- CM level of specificity. Instead, ICD-10-PCS provides a standardized level of specificity that can be predicted across the system.

Diagnosis Information Excluded

Another key feature of ICD-10-PCS is that information pertaining to a diagnosis is excluded from the code descriptions.

ICD-9-CM often contains information about the diagnosis in its procedure codes. Adding diagnosis information limits the flexibility and functionality of a procedure coding system. It has the effect of placing a code "off limits" because the diagnosis in the medical record does not match the diagnosis in the procedure code description. The code cannot be used even though the procedural part of the code description precisely matches the procedure performed.

Diagnosis information is not contained in any ICD-10-PCS code. The diagnosis codes, not the procedure codes, will specify the reason the procedure is performed.

NOS Code Options Restricted

ICD-9-CM often designates codes as "unspecified" or "not otherwise specified" codes. By contrast, the standardized level of specificity designed into ICD-10-PCS restricts the use of broadly applicable NOS or unspecified code options in the system. A minimal level of specificity is required to construct a valid code.

In ICD-10-PCS, each character defines information about the procedure and all seven characters must contain a specific value obtained from a single row of a table to build a valid code. Even values such as the sixth-character value Z, No Device and the seventh-character value Z, No Qualifier, provide important information about the procedure performed.

Limited NEC Code Options

ICD-9-CM often designates codes as "not elsewhere classified" or "other specified" versions of a procedure throughout the code set. NEC options are also provided in ICD-10-PCS, but only for specific, limited use.

In the Medical and Surgical section, two significant "not elsewhere classified" options are the root operation value Q, Repair and the device value Y, Other Device.

The root operation Repair is a true NEC value. It is used only when the procedure performed is not one of the other root operations in the Medical and Surgical section.

Other Device, on the other hand, is intended to be used to temporarily define new devices that do not have a specific value assigned, until one can be added to the system. No categories of medical or surgical devices are permanently classified to Other Device.

ICD-10-PCS Applications

ICD-10-PCS code structure results in qualities that optimize the performance of the system in electronic applications, and maximize the usefulness of the coded healthcare data. These qualities include

- Optimal search capability
- Consistent character definitions
- Consistent values wherever possible
- Code readability

Some have argued that, in the world of the electronic health record, the classification system as we know it is outmoded, that classification doesn't matter because a computer is able to find a code with equal ease whether the code has been generated at random or is part of a classification scheme. While this may be true from an IT perspective, assignment of randomly generated code numbers makes it impossible to aggregate data according to related ranges of codes. This is a critical capability for providers, payers, and researchers to make meaningful use of the data.

Optimal Search Capability

ICD-10-PCS is designed for maximum versatility in the ability to aggregate coded data. Values belonging to the same character as defined in a section or sections can be easily compared, since they occupy the same position in a code. This provides a high degree of flexibility and functionality for data mining.

For example, the body part value 6, Stomach, retains its meaning for all codes in the Medical and Surgical section that define procedures performed on the stomach. Because the body part value is dependent for its meaning on the body system in which it

is found, the body system value D, Gastrointestinal, must also be included in the search.

A person wishing to examine data regarding all medical and surgical procedures performed on the stomach could do so simply by searching the code range below.

```
0D*6***
```

Consistent Characters and Values

In the previous example, the value 6 means Stomach only when the body system value is D, Gastrointestinal. In many other cases, values retain their meaning across a much broader range of codes. This provides consistency and readability.

For example, the value 0 in the fifth character defines the approach Open and the value 3 in the fifth character defines the approach Percutaneous across sections 0 through 4 and 7 through 9, where applicable. As a result, all open and percutaneous procedures represented by codes in sections 0-4 and 7-9 can be compared based on a single character—approach—by conducting a query on the code ranges below.

```
[0 through 4,7 through 9]***0** vs. [0 through 4,7 through 9]***3**
```

Searches can be progressively refined by adding specific values. For example, one could search on a body system value or range of body system values, plus a body part value or range of body part values, plus a root operation value or range of root operation values.

To refine the search above, one could add the body system value for Gastrointestinal and the body part value for Stomach to limit the search to open vs. percutaneous procedures performed on the stomach:

```
0D*60** vs. 0D*63**
```

To refine the search even further and limit the comparison to open and percutaneous biopsies of the stomach, one could add the third-character value for the root operation Excision and the seventh-character qualifier Diagnostic, as below.

```
0DB60*X vs. 0DB63*X
```

Stability of characters and values across vast ranges of codes provides the maximum degree of functionality and flexibility for the collection and analysis of data. The search capabilities demonstrated above function equally well for all uses of healthcare data: investigating quality of care, resource utilization, risk management, conducting research, determining reimbursement, and many others.

Because the character definition is consistent, and only the individual values assigned to that character differ as needed, meaningful comparisons of data over time can be conducted across a virtually infinite range of procedures.

Code Readability

ICD-10-PCS resembles a language in the sense that it is made up of semi- independent values combined by following the rules of the system, much the way a sentence is formed by combining words and following the rules of grammar and syntax. As with words in their context, the meaning of any single value is a combination of its position in the code and any preceding values on which it may be dependent.

For example, in the Medical and Surgical section, a body part value is always dependent for its meaning on the body system in which it is found. It cannot stand alone as a letter or a number and be meaningful. A fourth-character value of 6 by itself can mean 31 different things, but a fourth-character value of 6 in the context of a second-character value of D means one thing only—Stomach.

On the other hand, a root operation value is not dependent on any character but the section for its meaning, and identifies a single consistent objective wherever the third character is defined as root operation. For example, the third-character value T identifies the root operation Resection in both the Medical and Surgical and Obstetrics sections.

The approach value also identifies a single consistent approach wherever the fifth character is defined as approach. The fifth-character value 3 identifies the approach Percutaneous in the Medical and Surgical section, the Obstetrics section, the Administration section, and others.

The sixth-character device value or seventh-character qualifier value identifies the same device or qualifier in the context of the body system where it is found. Although there may be consistencies across body systems or within whole sections, this is not true in all cases.

Values in their designated context have a precise meaning, like words in a language. As seen in the code example which began this overview, 0LB50ZZ represents the text description of the specific procedure "Excision of right lower arm and wrist tendon, open approach." Since ICD-10-PCS values in context have a single, precise meaning, a complete, valid code can be read and understood without its accompanying text description, much like one would read a sentence.

Procedures in the Medical and Surgical Section – Root Operation Groups

This section provides reference material for the root operations in the Medical and Surgical section of ICD-10-PCS. The vast majority of codes reported in an inpatient setting are found in this section.

First, a table presents all root operations in the Medical and Surgical section, organized into logical groups. Following the table are definitions of each root operation, presented in the order shown in the table. Material on each root operation includes

- Definition, explanation, Illustrations and examples of the root operation
- Coding notes as needed
- A representative procedure excerpt for each root operation, followed by the correct code for the procedure. The code is provided in table excerpt format, along with explanatory notes as needed.
- Coding exercises that provide example procedures and their corresponding ICD-10-PCS codes, with explanatory notes as needed

Root Operation Groups

The Medical and Surgical root operations are divided into groups that share similar attributes. These groups, and the root operations in each, are listed in the table below. Subsequent pages of this section provide a definition of each root operation in a group.

Root operation	What operation does	Objective of procedure	Procedure site	Example
Alteration	Includes other objectives	Modifying body part for cosmetic purposes without affecting function	Some/all of a body part	Face lift
Bypass	Alters the diameter/route of a tubular body part	Altering route of passage	Tubular body part	Coronary artery bypass graft (CABG)
Change	Always involves a device	Exchanging device w/out cutting/puncturing	In/on a body part	Drainage tube change
Control	Includes other repairs	Stopping/attempting to stop postprocedural bleed	Anatomical region	Post-prostatectomy bleeding
Creation	Includes other objectives	Making new structure for sex change operation	Perineum	Artificial vagina/penis
Destruction	Takes out some/all of a body part	Eradicating without replacement	Some/all of a body part	Fulguration of endometrium
Detachment	Takes out some/all of a body part	Cutting out/off without replacement	Extremity only, any level	Amputation above elbow
Dilation	Alters the diameter/route of a tubular body part	Expanding orifice/lumen	Tubular body part	Percutaneous transluminal coronary angioplasty (PTCA)
Division	Involves cutting or separation only	Cutting into/separating a body part	Within a body part	Neurotomy
Drainage	Takes out solids/fluids/gases from a body part	Taking/letting out fluids/gases	Within a body part	Incision and drainage
Excision	Takes out some/all of a body part	Cutting out/off without replacement	Some of a body part	Breast lumpectomy
Extirpation	Takes out solids/fluids/gases from a body part	Taking/cutting out solid matter	Within a body part	Thrombectomy
Extraction	Takes out some/all of a body part	Pulling out or off without replacement	Some/all of a body part	Suction D&C
Fragmentation	Takes out solids/fluids/gases from a body part	Breaking solid matter into pieces	Within a body part	Lithotripsy
Fusion	Includes other objectives	Rendering joint immobile	Joint	Spinal fusion
Insertion	Always involves a device	Putting in non-biological device	In/on a body part	Central line insertion
Inspection	Involves examination only	Visual/manual exploration	Some/all of a body part	Diagnostic cystoscopy
Map	Involves examination only	Locating electrical impulses/functional areas	Brain/cardiac conduction mechanism	Cardiac mapping
Occlusion	Alters the diameter/route of a tubular body part	Completely closing orifice/lumen	Tubular body part	Fallopian tube ligation
Reattachment	Puts in/puts back or move some/all of a body part	Putting back a detached body part	Some/all of a body part	Reattach severed finger
Release	Involves cutting or separation only	Freeing a body part from constraint	Around a body part	Adhesiolysis
Removal	Always involves a device	Taking out device	In/on a body part	Central line removal
Repair	Includes other repairs	Restoring body part to its normal structure	Some/all of a body part	Suture laceration
Replacement	Always involves a device	Putting in device that replaces a body part	Some/all of a body part	Total hip replacement
Reposition	Puts in/puts back or move some/all of a body part	Moving, to normal or other suitable location	Some/all of a body part	Move undescended testicle
Resection	Takes out some/all of a body part	Cutting out/off without replacement	All of a body part	Total mastectomy
Restriction	Alters the diameter/route of a tubular body part	Partially closing orifice/lumen	Tubular body part	Gastroesophageal fundoplication
Revision	Always involves a device	Correcting a malfunctioning/displaced device	In/on a body part	Revision of pacemaker insertion
Supplement	Always involves a device	Putting in device that reinforces or augments a body part	In/on a body part	Abdominal wall herniorrhaphy using mesh
Transfer	Puts in/puts back or move some/all of a body part	Moving, to function for a similar body part	Some/all of a body part	Skin transfer flap
Transplantation	Puts in/puts back or move some/all of a body part	Putting in a living body part from a person/animal	Some/all of a body part	Kidney transplant

Root operations that take out some or all of a body part

The following root operations represent procedures for taking out or otherwise eradicating some or all of a body part. These root operations are listed below and described in detail in the pages that follow.

Objective of procedure

- Excision: Cutting out/off without replacement
- Resection: Cutting out/off without replacement
- Detachment: Cutting out/off without replacement
- Destruction: Eradicating without replacement
- Extraction: Pulling out or off without replacement

Site of procedure

- Excision: Some of a body part
- Resection: All of a body part
- Detachment: Extremity only, any level
- Destruction: Some/all of a body part
- Extraction: Some/all of a body part

Example

- Excision: Breast lumpectomy
- Resection: Total mastectomy
- Detachment: Amputation above elbow
- Destruction: Fulguration of endometrium
- Extraction: Suction D&C

Excision—Root operation B

Definition: Cutting out or off, without replacement, a portion of a body part

Explanation: The qualifier Diagnostic is used to identify excision procedures that are biopsies

Examples: Partial nephrectomy (Illustration 1), liver biopsy

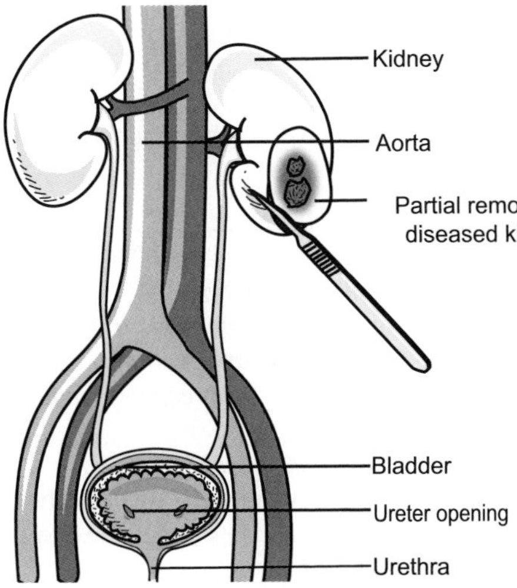

Illustration 1

Excision is coded when a portion of a body part is cut out or off using a sharp instrument. All root operations that employ cutting to accomplish the objective allow the use of any sharp instrument, including but not limited to

- Scalpel
- Wire
- Scissors
- Bone saw
- Electrocautery tip

Coding note: Bone marrow and endometrial biopsies

Bone marrow and endometrial biopsies are not coded to the root operation excision. They are coded to Extraction, with the qualifier Diagnostic .

Example: Excision of sebaceous cyst (right buttock)

...the patient was brought in the room and placed on the table in jack knife, prone position and a spinal block was used for anesthesia. She was prepped and draped in the usual sterile manner. A digital rectal examination was performed and we did not notice any communication between mass and rectum. The mass was palpated and a radial transverse incision was made over the mass.

Using blunt and sharp dissection the top of the mass was identified and shown to be a sebaceous cyst. The sebaceous cyst was freed from the surrounding tissue using blunt dissection. The entire cyst was removed. Hemostasis was obtained and the skin was closed using 5-0 Dexon interrupted sutures...

Character 1 Section	Character 2 Body System	Character 3 Root Operation	Character 4 Body Part	Character 5 Approach	Character 6 Device	Character 7 Qualifier
Medical and Surgical	Skin	Excision	Buttock	External	No Device	No Qualifier
0	H	B	8	X	Z	Z

Coding exercises

Using the ICD-10-PCS Tables, construct the code that accurately represents the procedure performed.

1. Excision of malignant melanoma from skin of right ear (Illustration 2): 0HB2XZZ

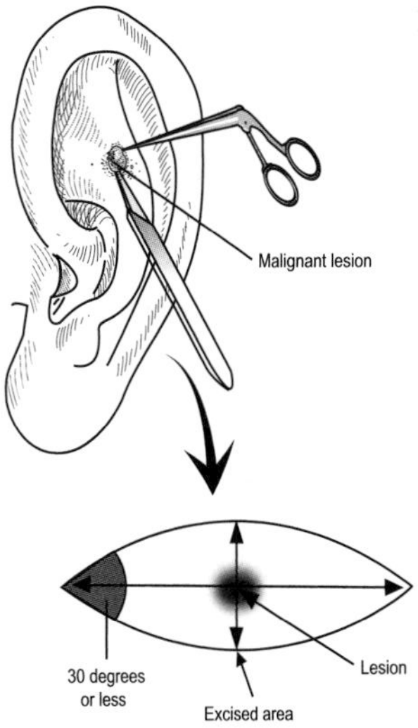

Illustration 2

2. Laparoscopy with excision of endometrial implant from left ovary: 0UB14ZZ
3. Percutaneous needle core biopsy of right kidney: 0TB03ZX
4. EGD with gastric biopsy: 0DB68ZX
5. Laparotomy with wedge resection of left lateral segment of liver: 0FB20ZZ
6. Excision of basal cell carcinoma of lower lip: 0CB1XZZ
7. Open excision of tail of pancreas; 0FBG0ZZ
8. Percutaneous biopsy of right gastrocnemius muscle: 0KBS3ZX
9. Sigmoidoscopy with sigmoid polypectomy: 0DBN8ZZ
10. Open excision of lesion from right Achilles tendon: 0LBN0ZZ
11. Laparoscopic vertical sleeve gastrectomy: 0DB64Z3

Resection—Root operation T

Definition: Cutting out or off, without replacement, all of a body part

Explanation: N/A

Examples: Total nephrectomy (Illustration 3), total lobectomy of lung

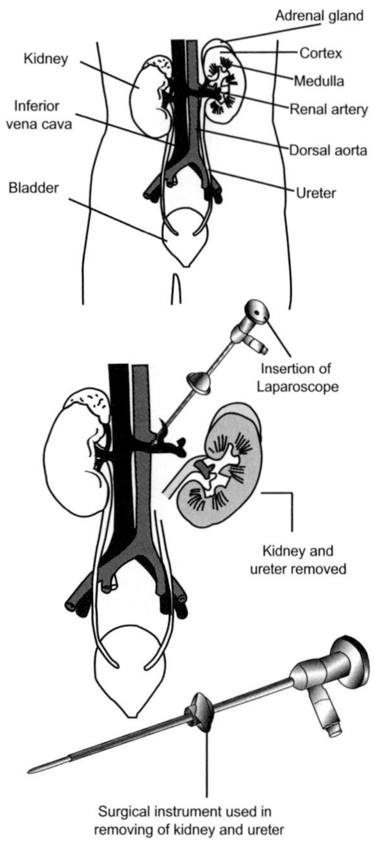

Illustration 3

Resection is similar to Excision (except Resection includes all of a body part, or any subdivision of a body part that has its own body part value in ICD-10-PCS, while Excision includes only a portion of a body part.

Coding note: Lymph nodes

When an entire lymph node chain is cut out, the appropriate root operation is Resection. When a lymph node(s) is cut out, the root operation is Excision.

Example: Right hemicolectomy

...a vertical midline incision was used to enter the abdominal cavity. There was noted to be a mass in the region of the cecum. The mass was easily mobilized and it was felt that a right hemicolectomy was indicated. The right colon was mobilized by incising the white line of Toldt and reflecting colon medially. The loose tissue was taken down bluntly with a hand and adhesions were taken down sharply.

The colon was mobilized to the left end up to the level of the hepatic flexure. The mesentery was incised sharply with a knife and down to the level of the root of the mesentery. The mesentery of the right colon and the distal ileum was then taken down between Kellys and tied with #2-0 silk, down to the level of the takeoff vessels.

After removing the right colon specimen off the field, a primary anastomosis was planned...

Character 1 Section	Character 2 Body System	Character 3 Root Operation	Character 4 Body Part	Character 5 Approach	Character 6 Device	Character 7 Qualifier
Medical and Surgical	Gastrointestinal System	Resection	Large Intestine, Rt	Open	No Device	No Qualifier
0	D	T	F	0	Z	Z

Coding note: Anastomotic technique

Adjunct information about the anastomotic technique used to complete a colectomy procedure (e.g., side to end) is not specified in ICD-10-PCS. Only the specific Excision or Resection code is assigned.

Coding exercises

Using the ICD-10-PCS Tables, construct the code that accurately represents the procedure performed.

1. *Open resection of cecum: 0DTH0ZZ*
2. *Total excision of pituitary gland, open: 0GT00ZZ*
3. *Explantation of left failed kidney, open: 0TT10ZZ*
4. *Open left axillary total lymphadenectomy: 07T60ZZ (Resection is coded for cutting out a chain of lymph nodes.)*
5. *Laparoscopic-assisted vaginal hysterectomy, supracervical resection: 0UT9FZZ*
6. *Right total mastectomy, open : 0HTT0ZZ*
7. Open resection of papillary muscle: 02TD0ZZ (The papillary muscle refers to the heart and is found in the Heart and Great Vessels body system.)
8. Total retropubic prostatectomy, open: 0VT00ZZ
9. Laparoscopic cholecystectomy : 0FT44ZZ
10. Endoscopic bilateral total maxillary sinusectomy: 09TQ4ZZ, 09TR4ZZ

Detachment—Root operation 6

Definition: Cutting off all or part of the upper or lower extremities

Explanation: The body part value is the site of the detachment, with a qualifier if applicable to further specify the level where the extremity was detached

Examples: Below knee amputation (Illustration 4), disarticulation of shoulder

Detachment represents a narrow range of procedures; it is used exclusively for amputation procedures. Detachment procedure codes are found only in body systems X Anatomical Regions, Upper Extremities and Y Anatomical Regions, Lower Extremities, because amputations are performed on the extremities, across overlapping body layers, and so could not be coded to a specific musculoskeletal body system such as the bones or joints.

Detachment qualifiers

The specific qualifiers used for Detachment are dependent on the body part value in the upper and lower extremities body systems. The table information below defines the meaning of the qualifiers used in both the upper and lower extremities.

Upper arm and upper leg

- Qualifier 1 High: Amputation at the proximal portion of the shaft of the humerus or femur
- Qualifier 2 Mid: Amputation at the middle portion of the shaft of the humerus or femur
- Qualifier 3 Low: Amputation at the distal portion of the shaft of the humerus or femur

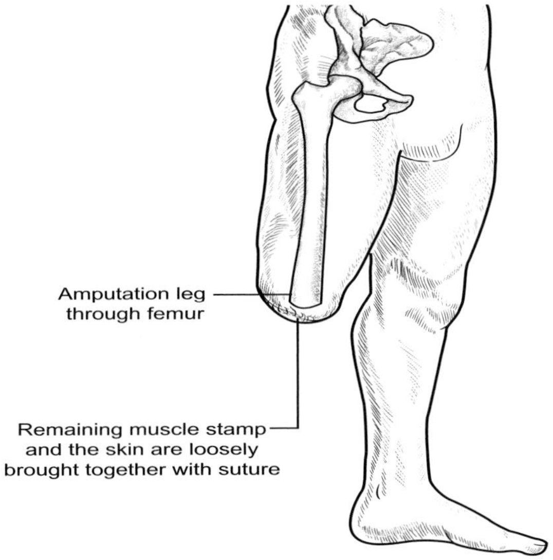

Illustration 4

Hand and foot

Complete: Amputation through the carpometacarpal joint of the hand, or through the tarsal-metatarsal joint of the foot

Partial: Amputation anywhere along the shaft or head of the metacarpal bone of the hand (Illustration 5), or of the metatarsal bone of the foot

- Qualifier 0 Complete
- Qualifier 4 Complete 1st Ray
- Qualifier 5 Complete 2nd Ray
- Qualifier 6 Complete 3rd Ray
- Qualifier 7 Complete 4th Ray
- Qualifier 8 Complete 5th Ray
- Qualifier 9 Partial 1st Ray
- Qualifier B Partial 2nd Ray
- Qualifier C Partial 3rd Ray
- Qualifier D Partial 4th Ray
- Qualifier F Partial 5th Ray

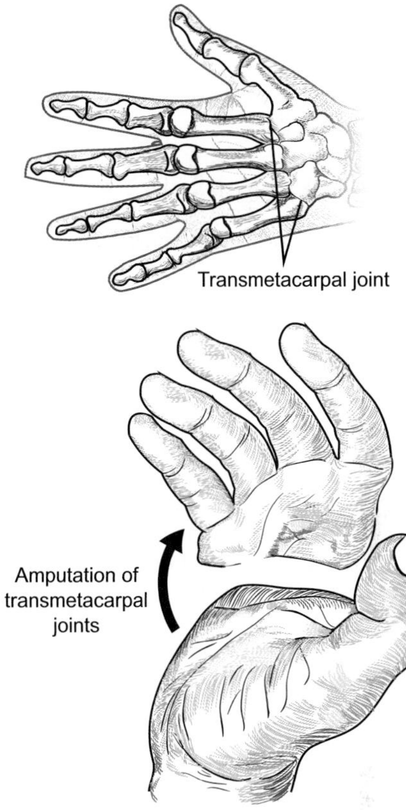

Illustration 5

Thumb, finger, or toe

- Qualifier 0 Complete: Amputation at the metacarpophalangeal/metatarsal-phalangeal joint
- Qualifier 1 High: Amputation anywhere along the proximal phalanx
- Qualifier 2 Mid: Amputation through the proximal interphalangeal joint or anywhere along the middle phalanx
- Qualifier 3 Low: Amputation through the distal interphalangeal joint or anywhere along the distal phalanx

Example: Fifth toe ray amputation

...a semi- elliptical incision was made around the base of the left toe with a #15 blade without difficulty. Careful sharp dissection was made down to the bone, and care was taken to avoid the fourth toe's neurovascular bundle. There was obvious osteomyelitis of the proximal phalanx of the fifth toe and the toe itself was disarticulated, the proximal head of the fifth lower extremity metatarsal, without difficulty. Specimens were sent to pathology for culture and examination.

Next, both sharp and blunt dissection were used to adequately expose the head of the fifth metatarsal, and this was done without difficulty. A small rongeur was then used to remove the head of the fifth metatarsal, and soft spongy bone was felt beneath this area.

Examination of the patient's x-rays revealed that there was an area of cortical lucency at the base of the head of the fifth metatarsal, and the decision was made to extend the amputation to the midshaft of the fifth metatarsal, and this was done without difficulty using a rongeur. The wound was then flushed with normal saline, and bleeding viable tissue was observed throughout the wound. There was adequate flap coverage of the remaining fifth metatarsal...

Character 1 Section	Character 2 Body System	Character 3 Root Operation	Character 4 Body Part	Character 5 Approach	Character 6 Device	Character 7 Qualifier
Medical and Surgical	Lower Extremities	Detachment	Foot, Left	Open	No Device	Partial 5th Ray
0	Y	6	N	0	Z	F

Coding exercises

Using the ICD-10-PCS Tables, construct the code that accurately represents the procedure performed.

1. Amputation at right elbow level: 0X6B0ZZ
2. Right below-knee amputation, proximal tibia/fibula: 0Y6H0Z1 (The qualifier High here means the portion of the tib/fib closest to the knee.)
3. Fifth ray carpometacarpal joint amputation, left hand: 0X6K0Z8 (A Complete ray amputation is through the carpometacarpal joint.)
4. Right leg and hip amputation through ischium: 0Y620ZZ (The Hindquarter body part includes amputation along any part of the hip bone.)
5. DIP joint amputation of right thumb: 0X6L0Z3 (The qualifier Low here means through the distal interphalangeal joint,)
6. Right wrist joint amputation: 0X6J0Z0 (Amputation at the wrist joint is actually complete amputation of the hand.)
7. Trans-metatarsal amputation of foot at left big toe: 0Y6N0Z9 (A Partial amputation is through the shaft of the metatarsal bone.)
8. Mid-shaft amputation, right humerus: 0X680Z2
9. Left fourth toe amputation, mid-proximal phalanx: 0Y6W0Z1 (The qualifier High here means anywhere along the proximal phalanx.)
10. Right above-knee amputation, distal femur : 0Y6C0Z3
11. Right forequarter amputation: 0X600ZZ Detachment at Right Forequarter, Open Approach. (The Forequarter body part includes amputation along any part of the scapula and clavicle.)

Coding note: Qualifier value

The surgeon uses the word "toe" to describe the amputation, but the operative report says he extends the amputation to the midshaft of the fifth metatarsal, which is the foot, so the qualifier is Partial 5th Ray.

Destruction—Root operation 5

Definition: Physical eradication of all or a portion of a body part by the direct use of energy, force or a destructive agent

Explanation: None of the body part is physically taken out

Examples: Fulguration of rectal polyp, cautery of skin lesion

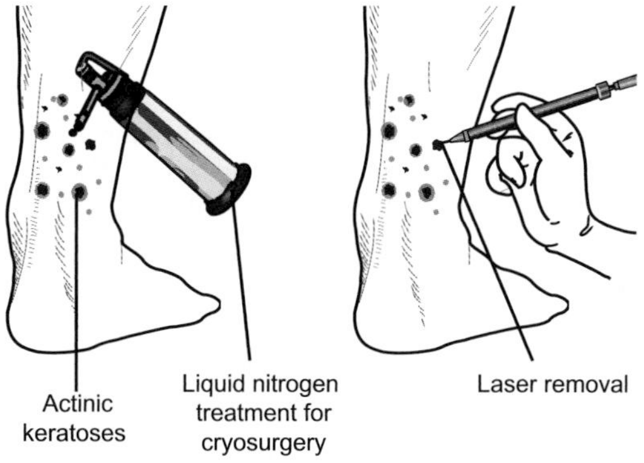

Illustration 6

Destruction "takes out" a body part in the sense that it obliterates the body part so it is no longer there. This root operation defines a broad range of common procedures, since it can be used anywhere in the body to treat a variety of conditions (Illustrations 6, 7), including:

- Skin and genital warts
- Nasal and colon polyps
- Esophageal varices
- Endometrial implants
- Nerve lesions

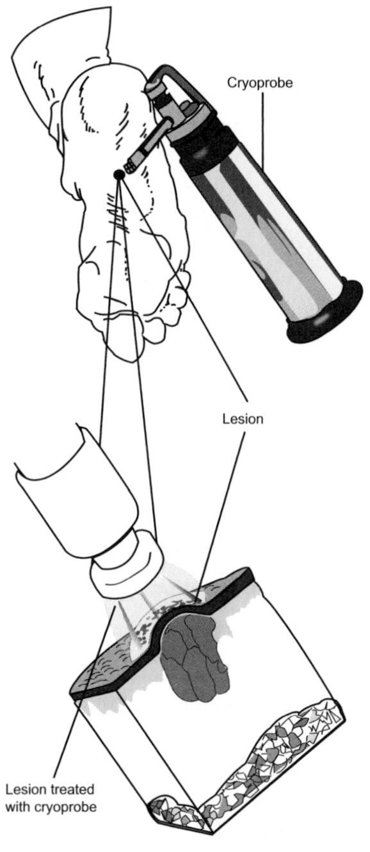

Illustration 7

Example: Radiofrequency coagulation of the trigeminal nerve

...The right cheek was infiltrated dermally with Xylocaine, and a small nick in the skin 2.5 cm lateral to the corner of the mouth was performed with an 18 gauge needle. The radiofrequency needle with 2 mm exposed tip was then introduced using the known anatomical landmarks and under lateral fluoroscopy guidance into the foramen ovale.

Confirmation of the placement of the needle was done by the patient grimacing to pain and by the lateral x-ray. The first treatment, 90 seconds in length, was administered with the tip of the needle 3 mm below the clival line at a temperature of 75 degrees C.

The needle was then advanced further to the mid clival line and another treatment of similar strength and duration was also administered. Finally the third and last treatment was administered with the tip of the needle about 3 cm above the line. The needle was removed. The patient tolerated the procedure well...

Character 1 Section	Character 2 Body System	Character 3 Root Operation	Character 4 Body Part	Character 5 Approach	Character 6 Device	Character 7 Qualifier
Medical and Surgical	Central Nervous	Destruction	Trigeminal Nerve	Percutaneous	No Device	No Qualifier
0	0	5	K	3	Z	Z

Coding note: Approach value

The small nick in the skin does not constitute an open approach. It was made to accommodate the radiofrequency needle. The needle was advanced all the way to the operative site, so the correct approach value is Percutaneous.

Coding exercises

Using the ICD-10-PCS Tables, construct the code that accurately represents the procedure performed.

1. Cryotherapy of wart on left hand: 0H5GXZZ
2. Percutaneous radiofrequency ablation of right vocal cord lesion: 0C5T3ZZ
3. Left heart catheterization with laser destruction of arrhythmogenic focus, A-V node: 02583ZZ
4. Cautery of nosebleed: 095KXZZ
5. Transurethral endoscopic laser ablation of prostate: 0V508ZZ
6. Cautery of oozing varicose vein, left calf: 065Y3ZZ (The approach is coded Percutaneous because that is the normal route to a vein. No mention is made of approach, because likely the skin has eroded at that spot.)
7. Laparoscopy with destruction of endometriosis, bilateral ovaries: 0U524ZZ
8. Laser coagulation of right retinal vessel hemorrhage, percutaneous: 085G3ZZ (The Retinal Vessel body part values are in the Eye body system.)
9. Thoracoscopy with mechanical abrasion and application of talc for pleurodesis: 0B5P4ZZ

Extraction—Root operation D

Definition: Pulling or stripping out or off all or a portion of a body part by the use of force

Explanation: The qualifier Diagnostic is used to identify extraction procedures that are biopsies

Examples: Dilation and curettage, vein stripping (Illustration 8):

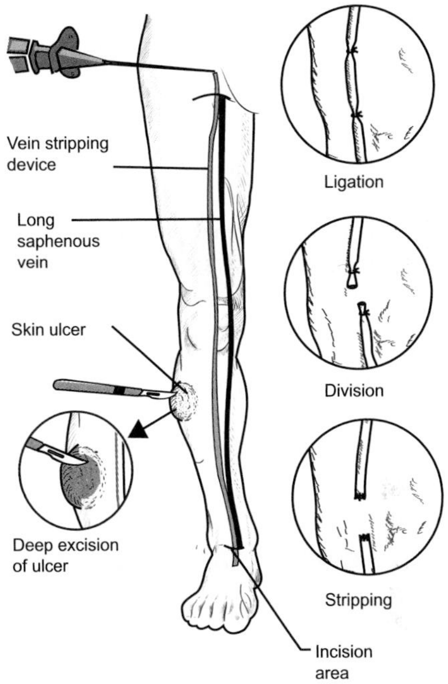

Illustration 8 - Examples of excision and of stripping

Extraction is coded when the method employed to take out the body part is pulling or stripping. Minor cutting, such as that used in vein stripping procedures, is included in Extraction if the objective of the procedure is nevertheless met by pulling or stripping. As with all applicable ICD-10-PCS codes, cutting used to reach the procedure site is specified in the approach value.

Example: Suction dilation & curettage

...after induction of general anesthesia the patient was placed in the dorsal lithotomy position and appropriately prepped and draped. Successive dilators were placed until the cervix was adequate for insertion of the suction cannula.

Suction cannula was placed and suction curettage performed with no residual endometrial lining.
The tissue was sent to pathology to rule out endometrial cancer...

Character 1 Section	Character 2 Body System	Character 3 Root Operation	Character 4 Body Part	Character 5 Approach	Character 6 Device	Character 7 Qualifier
Medical and Surgical	Female Reproductive	Extraction	Endometrium	Via Nat./ Artif. Opening	No Device	Diagnostic
0	U	D	B	7	Z	X

Coding exercises

Using the ICD-10-PCS Tables, construct the code that accurately represents the procedure performed.

1. Forceps total mouth extraction, upper and lower teeth: 0CDWXZ2, 0CDXXZ2
2. Removal of left thumbnail: 0HDQXZZ (No separate body part value is given for thumbnail, so this is coded to Fingernail.)
3. Extraction of right intraocular lens without replacement, percutaneous: 08DJ3ZZ
4. Laparoscopy with needle aspiration of ova for in-vitro fertilization: 0UDN4ZZ
5. Non-excisional debridement of skin ulcer, right foot: 0HDMXZZ
6. Open stripping of abdominal fascia, right side: 0JD80ZZ
7. Hysteroscopy with D&C, diagnostic: 0UDB8ZX
8. Liposuction for medical purposes, left upper arm: 0JDF3ZZ (The Percutaneous approach is inherent in the liposuction technique.)
9. Removal of tattered right ear drum fragments with tweezers: 09D77ZZ
10. Microincisional phlebectomy of spider veins, right lower leg: 06DY3ZZ

Root operations that take out solids/fluids/gases from a body part

The following root operations represent procedures for taking out or otherwise eradicating solids, fluids, or gases from a body part. These root operations are listed below and described in detail in the pages that follow.

Objective of procedure

- Drainage: Taking/letting out fluids/gases
- Extirpation: Taking/cutting out solid matter
- Fragmentation: Breaking solid matter into pieces

Site of procedure

- Drainage: Within a body part
- Extirpation: Within a body part
- Fragmentation: Within a body part

Example

- Drainage: Incision and drainage
- Extirpation: Thrombectomy
- Fragmentation: Lithotripsy

Drainage—Root operation 9

Definition: Taking or letting out fluids and/or gases from a body part

Explanation: The qualifier Diagnostic is used to identify drainage procedures that are biopsies

Examples: Thoracentesis, incision and drainage

The root operation Drainage is coded for both diagnostic and therapeutic drainage procedures. When drainage is accomplished by putting in a catheter, the device value Drainage Device is coded in the sixth character.

Example: Urinary nephrostomy catheter placement

...using fluoroscopy and sterile technique a needle was placed through the skin into a markedly dilated right renal collecting system. Guidewire was inserted and an 8 French locking catheter was positioned with the dilated right renal pelvis. It was attached to a bag and immediate drainage of urine was evident...

Character 1 Section	Character 2 Body System	Character 3 Root Operation	Character 4 Body Part	Character 5 Approach	Character 6 Device	Character 7 Qualifier
Medical and Surgical	Urinary	Drainage	Kidney Pelvis, Right	Percutaneous	Drainage Device	No Qualifier
0	T	9	3	3	0	Z

Coding exercises

Using the ICD-10-PCS Tables, construct the code that accurately represents the procedure performed.

1. Routine Foley catheter placement: 0T9B70Z
2. Incision and drainage of external anal abscess: 0D9QXZZ
3. Percutaneous drainage of ascites: 0W9G3ZZ (This is drainage of the cavity and not the peritoneal membrane itself.)
4. Laparoscopy with left ovarian cystotomy and drainage: 0U914ZZ
5. Laparotomy with drain placement for liver abscess, right lobe: 0F9100Z
6. Right knee arthrotomy with drain placement: 0S9C00Z
7. Thoracentesis of left pleural effusion: 0W9B3ZZ (This is drainage of the pleural cavity.)
8. Phlebotomy of left median cubital vein for polycythemia vera: 059C3ZZ (The median cubital vein is a branch of the basilic vein.)
9. Percutaneous chest tube placement for right pneumothorax: 0W9930Z
10. Endoscopic drainage of left ethmoid sinus: 099V4ZZ
11. External ventricular CSF drainage catheter placement via burr hole: 009630Z

Extirpation—Root operation C

Definition: Taking or cutting out solid matter from a body part

Explanation: The solid matter may be an abnormal byproduct of a biological function or a foreign body; it may be imbedded in a body part or in the lumen of a tubular body part. The solid matter may or may not have been previously broken into pieces.

Examples: Thrombectomy, endarterectomy, choledocholithotomy

Extirpation represents a range of procedures where the body part itself is not the focus of the procedure. Instead, the objective is to remove solid material such as a foreign body, thrombus, or calculus from the body part.

Example: De-clotting of AV dialysis graft

...the right upper extremity was properly prepped and draped. Local anesthesia was used to explore the graft. A transverse incision in the previous site of the incision, 1 cm below the elbow crease, was performed. The venous limb of the graft was dissected free up to the venous anastomosis.

A small incision on the graft was performed. Then a #3 Fogarty catheter was passed on the venous side. The cephalic vein was found obstructed, not on the anastomotic site, but about 4 cm proximal to the anastomosis. A large number of clots were extracted. After the embolectomy a good back flow from the venous side was obtained.

Then the embolectomy was performed throughout the limb on the arterial side. More clots were extracted and a good arterial flow was obtained.

The procedure was concluded, closing the incision on the graft with 6-0 prolene®...

Character 1 Section	Character 2 Body System	Character 3 Root Operation	Character 4 Body Part	Character 5 Approach	Character 6 Device	Character 7 Qualifier
Medical and Surgical	Upper Veins	Extirpation	Cephalic Vein, Right	Open	No Device	No Qualifier
0	5	C	D	0	Z	Z

Coding note: body part value

Do not code separate body parts based on the words "venous side" and "arterial side" in the procedure report. They refer to the two ends of the cephalic vein used to create the fistula.

Coding exercises

Using the ICD-10-PCS Tables, construct the code that accurately represents the procedure performed.

1. Removal of foreign body, right cornea: 08C8XZZ
2. Percutaneous mechanical thrombectomy, left brachial artery: 03C83ZZ
3. Esophagogastroscopy with removal of bezoar from stomach: 0DC68ZZ
4. Foreign body removal, skin of left thumb: 0HCGXZZ (There is no specific value for thumb skin, so the procedure is coded to the hand.)
5. Transurethral cystoscopy with removal of bladder stone: 0TCB8ZZ
6. Forceps removal of foreign body in right nostril: 09CKXZZ (Nostril is coded to the Nose body part value.)
7. Laparoscopy with excision of old suture from mesentery: 0DCV4ZZ
8. Incision and removal of right lacrimal duct stone: 08CX0ZZ
9. Non-incisional removal of intraluminal foreign body from vagina: 0UCG7ZZ (The approach External is also a possibility. It is assumed here that since the patient went to the doctor to have the object removed, that it was not in the vaginal orifice.)
10. Right common carotid endarterectomy, open: 03CH0ZZ

Fragmentation—Root operation F

Definition: Breaking solid matter in a body part into pieces

Explanation: The Physical force (e.g., manual, ultrasonic) applied directly or indirectly is used to break the solid matter into pieces. The solid matter may be an abnormal byproduct of a biological function or a foreign body. The pieces of solid matter are not taken out.

Examples: Extracorporeal shockwave lithotripsy (Illustration 9), transurethral lithotripsy

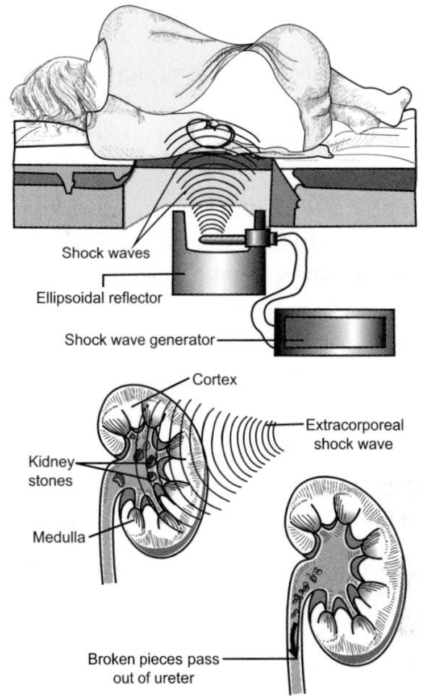

Illustration 9

Fragmentation is coded for procedures to break up, but not remove, solid material such as a calculus or foreign body. This root operation includes both direct and extracorporeal Fragmentation procedures.

ESWL of left kidney

With the patient having been identified, under satisfactory IV sedation and using the MFL 1000 for extracorporeal shock wave lithotripsy, 1000 shocks were delivered to the stone in the lower pole of the left kidney, and 800 shocks were delivered to the stone in the upper pole of the same, with change in shape and density of the stone indicating fragmentation. The patient tolerated the procedure well...

Character 1 Section	Character 2 Body System	Character 3 Root Operation	Character 4 Body Part	Character 5 Approach	Character 6 Device	Character 7 Qualifier
Medical and Surgical	Urinary	Fragment.	Kidney Pelvis, Left	External	No Device	No Qualifier
0	T	F	4	X	Z	Z

Coding exercises

Using the ICD-10-PCS Tables, construct the code that accurately represents the procedure performed.

1. Extracorporeal shock-wave lithotripsy (ESWL), bilateral ureters: 0TF6XZZ, 0TF7XZZ (The bilateral ureter body part value is not available for the root operation Fragmentation, so the procedures are coded separately.)
2. Endoscopic Retrograde Cholangiopancreatography (ERCP) with lithotripsy of common bile duct stone: 0FF98ZZ (ERCP is performed through the mouth to the biliary system via the duodenum, so the approach value is Via Natural or Artificial Opening Endoscopic.)
3. Thoracotomy with crushing of pericardial calcifications: 02FN0ZZ
4. Transurethral cystoscopy with fragmentation of bladder calculus: 0TFB8ZZ
5. Hysteroscopy with intraluminal lithotripsy of left fallopian tube calcification: 0UF68ZZ

Root operations involving cutting or separation only

The following root operations represent procedures that cut or separate a body part. These root operations are listed below and described in detail in the pages that follow.

Objective of procedure

- Division: Cutting into/separating a body part
- Release: Freeing a body part from constraint

Site of procedure

- Division: Within a body part
- Release: Around a body part

Example

- Division: Neurotomy
- Release: Adhesiolysis

Division—Root operation 8

Definition: Cutting into a body part without draining fluids and/or gases from the body part in order to separate or transect a body part

Explanation: All or a portion of the body part is separated into two or more portions

Examples: Spinal cordotomy, osteotomy

The root operation Division is coded when the objective of the procedure is to cut into, transect, or otherwise separate all or a portion of a body part. When the objective is to cut or separate the area around a body part, the attachments to a body part, or between subdivisions of a body part that are causing abnormal constraint, then the root operation Release is coded instead.

Example: Anal sphincterotomy

Manual examination of the rectum and anus was done, and examination showed that the patient has an anterior anal fissure. For that reason, lateral sphincterotomy was done at the 3 o'clock position using the closed approach, dividing only the internal sphincter using the #11 blade...

Character 1 Section	Character 2 Body System	Character 3 Root Operation	Character 4 Body Part	Character 5 Approach	Character 6 Device	Character 7 Qualifier
Medical and Surgical	Gastrointestinal System	Division	Anal Sphincter	Percutaneous	No Device	No Qualifier
0	D	8	R	3	Z	Z

Coding note: Approach value

This is coded to the Percutaneous approach, because the procedure report says that the sphincterotomy was done using the closed approach, dividing only the internal sphincter.

Coding exercises

Using the ICD-10-PCS Tables, construct the code that accurately represents the procedure performed.

1. Division of right foot tendon, percutaneous: 0L8V3ZZ
2. Left heart catheterization with division of bundle of HIS: 02883ZZ
3. Open osteotomy of capitate, left hand: 0P8N0ZZ (The capitate is one of the carpal bones of the hand.)
4. EGD with esophagotomy of esophagogastric junction: 0D848ZZ
5. Sacral rhizotomy for pain control, percutaneous: 018R3ZZ

Release—Root operation N

Definition: Freeing a body part from an abnormal physical constraint by cutting or by use of force

Explanation: Some of the restraining tissue may be taken out but none of the body part is taken out

Examples: Adhesiolysis, carpal tunnel release

The objective of procedures represented in the root operation Release is to free a body part from abnormal constraint. Release procedures are coded to the body part being freed. The procedure can be performed on the area around a body part, on the attachments to a body part, or between subdivisions of a body part that are causing the abnormal constraint.

Example: Release of median nerve

...the right arm was scrubbed with Betadine and prepped and draped in the usual sterile fashion. A well-padded tourniquet was fixed to the right proximal arm but not inflated until after draping. After draping, the right arm was exsanguinated with a combination of elevation and an Esmarch bandage, placing a sponge in the palm. The tourniquet was inflated to 250.

A transverse incision was made at the level of the proximal wrist crease between the palmaris longus and the flexor carpi ulnaris sharply through the skin with a knife, and subcutaneous tissue was dissected by blunt spreading.

The volar fascia was identified and a transverse incision was made sharply with a knife. The flat synovial retractor was pushed through the underneath of the transverse carpal ligament, removing synovium from beneath the ligament.

The entire carpal tunnel and the fat pad distally was visualized. The blade was inserted into the carpal tunnel, was elevated at the distal edge of the transverse carpal ligament, and was pulled proximally, spreading and cutting through the transverse carpal ligament.

It was visualized that the entire median nerve had been released, and that configuration of the end of the transverse carpal ligament was a rectangle, denoting that both the deep and the superficial fibers had been cut.

The wound was then copiously irrigated with saline...

Character 1 Section	Character 2 Body System	Character 3 Root Operation	Character 4 Body Part	Character 5 Approach	Character 6 Device	Character 7 Qualifier
Medical and Surgical	Peripheral Nervous	Release	Median Nerve	Open	No Device	No Qualifier
0	1	N	5	0	Z	Z

Coding note: body part value

The body part value assigned is the structure released and not the structure cut to obtain the release, where the two differ. The transverse carpal ligament was cut to release the median nerve and not for its own sake.

Coding exercises

Using the ICD-10-PCS Tables, construct the code that accurately represents the procedure performed.

1. Laparotomy with exploration and adhesiolysis of right ureter: 0TN60ZZ
2. Incision of scar contracture, right elbow: 0HNDXZZ (The skin of the elbow region is coded to the lower arm.)
3. Frenulotomy for treatment of tongue-tie syndrome: 0CN7XZZ (The frenulum is coded to the body part value Tongue.)
4. Right shoulder arthroscopy with coracoacromial ligament release: 0MN14ZZ
5. Mitral valvulotomy for release of fused leaflets, open approach: 02NG0ZZ
6. Percutaneous left Achilles tendon release: 0LNP3ZZ
7. Laparoscopy with lysis of peritoneal adhesions: 0DNW4ZZ
8. Manual rupture of right shoulder joint adhesions under general anesthesia: 0RNJXZZ
9. Open posterior tarsal tunnel release: 01NG0ZZ (The nerve released in the posterior tarsal tunnel is the tibial nerve.)
10. Laparoscopy with freeing of left ovary and fallopian tube: 0UN14ZZ, 0UN64ZZ

Root operations that put in/put back or move some/all of a body part

The following root operations represent procedures that put in/put back or move some/all of a body part. These root operations are listed below and described in detail in the pages that follow.

Objective of procedure

- Transplantation: Putting in a living body part from a person/animal
- Reattachment: Putting back a detached body part
- Transfer: Moving a body part to function for a similar body part
- Reposition: Moving a body part to normal or other suitable location

Site of procedure

- Transplantation: Some/all of a body part
- Reattachment: Some/all of a body part
- Transfer: Some/all of a body part
- Reposition: Some/all of a body part

Example

- Transplantation: Kidney transplant
- Reattachment: Reattach finger
- Transfer: Skin transfer flap
- Reposition: Move undescended testicle

Transplantation—Root operation Y

Definition: Putting in or on all or a portion of a living body part taken from another individual or animal to physically take the place and/or function of all or a portion of a similar body part

Explanation: The native body part may or may not be taken out, and the transplanted body part may take over all or a portion of its function

Examples: Kidney transplant, heart transplant

A small number of procedures is represented in the root operation Transplantation and includes only the body parts currently being transplanted. Qualifier values specify the genetic compatibility of the body part transplanted.

Example: Right kidney transplant (syngeneic)

...the abdomen was sterilely prepped and draped in the usual fashion and incision in the right flank, the Gibson technique, performed. In doing so the right pelvis was entered and Bookwalter retractor appropriately positioned to provide exposure of the external iliac artery and vein.

The artery was placed on vessel loop retraction. We then proceeded with the kidney transplant, and the kidney which was trimmed on the back table was brought into the field. The right renal vein was cut short without reconstruction of the inferior vena cava, and single ureter was identified. Kidney was brought up and an end- to-end anastomosis was performed in the usual fashion with 5-0 Prolene® between donor renal vein and external iliac vein on the right.

The long renal artery was brought into view, and end-to-side anastomosis performed in the usual fashion with 5-0 Prolene®.

We then turned our attention to performing the neoureterocystostomy after appropriate positioning of the graft and evaluation of the vessels.

After the anastomosis was completed there was no evidence of leak. A Blake drain was brought out through a stab incision and the tip of the drain placed near the neoureterocystostomy and both wounds were closed. The infrainguinal wound was closed with running 3-0 Vicryl® and the kidney transplant wound was closed with #1 PDS...

Character 1 Section	Character 2 Body System	Character 3 Root Operation	Character 4 Body Part	Character 5 Approach	Character 6 Device	Character 7 Qualifier
Medical and Surgical	Urinary	Transplant.	Kidney, Right	Open	No Device	Syngeneic
0	T	Y	0	0	Z	1

Coding note: bone marrow transplant

Bone marrow transplant procedures are coded in section 3 Administration to the root operation 2 Transfusion.

Coding exercises

Using the ICD-10-PCS Tables, construct the code that accurately represents the procedure performed.

1. Liver transplant with donor matched liver: 0FY00Z0
2. Orthotopic heart transplant using porcine heart: 02YA0Z2 (The donor heart comes from an animal (pig), so the qualifier value is Zooplastic.)
3. Right lung transplant, open, using organ donor match: 0BYK0Z0
4. Transplant of large intestine, organ donor match: 0DYE0Z0
5. Left kidney/pancreas organ bank transplant: 0FYG0Z0, 0TY10Z0

Reattachment—Root operation M

Definition: Putting back in or on all or a portion of a separated body part to its normal location or other suitable location

Explanation: Vascular circulation and nervous pathways may or may not be reestablished

Examples: Reattachment of hand, reattachment of avulsed kidney

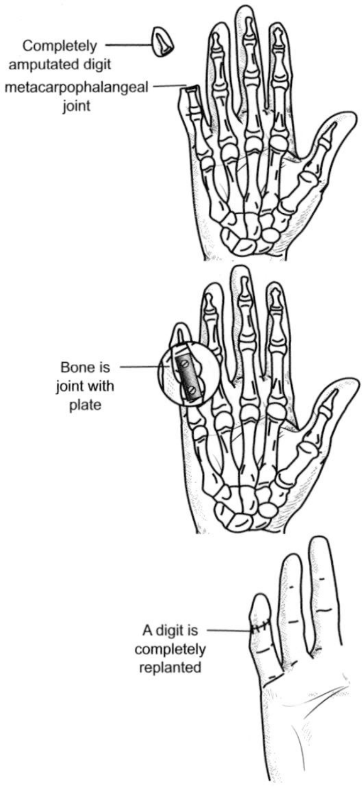

Illustration 10

Procedures coded to Reattachment include putting back a body part that has been cut off or avulsed. Nerves and blood vessels may or may not be reconnected in a Reattachment procedure.

Example: Complex reattachment, left index finger (Illustration 10) - Example shows right 5th digit reattachment

A sharp debridement of grossly contaminated tissue was carried out. It was noted that the extensor mechanism distal to the PIP joint had been lost. There were circumferential lacerations about the finger, save for a cutaneous bridge and ulnar vascular pedicle present at the PIP level.

Nonviable bony fragments were removed and then the distal portion of the PIP joint was reshaped with removal of cartilage using double-rongeurs. It was noted that the fractures through the proximal phalanx extended longitudinally. Stabilization was then carried out, with 0.062 K-wire brought down through the distal finger, out through the fingertip, and then back into the proximal phalanx centrally.

The A2 pulley was restored, using figure of eight interrupted sutures of 4 and 5-0 Vicryl®, reapproximating the flexor tendons. The extensor mechanisms and tendons were repaired using 4 and 5-0 Vicryl®, and anchored to the periosteum on the middle phalanx. A digital nerve was then carried out on the radial aspect of the digit at the PIP joint level using interrupted sutures of 9-0 Ethilon beneath the microscope.

At this point, the skin was trimmed, removing skin margins, and then multiple lacerations were closed with 5-0 Prolene®...

Character 1 Section	Character 2 Body System	Character 3 Root Operation	Character 4 Body Part	Character 5 Approach	Character 6 Device	Character 7 Qualifier
Medical and Surgical	Upper Extremities	Reattachment	Index Finger, Left	Open	No Device	No Qualifier
0	X	M	P	0	Z	Z

Coding exercises

Using the ICD-10-PCS Tables, construct the code that accurately represents the procedure performed.

1. Replantation of avulsed scalp: 0HM0XZZ
2. Reattachment of severed right ear: 09M0XZZ
3. Reattachment of traumatic left gastrocnemius avulsion, open: 0KMT0ZZ
4. Closed replantation of three avulsed teeth, lower jaw: 0CMXXZ1
5. Reattachment of severed left hand: 0XMK0ZZ

Transfer—Root operation X

Definition: Moving, without taking out, all or a portion of a body part to another location to take over the function of all or a portion of a body part

Explanation: The body part transferred remains connected to its vascular and nervous supply

Examples: Tendon transfer, skin pedicle flap transfer

The root operation Transfer is used to represent procedures where a body part is moved to another location without disrupting its

vascular and nervous supply. In the body systems that classify the subcutaneous tissue, fascia and muscle body parts, qualifiers can be used to specify when more than one tissue layer was used in the transfer procedure, such as a musculocutaneous flap transfer.

Example: Fasciocutaneous flap from scalp to cheek

...development of the plane of dissection was completed into the superficial temporal fascia. Development of subgaleal dissection posteriorly was then completed, a distance of 7-8 cm, with hemostasis by electrocautery.

The flaps were advanced to the cheek defect and secured with 2-0 inverted PDS sutures and 3-0 inverted Monocryl...

Character 1 Section	Character 2 Body System	Character 3 Root Operation	Character 4 Body Part	Character 5 Approach	Character 6 Device	Character 7 Qualifier
Medical and Surgical	Subcu. Tissue and Fascia	Transfer	Scalp	Open	No Device	Skin, Subcu. and Fascia
0	J	X	0	0	Z	C

Coding note: body system value

For procedures involving transfer of tissue layers such as skin, fascia and muscle, the procedure is coded to the body system value that describes the deepest tissue layer in the flap. When the tissue transferred is composed of more than one tissue layer, the qualifier can be used to describe the other tissue layers, if any, being transferred.

For transfer procedures classified to other body systems such as peripheral nervous system, the body part value specifies the body part that is the source of the transfer ("from"). Where qualifiers are available, they specify the destination of the transfer ("to").

Coding exercises

Using the ICD-10-PCS Tables, construct the code that accurately represents the procedure performed.

1. Right open palmaris longus tendon transfer: 0LX70ZZ
2. Endoscopic radial to median nerve transfer: 01X64Z5
3. Fasciocutaneous flap closure of left thigh, open: 0JXM0ZC (The qualifier identifies the body layers in addition to fascia included in the procedure.)
4. Transfer left index finger to left thumb position, open: 0XXP0ZM
5. Percutaneous fascia transfer to fill defect, anterior neck: 0JX43ZZ
6. Trigeminal to facial nerve transfer, percutaneous endoscopic: 00XK4ZM
7. Endoscopic left leg flexor hallucis longus tendon transfer: 0LXP4ZZ
8. Right scalp advancement flap to right temple: 0HX0XZZ
9. Bilateral TRAM pedicle flap reconstruction status post mastectomy, muscle only, open: 0KXK0Z6, 0KXL0Z6 (The transverse rectus abdominis muscle (TRAM) flap is coded for each flap developed.)
10. Skin transfer flap closure of complex open wound, left lower back: 0HX6XZZ

Reposition—Root operation S

Definition: Moving to its normal location or other suitable location all or a portion of a body part

Explanation: The body part is moved to a new location from an abnormal location, or from a normal location where it is not functioning correctly. The body part may or may not be cut out or off to be moved to the new location

Examples: Reposition of undescended testicle, fracture reduction

Reposition represents procedures for moving a body part to a new location. The range of Reposition procedures includes moving a body part to its normal location, or moving a body part to a new location to enhance its ability to function.

Example: Reposition of undescended right testicle from pelvic region to scrotum

...Following satisfactory induction of general anesthesia, an incision was made in the inguinal region and dissection carried down to the pelvic cavity, where the right testis was located and mobilized.

The spermatic cord was located and freed from surrounding tissue, and its length judged to be sufficient.

A one centimeter incision was made in the scrotum and a pouch created in the usual fashion. The right testicle was mobilized down through the inguinal canal into the scrotum, and stitched in place.

Meticulous hemostasis was obtained, and the incisions closed in layers...

Character 1 Section	Character 2 Body System	Character 3 Root Operation	Character 4 Body Part	Character 5 Approach	Character 6 Device	Character 7 Qualifier
Medical and Surgical	Male Reproductive	Reposition	Testis, Right	Open	No Device	No Qualifier
0	V	S	9	0	Z	Z

Coding exercises

Using the ICD-10-PCS Tables, construct the code that accurately represents the procedure performed.

1. Open fracture reduction, right tibia: 0QSG0ZZ
2. Laparoscopy with gastropexy for malrotation: 0DS64ZZ
3. Left knee arthroscopy with reposition of anterior cruciate ligament: 0MSP4ZZ
4. Open transposition of ulnar nerve: 01S40ZZ
5. Closed reduction with percutaneous internal fixation of right femoral neck fracture: 0QS634Z

Root operations that alter the diameter/route of a tubular body part

The following root operations represent procedures that alter the diameter or route of a tubular body part. Tubular body parts are defined in ICD-10- PCS as those hollow body parts that provide a route of passage for solids, liquids, or gases.

They include the cardiovascular system, and body parts such as those contained in the gastrointestinal tract, genitourinary tract, biliary tract, and respiratory tract.

These root operations are listed below and described in detail in the pages that follow.

Objective of procedure

- Restriction: Partially closing orifice/lumen
- Occlusion: Completely closing orifice/lumen
- Dilation: Expanding orifice/lumen
- Bypass: Altering route of passage

Site of procedure

- Restriction: Tubular body part
- Occlusion: Tubular body part
- Dilation: Tubular body part
- Bypass: Tubular body part

Example

- Restriction: Gastroesophageal fundoplication
- Occlusion: Fallopian tube ligation
- Dilation: Percutaneous transluminal coronary angioplasty (PTCA)
- Bypass: Coronary artery bypass graft (CABG)

Restriction—Root operation V

Definition: Partially closing an orifice or the lumen of a tubular body part

Explanation: The orifice can be a natural orifice or an artificially created orifice

Examples: Esophagogastric fundoplication, cervical cerclage

The root operation Restriction is coded when the objective of the procedure is to narrow the diameter of a tubular body part or orifice. Restriction includes both intraluminal or extraluminal methods for narrowing the diameter.

Example: Laparoscopic gastroesophageal fundoplication

...Insufflation was accomplished through a 5 mm infraumbilical incision. Five separate 5 mm ports were placed under direct visualization other than the initial port. Laparoscopy revealed a large hiatal hernia. Electrocautery was used to free up adhesions from the hernia sac to the stomach.

Next, the fundus which had been mobilized was brought down into the stomach and it was felt there was enough mobilization to perform a fundoplication. A generous loose fundoplication was then performed by wrapping the fundus around the esophagus. Interrupted 0 Ethibond sutures were used to secure the stomach in this fashion.

There was generally good hemostasis throughout the case. All instruments were removed and ports closed...

Character 1 Section	Character 2 Body System	Character 3 Root Operation	Character 4 Body Part	Character 5 Approach	Character 6 Device	Character 7 Qualifier
Medical and Surgical	Gastrointestinal System	Restriction	Esophagogast Junction	Percutaneous Endoscopic	No Device	No Qualifier
0	D	V	4	4	Z	Z

Coding exercises

Using the ICD-10-PCS Tables, construct the code that accurately represents the procedure performed.

1. Cervical cerclage using Shirodkar technique: 0UVC7ZZ
2. Thoracotomy with banding of left pulmonary artery using extraluminal device: 02VR0CZ
3. Restriction of thoracic duct with intraluminal stent, percutaneous: 07VK3DZ
4. Craniotomy with clipping of cerebral aneurysm: 03VG0CZ (A clip is placed lengthwise on the outside wall of the widened portion of the vessel.)
5. Non-incisional, trans-nasal placement of restrictive stent in right lacrimal duct: 08VX7DZ
6. Catheter-based temporary restriction of blood flow in abdominal aorta for treatment of cerebral ischemia: 04V03DJ

Occlusion—Root operation L

Definition: Completely closing an orifice or the lumen of a tubular body part

Explanation: The orifice can be a natural orifice or an artificially created orifice

Examples: Fallopian tube ligation, ligation of inferior vena cava

The root operation Occlusion is coded when the objective of the procedure is to close off a tubular body part or orifice. Occlusion includes both intraluminal or extraluminal methods of closing off the body part. Division of the tubular body part prior to closing it is an integral part of the Occlusion procedure.

Example: Uterine artery embolization

...catheter was advanced over a 0.18 Terumo gold guidewire and advanced several centimeters superselectively into the left uterine artery. Contrast injection was performed here, confirming filling of the uterine artery and subsequent opacification of large vascular structures in the uterus compatible with uterine fibroids.

A syringe and a half of 500-700 micron biospheres was then instilled slowly through the catheter, and at the conclusion of this infusion there was cessation of flow through the uterine artery.

The catheter was then removed and hemostasis achieved...

Character 1 Section	Character 2 Body System	Character 3 Root Operation	Character 4 Body Part	Character 5 Approach	Character 6 Device	Character 7 Qualifier
Medical and Surgical	Lower Arteries	Occlusion	Internal Iliac Artery, Left	Percutaneous	Intraluminal Device	Uterine Artery, Left
0	4	L	F	3	D	U

Coding exercises

Using the ICD-10-PCS Tables, construct the code that accurately represents the procedure performed.

1. Percutaneous ligation of esophageal vein: 06L33ZZ
2. Percutaneous embolization of left internal carotid-cavernous fistula: 03LL3DZ

3. Laparoscopy with bilateral occlusion of fallopian tubes using Hulka extraluminal clips: 0UL74CZ
4. Open suture ligation of failed AV graft, left brachial artery: 03L80ZZ
5. Percutaneous embolization of vascular supply, intracranial meningioma: 03LG3DZ
6. Percutaneous embolization of right uterine artery, using coils: 04LE3DT
7. Open occlusion of left atrial appendage, using extraluminal pressure clips: 02L70CK
8. Percutaneous suture exclusion of left atrial appendage, via femoral artery access: 02L73ZK

Dilation—Root operation 7

Definition: Expanding an orifice or the lumen of a tubular body part

Explanation: The orifice can be a natural orifice or an artificially created orifice. Accomplished by stretching a tubular body part using intraluminal pressure or by cutting part of the orifice or wall of the tubular body part

Examples: Percutaneous transluminal angioplasty, pyloromyotomy

The root operation Dilation is coded when the objective of the procedure is to enlarge the diameter of a tubular body part or orifice. Dilation includes both intraluminal or extraluminal methods of enlarging the diameter. A device placed to maintain the new diameter is an integral part of the Dilation procedure, and is coded to a sixth-character device value in the Dilation procedure code.

Example: PTCA of left anterior descending

...under 1% Lidocaine local anesthesia, the right femoral artery was entered by the Seldinger technique and a #7 French sheath was placed. A Judkins left guiding catheter was advanced to the left coronary ostium and using a .014 Entrée wire and a 2.5 x 30 mm Panther balloon, it was easily placed across the lesion in the left anterior descending.

The balloon was inflated times two for five minutes for up to 9 atmospheres. Angiography demonstrated an excellent result...

Character 1 Section	Character 2 Body System	Character 3 Root Operation	Character 4 Body Part	Character 5 Approach	Character 6 Device	Character 7 Qualifier
Medical and Surgical	Heart and Gr.Vessels	Dilation	Coronary Art., One Site	Percutaneous	No Device	No Qualifier
0	2	7	0	3	Z	Z

Coding exercises

Using the ICD-10-PCS Tables, construct the code that accurately represents the procedure performed.

1. ERCP with balloon dilation of common bile duct: 0F798ZZ
2. PTCA of two coronary arteries, LAD with stent placement, RCA with no stent: 02703DZ, 02703ZZ
(A separate procedure is coded for each artery dilated, since the device value differs for each artery.)
3. Cystoscopy with intraluminal dilation of bladder neck stricture: 0T7C8ZZ
4. Open dilation of old anastomosis, left femoral artery: 047L0ZZ
5. Dilation of upper esophageal stricture, direct visualization, with Bougie sound: 0D717ZZ
6. PTA of right brachial artery stenosis: 03773ZZ
7. Trans-nasal dilation and stent placement in right lacrimal duct: 087X7DZ
8. Hysteroscopy with balloon dilation of bilateral fallopian tubes: 0U778ZZ
9. Tracheoscopy with intraluminal dilation of tracheal stenosis: 0B718ZZ
10. Cystoscopy with dilation of left ureteral stricture, with stent placement: 0T778DZ

Bypass—Root operation 1

Definition: Altering the route of passage of the contents of a tubular body part

Explanation: Rerouting contents of a body part to a downstream area of the normal route, to a similar route and body part, or to an abnormal route and dissimilar body part. Includes one or more anastomoses, with or without the use of a device

Examples: Coronary artery bypass (Illustration 11), colostomy formation

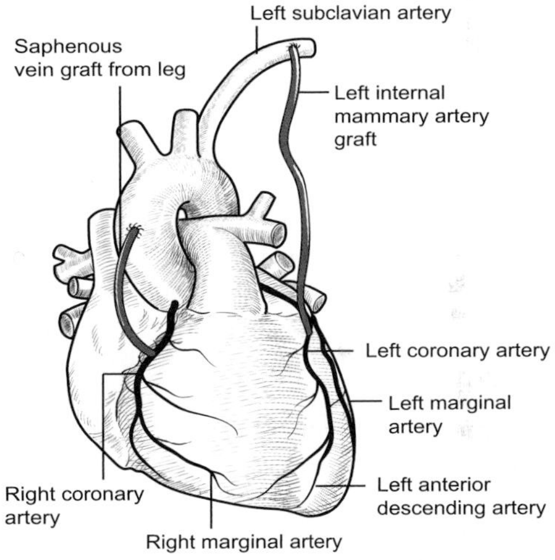

Illustration 11

Bypass is coded when the objective of the procedure is to reroute the contents of a tubular body part. The range of Bypass procedures includes normal routes such as those made in coronary artery bypass procedures, and abnormal routes such as those made in colostomy formation procedures.

Example: Aorto-bifemoral bypass graft

...the patient was prepped and draped, and groin incisions were opened. The common femoral vein and its branches were isolated and Teflon tapes were placed around the vessels.

The aorta and iliacs were mobilized. Bleeding points were controlled with electrocautery and Ligaclip® devices. Tapes were placed around

the vessel, the vessel measured, and the aorta was found to be 12 mm. A 12 x 7 bifurcated Microvelour® graft was then preclotted with the patient's own blood.

An end-to-end anastomosis was made on the aorta and the graft using a running suture of 2-0 Prolene®. The limbs were taken down through tunnels noting that the ureters were anterior, and at this point an end- to-side anastomosis was made between the graft and the femoral arteries with running suture of 4-0 Prolene®.

The inguinal incisions were closed...

Character 1 Section	Character 2 Body System	Character 3 Root Operation	Character 4 Body Part	Character 5 Approach	Character 6 Device	Character 7 Qualifier
Medical and Surgical	Lower Arteries	Bypass	Abdominal Aorta	Open	Synthetic Substitute	Bil. Femoral Arteries
0	4	1	0	0	J	K

Coding exercises

Using the ICD-10-PCS Tables, construct the code that accurately represents the procedure performed.

1. Open gastric bypass with Roux-en-Y limb to jejunum: 0D160ZA
2. Right temporal artery to intracranial artery bypass using Gore-Tex® graft, open: 031S0JG
3. Tracheostomy formation with tracheostomy tube placement, percutaneous: 0B113F4
4. PICVA (Percutaneous in-situ coronary venous arterialization) of single coronary artery: 02103D4
5. Open left femoral-popliteal artery bypass using cadaver vein graft: 041L0KL
6. Shunting of intrathecal cerebrospinal fluid to peritoneal cavity using synthetic shunt: 00160J6
7. Colostomy formation, open, transverse colon to abdominal wall: 0D1L0Z4
8. Open urinary diversion, left ureter, using ileal conduit to skin: 0T170ZC
9. CABG of LAD using left internal mammary artery, open off-bypass: 02100Z9
10. Open pleuroperitoneal shunt, right pleural cavity, using synthetic device: 0W190JG
11. Percutaneous placement of ventriculoperitoneal shunt for treatment of hydrocephalus: 00163J6

Root operations that always involve a device

The following root operations represent procedures that always involve a device. These root operations are listed below and described in detail in the pages that follow.

Objective of procedure

- Insertion: Putting in non-biological device
- Replacement: Putting in device that replaces a body part
- Supplement: Putting in device that reinforces or augments a body part
- Change: Exchanging device w/out cutting/puncturing
- Removal: Taking out device
- Revision: Correcting a malfunctioning/displaced device

Site of procedure

- Insertion: In/on a body part
- Replacement: Some/all of a body part
- Supplement: In/on a body part
- Change: In/on a body part
- Removal: In/on a body part
- Revision: In/on a body part

Example

- Insertion: Central line insertion
- Replacement: Total hip replacement
- Supplement: Abdominal wall herniorrhaphy using mesh
- Change: Drainage tube change
- Removal: Central line removal
- Revision: Revision of pacemaker insertion

Insertion—Root operation H

Definition: Putting in a non-biological device that monitors, assists, performs or prevents a physiological function but does not physically take the place of a body part

Explanation: N/A

Examples: Insertion of radioactive implant, insertion of central venous catheter (Illustration 12)

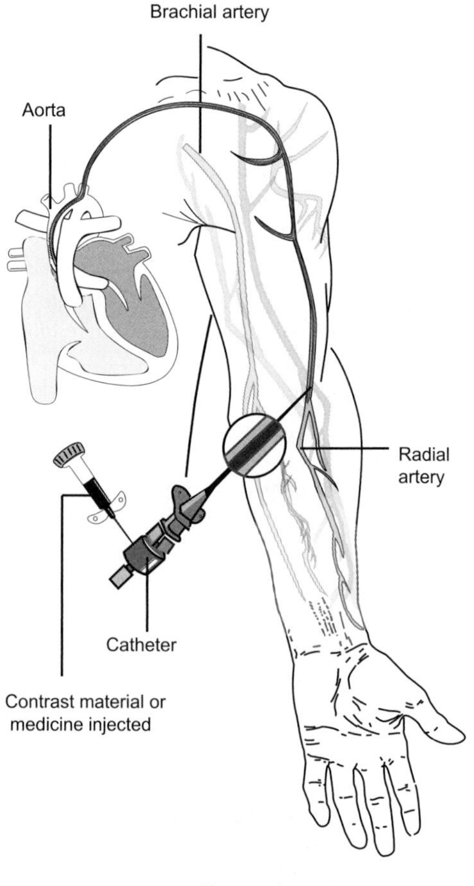

Illustration 12

The root operation Insertion represents those procedures where the sole objective is to put in a device without doing anything else to a body part. Procedures typical of those coded to Insertion include putting in a vascular catheter, a pacemaker lead, or a tissue expander.

Example: Placement of totally implanted central venous access device

...the right chest and neck were prepped and draped in the usual manner and 10 cc's of 1% Lidocaine were injected in the right infraclavicular area.

The right subclavian vein was then punctured and a wire was passed through the needle into the superior vena cava. This was documented by fluoroscopy. Introducer kit was introduced into the subclavian vein and the Port-a-Cath® was placed through the introducer and by fluoroscopy was placed down to the superior vena cava.

The pocket was then made over the right pectoralis major muscle, superior to the breast, and the Port-a-Cath® reservoir was placed into this pocket and tacked down with #0 Prolene® sutures.

The catheter was then tunneled through a subcutaneous tunnel to this receptacle. Hemostasis was achieved and the subcutaneous tissue closed...

Character 1 Section	Character 2 Body System	Character 3 Root Operation	Character 4 Body Part	Character 5 Approach	Character 6 Device	Character 7 Qualifier
Medical and Surgical	Subcu.Tissue and Fascia	Insertion	Chest	Percutaneous	Vascular Access Dev	No Qualifier
0	J	H	6	3	X	Z

Character 1 Section	Character 2 Body System	Character 3 Root Operation	Character 4 Body Part	Character 5 Approach	Character 6 Device	Character 7 Qualifier
Medical and Surgical	Heart and Great Vessels	Insertion	Superior Vena Cava	Percutaneous	Infusion Device	No Qualifier
0	2	H	V	3	3	Z

Coding note: imaging guidance

Imaging guidance done to assist in the performance of a procedure can be coded separately in the Imaging section, if desired. (Section B)

Coding exercises

Using the ICD-10-PCS Tables, construct the code that accurately represents the procedure performed.

1. End-of -life replacement of spinal neurostimulator generator, multiple array, in lower abdomen: 0JH80DZ (Taking out the old generator is coded separately to the root operation Removal.)
2. Percutaneous replacement of broken pacemaker lead in left atrium: 02H73JZ (Taking out the broken pacemaker lead is coded separately to the root operation Removal.)
3. Open placement of dual chamber pacemaker generator in chest wall: 0JH606Z
4. Percutaneous placement of venous central line in right internal jugular, with tip in Superior Vena Cava: 02HV33Z
5. Open insertion of multiple channel cochlear implant, left ear: 09HE06Z
6. Percutaneous placement of Swan-Ganz catheter in pulmonary trunk: 02HP32Z (The Swan-Ganz catheter is coded to the device value Monitoring Device because it monitors pulmonary artery output.)
7. Bronchoscopy with insertion of brachytherapy seeds, right main bronchus: 0BH081Z
8. Open placement of bone growth stimulator, left femoral shaft: 0QHY0MZ
9. Cystoscopy with placement of brachytherapy seeds in prostate gland: 0VH081Z
10. Percutaneous insertion of Greenfield IVC filter: 06H03DZ

Replacement—Root operation R

Definition: Putting in or on biological or synthetic material that physically takes the place and/or function of all or a portion of a body part

Explanation: The body part may have been taken out or replaced, or may be taken out, physically eradicated, or rendered nonfunctional during the Replacement procedure. A Removal procedure is coded for taking out the device used in a previous replacement procedure.

Examples: Total hip replacement (Illustration 13), bone graft, free skin graft

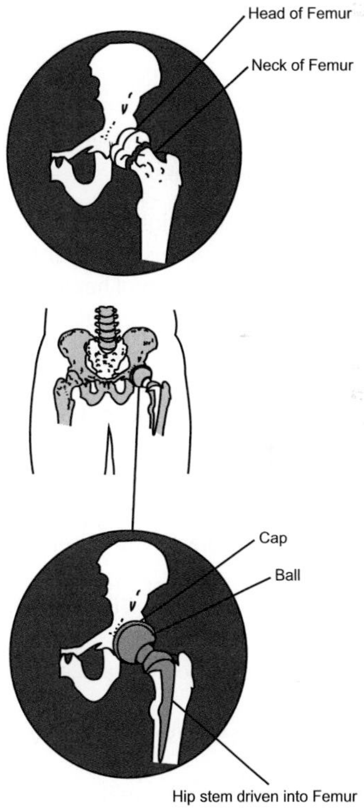

Illustration 13

The objective of procedures coded to the root operation Replacement is to put in a device that takes the place of some or all of a body part. Replacement encompasses a wide range of procedures, from joint replacements to grafts of all kinds.

Example: Prosthetic lens implantation

...a superior peritomy was made on the left eye and adequate hemostasis was achieved using eraser cautery. A posterior one-half

thickness groove was placed posterior to the blue line. This was beveled forward toward clear cornea.

The anterior chamber was entered at the 11:30 position with a blade. The eye was filled with viscoelastic substance. A can-opener type capsulotomy was performed with a cystitome. Hydrodissection was carried out and the lens was rocked gently with a cystitome to loosen it from the cortex.

The wound was then opened with corneal scleral scissors. The lens was prolapsed in the anterior chamber and removed. The anterior chamber was then temporarily closed with 8-0 Vicryl® sutures and cortical clean-up was performed.

One of the sutures was removed and a posterior chamber intraocular lens (Alcon model #MZ50BD) was inspected, rinsed, and placed into a capsular bag. Miochol was then instilled into the anterior chamber. The conjunctiva was pulled over the incision and cauterized into place...

Character 1 Section	Character 2 Body System	Character 3 Root Operation	Character 4 Body Part	Character 5 Approach	Character 6 Device	Character 7 Qualifier
Medical and Surgical	Eye	Replacement	Lens, Left	Percutaneous	Synthetic Substitute	No Qualifier
0	8	R	K	3	J	Z

Coding exercises

Using the ICD-10-PCS Tables, construct the code that accurately represents the procedure performed.

1. Full-thickness skin graft to right lower arm, autograft (do not code graft harvest for this exercise): 0HRDX73
2. Excision of necrosed left femoral head with bone bank bone graft to fill the defect, open: 0QR70KZ
3. Penetrating keratoplasty of right cornea with donor matched cornea, percutaneous approach: 08R83KZ
4. Bilateral mastectomy with concomitant saline breast implants, open: 0HRV0JZ
5. Excision of abdominal aorta with Gore-Tex® graft replacement, open: 04R00JZ
6. Total right knee arthroplasty with insertion of total knee prosthesis: 0SRC0JZ
7. Bilateral mastectomy with free TRAM flap reconstruction: 0HRV076
8. Tenonectomy with graft to right ankle using cadaver graft, open: 0LRS0KZ
9. Mitral valve replacement using porcine valve, open: 02RG08Z
10. Percutaneous phacoemulsification of right eye cataract with prosthetic lens insertion: 08RJ3JZ
11. Transcatheter replacement of pulmonary valve using of bovine jugular vein valve: 02RH38Z
12. Total left hip replacement using ceramic on ceramic prosthesis, without bone cement: 0SRB03A

Supplement—Root operation U

Definition: Putting in or on biologic or synthetic material that physically reinforces and/or augments the function a portion of a body part

Explanation: The biological material is non-living, or is living and from the same individual. The body part may have been previously replaced, and the Supplement procedure is performed to physically reinforce and/or augment the function of the replaced body part.

Examples: Herniorrhaphy using mesh (Illustration 14), free nerve graft, mitral valve ring annuloplasty, put a new acetabular liner in a previous hip replacement

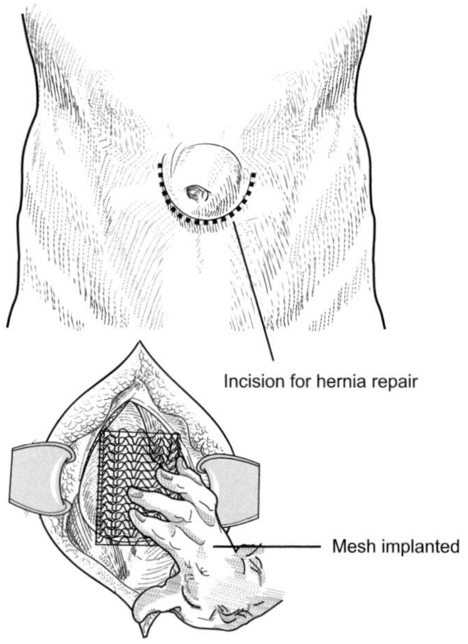

Illustration 14

The objective of procedures coded to the root operation Supplement is to put in a device that reinforces or augments the functions of some or all of a body part. The body part may have been taken out during a previous procedure, but is not taken out as part of the Supplement procedure. Supplement includes a wide range of procedures, from hernia repairs using mesh reinforcement to heart valve annuloplasties and grafts such as nerve grafts that supplement but do not physically take the place of the existing body part.

Example: Posterior colporrhaphy with Gynemesh

...attention was then turned to the posterior wall. Two Allis clamps were placed at the mucocutaneous junction in the region of the fourchette, and another clamp was placed at the apex of the rectocele.

The tissue between the distal clamps and the fourchette was excised, and carefully measured so that the introitus would be a 3- finger introitus The posterior vaginal mucosa was then incised in the midline by sharp and blunt dissection. The mucosa was then dissected to the level at the Allis clamp at the apex of the rectocele, and dissected with blunt and sharp dissection from the underlying tissue. The rectocele was then imbricated using mattress sutures of 2-0 Vicryl®, and the area of the levator ani reinforced with Gynemesh.

Two sutures of 2- 0 Vicryl® were taken in the levator ani muscle, the excess posterior vaginal mucosa excised, and then closed with interrupted sutures of 2-0 Vicryl®.

The perineal muscles were then approximated in the midline in layers, using 2-0 Vicryl®, after which the perineal skin was approximated using interrupted sutures of 2-0 Vicryl®...

Character 1 Section	Character 2 Body System	Character 3 Root Operation	Character 4 Body Part	Character 5 Approach	Character 6 Device	Character 7 Qualifier
Medical and Surgical	Subcutaneous Tissue and Fascia	Supplement	Pelvic Region	Open	Synthetic Substitute	No Qualifier
0	J	U	C	0	J	Z

Coding exercises

Using the ICD-10-PCS Tables, construct the code that accurately represents the procedure performed.

1. Aortic valve annuloplasty using ring, open: 02UF0JZ
2. Laparoscopic repair of left inguinal hernia with Marlex® plug: 0YU64JZ
3. Autograft nerve graft to right median nerve, percutaneous endoscopic (do not code graft harvest for this exercise): 01U547Z
4. Exchange of liner in femoral component of previous left hip replacement, open approach: 0SUS09Z (Taking out the old liner is coded separately to the root operation Removal.)
5. Anterior colporrhaphy with polypropylene mesh reinforcement, open approach: 0JUC0JZ
6. Implantation of CorCap® cardiac support device, open approach: 02UA0JZ
7. Abdominal wall herniorrhaphy, open, using synthetic mesh: 0WUF0JZ
8. Tendon graft to strengthen injured left shoulder using autograft, open (do not code graft harvest for this exercise): 0LU207Z
9. Onlay lamellar keratoplasty of left cornea using autograft, external approach: 08U9X7Z
10. Resurfacing procedure on right femoral head, open approach: 0SUR0BZ

Change—Root operation 2

Definition: Taking out or off a device from a body part and putting back an identical or similar device in or on the same body part without cutting or puncturing the skin or a mucous membrane

Explanation: All Change procedures are coded using the approach External

Examples: Urinary catheter change (Illustration 15), gastrostomy tube change

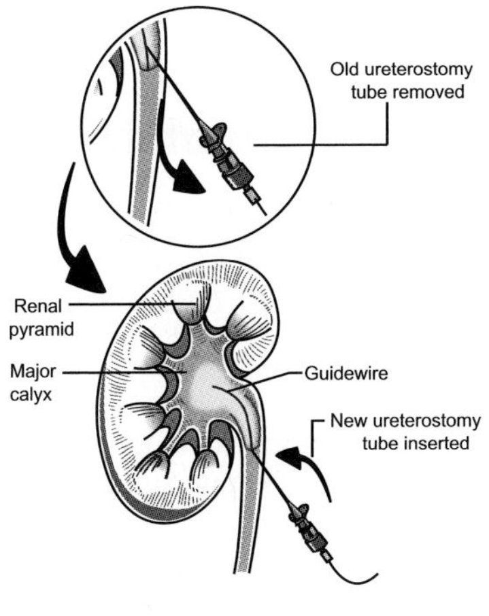

Illustration 15

The root operation Change represents only those procedures where a similar device is exchanged without making a new incision or puncture. Typical Change procedures include exchange of drainage devices and feeding devices.

Coding note: Change

In the root operation Change, general body part values are used when the specific body part value is not in the table.

Example: Percutaneous endoscopic gastrostomy (PEG) tube exchange

Character 1 Section	Character 2 Body System	Character 3 Root Operation	Character 4 Body Part	Character 5 Approach	Character 6 Device	Character 7 Qualifier
Medical and Surgical	Gastrointestinal System	Change	Upper Intest. Tract	External	Feeding Device	No Qualifier
0	D	2	0	X	U	Z

Coding exercises

Using the ICD-10-PCS Tables, construct the code that accurately represents the procedure performed.

1. Exchange of drainage tube from right hip joint: 0S2YX0Z
2. Tracheostomy tube exchange: 0B21XFZ
3. Change chest tube for left pneumothorax: 0W2BX0Z
4. Exchange of cerebral ventriculostomy drainage tube: 0020X0Z
5. Foley urinary catheter exchange: 0T2BX0Z (This is coded to Drainage Device because urine is being drained.)

Removal—Root operation P

Definition: Taking out or off a device from a body part

Explanation: If a device is taken out and a similar device put in without cutting or puncturing the skin or mucous membrane, the procedure is coded to the root operation Change. Otherwise, the procedure for taking out a device is coded to the root operation Removal.

Examples: Drainage tube removal, cardiac pacemaker removal

Removal represents a much broader range of procedures than those for removing the devices contained in the root operation Insertion. A procedure to remove a device is coded to Removal if it is not an integral part of another root operation, and regardless of the approach or the original root operation by which the device was put in.

Coding note: Removal

In the root operation Removal, general body part values are used when the specific body part value is not in the table

Example: Removal of right forearm external fixator

...the right upper extremity was prepped and draped in a sterile fashion. A tourniquet was placed at 250 mm of pressure.

The external fixator was removed using the appropriate wrench. The four pins in the ulna were then removed manually, as well as with the drill. The wounds were irrigated with antibiotic solution and a sterile dressing applied...

Character 1 Section	Character 2 Body System	Character 3 Root Operation	Character 4 Body Part	Character 5 Approach	Character 6 Device	Character 7 Qualifier
Medical and Surgical	Upper Bones	Removal	Ulna, Right	External	External Fixation	No Qualifier
0	P	P	K	X	5	Z

Coding exercises

Using the ICD-10-PCS Tables, construct the code that accurately represents the procedure performed.

1. Open removal of lumbar sympathetic neurostimulator: 01PY0MZ
2. Non-incisional removal of Swan-Ganz catheter from right pulmonary artery: 02PYX2Z
3. Laparotomy with removal of pancreatic drain: 0FPG00Z
4. Extubation, endotracheal tube: 0BP1XDZ
5. Non-incisional PEG tube removal: 0DP6XUZ
6. Transvaginal removal of brachytherapy seeds: 0UPH71Z
7. Incision with removal of K-wire fixation, right first metatarsal: 0QPN04Z
8. Cystoscopy with retrieval of left ureteral stent: 0TP98DZ
9. Removal of nasogastric drainage tube for decompression: 0DP6X0Z
10. Removal of external fixator, left radial fracture: 0PPJX5Z

Revision—Root operation W

Definition: Correcting, to the extent possible, a portion of a malfunctioning device or the position of a displaced device

Explanation: Revision can include correcting a malfunctioning device by taking out and/or putting in part of the device

Examples: Adjustment of pacemaker lead, adjustment of hip prosthesis (Illustration 16)

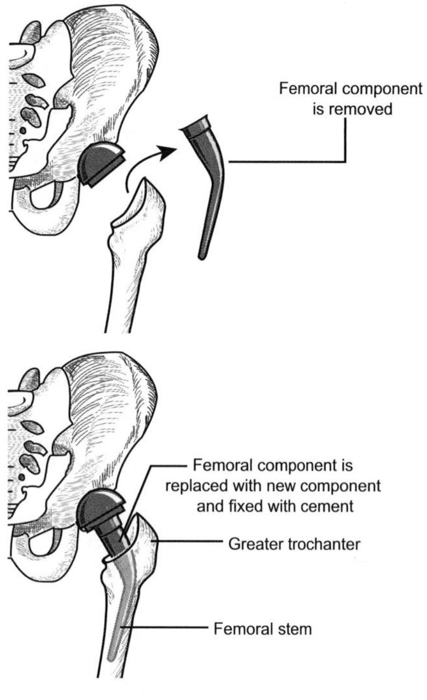

Illustration 16

Revision is coded when the objective of the procedure is to correct the position or function of a previously placed device, without taking the entire device out and putting a whole new device in its place. A complete re-do of a procedure is coded to the root operation performed.

Coding note: Revision

In the root operation Revision, general body part values are used when the specific body part value is not in the table.

Example: Revision of artificial anal sphincter

...Proceeding through a suprapubic incision, this was then extended after injecting local anesthetic, thereby exposing the underlying tubing, which was then delivered through the suprapubic region.

Meticulous hemostasis was achieved using electrocautery. At that point the pump device was then repositioned in the left lower quadrant abdominal wall region. The tubing was reinserted using dilators, and the skin reapproximated using 2-0 Vicryl® sutures. Sterile dressing was then applied...

Character 1 Section	Character 2 Body System	Character 3 Root Operation	Character 4 Body Part	Character 5 Approach	Character 6 Device	Character 7 Qualifier
Medical and Surgical	Gastrointestinal System	Revision	Anus	Open	Artificial Sphincter	No Qualifier
0	D	W	Q	0	L	Z

Coding exercises

Using the ICD-10-PCS Tables, construct the code that accurately represents the procedure performed.

1. Trimming and reanastomosis of stenosed femorofemoral synthetic bypass graft, open: 04WY0JZ
2. Open revision of right hip replacement, with recementing of the prosthesis: 0SW90JZ
3. Adjustment of position, pacemaker lead in left ventricle, percutaneous: 02WA3MZ
4. Taking out loose screw and putting larger screw in fracture repair plate, left tibia: 0QWH04Z
5. Revision of totally implantable VAD port placement in chest wall, causing patient discomfort, open: 0JWT0XZ

Root operations involving examination only

The table below lists the root operations that involve examination of a body part. Each is described in detail in the pages that follow.

Objective of procedure

- Inspection: Visual/manual exploration
- Map: Location electrical impulses/functional areas

Site of procedure

- Inspection: Some/all of a body part
- Map: Brain/cardiac conduction mechanism

Example

- Inspection: Diagnostic cystoscopy
- Map: Cardiac mapping

Inspection—Root operation J

Definition: Visually and/or manually exploring a body part

Explanation: Visual exploration may be performed with or without optical instrumentation. Manual exploration may be performed directly or through intervening body layers

Examples: Diagnostic arthroscopy, exploratory laparotomy

The root operation Inspection represents procedures where the sole objective is to examine a body part. Procedures that are discontinued without any other root operation being performed are also coded to Inspection.

Example: Diagnostic colposcopy with examination of cervix

...Colposcopy was done which revealed pseudo-white areas at 2 o'clock and 6 o'clock on the cervix, with abnormal cells and irregular white borders noted on both...

Character 1 Section	Character 2 Body System	Character 3 Root Operation	Character 4 Body Part	Character 5 Approach	Character 6 Device	Character 7 Qualifier
Medical and Surgical	Female Reproductive	Inspection	Uterus and Cervix	Via Nat./ Artif. Opening Endo	No Device	No Qualifier
0	U	J	D	8	Z	Z

Coding exercises

Using the ICD-10-PCS Tables, construct the code that accurately represents the procedure performed.

1. Thoracotomy with exploration of right pleural cavity: 0WJ90ZZ
2. Diagnostic laryngoscopy: 0CJS8ZZ
3. Exploratory arthrotomy of left knee: 0SJD0ZZ
4. Colposcopy with diagnostic hysteroscopy: 0UJD8ZZ
5. Digital rectal exam: 0DJD7ZZ
6. Diagnostic arthroscopy of right shoulder: 0RJJ4ZZ
7. EGD (esophagogastroduodenoscopy) 0DJ08ZZ
8. Laparotomy with palpation of liver: 0FJ00ZZ
9. Transurethral diagnostic cystoscopy: 0TJB8ZZ
10. Colonoscopy, discontinued at sigmoid colon: 0DJD8ZZ

Map—Root operation K

Definition: Locating the route of passage of electrical impulses and/or locating functional areas in a body part

Explanation: Applicable only to the cardiac conduction mechanism and the central nervous system

Examples: Cardiac mapping, cortical mapping

Mapping represents a very narrow range of procedures. Procedures include only cardiac mapping and cortical mapping

Example: Cardiac mapping

...under sterile technique arterial sheath was placed in the right femoral artery. The electrical catheter was advanced up the aorta and into the left atrium under fluoroscopic guidance and mapping commenced. After adequate recordings were obtained the catheter was withdrawn and hemostasis achieved with manual pressure on the right femoral artery...

Character 1 Section	Character 2 Body System	Character 3 Root Operation	Character 4 Body Part	Character 5 Approach	Character 6 Device	Character 7 Qualifier
Medical and Surgical	Heart and Gr. Vessels	Map	Conduction Mechanism	Percutaneous	No Device	No Qualifier
0	2	K	8	3	Z	Z

Coding exercises

Using the ICD-10-PCS Tables, construct the code that accurately represents the procedure performed.

1. Percutaneous mapping of basal ganglia: 00K83ZZ
2. Heart catheterization with cardiac mapping: 02K83ZZ
3. Intraoperative whole brain mapping via craniotomy: 00K00ZZ
4. Mapping of left cerebral hemisphere, percutaneous endoscopic: 00K74ZZ
5. Intraoperative cardiac mapping during open heart surgery: 02K80ZZ

Root operations that define other repairs

The table below lists the root operations that define other repairs. Control describes the effort to locate and stop postprocedural hemorrhage. Repair is described in detail in the pages that follow.

Objective of procedure

- Control: Stopping/attempting to stop postprocedural bleed
- Repair: Restoring body part to its normal structure

Site of procedure

- Control: Anatomical region
- Repair: Some/all of a body part

Example

- Control: Post-prostatectomy bleeding control
- Repair: Suture laceration

Control—Root operation 3

Definition: Stopping, or attempting to stop, postprocedural bleeding (Illustration 17)

Explanation: The site of the bleeding is coded as an anatomical region and not to a specific body part

Examples: Control of post-prostatectomy hemorrhage, control of post-tonsillectomy hemorrhage

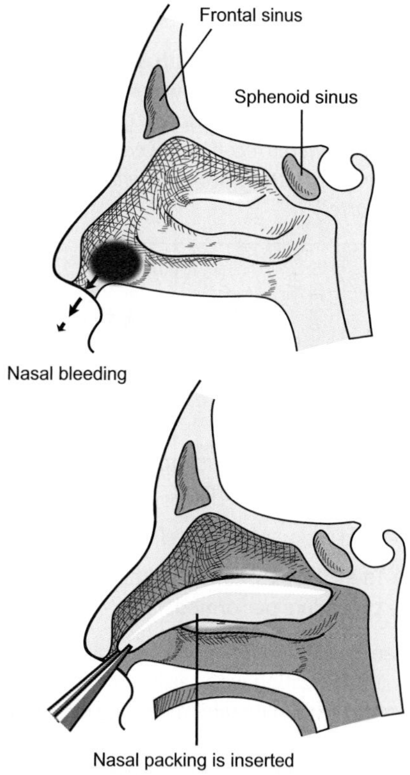

Illustration 17 - Example shows control of nasal hemorrhage

Control is used to represent a small range of procedures performed to treat postprocedural bleeding. If performing Bypass, Detachment, Excision, Extraction, Reposition, Replacement, or Resection is required to stop the bleeding, then Control is not coded separately.

Coding note: Control

Control includes irrigation or evacuation of hematoma done at the operative site. Both irrigation and evacuation may be necessary to clear the operative field and effectively stop the bleeding.

Example: Re-opening of laparotomy site with ligation of arterial bleeder

Character 1 Section	Character 2 Body System	Character 3 Root Operation	Character 4 Body Part	Character 5 Approach	Character 6 Device	Character 7 Qualifier
Medical and Surgical	Anatomical Regions, Gen.	Control	Peritoneal Cavity	Open	No Device	No Qualifier
0	W	3	G	0	Z	Z

Coding exercises

Using the ICD-10-PCS Tables, construct the code that accurately represents the procedure performed.

1. Hysteroscopy with cautery of post-hysterectomy oozing and evacuation of clot: 0W3R8ZZ
2. Open exploration and ligation of post-op arterial bleeder, left forearm: 0X3F0ZZ
3. Control of post-operative retroperitoneal bleeding via laparotomy: 0W3H0ZZ
4. Reopening of thoracotomy site with drainage and control of post-op hemopericardium: 0W3D0ZZ
5. Arthroscopy with drainage of hemarthrosis at previous operative site, right knee: 0Y3F4ZZ

Repair—Root operation Q

Definition: Restoring, to the extent possible, a body part to its normal anatomic structure and function

Explanation: Used only when the method to accomplish the repair is not one of the other root operations

Examples: Herniorrhaphy, suture of laceration

The root operation Repair represents a broad range of procedures for restoring the anatomic structure of a body part such as suture of lacerations. Repair also functions as the "not elsewhere classified (NEC)" root operation, to be used when the procedure performed does not meet the definition of one of the other root operations.

Example: Left open inguinal herniorrhaphy

...an incision in the left groin extending on the skin from the internal to the external inguinal ring was made. The external oblique aponeurosis was exposed.

The hernia sac was then ligated at the internal ring with non-dissolving sutures. A hernia repair was then performed. The internal oblique fascia was sutured in interrupted stitches to the iliopubic fascia. The spermatic cord was then returned to its anatomical position.

The external oblique aponeurosis was then repaired in interrupted sutures. Complete hemostasis was obtained, and the skin closed...

Character 1 Section	Character 2 Body System	Character 3 Root Operation	Character 4 Body Part	Character 5 Approach	Character 6 Device	Character 7 Qualifier
Medical and Surgical	Lower Extremities	Repair	Inguinal Region, Left	Open	No Device	No Qualifier
0	Y	Q	6	0	Z	Z

Coding exercises

Using the ICD-10-PCS Tables, construct the code that accurately represents the procedure performed.

1. Suture repair of left radial nerve laceration: 01Q60ZZ (The approach value is Open, though the surgical exposure may have been created by the wound itself.)
2. Laparotomy with suture repair of blunt force duodenal laceration: 0DQ90ZZ
3. Perineoplasty with repair of old obstetric laceration, open: 0WQN0ZZ
4. Suture repair of right biceps tendon laceration, open: 0LQ30ZZ
5. Closure of abdominal wall stab wound: 0WQF0ZZ

Root operations that define other objectives

The last three root operations in the Medical and Surgical section, Fusion, Alteration, and Creation, describe procedures performed for three distinct reasons. Beyond that they have little in common. A Fusion procedure puts a dysfunctional joint out of service rather than restoring function to the joint. Alteration encompasses a whole range of procedures that share only the fact that they are done to improve the way the patient looks. Creation represents only two very specific sex change operations.

Objective of procedure

- Fusion: Rendering joint immobile
- Alteration: Modifying body part for cosmetic purposes without affecting function
- Creation: Making new structure for sex change operation

Site of procedure

- Fusion: Joint
- Alteration: Some/all of a body part
- Creation: Perineum

Example

- Fusion: Spinal fusion
- Alteration: Face lift
- Creation: Artificial vagina/penis

Fusion—Root operation G

Definition: Joining together portions of an articular body part rendering the articular body part immobile

Explanation: The body part is joined together by fixation device, bone graft, or other means

Examples: Spinal fusion, ankle arthrodesis

A limited range of procedures is represented in the root operation Fusion, because fusion procedures are by definition only performed on the joints. Qualifier values are used to specify whether a vertebral joint fusion uses an anterior or posterior approach, and whether the anterior or posterior column of the spine is fused.

Example: Anterior cervical fusion C-2 through C-4 with bone bank graft

...after skull tong traction was applied, incision was made in the left neck, and Gardner retractors placed to separate the intervertebral muscles at the C-2 through C-4 levels.

Using the drill, a trough was incised on the anterior surface of the C-2 vertebra, and the C-2/C-3 space evacuated with a rongeur, and the accompanying cartilage removed. This procedure was then repeated at the C-3/C-4 level.

Bone bank patella strut graft was trimmed with a saw and fashioned to fit the C-2/C-3 interspace. After adequate adjustments in the size and shape had been made, the graft was tapped securely into place. The procedure was repeated for the C-3/C-4 level.

X-rays revealed good alignment and final position. Traction was gradually decreased to maintain position. Retractors were removed and the fascia was reapproximated with 0 Vicryl®...

Character 1 Section	Character 2 Body System	Character 3 Root Operation	Character 4 Body Part	Character 5 Approach	Character 6 Device	Character 7 Qualifier
Medical and Surgical	Upper Joints	Fusion	Cervical Jt, 2 or More	Open	Nonautolog Tissue Subst	Ant Approach Ant Column
0	R	G	2	0	K	0

Coding exercises

Using the ICD-10-PCS Tables, construct the code that accurately represents the procedure performed.

1. Radiocarpal fusion of left hand with internal fixation, open: 0RGP04Z
2. Posterior spinal fusion at L1-L3 level with BAK® cage interbody fusion device, open: 0SG10AJ
3. Intercarpal fusion of right hand with bone bank bone graft, open: 0RGQ0KZ
4. Sacrococcygeal fusion with bone graft from same operative site, open: 0SG507Z
5. Interphalangeal fusion of left great toe, percutaneous pin fixation: 0SGQ34Z

Alteration—Root operation 0

Definition: Modifying the natural anatomic structure of a body part without affecting the function of the body part

Explanation: Principal purpose is to improve appearance

Examples: Face lift, breast augmentation

Alteration is coded for all procedures performed solely to improve appearance. All methods, approaches, and devices used for the objective of improving appearance are coded here.

Coding note: Alteration

Because some surgical procedures can be performed for either medical or cosmetic purposes, coding for Alteration requires diagnostic confirmation that the surgery is in fact performed to improve appearance.

Example: Cosmetic blepharoplasty

...attention was turned to the redundant upper eyelid skin. The ellipse of skin as marked preoperatively was excised bilaterally.

The medial and lateral fat compartments were open bilaterally. The medial compartment had severe fatty excess and periorbital fat herniation. This was resected. The lateral fat compartment was opened and the lateral fat tailored as well.

Subdermal closure was performed with interrupted 3-0 sutures bilaterally. The skin was closed...

Character 1 Section	Character 2 Body System	Character 3 Root Operation	Character 4 Body Part	Character 5 Approach	Character 6 Device	Character 7 Qualifier
Medical and Surgical	Eye	Alteration	Upper Eyelid, Left	Open	No Device	No Qualifier
0	8	0	P	0	Z	Z

Character 1 Section	Character 2 Body System	Character 3 Root Operation	Character 4 Body Part	Character 5 Approach	Character 6 Device	Character 7 Qualifier
Medical and Surgical	Eye	Alteration	Upper Eyelid, Right	Open	No Device	No Qualifier
0	8	0	N	0	Z	Z

Coding exercises

Using the ICD-10-PCS Tables, construct the code that accurately represents the procedure performed.

1. Cosmetic face lift, open, no other information available: 0W020ZZ
2. Bilateral breast augmentation with silicone implants, open: 0H0V0JZ
3. Cosmetic rhinoplasty with septal reduction and tip elevation using local tissue graft, open: 090K07Z
4. Abdominoplasty (tummy tuck), open: 0W0F0ZZ
5. Liposuction of bilateral thighs: 0J0L3ZZ, 0J0M3ZZ

Creation—Root operation 4

Definition: Making a new genital structure that does not physically take the place of a body part

Explanation: Used only for sex change operations

Examples: Creation of vagina in a male, creation of penis in a female

Creation is used to represent a very narrow range of procedures. Only the procedures performed for sex change operations are included here.

Coding note: Harvesting autograft tissue

If a separate procedure is performed to harvest autograft tissue, it is coded to the appropriate root operation in addition to the primary procedure.

Example: Creating a vagina in a male patient using autograft

Character 1 Section	Character 2 Body System	Character 3 Root Operation	Character 4 Body Part	Character 5 Approach	Character 6 Device	Character 7 Qualifier
Medical and Surgical	Anatomical Regions, Gen.	Creation	Perineum, Male	Open	Autolog. Tissue Subst.	Vagina
0	W	4	M	0	7	0

Coding exercises

Using the ICD-10-PCS Tables, construct the code that accurately represents the procedure performed.

1. Creation of penis in female patient using tissue bank donor graft: 0W4N0K1
2. Creation of vagina in male patient using synthetic material: 0W4M0J0

Procedures in the Medical and Surgical-related Sections

Obstetrics—Section 1

The Obstetrics section follows the same conventions established in the Medical and Surgical section, with all seven characters retaining the same meaning, as shown in this example of a low forceps extraction.

Character 1 Section	Character 2 Body System	Character 3 Root Operation	Character 4 Body Part	Character 5 Approach	Character 6 Device	Character 7 Qualifier
Obstetrics	Pregnancy	Extraction	Products of Conception	Via Nat./Artif. Opening	No Device	Low Forceps
1	0	D	0	7	Z	3

Root operations

There are twelve root operations in the Obstetrics section. Ten of these are also found in the Medical and Surgical section.

For the complete list of root operations and their definitions, please refer to ICD-10-PCS definitions

The two root operations unique to Obstetrics are defined below:

- A – Abortion: Artificially terminating a pregnancy
- E – Delivery: Assisting the passage of the products of conception from the genital canal

Coding note: Abortion

Abortion is subdivided according to whether an additional device such as a laminaria or abortifacient is used, or whether the abortion was performed by mechanical means.

If either a laminaria or abortifacient is used, then the approach is Via Natural or Artificial Opening.

All other abortion procedures are those done by mechanical means (the products of conception are physically removed using instrumentation), and the device value is Z, No Device.

Example: Transvaginal abortion using vacuum aspiration technique

Character 1 Section	Character 2 Body System	Character 3 Root Operation	Character 4 Body Part	Character 5 Approach	Character 6 Device	Character 7 Qualifier
Obstetrics	Pregnancy	Abortion	Products of Conception	Via Nat./Artif. Opening	No Device	Vacuum
1	0	A	0	7	Z	6

Coding note: Delivery

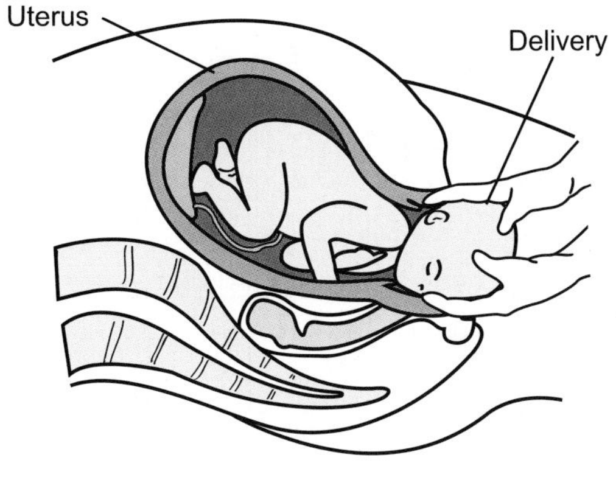

Illustration 18

Delivery applies only to manually-assisted, vaginal delivery (Illustration 18) and is defined as assisting the passage of the products of conception from the genital canal. Cesarean deliveries are coded in this section to the root operation Extraction.

Example: Manually-assisted delivery

Character 1 Section	Character 2 Body System	Character 3 Root Operation	Character 4 Body Part	Character 5 Approach	Character 6 Device	Character 7 Qualifier
Obstetrics	Pregnancy	Delivery	Products of Conception	External	No Device	No Qualifier
1	0	E	0	X	Z	Z

Coding exercises

Using the ICD-10-PCS Tables, construct the code that accurately represents the procedure performed.

1. Abortion by dilation and evacuation following laminaria insertion: 10A07ZW
2. Manually assisted spontaneous abortion: 10E0XZZ (Since the pregnancy was not artificially terminated, this is coded to Delivery, because it captures the procedure objective. The fact that it was an abortion will be identified in the diagnosis code.)
3. Abortion by abortifacient insertion: 10A07ZX
4. Bimanual pregnancy examination: 10J07ZZ
5. Extraperitoneal c-section, low transverse incision: 10D00Z2
6. Fetal spinal tap, percutaneous: 10903ZA
7. Fetal kidney transplant, laparoscopic: 10Y04ZS
8. Open in utero repair of congenital diaphragmatic hernia: 10Q00ZK (Diaphragm is classified to the Respiratory body system in the Medical and Surgical section.)
9. Laparoscopy with total excision of tubal pregnancy: 10T24ZZ
10. Transvaginal removal of fetal monitoring electrode: 10P073Z

Placement—Section 2

The Placement section follows the same conventions established in the Medical and Surgical section, with all seven characters retaining the same meaning, as in the example of cast change on the right forearm below.

Character 1 Section	Character 2 Body System	Character 3 Root Operation	Character 4 Body Region	Character 5 Approach	Character 6 Device	Character 7 Qualifier
Placement	Anatomical Regions	Change	Lower Arm, Right	External	Cast	No Qualifier
2	W	0	C	X	2	Z

Root operations

The root operations in the Placement section include only those procedures performed without making an incision or a puncture.

- 0 – Change: Taking out or off a device from a body region and putting back an identical or similar device in or on the same body region without cutting or puncturing the skin or a mucous membrane
- 1 – Compression: Putting pressure on a body region
- 2 – Dressing: Putting material on a body region for protection
- 3 – Immobilization: Limiting or preventing motion of a body region
- 4 – Packing: Putting material in a body region
- 5 – Removal: Taking out or off a device from a body region
- 6 – Traction: Exerting a pulling force on a body region in a distal direction

Example: Change of vaginal packing

Character 1 Section	Character 2 Body System	Character 3 Root Operation	Character 4 Body Region	Character 5 Approach	Character 6 Device	Character 7 Qualifier
Placement	Anatomical Orifices	Change	Female Genital Tract	External	Packing Material	No Qualifier
2	Y	0	4	X	5	Z

Example: Placement of pressure dressing on abdominal wall

Character 1 Section	Character 2 Body System	Character 3 Root Operation	Character 4 Body Region	Character 5 Approach	Character 6 Device	Character 7 Qualifier
Placement	Anatomical Regions	Compression	Abdominal Wall	External	Pressure Dressing	No Qualifier
2	W	1	3	X	6	Z

Example: Application of sterile dressing to head wound

Character 1 Section	Character 2 Body System	Character 3 Root Operation	Character 4 Body Region	Character 5 Approach	Character 6 Device	Character 7 Qualifier
Placement	Anatomical Regions	Dressing	Head	External	Bandage	No Qualifier
2	W	2	0	X	4	Z

Coding note: Immobilization

The procedures to fit a device, such as splints and braces, as described in F0DZ6EZ and F0DZ7EZ, apply only to the rehabilitation setting. Splints and braces placed in other inpatient settings are coded to Immobilization, table 2W3 in the Placement section.

Example: Placement of splint on left finger

Character 1 Section	Character 2 Body System	Character 3 Root Operation	Character 4 Body Region	Character 5 Approach	Character 6 Device	Character 7 Qualifier
Placement	Anatomical Regions	Immobilization	Finger, Left	External	Splint	No Qualifier
2	W	3	K	X	1	Z

Example: Placement of nasal packing

Character 1 Section	Character 2 Body System	Character 3 Root Operation	Character 4 Body Region	Character 5 Approach	Character 6 Device	Character 7 Qualifier
Placement	Anatomical Orifices	Packing	Nasal	External	Packing Material	No Qualifier
2	Y	4	1	X	5	Z

Example: Removal of stereotactic head frame

Character 1 Section	Character 2 Body System	Character 3 Root Operation	Character 4 Body Region	Character 5 Approach	Character 6 Device	Character 7 Qualifier
Placement	Anatomical Regions	Removal	Head	External	Stereotactic Apparatus	No Qualifier
2	W	5	0	X	Y	Z

Coding note: Traction

Traction in this section includes only the task performed using a mechanical traction apparatus. Manual traction performed by a physical therapist is coded to Manual Therapy Techniques in section F, Physical Rehabilitation and Diagnostic Audiology.

Example: Lumbar traction using motorized split-traction table

Character 1 Section	Character 2 Body System	Character 3 Root Operation	Character 4 Body Region	Character 5 Approach	Character 6 Device	Character 7 Qualifier
Placement	Anatomical Regions	Traction	Back	External	Traction Apparatus	No Qualifier
2	W	6	5	X	0	Z

Coding exercises

Using the ICD-10-PCS Tables, construct the code that accurately represents the procedure performed.

1. Placement of packing material, right ear: 2Y42X5Z
2. Mechanical traction of entire left leg: 2W6MX0Z
3. Removal of splint, right shoulder: 2W5AX1Z
4. Placement of neck brace: 2W32X3Z
5. Change of vaginal packing: 2Y04X5Z
6. Packing of wound, chest wall: 2W44X5Z
7. Sterile dressing placement to left groin region: 2W27X4Z
8. Removal of packing material from pharynx: 2Y50X5Z
9. Placement of intermittent pneumatic compression device, covering entire right arm: 2W18X7Z
10. Exchange of pressure dressing to left thigh: 2W0PX6Z

Administration—Section 3

The Administration section includes infusions, injections, and transfusions, as well as other related procedures, such as irrigation and tattooing. All codes in this section define procedures where a diagnostic or therapeutic substance is given to the patient, as in the platelet transfusion example below.

Character 1 Section	Character 2 Body System	Character 3 Root Operation	Character 4 Body System	Character 5 Approach	Character 6 Substance	Character 7 Qualifier
Administration	Circulatory	Transfusion	Central Vein	Percutaneous	Platelets	Nonautologous
3	0	2	4	3	R	1

Root operations

Root operations in this section are classified according to the broad category of substance administered. If the substance given is a blood product or a cleansing substance, then the procedure is coded to Transfusion and Irrigation respectively. All the other substances administered, such as anti-neoplastic substances, are coded to the root operation Introduction.

- 0 – Introduction: Putting in or on a therapeutic, diagnostic, nutritional, physiological, or prophylactic substance except blood or blood products
- 1 – Irrigation: Putting in or on a cleansing substance
- 2 – Transfusion: Putting in blood or blood products

Example: Nerve block injection to median nerve

Character 1 Section	Character 2 Body System	Character 3 Root Operation	Character 4 Body System	Character 5 Approach	Character 6 Substance	Character 7 Qualifier
Administration	Phys. Sys. & Anat. Regions	Introduction	Peripheral Nerves	Percutaneous	Regional Anesthetic	No Qualifier
3	E	0	T	3	C	Z

Example: Flushing of eye

Character 1 Section	Character 2 Body System	Character 3 Root Operation	Character 4 Body System	Character 5 Approach	Character 6 Substance	Character 7 Qualifier
Administration	Phys. Sys. & Anat. Regions	Irrigation	Eye	External	Irrigating Substance	No Qualifier
3	E	1	C	X	8	Z

Example: Transfusion of cell saver red cells into central venous line

Character 1 Section	Character 2 Body System	Character 3 Root Operation	Character 4 Body System	Character 5 Approach	Character 6 Substance	Character 7 Qualifier
Administration	Circulatory	Transfusion	Central Vein	Percutaneous	Red Blood Cells	Autologous
3	0	2	4	3	N	0

Coding exercises

Using the ICD-10-PCS Tables, construct the code that accurately represents the procedure performed.

1. Peritoneal dialysis via indwelling catheter: 3E1M39Z
2. Transvaginal artificial insemination: 3E0P7LZ
3. Infusion of total parenteral nutrition via central venous catheter: 3E0436Z
4. Esophagogastroscopy with Botox® injection into esophageal sphincter: 3E0G8GC (Botulinum toxin is a paralyzing agent with temporary effects; it does not sclerose or destroy the nerve.)
5. Percutaneous irrigation of knee joint: 3E1U38Z
6. Systemic infusion of recombinant tissue plasminogen activator (r-tPA) via peripheral venous catheter: 3E03317
7. Transfusion of antihemophilic factor, (nonautologous) via arterial central line: 30263V1
8. Transabdominal in-vitro fertilization, implantation of donor ovum: 3E0P3Q1
9. Autologous bone marrow transplant via central venous line: 30243G0
10. Implantation of anti-microbial envelope with cardiac defibrillator placement, open: 3E0102A

Measurement and Monitoring—Section 4

There are two root operations in this section, and they differ in only one respect: Measurement defines one procedure and Monitoring defines a series of procedures.

Root operations

Measurement describes a single level taken, while Monitoring describes a series of levels obtained at intervals. For example,

- A single temperature reading is considered Measurement.
- Temperature taken every half hour for 8 hours is considered Monitoring.

Instead of defining a device, the sixth character defines the physiological or physical function being tested.

- 0 – Measurement: Determining the level of a physiological or physical function at a point in time
- 1 – Monitoring: Determining the level of a physiological or physical function repetitively over a period of time

Example: External electrocardiogram (EKG), single reading

Character 1 Section	Character 2 Body System	Character 3 Root Operation	Character 4 Body System	Character 5 Approach	Character 6 Function	Character 7 Qualifier
Measurement & Monitoring	Physiological Systems	Measurement	Cardiac	External	Electrical Activity	No Qualifier
4	A	0	2	X	4	Z

Example: Urinary pressure monitoring

Character 1 Section	Character 2 Body System	Character 3 Root Operation	Character 4 Body System	Character 5 Approach	Character 6 Device	Character 7 Qualifier
Measurement & Monitoring	Physiological Systems	Monitoring	Urinary	Via Nat./Artif. Opening	Pressure	No Qualifier
4	A	1	D	7	B	Z

Coding exercises

Using the ICD-10-PCS Tables, construct the code that accurately represents the procedure performed.

1. Cardiac stress test, single measurement: 4A02XM4
2. EGD with biliary flow measurement: 4A0C85Z
3. Right and left heart cardiac catheterization with bilateral sampling and pressure measurements: 4A023N8
4. Peripheral venous pulse, external, single measurement: 4A04XJ1
5. Holter monitoring: 4A12X45
6. Respiratory rate, external, single measurement: 4A09XCZ
7. Fetal heart rate monitoring, transvaginal: 4A1H7CZ
8. Visual mobility test, single measurement: 4A07X7Z
9. Left ventricular cardiac output monitoring from pulmonary artery wedge (Swan-Ganz) catheter: 4A1239Z
10. Olfactory acuity test, single measurement: 4A08X0Z

Extracorporeal Assistance and Performance—Section 5

This section includes procedures performed in a critical care setting, such as mechanical ventilation and cardioversion. It also includes other procedures, such as hemodialysis and hyperbaric oxygen treatment. These procedures all use equipment to support a physiological function in some way, whether it is breathing, circulating the blood, or restoring the natural rhythm of the heart.

The fifth and sixth characters in this section define duration and function respectively. These characters describe the duration of the procedure and the body function being acted upon, rather than the approach and device used.

Root operations

Assistance and Performance are two variations of the same kinds of procedures, varying only in the degree of control exercised over the physiological function.

- 0 – Assistance: Taking over a portion of a physiological function by extracorporeal means
- 1 – Performance: Completely taking over a physiological function by extracorporeal means
- 2 – Restoration: Returning, or attempting to return, a physiological function to its original state by extracorporeal means

Coding note: Assistance

Assistance defines procedures that support a physiological function but do not take complete control of it, such as intra-aortic balloon pump to support cardiac output and hyperbaric oxygen treatment.

Example: Hyperbaric oxygenation of wound

Character 1 Section	Character 2 Body System	Character 3 Root Operation	Character 4 Body System	Character 5 Duration	Character 6 Function	Character 7 Qualifier
Extracorp. Assistance & Performance	Physiological Systems	Assistance	Circulatory	Intermittent	Oxygenation	Hyperbaric
5	A	0	5	1	2	1

Coding note: Performance

Performance defines procedures where complete control is exercised over a physiological function, such as total mechanical ventilation, cardiac pacing, and cardiopulmonary bypass.

Example: Cardiopulmonary bypass in conjunction with CABG

Character 1 Section	Character 2 Body System	Character 3 Root Operation	Character 4 Body System	Character 5 Duration	Character 6 Function	Character 7 Qualifier
Extracorp. Assistance & Performance	Physiological Systems	Performance	Cardiac	Continuous	Output	No Qualifier
5	A	1	2	2	1	Z

Coding note: Restoration

Restoration defines only external cardioversion and defibrillation procedures. Failed cardioversion procedures are also included in the definition of Restoration, and are coded the same as successful procedures.

Example: Attempted cardiac defibrillation, unsuccessful

Character 1 Section	Character 2 Body System	Character 3 Root Operation	Character 4 Body System	Character 5 Duration	Character 6 Function	Character 7 Qualifier
Extracorp. Assist. and Performance	Physiological	Restoration	Cardiac	Single	Rhythm	No Qualifier
5	A	2	2	0	4	Z

Coding exercises

Using the ICD-10-PCS Tables, construct the code that accurately represents the procedure performed.

1. Intermittent mechanical ventilation, 16 hours: 5A1935Z
2. Liver dialysis, single encounter: 5A1C00Z
3. Cardiac countershock with successful conversion to sinus rhythm: 5A2204Z
4. IPPB (intermittent positive pressure breathing) for mobilization of secretions, 22 hours: 5A09358
5. Renal dialysis, series of encounters: 5A1D60Z
6. IABP (intra-aortic balloon pump) continuous: 5A02210
7. Intra-operative cardiac pacing, continuous: 5A1223Z
8. ECMO (extracorporeal membrane oxygenation), continuous: 5A15223
9. Controlled mechanical ventilation (CMV), 45 hours: 5A1945Z
10. Pulsatile compression boot with intermittent inflation: 5A02115 (This is coded to the function value Cardiac Output, because the purpose of such compression devices is to return blood to the heart faster.)

Extracorporeal Therapies—Section 6

Section 6, Extracorporeal Therapies, describes other extracorporeal procedures that are not defined by Assistance and Performance in section 5 Examples are bili-lite phototherapy, apheresis, and whole body hypothermia.

The second character contains a single general body system choice, Physiological Systems, as in the phototherapy example below. The sixth character is defined as a qualifier, but contains no specific qualifier values. The seventh-character qualifier identifies various blood components separated out in pheresis procedures.

Character 1 Section	Character 2 Body System	Character 3 Root Operation	Character 4 Body System	Character 5 Duration	Character 6 Qualifier	Character 7 Qualifier
Extracorp. Therapies	Physiological Systems	Phototherapy	Skin	Single	No Qualifier	No Qualifier
6	A	6	0	0	Z	Z

Root operations

The meaning of each root operation is consistent with the term as used in the medical community. Decompression and Hyperthermia have a more specialized meaning. All are defined in the table below.

- 0 – Atmospheric Control: Extracorporeal control of atmospheric pressure and composition
- 1 – Decompression: Extracorporeal elimination of undissolved gas from body fluids
- 2 – Electromagnetic Therapy: Extracorporeal treatment by electromagnetic rays
- 3 – Hyperthermia: Extracorporeal raising of body temperature
- 4 – Hypothermia: Extracorporeal lowering of body temperature
- 5 – Pheresis: Extracorporeal separation of blood products
- 6 – Phototherapy: Extracorporeal treatment by light rays
- 7 – Ultrasound Therapy: Extracorporeal treatment by ultrasound
- 8 – Ultraviolet Light Therapy: Extracorporeal treatment by ultraviolet light
- 9 – Shock Wave Therapy: Extracorporeal treatment by shock waves

Coding note: Decompression

Decompression describes a single type of procedure—treatment for decompression sickness (the bends) in a hyperbaric chamber.

Example: Hyperbaric decompression treatment, single

Character 1 Section	Character 2 Body System	Character 3 Root Operation	Character 4 Body System	Character 5 Duration	Character 6 Qualifier	Character 7 Qualifier
Extracorp. Therapies	Physiological Systems	Decompression	Circulatory	Single	No Qualifier	No Qualifier
6	A	1	5	0	Z	Z

Coding note: Hyperthermia

Hyperthermia is used both to treat temperature imbalance, and as an adjunct radiation treatment for cancer. When performed to treat temperature imbalance, the procedure is coded to this section.

When performed for cancer treatment, whole-body hyperthermia is classified as a modality qualifier in section D, Radiation Therapy.

Example: Whole body hypothermia treatment for temperature imbalance, series

Character 1 Section	Character 2 Body System	Character 3 Root Operation	Character 4 Body System	Character 5 Duration	Character 6 Qualifier	Character 7 Qualifier
Extracorp. Therapies	Physiological Systems	Hypothermia	None	Multiple	No Qualifier	No Qualifier
6	A	4	Z	1	Z	Z

Coding note: Pheresis

Pheresis is used in medical practice for two main purposes: to treat diseases where too much of a blood component is produced, such as leukemia, or to remove a blood product such as platelets from a donor, for transfusion into a patient who needs them.

Example: Therapeutic leukapheresis, single treatment

Character 1 Section	Character 2 Body System	Character 3 Root Operation	Character 4 Body System	Character 5 Duration	Character 6 Qualifier	Character 7 Qualifier
Extracorp. Therapies	Physiological Systems	Pheresis	Circulatory	Single	No Qualifier	Leukocytes
6	A	5	5	0	Z	1

Coding note: Phototherapy

Phototherapy to the circulatory system means exposing the blood to light rays outside the body, using a machine that recirculates the blood and returns it to the body after phototherapy.

Example: Phototherapy of circulatory system, series treatment

Character 1 Section	Character 2 Body System	Character 3 Root Operation	Character 4 Body System	Character 5 Duration	Character 6 Qualifier	Character 7 Qualifier
Extracorp. Therapies	Physiological Systems	Phototherapy	Circulatory	Multiple	No Qualifier	No Qualifier
6	A	6	5	1	Z	Z

Example: Ultraviolet light phototherapy, series treatment

Character 1 Section	Character 2 Body System	Character 3 Root Operation	Character 4 Body System	Character 5 Duration	Character 6 Qualifier	Character 7 Qualifier
Extracorp. Therapies	Physiological Systems	UV Light Phototherapy	Skin	Multiple	No Qualifier	No Qualifier
6	A	8	0	1	Z	Z

Coding exercises

Using the ICD-10-PCS Tables, construct the code that accurately represents the procedure performed.

1. Donor thrombocytapheresis, single encounter: 6A550Z2
2. Bili-lite phototherapy, series treatment: 6A651ZZ
3. Whole body hypothermia, single treatment: 6A4Z0ZZ
4. Circulatory phototherapy, single encounter: 6A650ZZ
5. Shock wave therapy of plantar fascia, single treatment: 6A930ZZ
6. Antigen-free air conditioning, series treatment: 6A0Z1ZZ
7. TMS (transcranial magnetic stimulation), series treatment: 6A221ZZ
8. Therapeutic ultrasound of peripheral vessels, single treatment: 6A750ZZ
9. Plasmapheresis, series treatment: 6A551Z3
10. Extracorporeal electromagnetic stimulation (EMS) for urinary incontinence, single treatment: 6A210ZZ

Osteopathic—Section 7

Osteopathic, is one of the smallest sections in ICD-10-PCS. There is a single body system, Anatomical Regions, and a single root operation, Treatment.

The sixth- character methods such as Lymphatic Pump and Fascial Release are not explicitly defined in ICD-10-PCS, and rely on the standard definitions as used in this specialty.

0 – Treatment: Manual treatment to eliminate or alleviate somatic dysfunction and related disorders

Example: Fascial release of abdomen, osteopathic treatment

Character 1 Section	Character 2 Body System	Character 3 Root Operation	Character 4 Body System	Character 5 Approach	Character 6 Method	Character 7 Qualifier
Osteopathic	Anatomical Regions	Treatment	Abdomen	External	Fascial Release	No Qualifier
7	W	0	9	X	1	Z

Example: General osteopathic mobilization of legs

Character 1 Section	Character 2 Body System	Character 3 Root Operation	Character 4 Body System	Character 5 Approach	Character 6 Method	Character 7 Qualifier
Osteopathic	Anatomical Regions	Treatment	Lower Extremities	External	General Mobilization	No Qualifier
7	W	0	6	X	2	Z

Coding exercises

Using the ICD-10-PCS Tables, construct the code that accurately represents the procedure performed.

1. Isotonic muscle energy treatment of right leg: 7W06X8Z
2. Low velocity-high amplitude osteopathic treatment of head: 7W00X5Z
3. Lymphatic pump osteopathic treatment of left axilla: 7W07X6Z
4. Indirect osteopathic treatment of sacrum: 7W04X4Z
5. Articulatory osteopathic treatment of cervical region: 7W01X0Z

Other Procedures—Section 8

The Other Procedures section contains codes for procedures not included in the other medical and surgical-related sections. A single root operation, Other Procedures, is defined below.

0 – Other Procedures: Methodologies which attempt to remediate or cure a disorder or disease

There are relatively few procedure codes in this section, for nontraditional, whole body therapies including acupuncture and meditation. There is also a code for the fertilization portion of an in-vitro fertilization procedure.

Example: Acupuncture

Character 1 Section	Character 2 Body System	Character 3 Root Operation	Character 4 Body System	Character 5 Approach	Character 6 Method	Character 7 Qualifier
Other Procedures	Phys. Sys. & Anat. Regions	Other Procedures	Integ. Sys. & Breast	Percutaneous	Acupuncture	No Qualifier
8	E	0	H	3	0	Z

Example: Yoga therapy

Character 1 Section	Character 2 Body System	Character 3 Root Operation	Character 4 Body System	Character 5 Approach	Character 6 Method	Character 7 Qualifier
Other Procedures	Phys. Sys. & Anat. Regions	Other Procedures	None	External	Other Method	Yoga Therapy
8	E	0	Z	X	Y	4

Coding exercises

Using the ICD-10-PCS Tables, construct the code that accurately represents the procedure performed.

1. Near infrared spectroscopy of leg vessels: 8E023DZ
2. CT computer assisted sinus surgery: 8E09XBG (The primary procedure is coded separately.)
3. Suture removal, abdominal wall: 8E0WXY8
4. Isolation after infectious disease exposure: 8E0ZXY6
5. Robotic assisted open prostatectomy: 8E0W0CZ (The primary procedure is coded separately.)

Chiropractic—Section 9

The Chiropractic section consists of a single body system, Anatomical Regions, and a single root operation, Manipulation, defined below.

- B – Manipulation: Manual procedure that involves a directed thrust to move a joint past the physiological range of motion, without exceeding the anatomical limit

Example: Chiropractic treatment of cervical spine, short lever specific contact

Character 1 Section	Character 2 Body System	Character 3 Root Operation	Character 4 Body System	Character 5 Approach	Character 6 Method	Character 7 Qualifier
Chiropractic	Anatomical Regions	Manipulation	Cervical	External	Short Lever Sp. Contact	No Qualifier
9	W	B	1	X	H	Z

Example: Non-manual chiropractic manipulation of pelvis

Character 1 Section	Character 2 Body System	Character 3 Root Operation	Character 4 Body System	Character 5 Approach	Character 6 Method	Character 7 Qualifier
Chiropractic	Anatomical Regions	Manipulation	Pelvis	External	Non-Manual	No Qualifier
9	W	B	5	X	B	Z

Coding exercises

Using the ICD-10-PCS Tables, construct the code that accurately represents the procedure performed.

1. Chiropractic treatment of lumbar region using long lever specific contact: 9WB3XGZ
2. Chiropractic manipulation of abdominal region, indirect visceral: 9WB9XCZ
3. Chiropractic extra-articular treatment of hip region: 9WB6XDZ
4. Chiropractic treatment of sacrum using long and short lever specific contact: 9WB4XJZ
5. Mechanically-assisted chiropractic manipulation of head: 9WB0XKZ

Procedures in the Ancillary Sections

Imaging—Section B

Imaging follows the same conventions established in the Medical and Surgical, for the section, body system, and body part characters. However, the third and fourth characters introduce definitions not used in previous sections.

- Third character defines procedure by root type, instead of root operation.
- Fifth character defines contrast if used.
- Sixth character is a qualifier that specifies an image taken without contrast followed by one with contrast.
- Seventh character is a qualifier that is not specified in this section.

Root types

The Imaging root types are defined below:

- 0 – Plain Radiography: Planar display of an image developed from the capture of external ionizing radiation on photographic or photoconductive plate
- 1 – Fluoroscopy: Single plane or bi-plane real time display of an image developed from the capture of external ionizing radiation on a fluorescent screen. The image may also be stored by either digital or analog means
- 2 – Computerized Tomography (CT scan): Computer reformatted digital display of multiplanar images developed from the capture of multiple exposures of external ionizing radiation
- 3 – Magnetic Resonance Imaging (MRI): Computer reformatted digital display of multiplanar images developed from the capture of radio-frequency signals emitted by nuclei in a body site excited within a magnetic field
- 4 – Ultrasonography: Real time display of images of anatomy or flow information developed from the capture of reflected and attenuated high frequency sound waves

Example: X-ray of right clavicle, limited study

Character 1 Section	Character 2 Body System	Character 3 Root Type	Character 4 Body Part	Character 5 Contrast	Character 6 Qualifier	Character 7 Qualifier
Imaging	Non-axial Upper Bones	Plain Radiography	Clavicle, Right	None	None	None
B	P	0	4	Z	Z	Z

Example: Fluoroscopy of renal dialysis shunt using CO2 contrast

Character 1 Section	Character 2 Body System	Character 3 Root Type	Character 4 Body Part	Character 5 Contrast	Character 6 Qualifier	Character 7 Qualifier
Imaging	Veins	Fluoroscopy	Dialysis Shunt/Fistula	Other Contrast	None	None
B	5	1	W	Y	Z	Z

Example: CT of brain without contrast followed by high osmolar contrast

Character 1 Section	Character 2 Body System	Character 3 Root Type	Character 4 Body Part	Character 5 Contrast	Character 6 Qualifier	Character 7 Qualifier
Imaging	Central Nervous	Computerized Tomography	Brain	High Osmolar	Unenhanced and Enhanced	None
B	0	2	0	0	0	Z

Example: MRI of liver using gadoteridol

Character 1 Section	Character 2 Body System	Character 3 Root Type	Character 4 Body Part	Character 5 Contrast	Character 6 Qualifier	Character 7 Qualifier
Imaging	Hepatobiliary & Pancreas	Magnetic Resonance Imaging	Liver	Other Contrast	None	None
B	F	3	5	Y	Z	Z

Example: Ultrasound of prostate gland

Character 1 Section	Character 2 Body System	Character 3 Root Type	Character 4 Body Part	Character 5 Contrast	Character 6 Qualifier	Character 7 Qualifier
Imaging	Male Reproductive	Ultrasonography	Prostate and Seminal Vesicles	None	None	None
B	V	4	9	Z	Z	Z

Coding exercises

Using the ICD-10-PCS Tables, construct the code that accurately represents the procedure performed.

1. Non-contrast CT of abdomen and pelvis: BW21ZZZ
2. Intravascular ultrasound, left subclavian artery: B342ZZ3
3. Fluoroscopic guidance for insertion of central venous catheter in SVC, low osmolar contrast: B5181ZA
4. Endoluminal ultrasound of gallbladder and bile ducts: BF43ZZZ
5. Left ventriculography using low osmolar contrast: B2151ZZ
6. Esophageal videofluoroscopy study with oral barium contrast: BD11YZZ
7. Portable X-ray study of right radius/ulna shaft, standard series: BP0JZZZ
8. Routine fetal ultrasound, second trimester twin gestation: BY4DZZZ
9. CT scan of bilateral lungs, high osmolar contrast with densitometry: BB240ZZ
10. Fluoroscopic guidance for percutaneous transluminal angioplasty (PTA) of left common femoral artery, low osmolar contrast: B41G1ZZ

Nuclear Medicine—Section C

Nuclear Medicine is organized like the Imaging section. The only significant difference is that the fifth character defines the radionuclide instead of the contrast material used in the procedure, as described below.

- The fifth character specifies the radionuclide, the radiation source used in the procedure. Choices are applicable for the root procedure type.
- The sixth and seventh characters are qualifiers, and are not specified in this section.

Root types

The third character classifies the procedure by root type instead of by root operation.

- 1 – Planar Nuclear Medicine Imaging: Introduction of radioactive materials into the body for single plane display of images developed from the capture of radioactive emissions
- 2 – Tomographic (Tomo®) Nuclear Medicine Imaging: Introduction of radioactive materials into the body for three-dimensional display of images developed from the capture of radioactive emissions
- 3 – Positron Emission Tomography (PET): Introduction of radioactive materials into the body for three-dimensional display of images developed from the simultaneous capture, 180 degrees apart, of radioactive emissions
- 4 – Nonimaging Nuclear Medicine Uptake: Introduction of radioactive materials into the body for measurements of organ function, from the detection of radioactive emissions
- 5 – Nonimaging Nuclear Medicine Probe: Introduction of radioactive materials into the body for the study of distribution and fate of certain substances by the detection of radioactive emissions from an external source
- 6 – Nonimaging Nuclear medicine Assay: Introduction of radioactive materials into the body for the study of body fluids and blood elements, by the detection of radioactive emissions
- 7 – Systemic Nuclear Medicine Therapy: Introduction of unsealed radioactive materials into the body for treatment

Example: Adenosine sestamibi (technetium) planar scan of heart muscle at rest

Character 1 Section	Character 2 Body System	Character 3 Root Type	Character 4 Body Part	Character 5 Radionuclide	Character 6 Qualifier.	Character 7 Qualifier
Nuclear Medicine	Heart	Planar Nuclear Imaging	Myocardium	Technetium 99m	None	None
C	2	1	G	1	Z	Z

Example: Technetium tomo® scan of liver

Character 1 Section	Character 2 Body System	Character 3 Root Type	Character 4 Body Part	Character 5 Radionuclide	Character 6 Qualifier.	Character 7 Qualifier
Nuclear Medicine	Hepatobiliary and Pancreas	Tomo Nuclear Imaging	Liver	Technetium 99m	None	None
C	F	2	5	1	Z	Z

Coding exercises

Using the ICD-10-PCS Tables, construct the code that accurately represents the procedure performed.

1. Tomo® scan of right and left heart, unspecified radiopharmaceutical, qualitative gated rest: C226YZZ
2. Technetium pentetate assay of kidneys, ureters, and bladder: CT631ZZ
3. Uniplanar scan of spine using technetium oxidronate, with first pass study: CP151ZZ
4. Thallous chloride tomographic scan of bilateral breasts: CH22SZZ
5. PET scan of myocardium using rubidium: C23GQZZ
6. Gallium citrate scan of head and neck, single plane imaging: CW1BLZZ
7. Xenon gas nonimaging probe of brain: C050VZZ
8. Upper GI scan, radiopharmaceutical unspecified, for gastric emptying: CD15YZZ
9. Carbon 11 PET scan of brain with quantification: C030BZZ
10. Iodinated albumin nuclear medicine assay, blood plasma volume study: C763HZZ

Radiation Therapy—Section D

Radiation Therapy contains the radiation procedures performed for cancer treatment. Character meanings are described below.

- Third character defines root type, which is the basic modality.
- Fifth character further specifies treatment modality.
- Sixth character defines the radioactive isotope used, if applicable.
- Seventh character is a qualifier, and is not specified in this section.

Root type

The third character defines the treatment modality as root type. Examples are Brachytherapy and Stereotactic Radiosurgery. Four different root types are used in this section, as listed below.

- 0: Beam Radiation
- 1: Brachytherapy
- 2: Stereotactic Radiosurgery
- Y: Other Radiation

Example: LDR Brachytherapy of cervix using Iridium 192

Character 1 Section	Character 2 Body System	Character 3 Root Type	Character 4 Body Part	Character 5 Modal. Qualifier	Character 6 Isotope	Character 7 Qualifier
Radiation Therapy	Female Reproductive	Brachy-therapy	Cervix	LDR Brachytherapy	Iridium 192	None
D	U	1	1	B	8	Z

Example: Intraoperative radiation therapy (IORT) of bladder

Character 1 Section	Character 2 Body Sys	Character 3 Root Type	Character 4 Body Part	Character 5 Modal. Qualifier	Character 6 Isotope	Character 7 Qualifier
Radiation Therapy	Urinary System	Other Radiation	Bladder	IORT	None	None
D	T	Y	2	C	Z	Z

Coding exercises

Using the ICD-10-PCS Tables, construct the code that accurately represents the procedure performed.

1. Plaque radiation of left eye, single port: D8Y0FZZ
2. 8 MeV photon beam radiation to brain: D0011ZZ
3. IORT of colon, 3 ports: DDY5CZZ
4. HDR Brachytherapy of prostate using Palladium 103: DV109BZ
5. Electron radiation treatment of right breast, custom device: DM013ZZ
6. Hyperthermia oncology treatment of pelvic region: DWY68ZZ
7. Contact radiation of tongue: D9Y57ZZ
8. Heavy particle radiation treatment of pancreas, four risk sites: DF034ZZ
9. LDR brachytherapy to spinal cord using iodine: D016B9Z
10. Whole body Phosphorus 32 administration with risk to hematopoietic system: DWY5GFZ

Physical Rehabilitation and Diagnostic Audiology—Section F

Physical Rehabilitation and Diagnostic Audiology contains character definitions unlike the other sections in ICD-10-PCS. They are described below.

- Second character is a section qualifier that specifies whether the procedure is a rehabilitation or diagnostic audiology procedure.
- Third character defines the general procedure root type.
- Fourth character defines the body system and body region combined, where applicable.
- Fifth character further specifies the procedure type.
- Sixth character specifies the equipment used, if any.

Root types

This section uses the third character to classify procedures into 14 root types. They are defined in the table below.

- 0 – Speech Assessment: Measurement of speech and related functions
- 1 – Motor and/or Nerve Function Assessment: Measurement of motor, nerve, and related functions
- 2 – Activities of Daily Living Assessment: Measurement of functional level for activities of daily living
- 3 – Hearing Assessment: Measurement of hearing and related functions
- 4 – Hearing Aid Assessment: Measurement of the appropriateness and/or effectiveness of a hearing device
- 5 – Vestibular Assessment: Measurement of the vestibular system and related functions
- 6 – Speech Treatment: Application of techniques to improve, augment, or compensate for speech and related functional impairment
- 7 – Motor Treatment: Exercise or activities to increase or facilitate motor function
- 8 – Activities of Daily Living Treatment: Exercise or activities to facilitate functional competence for activities of daily living
- 9 – Hearing Treatment: Application of techniques to improve, augment, or compensate for hearing and related functional impairment
- B – Cochlear Implant Treatment: Application of techniques to improve the communication abilities of individuals with cochlear implant
- C – Vestibular Treatment: Application of techniques to improve, augment, or compensate for vestibular and related functional impairment
- D – Device Fitting: Fitting of a device designed to facilitate or support achievement of a higher level of function
- F – Caregiver Training: Training in activities to support patient's optimal level of function

Coding note: Treatment

Treatment procedures include swallowing dysfunction exercises, bathing and showering techniques, wound management, gait training, and a host of activities typically associated with rehabilitation.

Example: Wound care treatment of left calf ulcer using pulsatile lavage

Character 1 Section	Character 2 Section Qualifier	Character 3 Root Type	Character 4 Body System & Region	Character 5 Type Qualifier	Character 6 Equipment	Character 7 Qualifier
Rehabilitation & Diagnostic Audiology	Rehabilitation	Activities of Daily Living Treatment	Musculoskel. Lower Extremity	Wound Management	Physical Agents	None
F	0	8	L	5	B	Z

Coding note: Assessment

Assessments are further classified into more than 100 different tests or methods. The majority of these focus on the faculties of hearing and speech, but others focus on various aspects of body function, and on the patient's quality of life, such as muscle performance, neuromotor development, and reintegration skills.

Example: Articulation and phonology assessment using spectrograph

Character 1 Section	Character 2 Section Qualifier	Character 3 Root Type	Character 4 Body System & Region	Character 5 Type Qualifier	Character 6 Equipment	Character 7 Qualifier
Rehabilitation & Diagnostic Audiology	Rehabilitation	Speech Assessment	None	Articulation/ Phonology	Speech Analysis	None
F	0	0	Z	9	Q	Z

Coding note: Device Fitting

The fifth character used in Device Fitting procedures describes the device being fitted rather than the method used to fit the device. Where definitions of devices are provided, they are located in the definitions portion of the ICD-10-PCS Tables and Index, under section F, character 5.

Example: Individual fitting of moveable brace, right knee

Character 1 Section	Character 2 Section Qualifier	Character 3 Root Type	Character 4 Body System & Region	Character 5 Type Qualifier	Character 6 Equipment	Character 7 Qualifier
Rehabilitation & Diagnostic Audiology	Rehabilitation	Device Fitting	None	Dynamic Orthosis	Orthosis	None
F	0	D	Z	6	E	Z

Coding note: Caregiver Training

Caregiver Training is divided into eighteen different broad subjects taught to help a caregiver provide proper patient care.

Example: Caregiver training in feeding, no special equipment used

Character 1 Section	Character 2 Section Qualifier	Character 3 Root Type	Character 4 Body System & Region	Character 5 Type Qualifier	Character 6 Equipment	Character 7 Qualifier
Rehabilitation & Diagnostic Audiology	Rehabilitation	Caregiver Training	None	Feeding and Eating	None	None
F	0	F	Z	2	Z	Z

Coding exercises

Using the ICD-10-PCS Tables, construct the code that accurately represents the procedure performed.

1. Bekesy assessment using audiometer: F13Z31Z
2. Individual fitting of left eye prosthesis: F0DZ8UZ
3. Physical therapy for range of motion and mobility, patient right hip, no special equipment: F07L0ZZ
4. Bedside swallow assessment using assessment kit: F00ZHYZ
5. Caregiver training in airway clearance techniques: F0FZ8ZZ
6. Application of short arm cast in rehabilitation setting: F0DZ7EZ (Inhibitory cast is listed in the equipment reference table under E, Orthosis.)
7. Verbal assessment of patient's pain level: F02ZFZZ
8. Caregiver training in communication skills using manual communication board: F0FZJMZ (Manual communication board is listed in the equipment reference table under M, Augmentative/Alternative Communication.)
9. Group musculoskeletal balance training exercises, whole body, no special equipment : F07M6ZZ (Balance training is included in the Motor Treatment reference table under Therapeutic Exercise.)
10. Individual therapy for auditory processing using tape recorder: F09Z2KZ (Tape recorder is listed in the equipment reference table under Audiovisual Equipment.)

Mental Health—Section G

Mental Health contains specific values in the third and fourth characters to describe mental health procedures. The remaining characters function as placeholders only. Character meanings are described below.

- Third character describes the mental health procedure root type.
- Fourth character further specifies the procedure type as needed.
- Second, fifth, sixth, and seventh characters do not convey specific information about the procedure. The value Z functions as a placeholder in these characters.

Root Type

The third character describes the mental health root type. There are 11 root type values in this section, as listed in the table below.

- 1: Psychological Tests
- 2: Crisis Intervention
- 5: Individual Psychotherapy
- 6: Counseling
- 7: Family Psychotherapy
- B: Electroconvulsive Therapy
- C: Biofeedback
- F: Hypnosis
- G: Narcosynthesis
- H: Group Therapy
- J: Light Therapy

Example: Galvanic skin response (GSR) biofeedback

Character 1 Section	Character 2 Body System	Character 3 Root Type	Character 4 Type Qualifier	Character 5 Qualifier	Character 6 Qualifier	Character 7 Qualifier
Mental Health	None	Biofeedback	Other Biofeedback	None	None	None
G	Z	C	9	Z	Z	Z

Coding exercises

Using the ICD-10-PCS Tables, construct the code that accurately represents the procedure performed.

1. Cognitive-behavioral psychotherapy, individual: GZ58ZZZ
2. Narcosynthesis: GZGZZZZ
3. Light therapy: GZJZZZZ
4. ECT (Electroconvulsive therapy), unilateral, multiple seizure: GZB1ZZZ
5. Crisis intervention: GZ2ZZZZ
6. Neuropsychological testing: GZ13ZZZ
7. Hypnosis: GZFZZZZ
8. Developmental testing: GZ10ZZZ
9. Vocational counseling: GZ61ZZZ
10. Family psychotherapy: GZ72ZZZ

Substance Abuse Treatment—Section H

Substance Abuse Treatment is structured like a smaller version of the Mental Health section. Character meanings are described below.

- Third character describes the root type.
- Fourth character is a qualifier that further classifies the root type.
- Second, fifth, sixth, and seventh characters do not convey specific information about the procedure. The value Z functions as a placeholder in these characters.

There are seven different root type values classified in this section, as listed in the following table.

- 2: Detoxification Services
- 3: Individual Counseling
- 4: Group Counseling
- 5: Individual Psychotherapy
- 6: Family Counseling
- 8: Medication Management
- 9: Pharmacotherapy

Example: Pharmacotherapy treatment with Antabuse for alcohol addiction

Character 1 Section	Character 2 Body System	Character 3 Root Type	Character 4 Type Qualifier	Character 5 Qualifier	Character 6 Qualifier	Character 7 Qualifier
Substance Abuse Trmnt.	None	Pharmacotherapy	Antabuse	None	None	None
H	Z	9	3	Z	Z	Z

Coding exercises

Using the ICD-10-PCS Tables, construct the code that accurately represents the procedure performed.

1. Naltrexone treatment for drug dependency: HZ94ZZZ
2. Substance abuse treatment family counseling: HZ63ZZZ
3. Medication monitoring of patient on methadone maintenance: HZ81ZZZ
4. Individual interpersonal psychotherapy for drug abuse: HZ54ZZZ
5. Patient in for alcohol detoxification treatment: HZ2ZZZZ
6. Group motivational counseling: HZ47ZZZ
7. Individual 12-step psychotherapy for substance abuse: HZ53ZZZ
8. Post-test infectious disease counseling for IV drug abuser: HZ3CZZZ
9. Psychodynamic psychotherapy for drug dependent patient: HZ5CZZZ
10. Group cognitive-behavioral counseling for substance abuse: HZ42ZZZ

New Technology–Section X

Section X New Technology is the section in ICD-10-PCS for codes that uniquely identify procedures requested via the New Technology Application Process, and for codes that capture new technologies not currently classified in ICD-10-PCS.

This section may include codes for medical and surgical procedures, medical and surgical- related procedures, or ancillary procedures designated as new technology.

In section X, the seven characters are defined as follows:

- First character: section (X)
- Second character: body system
- Third character: operation
- Fourth character: body part
- Fifth character: approach
- Sixth character: device/substance/technology
- Seventh character: new technology group

The New Technology section includes infusions of new technology drugs, and can potentially include a wide range of other new technology medical, surgical and ancillary procedures. The example below is for infusion of a new technology drug.

Example New Technology

Character 1 Section	Character 2 Body System	Character 3 Root Operation	Character 4 Body Part	Character 5 Approach	Character 6 Device/ Substance/ Technology	Character 7 Qualifier
New Technology	Anatomical Regions	Introduction	Central Vein	Percutaneous	Ceftazidime-Avibactam Anti-infective	New Technology Group 1
X	W	0	4	3	2	1

Coding note: Seventh Character New Technology Group

In ICD-10-PCS, the type of information specified in the seventh character is called the qualifier, and the information specified depends on the section. In this section, the seventh character is used exclusively to indicate the new technology group.

The New Technology Group is a number or letter that changes each year that new technology codes are added to the system. For

example, Section X codes added for the first year have the seventh character value 1, New Technology Group 1, and the next year that Section X codes are added have the seventh character value 2 New Technology Group 2, and so on.

Changing the seventh character New Technology Group to a unique value every year that there are new codes in this section allows the ICD-10-PCS to "recycle" the values in the third, fourth, and sixth characters as needed. This avoids the creation of duplicate codes, because the root operation, body part and device/substance/technology values can specify a different meaning with every new technology group, if needed. Having a unique value for the New Technology Group maximizes the flexibility and capacity of section X over its lifespan, and allows it to evolve as medical technology evolves.

Body system values

Second character body systems in this section do not change from year to year. They are a fixed set of values that combine the uses of body system, body region, and physiological system as specified in other sections in ICD-10-PCS. As a result, the second character body system values are broader values. This allows body part values to be as general or specific as they need to be to efficiently represent the body part applicable to a new technology.

Root operations

Third character root operations in this section use the same root operation values as their counterparts in other sections of ICD-10-PCS. The example above uses the root operation value Introduction. This root operation has the same definition as its counterpart in section 3 of ICD-10-PCS, as given below.

- 0 – Introduction: Putting in or on a therapeutic, diagnostic, nutritional, physiological, or prophylactic substance except blood or blood products

Body part values

Fourth character body part values in this section use the same body part values as their closest counterparts in other sections of ICD-10-PCS. The example above uses the body part value 4 Central Vein. This is its closest counterpart in section 3 of ICD-10-PCS.

Device/Substance/Technology values

In this section, the sixth character contains a general description of the key feature of the new technology. The example above uses the device/substance/technology value 2 ceftazidime-avibactam Anti-infective.

Coding exercises

Using the ICD-10-PCS Tables, construct the code that accurately represents the procedure performed.

1. Infusion of ceftazidime via peripheral venous catheter: XW03321

This page intentionally left blank

ICD-10-PCS Official Guidelines for Coding and Reporting

The Centers for Medicare and Medicaid Services (CMS) and the National Center for Health Statistics (NCHS), two departments within the U.S. Federal Government's Department of Health and Human Services (DHHS) provide the following guidelines for coding and reporting using the International Classification of Diseases, 10th Revision, Procedure Coding System (ICD-10-PCS). These guidelines should be used as a companion document to the official version of the ICD-10-PCS as published on the CMS website. The ICD-10-PCS is a procedure classification published by the United States for classifying procedures performed in hospital inpatient health care settings.

These guidelines have been approved by the four organizations that make up the Cooperating Parties for the ICD-10-PCS: the American Hospital Association (AHA), the American Health Information Management Association (AHIMA), CMS, and NCHS.

These guidelines are a set of rules that have been developed to accompany and complement the official conventions and instructions provided within the ICD-10-PCS itself. The instructions and conventions of the classification take precedence over guidelines. These guidelines are based on the coding and sequencing instructions in the Tables, Index and Definitions of ICD-10-PCS, but provide additional instruction. Adherence to these guidelines when assigning ICD-10-PCS procedure codes is required under the Health Insurance Portability and Accountability Act (HIPAA). The procedure codes have been adopted under HIPAA for hospital inpatient healthcare settings. A joint effort between the healthcare provider and the coder is essential to achieve complete and accurate documentation, code assignment, and reporting of diagnoses and procedures. These guidelines have been developed to assist both the healthcare provider and the coder in identifying those procedures that are to be reported. The importance of consistent, complete documentation in the medical record cannot be overemphasized. Without such documentation accurate coding cannot be achieved.

Table of Contents

Conventions

A1

ICD-10-PCS codes are composed of seven characters. Each character is an axis of classification that specifies information about the procedure performed. Within a defined code range, a character specifies the same type of information in that axis of classification.

Example: The fifth axis of classification specifies the approach in sections 0 through 4 and 7 through 9 of the system.

A2

One of 34 possible values can be assigned to each axis of classification in the seven-character code: they are the numbers 0 through 9 and the alphabet (except I and O because they are easily confused with the numbers 1 and 0). The number of unique values used in an axis of classification differs as needed.

Example: Where the fifth axis of classification specifies the approach, seven different approach values are currently used to specify the approach.

A3

The valid values for an axis of classification can be added to as needed.

Example: If a significantly distinct type of device is used in a new procedure, a new device value can be added to the system.

A4

As with words in their context, the meaning of any single value is a combination of its axis of classification and any preceding values on which it may be dependent.

Example: The meaning of a body part value in the Medical and Surgical section is always dependent on the body system value. The body part value 0 in the Central Nervous body system specifies Brain and the body part value 0 in the Peripheral Nervous body system specifies Cervical Plexus.

A5

As the system is expanded to become increasingly detailed, over time more values will depend on preceding values for their meaning.

Example: In the Lower Joints body system, the device value 3 in the root operation Insertion specifies Infusion Device and the device value 3 in the root operation Replacement specifies Ceramic Synthetic Substitute.

A6

The purpose of the alphabetic index is to locate the appropriate table that contains all information necessary to construct a procedure code. The PCS Tables should always be consulted to find the most appropriate valid code.

A7

is not required to consult the index first before proceeding to the tables to complete the code. A valid code may be chosen directly from the tables.

A8

All seven characters must be specified to be a valid code. If the documentation is incomplete for coding purposes, the physician should be queried for the necessary information.

A9

Within a PCS table, valid codes include all combinations of choices in characters 4 through 7 contained in the same row of the table. In the example below, 0JHT3VZ is a valid code, and 0JHW3VZ is *not* a valid code.

Section: 0 Medical and Surgical

Body System: J Subcutaneous Tissue and Fascia

Operation: H Insertion: Putting in a nonbiological appliance that monitors, assists, performs, or prevents a physiological function but does not physically take the place of a body part

Body Part	Approach	Device	Qualifier
S Subcutaneous Tissue and Fascia, Head and Neck V Subcutaneous Tissue and Fascia, Upper Extremity W Subcutaneous Tissue and Fascia, Lower Extremity	0 Open 3 Percutaneous	1 Radioactive Element 3 Infusion Device	Z No Qualifier
T Subcutaneous Tissue and Fascia, Trunk	0 Open 3 Percutaneous	1 Radioactive Element 3 Infusion Device V Infusion Pump	Z No Qualifier

A10
"And," when used in a code description, means "and/or."

Example: Lower Arm and Wrist Muscle means lower arm and/or wrist muscle.

A11
Many of the terms used to construct PCS codes are defined within the system. It is the coder's responsibility to determine what the documentation in the medical record equates to in the PCS definitions. The physician is not expected to use the terms used in PCS code descriptions, nor is the coder required to query the physician when the correlation between the documentation and the defined PCS terms is clear.

Example: When the physician documents "partial resection" the coder can independently correlate "partial resection" to the root operation Excision without querying the physician for clarification.

Medical and Surgical Section Guidelines (section 0)

B2. Body System

General guidelines

B2.1a
The procedure codes in the general anatomical regions body systems can be used when the procedure is performed on an anatomical region rather than a specific body part (e.g., root operations Control and Detachment, Drainage of a body cavity) or on the rare occasion when no information is available to support assignment of a code to a specific body part.

Example: Control of postoperative hemorrhage is coded to the root operation Control found in the general anatomical regions body systems.
Chest tube drainage of the pleural cavity is coded to the root operation Drainage found in the general anatomical regions body systems. Suture repair of the abdominal wall is coded to the root operation Repair in the general anatomical regions body system.

B2.1b
Where the general body part values "upper" and "lower" are provided as an option in the Upper Arteries, Lower Arteries, Upper Veins, Lower Veins, Muscles and Tendons body systems, "upper" or "lower "specifies body parts located above or below the diaphragm respectively.

Example: Vein body parts above the diaphragm are found in the Upper Veins body system; vein body parts below the diaphragm are found in the Lower Veins body system.

B3. Root Operation

General guidelines

B3.1a
In order to determine the appropriate root operation, the full definition of the root operation as contained in the PCS Tables must be applied.

B3.1b
Components of a procedure specified in the root operation definition and explanation are not coded separately. Procedural steps necessary to reach the operative site and close the operative site, including anastomosis of a tubular body part, are also not coded separately

Examples: Resection of a joint as part of a joint replacement procedure is included in the root operation definition of Replacement and is not coded separately.

Laparotomy performed to reach the site of an open liver biopsy is not coded separately. In a resection of sigmoid colon with anastomosis of descending colon to rectum, the anastomosis is not coded separately.

Multiple procedures

B3.2
During the same operative episode, multiple procedures are coded if:

a. The same root operation is performed on different body parts as defined by distinct values of the body part character.
   Examples: Diagnostic excision of liver and pancreas are coded separately.

   Excision of lesion in the ascending colon and excision of lesion in the transverse colon are coded separately.

b. The same root operation is repeated in multiple body parts, and those body parts are separate and distinct body parts classified to a single ICD-10-PCS body part value.
   Examples: Excision of the sartorius muscle and excision of the gracilis muscle are both included in the upper leg muscle body part value, and multiple procedures are coded.

   Extraction of multiple toenails are coded separately.

c. Multiple root operations with distinct objectives are performed on the same body part.
   Example: Destruction of sigmoid lesion and bypass of sigmoid colon are coded separately.

d. The intended root operation is attempted using one approach, but is converted to a different approach.
   Example: Laparoscopic cholecystectomy converted to an open cholecystectomy is coded as percutaneous endoscopic Inspection and open Resection.

Discontinued procedures

B3.3
If the intended procedure is discontinued, code the procedure to the root operation performed. If a procedure is discontinued before any other root operation is performed, code the root operation Inspection of the body part or anatomical region inspected.

Example: A planned aortic valve replacement procedure is discontinued after the initial thoracotomy and before any incision is made in the heart muscle, when the patient becomes hemodynamically unstable. This procedure is coded as an open Inspection of the mediastinum.

Biopsy procedures

B3.4a
Biopsy procedures are coded using the root operations Excision, Extraction, or Drainage and the qualifier Diagnostic.
Examples: Fine needle aspiration biopsy of fluid in the lung is coded to the root operation Drainage with the qualifier Diagnostic. Biopsy of bone marrow is coded to the root operation Extraction with the qualifier Diagnostic. Lymph node sampling for biopsy is coded to the root operation Excision with the qualifier Diagnostic.

Biopsy followed by more definitive treatment

B3.4b
If a diagnostic Excision, Extraction, or Drainage procedure (biopsy) is followed by a more definitive procedure, such as Destruction, Excision or Resection at the same procedure site, both the biopsy and the more definitive treatment are coded.

Example: Biopsy of breast followed by partial mastectomy at the same procedure site, both the biopsy and the partial mastectomy procedure are coded.

Overlapping body layers

B3.5
If the root operations Excision, Repair or Inspection are performed on overlapping layers of the musculoskeletal system, the body part specifying the deepest layer is coded.
Example : Excisional debridement that includes skin and subcutaneous tissue and muscle is coded to the muscle body part.

Bypass procedures

B3.6a
Bypass procedures are coded by identifying the body part bypassed "from" and the body part bypassed "to." The fourth character body part specifies the body part bypassed from, and the qualifier specifies the body part bypassed to.

Example: Bypass from stomach to jejunum, stomach is the body part and jejunum is the qualifier.

B3.6b
Coronary artery bypass procedures are coded differently than other bypass procedures as described in the previous guideline. Rather than identifying the body part bypassed from, the body part identifies the number of coronary arteries bypassed to, and the qualifier specifies the vessel bypassed from.

Example: Aortocoronary artery bypass of the left anterior descending coronary artery and the obtuse marginal coronary artery is classified in the body part axis of classification as two coronary arteries, and the qualifier specifies the aorta as the body part bypassed from.

B3.6c
If multiple coronary arteries are bypassed, a separate procedure is coded for each coronary artery that uses a different device and/or qualifier.

Example: Aortocoronary artery bypass and internal mammary coronary artery bypass are coded separately.

Control vs. more definitive root operations

B3.7
The root operation Control is defined as, "Stopping, or attempting to stop, postprocedural or other acute bleeding." If an attempt to stop postprocedural or other acute bleeding is initially unsuccessful, and to stop the bleeding requires performing any of the definitive root operations Bypass, Detachment, Excision, Extraction, Reposition, Replacement, or Resection, then that root operation is coded instead of Control.

Example: Resection of spleen to stop bleeding is coded to Resection instead of Control.

Excision vs. Resection

B3.8
PCS contains specific body parts for anatomical subdivisions of a body part, such as lobes of the lungs or liver and regions of the intestine. Resection of the specific body part is coded whenever all of the body part is cut out or off, rather than coding Excision of a less specific body part.

Example: Left upper lung lobectomy is coded to Resection of Upper Lung Lobe, Left rather than Excision of Lung, Left.

Excision for graft

B3.9
If an autograft is obtained from a different procedure site in order to complete the objective of the procedure, a separate procedure is coded.

Example: Coronary bypass with excision of saphenous vein graft, excision of saphenous vein is coded separately.

Fusion procedures of the spine

B3.10a
The body part coded for a spinal vertebral joint(s) rendered immobile by a spinal fusion procedure is classified by the level of the spine (e.g. thoracic). There are distinct body part values for a single vertebral joint and for multiple vertebral joints at each spinal level.

Example: Body part values specify Lumbar Vertebral Joint, Lumbar Vertebral Joints, 2 or More and Lumbosacral Vertebral Joint.

B3.10b
If multiple vertebral joints are fused, a separate procedure is coded for each vertebral joint that uses a different device and/or qualifier.

Example: Fusion of lumbar vertebral joint, posterior approach, anterior column and fusion of lumbar vertebral joint, posterior approach, posterior column are coded separately.

B3.10c
Combinations of devices and materials are often used on a vertebral joint to render the joint immobile. When combinations of devices are used on the same vertebral joint, the device value coded for the procedure is as follows:

- If an interbody fusion device is used to render the joint immobile (alone or containing other material like bone graft), the procedure is coded with the device value Interbody Fusion Device
- If bone graft is the *only* device used to render the joint immobile, the procedure is coded with the device value Nonautologous Tissue Substitute or Autologous Tissue Substitute
- If a mixture of autologous and nonautologous bone graft (with or without biological or synthetic extenders or binders) is used to render the joint immobile, code the procedure with the device value Autologous Tissue Substitute

Examples: Fusion of a vertebral joint using a cage style interbody fusion device containing morselized bone graft is coded to the device Interbody Fusion Device.

Fusion of a vertebral joint using a bone dowel interbody fusion device made of cadaver bone and packed with a mixture of local morselized bone and demineralized bone matrix is coded to the device Interbody Fusion Device.
Fusion of a vertebral joint using both autologous bone graft and bone bank bone graft is coded to the device Autologous Tissue Substitute.

Inspection procedures

B3.11a
Inspection of a body part(s) performed in order to achieve the objective of a procedure is not coded separately.

Example: Fiberoptic bronchoscopy performed for irrigation of bronchus, only the irrigation procedure is coded.

B3.11b
If multiple tubular body parts are inspected, the most distal body part (the body part furthest from the starting point of the inspection) is coded. If multiple non-tubular body parts in a region are inspected, the body part that specifies the entire area inspected is coded.

Examples: Cystoureteroscopy with inspection of bladder and ureters is coded to the ureter body part value.

Exploratory laparotomy with general inspection of abdominal contents is coded to the peritoneal cavity body part value.

B3.11c
When both an Inspection procedure and another procedure are performed on the same body part during the same episode, if the Inspection procedure is performed using a different approach than the other procedure, the Inspection procedure is coded separately.

Example: Endoscopic Inspection of the duodenum is coded separately when open Excision of the duodenum is performed during the same procedural episode.

Occlusion vs. Restriction for vessel embolization procedures

B3.12
If the objective of an embolization procedure is to completely close a vessel, the root operation Occlusion is coded. If the objective of an embolization procedure is to narrow the lumen of a vessel, the root operation Restriction is coded.

Examples : Tumor embolization is coded to the root operation Occlusion, because the objective of the procedure is to cut off the blood supply to the vessel.

Embolization of a cerebral aneurysm is coded to the root operation Restriction, because the objective of the procedure is not to close off the vessel entirely, but to narrow the lumen of the vessel at the site of the aneurysm where it is abnormally wide.

Release procedures

B3.13
In the root operation Release, the body part value coded is the body part being freed and not the tissue being manipulated or cut to free the body part.

Example: Lysis of intestinal adhesions is coded to the specific intestine body part value.

Release vs. Division

B3.14
If the sole objective of the procedure is freeing a body part without cutting the body part, the root operation is Release. If the sole objective of the procedure is separating or transecting a body part, the root operation is Division.

Examples: Freeing a nerve root from surrounding scar tissue to relieve pain is coded to the root operation Release. Severing a nerve root to relieve pain is coded to the root operation Division.

Reposition for fracture treatment

B3.15
Reduction of a displaced fracture is coded to the root operation Reposition and the application of a cast or splint in conjunction with the Reposition procedure is not coded separately. Treatment of a nondisplaced fracture is coded to the procedure performed.

Examples: Casting of a nondisplaced fracture is coded to the root operation Immobilization in the Placement section.
Putting a pin in a nondisplaced fracture is coded to the root operation Insertion.

Transplantation vs. Administration

B3.16
Putting in a mature and functioning living body part taken from another individual or animal is coded to the root operation Transplantation. Putting in autologous or nonautologous cells is coded to the Administration section.

Example: Putting in autologous or nonautologous bone marrow, pancreatic islet cells or stem cells is coded to the Administration section.

B4. Body Part

General guidelines

B4.1a
If a procedure is performed on a portion of a body part that does not have a separate body part value, code the body part value corresponding to the whole body part.

Example: A procedure performed on the alveolar process of the mandible is coded to the mandible body part.

B4.1b
If the prefix "peri" is combined with a body part to identify the site of the procedure, and the site of the procedure is not further specified, then the procedure is coded to the body part named. This guideline applies only when a more specific body part value is not available.

Example: A procedure site identified as perirenal is coded to the kidney body part when the site of the procedure is not further specified.

A procedure site described in the documentation as periurethral and the documentation also indicates that it is the vulvar tissue and not the urethral tissue that is the site of the procedure, then the procedure is coded to the vulva body part.

Branches of body parts

B4.2
Where a specific branch of a body part does not have its own body part value in PCS, the body part is typically coded to the closest proximal branch that has a specific body part value. In the cardiovascular body systems, if a general body part is available in the correct root operation table, and coding to a proximal branch would require assigning a code in a different body system, the procedure is coded using the general body part value.

Example : A procedure performed on the mandibular branch of the trigeminal nerve is coded to the trigeminal nerve body part value. Occlusion of the bronchial artery is coded to the body part value Upper Artery in the body system Upper Arteries, and not to the body part value Thoracic Aorta, Descending in the body system Heart and Great Vessels.

Bilateral body part values

B4.3
Bilateral body part values are available for a limited number of body parts. If the identical procedure is performed on contralateral body parts, and a bilateral body part value exists for that body part, a single procedure is coded using the bilateral body part value. If no bilateral body part value exists, each procedure is coded separately using the appropriate body part value.

Example : The identical procedure performed on both fallopian tubes is coded once using the body part value Fallopian Tube, Bilateral.

The identical procedure performed on both knee joints is coded twice using the body part values Knee Joint, Right and Knee Joint, Left.

Coronary arteries

B4.4
The coronary arteries are classified as a single body part that is further specified by number of arteries treated. One procedure code specifying multiple arteries is used when the same procedure is performed, including the same device and qualifier values.

Examples: Angioplasty of two distinct coronary arteries with placement of two stents is coded as Dilation of Coronary Artery, Two Arteries with Two Intraluminal Devices.

Angioplasty of two distinct coronary arteries, one with stent placed and one without, is coded separately as Dilation of Coronary Artery, One Artery with Intraluminal Device, and Dilation of Coronary Artery, One Artery with no device.

Tendons, ligaments, bursae and fascia near a joint

B4.5
Procedures performed on tendons, ligaments, bursae and fascia supporting a joint are coded to the body part in the respective body system that is the focus of the procedure. Procedures performed on joint structures themselves are coded to the body part in the joint body systems.

Example: Repair of the anterior cruciate ligament of the knee is coded to the knee bursa and ligament body part in the bursae and ligaments body system.

Knee arthroscopy with shaving of articular cartilage is coded to the knee joint body part in the Lower Joints body system.

Skin, subcutaneous tissue and fascia overlying a joint

B4.6
If a procedure is performed on the skin, subcutaneous tissue or fascia overlying a joint, the procedure is coded to the following body part:

- Shoulder is coded to Upper Arm
- Elbow is coded to Lower Arm
- Wrist is coded to Lower Arm
- Hip is coded to Upper Leg
- Knee is coded to Lower Leg
- Ankle is coded to Foot

Fingers and toes

B4.7
If a body system does not contain a separate body part value for fingers, procedures performed on the fingers are coded to the body part value for the hand. If a body system does not contain a separate body part value for toes, procedures performed on the toes are coded to the body part value for the foot.

Example: Excision of finger muscle is coded to one of the hand muscle body part values in the Muscles body system.

Upper and lower intestinal tract

B4.8
In the Gastrointestinal body system, the general body part values Upper Intestinal Tract and Lower Intestinal Tract are provided as an option for the root operations Change, Inspection, Removal and Revision. Upper Intestinal Tract includes the portion of the gastrointestinal tract from the esophagus down to and including the duodenum, and Lower Intestinal Tract includes the portion of the gastrointestinal tract from the jejunum down to and including the rectum and anus.

Example: In the root operation Change table, change of a device in the jejunum is coded using the body part Lower Intestinal Tract.

B5. Approach

Open approach with percutaneous endoscopic assistance

B5.2
Procedures performed using the open approach with percutaneous endoscopic assistance are coded to the approach Open.

Example: Laparoscopic-assisted sigmoidectomy is coded to the approach Open.

External approach

B5.3a
Procedures performed within an orifice on structures that are visible without the aid of any instrumentation are coded to the approach External.

Example: Resection of tonsils is coded to the approach External.

B5.3b
Procedures performed indirectly by the application of external force through the intervening body layers are coded to the approach External.

Example: Closed reduction of fracture is coded to the approach External.

Percutaneous procedure via device

B5.4
Procedures performed percutaneously via a device placed for the procedure are coded to the approach Percutaneous.

Example : Fragmentation of kidney stone performed via percutaneous nephrostomy is coded to the approach Percutaneous.

B6. Device

General guidelines

B6.1a
A device is coded only if a device remains after the procedure is completed. If no device remains, the device value No Device is coded.

B6.1b
Materials such as sutures, ligatures, radiological markers and temporary post-operative wound drains are considered integral to the performance of a procedure and are not coded as devices.

B6.1c
Procedures performed on a device only and not on a body part are specified in the root operations Change, Irrigation, Removal and Revision, and are coded to the procedure performed.

Example: Irrigation of percutaneous nephrostomy tube is coded to the root operation Irrigation of indwelling device in the Administration section.

Drainage device

B6.2
A separate procedure to put in a drainage device is coded to the root operation Drainage with the device value Drainage Device.

Obstetric Section Guidelines (section 1)

C. Obstetrics Section

Products of conception

C1
Procedures performed on the products of conception are coded to the Obstetrics section. Procedures performed on the pregnant female other than the products of conception are coded to the appropriate root operation in the Medical and Surgical section.

Example: Amniocentesis is coded to the products of conception body part in the Obstetrics section. Repair of obstetric urethral laceration is coded to the urethra body part in the Medical and Surgical section.

Procedures following delivery or abortion

C2
Procedures performed following a delivery or abortion for curettage of the endometrium or evacuation of retained products of conception are all coded in the Obstetrics section, to the root operation Extraction and the body part Products of Conception, Retained. Diagnostic or therapeutic dilation and curettage performed during times other than the postpartum or post-abortion period are all coded in the Medical and Surgical section, to the root operation Extraction and the body part Endometrium.

New Technology Section Guidelines (section X)

D. New Technology Section

General guidelines

D1
Section X codes are standalone codes. They are not supplemental codes. Section X codes fully represent the specific procedure described in the code title, and do not require any additional codes from other sections of ICD-10-PCS. When section X contains a code title which describes a specific new technology procedure, only that X code is reported for the procedure. There is no need to report a broader, non-specific code in another section of ICD-10-PCS.

Example: XW04321 Introduction of ceftazidime-avibactam anti-infective into Central Vein, Percutaneous Approach, New Technology Group 1, can be coded to indicate that ceftazidime-avibactam anti-infective was administered via a central vein. A separate code from table 3E0 in the Administration section of ICD-10-PCS is not coded in addition to this code.

Selection of Principal Procedure

The following instructions should be applied in the selection of principal procedure and clarification on the importance of the relation to the principal diagnosis when more than one procedure is performed:

1. Procedure performed for definitive treatment of both principal diagnosis and secondary diagnosis
   a. Sequence procedure performed for definitive treatment most related to principal diagnosis as principal procedure.

2. Procedure performed for definitive treatment and diagnostic procedures performed for both principal diagnosis and secondary diagnosis.
   a. Sequence procedure performed for definitive treatment most related to principal diagnosis as principal procedure

3. A diagnostic procedure was performed for the principal diagnosis and a procedure is performed for definitive treatment of a secondary diagnosis.
   a. Sequence diagnostic procedure as principal procedure, since the procedure most related to the principal diagnosis takes precedence.

4. No procedures performed that are related to principal diagnosis; procedures performed for definitive treatment and diagnostic procedures were performed for secondary diagnosis
   a. Sequence procedure performed for definitive treatment of secondary diagnosis as principal procedure, since there are no procedures (definitive or nondefinitive treatment) related to principal diagnosis.

Anatomical Illustrations

Circulatory System — Arteries and Veins

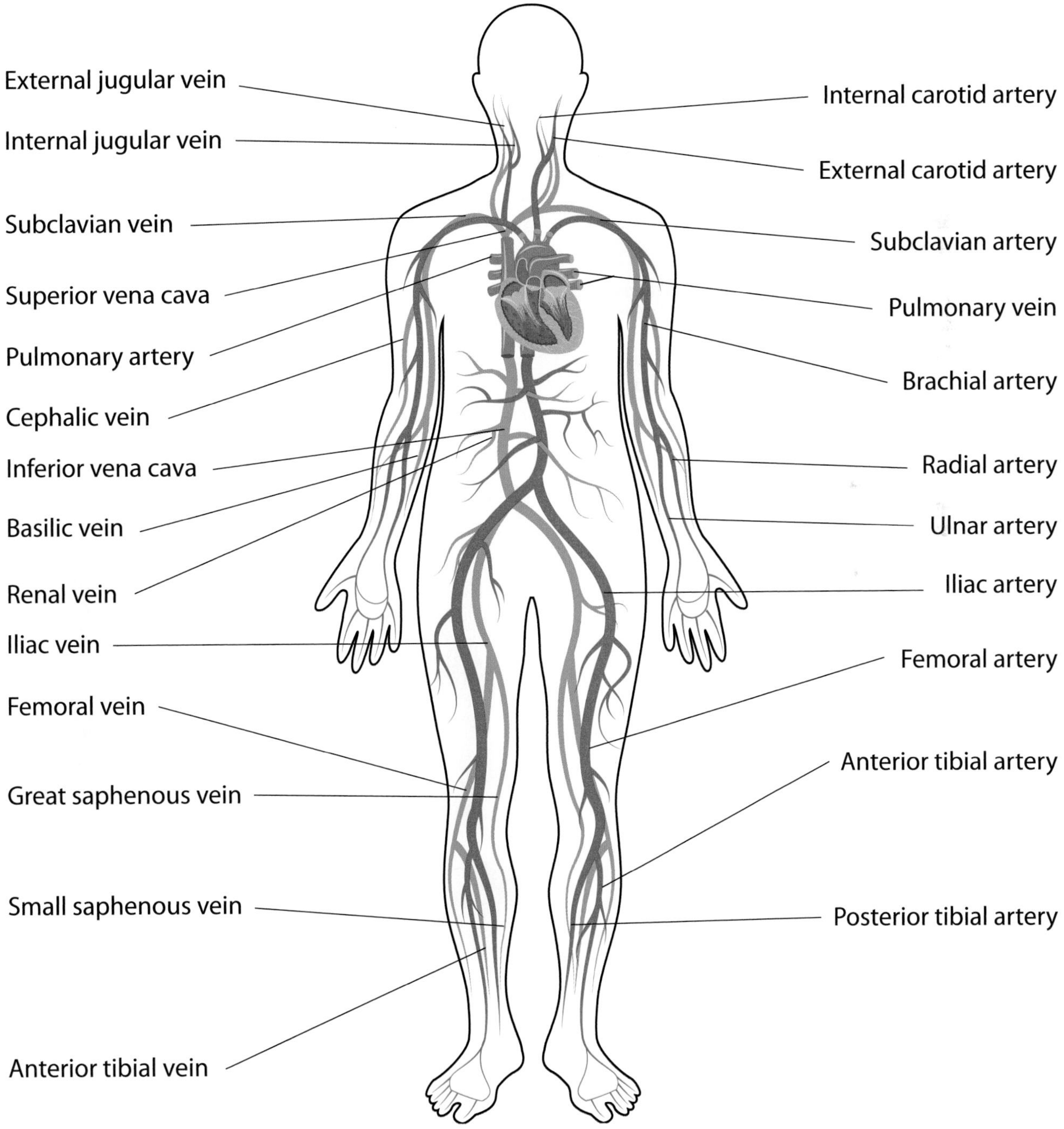

Circulatory System — Artery and Vein Anatomy

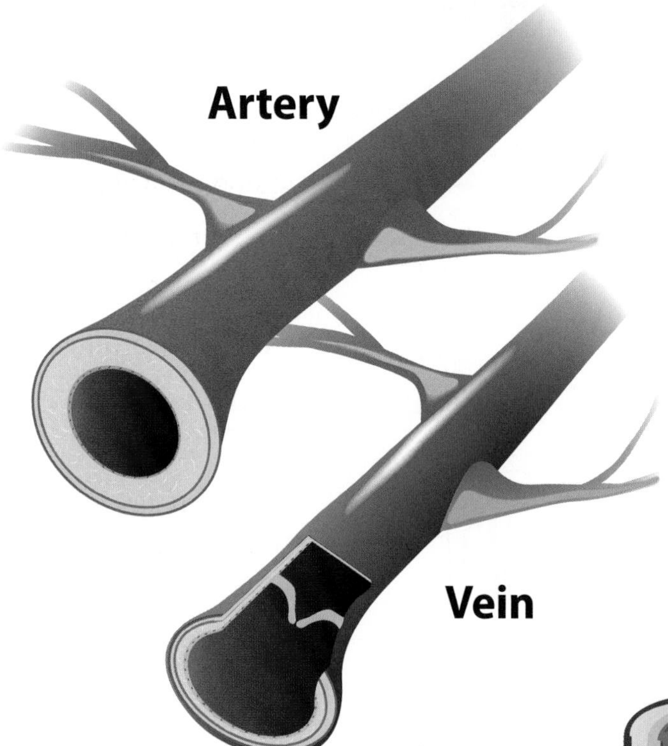

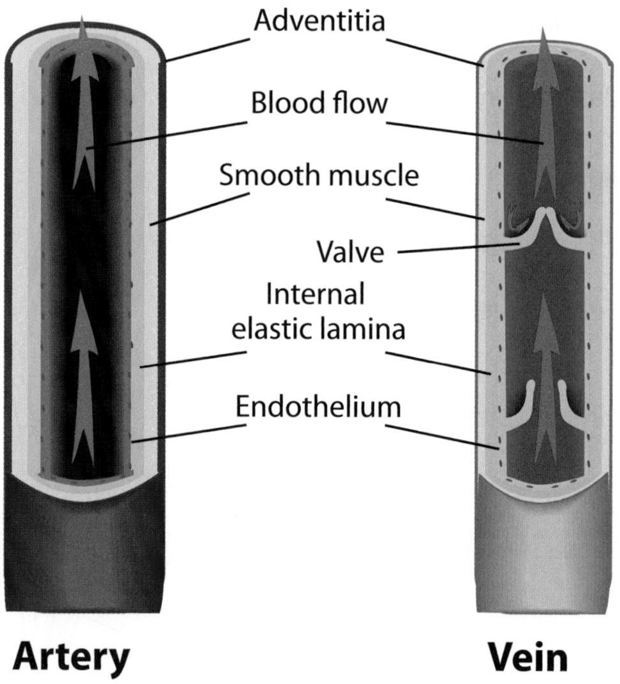

Circulatory System — Heart Anatomy and Cardiac Cycle

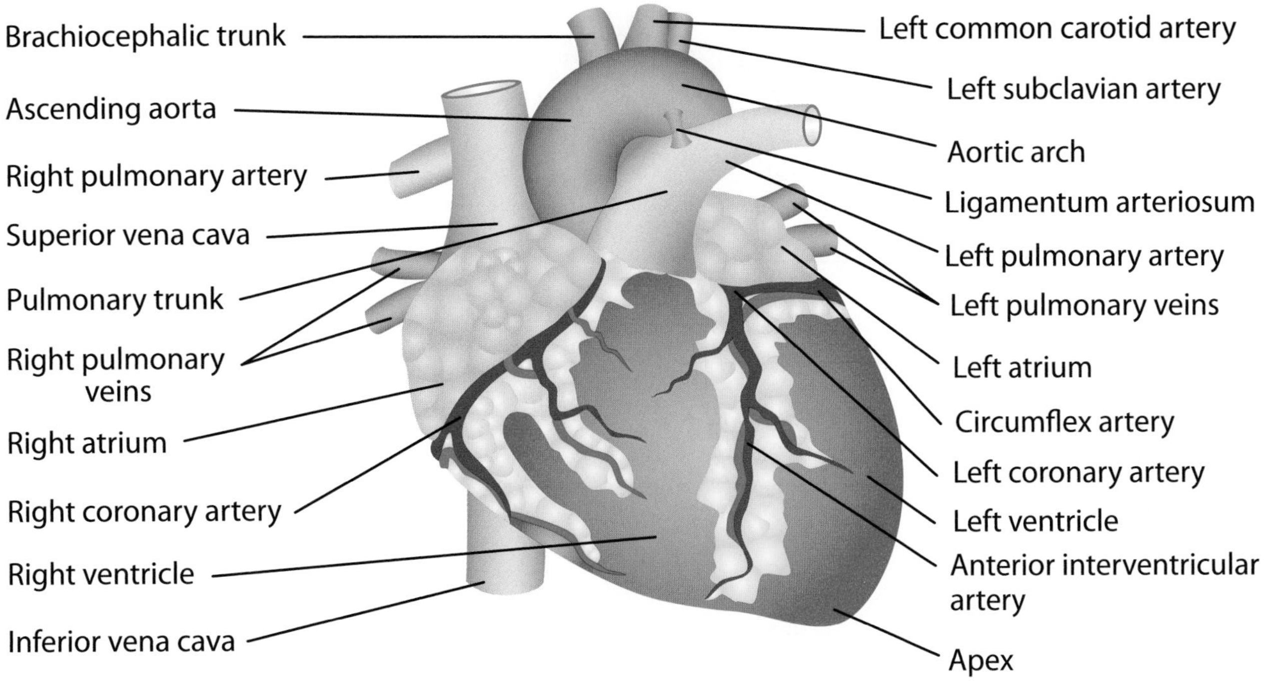

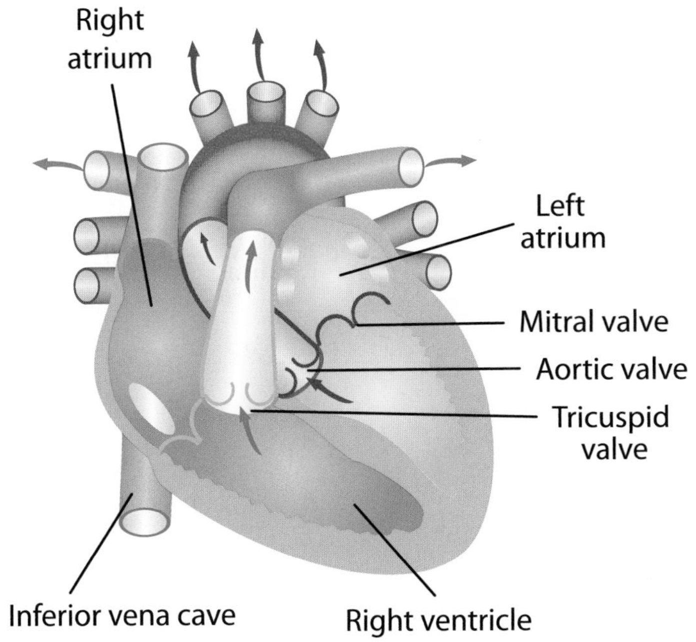

Diastole Ventricular Relaxation and Filling

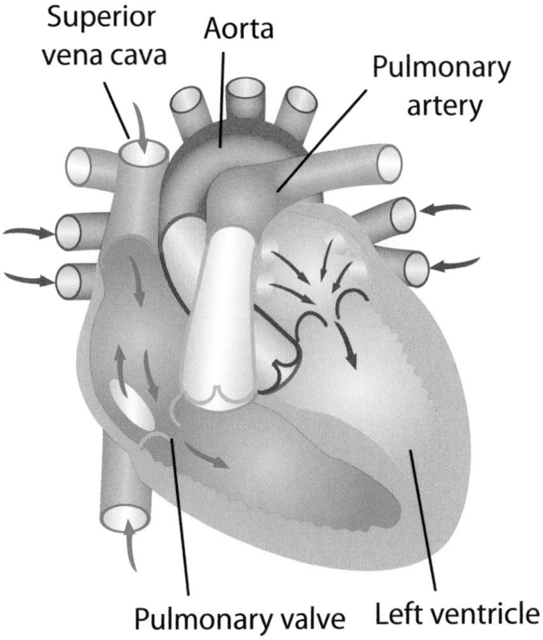

Systole Ventricular Contraction and Ejection

Digestive System — Digestive Organs

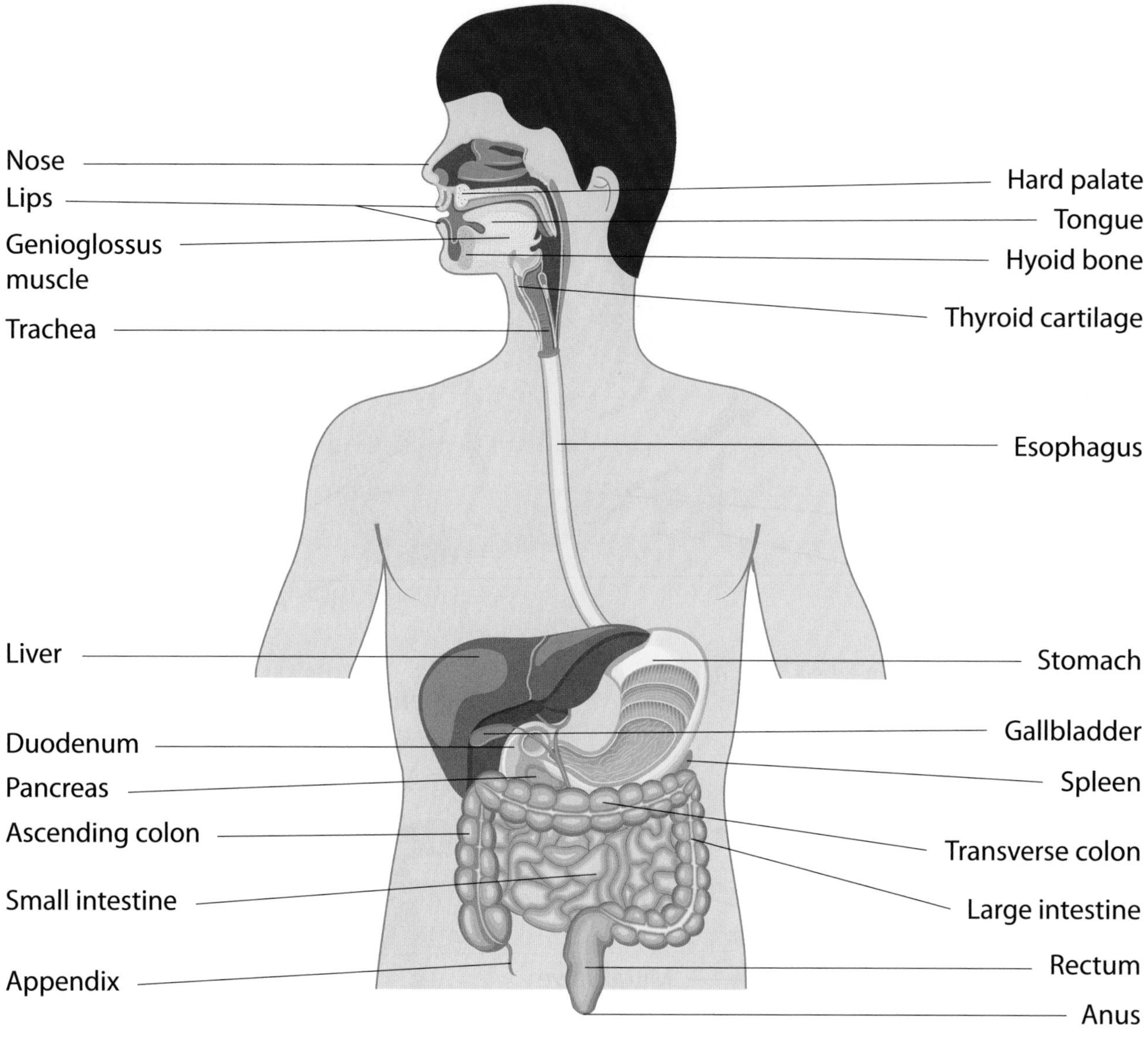

Digestive System — Large Intestine Anatomy

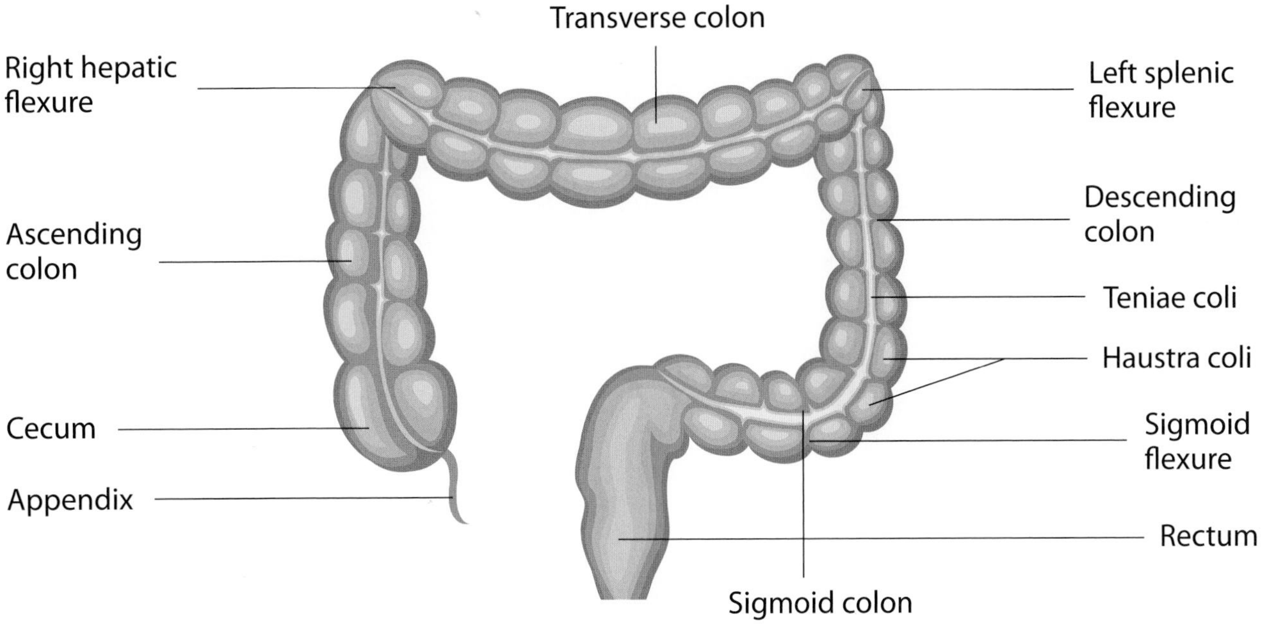

Rectum Anatomy

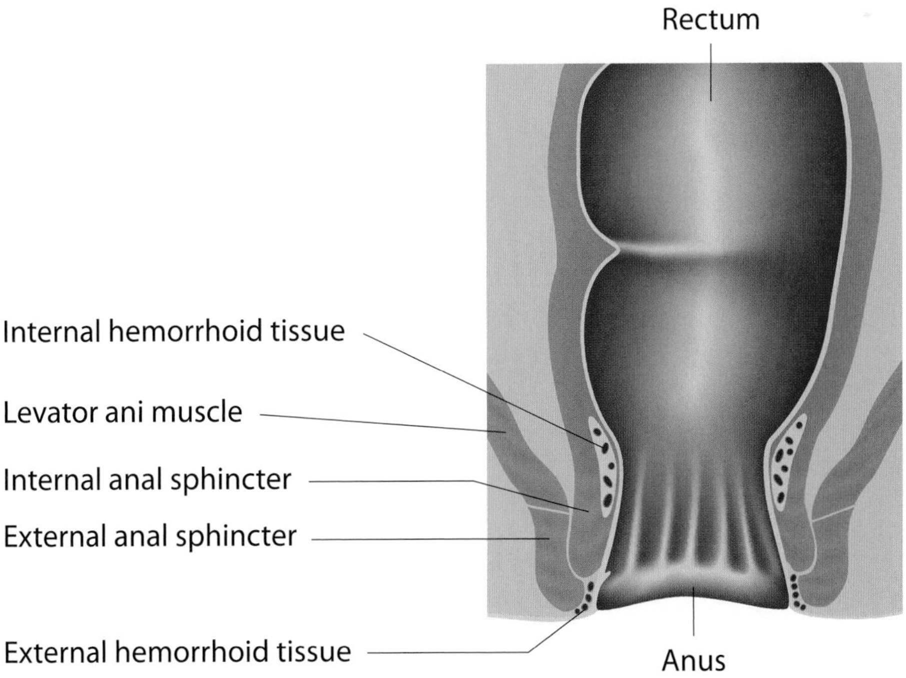

Digestive System — Liver Anatomy

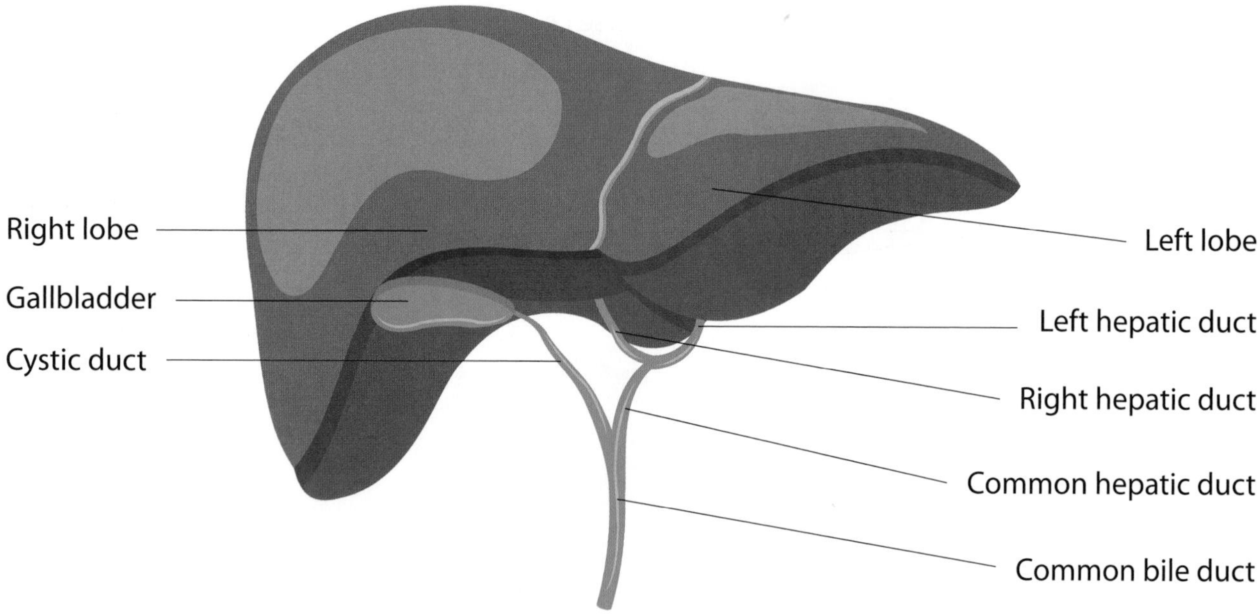

Pancreas Anatomy

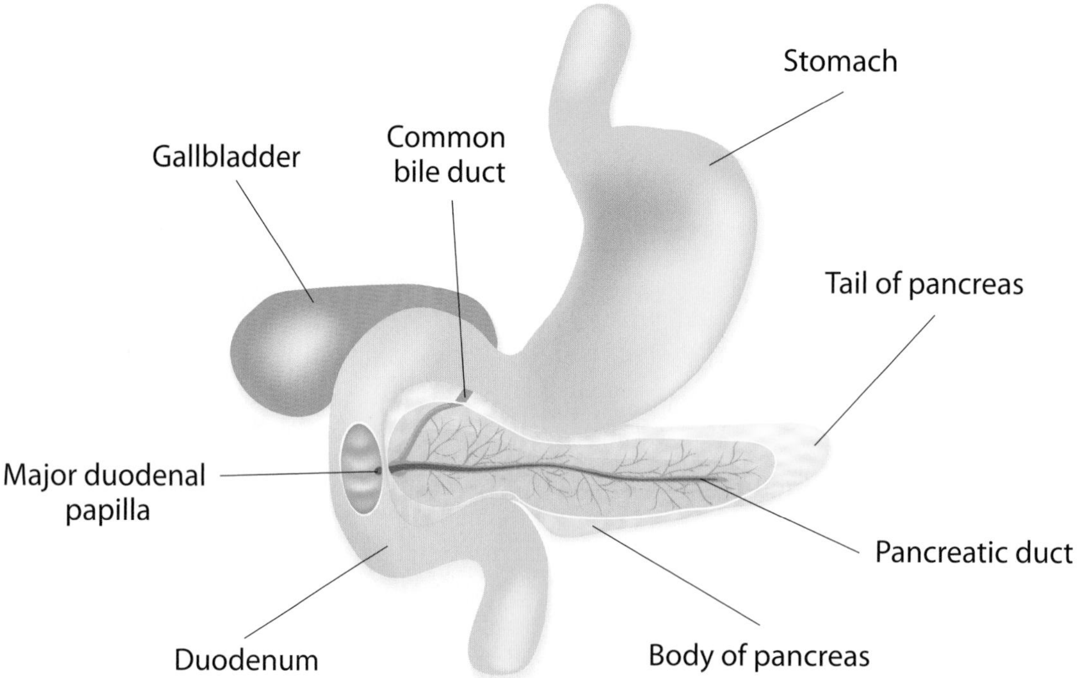

Digestive System — Mouth Anatomy

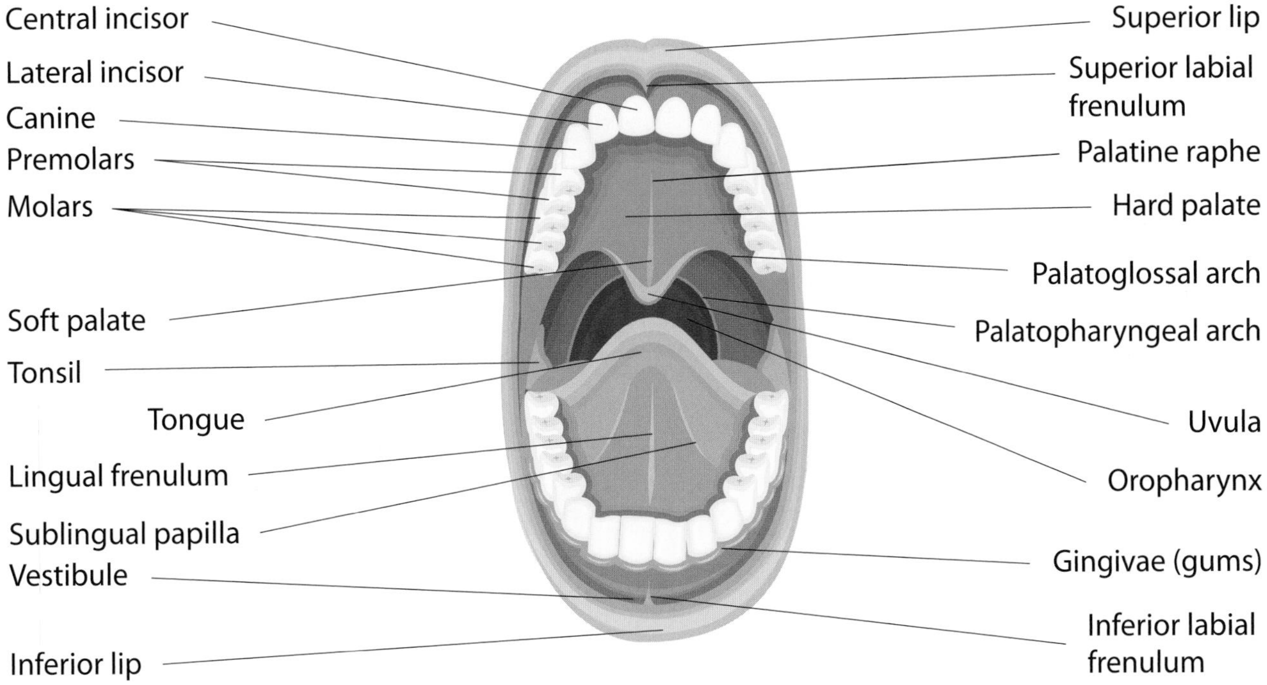
Central incisor
Lateral incisor
Canine
Premolars
Molars
Soft palate
Tonsil
Tongue
Lingual frenulum
Sublingual papilla
Vestibule
Inferior lip
Superior lip
Superior labial frenulum
Palatine raphe
Hard palate
Palatoglossal arch
Palatopharyngeal arch
Uvula
Oropharynx
Gingivae (gums)
Inferior labial frenulum

Tongue Anatomy

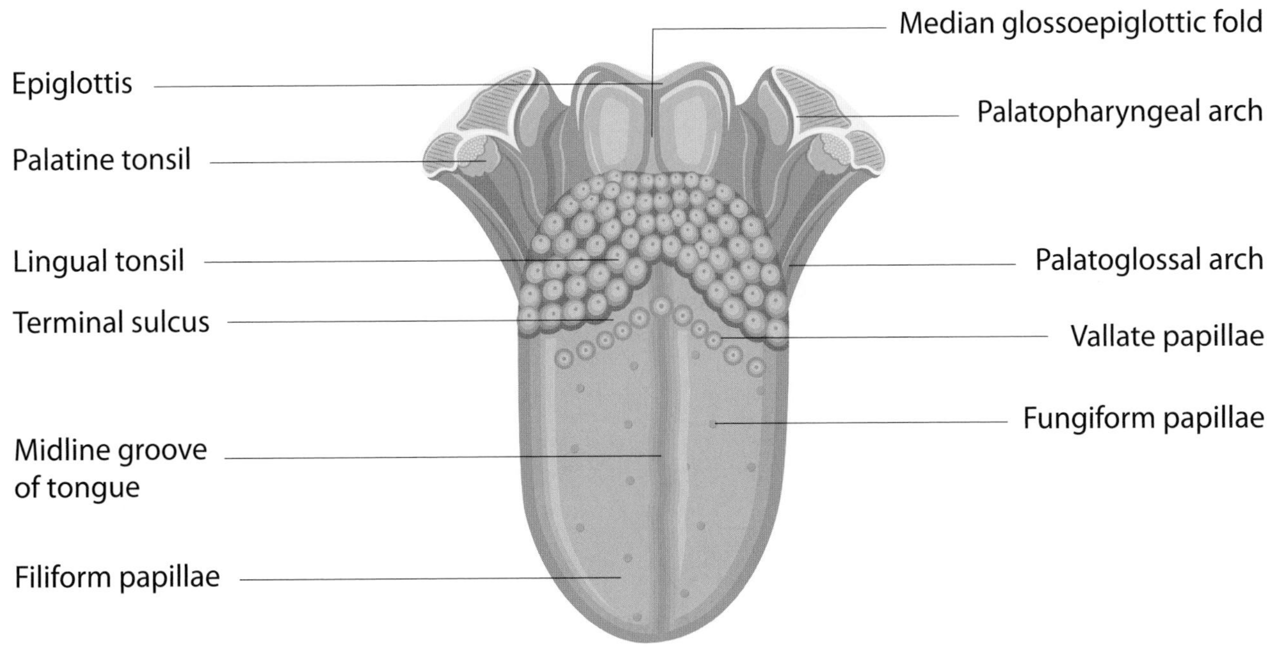
Epiglottis
Palatine tonsil
Lingual tonsil
Terminal sulcus
Midline groove of tongue
Filiform papillae
Median glossoepiglottic fold
Palatopharyngeal arch
Palatoglossal arch
Vallate papillae
Fungiform papillae

Digestive System — Small Intestine Anatomy

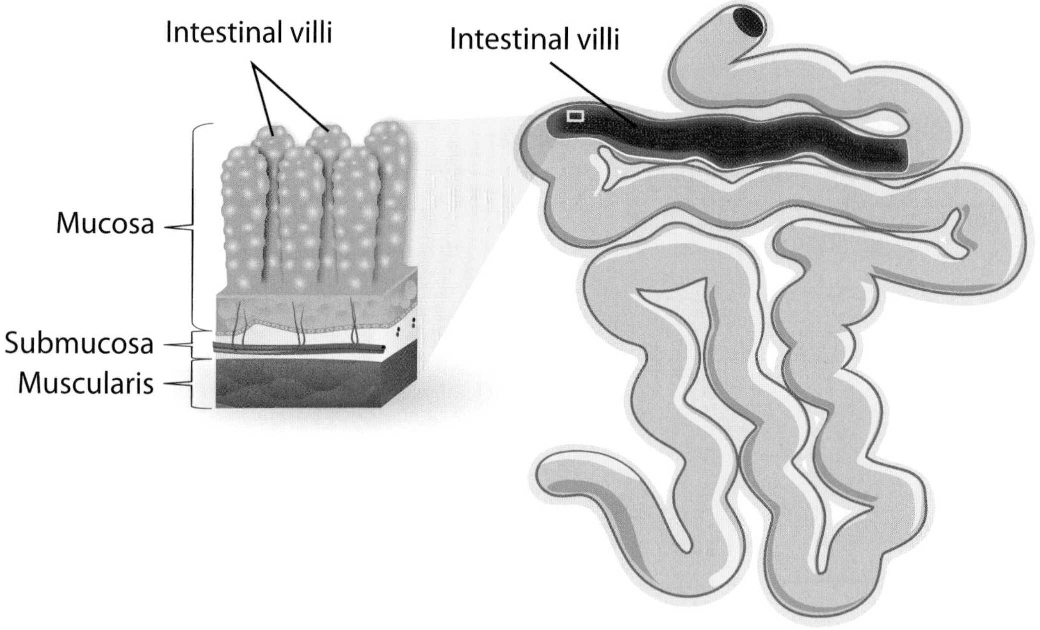

Stomach Anatomy

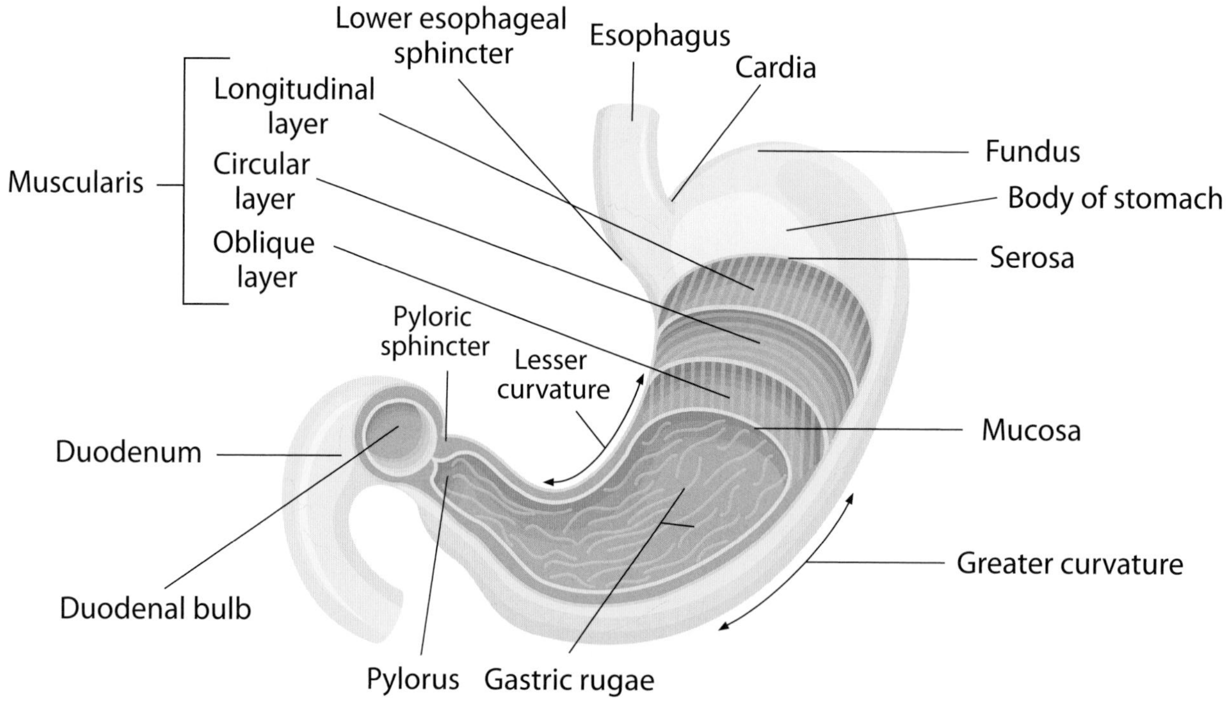

Ear — Ear Anatomy

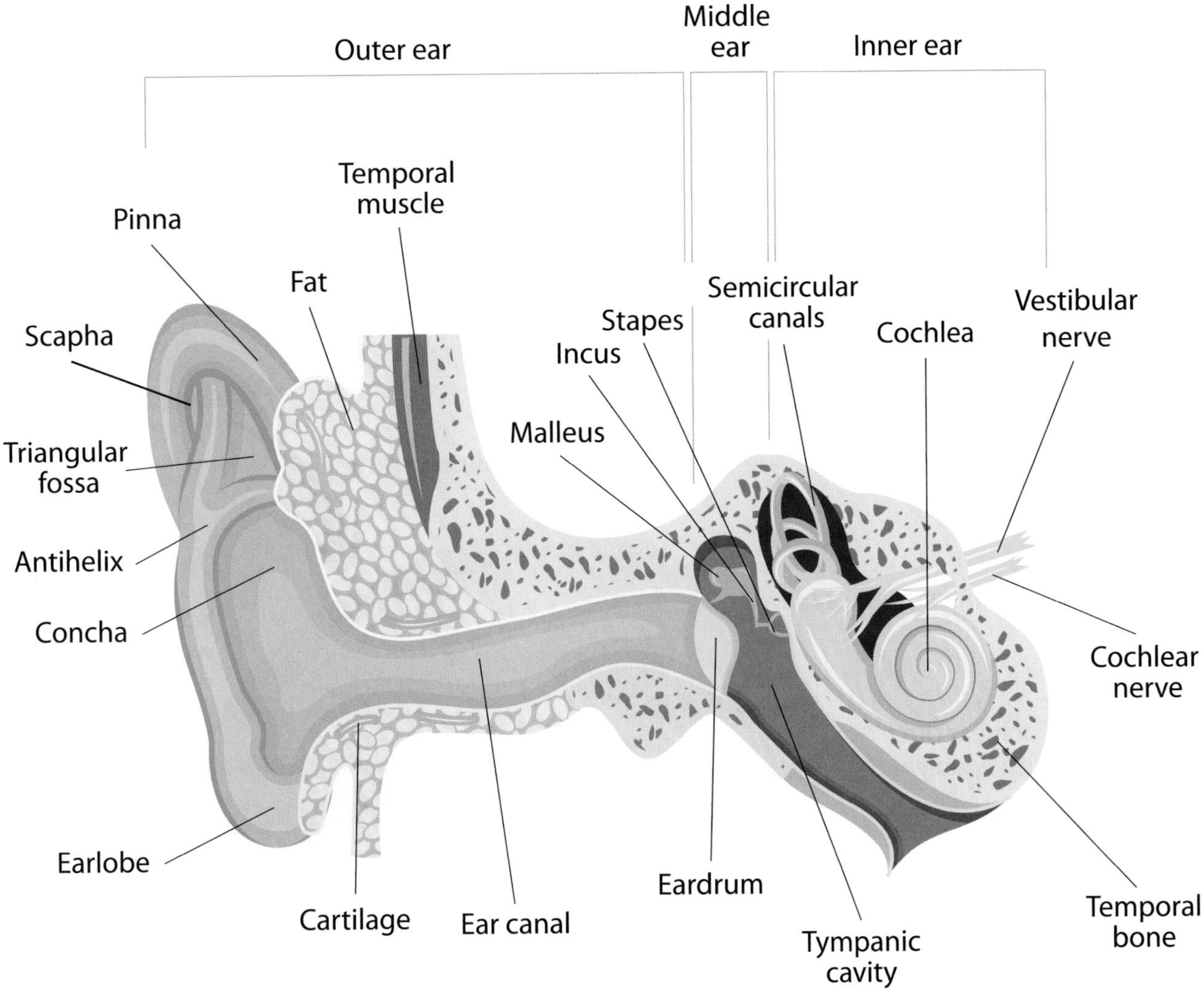

Ear — Cochlea Anatomy (Inner Ear)

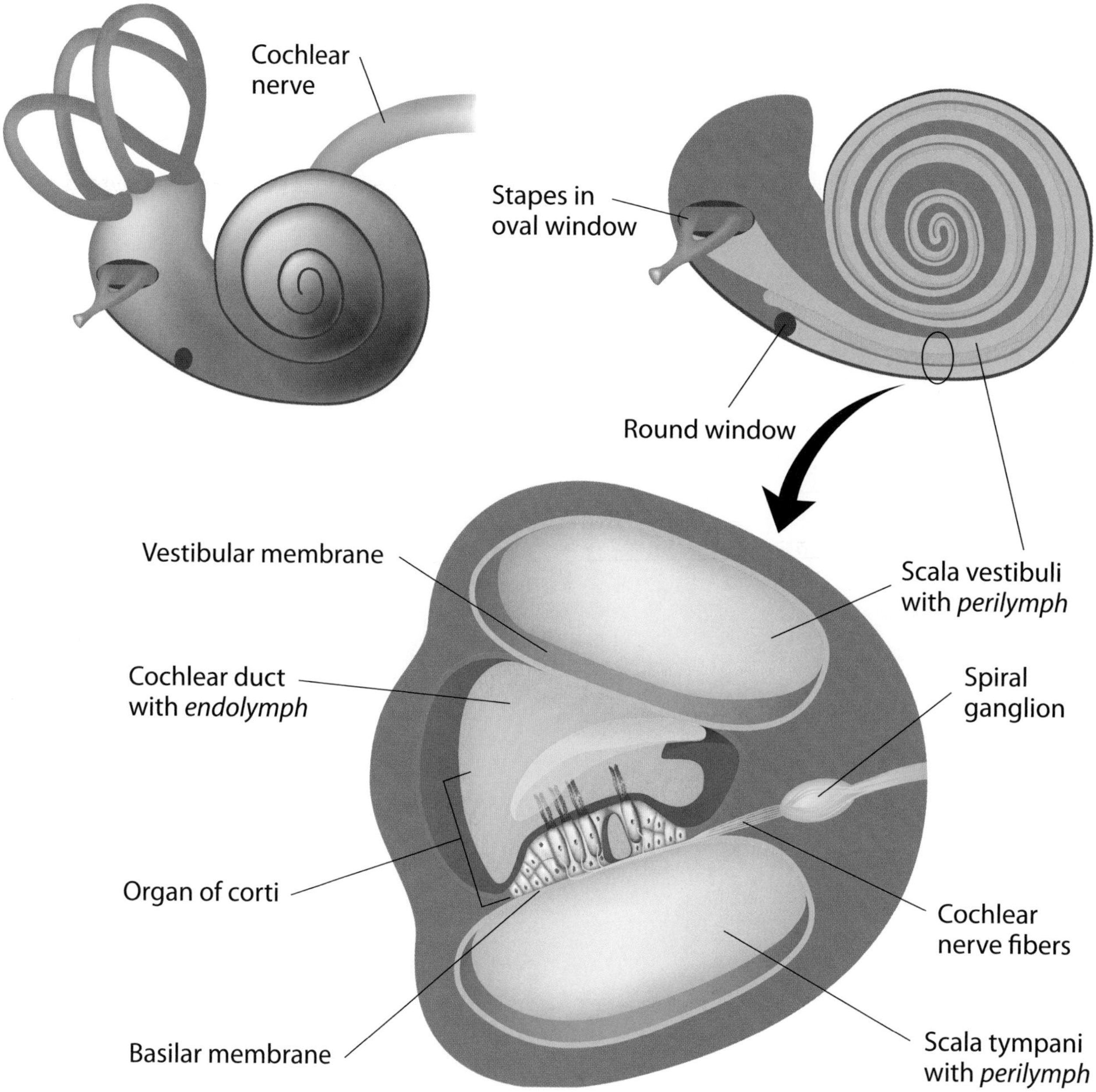

Endocrine System — Endocrine Anatomy

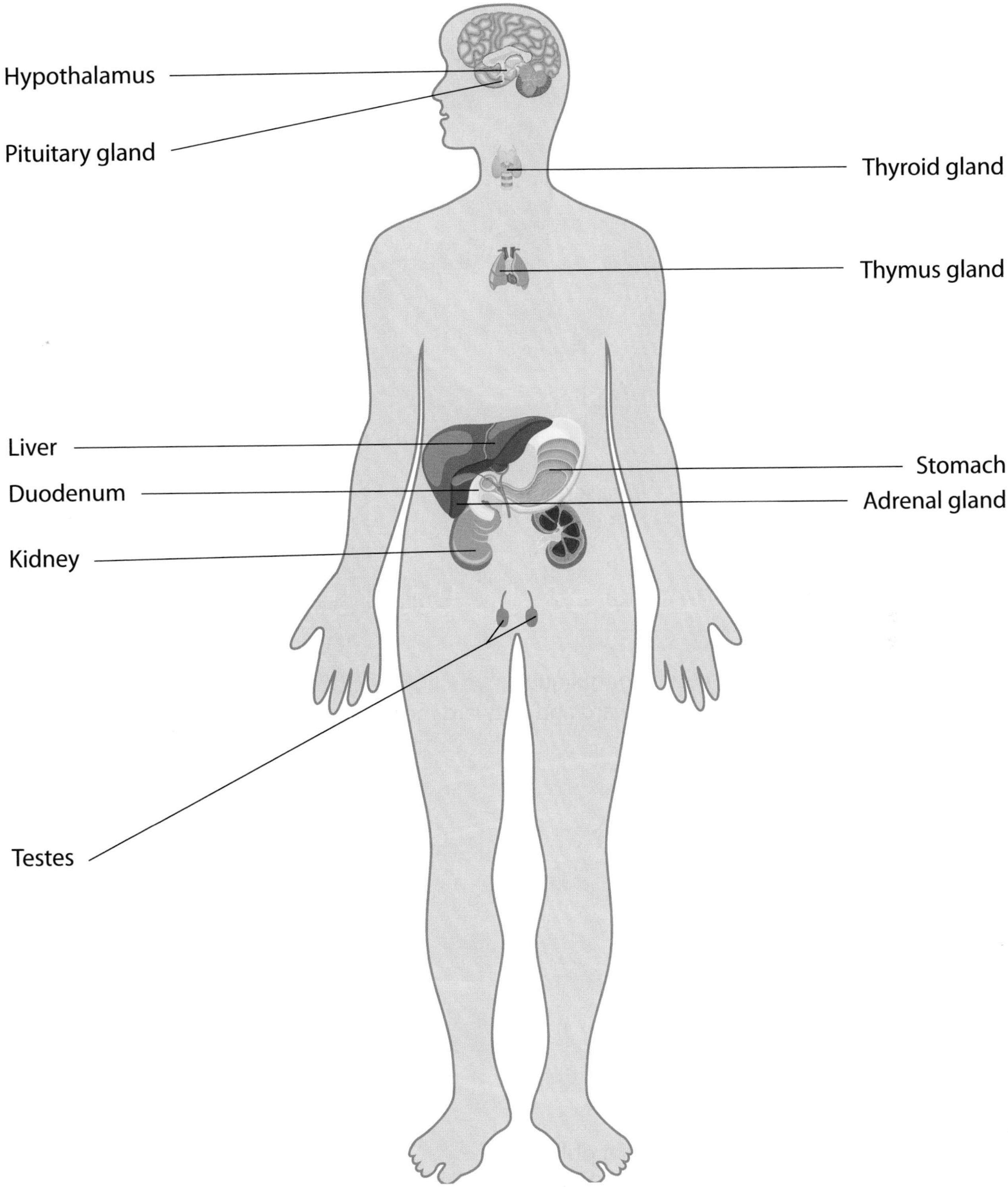

Eye — Eye Anatomy

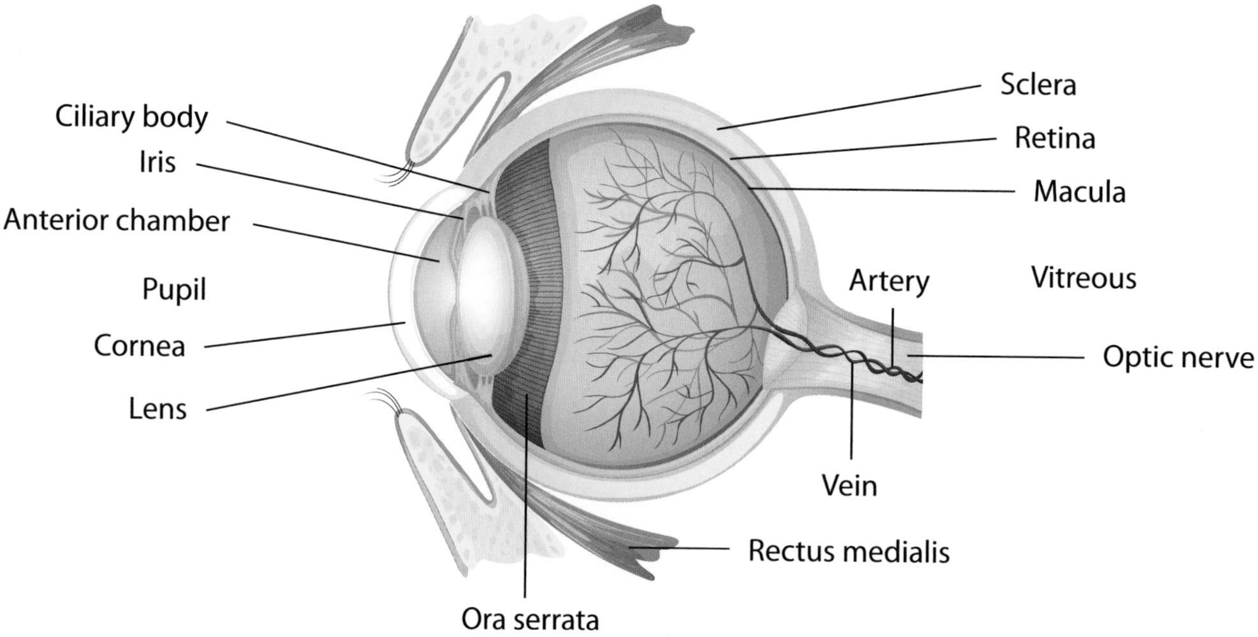
Ciliary body
Iris
Anterior chamber
Pupil
Cornea
Lens
Sclera
Retina
Macula
Artery
Vitreous
Optic nerve
Vein
Rectus medialis
Ora serrata

Muscles of the Eye

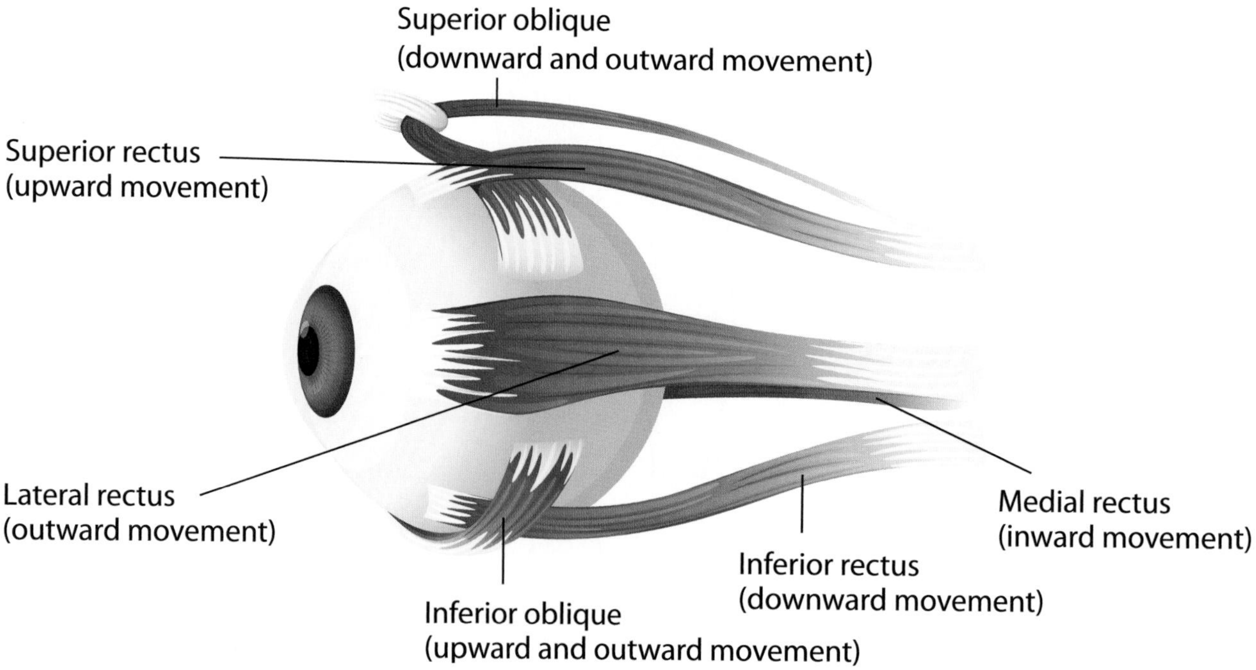
Superior oblique
(downward and outward movement)
Superior rectus
(upward movement)
Lateral rectus
(outward movement)
Medial rectus
(inward movement)
Inferior rectus
(downward movement)
Inferior oblique
(upward and outward movement)

Female Reproductive System — Breast Anatomy

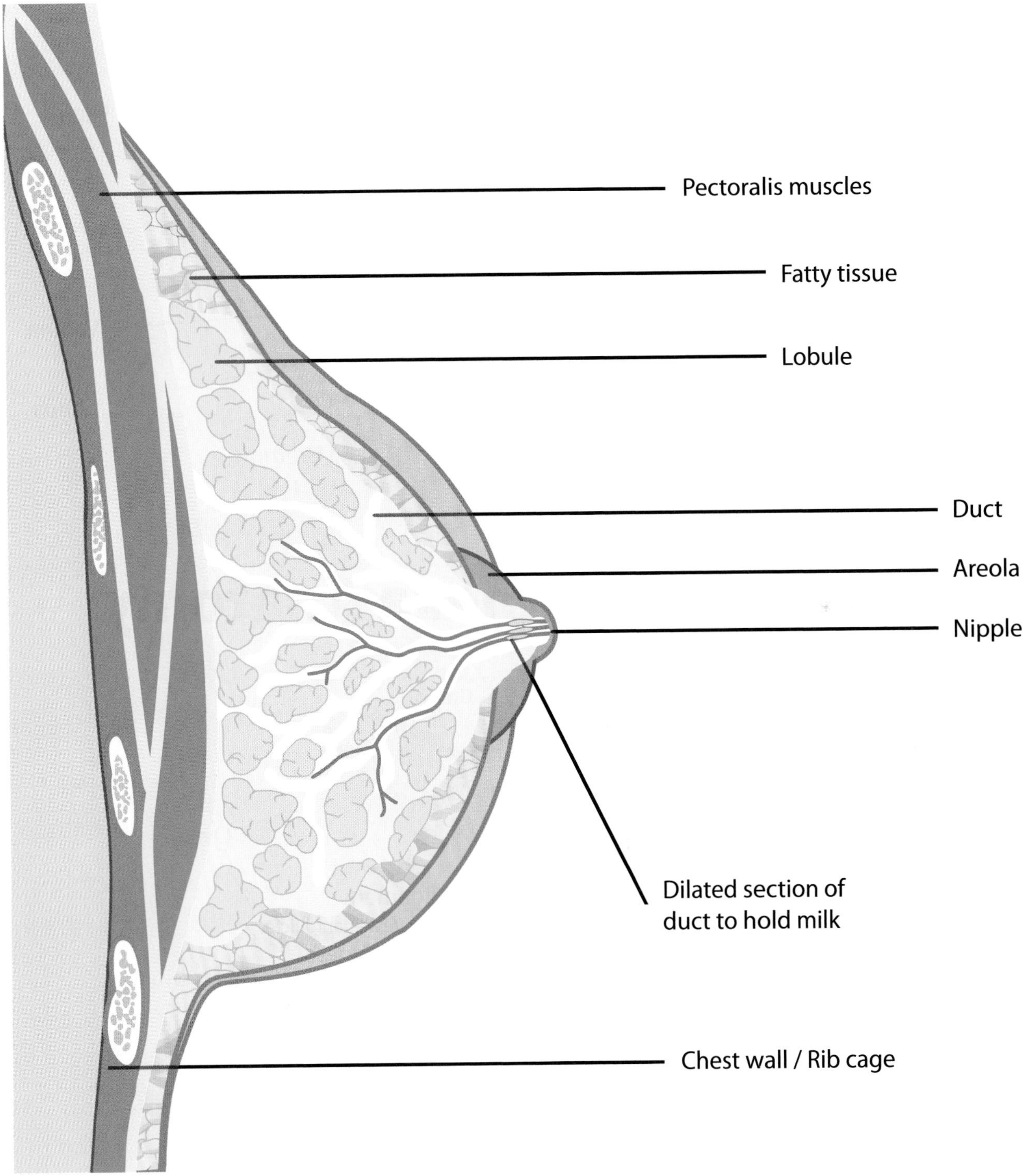

Female Reproductive System — Female Reproductive Anatomy

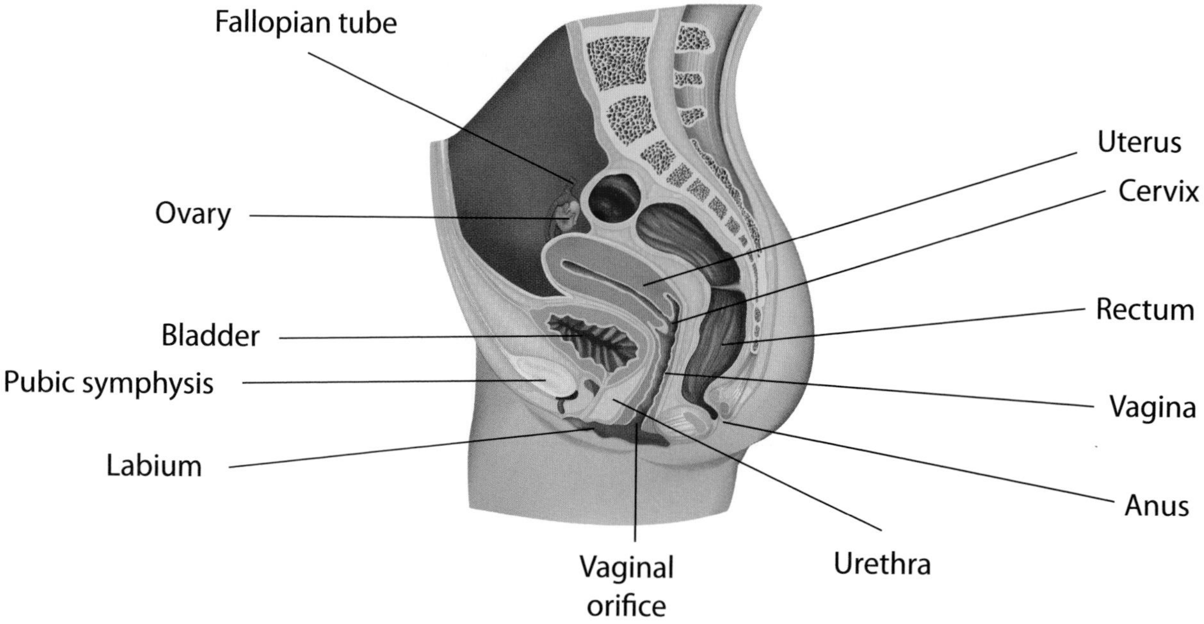

Uterus and Adnexa Anatomy

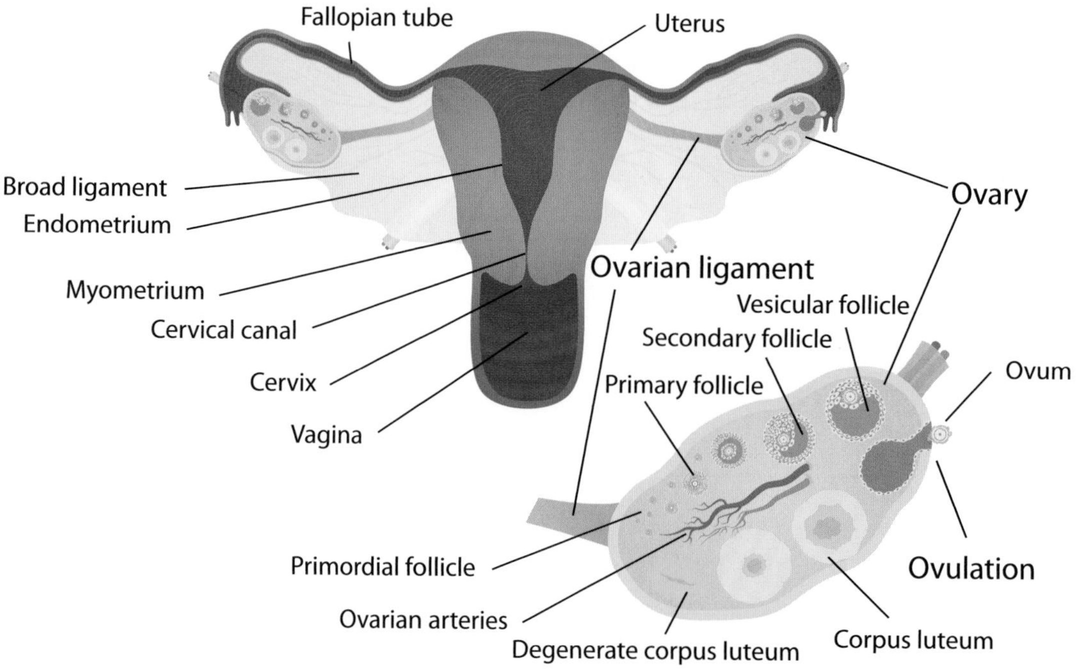

Female Reproductive System — Perineum Anatomy

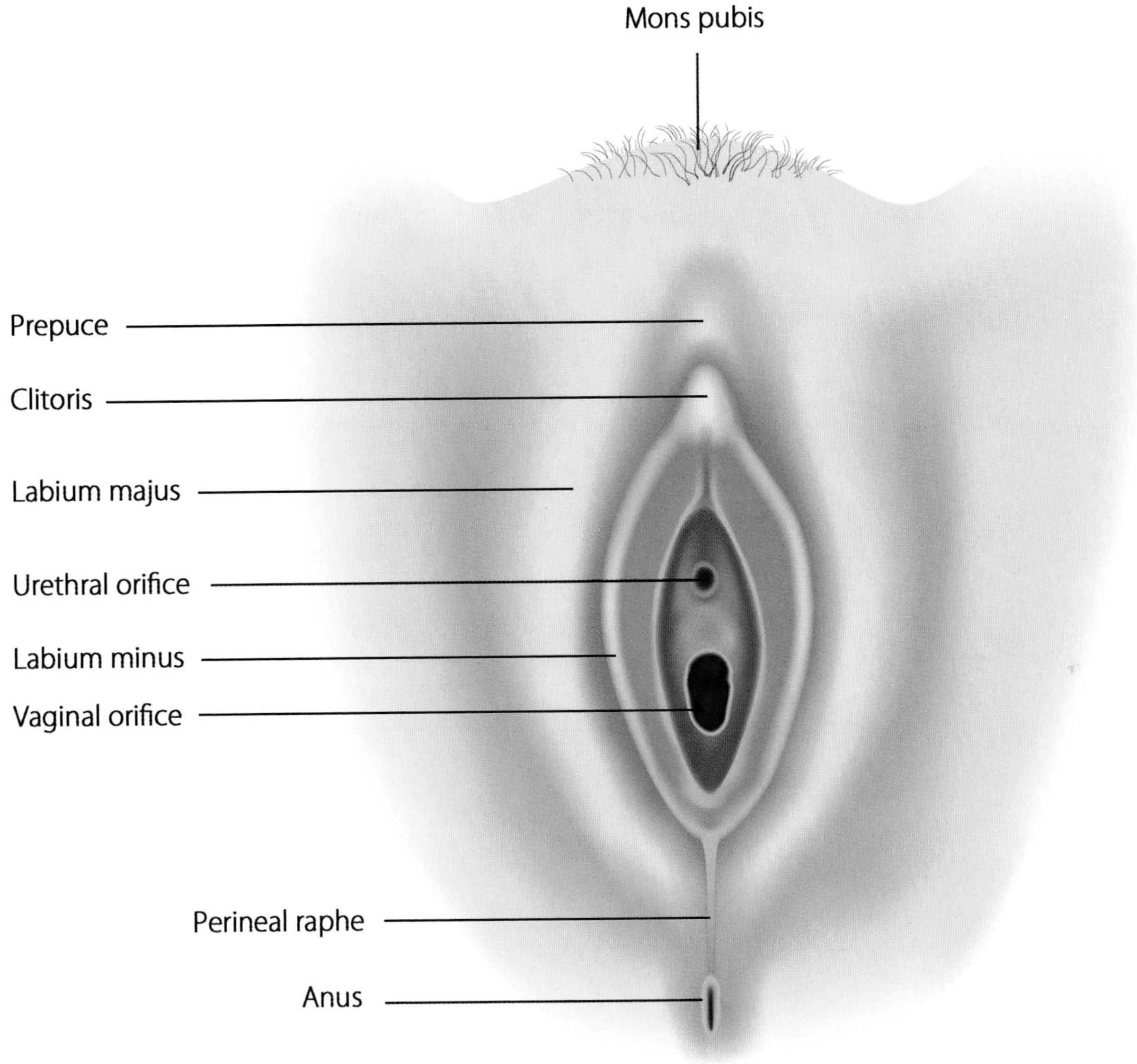

Integumentary System — Skin Anatomy

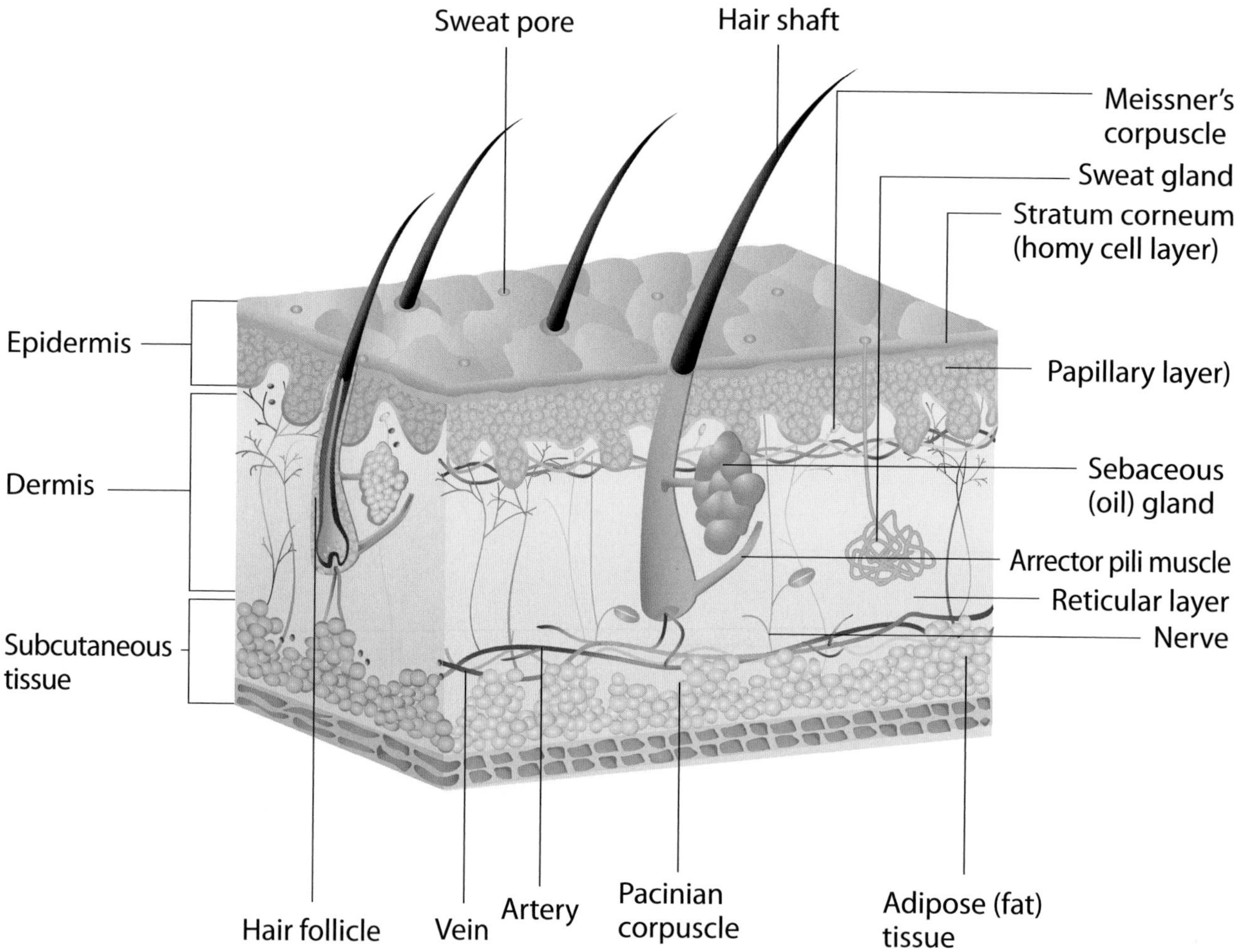

Lymphatic System — Lymphatic Anatomy

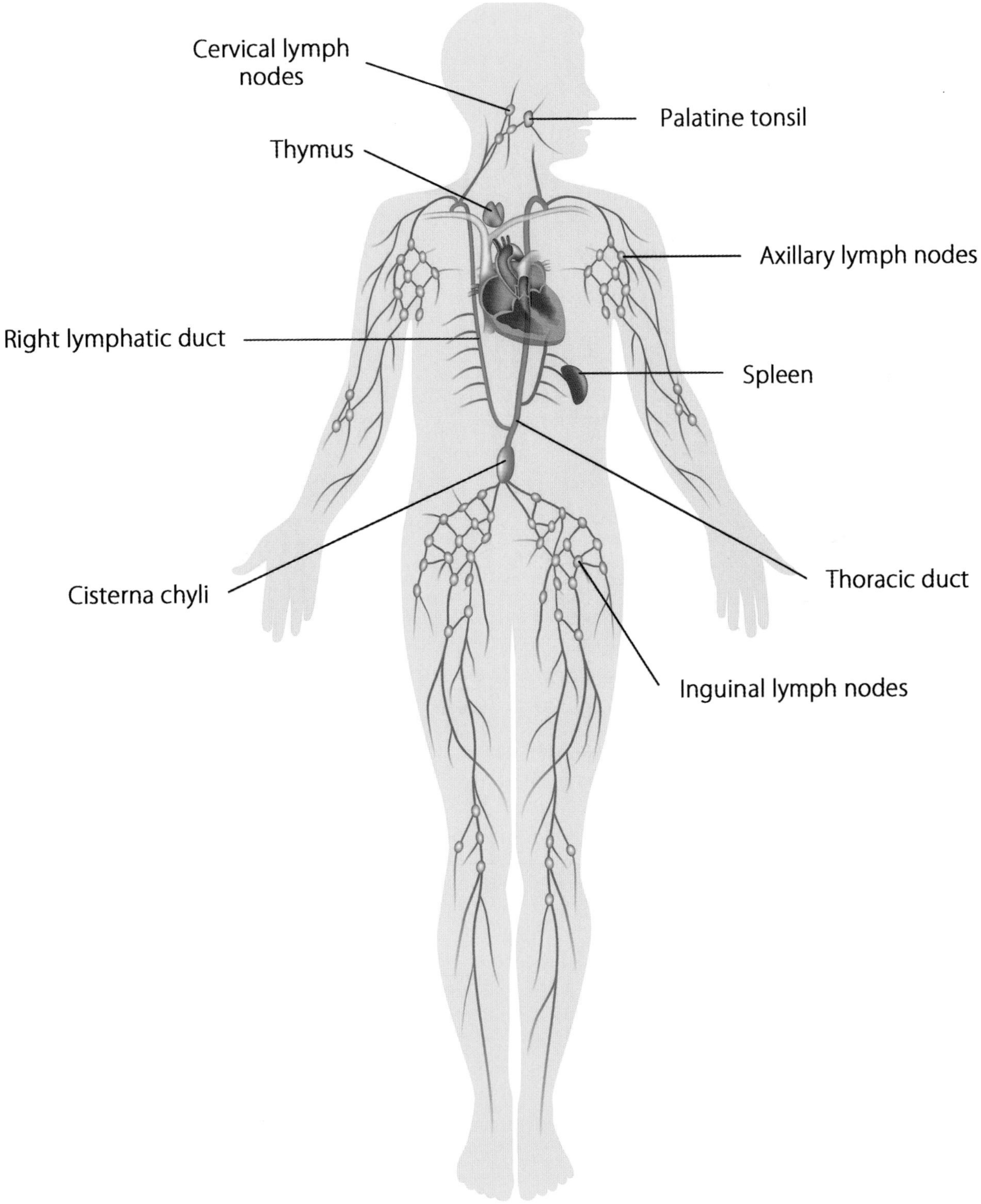

Lymphatic System — Humoral Immunity

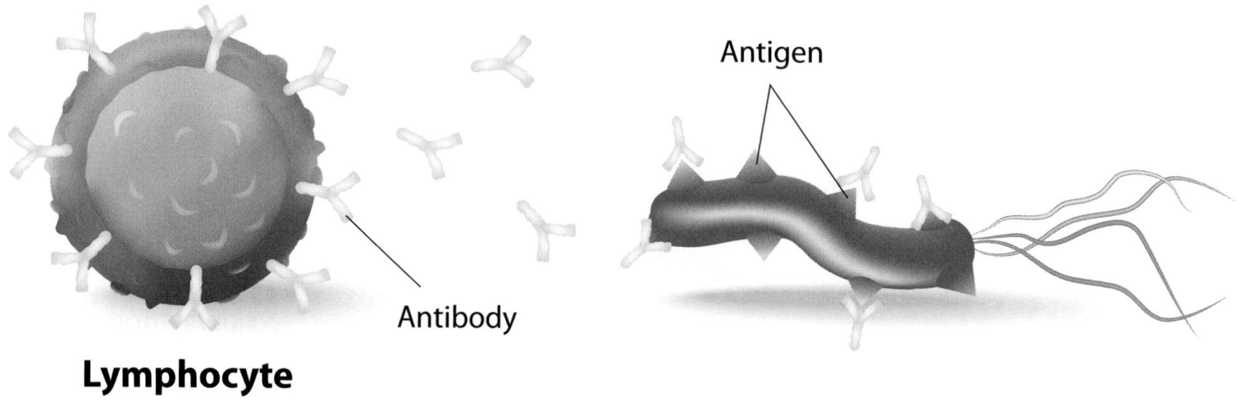

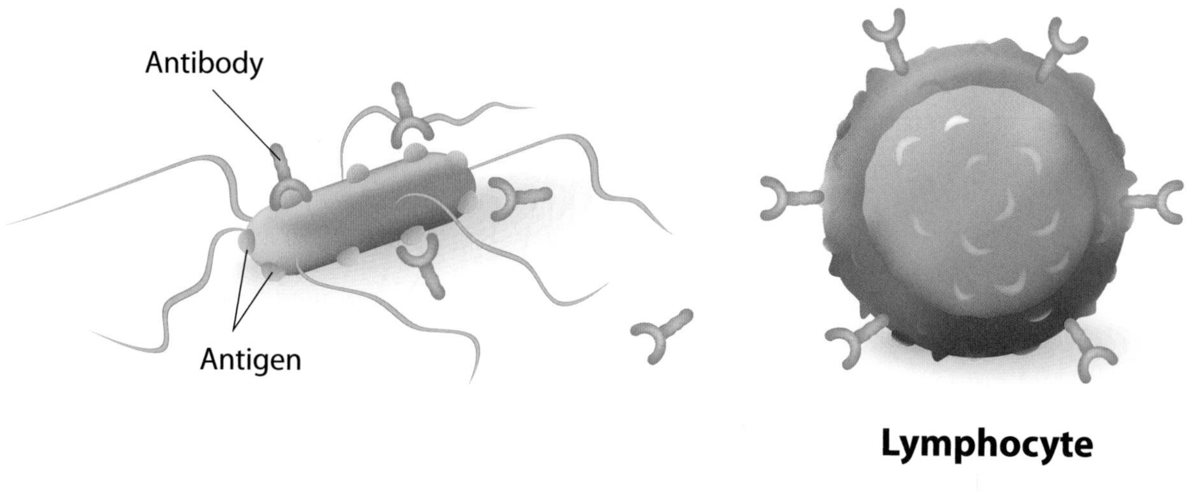

Lymphatic System — Lymph Node Anatomy

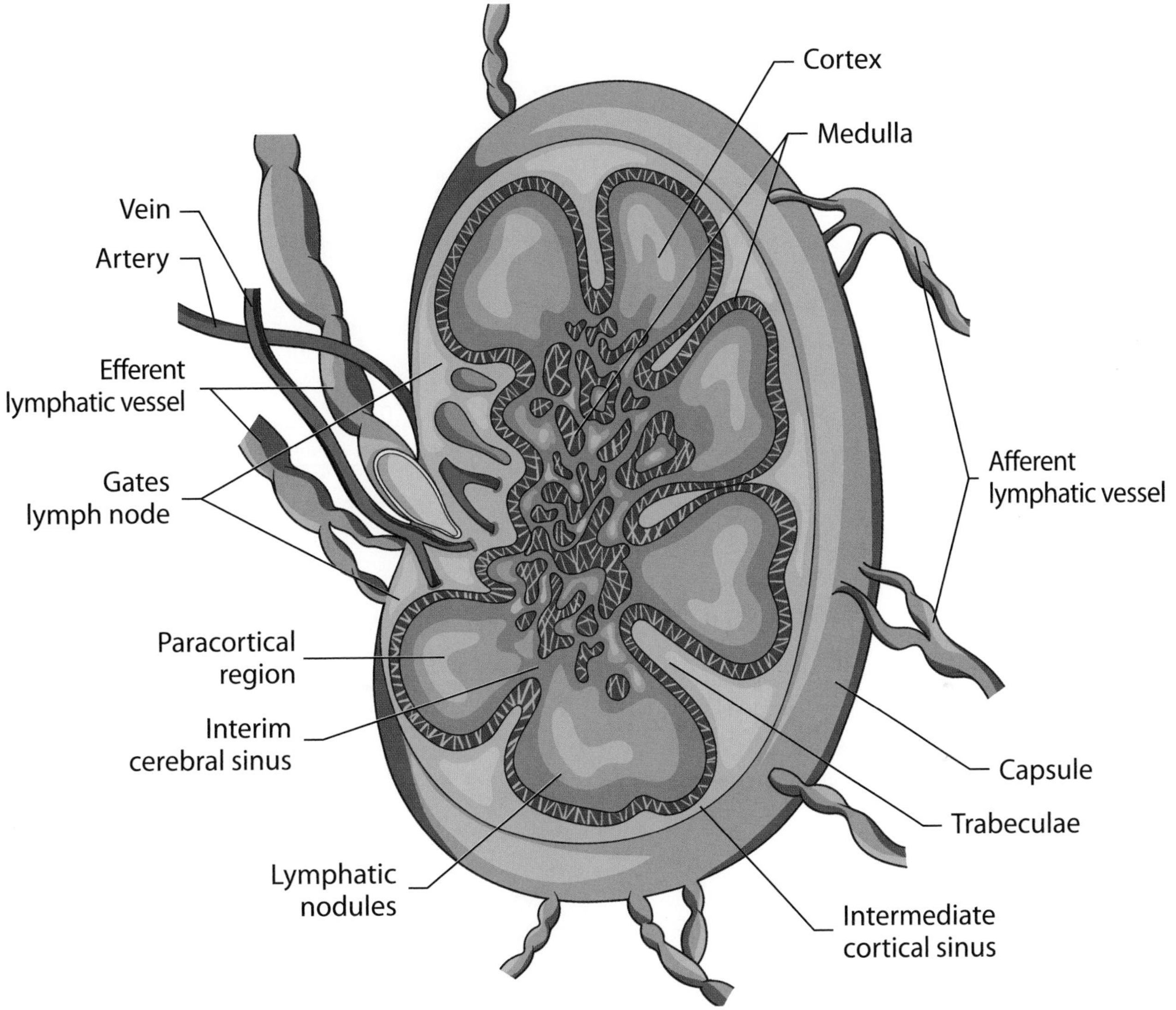

Male Reproductive System — Male Reproductive Anatomy

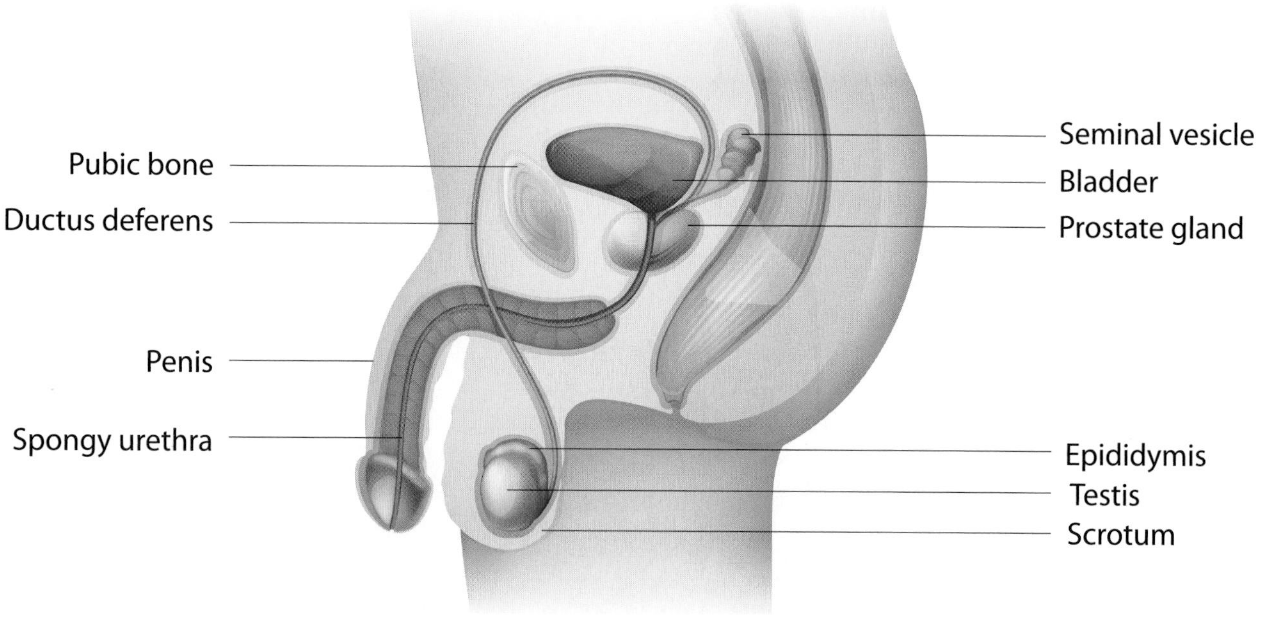

Testicle Anatomy

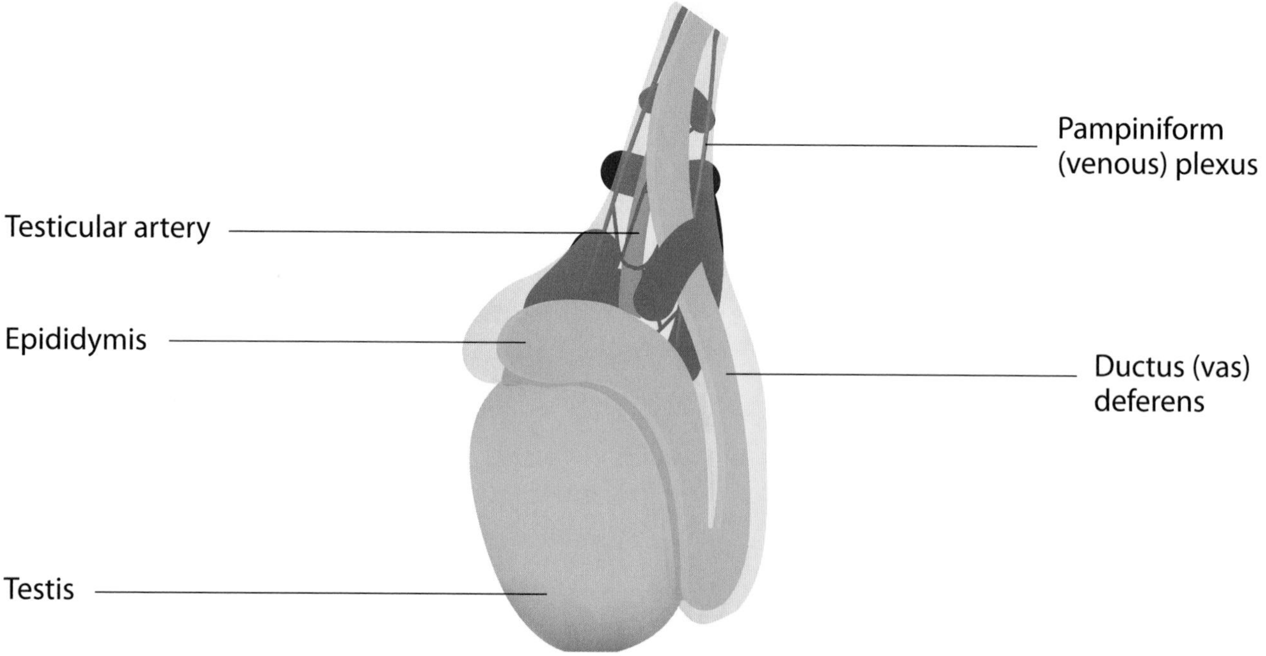

Male Reproductive System — Penis Anatomy

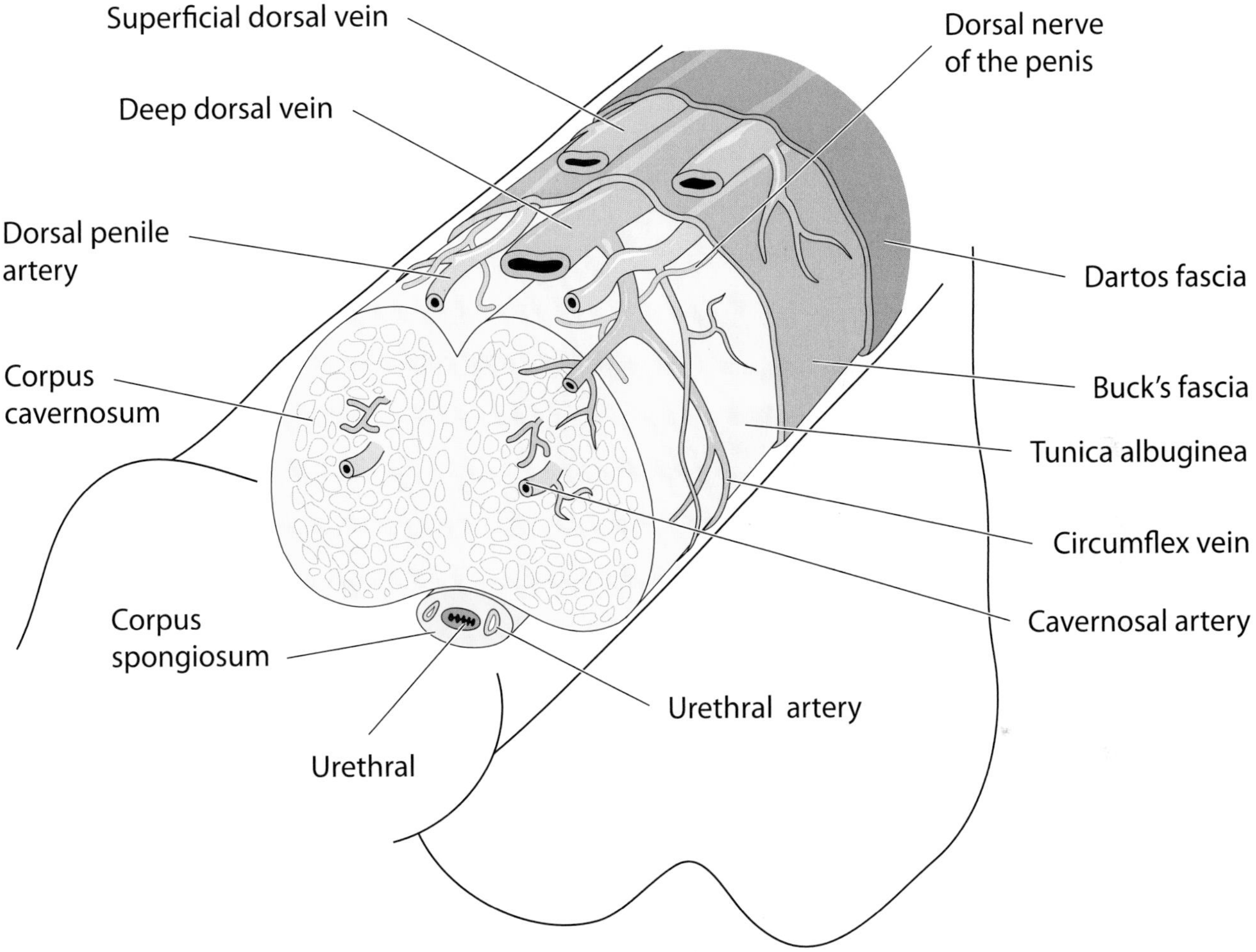

Muscular System — Muscle Anatomy

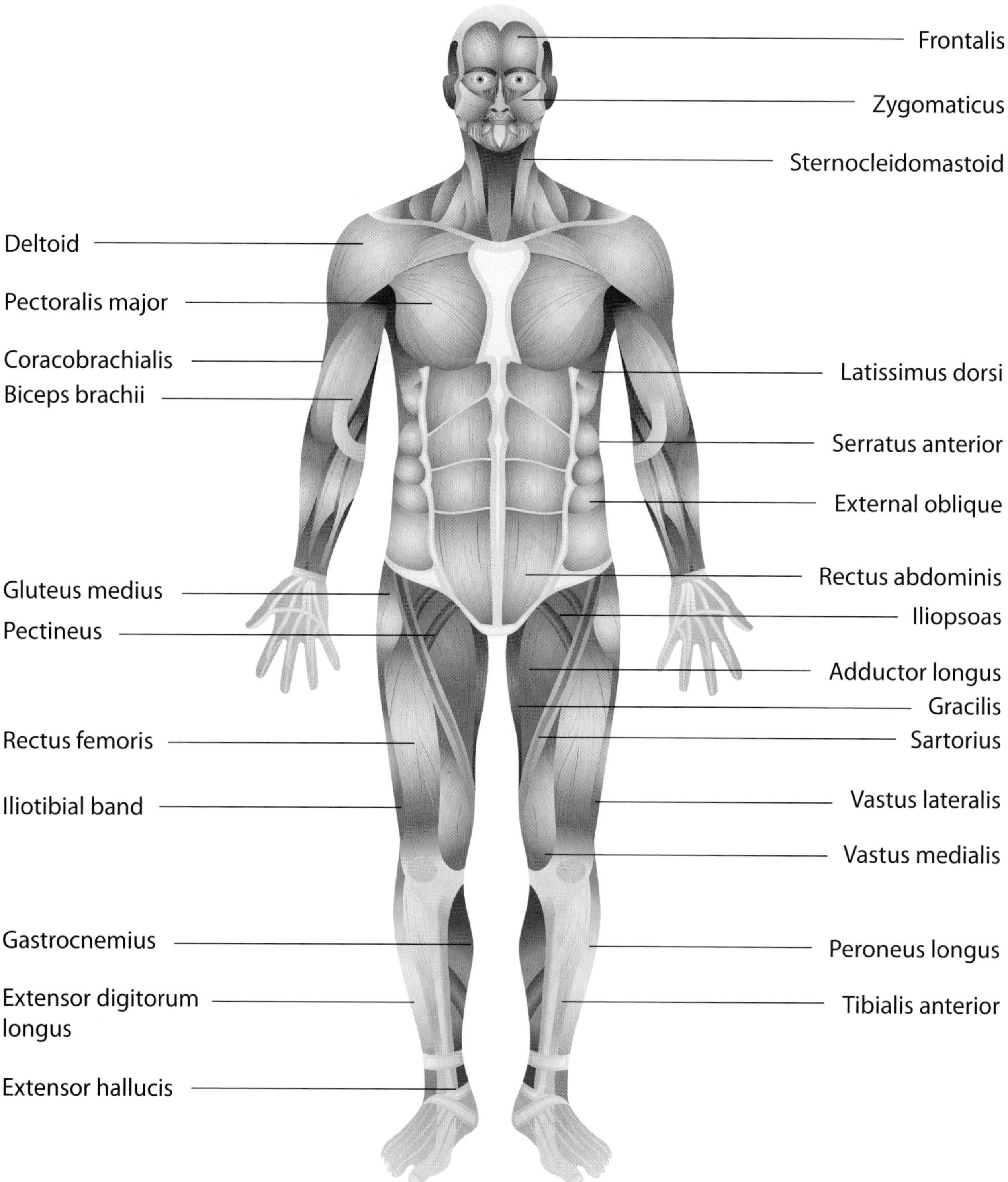
Frontalis
Zygomaticus
Sternocleidomastoid
Deltoid
Pectoralis major
Coracobrachialis
Biceps brachii
Latissimus dorsi
Serratus anterior
External oblique
Rectus abdominis
Gluteus medius
Pectineus
Iliopsoas
Adductor longus
Gracilis
Sartorius
Rectus femoris
Iliotibial band
Vastus lateralis
Vastus medialis
Gastrocnemius
Peroneus longus
Extensor digitorum longus
Tibialis anterior
Extensor hallucis

Muscular System — Forearm Muscles (right arm, posterior compartment)

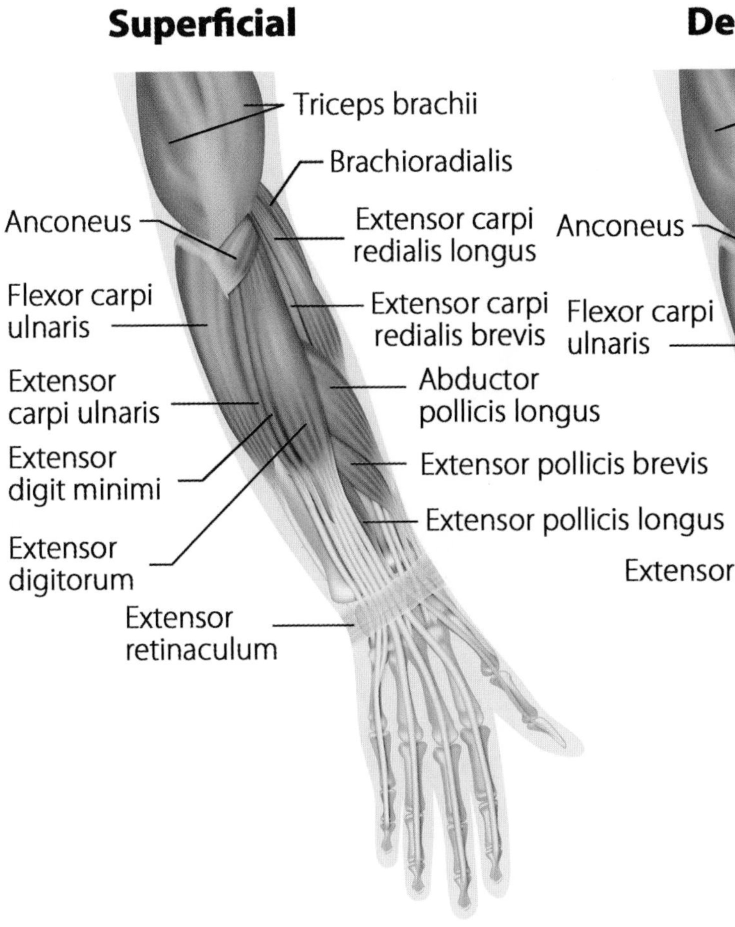
Superficial
Triceps brachii
Brachioradialis
Anconeus
Extensor carpi redialis longus
Flexor carpi ulnaris
Extensor carpi redialis brevis
Extensor carpi ulnaris
Abductor pollicis longus
Extensor digit minimi
Extensor pollicis brevis
Extensor pollicis longus
Extensor digitorum
Extensor retinaculum

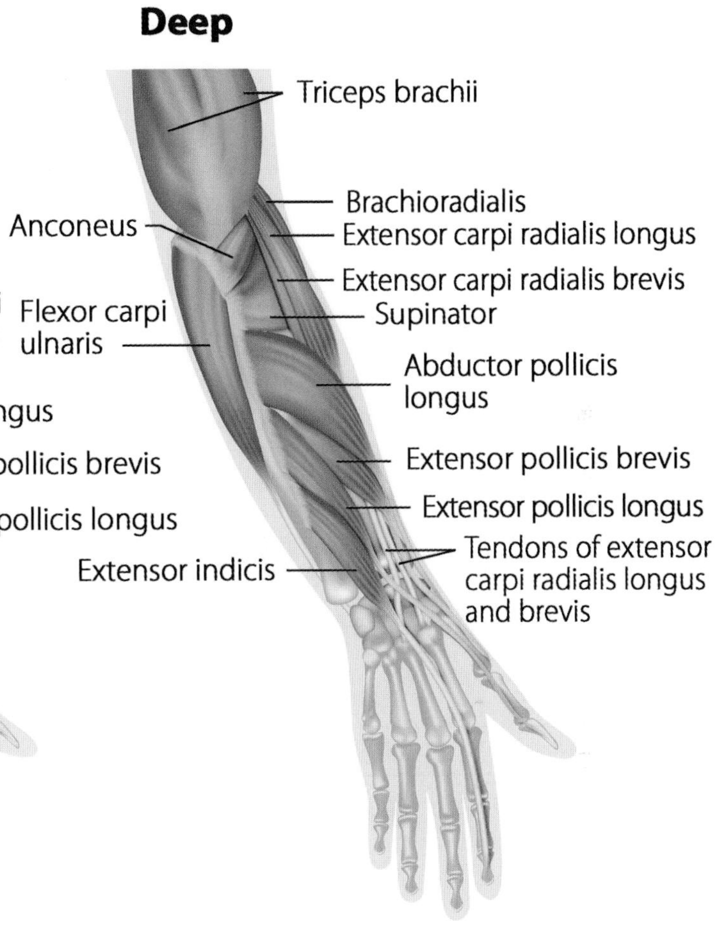
Deep
Triceps brachii
Brachioradialis
Anconeus
Extensor carpi radialis longus
Extensor carpi radialis brevis
Supinator
Flexor carpi ulnaris
Abductor pollicis longus
Extensor pollicis brevis
Extensor pollicis longus
Tendons of extensor carpi radialis longus and brevis
Extensor indicis

Muscular System — Knee Joint Anatomy

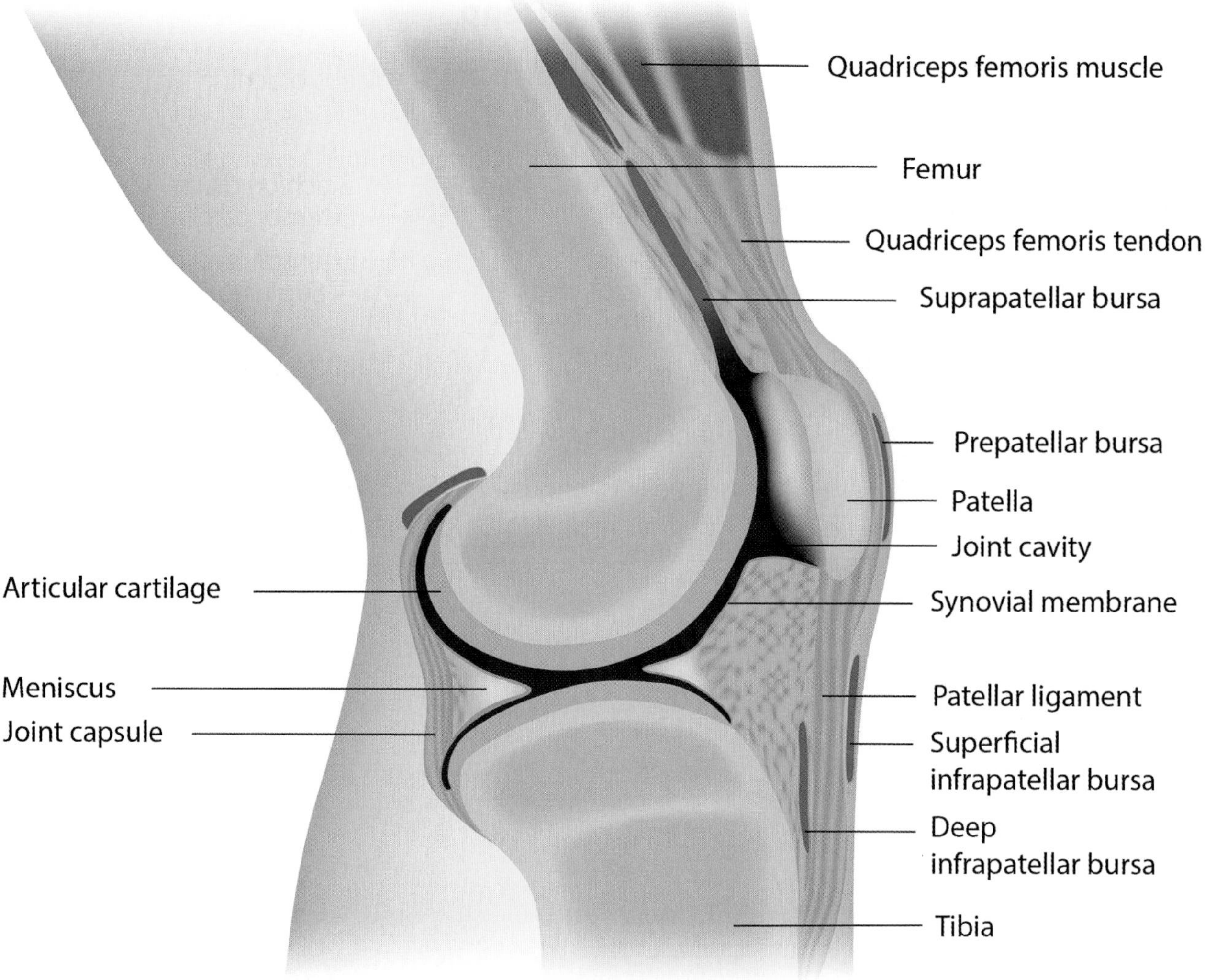

Muscular System — Shoulder (Rotator Cuff) Muscles

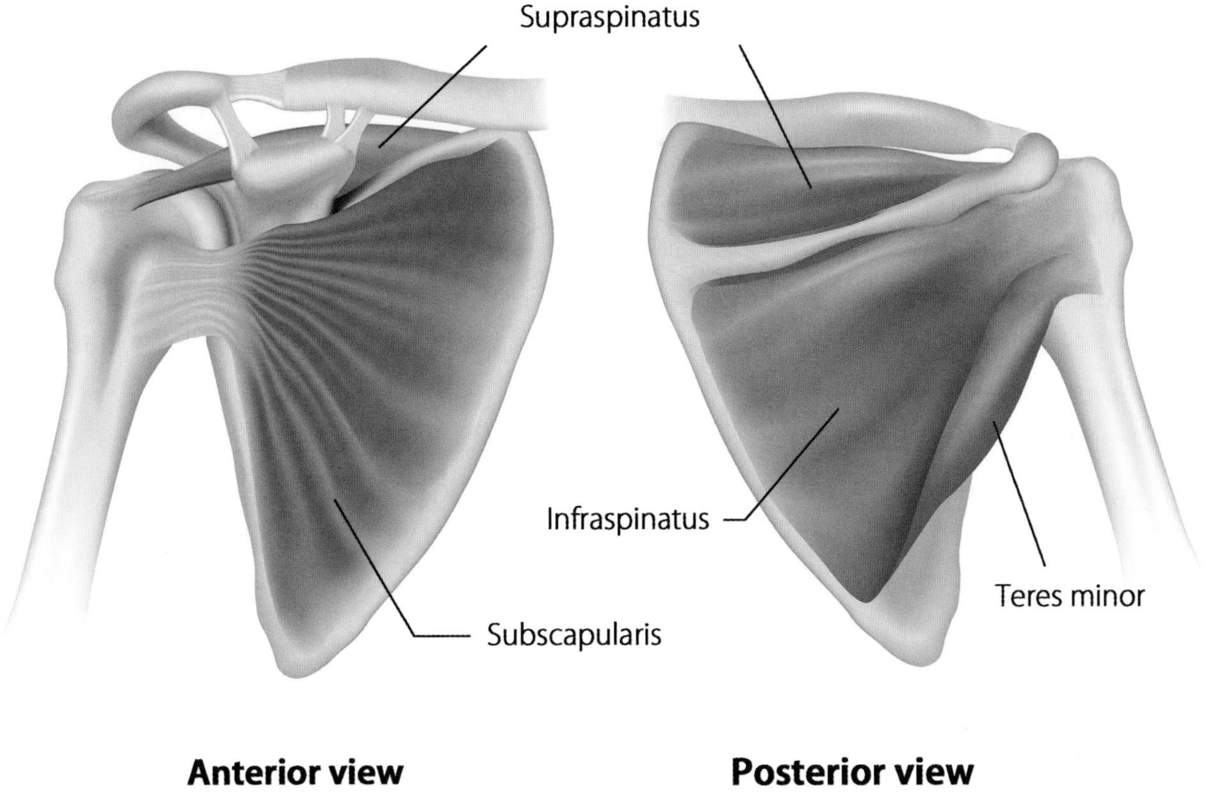

Nervous System — Nervous System Anatomy

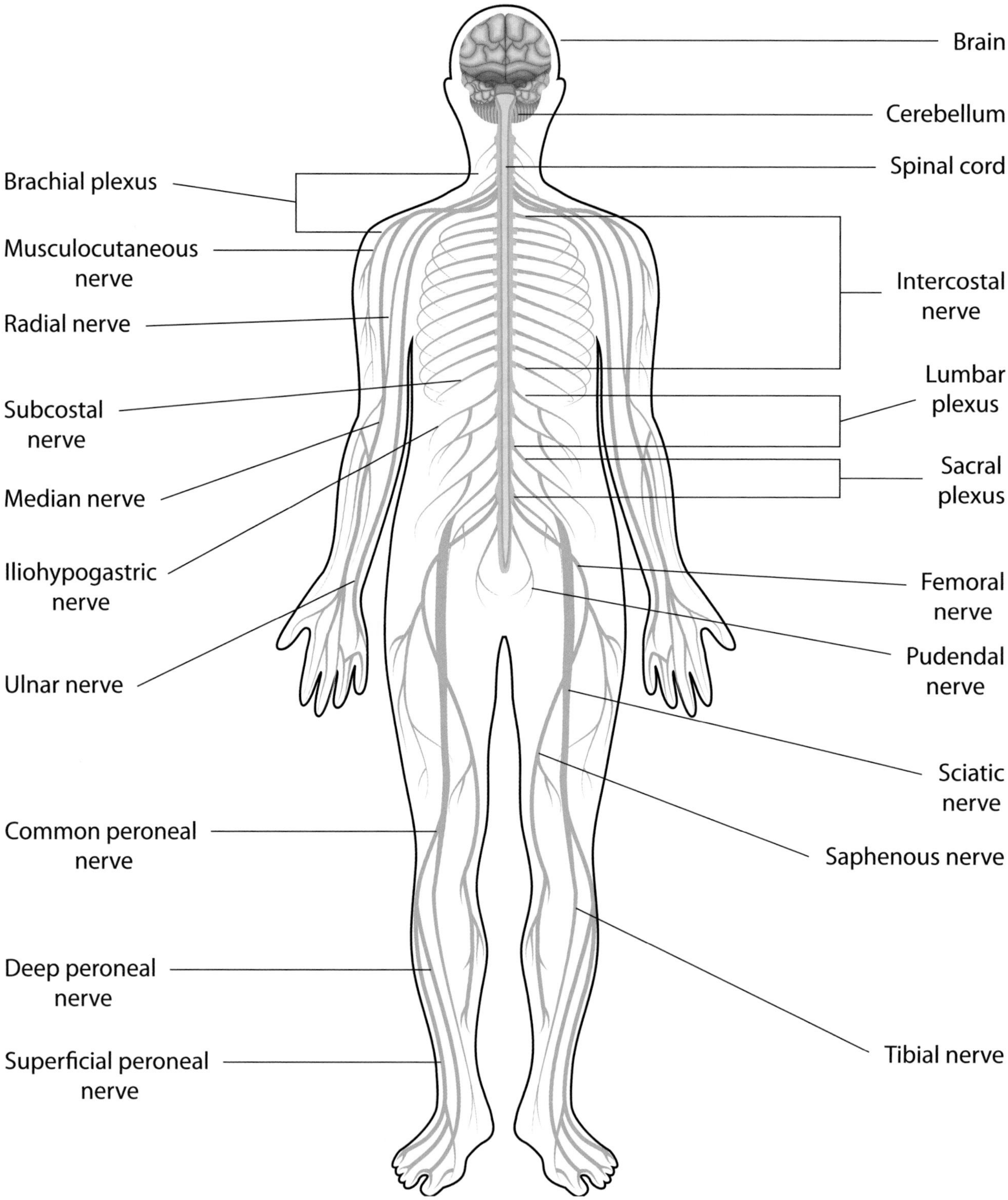

Nervous System — Brain Anatomy

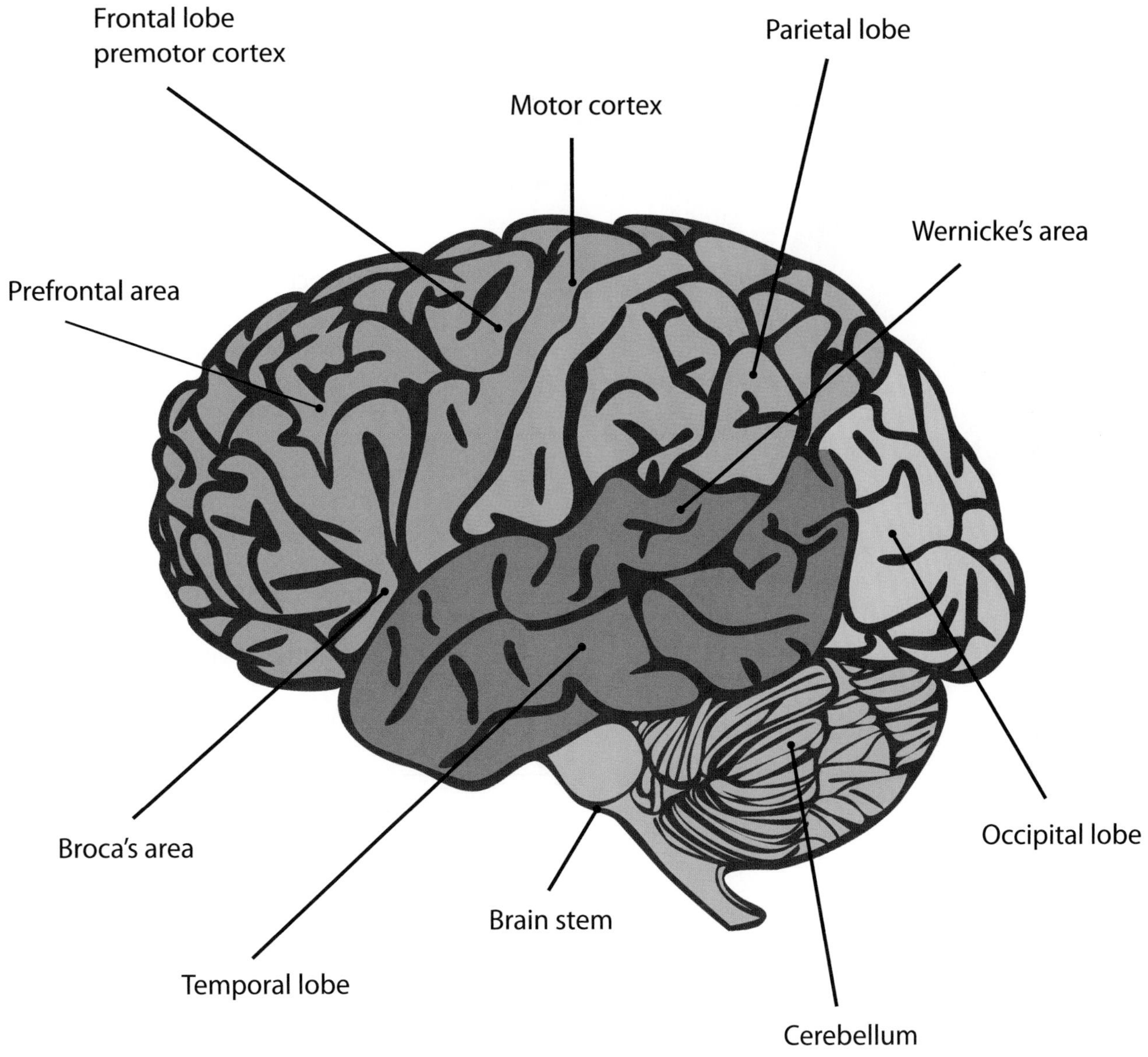

Nervous System — Cranial Nerves

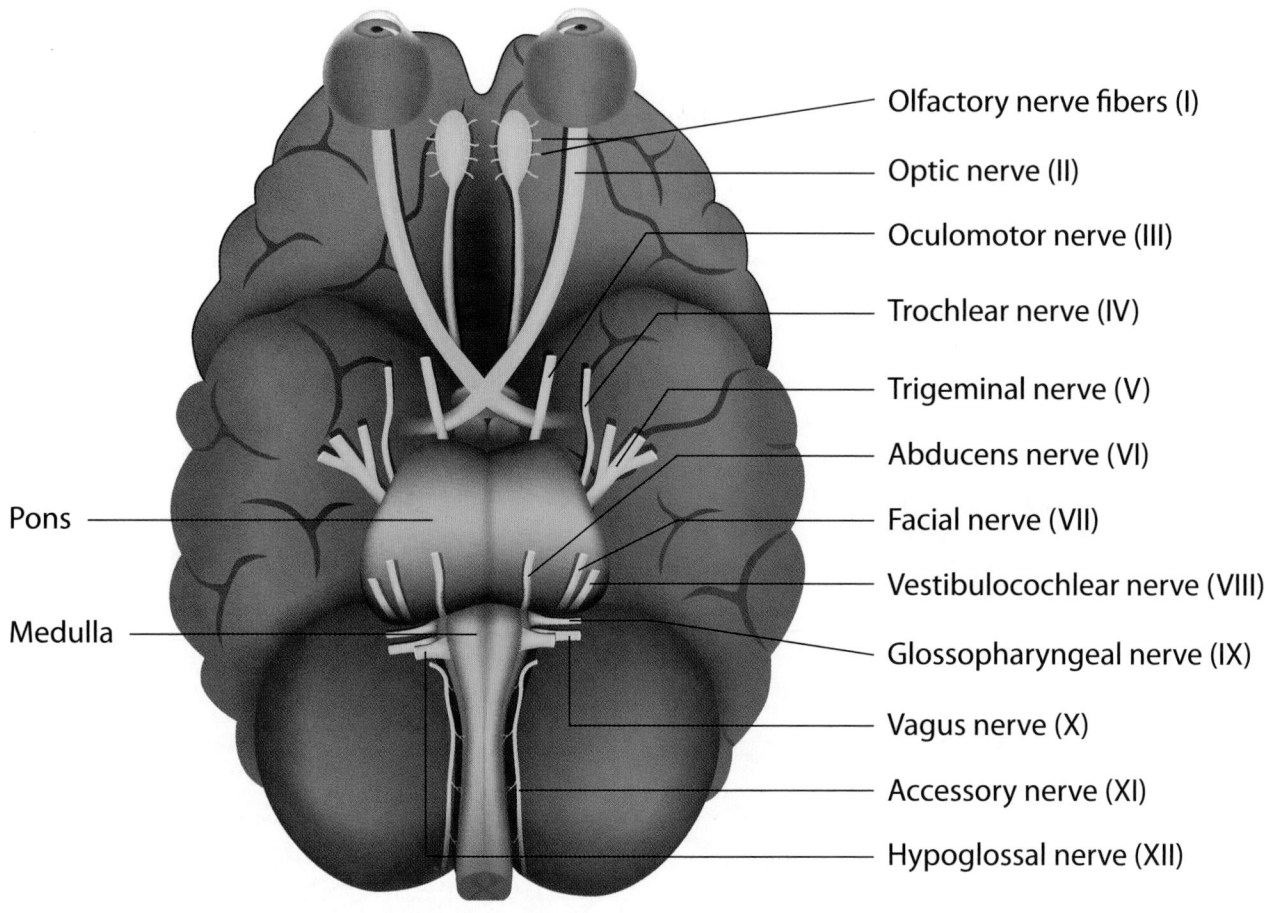

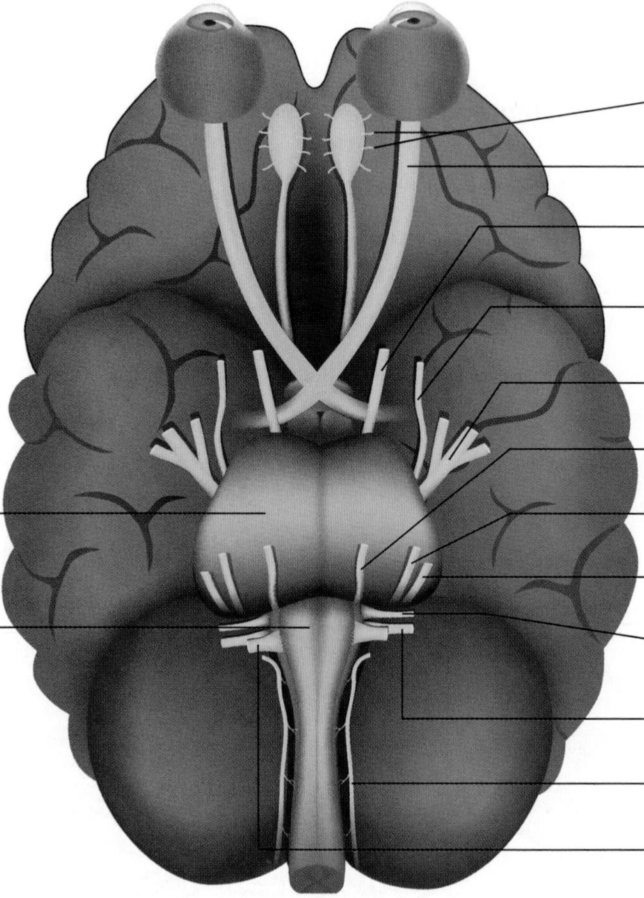

Nervous System — Nerve Anatomy

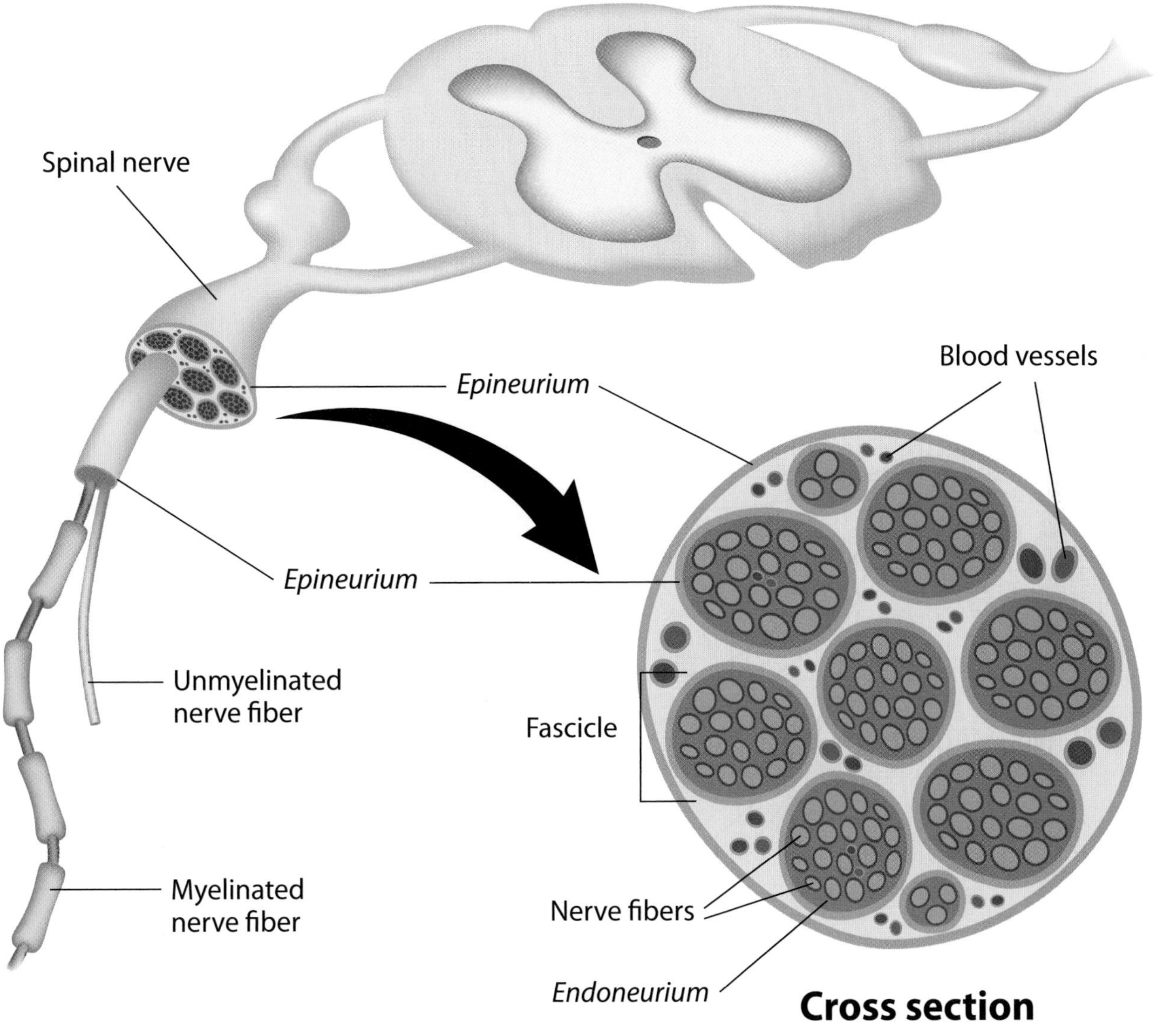

Nervous System — Parasympathetic System Anatomy

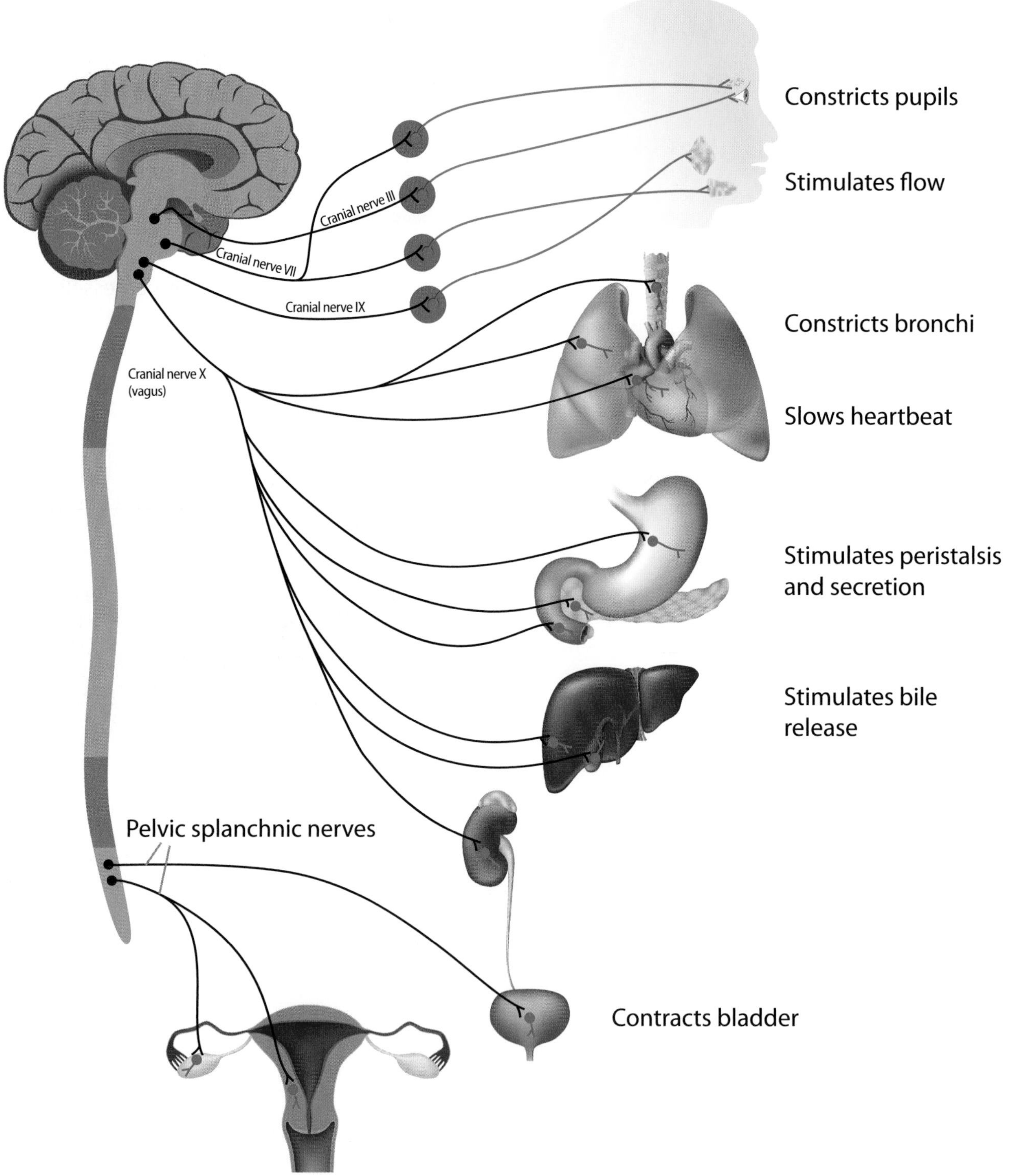

Nervous System — Sympathetic System Anatomy

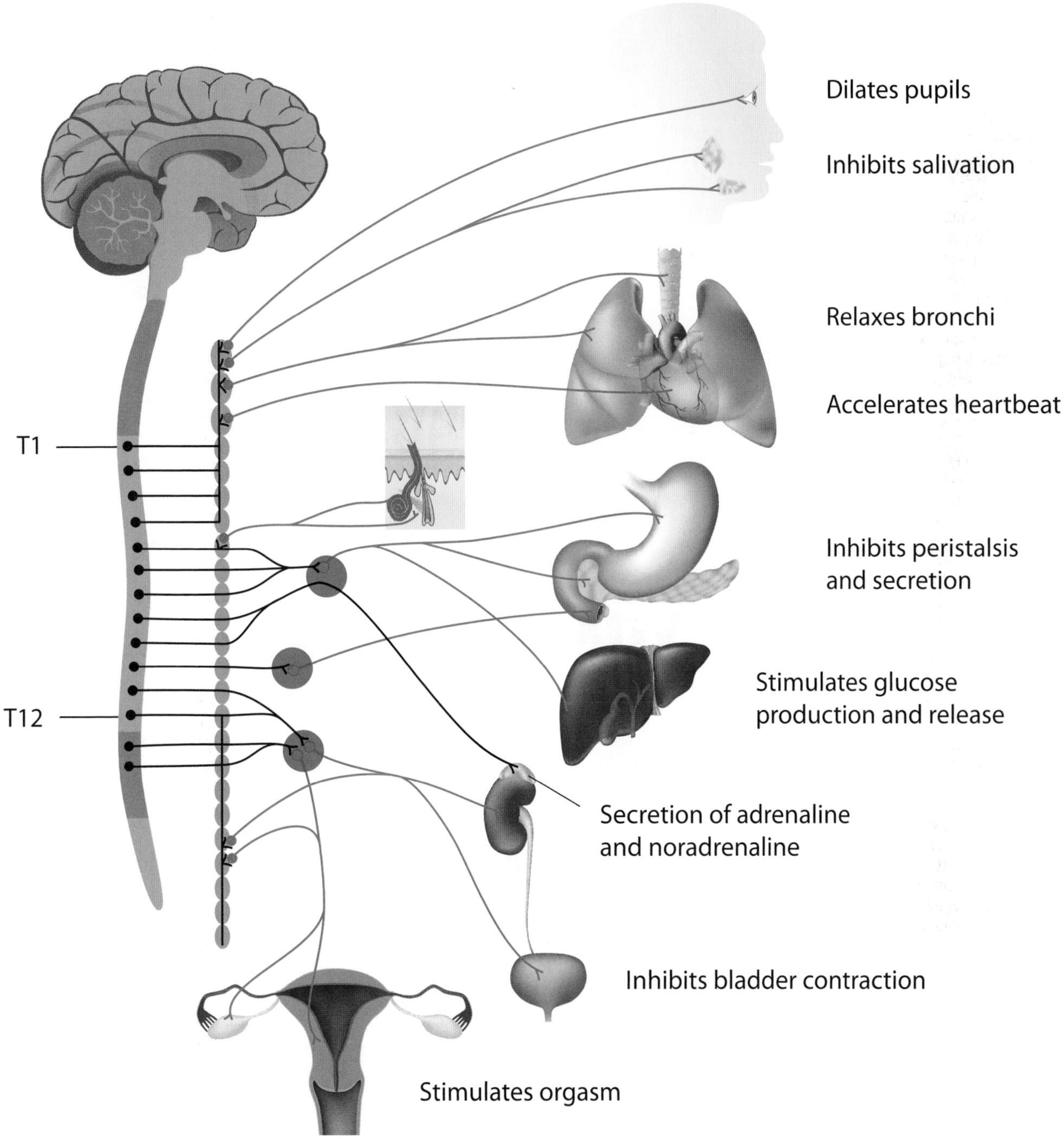

Respiratory System — Respiratory Anatomy

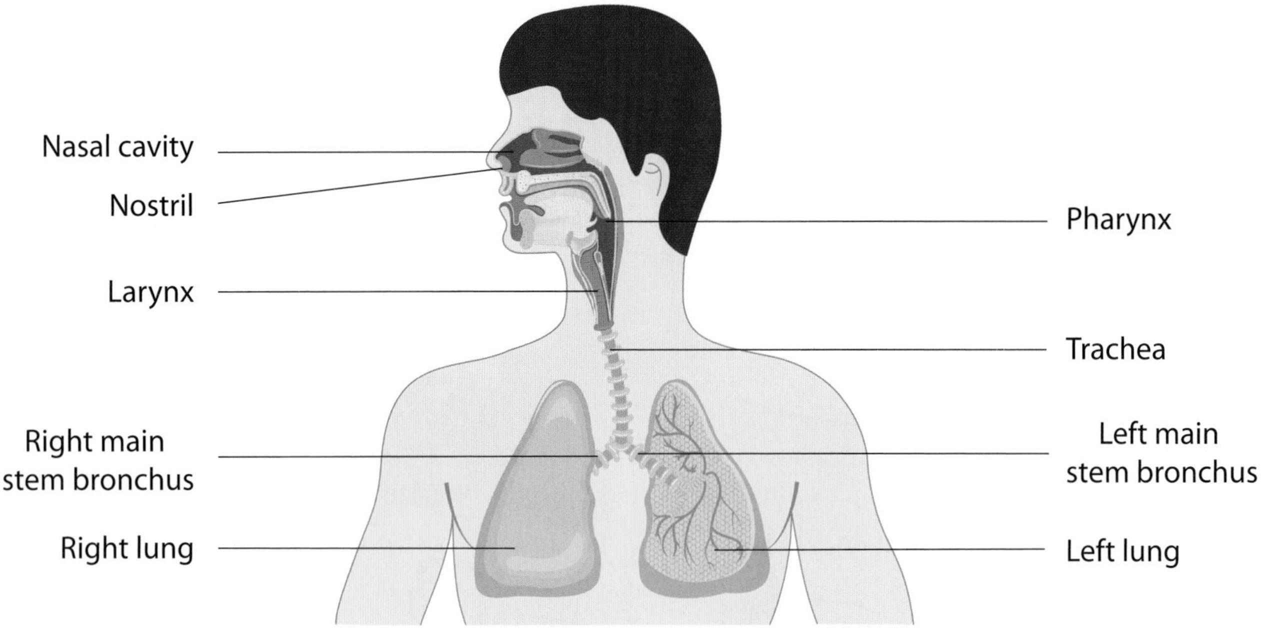

Larynx Anatomy

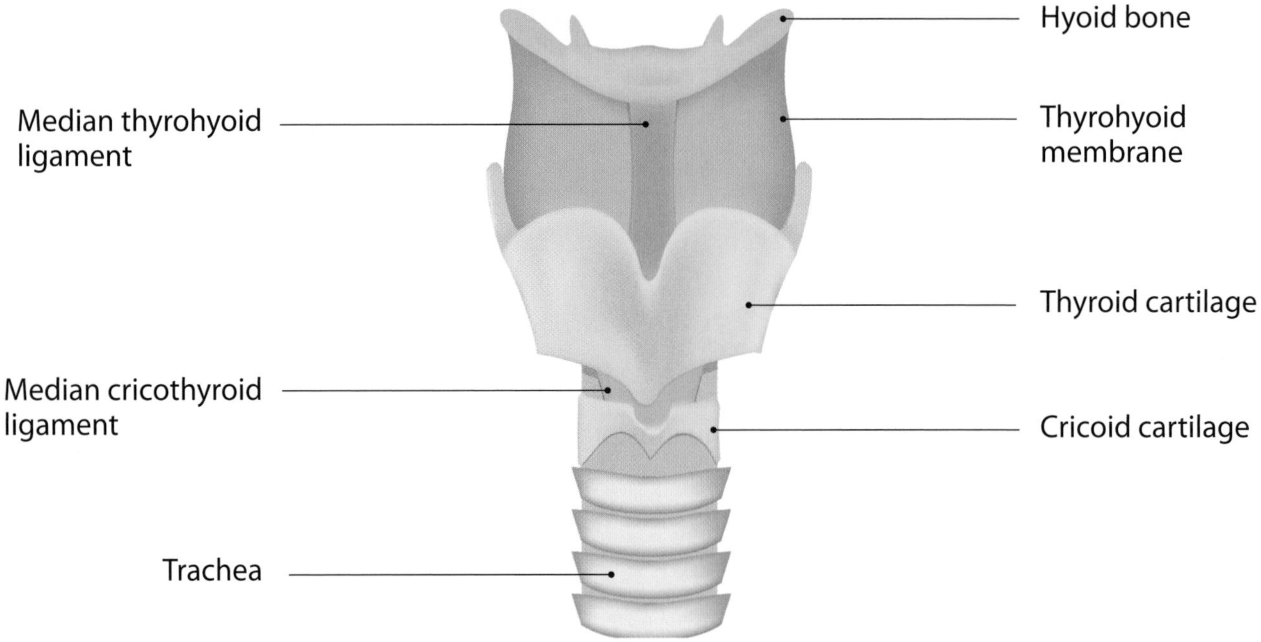

Respiratory System — Lung Anatomy

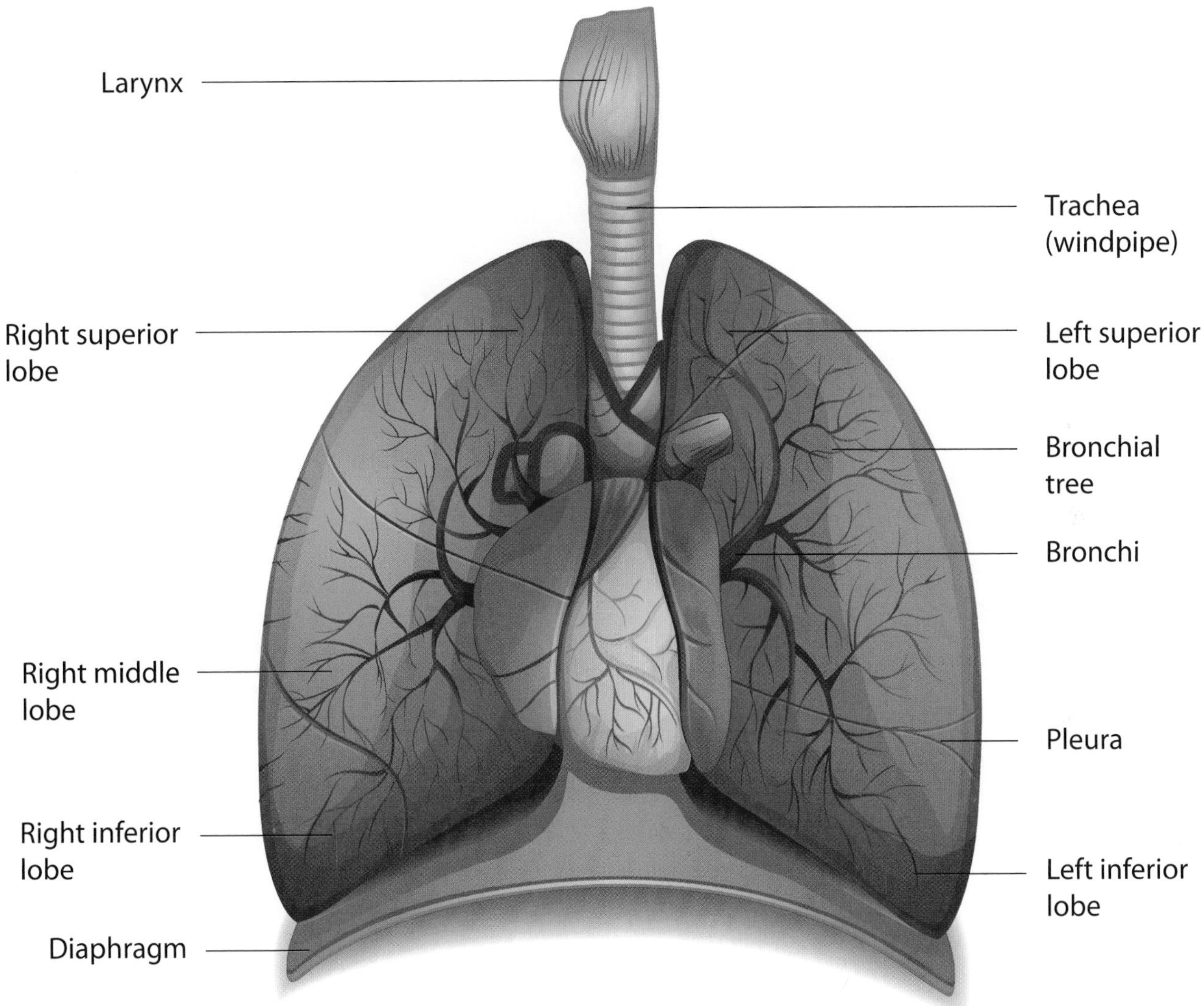

Respiratory System — Lung Anatomy and Function

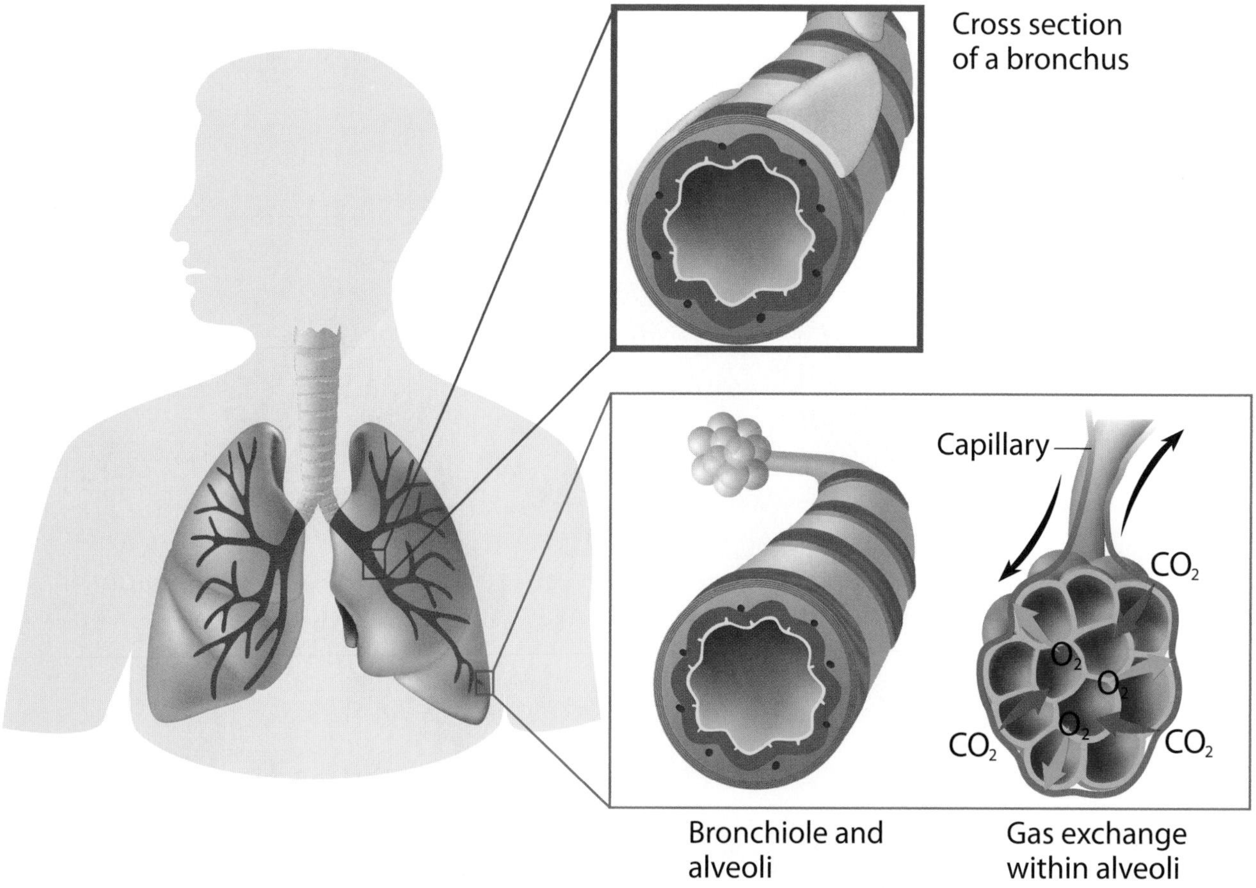

Respiratory System — Nose Anatomy

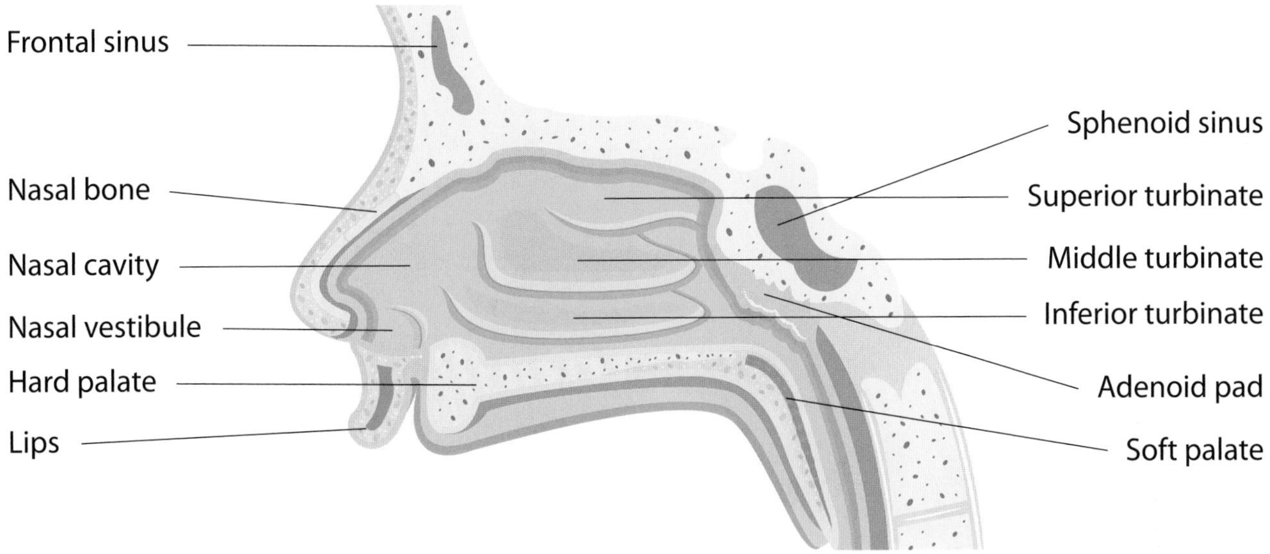

Sinus Anatomy

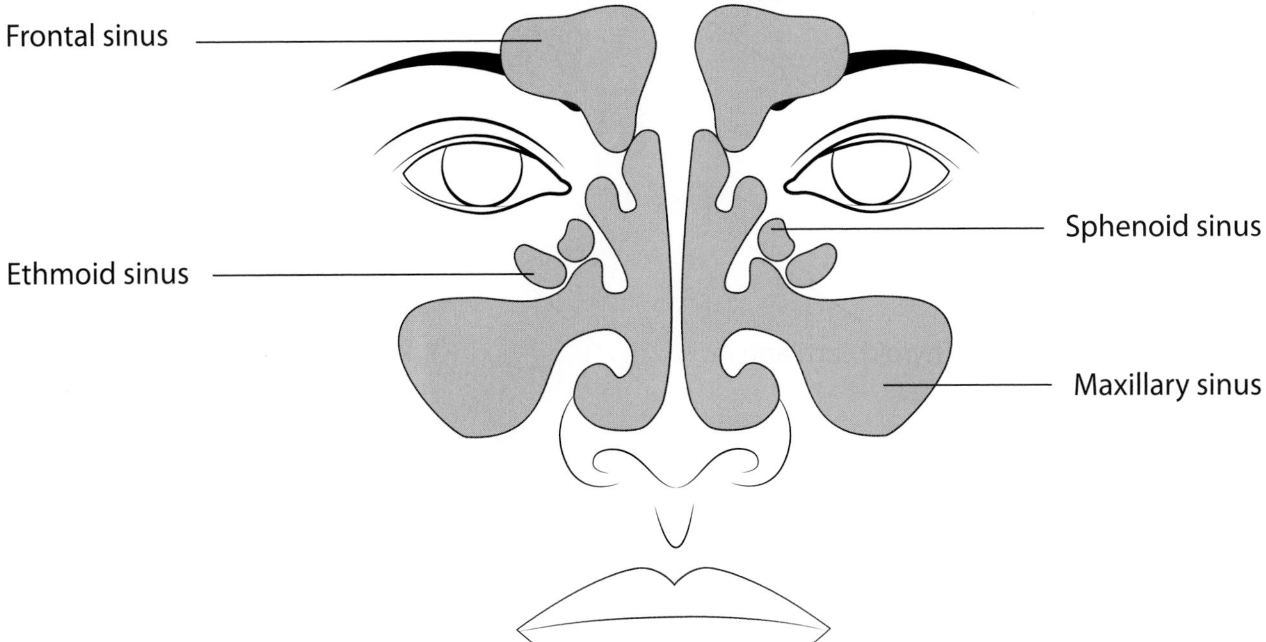

Respiratory System — Throat Anatomy

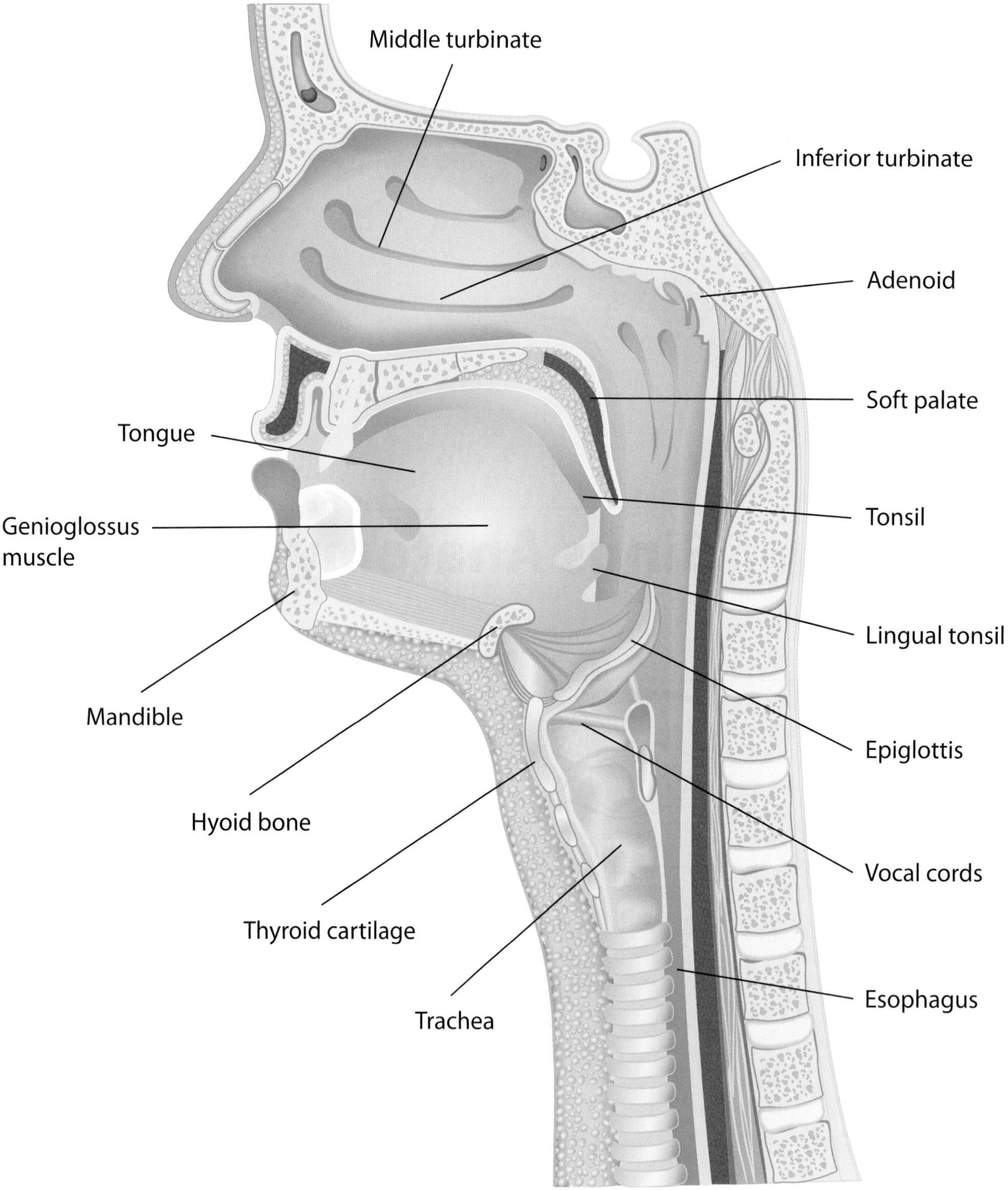

Skeletal System — Skeletal Anatomy

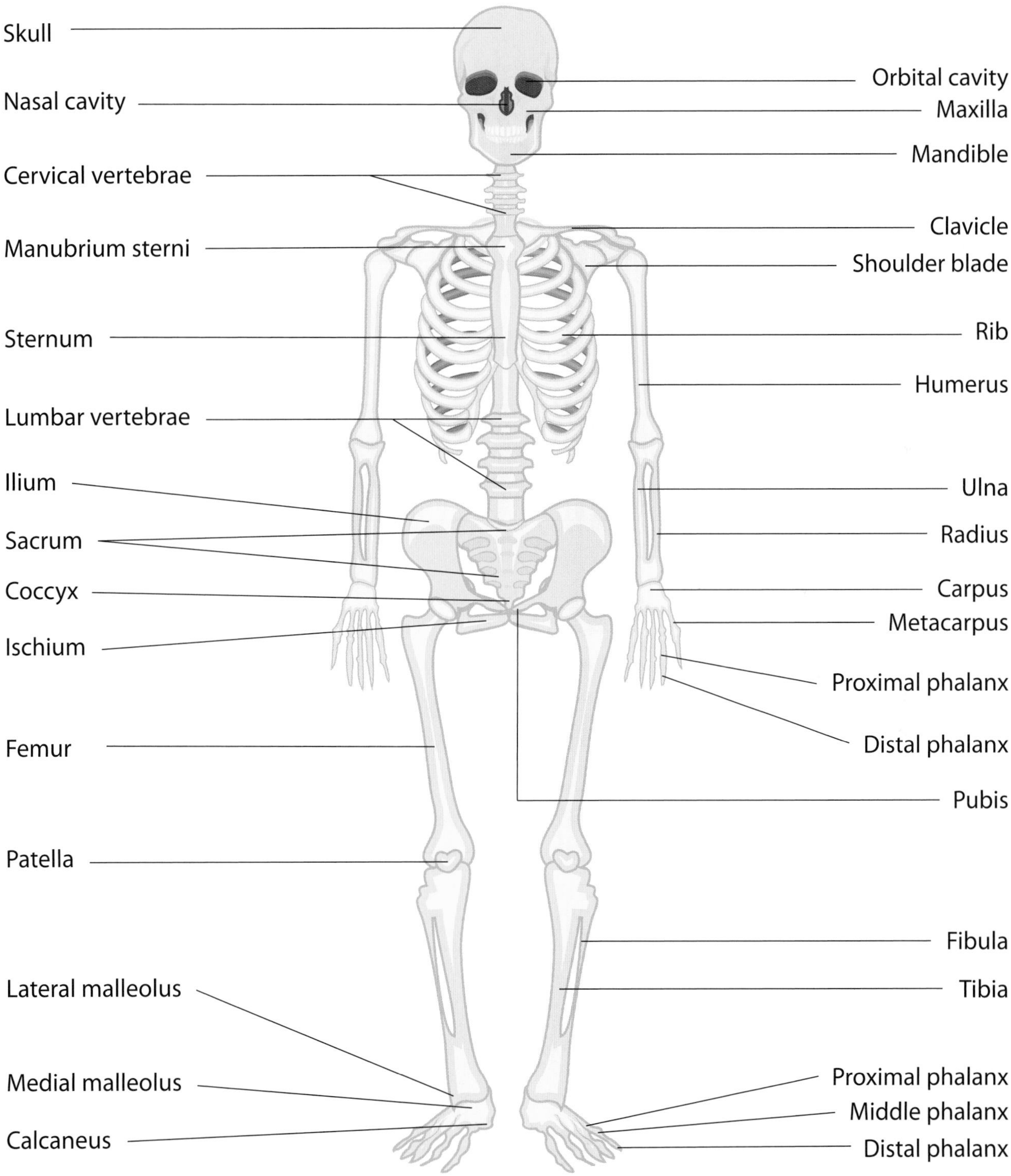
Skull
Nasal cavity
Cervical vertebrae
Manubrium sterni
Sternum
Lumbar vertebrae
Ilium
Sacrum
Coccyx
Ischium
Femur
Patella
Lateral malleolus
Medial malleolus
Calcaneus
Orbital cavity
Maxilla
Mandible
Clavicle
Shoulder blade
Rib
Humerus
Ulna
Radius
Carpus
Metacarpus
Proximal phalanx
Distal phalanx
Pubis
Fibula
Tibia
Proximal phalanx
Middle phalanx
Distal phalanx

Skeletal System — Bone Structure

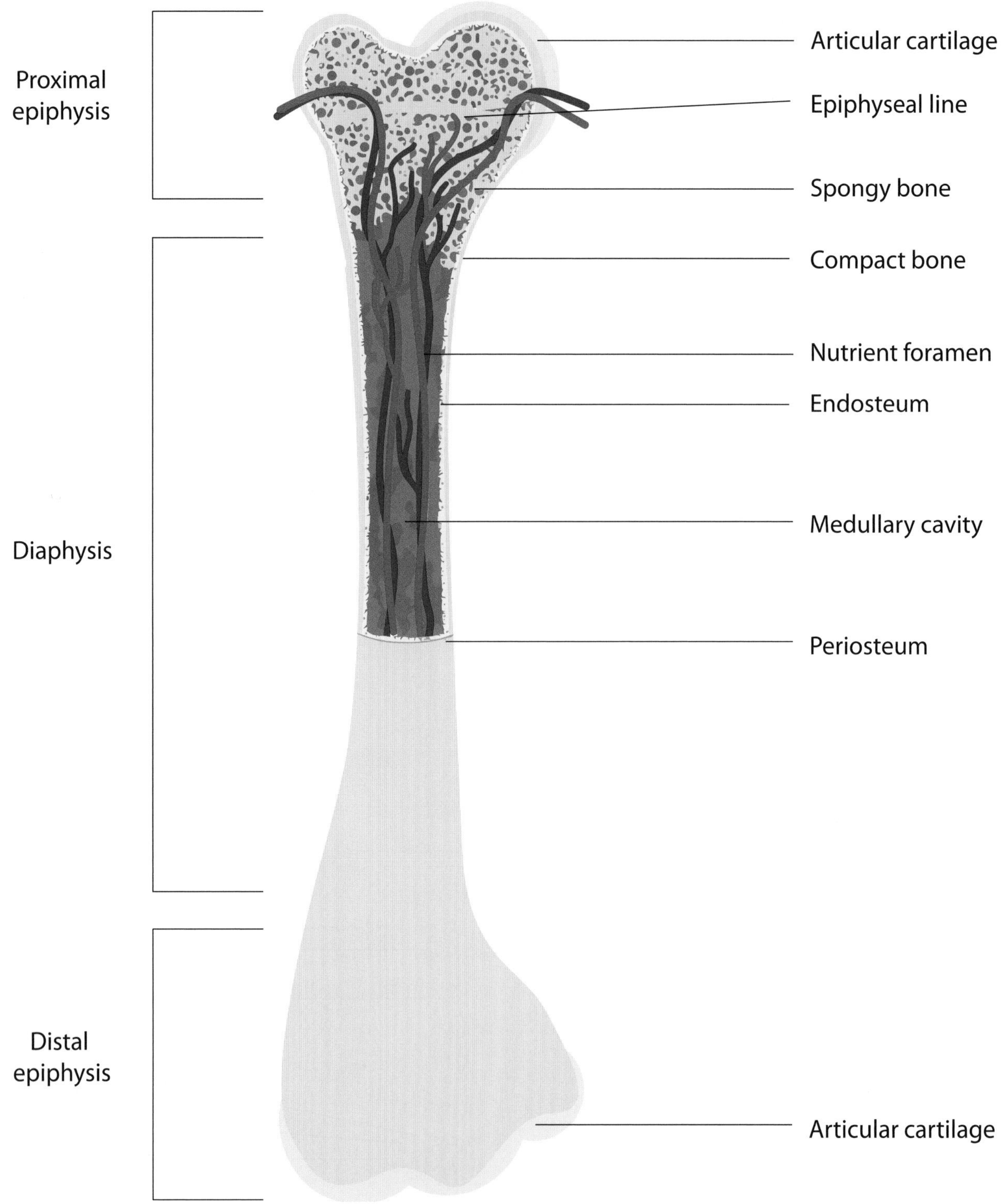

Skeletal System — Cervical, Thoracic, and Lumbar Spine

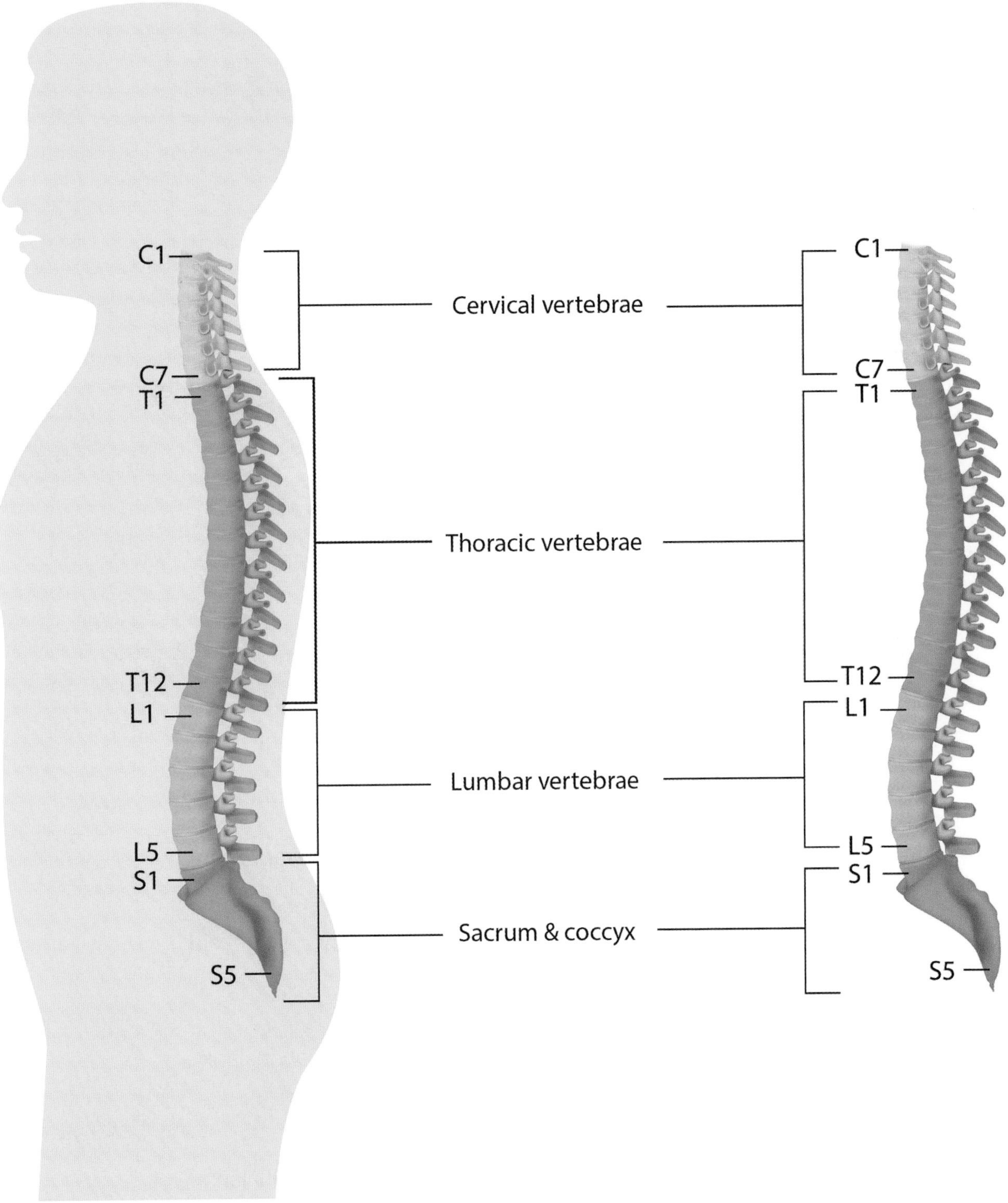

Skeletal System — Foot Bones (right foot, lateral view)

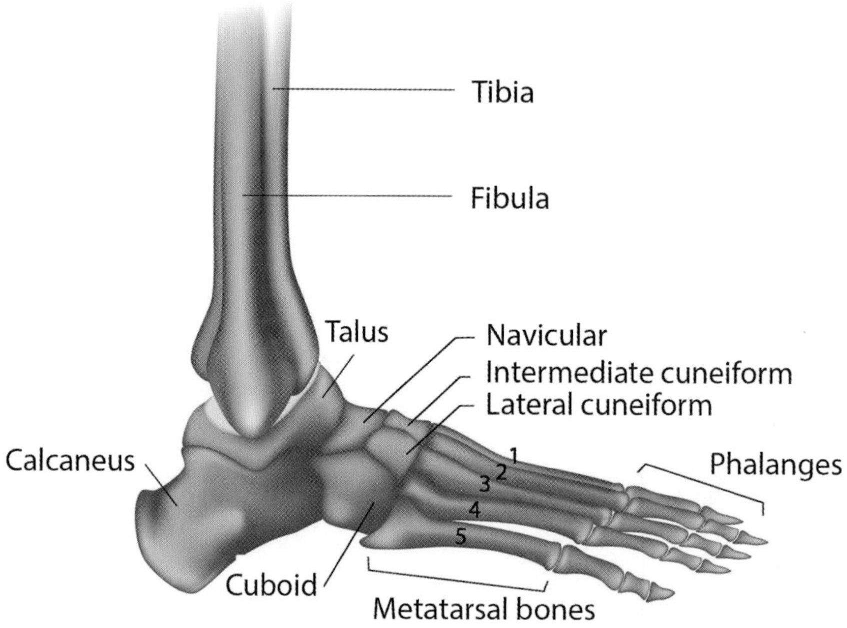

Hand Bones

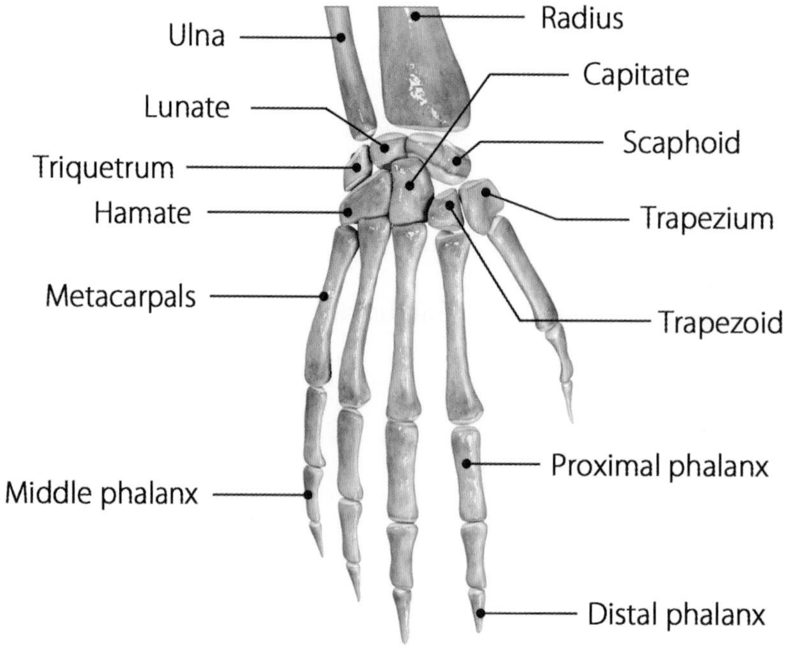

Skeletal System — Skull Anatomy

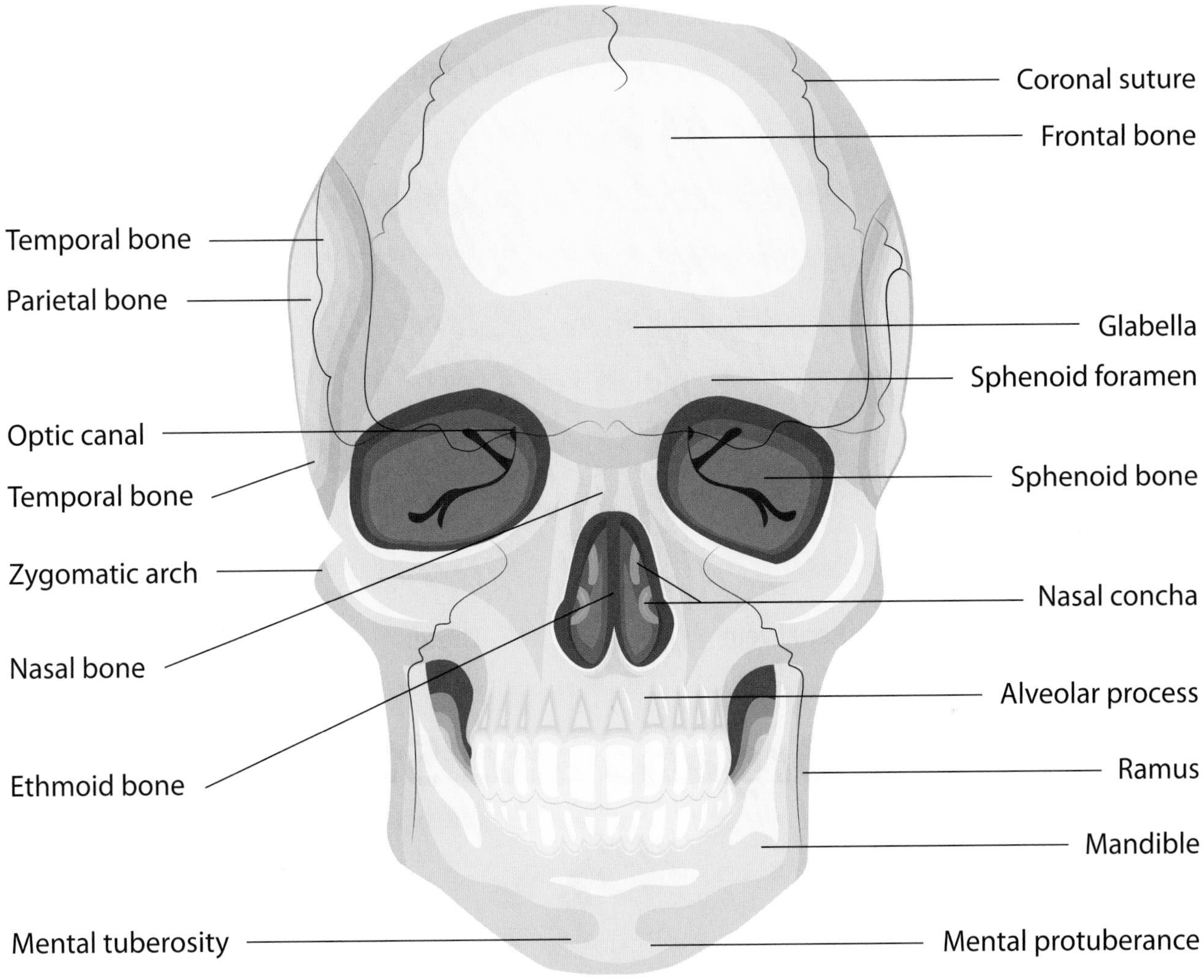

Urinary System — Kidney Anatomy

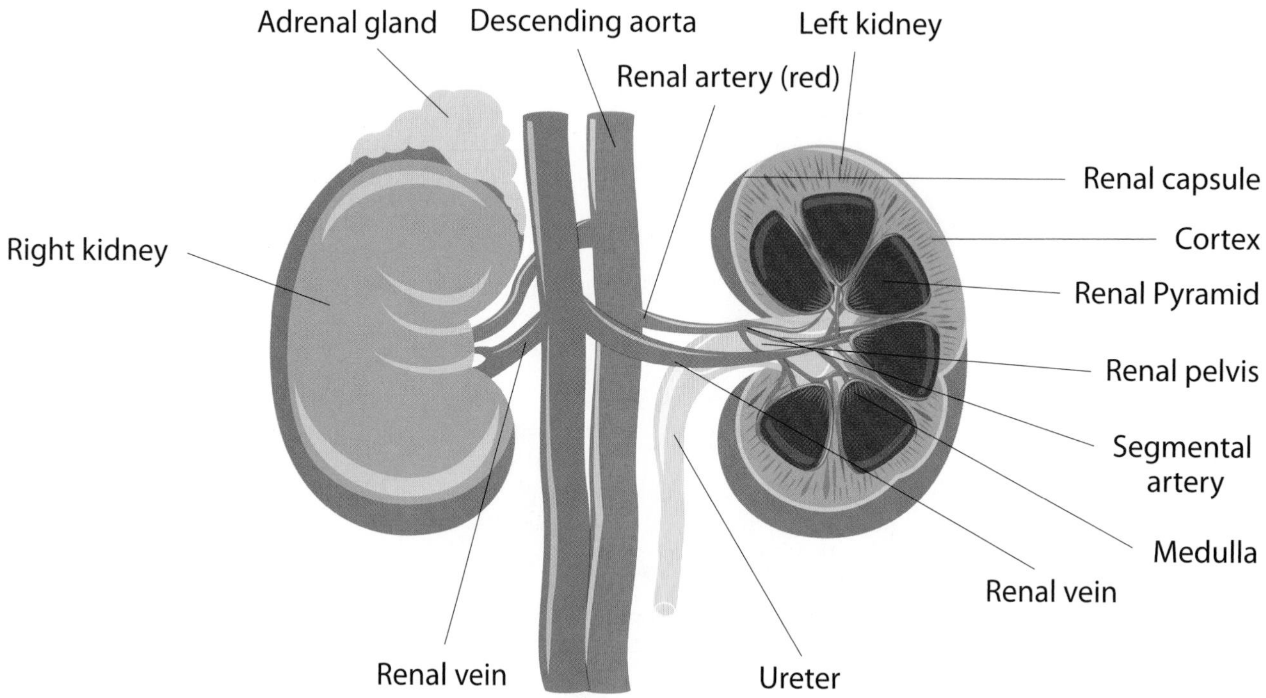

Urinary Organs and Structures

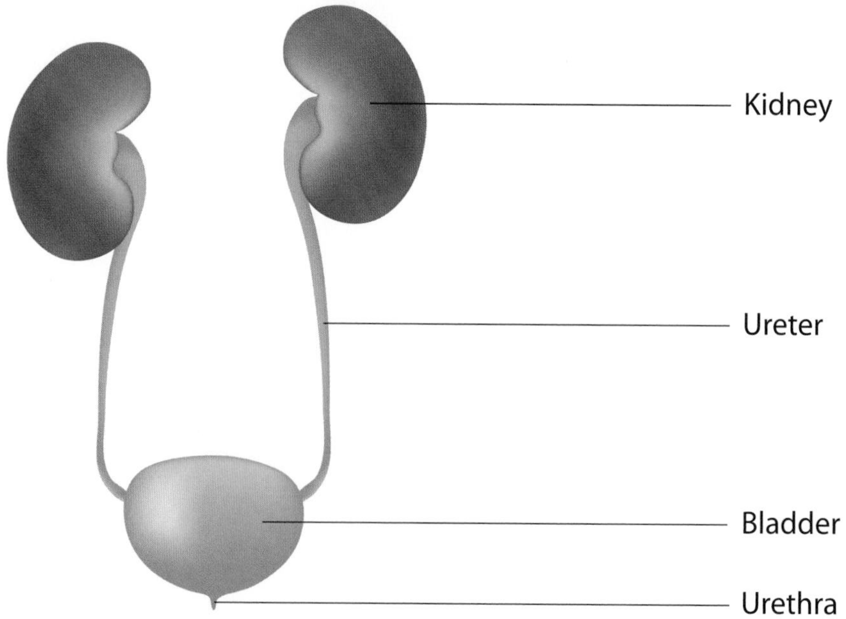

ICD-10-PCS Index

3

A

- **Arachnoid mater, intracranial** *use* Cerebral Meninges
- **Arachnoid mater, spinal** *use* Spinal Meninges
- **Arcuate artery**
  - *use* Foot Artery, Right
  - *use* Foot Artery, Left
- **Areola**
  - *use* Nipple, Right
  - *use* Nipple, Left
- **AROM (artificial rupture of membranes)** 10907ZC
- **Arterial canal (duct)** *use* Pulmonary Artery, Left
- **Arterial pulse tracing** *see* Measurement, Arterial 4A03
- **Arteriectomy**
  - *see* Excision, Heart and Great Vessels 02B
  - *see* Excision, Upper Arteries 03B
  - *see* Excision, Lower Arteries 04B
- **Arteriography**
  - *see* Plain Radiography, Heart B20
  - *see* Fluoroscopy, Heart B21
  - *see* Plain Radiography, Upper Arteries B30
  - *see* Fluoroscopy, Upper Arteries B31
  - *see* Plain Radiography, Lower Arteries B40
  - *see* Fluoroscopy, Lower Arteries B41
- **Arterioplasty**
  - *see* Repair, Heart and Great Vessels 02Q
  - *see* Replacement, Heart and Great Vessels 02R
  - *see* Supplement, Heart and Great Vessels 02U
  - *see* Repair, Upper Arteries 03Q
  - *see* Replacement, Upper Arteries 03R
  - *see* Supplement, Upper Arteries 03U
  - *see* Repair, Lower Arteries 04Q
  - *see* Replacement, Lower Arteries 04R
  - *see* Supplement, Lower Arteries 04U
- **Arteriorrhaphy**
  - *see* Repair, Heart and Great Vessels 02Q
  - *see* Repair, Upper Arteries 03Q
  - *see* Repair, Lower Arteries 04Q
- **Arterioscopy**
  - *see* Inspection, Great Vessel 02JY
  - *see* Inspection, Artery, Upper 03JY
  - *see* Inspection, Artery, Lower 04JY
- **Arthrectomy**
  - *see* Excision, Upper Joints 0RB
  - *see* Resection, Upper Joints 0RT
  - *see* Excision, Lower Joints 0SB
  - *see* Resection, Lower Joints 0ST
- **Arthrocentesis**
  - *see* Drainage, Upper Joints 0R9
  - *see* Drainage, Lower Joints 0S9
- **Arthrodesis**
  - *see* Fusion, Upper Joints 0RG
  - *see* Fusion, Lower Joints 0SG
- **Arthrography**
  - *see* Plain Radiography, Skull and Facial Bones BN0
  - *see* Plain Radiography, Non-Axial Upper Bones BP0
  - *see* Plain Radiography, Non-Axial Lower Bones BQ0
- **Arthrolysis**
  - *see* Release, Upper Joints 0RN
  - *see* Release, Lower Joints 0SN
- **Arthropexy**
  - *see* Repair, Upper Joints 0RQ
  - *see* Reposition, Upper Joints 0RS
  - *see* Repair, Lower Joints 0SQ
  - *see* Reposition, Lower Joints 0SS
- **Arthroplasty**
  - *see* Repair, Upper Joints 0RQ
  - *see* Replacement, Upper Joints 0RR
  - *see* Supplement, Upper Joints 0RU
  - *see* Repair, Lower Joints 0SQ
- **Arthroplasty** — *continued*
  - *see* Replacement, Lower Joints 0SR
  - *see* Supplement, Lower Joints 0SU
- **Arthroscopy**
  - *see* Inspection, Upper Joints 0RJ
  - *see* Inspection, Lower Joints 0SJ
- **Arthrotomy**
  - *see* Drainage, Upper Joints 0R9
  - *see* Drainage, Lower Joints 0S9
- **Artificial anal sphincter (AAS)** *use* Artificial Sphincter in Gastrointestinal System
- **Artificial bowel sphincter (neosphincter)** *use* Artificial Sphincter in Gastrointestinal System
- **Artificial Sphincter**
  - Insertion of device in
    - Anus 0DHQ
    - Bladder 0THB
    - Bladder Neck 0THC
    - Urethra 0THD
  - Removal of device from
    - Anus 0DPQ
    - Bladder 0TPB
    - Urethra 0TPD
  - Revision of device in
    - Anus 0DWQ
    - Bladder 0TWB
    - Urethra 0TWD
- **Artificial urinary sphincter (AUS)** *use* Artificial Sphincter in Urinary System
- **Aryepiglottic fold** *use* Larynx
- **Arytenoid cartilage** *use* Larynx
- **Arytenoid muscle**
  - *use* Neck Muscle, Right
  - *use* Neck Muscle, Left
- **Arytenoidectomy** *see* Excision, Larynx 0CBS
- **Arytenoidopexy** *see* Repair, Larynx 0CQS
- **Ascenda Intrathecal Catheter** *use* Infusion Device
- **Ascending aorta** *use* Thoracic Aorta, Ascending/Arch
- **Ascending palatine artery** *use* Face Artery
- **Ascending pharyngeal artery**
  - *use* External Carotid Artery, Right
  - *use* External Carotid Artery, Left
- **Aspiration, fine needle**
  - fluid or gas *see* Drainage
  - tissue *see* Excision
- **Assessment**
  - Activities of daily living *see* Activities of Daily Living Assessment, Rehabilitation F02
  - Hearing *see* Hearing Assessment, Diagnostic Audiology F13
  - Hearing aid *see* Hearing Aid Assessment, Diagnostic Audiology F14
  - intravascular perfusion, using indocyanine green (ICG) dye *see* Monitoring, Physiological Systems 4A1
  - Motor function *see* Motor Function Assessment, Rehabilitation F01
  - Nerve function *see* Motor Function Assessment, Rehabilitation F01
  - Speech *see* Speech Assessment, Rehabilitation F00
  - Vestibular *see* Vestibular Assessment, Diagnostic Audiology F15
  - Vocational *see* Activities of Daily Living Treatment, Rehabilitation F08
- **Assistance**
  - Cardiac
    - Continuous
      - Balloon Pump 5A02210
      - Impeller Pump 5A0221D
      - Other Pump 5A02216
      - Pulsatile Compression 5A02215
    - Intermittent
- **Assistance** — *continued*
  - Cardiac — *continued*
      - Balloon Pump 5A02110
      - Impeller Pump 5A0211D
      - Other Pump 5A02116
      - Pulsatile Compression 5A02115
  - Circulatory
    - Continuous
      - Hyperbaric 5A05221
      - Supersaturated 5A0522C
    - Intermittent
      - Hyperbaric 5A05121
      - Supersaturated 5A0512C
  - Respiratory
    - 24-96 Consecutive Hours
      - Continuous Negative Airway Pressure 5A09459
      - Continuous Positive Airway Pressure 5A09457
      - Intermittent Negative Airway Pressure 5A0945B
      - Intermittent Positive Airway Pressure 5A09458
      - No Qualifier 5A0945Z
    - Greater than 96 Consecutive Hours
      - Continuous Negative Airway Pressure 5A09559
      - Continuous Positive Airway Pressure 5A09557
      - Intermittent Negative Airway Pressure 5A0955B
      - Intermittent Positive Airway Pressure 5A09558
      - No Qualifier 5A0955Z
    - Less than 24 Consecutive Hours
      - Continuous Negative Airway Pressure 5A09359
      - Continuous Positive Airway Pressure 5A09357
      - Intermittent Negative Airway Pressure 5A0935B
      - Intermittent Positive Airway Pressure 5A09358
      - No Qualifier 5A0935Z
- **Assurant (Cobalt)® stent** *use* Intraluminal Device
- **Atherectomy**
  - *see* Extirpation, Heart and Great Vessels 02C
  - *see* Extirpation, Upper Arteries 03C
  - *see* Extirpation, Lower Arteries 04C
- **Atlantoaxial joint** *use* Cervical Vertebral Joint
- **Atmospheric Control** 6A0Z
- **Atrioseptoplasty**
  - *see* Repair, Heart and Great Vessels 02Q
  - *see* Replacement, Heart and Great Vessels 02R
  - *see* Supplement, Heart and Great Vessels 02U
- **Atrioventricular node** *use* Conduction Mechanism
- **Atrium dextrum cordis** *use* Atrium, Right
- **Atrium pulmonale** *use* Atrium, Left
- **Attain Ability® lead**
  - *use* Cardiac Lead, Pacemaker in 02H
  - *use* Cardiac Lead, Defibrillator in 02H
- **Attain StarFix® (OTW) lead**
  - *use* Cardiac Lead, Pacemaker in 02H
  - *use* Cardiac Lead, Defibrillator in 02H
- **Audiology, diagnostic**
  - *see* Hearing Assessment, Diagnostic Audiology F13
  - *see* Hearing Aid Assessment, Diagnostic Audiology F14
  - *see* Vestibular Assessment, Diagnostic Audiology F15
- **Audiometry** *see* Hearing Assessment, Diagnostic Audiology F13

B

D

Drainage — *continued*
Joint — *continued*
Tarsal
Left 0S9J
Right 0S9H
Temporomandibular
Left 0R9D
Right 0R9C
Thoracic Vertebral 0R96
Thoracolumbar Vertebral 0R9A
Toe Phalangeal
Left 0S9Q
Right 0S9P
Wrist
Left 0R9P
Right 0R9N
Kidney
Left 0T91
Right 0T90
Kidney Pelvis
Left 0T94
Right 0T93
Knee Region
Left 0Y9G
Right 0Y9F
Larynx 0C9S
Leg
Lower
Left 0Y9J
Right 0Y9H
Upper
Left 0Y9D
Right 0Y9C
Lens
Left 089K
Right 089J
Lip
Lower 0C91
Upper 0C90
Liver 0F90
Left Lobe 0F92
Right Lobe 0F91
Lung
Bilateral 0B9M
Left 0B9L
Lower Lobe
Left 0B9J
Right 0B9F
Middle Lobe, Right 0B9D
Right 0B9K
Upper Lobe
Left 0B9G
Right 0B9C
Lung Lingula 0B9H
Lymphatic
Aortic 079D
Axillary
Left 0796
Right 0795
Head 0790
Inguinal
Left 079J
Right 079H
Internal Mammary
Left 0799
Right 0798
Lower Extremity
Left 079G
Right 079F
Mesenteric 079B
Neck
Left 0792
Right 0791
Pelvis 079C
Thoracic Duct 079K
Thorax 0797
Upper Extremity

Drainage — *continued*
Lymphatic — *continued*
Left 0794
Right 0793
Mandible
Left 0N9V
Right 0N9T
Maxilla
Left 0N9S
Right 0N9R
Mediastinum 0W9C
Medulla Oblongata 009D
Mesentery 0D9V
Metacarpal
Left 0P9Q
Right 0P9P
Metatarsal
Left 0Q9P
Right 0Q9N
Muscle
Abdomen
Left 0K9L
Right 0K9K
Extraocular
Left 089M
Right 089L
Facial 0K91
Foot
Left 0K9W
Right 0K9V
Hand
Left 0K9D
Right 0K9C
Head 0K90
Hip
Left 0K9P
Right 0K9N
Lower Arm and Wrist
Left 0K9B
Right 0K99
Lower Leg
Left 0K9T
Right 0K9S
Neck
Left 0K93
Right 0K92
Perineum 0K9M
Shoulder
Left 0K96
Right 0K95
Thorax
Left 0K9J
Right 0K9H
Tongue, Palate, Pharynx 0K94
Trunk
Left 0K9G
Right 0K9F
Upper Arm
Left 0K98
Right 0K97
Upper Leg
Left 0K9R
Right 0K9Q
Nasopharynx 099N
Neck 0W96
Nerve
Abdominal Sympathetic 019M
Abducens 009L
Accessory 009R
Acoustic 009N
Brachial Plexus 0193
Cervical 0191
Cervical Plexus 0190
Facial 009M
Femoral 019D
Glossopharyngeal 009P
Head and Neck Sympathetic 019K

Drainage — *continued*
Nerve — *continued*
Hypoglossal 009S
Lumbar 019B
Lumbar Plexus 0199
Lumbar Sympathetic 019N
Lumbosacral Plexus 019A
Median 0195
Oculomotor 009H
Olfactory 009F
Optic 009G
Peroneal 019H
Phrenic 0192
Pudendal 019C
Radial 0196
Sacral 019R
Sacral Plexus 019Q
Sacral Sympathetic 019P
Sciatic 019F
Thoracic 0198
Thoracic Sympathetic 019L
Tibial 019G
Trigeminal 009K
Trochlear 009J
Ulnar 0194
Vagus 009Q
Nipple
Left 0H9X
Right 0H9W
Nose 099K
Omentum
Greater 0D9S
Lesser 0D9T
Oral Cavity and Throat 0W93
Orbit
Left 0N9Q
Right 0N9P
Ovary
Bilateral 0U92
Left 0U91
Right 0U90
Palate
Hard 0C92
Soft 0C93
Pancreas 0F9G
Para-aortic Body 0G99
Paraganglion Extremity 0G9F
Parathyroid Gland 0G9R
Inferior
Left 0G9P
Right 0G9N
Multiple 0G9Q
Superior
Left 0G9M
Right 0G9L
Patella
Left 0Q9F
Right 0Q9D
Pelvic Cavity 0W9J
Penis 0V9S
Pericardial Cavity 0W9D
Perineum
Female 0W9N
Male 0W9M
Peritoneal Cavity 0W9G
Peritoneum 0D9W
Phalanx
Finger
Left 0P9V
Right 0P9T
Thumb
Left 0P9S
Right 0P9R
Toe
Left 0Q9R
Right 0Q9Q
Pharynx 0C9M

Drainage — *continued*
Pineal Body 0G91
Pleura
Left 0B9P
Right 0B9N
Pleural Cavity
Left 0W9B
Right 0W99
Pons 009B
Prepuce 0V9T
Products of Conception
Amniotic Fluid
Diagnostic 1090
Therapeutic 1090
Fetal Blood 1090
Fetal Cerebrospinal Fluid 1090
Fetal Fluid, Other 1090
Fluid, Other 1090
Prostate 0V90
Radius
Left 0P9J
Right 0P9H
Rectum 0D9P
Retina
Left 089F
Right 089E
Retinal Vessel
Left 089H
Right 089G
Retroperitoneum 0W9H
Rib
Left 0P92
Right 0P91
Sacrum 0Q91
Scapula
Left 0P96
Right 0P95
Sclera
Left 0897
Right 0896
Scrotum 0V95
Septum, Nasal 099M
Shoulder Region
Left 0X93
Right 0X92
Sinus
Accessory 099P
Ethmoid
Left 099V
Right 099U
Frontal
Left 099T
Right 099S
Mastoid
Left 099C
Right 099B
Maxillary
Left 099R
Right 099Q
Sphenoid
Left 099X
Right 099W
Skin
Abdomen 0H97
Back 0H96
Buttock 0H98
Chest 0H95
Ear
Left 0H93
Right 0H92
Face 0H91
Foot
Left 0H9N
Right 0H9M
Genitalia 0H9A
Hand
Left 0H9G

Drainage — *continued*
Skin — *continued*
Right 0H9F
Lower Arm
Left 0H9E
Right 0H9D
Lower Leg
Left 0H9L
Right 0H9K
Neck 0H94
Perineum 0H99
Scalp 0H90
Upper Arm
Left 0H9C
Right 0H9B
Upper Leg
Left 0H9J
Right 0H9H
Skull 0N90
Spinal Canal 009U
Spinal Cord
Cervical 009W
Lumbar 009Y
Thoracic 009X
Spinal Meninges 009T
Spleen 079P
Sternum 0P90
Stomach 0D96
Pylorus 0D97
Subarachnoid Space 0095
Subcutaneous Tissue and Fascia
Abdomen 0J98
Back 0J97
Buttock 0J99
Chest 0J96
Face 0J91
Foot
Left 0J9R
Right 0J9Q
Hand
Left 0J9K
Right 0J9J
Lower Arm
Left 0J9H
Right 0J9G
Lower Leg
Left 0J9P
Right 0J9N
Neck
Anterior 0J94
Posterior 0J95
Pelvic Region 0J9C
Perineum 0J9B
Scalp 0J90
Upper Arm
Left 0J9F
Right 0J9D
Upper Leg
Left 0J9M
Right 0J9L
Subdural Space 0094
Tarsal
Left 0Q9M
Right 0Q9L
Tendon
Abdomen
Left 0L9G
Right 0L9F
Ankle
Left 0L9T
Right 0L9S
Foot
Left 0L9W
Right 0L9V
Hand
Left 0L98
Right 0L97

Drainage — *continued*
Tendon — *continued*
Head and Neck 0L90
Hip
Left 0L9K
Right 0L9J
Knee
Left 0L9R
Right 0L9Q
Lower Arm and Wrist
Left 0L96
Right 0L95
Lower Leg
Left 0L9P
Right 0L9N
Perineum 0L9H
Shoulder
Left 0L92
Right 0L91
Thorax
Left 0L9D
Right 0L9C
Trunk
Left 0L9B
Right 0L99
Upper Arm
Left 0L94
Right 0L93
Upper Leg
Left 0L9M
Right 0L9L
Testis
Bilateral 0V9C
Left 0V9B
Right 0V99
Thalamus 0099
Thymus 079M
Thyroid Gland 0G9K
Left Lobe 0G9G
Right Lobe 0G9H
Tibia
Left 0Q9H
Right 0Q9G
Toe Nail 0H9R
Tongue 0C97
Tonsils 0C9P
Tooth
Lower 0C9X
Upper 0C9W
Trachea 0B91
Tunica Vaginalis
Left 0V97
Right 0V96
Turbinate, Nasal 099L
Tympanic Membrane
Left 0998
Right 0997
Ulna
Left 0P9L
Right 0P9K
Ureter
Left 0T97
Right 0T96
Ureters, Bilateral 0T98
Urethra 0T9D
Uterine Supporting Structure 0U94
Uterus 0U99
Uvula 0C9N
Vagina 0U9G
Vas Deferens
Bilateral 0V9Q
Left 0V9P
Right 0V9N
Vein
Axillary
Left 0598
Right 0597

E

Excision — *continued*
Artery — *continued*
Right 03BH
Common Iliac
Left 04BD
Right 04BC
External Carotid
Left 03BN
Right 03BM
External Iliac
Left 04BJ
Right 04BH
Face 03BR
Femoral
Left 04BL
Right 04BK
Foot
Left 04BW
Right 04BV
Gastric 04B2
Hand
Left 03BF
Right 03BD
Hepatic 04B3
Inferior Mesenteric 04BB
Innominate 03B2
Internal Carotid
Left 03BL
Right 03BK
Internal Iliac
Left 04BF
Right 04BE
Internal Mammary
Left 03B1
Right 03B0
Intracranial 03BG
Lower 04BY
Peroneal
Left 04BU
Right 04BT
Popliteal
Left 04BN
Right 04BM
Posterior Tibial
Left 04BS
Right 04BR
Pulmonary
Left 02BR
Right 02BQ
Pulmonary Trunk 02BP
Radial
Left 03BC
Right 03BB
Renal
Left 04BA
Right 04B9
Splenic 04B4
Subclavian
Left 03B4
Right 03B3
Superior Mesenteric 04B5
Temporal
Left 03BT
Right 03BS
Thyroid
Left 03BV
Right 03BU
Ulnar
Left 03BA
Right 03B9
Upper 03BY
Vertebral
Left 03BQ
Right 03BP
Atrium
Left 02B7
Right 02B6

Excision — *continued*
Auditory Ossicle
Left 09BA0Z
Right 09B90Z
Axilla
Left 0XB5
Right 0XB4
Back
Lower 0WBL
Upper 0WBK
Basal Ganglia 00B8
Bladder 0TBB
Bladder Neck 0TBC
Bone
Ethmoid
Left 0NBG
Right 0NBF
Frontal
Left 0NB2
Right 0NB1
Hyoid 0NBX
Lacrimal
Left 0NBJ
Right 0NBH
Nasal 0NBB
Occipital
Left 0NB8
Right 0NB7
Palatine
Left 0NBL
Right 0NBK
Parietal
Left 0NB4
Right 0NB3
Pelvic
Left 0QB3
Right 0QB2
Sphenoid
Left 0NBD
Right 0NBC
Temporal
Left 0NB6
Right 0NB5
Zygomatic
Left 0NBN
Right 0NBM
Brain 00B0
Breast
Bilateral 0HBV
Left 0HBU
Right 0HBT
Supernumerary 0HBY
Bronchus
Lingula 0BB9
Lower Lobe
Left 0BBB
Right 0BB6
Main
Left 0BB7
Right 0BB3
Middle Lobe, Right 0BB5
Upper Lobe
Left 0BB8
Right 0BB4
Buccal Mucosa 0CB4
Bursa and Ligament
Abdomen
Left 0MBJ
Right 0MBH
Ankle
Left 0MBR
Right 0MBQ
Elbow
Left 0MB4
Right 0MB3
Foot
Left 0MBT

Excision — *continued*
Bursa and Ligament — *continued*
Right 0MBS
Hand
Left 0MB8
Right 0MB7
Head and Neck 0MB0
Hip
Left 0MBM
Right 0MBL
Knee
Left 0MBP
Right 0MBN
Lower Extremity
Left 0MBW
Right 0MBV
Perineum 0MBK
Shoulder
Left 0MB2
Right 0MB1
Thorax
Left 0MBG
Right 0MBF
Trunk
Left 0MBD
Right 0MBC
Upper Extremity
Left 0MBB
Right 0MB9
Wrist
Left 0MB6
Right 0MB5
Buttock
Left 0YB1
Right 0YB0
Carina 0BB2
Carotid Bodies, Bilateral 0GB8
Carotid Body
Left 0GB6
Right 0GB7
Carpal
Left 0PBN
Right 0PBM
Cecum 0DBH
Cerebellum 00BC
Cerebral Hemisphere 00B7
Cerebral Meninges 00B1
Cerebral Ventricle 00B6
Cervix 0UBC
Chest Wall 0WB8
Chordae Tendineae 02B9
Choroid
Left 08BB
Right 08BA
Cisterna Chyli 07BL
Clavicle
Left 0PBB
Right 0PB9
Clitoris 0UBJ
Coccygeal Glomus 0GBB
Coccyx 0QBS
Colon
Ascending 0DBK
Descending 0DBM
Sigmoid 0DBN
Transverse 0DBL
Conduction Mechanism 02B8
Conjunctiva
Left 08BTXZ
Right 08BSXZ
Cord
Bilateral 0VBH
Left 0VBG
Right 0VBF
Cornea
Left 08B9XZ
Right 08B8XZ

Excision — *continued*
Leg
Lower
Left 0YBJ
Right 0YBH
Upper
Left 0YBD
Right 0YBC
Lens
Left 08BK3Z
Right 08BJ3Z
Lip
Lower 0CB1
Upper 0CB0
Liver 0FB0
Left Lobe 0FB2
Right Lobe 0FB1
Lung
Bilateral 0BBM
Left 0BBL
Lower Lobe
Left 0BBJ
Right 0BBF
Middle Lobe, Right 0BBD
Right 0BBK
Upper Lobe
Left 0BBG
Right 0BBC
Lung Lingula 0BBH
Lymphatic
Aortic 07BD
Axillary
Left 07B6
Right 07B5
Head 07B0
Inguinal
Left 07BJ
Right 07BH
Internal Mammary
Left 07B9
Right 07B8
Lower Extremity
Left 07BG
Right 07BF
Mesenteric 07BB
Neck
Left 07B2
Right 07B1
Pelvis 07BC
Thoracic Duct 07BK
Thorax 07B7
Upper Extremity
Left 07B4
Right 07B3
Mandible
Left 0NBV
Right 0NBT
Maxilla
Left 0NBS
Right 0NBR
Mediastinum 0WBC
Medulla Oblongata 00BD
Mesentery 0DBV
Metacarpal
Left 0PBQ
Right 0PBP
Metatarsal
Left 0QBP
Right 0QBN
Muscle
Abdomen
Left 0KBL
Right 0KBK
Extraocular
Left 08BM
Right 08BL
Facial 0KB1

Excision — *continued*
Muscle — *continued*
Foot
Left 0KBW
Right 0KBV
Hand
Left 0KBD
Right 0KBC
Head 0KB0
Hip
Left 0KBP
Right 0KBN
Lower Arm and Wrist
Left 0KBB
Right 0KB9
Lower Leg
Left 0KBT
Right 0KBS
Neck
Left 0KB3
Right 0KB2
Papillary 02BD
Perineum 0KBM
Shoulder
Left 0KB6
Right 0KB5
Thorax
Left 0KBJ
Right 0KBH
Tongue, Palate, Pharynx 0KB4
Trunk
Left 0KBG
Right 0KBF
Upper Arm
Left 0KB8
Right 0KB7
Upper Leg
Left 0KBR
Right 0KBQ
Nasopharynx 09BN
Neck 0WB6
Nerve
Abdominal Sympathetic 01BM
Abducens 00BL
Accessory 00BR
Acoustic 00BN
Brachial Plexus 01B3
Cervical 01B1
Cervical Plexus 01B0
Facial 00BM
Femoral 01BD
Glossopharyngeal 00BP
Head and Neck Sympathetic 01BK
Hypoglossal 00BS
Lumbar 01BB
Lumbar Plexus 01B9
Lumbar Sympathetic 01BN
Lumbosacral Plexus 01BA
Median 01B5
Oculomotor 00BH
Olfactory 00BF
Optic 00BG
Peroneal 01BH
Phrenic 01B2
Pudendal 01BC
Radial 01B6
Sacral 01BR
Sacral Plexus 01BQ
Sacral Sympathetic 01BP
Sciatic 01BF
Thoracic 01B8
Thoracic Sympathetic 01BL
Tibial 01BG
Trigeminal 00BK
Trochlear 00BJ
Ulnar 01B4
Vagus 00BQ

Excision — *continued*
Nipple
Left 0HBX
Right 0HBW
Nose 09BK
Omentum
Greater 0DBS
Lesser 0DBT
Orbit
Left 0NBQ
Right 0NBP
Ovary
Bilateral 0UB2
Left 0UB1
Right 0UB0
Palate
Hard 0CB2
Soft 0CB3
Pancreas 0FBG
Para-aortic Body 0GB9
Paraganglion Extremity 0GBF
Parathyroid Gland 0GBR
Inferior
Left 0GBP
Right 0GBN
Multiple 0GBQ
Superior
Left 0GBM
Right 0GBL
Patella
Left 0QBF
Right 0QBD
Penis 0VBS
Pericardium 02BN
Perineum
Female 0WBN
Male 0WBM
Peritoneum 0DBW
Phalanx
Finger
Left 0PBV
Right 0PBT
Thumb
Left 0PBS
Right 0PBR
Toe
Left 0QBR
Right 0QBQ
Pharynx 0CBM
Pineal Body 0GB1
Pleura
Left 0BBP
Right 0BBN
Pons 00BB
Prepuce 0VBT
Prostate 0VB0
Radius
Left 0PBJ
Right 0PBH
Rectum 0DBP
Retina
Left 08BF3Z
Right 08BE3Z
Retroperitoneum 0WBH
Rib
Left 0PB2
Right 0PB1
Sacrum 0QB1
Scapula
Left 0PB6
Right 0PB5
Sclera
Left 08B7XZ
Right 08B6XZ
Scrotum 0VB5
Septum
Atrial 02B5

Excision — *continued*
Septum — *continued*
Nasal 09BM
Ventricular 02BM
Shoulder Region
Left 0XB3
Right 0XB2
Sinus
Accessory 09BP
Ethmoid
Left 09BV
Right 09BU
Frontal
Left 09BT
Right 09BS
Mastoid
Left 09BC
Right 09BB
Maxillary
Left 09BR
Right 09BQ
Sphenoid
Left 09BX
Right 09BW
Skin
Abdomen 0HB7XZ
Back 0HB6XZ
Buttock 0HB8XZ
Chest 0HB5XZ
Ear
Left 0HB3XZ
Right 0HB2XZ
Face 0HB1XZ
Foot
Left 0HBNXZ
Right 0HBMXZ
Genitalia 0HBAXZ
Hand
Left 0HBGXZ
Right 0HBFXZ
Lower Arm
Left 0HBEXZ
Right 0HBDXZ
Lower Leg
Left 0HBLXZ
Right 0HBKXZ
Neck 0HB4XZ
Perineum 0HB9XZ
Scalp 0HB0XZ
Upper Arm
Left 0HBCXZ
Right 0HBBXZ
Upper Leg
Left 0HBJXZ
Right 0HBHXZ
Skull 0NB0
Spinal Cord
Cervical 00BW
Lumbar 00BY
Thoracic 00BX
Spinal Meninges 00BT
Spleen 07BP
Sternum 0PB0
Stomach 0DB6
Pylorus 0DB7
Subcutaneous Tissue and Fascia
Abdomen 0JB8
Back 0JB7
Buttock 0JB9
Chest 0JB6
Face 0JB1
Foot
Left 0JBR
Right 0JBQ
Hand
Left 0JBK

Excision — *continued*
Subcutaneous Tissue — *continued*
Right 0JBJ
Lower Arm
Left 0JBH
Right 0JBG
Lower Leg
Left 0JBP
Right 0JBN
Neck
Anterior 0JB4
Posterior 0JB5
Pelvic Region 0JBC
Perineum 0JBB
Scalp 0JB0
Upper Arm
Left 0JBF
Right 0JBD
Upper Leg
Left 0JBM
Right 0JBL
Tarsal
Left 0QBM
Right 0QBL
Tendon
Abdomen
Left 0LBG
Right 0LBF
Ankle
Left 0LBT
Right 0LBS
Foot
Left 0LBW
Right 0LBV
Hand
Left 0LB8
Right 0LB7
Head and Neck 0LB0
Hip
Left 0LBK
Right 0LBJ
Knee
Left 0LBR
Right 0LBQ
Lower Arm and Wrist
Left 0LB6
Right 0LB5
Lower Leg
Left 0LBP
Right 0LBN
Perineum 0LBH
Shoulder
Left 0LB2
Right 0LB1
Thorax
Left 0LBD
Right 0LBC
Trunk
Left 0LBB
Right 0LB9
Upper Arm
Left 0LB4
Right 0LB3
Upper Leg
Left 0LBM
Right 0LBL
Testis
Bilateral 0VBC
Left 0VBB
Right 0VB9
Thalamus 00B9
Thymus 07BM
Thyroid Gland
Left Lobe 0GBG
Right Lobe 0GBH
Tibia

Excision — *continued*
Tibia — *continued*
Left 0QBH
Right 0QBG
Toe Nail 0HBRXZ
Tongue 0CB7
Tonsils 0CBP
Tooth
Lower 0CBX
Upper 0CBW
Trachea 0BB1
Tunica Vaginalis
Left 0VB7
Right 0VB6
Turbinate, Nasal 09BL
Tympanic Membrane
Left 09B8
Right 09B7
Ulna
Left 0PBL
Right 0PBK
Ureter
Left 0TB7
Right 0TB6
Urethra 0TBD
Uterine Supporting Structure 0UB4
Uterus 0UB9
Uvula 0CBN
Vagina 0UBG
Valve
Aortic 02BF
Mitral 02BG
Pulmonary 02BH
Tricuspid 02BJ
Vas Deferens
Bilateral 0VBQ
Left 0VBP
Right 0VBN
Vein
Axillary
Left 05B8
Right 05B7
Azygos 05B0
Basilic
Left 05BC
Right 05BB
Brachial
Left 05BA
Right 05B9
Cephalic
Left 05BF
Right 05BD
Colic 06B7
Common Iliac
Left 06BD
Right 06BC
Coronary 02B4
Esophageal 06B3
External Iliac
Left 06BG
Right 06BF
External Jugular
Left 05BQ
Right 05BP
Face
Left 05BV
Right 05BT
Femoral
Left 06BN
Right 06BM
Foot
Left 06BV
Right 06BT
Gastric 06B2
Greater Saphenous
Left 06BQ

Excision — *continued*
- Vein — *continued*
  - Right 06BP
  - Hand
    - Left 05BH
    - Right 05BG
  - Hemiazygos 05B1
  - Hepatic 06B4
  - Hypogastric
    - Left 06BJ
    - Right 06BH
  - Inferior Mesenteric 06B6
  - Innominate
    - Left 05B4
    - Right 05B3
  - Internal Jugular
    - Left 05BN
    - Right 05BM
  - Intracranial 05BL
  - Lesser Saphenous
    - Left 06BS
    - Right 06BR
  - Lower 06BY
  - Portal 06B8
  - Pulmonary
    - Left 02BT
    - Right 02BS
  - Renal
    - Left 06BB
    - Right 06B9
  - Splenic 06B1
  - Subclavian
    - Left 05B6
    - Right 05B5
  - Superior Mesenteric 06B5
  - Upper 05BY
  - Vertebral
    - Left 05BS
    - Right 05BR
- Vena Cava
  - Inferior 06B0
  - Superior 02BV
- Ventricle
  - Left 02BL
  - Right 02BK
- Vertebra
  - Cervical 0PB3
  - Lumbar 0QB0
  - Thoracic 0PB4
- Vesicle
  - Bilateral 0VB3
  - Left 0VB2
  - Right 0VB1
- Vitreous
  - Left 08B53Z
  - Right 08B43Z
- Vocal Cord
  - Left 0CBV
  - Right 0CBT
- Vulva 0UBM
- Wrist Region
  - Left 0XBH
  - Right 0XBG

EXCLUDER® AAA Endoprosthesis
- *use* Intraluminal Device, Branched or Fenestrated, One or Two Arteries in 04V
- *use* Intraluminal Device, Branched or Fenestrated, Three or More Arteries in 04V
- *use* Intraluminal Device

EXCLUDER® IBE Endoprosthesis *use* Intraluminal Device, Branched or Fenestrated, One or Two Arteries in 04V

Exclusion, Left atrial appendage (LAA) *see* Occlusion, Atrium, Left 02L7

Exercise, rehabilitation *see* Motor Treatment, Rehabilitation F07

Exploration *see* Inspection

Express® (LD) Premounted Stent System *use* Intraluminal Device

Express® Biliary SD Monorail® Premounted Stent System *use* Intraluminal Device

Express® SD Renal Monorail® Premounted Stent System *use* Intraluminal Device

Extensor carpi radialis muscle
- *use* Lower Arm and Wrist Muscle, Right
- *use* Lower Arm and Wrist Muscle, Left

Extensor carpi ulnaris muscle
- *use* Lower Arm and Wrist Muscle, Right
- *use* Lower Arm and Wrist Muscle, Left

Extensor digitorum brevis muscle
- *use* Foot Muscle, Right
- *use* Foot Muscle, Left

Extensor digitorum longus muscle
- *use* Lower Leg Muscle, Right
- *use* Lower Leg Muscle, Left

Extensor hallucis brevis muscle
- *use* Foot Muscle, Right
- *use* Foot Muscle, Left

Extensor hallucis longus muscle
- *use* Lower Leg Muscle, Right
- *use* Lower Leg Muscle, Left

External anal sphincter *use* Anal Sphincter

External auditory meatus
- *use* External Auditory Canal, Right
- *use* External Auditory Canal, Left

External fixator
- *use* External Fixation Device in Head and Facial Bones
- *use* External Fixation Device in Upper Bones
- *use* External Fixation Device in Lower Bones
- *use* External Fixation Device in Upper Joints
- *use* External Fixation Device in Lower Joints

External maxillary artery *use* Face Artery

External naris *use* Nose

External oblique aponeurosis *use* Subcutaneous Tissue and Fascia, Trunk

External oblique muscle
- *use* Abdomen Muscle, Right
- *use* Abdomen Muscle, Left

External popliteal nerve *use* Peroneal Nerve

External pudendal artery
- *use* Femoral Artery, Right
- *use* Femoral Artery, Left

External pudendal vein
- *use* Greater Saphenous Vein, Right
- *use* Greater Saphenous Vein, Left

External urethral sphincter *use* Urethra

Extirpation
- Acetabulum
  - Left 0QC5
  - Right 0QC4
- Adenoids 0CCQ
- Ampulla of Vater 0FCC
- Anal Sphincter 0DCR
- Anterior Chamber
  - Left 08C3
  - Right 08C2
- Anus 0DCQ
- Aorta
  - Abdominal 04C0
  - Thoracic
    - Ascending/Arch 02CX
    - Descending 02CW
- Aortic Body 0GCD
- Appendix 0DCJ
- Artery
  - Anterior Tibial
    - Left 04CQ
    - Right 04CP
  - Axillary

Extirpation — *continued*
- Artery — *continued*
    - Left 03C6
    - Right 03C5
  - Brachial
    - Left 03C8
    - Right 03C7
  - Celiac 04C1
  - Colic
    - Left 04C7
    - Middle 04C8
    - Right 04C6
  - Common Carotid
    - Left 03CJ
    - Right 03CH
  - Common Iliac
    - Left 04CD
    - Right 04CC
  - Coronary
    - Four or More Arteries 02C3
    - One Artery 02C0
    - Three Arteries 02C2
    - Two Arteries 02C1
  - External Carotid
    - Left 03CN
    - Right 03CM
  - External Iliac
    - Left 04CJ
    - Right 04CH
  - Face 03CR
  - Femoral
    - Left 04CL
    - Right 04CK
  - Foot
    - Left 04CW
    - Right 04CV
  - Gastric 04C2
  - Hand
    - Left 03CF
    - Right 03CD
  - Hepatic 04C3
  - Inferior Mesenteric 04CB
  - Innominate 03C2
  - Internal Carotid
    - Left 03CL
    - Right 03CK
  - Internal Iliac
    - Left 04CF
    - Right 04CE
  - Internal Mammary
    - Left 03C1
    - Right 03C0
  - Intracranial 03CG
  - Lower 04CY
  - Peroneal
    - Left 04CU
    - Right 04CT
  - Popliteal
    - Left 04CN
    - Right 04CM
  - Posterior Tibial
    - Left 04CS
    - Right 04CR
  - Pulmonary
    - Left 02CR
    - Right 02CQ
  - Pulmonary Trunk 02CP
  - Radial
    - Left 03CC
    - Right 03CB
  - Renal
    - Left 04CA
    - Right 04C9
  - Splenic 04C4
  - Subclavian
    - Left 03C4
    - Right 03C3

F

Fusion — *continued*
Thoracic Vertebral — *continued*
Interbody Fusion Device, Nanotextured Surface XRG6092
Thoracolumbar Vertebral 0RGA
Interbody Fusion Device, Nanotextured Surface XRGA092
Toe Phalangeal
Left 0SGQ
Right 0SGP
Wrist
Left 0RGP
Right 0RGN
Fusion screw (compression)(lag)(locking)
use Internal Fixation Device in Upper Joints
use Internal Fixation Device in Lower Joints

G

Gait training *see* Motor Treatment, Rehabilitation F07
Galea aponeurotica *use* Subcutaneous Tissue and Fascia, Scalp
Ganglion impar (ganglion of Walther) *use* Sacral Sympathetic Nerve
Ganglionectomy
Destruction of lesion *see* Destruction
Excision of lesion *see* Excision
Gasserian ganglion *use* Trigeminal Nerve
Gastrectomy
Partial *see* Excision, Stomach 0DB6
Total *see* Resection, Stomach 0DT6
Vertical (sleeve) *see* Excision, Stomach 0DB6
Gastric electrical stimulation (GES) lead *use* Stimulator Lead in Gastrointestinal System
Gastric lymph node *use* Lymphatic, Aortic
Gastric pacemaker lead *use* Stimulator Lead in Gastrointestinal System
Gastric plexus *use* Abdominal Sympathetic Nerve
Gastrocnemius muscle
use Lower Leg Muscle, Right
use Lower Leg Muscle, Left
Gastrocolic ligament *use* Greater Omentum
Gastrocolic omentum *use* Greater Omentum
Gastrocolostomy
see Bypass, Gastrointestinal System 0D1
see Drainage, Gastrointestinal System 0D9
Gastroduodenal artery *use* Hepatic Artery
Gastroduodenectomy
see Excision, Gastrointestinal System 0DB
see Resection, Gastrointestinal System 0DT
Gastroduodenoscopy 0DJ08ZZ
Gastroenteroplasty
see Repair, Gastrointestinal System 0DQ
see Supplement, Gastrointestinal System 0DU
Gastroenterostomy
see Bypass, Gastrointestinal System 0D1
see Drainage, Gastrointestinal System 0D9
Gastroesophageal (GE) junction *use* Esophagogastric Junction
Gastrogastrostomy
see Bypass, Stomach 0D16
see Drainage, Stomach 0D96
Gastrohepatic omentum *use* Lesser Omentum
Gastrojejunostomy
see Bypass, Stomach 0D16
see Drainage, Stomach 0D96
Gastrolysis *see* Release, Stomach 0DN6
Gastropexy
see Repair, Stomach 0DQ6
see Reposition, Stomach 0DS6
Gastrophrenic ligament *use* Greater Omentum
Gastroplasty
see Repair, Stomach 0DQ6
see Supplement, Stomach 0DU6
Gastroplication *see* Restriction, Stomach 0DV6
Gastropylorectomy *see* Excision, Gastrointestinal System 0DB
Gastrorrhaphy *see* Repair, Stomach 0DQ6
Gastroscopy 0DJ68ZZ
Gastrosplenic ligament *use* Greater Omentum
Gastrostomy
see Bypass, Stomach 0D16
see Drainage, Stomach 0D96
Gastrotomy *see* Drainage, Stomach 0D96
Gemellus muscle
use Hip Muscle, Right
use Hip Muscle, Left
Geniculate ganglion *use* Facial Nerve
Geniculate nucleus *use* Thalamus
Genioglossus muscle *use* Tongue, Palate, Pharynx Muscle
Genioplasty *see* Alteration, Jaw, Lower 0W05
Genitofemoral nerve *use* Lumbar Plexus
Gingivectomy *see* Excision, Mouth and Throat 0CB
Gingivoplasty
see Repair, Mouth and Throat 0CQ
see Replacement, Mouth and Throat 0CR
see Supplement, Mouth and Throat 0CU
Glans penis *use* Prepuce
Glenohumeral joint
use Shoulder Joint, Right
use Shoulder Joint, Left
Glenohumeral ligament
use Shoulder Bursa and Ligament, Right
use Shoulder Bursa and Ligament, Left
Glenoid fossa (of scapula)
use Glenoid Cavity, Right
use Glenoid Cavity, Left
Glenoid ligament (labrum)
use Shoulder Joint, Right
use Shoulder Joint, Left
Globus pallidus *use* Basal Ganglia
Glomectomy
see Excision, Endocrine System 0GB
see Resection, Endocrine System 0GT
Glossectomy
see Excision, Tongue 0CB7
see Resection, Tongue 0CT7
Glossoepiglottic fold *use* Epiglottis
Glossopexy
see Repair, Tongue 0CQ7
see Reposition, Tongue 0CS7
Glossoplasty
see Repair, Tongue 0CQ7
see Replacement, Tongue 0CR7
see Supplement, Tongue 0CU7
Glossorrhaphy *see* Repair, Tongue 0CQ7
Glossotomy *see* Drainage, Tongue 0C97
Glottis *use* Larynx
Gluteal Artery Perforator Flap
Bilateral 0HRV079
Left 0HRU079
Right 0HRT079
Gluteal lymph node *use* Lymphatic, Pelvis
Gluteal vein
use Hypogastric Vein, Right
use Hypogastric Vein, Left
Gluteus maximus muscle
use Hip Muscle, Right
use Hip Muscle, Left
Gluteus medius muscle
use Hip Muscle, Right
use Hip Muscle, Left
Gluteus minimus muscle
use Hip Muscle, Right
use Hip Muscle, Left
GORE EXCLUDER® AAA Endoprosthesis
use Intraluminal Device, Branched or Fenestrated, One or Two Arteries in 04V
use Intraluminal Device, Branched or Fenestrated, Three or More Arteries in 04V
use Intraluminal Device
GORE EXCLUDER® IBE Endoprosthesis *use* Intraluminal Device, Branched or Fenestrated, One or Two Arteries in 04V
GORE TAG® Thoracic Endoprosthesis *use* Intraluminal Device
GORE® DUALMESH® *use* Synthetic Substitute
Gracilis muscle
use Upper Leg Muscle, Right
use Upper Leg Muscle, Left
Graft
see Replacement
see Supplement
Great auricular nerve *use* Cervical Plexus
Great cerebral vein *use* Intracranial Vein
Great saphenous vein
use Greater Saphenous Vein, Right
use Greater Saphenous Vein, Left
Greater alar cartilage *use* Nose
Greater occipital nerve *use* Cervical Nerve
Greater splanchnic nerve *use* Thoracic Sympathetic Nerve
Greater superficial petrosal nerve *use* Facial Nerve
Greater trochanter
use Upper Femur, Right
use Upper Femur, Left
Greater tuberosity
use Humeral Head, Right
use Humeral Head, Left
Greater vestibular (Bartholin's) gland *use* Vestibular Gland
Greater wing
use Sphenoid Bone, Right
use Sphenoid Bone, Left
Guedel airway *use* Intraluminal Device, Airway in Mouth and Throat
Guidance, catheter placement
EKG *see* Measurement, Physiological Systems 4A0
Fluoroscopy *see* Fluoroscopy, Veins B51
Ultrasound *see* Ultrasonography, Veins B54

H

Hallux
use 1st Toe, Right
use 1st Toe, Left
Hamate bone
use Carpal, Right
use Carpal, Left
Hancock® Bioprosthesis (aortic) (mitral) valve *use* Zooplastic Tissue in Heart and Great Vessels
Hancock® Bioprosthetic Valved Conduit *use* Zooplastic Tissue in Heart and Great Vessels
Harvesting, stem cells *see* Pheresis, Circulatory 6A55
Head of fibula
use Fibula, Right
use Fibula, Left
Hearing Aid Assessment F14Z
Hearing Assessment F13Z
Hearing Device
Bone Conduction
Left 09HE
Right 09HD

I

J

K

L

M

N

O

P

Q

R

Resection — *continued*
Femur — *continued*
Left 0QTC0ZZ
Right 0QTB0ZZ
Upper
Left 0QT70ZZ
Right 0QT60ZZ
Fibula
Left 0QTK0ZZ
Right 0QTJ0ZZ
Finger Nail 0HTQXZZ
Gallbladder 0FT4
Gland
Adrenal
Bilateral 0GT4
Left 0GT2
Right 0GT3
Lacrimal
Left 08TW
Right 08TV
Minor Salivary 0CTJ0ZZ
Parotid
Left 0CT90ZZ
Right 0CT80ZZ
Pituitary 0GT0
Sublingual
Left 0CTF0ZZ
Right 0CTD0ZZ
Submaxillary
Left 0CTH0ZZ
Right 0CTG0ZZ
Vestibular 0UTL
Glenoid Cavity
Left 0PT80ZZ
Right 0PT70ZZ
Glomus Jugulare 0GTC
Humeral Head
Left 0PTD0ZZ
Right 0PTC0ZZ
Humeral Shaft
Left 0PTG0ZZ
Right 0PTF0ZZ
Hymen 0UTK
Ileocecal Valve 0DTC
Ileum 0DTB
Intestine
Large 0DTE
Left 0DTG
Right 0DTF
Small 0DT8
Iris
Left 08TD3ZZ
Right 08TC3ZZ
Jejunum 0DTA
Joint
Acromioclavicular
Left 0RTH0ZZ
Right 0RTG0ZZ
Ankle
Left 0STG0ZZ
Right 0STF0ZZ
Carpal
Left 0RTR0ZZ
Right 0RTQ0ZZ
Cervicothoracic Vertebral 0RT40ZZ
Coccygeal 0ST60ZZ
Elbow
Left 0RTM0ZZ
Right 0RTL0ZZ
Finger Phalangeal
Left 0RTX0ZZ
Right 0RTW0ZZ
Hip
Left 0STB0ZZ
Right 0ST90ZZ
Knee
Left 0STD0ZZ

Resection — *continued*
Joint — *continued*
Right 0STC0ZZ
Metacarpocarpal
Left 0RTT0ZZ
Right 0RTS0ZZ
Metacarpophalangeal
Left 0RTV0ZZ
Right 0RTU0ZZ
Metatarsal-Phalangeal
Left 0STN0ZZ
Right 0STM0ZZ
Metatarsal-Tarsal
Left 0STL0ZZ
Right 0STK0ZZ
Sacrococcygeal 0ST50ZZ
Sacroiliac
Left 0ST80ZZ
Right 0ST70ZZ
Shoulder
Left 0RTK0ZZ
Right 0RTJ0ZZ
Sternoclavicular
Left 0RTF0ZZ
Right 0RTE0ZZ
Tarsal
Left 0STJ0ZZ
Right 0STH0ZZ
Temporomandibular
Left 0RTD0ZZ
Right 0RTC0ZZ
Toe Phalangeal
Left 0STQ0ZZ
Right 0STP0ZZ
Wrist
Left 0RTP0ZZ
Right 0RTN0ZZ
Kidney
Left 0TT1
Right 0TT0
Kidney Pelvis
Left 0TT4
Right 0TT3
Kidneys, Bilateral 0TT2
Larynx 0CTS
Lens
Left 08TK3ZZ
Right 08TJ3ZZ
Lip
Lower 0CT1
Upper 0CT0
Liver 0FT0
Left Lobe 0FT2
Right Lobe 0FT1
Lung
Bilateral 0BTM
Left 0BTL
Lower Lobe
Left 0BTJ
Right 0BTF
Middle Lobe, Right 0BTD
Right 0BTK
Upper Lobe
Left 0BTG
Right 0BTC
Lung Lingula 0BTH
Lymphatic
Aortic 07TD
Axillary
Left 07T6
Right 07T5
Head 07T0
Inguinal
Left 07TJ
Right 07TH
Internal Mammary
Left 07T9

Resection — *continued*
Lymphatic — *continued*
Right 07T8
Lower Extremity
Left 07TG
Right 07TF
Mesenteric 07TB
Neck
Left 07T2
Right 07T1
Pelvis 07TC
Thoracic Duct 07TK
Thorax 07T7
Upper Extremity
Left 07T4
Right 07T3
Mandible
Left 0NTV0ZZ
Right 0NTT0ZZ
Maxilla
Left 0NTS0ZZ
Right 0NTR0ZZ
Metacarpal
Left 0PTQ0ZZ
Right 0PTP0ZZ
Metatarsal
Left 0QTP0ZZ
Right 0QTN0ZZ
Muscle
Abdomen
Left 0KTL
Right 0KTK
Extraocular
Left 08TM
Right 08TL
Facial 0KT1
Foot
Left 0KTW
Right 0KTV
Hand
Left 0KTD
Right 0KTC
Head 0KT0
Hip
Left 0KTP
Right 0KTN
Lower Arm and Wrist
Left 0KTB
Right 0KT9
Lower Leg
Left 0KTT
Right 0KTS
Neck
Left 0KT3
Right 0KT2
Papillary 02TD
Perineum 0KTM
Shoulder
Left 0KT6
Right 0KT5
Thorax
Left 0KTJ
Right 0KTH
Tongue, Palate, Pharynx 0KT4
Trunk
Left 0KTG
Right 0KTF
Upper Arm
Left 0KT8
Right 0KT7
Upper Leg
Left 0KTR
Right 0KTQ
Nasopharynx 09TN
Nipple
Left 0HTXXZZ
Right 0HTWXZZ

Restriction — *continued*
- Artery — *continued*
  - Right 04VH
  - Face 03VR
  - Femoral
    - Left 04VL
    - Right 04VK
  - Foot
    - Left 04VW
    - Right 04VV
  - Gastric 04V2
  - Hand
    - Left 03VF
    - Right 03VD
  - Hepatic 04V3
  - Inferior Mesenteric 04VB
  - Innominate 03V2
  - Internal Carotid
    - Left 03VL
    - Right 03VK
  - Internal Iliac
    - Left 04VF
    - Right 04VE
  - Internal Mammary
    - Left 03V1
    - Right 03V0
  - Intracranial 03VG
  - Lower 04VY
  - Peroneal
    - Left 04VU
    - Right 04VT
  - Popliteal
    - Left 04VN
    - Right 04VM
  - Posterior Tibial
    - Left 04VS
    - Right 04VR
  - Pulmonary
    - Left 02VR
    - Right 02VQ
  - Pulmonary Trunk 02VP
  - Radial
    - Left 03VC
    - Right 03VB
  - Renal
    - Left 04VA
    - Right 04V9
  - Splenic 04V4
  - Subclavian
    - Left 03V4
    - Right 03V3
  - Superior Mesenteric 04V5
  - Temporal
    - Left 03VT
    - Right 03VS
  - Thyroid
    - Left 03VV
    - Right 03VU
  - Ulnar
    - Left 03VA
    - Right 03V9
  - Upper 03VY
  - Vertebral
    - Left 03VQ
    - Right 03VP
- Bladder 0TVB
- Bladder Neck 0TVC
- Bronchus
  - Lingula 0BV9
  - Lower Lobe
    - Left 0BVB
    - Right 0BV6
  - Main
    - Left 0BV7
    - Right 0BV3
  - Middle Lobe, Right 0BV5
  - Upper Lobe

Restriction — *continued*
- Bronchus — *continued*
    - Left 0BV8
    - Right 0BV4
- Carina 0BV2
- Cecum 0DVH
- Cervix 0UVC
- Cisterna Chyli 07VL
- Colon
  - Ascending 0DVK
  - Descending 0DVM
  - Sigmoid 0DVN
  - Transverse 0DVL
- Duct
  - Common Bile 0FV9
  - Cystic 0FV8
  - Hepatic
    - Left 0FV6
    - Right 0FV5
  - Lacrimal
    - Left 08VY
    - Right 08VX
  - Pancreatic 0FVD
    - Accessory 0FVF
  - Parotid
    - Left 0CVC
    - Right 0CVB
- Duodenum 0DV9
- Esophagogastric Junction 0DV4
- Esophagus 0DV5
  - Lower 0DV3
  - Middle 0DV2
  - Upper 0DV1
- Heart 02VA
- Ileocecal Valve 0DVC
- Ileum 0DVB
- Intestine
  - Large 0DVE
    - Left 0DVG
    - Right 0DVF
  - Small 0DV8
- Jejunum 0DVA
- Kidney Pelvis
  - Left 0TV4
  - Right 0TV3
- Lymphatic
  - Aortic 07VD
  - Axillary
    - Left 07V6
    - Right 07V5
  - Head 07V0
  - Inguinal
    - Left 07VJ
    - Right 07VH
  - Internal Mammary
    - Left 07V9
    - Right 07V8
  - Lower Extremity
    - Left 07VG
    - Right 07VF
  - Mesenteric 07VB
  - Neck
    - Left 07V2
    - Right 07V1
  - Pelvis 07VC
  - Thoracic Duct 07VK
  - Thorax 07V7
  - Upper Extremity
    - Left 07V4
    - Right 07V3
- Rectum 0DVP
- Stomach 0DV6
  - Pylorus 0DV7
- Trachea 0BV1
- Ureter
  - Left 0TV7
  - Right 0TV6

Restriction — *continued*
- Urethra 0TVD
- Vein
  - Axillary
    - Left 05V8
    - Right 05V7
  - Azygos 05V0
  - Basilic
    - Left 05VC
    - Right 05VB
  - Brachial
    - Left 05VA
    - Right 05V9
  - Cephalic
    - Left 05VF
    - Right 05VD
  - Colic 06V7
  - Common Iliac
    - Left 06VD
    - Right 06VC
  - Esophageal 06V3
  - External Iliac
    - Left 06VG
    - Right 06VF
  - External Jugular
    - Left 05VQ
    - Right 05VP
  - Face
    - Left 05VV
    - Right 05VT
  - Femoral
    - Left 06VN
    - Right 06VM
  - Foot
    - Left 06VV
    - Right 06VT
  - Gastric 06V2
  - Greater Saphenous
    - Left 06VQ
    - Right 06VP
  - Hand
    - Left 05VH
    - Right 05VG
  - Hemiazygos 05V1
  - Hepatic 06V4
  - Hypogastric
    - Left 06VJ
    - Right 06VH
  - Inferior Mesenteric 06V6
  - Innominate
    - Left 05V4
    - Right 05V3
  - Internal Jugular
    - Left 05VN
    - Right 05VM
  - Intracranial 05VL
  - Lesser Saphenous
    - Left 06VS
    - Right 06VR
  - Lower 06VY
  - Portal 06V8
  - Pulmonary
    - Left 02VT
    - Right 02VS
  - Renal
    - Left 06VB
    - Right 06V9
  - Splenic 06V1
  - Subclavian
    - Left 05V6
    - Right 05V5
  - Superior Mesenteric 06V5
  - Upper 05VY
  - Vertebral
    - Left 05VS
    - Right 05VR

ICD-10-PCS Index
Revision of device - Robotic assisted procedure

Revision of device — *continued*
Joint — *continued*
Right 0SW7
Shoulder
Left 0RWK
Right 0RWJ
Sternoclavicular
Left 0RWF
Right 0RWE
Tarsal
Left 0SWJ
Right 0SWH
Temporomandibular
Left 0RWD
Right 0RWC
Thoracic Vertebral 0RW6
Thoracolumbar Vertebral 0RWA
Toe Phalangeal
Left 0SWQ
Right 0SWP
Wrist
Left 0RWP
Right 0RWN
Kidney 0TW5
Larynx 0CWS
Lens
Left 08WK
Right 08WJ
Liver 0FW0
Lung
Left 0BWL
Right 0BWK
Lymphatic 07WN
Thoracic Duct 07WK
Mediastinum 0WWC
Mesentery 0DWV
Metacarpal
Left 0PWQ
Right 0PWP
Metatarsal
Left 0QWP
Right 0QWN
Mouth and Throat 0CWY
Muscle
Extraocular
Left 08WM
Right 08WL
Lower 0KWY
Upper 0KWX
Neck 0WW6
Nerve
Cranial 00WE
Peripheral 01WY
Nose 09WK
Omentum 0DWU
Ovary 0UW3
Pancreas 0FWG
Parathyroid Gland 0GWR
Patella
Left 0QWF
Right 0QWD
Pelvic Cavity 0WWJ
Penis 0VWS
Pericardial Cavity 0WWD
Perineum
Female 0WWN
Male 0WWM
Peritoneal Cavity 0WWG
Peritoneum 0DWW
Phalanx
Finger
Left 0PWV
Right 0PWT
Thumb
Left 0PWS
Right 0PWR
Toe

Revision of device — *continued*
Phalanx — *continued*
Left 0QWR
Right 0QWQ
Pineal Body 0GW1
Pleura 0BWQ
Pleural Cavity
Left 0WWB
Right 0WW9
Prostate and Seminal Vesicles 0VW4
Radius
Left 0PWJ
Right 0PWH
Respiratory Tract 0WWQ
Retroperitoneum 0WWH
Rib
Left 0PW2
Right 0PW1
Sacrum 0QW1
Scapula
Left 0PW6
Right 0PW5
Scrotum and Tunica Vaginalis 0VW8
Septum
Atrial 02W5
Ventricular 02WM
Sinus 09WY
Skin 0HWPX
Skull 0NW0
Spinal Canal 00WU
Spinal Cord 00WV
Spleen 07WP
Sternum 0PW0
Stomach 0DW6
Subcutaneous Tissue and Fascia
Head and Neck 0JWS
Lower Extremity 0JWW
Trunk 0JWT
Upper Extremity 0JWV
Tarsal
Left 0QWM
Right 0QWL
Tendon
Lower 0LWY
Upper 0LWX
Testis 0VWD
Thymus 07WM
Thyroid Gland 0GWK
Tibia
Left 0QWH
Right 0QWG
Toe Nail 0HWRX
Trachea 0BW1
Tracheobronchial Tree 0BW0
Tympanic Membrane
Left 09W8
Right 09W7
Ulna
Left 0PWL
Right 0PWK
Ureter 0TW9
Urethra 0TWD
Uterus and Cervix 0UWD
Vagina and Cul-de-sac 0UWH
Valve
Aortic 02WF
Mitral 02WG
Pulmonary 02WH
Tricuspid 02WJ
Vas Deferens 0VWR
Vein
Azygos 05W0
Innominate
Left 05W4
Right 05W3
Lower 06WY
Upper 05WY
Vertebra

Revision of device — *continued*
Cervical 0PW3
Lumbar 0QW0
Thoracic 0PW4
Vulva 0UWM
Revo MRI™ SureScan® pacemaker *use* Pacemaker, Dual Chamber in 0JH
rhBMP-2 *use* Recombinant Bone Morphogenetic Protein
Rheos® System device *use* Stimulator Generator in Subcutaneous Tissue and Fascia
Rheos® System lead *use* Stimulator Lead in Upper Arteries
Rhinopharynx *use* Nasopharynx
Rhinoplasty
see Alteration, Nose 090K
see Repair, Nose 09QK
see Replacement, Nose 09RK
see Supplement, Nose 09UK
Rhinorrhaphy *see* Repair, Nose 09QK
Rhinoscopy 09JKXZZ
Rhizotomy
see Division, Central Nervous System 008
see Division, Peripheral Nervous System 018
Rhomboid major muscle
use Trunk Muscle, Right
use Trunk Muscle, Left
Rhomboid minor muscle
use Trunk Muscle, Right
use Trunk Muscle, Left
Rhythm electrocardiogram *see* Measurement, Cardiac 4A02
Rhytidectomy *see* Face lift
Right ascending lumbar vein *use* Azygos Vein
Right atrioventricular valve *use* Tricuspid Valve
Right auricular appendix *use* Atrium, Right
Right colic vein *use* Colic Vein
Right coronary sulcus *use* Heart, Right
Right gastric artery *use* Gastric Artery
Right gastroepiploic vein *use* Superior Mesenteric Vein
Right inferior phrenic vein *use* Inferior Vena Cava
Right inferior pulmonary vein *use* Pulmonary Vein, Right
Right jugular trunk *use* Lymphatic, Right Neck
Right lateral ventricle *use* Cerebral Ventricle
Right lymphatic duct *use* Lymphatic, Right Neck
Right ovarian vein *use* Inferior Vena Cava
Right second lumbar vein *use* Inferior Vena Cava
Right subclavian trunk *use* Lymphatic, Right Neck
Right subcostal vein *use* Azygos Vein
Right superior pulmonary vein *use* Pulmonary Vein, Right
Right suprarenal vein *use* Inferior Vena Cava
Right testicular vein *use* Inferior Vena Cava
Rima glottidis *use* Larynx
Risorius muscle *use* Facial Muscle
RNS® System lead *use* Neurostimulator Lead in Central Nervous System
RNS® system neurostimulator generator *use* Neurostimulator Generator in Head and Facial Bones
Robotic assisted procedure
Extremity
Lower 8E0Y
Upper 8E0X
Head and Neck Region 8E09
Trunk Region 8E0W

Revision of device - Robotic assisted procedure
ICD-10-PCS INDEX

S

ICD-10-PCS Index
Stereotactic Radiosurgery - Stimulator Generator

Stereotactic Radiosurgery — *continued*
Lung DB22
Lymphatics
Abdomen D726
Axillary D724
Inguinal D728
Neck D723
Pelvis D727
Thorax D725
Mediastinum DB26
Mouth D924
Nasopharynx D92D
Neck and Head DW21
Nerve, Peripheral D027
Nose D921
Other Photon
Abdomen DW23DZZ
Adrenal Gland DG22DZZ
Bile Ducts DF22DZZ
Bladder DT22DZZ
Bone Marrow D720DZZ
Brain D020DZZ
Brain Stem D021DZZ
Breast
Left DM20DZZ
Right DM21DZZ
Bronchus DB21DZZ
Cervix DU21DZZ
Chest DW22DZZ
Chest Wall DB27DZZ
Colon DD25DZZ
Diaphragm DB28DZZ
Duodenum DD22DZZ
Ear D920DZZ
Esophagus DD20DZZ
Eye D820DZZ
Gallbladder DF21DZZ
Gland
Adrenal DG22DZZ
Parathyroid DG24DZZ
Pituitary DG20DZZ
Thyroid DG25DZZ
Glands, Salivary D926DZZ
Head and Neck DW21DZZ
Ileum DD24DZZ
Jejunum DD23DZZ
Kidney DT20DZZ
Larynx D92BDZZ
Liver DF20DZZ
Lung DB22DZZ
Lymphatics
Abdomen D726DZZ
Axillary D724DZZ
Inguinal D728DZZ
Neck D723DZZ
Pelvis D727DZZ
Thorax D725DZZ
Mediastinum DB26DZZ
Mouth D924DZZ
Nasopharynx D92DDZZ
Neck and Head DW21DZZ
Nerve, Peripheral D027DZZ
Nose D921DZZ
Ovary DU20DZZ
Palate
Hard D928DZZ
Soft D929DZZ
Pancreas DF23DZZ
Parathyroid Gland DG24DZZ
Pelvic Region DW26DZZ
Pharynx D92CDZZ
Pineal Body DG21DZZ
Pituitary Gland DG20DZZ
Pleura DB25DZZ
Prostate DV20DZZ
Rectum DD27DZZ
Sinuses D927DZZ

Stereotactic Radiosurgery — *continued*
Other Photon — *continued*
Spinal Cord D026DZZ
Spleen D722DZZ
Stomach DD21DZZ
Testis DV21DZZ
Thymus D721DZZ
Thyroid Gland DG25DZZ
Tongue D925DZZ
Trachea DB20DZZ
Ureter DT21DZZ
Urethra DT23DZZ
Uterus DU22DZZ
Ovary DU20
Palate
Hard D928
Soft D929
Pancreas DF23
Parathyroid Gland DG24
Particulate
Abdomen DW23HZZ
Adrenal Gland DG22HZZ
Bile Ducts DF22HZZ
Bladder DT22HZZ
Bone Marrow D720HZZ
Brain D020HZZ
Brain Stem D021HZZ
Breast
Left DM20HZZ
Right DM21HZZ
Bronchus DB21HZZ
Cervix DU21HZZ
Chest DW22HZZ
Chest Wall DB27HZZ
Colon DD25HZZ
Diaphragm DB28HZZ
Duodenum DD22HZZ
Ear D920HZZ
Esophagus DD20HZZ
Eye D820HZZ
Gallbladder DF21HZZ
Gland
Adrenal DG22HZZ
Parathyroid DG24HZZ
Pituitary DG20HZZ
Thyroid DG25HZZ
Glands, Salivary D926HZZ
Head and Neck DW21HZZ
Ileum DD24HZZ
Jejunum DD23HZZ
Kidney DT20HZZ
Larynx D92BHZZ
Liver DF20HZZ
Lung DB22HZZ
Lymphatics
Abdomen D726HZZ
Axillary D724HZZ
Inguinal D728HZZ
Neck D723HZZ
Pelvis D727HZZ
Thorax D725HZZ
Mediastinum DB26HZZ
Mouth D924HZZ
Nasopharynx D92DHZZ
Neck and Head DW21HZZ
Nerve, Peripheral D027HZZ
Nose D921HZZ
Ovary DU20HZZ
Palate
Hard D928HZZ
Soft D929HZZ
Pancreas DF23HZZ
Parathyroid Gland DG24HZZ
Pelvic Region DW26HZZ
Pharynx D92CHZZ
Pineal Body DG21HZZ
Pituitary Gland DG20HZZ

Stereotactic Radiosurgery — *continued*
Particulate — *continued*
Pleura DB25HZZ
Prostate DV20HZZ
Rectum DD27HZZ
Sinuses D927HZZ
Spinal Cord D026HZZ
Spleen D722HZZ
Stomach DD21HZZ
Testis DV21HZZ
Thymus D721HZZ
Thyroid Gland DG25HZZ
Tongue D925HZZ
Trachea DB20HZZ
Ureter DT21HZZ
Urethra DT23HZZ
Uterus DU22HZZ
Pelvic Region DW26
Pharynx D92C
Pineal Body DG21
Pituitary Gland DG20
Pleura DB25
Prostate DV20
Rectum DD27
Sinuses D927
Spinal Cord D026
Spleen D722
Stomach DD21
Testis DV21
Thymus D721
Thyroid Gland DG25
Tongue D925
Trachea DB20
Ureter DT21
Urethra DT23
Uterus DU22
Sternoclavicular ligament
use Shoulder Bursa and Ligament, Right
use Shoulder Bursa and Ligament, Left
Sternocleidomastoid artery
use Thyroid Artery, Right
use Thyroid Artery, Left
Sternocleidomastoid muscle
use Neck Muscle, Right
use Neck Muscle, Left
Sternocostal ligament
use Thorax Bursa and Ligament, Right
use Thorax Bursa and Ligament, Left
Sternotomy
see Division, Sternum 0P80
see Drainage, Sternum 0P90
Stimulation, cardiac
Cardioversion 5A2204Z
Electrophysiologic testing *see* Measurement, Cardiac 4A02
Stimulator Generator
Insertion of device in
Abdomen 0JH8
Back 0JH7
Chest 0JH6
Multiple Array
Abdomen 0JH8
Back 0JH7
Chest 0JH6
Multiple Array Rechargeable
Abdomen 0JH8
Back 0JH7
Chest 0JH6
Removal of device from, Subcutaneous Tissue and Fascia, Trunk 0JPT
Revision of device in, Subcutaneous Tissue and Fascia, Trunk 0JWT
Single Array
Abdomen 0JH8
Back 0JH7
Chest 0JH6
Single Array Rechargeable
Abdomen 0JH8

Stereotactic Radiosurgery - Stimulator Generator
ICD-10-PCS INDEX

Supplement — *continued*
- Bone — *continued*
  - Left 0NU6
  - Right 0NU5
  - Zygomatic
    - Left 0NUN
    - Right 0NUM
- Breast
  - Bilateral 0HUV
  - Left 0HUU
  - Right 0HUT
- Bronchus
  - Lingula 0BU9
  - Lower Lobe
    - Left 0BUB
    - Right 0BU6
  - Main
    - Left 0BU7
    - Right 0BU3
  - Middle Lobe, Right 0BU5
  - Upper Lobe
    - Left 0BU8
    - Right 0BU4
- Buccal Mucosa 0CU4
- Bursa and Ligament
  - Abdomen
    - Left 0MUJ
    - Right 0MUH
  - Ankle
    - Left 0MUR
    - Right 0MUQ
  - Elbow
    - Left 0MU4
    - Right 0MU3
  - Foot
    - Left 0MUT
    - Right 0MUS
  - Hand
    - Left 0MU8
    - Right 0MU7
  - Head and Neck 0MU0
  - Hip
    - Left 0MUM
    - Right 0MUL
  - Knee
    - Left 0MUP
    - Right 0MUN
  - Lower Extremity
    - Left 0MUW
    - Right 0MUV
  - Perineum 0MUK
  - Shoulder
    - Left 0MU2
    - Right 0MU1
  - Thorax
    - Left 0MUG
    - Right 0MUF
  - Trunk
    - Left 0MUD
    - Right 0MUC
  - Upper Extremity
    - Left 0MUB
    - Right 0MU9
  - Wrist
    - Left 0MU6
    - Right 0MU5
- Buttock
  - Left 0YU1
  - Right 0YU0
- Carina 0BU2
- Carpal
  - Left 0PUN
  - Right 0PUM
- Cecum 0DUH
- Cerebral Meninges 00U1
- Chest Wall 0WU8
- Chordae Tendineae 02U9

Supplement — *continued*
- Cisterna Chyli 07UL
- Clavicle
  - Left 0PUB
  - Right 0PU9
- Clitoris 0UUJ
- Coccyx 0QUS
- Colon
  - Ascending 0DUK
  - Descending 0DUM
  - Sigmoid 0DUN
  - Transverse 0DUL
- Cord
  - Bilateral 0VUH
  - Left 0VUG
  - Right 0VUF
- Cornea
  - Left 08U9
  - Right 08U8
- Cul-de-sac 0UUF
- Diaphragm
  - Left 0BUS
  - Right 0BUR
- Disc
  - Cervical Vertebral 0RU3
  - Cervicothoracic Vertebral 0RU5
  - Lumbar Vertebral 0SU2
  - Lumbosacral 0SU4
  - Thoracic Vertebral 0RU9
  - Thoracolumbar Vertebral 0RUB
- Duct
  - Common Bile 0FU9
  - Cystic 0FU8
  - Hepatic
    - Left 0FU6
    - Right 0FU5
  - Lacrimal
    - Left 08UY
    - Right 08UX
  - Pancreatic 0FUD
    - Accessory 0FUF
- Duodenum 0DU9
- Dura Mater 00U2
- Ear
  - External
    - Bilateral 09U2
    - Left 09U1
    - Right 09U0
  - Inner
    - Left 09UE0
    - Right 09UD0
  - Middle
    - Left 09U60
    - Right 09U50
- Elbow Region
  - Left 0XUC
  - Right 0XUB
- Epididymis
  - Bilateral 0VUL
  - Left 0VUK
  - Right 0VUJ
- Epiglottis 0CUR
- Esophagogastric Junction 0DU4
- Esophagus 0DU5
  - Lower 0DU3
  - Middle 0DU2
  - Upper 0DU1
- Extremity
  - Lower
    - Left 0YUB
    - Right 0YU9
  - Upper
    - Left 0XU7
    - Right 0XU6
- Eye
  - Left 08U1
  - Right 08U0
- Eyelid

Supplement — *continued*
  - Lower
    - Left 08UR
    - Right 08UQ
  - Upper
    - Left 08UP
    - Right 08UN
- Face 0WU2
- Fallopian Tube
  - Left 0UU6
  - Right 0UU5
- Fallopian Tubes, Bilateral 0UU7
- Femoral Region
  - Bilateral 0YUE
  - Left 0YU8
  - Right 0YU7
- Femoral Shaft
  - Left 0QU9
  - Right 0QU8
- Femur
  - Lower
    - Left 0QUC
    - Right 0QUB
  - Upper
    - Left 0QU7
    - Right 0QU6
- Fibula
  - Left 0QUK
  - Right 0QUJ
- Finger
  - Index
    - Left 0XUP
    - Right 0XUN
  - Little
    - Left 0XUW
    - Right 0XUV
  - Middle
    - Left 0XUR
    - Right 0XUQ
  - Ring
    - Left 0XUT
    - Right 0XUS
- Foot
  - Left 0YUN
  - Right 0YUM
- Gingiva
  - Lower 0CU6
  - Upper 0CU5
- Glenoid Cavity
  - Left 0PU8
  - Right 0PU7
- Hand
  - Left 0XUK
  - Right 0XUJ
- Head 0WU0
- Heart 02UA
- Humeral Head
  - Left 0PUD
  - Right 0PUC
- Humeral Shaft
  - Left 0PUG
  - Right 0PUF
- Hymen 0UUK
- Ileocecal Valve 0DUC
- Ileum 0DUB
- Inguinal Region
  - Bilateral 0YUA
  - Left 0YU6
  - Right 0YU5
- Intestine
  - Large 0DUE
    - Left 0DUG
    - Right 0DUF
  - Small 0DU8
- Iris
  - Left 08UD
  - Right 08UC
- Jaw

Supplement — *continued*
Finger
Left 0PUV
Right 0PUT
Thumb
Left 0PUS
Right 0PUR
Toe
Left 0QUR
Right 0QUQ
Pharynx 0CUM
Prepuce 0VUT
Radius
Left 0PUJ
Right 0PUH
Rectum 0DUP
Retina
Left 08UF
Right 08UE
Retinal Vessel
Left 08UH
Right 08UG
Rib
Left 0PU2
Right 0PU1
Sacrum 0QU1
Scapula
Left 0PU6
Right 0PU5
Scrotum 0VU5
Septum
Atrial 02U5
Nasal 09UM
Ventricular 02UM
Shoulder Region
Left 0XU3
Right 0XU2
Skull 0NU0
Spinal Meninges 00UT
Sternum 0PU0
Stomach 0DU6
Pylorus 0DU7
Subcutaneous Tissue and Fascia
Abdomen 0JU8
Back 0JU7
Buttock 0JU9
Chest 0JU6
Face 0JU1
Foot
Left 0JUR
Right 0JUQ
Hand
Left 0JUK
Right 0JUJ
Lower Arm
Left 0JUH
Right 0JUG
Lower Leg
Left 0JUP
Right 0JUN
Neck
Anterior 0JU4
Posterior 0JU5
Pelvic Region 0JUC
Perineum 0JUB
Scalp 0JU0
Upper Arm
Left 0JUF
Right 0JUD
Upper Leg
Left 0JUM
Right 0JUL
Tarsal
Left 0QUM
Right 0QUL
Tendon

Supplement — *continued*
Abdomen
Left 0LUG
Right 0LUF
Ankle
Left 0LUT
Right 0LUS
Foot
Left 0LUW
Right 0LUV
Hand
Left 0LU8
Right 0LU7
Head and Neck 0LU0
Hip
Left 0LUK
Right 0LUJ
Knee
Left 0LUR
Right 0LUQ
Lower Arm and Wrist
Left 0LU6
Right 0LU5
Lower Leg
Left 0LUP
Right 0LUN
Perineum 0LUH
Shoulder
Left 0LU2
Right 0LU1
Thorax
Left 0LUD
Right 0LUC
Trunk
Left 0LUB
Right 0LU9
Upper Arm
Left 0LU4
Right 0LU3
Upper Leg
Left 0LUM
Right 0LUL
Testis
Bilateral 0VUC0
Left 0VUB0
Right 0VU90
Thumb
Left 0XUM
Right 0XUL
Tibia
Left 0QUH
Right 0QUG
Toe
1st
Left 0YUQ
Right 0YUP
2nd
Left 0YUS
Right 0YUR
3rd
Left 0YUU
Right 0YUT
4th
Left 0YUW
Right 0YUV
5th
Left 0YUY
Right 0YUX
Tongue 0CU7
Trachea 0BU1
Tunica Vaginalis
Left 0VU7
Right 0VU6
Turbinate, Nasal 09UL
Tympanic Membrane
Left 09U8
Right 09U7
Ulna

Supplement — *continued*
Left 0PUL
Right 0PUK
Ureter
Left 0TU7
Right 0TU6
Urethra 0TUD
Uterine Supporting Structure 0UU4
Uvula 0CUN
Vagina 0UUG
Valve
Aortic 02UF
Mitral 02UG
Pulmonary 02UH
Tricuspid 02UJ
Vas Deferens
Bilateral 0VUQ
Left 0VUP
Right 0VUN
Vein
Axillary
Left 05U8
Right 05U7
Azygos 05U0
Basilic
Left 05UC
Right 05UB
Brachial
Left 05UA
Right 05U9
Cephalic
Left 05UF
Right 05UD
Colic 06U7
Common Iliac
Left 06UD
Right 06UC
Esophageal 06U3
External Iliac
Left 06UG
Right 06UF
External Jugular
Left 05UQ
Right 05UP
Face
Left 05UV
Right 05UT
Femoral
Left 06UN
Right 06UM
Foot
Left 06UV
Right 06UT
Gastric 06U2
Greater Saphenous
Left 06UQ
Right 06UP
Hand
Left 05UH
Right 05UG
Hemiazygos 05U1
Hepatic 06U4
Hypogastric
Left 06UJ
Right 06UH
Inferior Mesenteric 06U6
Innominate
Left 05U4
Right 05U3
Internal Jugular
Left 05UN
Right 05UM
Intracranial 05UL
Lesser Saphenous
Left 06US
Right 06UR
Lower 06UY

T

U

V

W

X

Y

Z

ICD-10-PCS Tables

Central Nervous System 001-00X

0 Medical and Surgical
0 Central Nervous System
1 Bypass: Altering the route of passage of the contents of a tubular body part

Body Part Character 4	Approach Character 5	Device Character 6	Qualifier Character 7
6 Cerebral Ventricle	**0** Open **3** Percutaneous	**7** Autologous Tissue Substitute **J** Synthetic Substitute **K** Nonautologous Tissue Substitute	**0** Nasopharynx **1** Mastoid Sinus **2** Atrium **3** Blood Vessel **4** Pleural Cavity **5** Intestine **6** Peritoneal Cavity **7** Urinary Tract **8** Bone Marrow **B** Cerebral Cisterns
U Spinal Canal	**0** Open **3** Percutaneous	**7** Autologous Tissue Substitute **J** Synthetic Substitute **K** Nonautologous Tissue Substitute	**4** Pleural Cavity **6** Peritoneal Cavity **7** Urinary Tract **9** Fallopian Tube

0 Medical and Surgical
0 Central Nervous System
2 Change: Taking out or off a device from a body part and putting back an identical or similar device in or on the same body part without cutting or puncturing the skin or a mucous membrane

Body Part Character 4	Approach Character 5	Device Character 6	Qualifier Character 7
0 Brain ⃠ **E** Cranial Nerve ⃠ **U** Spinal Canal ⃠	**X** External	**0** Drainage Device **Y** Other Device	**Z** No Qualifier

⃠ 0020X0Z 0020XYZ 002EX0Z 002EXYZ 002UX0Z 002UXYZ

0 Medical and Surgical
0 Central Nervous System
5 Destruction: Physical eradication of all or a portion of a body part by the direct use of energy, force, or a destructive agent

Body Part Character 4	Approach Character 5	Device Character 6	Qualifier Character 7
0 Brain	**0** Open	**Z** No Device	**Z** No Qualifier
1 Cerebral Meninges	**3** Percutaneous		
2 Dura Mater	**4** Percutaneous Endoscopic		
6 Cerebral Ventricle			
7 Cerebral Hemisphere			
8 Basal Ganglia			
9 Thalamus			
A Hypothalamus			
B Pons			
C Cerebellum			
D Medulla Oblongata			
F Olfactory Nerve ⦸			
G Optic Nerve ⦸			
H Oculomotor Nerve ⦸			
J Trochlear Nerve ⦸			
K Trigeminal Nerve ⦸			
L Abducens Nerve ⦸			
M Facial Nerve ⦸			
N Acoustic Nerve ⦸			
P Glossopharyngeal Nerve ⦸			
Q Vagus Nerve ⦸			
R Accessory Nerve ⦸			
S Hypoglossal Nerve ⦸			
T Spinal Meninges			
W Cervical Spinal Cord			
X Thoracic Spinal Cord			
Y Lumbar Spinal Cord			

⦸ 005F0ZZ 005F3ZZ 005F4ZZ 005G0ZZ 005G3ZZ 005G4ZZ 005H0ZZ 005H3ZZ 005H4ZZ 005J0ZZ 005J3ZZ 005J4ZZ 005K0ZZ 005K3ZZ 005K4ZZ 005L0ZZ 005L3ZZ 005L4ZZ 005M0ZZ 005M3ZZ 005M4ZZ 005N0ZZ 005N3ZZ 005N4ZZ 005P0ZZ 005P3ZZ 005P4ZZ 005Q0ZZ 005Q3ZZ 005Q4ZZ 005R0ZZ 005R3ZZ 005R4ZZ 005S0ZZ 005S3ZZ 005S4ZZ

0 Medical and Surgical
0 Central Nervous System
8 Division: Cutting into a body part, without draining fluids and/or gases from the body part, in order to separate or transect a body part

Body Part Character 4	Approach Character 5	Device Character 6	Qualifier Character 7
0 Brain	**0** Open	**Z** No Device	**Z** No Qualifier
7 Cerebral Hemisphere	**3** Percutaneous		
8 Basal Ganglia	**4** Percutaneous Endoscopic		
F Olfactory Nerve			
G Optic Nerve			
H Oculomotor Nerve			
J Trochlear Nerve			
K Trigeminal Nerve			
L Abducens Nerve			
M Facial Nerve			
N Acoustic Nerve			
P Glossopharyngeal Nerve			
Q Vagus Nerve			
R Accessory Nerve			
S Hypoglossal Nerve			
W Cervical Spinal Cord			
X Thoracic Spinal Cord			
Y Lumbar Spinal Cord			

LC Limited Coverage NC Noncovered HAC HAC Associated Procedure CC Combination Cluster - See Appendix G for code lists
DRG Non-OR-Affecting MS-DRG Assignment ⦸ Non-OR-Not Affecting MS-DRG Assignment New/Revised Text in **Orange** ♂ Male ♀ Female

0 Medical and Surgical
0 Central Nervous System
9 Drainage: Taking or letting out fluids and/or gases from a body part

Body Part Character 4	Approach Character 5	Device Character 6	Qualifier Character 7
0 Brain **1** Cerebral Meninges ⊘ **2** Dura Mater ⊘ **3** Epidural Space **4** Subdural Space ⊘ **5** Subarachnoid Space ⊘ **6** Cerebral Ventricle **7** Cerebral Hemisphere **8** Basal Ganglia **9** Thalamus **A** Hypothalamus **B** Pons **C** Cerebellum **D** Medulla Oblongata **F** Olfactory Nerve **G** Optic Nerve **H** Oculomotor Nerve **J** Trochlear Nerve **K** Trigeminal Nerve **L** Abducens Nerve **M** Facial Nerve **N** Acoustic Nerve **P** Glossopharyngeal Nerve **Q** Vagus Nerve **R** Accessory Nerve **S** Hypoglossal Nerve **T** Spinal Meninges **U** Spinal Canal ⊘ **W** Cervical Spinal Cord **X** Thoracic Spinal Cord **Y** Lumbar Spinal Cord	**0** Open **3** Percutaneous **4** Percutaneous Endoscopic	**0** Drainage Device	**Z** No Qualifier
0 Brain ⊘ **1** Cerebral Meninges ⊘ **2** Dura Mater ⊘ **3** Epidural Space ⊘ **4** Subdural Space ⊘ **5** Subarachnoid Space ⊘ **6** Cerebral Ventricle ⊘ **7** Cerebral Hemisphere ⊘ **8** Basal Ganglia ⊘ **9** Thalamus ⊘ **A** Hypothalamus ⊘ **B** Pons ⊘ **C** Cerebellum ⊘ **D** Medulla Oblongata ⊘ **F** Olfactory Nerve ⊘ **G** Optic Nerve ⊘ **H** Oculomotor Nerve ⊘ **J** Trochlear Nerve ⊘ **K** Trigeminal Nerve ⊘ **L** Abducens Nerve ⊘ **M** Facial Nerve ⊘ **N** Acoustic Nerve ⊘ **P** Glossopharyngeal Nerve ⊘ **Q** Vagus Nerve ⊘ **R** Accessory Nerve ⊘ **S** Hypoglossal Nerve ⊘ **T** Spinal Meninges **U** Spinal Canal ⊘ **W** Cervical Spinal Cord **X** Thoracic Spinal Cord **Y** Lumbar Spinal Cord	**0** Open **3** Percutaneous **4** Percutaneous Endoscopic	**Z** No Device	**X** Diagnostic **Z** No Qualifier

⊘ 00903ZX 00904ZX 009130Z 00913ZX 00913ZZ 009140Z 00914ZX 00914ZZ 009230Z 00923ZX 00923ZZ 009240Z 00924ZX
00924ZZ 00933ZX 00934ZX 009430Z 00943ZX 00943ZZ 009440Z 00944ZX 00944ZZ 009530Z 00953ZX 00953ZZ 009540Z
00954ZX 00954ZZ 00963ZX 00963ZZ 00964ZX 00964ZZ 00973ZX 00974ZX 00983ZX 00984ZX 00993ZX 00994ZX 009A3ZX
009A4ZX 009B3ZX 009B4ZX 009C3ZX 009C4ZX 009D3ZX 009D4ZX 009F3ZX 009F4ZX 009G3ZX 009G4ZX 009H3ZX 009H4ZX
009J3ZX 009J4ZX 009K3ZX 009K4ZX 009L3ZX 009L4ZX 009M3ZX 009M4ZX 009N3ZX 009N4ZX 009P3ZX 009P4ZX 009Q3ZX
009Q4ZX 009R3ZX 009R4ZX 009S3ZX 009S4ZX 009U30Z 009U3ZX 009U3ZZ 009U40Z 009U4ZX 009U4ZZ

LC Limited Coverage NC Noncovered HAC HAC Associated Procedure CC Combination Cluster - See Appendix G for code lists
DRG Non-OR-Affecting MS-DRG Assignment ⊘ Non-OR-Not Affecting MS-DRG Assignment New/Revised Text in **Orange** ♂ Male ♀ Female

0 Medical and Surgical
0 Central Nervous System
B Excision: Cutting out or off, without replacement, a portion of a body part

Body Part Character 4	Approach Character 5	Device Character 6	Qualifier Character 7
0 Brain ⃠ **1** Cerebral Meninges ⃠ **2** Dura Mater ⃠ **6** Cerebral Ventricle ⃠ **7** Cerebral Hemisphere ⃠ **8** Basal Ganglia ⃠ **9** Thalamus ⃠ **A** Hypothalamus ⃠ **B** Pons ⃠ **C** Cerebellum ⃠ **D** Medulla Oblongata ⃠ **F** Olfactory Nerve ⃠ **G** Optic Nerve ⃠ **H** Oculomotor Nerve ⃠ **J** Trochlear Nerve ⃠ **K** Trigeminal Nerve ⃠ **L** Abducens Nerve ⃠ **M** Facial Nerve ⃠ **N** Acoustic Nerve ⃠ **P** Glossopharyngeal Nerve ⃠ **Q** Vagus Nerve ⃠ **R** Accessory Nerve ⃠ **S** Hypoglossal Nerve ⃠ **T** Spinal Meninges **W** Cervical Spinal Cord **X** Thoracic Spinal Cord **Y** Lumbar Spinal Cord	**0** Open **3** Percutaneous **4** Percutaneous Endoscopic	**Z** No Device	**X** Diagnostic **Z** No Qualifier

⃠ 00B03ZX 00B04ZX 00B13ZX 00B14ZX 00B23ZX 00B24ZX 00B63ZX 00B64ZX 00B73ZX 00B74ZX 00B83ZX 00B84ZX 00B93ZX 00B94ZX 00BA3ZX 00BA4ZX 00BB3ZX 00BB4ZX 00BC3ZX 00BC4ZX 00BD3ZX 00BD4ZX 00BF3ZX 00BF4ZX 00BG3ZX 00BG4ZX 00BH3ZX 00BH4ZX 00BJ3ZX 00BJ4ZX 00BK3ZX 00BK4ZX 00BL3ZX 00BL4ZX 00BM3ZX 00BM4ZX 00BN3ZX 00BN4ZX 00BP3ZX 00BP4ZX 00BQ3ZX 00BQ4ZX 00BR3ZX 00BR4ZX 00BS3ZX 00BS4ZX

0 Medical and Surgical
0 Central Nervous System
C Extirpation: Taking or cutting out solid matter from a body part

Body Part Character 4	Approach Character 5	Device Character 6	Qualifier Character 7
0 Brain **1** Cerebral Meninges **2** Dura Mater **3** Epidural Space **4** Subdural Space **5** Subarachnoid Space **6** Cerebral Ventricle **7** Cerebral Hemisphere **8** Basal Ganglia **9** Thalamus **A** Hypothalamus **B** Pons **C** Cerebellum **D** Medulla Oblongata **F** Olfactory Nerve **G** Optic Nerve **H** Oculomotor Nerve **J** Trochlear Nerve **K** Trigeminal Nerve **L** Abducens Nerve **M** Facial Nerve **N** Acoustic Nerve **P** Glossopharyngeal Nerve **Q** Vagus Nerve **R** Accessory Nerve **S** Hypoglossal Nerve **T** Spinal Meninges **W** Cervical Spinal Cord **X** Thoracic Spinal Cord **Y** Lumbar Spinal Cord	**0** Open **3** Percutaneous **4** Percutaneous Endoscopic	**Z** No Device	**Z** No Qualifier

0 Medical and Surgical
0 Central Nervous System
D Extraction: Pulling or stripping out or off all or a portion of a body part by the use of force

Body Part Character 4	Approach Character 5	Device Character 6	Qualifier Character 7
1 Cerebral Meninges **2** Dura Mater **F** Olfactory Nerve **G** Optic Nerve **H** Oculomotor Nerve **J** Trochlear Nerve **K** Trigeminal Nerve **L** Abducens Nerve **M** Facial Nerve **N** Acoustic Nerve **P** Glossopharyngeal Nerve **Q** Vagus Nerve **R** Accessory Nerve **S** Hypoglossal Nerve **T** Spinal Meninges	**0** Open **3** Percutaneous **4** Percutaneous Endoscopic	**Z** No Device	**Z** No Qualifier

LC Limited Coverage NC Noncovered HAC HAC Associated Procedure CC Combination Cluster - See Appendix G for code lists
DRG Non-OR-Affecting MS-DRG Assignment ⊘ Non-OR-Not Affecting MS-DRG Assignment New/Revised Text in **Orange** ♂ Male ♀ Female

0 Medical and Surgical
0 Central Nervous System
F Fragmentation: Breaking solid matter in a body part into pieces

Body Part Character 4	Approach Character 5	Device Character 6	Qualifier Character 7
3 Epidural Space NC ⦸	**0** Open	**Z** No Device	**Z** No Qualifier
4 Subdural Space NC ⦸	**3** Percutaneous		
5 Subarachnoid Space NC ⦸	**4** Percutaneous Endoscopic		
6 Cerebral Ventricle NC ⦸	**X** External		
U Spinal Canal			

NC 00F3XZZ 00F4XZZ 00F5XZZ 00F6XZZ
⦸ 00F3XZZ 00F4XZZ 00F5XZZ 00F6XZZ

0 Medical and Surgical
0 Central Nervous System
H Insertion: Putting in a nonbiological appliance that monitors, assists, performs, or prevents a physiological function but does not physically take the place of a body part

Body Part Character 4	Approach Character 5	Device Character 6	Qualifier Character 7
0 Brain CC	**0** Open	**2** Monitoring Device	**Z** No Qualifier
6 Cerebral Ventricle CC	**3** Percutaneous	**3** Infusion Device	
E Cranial Nerve CC	**4** Percutaneous Endoscopic	**M** Neurostimulator Lead	
U Spinal Canal ⦸ CC			
V Spinal Cord ⦸ CC			

CC 00H00MZ 00H03MZ 00H04MZ 00H60MZ 00H63MZ 00H64MZ 00HE0MZ 00HE3MZ 00HE4MZ 00HU0MZ 00HU3MZ 00HU4MZ 00HV0MZ 00HV3MZ 00HV4MZ
⦸ 00HU03Z 00HU33Z 00HU43Z 00HV03Z 00HV33Z 00HV43Z

0 Medical and Surgical
0 Central Nervous System
J Inspection: Visually and/or manually exploring a body part

Body Part Character 4	Approach Character 5	Device Character 6	Qualifier Character 7
0 Brain ⦸	**0** Open	**Z** No Device	**Z** No Qualifier
E Cranial Nerve ⦸	**3** Percutaneous		
U Spinal Canal ⦸	**4** Percutaneous Endoscopic		
V Spinal Cord ⦸			

⦸ 00J03ZZ 00JE3ZZ 00JU3ZZ 00JV3ZZ

0 Medical and Surgical
0 Central Nervous System
K Map: Locating the route of passage of electrical impulses and/or locating functional areas in a body part

Body Part Character 4	Approach Character 5	Device Character 6	Qualifier Character 7
0 Brain	**0** Open	**Z** No Device	**Z** No Qualifier
7 Cerebral Hemisphere	**3** Percutaneous		
8 Basal Ganglia	**4** Percutaneous Endoscopic		
9 Thalamus			
A Hypothalamus			
B Pons			
C Cerebellum			
D Medulla Oblongata			

0 Medical and Surgical
0 Central Nervous System
N Release: Freeing a body part from an abnormal physical constraint by cutting or by the use of force

Body Part Character 4	Approach Character 5	Device Character 6	Qualifier Character 7
0 Brain **1** Cerebral Meninges **2** Dura Mater **6** Cerebral Ventricle **7** Cerebral Hemisphere **8** Basal Ganglia **9** Thalamus **A** Hypothalamus **B** Pons **C** Cerebellum **D** Medulla Oblongata **F** Olfactory Nerve **G** Optic Nerve **H** Oculomotor Nerve **J** Trochlear Nerve **K** Trigeminal Nerve **L** Abducens Nerve **M** Facial Nerve **N** Acoustic Nerve **P** Glossopharyngeal Nerve **Q** Vagus Nerve **R** Accessory Nerve **S** Hypoglossal Nerve **T** Spinal Meninges **W** Cervical Spinal Cord **X** Thoracic Spinal Cord **Y** Lumbar Spinal Cord	**0** Open **3** Percutaneous **4** Percutaneous Endoscopic	**Z** No Device	**Z** No Qualifier

0 Medical and Surgical
0 Central Nervous System
P Removal: Taking out or off a device from a body part

Body Part Character 4	Approach Character 5	Device Character 6	Qualifier Character 7
0 Brain **V** Spinal Cord	**0** Open **3** Percutaneous **4** Percutaneous Endoscopic	**0** Drainage Device **2** Monitoring Device **3** Infusion Device **7** Autologous Tissue Substitute **J** Synthetic Substitute **K** Nonautologous Tissue Substitute **M** Neurostimulator Lead	**Z** No Qualifier
0 Brain ⃠ **V** Spinal Cord ⃠	**X** External	**0** Drainage Device **2** Monitoring Device **3** Infusion Device **M** Neurostimulator Lead	**Z** No Qualifier
6 Cerebral Ventricle **U** Spinal Canal	**0** Open **3** Percutaneous **4** Percutaneous Endoscopic	**0** Drainage Device **2** Monitoring Device **3** Infusion Device **J** Synthetic Substitute **M** Neurostimulator Lead	**Z** No Qualifier
6 Cerebral Ventricle ⃠ **U** Spinal Canal ⃠	**X** External	**0** Drainage Device **2** Monitoring Device **3** Infusion Device **M** Neurostimulator Lead	**Z** No Qualifier
E Cranial Nerve	**0** Open **3** Percutaneous **4** Percutaneous Endoscopic	**0** Drainage Device **2** Monitoring Device **3** Infusion Device **7** Autologous Tissue Substitute **M** Neurostimulator Lead	**Z** No Qualifier
E Cranial Nerve ⃠	**X** External	**0** Drainage Device **2** Monitoring Device **3** Infusion Device **M** Neurostimulator Lead	**Z** No Qualifier

⃠ 00P0X0Z 00P0X2Z 00P0X3Z 00P0XMZ 00P6X0Z 00P6X3Z 00PEX0Z 00PEX2Z 00PEX3Z 00PUX0Z 00PUX2Z 00PUX3Z 00PUXMZ 00PVX0Z 00PVX2Z 00PVX3Z 00PVXMZ

0 Medical and Surgical
0 Central Nervous System
Q Repair: Restoring, to the extent possible, a body part to its normal anatomic structure and function

Body Part Character 4	Approach Character 5	Device Character 6	Qualifier Character 7
0 Brain **1** Cerebral Meninges **2** Dura Mater **6** Cerebral Ventricle **7** Cerebral Hemisphere **8** Basal Ganglia **9** Thalamus **A** Hypothalamus **B** Pons **C** Cerebellum **D** Medulla Oblongata **F** Olfactory Nerve **G** Optic Nerve **H** Oculomotor Nerve **J** Trochlear Nerve **K** Trigeminal Nerve **L** Abducens Nerve **M** Facial Nerve **N** Acoustic Nerve **P** Glossopharyngeal Nerve **Q** Vagus Nerve **R** Accessory Nerve **S** Hypoglossal Nerve **T** Spinal Meninges **W** Cervical Spinal Cord **X** Thoracic Spinal Cord **Y** Lumbar Spinal Cord	**0** Open **3** Percutaneous **4** Percutaneous Endoscopic	**Z** No Device	**Z** No Qualifier

0 Medical and Surgical
0 Central Nervous System
S Reposition: Moving to its normal location, or other suitable location, all or a portion of a body part

Body Part Character 4	Approach Character 5	Device Character 6	Qualifier Character 7
F Olfactory Nerve **G** Optic Nerve **H** Oculomotor Nerve **J** Trochlear Nerve **K** Trigeminal Nerve **L** Abducens Nerve **M** Facial Nerve **N** Acoustic Nerve **P** Glossopharyngeal Nerve **Q** Vagus Nerve **R** Accessory Nerve **S** Hypoglossal Nerve **W** Cervical Spinal Cord **X** Thoracic Spinal Cord **Y** Lumbar Spinal Cord	**0** Open **3** Percutaneous **4** Percutaneous Endoscopic	**Z** No Device	**Z** No Qualifier

0 Medical and Surgical
0 Central Nervous System
T Resection: Cutting out or off, without replacement, all of a body part

Body Part Character 4	Approach Character 5	Device Character 6	Qualifier Character 7
7 Cerebral Hemisphere	0 Open 3 Percutaneous 4 Percutaneous Endoscopic	Z No Device	Z No Qualifier

0 Medical and Surgical
0 Central Nervous System
U Supplement: Putting in or on biological or synthetic material that physically reinforces and/or augments the function of a portion of a body part

Body Part Character 4	Approach Character 5	Device Character 6	Qualifier Character 7
1 Cerebral Meninges 2 Dura Mater T Spinal Meninges	0 Open 3 Percutaneous 4 Percutaneous Endoscopic	7 Autologous Tissue Substitute J Synthetic Substitute K Nonautologous Tissue Substitute	Z No Qualifier
F Olfactory Nerve G Optic Nerve H Oculomotor Nerve J Trochlear Nerve K Trigeminal Nerve L Abducens Nerve M Facial Nerve N Acoustic Nerve P Glossopharyngeal Nerve Q Vagus Nerve R Accessory Nerve S Hypoglossal Nerve	0 Open 3 Percutaneous 4 Percutaneous Endoscopic	7 Autologous Tissue Substitute	Z No Qualifier

0 Medical and Surgical
0 Central Nervous System
W Revision: Correcting, to the extent possible, a portion of a malfunctioning device or the position of a displaced device

Body Part Character 4	Approach Character 5	Device Character 6	Qualifier Character 7
0 Brain ⦸ V Spinal Cord ⦸	0 Open 3 Percutaneous 4 Percutaneous Endoscopic X External	0 Drainage Device 2 Monitoring Device 3 Infusion Device 7 Autologous Tissue Substitute J Synthetic Substitute K Nonautologous Tissue Substitute M Neurostimulator Lead	Z No Qualifier
6 Cerebral Ventricle ⦸ U Spinal Canal ⦸	0 Open 3 Percutaneous 4 Percutaneous Endoscopic X External	0 Drainage Device 2 Monitoring Device 3 Infusion Device J Synthetic Substitute M Neurostimulator Lead	Z No Qualifier
E Cranial Nerve ⦸	0 Open 3 Percutaneous 4 Percutaneous Endoscopic X External	0 Drainage Device 2 Monitoring Device 3 Infusion Device 7 Autologous Tissue Substitute M Neurostimulator Lead	Z No Qualifier

⦸ 00W0X0Z 00W0X2Z 00W0X3Z 00W0X7Z 00W0XJZ 00W0XKZ 00W0XMZ 00W6X0Z 00W6X2Z 00W6X3Z 00W6XJZ 00W6XMZ 00WEX0Z 00WEX2Z 00WEX3Z 00WEX7Z 00WEXMZ 00WUX0Z 00WUX2Z 00WUX3Z 00WUXJZ 00WUXMZ 00WVX0Z 00WVX2Z 00WVX3Z 00WVX7Z 00WVXJZ 00WVXKZ 00WVXMZ

0 Medical and Surgical
0 Central Nervous System
X Transfer: Moving, without taking out, all or a portion of a body part to another location to take over the function of all or a portion of a body part

Body Part Character 4	Approach Character 5	Device Character 6	Qualifier Character 7
F Olfactory Nerve **G** Optic Nerve **H** Oculomotor Nerve **J** Trochlear Nerve **K** Trigeminal Nerve **L** Abducens Nerve **M** Facial Nerve **N** Acoustic Nerve **P** Glossopharyngeal Nerve **Q** Vagus Nerve **R** Accessory Nerve **S** Hypoglossal Nerve	**0** Open **4** Percutaneous Endoscopic	**Z** No Device	**F** Olfactory Nerve **G** Optic Nerve **H** Oculomotor Nerve **J** Trochlear Nerve **K** Trigeminal Nerve **L** Abducens Nerve **M** Facial Nerve **N** Acoustic Nerve **P** Glossopharyngeal Nerve **Q** Vagus Nerve **R** Accessory Nerve **S** Hypoglossal Nerve

Peripheral Nervous System 012-01X

0 Medical and Surgical
1 Peripheral Nervous System
2 Change: Taking out or off a device from a body part and putting back an identical or similar device in or on the same body part without cutting or puncturing the skin or a mucous membrane

Body Part Character 4	Approach Character 5	Device Character 6	Qualifier Character 7
Y Peripheral Nerve ⊘	**X** External	**0** Drainage Device **Y** Other Device	**Z** No Qualifier

⊘ 012YX0Z 012YXYZ

0 Medical and Surgical
1 Peripheral Nervous System
5 Destruction: Physical eradication of all or a portion of a body part by the direct use of energy, force, or a destructive agent

Body Part Character 4	Approach Character 5	Device Character 6	Qualifier Character 7
0 Cervical Plexus ⊘ **1** Cervical Nerve ⊘ **2** Phrenic Nerve ⊘ **3** Brachial Plexus ⊘ **4** Ulnar Nerve ⊘ **5** Median Nerve ⊘ **6** Radial Nerve ⊘ **8** Thoracic Nerve ⊘ **9** Lumbar Plexus ⊘ **A** Lumbosacral Plexus ⊘ **B** Lumbar Nerve ⊘ **C** Pudendal Nerve ⊘ **D** Femoral Nerve ⊘ **F** Sciatic Nerve ⊘ **G** Tibial Nerve ⊘ **H** Peroneal Nerve ⊘ **K** Head and Neck Sympathetic Nerve **L** Thoracic Sympathetic Nerve **M** Abdominal Sympathetic Nerve **N** Lumbar Sympathetic Nerve **P** Sacral Sympathetic Nerve **Q** Sacral Plexus ⊘ **R** Sacral Nerve ⊘	**0** Open **3** Percutaneous **4** Percutaneous Endoscopic	**Z** No Device	**Z** No Qualifier

⊘ 01500ZZ 01503ZZ 01504ZZ 01513ZZ 01520ZZ 01523ZZ 01524ZZ 01530ZZ 01533ZZ 01534ZZ 01540ZZ 01543ZZ 01544ZZ 01550ZZ 01553ZZ 01554ZZ 01560ZZ 01563ZZ 01564ZZ 01583ZZ 01590ZZ 01593ZZ 01594ZZ 015A0ZZ 015A3ZZ 015A4ZZ 015B3ZZ 015C0ZZ 015C3ZZ 015C4ZZ 015D0ZZ 015D3ZZ 015D4ZZ 015F0ZZ 015F3ZZ 015F4ZZ 015G0ZZ 015G3ZZ 015G4ZZ 015H0ZZ 015H3ZZ 015H4ZZ 015Q0ZZ 015Q3ZZ 015Q4ZZ 015R3ZZ

0 Medical and Surgical
1 Peripheral Nervous System
8 Division: Cutting into a body part, without draining fluids and/or gases from the body part, in order to separate or transect a body part

Body Part Character 4	Approach Character 5	Device Character 6	Qualifier Character 7
0 Cervical Plexus **1** Cervical Nerve **2** Phrenic Nerve **3** Brachial Plexus **4** Ulnar Nerve **5** Median Nerve **6** Radial Nerve **8** Thoracic Nerve **9** Lumbar Plexus **A** Lumbosacral Plexus **B** Lumbar Nerve **C** Pudendal Nerve **D** Femoral Nerve **F** Sciatic Nerve **G** Tibial Nerve **H** Peroneal Nerve **K** Head and Neck Sympathetic Nerve **L** Thoracic Sympathetic Nerve **M** Abdominal Sympathetic Nerve **N** Lumbar Sympathetic Nerve **P** Sacral Sympathetic Nerve **Q** Sacral Plexus **R** Sacral Nerve	**0** Open **3** Percutaneous **4** Percutaneous Endoscopic	**Z** No Device	**Z** No Qualifier

0 Medical and Surgical
1 Peripheral Nervous System
9 Drainage: Taking or letting out fluids and/or gases from a body part

Body Part Character 4	Approach Character 5	Device Character 6	Qualifier Character 7
0 Cervical Plexus ⊘ **1** Cervical Nerve ⊘ **2** Phrenic Nerve ⊘ **3** Brachial Plexus ⊘ **4** Ulnar Nerve ⊘ **5** Median Nerve ⊘ **6** Radial Nerve ⊘ **8** Thoracic Nerve ⊘ **9** Lumbar Plexus ⊘ **A** Lumbosacral Plexus ⊘ **B** Lumbar Nerve ⊘ **C** Pudendal Nerve ⊘ **D** Femoral Nerve ⊘ **F** Sciatic Nerve ⊘ **G** Tibial Nerve ⊘ **H** Peroneal Nerve ⊘ **K** Head and Neck Sympathetic Nerve ⊘ **L** Thoracic Sympathetic Nerve ⊘ **M** Abdominal Sympathetic Nerve ⊘ **N** Lumbar Sympathetic Nerve ⊘ **P** Sacral Sympathetic Nerve ⊘ **Q** Sacral Plexus ⊘ **R** Sacral Nerve ⊘	**0** Open **3** Percutaneous **4** Percutaneous Endoscopic	**0** Drainage Device	**Z** No Qualifier
0 Cervical Plexus ⊘ **1** Cervical Nerve ⊘ **2** Phrenic Nerve ⊘ **3** Brachial Plexus ⊘ **4** Ulnar Nerve ⊘ **5** Median Nerve ⊘ **6** Radial Nerve ⊘ **8** Thoracic Nerve ⊘ **9** Lumbar Plexus ⊘ **A** Lumbosacral Plexus ⊘ **B** Lumbar Nerve ⊘ **C** Pudendal Nerve ⊘ **D** Femoral Nerve ⊘ **F** Sciatic Nerve ⊘ **G** Tibial Nerve ⊘ **H** Peroneal Nerve ⊘ **K** Head and Neck Sympathetic Nerve ⊘ **L** Thoracic Sympathetic Nerve ⊘ **M** Abdominal Sympathetic Nerve ⊘ **N** Lumbar Sympathetic Nerve ⊘ **P** Sacral Sympathetic Nerve ⊘ **Q** Sacral Plexus ⊘ **R** Sacral Nerve ⊘	**0** Open **3** Percutaneous **4** Percutaneous Endoscopic	**Z** No Device	**X** Diagnostic **Z** No Qualifier

⊘ 019030Z 01903ZX 01903ZZ 01904ZX 019130Z 01913ZX 01913ZZ 01914ZX 019230Z 01923ZX 01923ZZ 01924ZX 019330Z 01933ZX 01933ZZ 01934ZX 019430Z 01943ZX 01943ZZ 01944ZX 019530Z 01953ZX 01953ZZ 01954ZX 019630Z 01963ZX 01963ZZ 01964ZX 019830Z 01983ZX 01983ZZ 01984ZX 019930Z 01993ZX 01993ZZ 01994ZX 019A30Z 019A3ZX 019A3ZZ 019A4ZX 019B30Z 019B3ZX 019B3ZZ 019B4ZX 019C30Z 019C3ZX 019C3ZZ 019C4ZX 019D30Z 019D3ZX 019D3ZZ 019D4ZX 019F30Z 019F3ZX 019F3ZZ 019F4ZX 019G30Z 019G3ZX 019G3ZZ 019G4ZX 019H30Z 019H3ZX 019H3ZZ 019H4ZX 019K30Z 019K3ZZ 019L30Z 019L3ZZ 019M30Z 019M3ZZ 019N30Z 019N3ZZ 019P30Z 019P3ZZ 019Q30Z 019Q3ZX 019Q3ZZ 019Q4ZX 019R30Z 019R3ZX 019R3ZZ 019R4ZX

0 Medical and Surgical
1 Peripheral Nervous System
B Excision: Cutting out or off, without replacement, a portion of a body part

Body Part Character 4	Approach Character 5	Device Character 6	Qualifier Character 7
0 Cervical Plexus ⦸	0 Open	Z No Device	X Diagnostic
1 Cervical Nerve ⦸	3 Percutaneous		Z No Qualifier
2 Phrenic Nerve ⦸	4 Percutaneous Endoscopic		
3 Brachial Plexus ⦸ CC			
4 Ulnar Nerve ⦸			
5 Median Nerve ⦸			
6 Radial Nerve ⦸			
8 Thoracic Nerve ⦸			
9 Lumbar Plexus ⦸			
A Lumbosacral Plexus ⦸			
B Lumbar Nerve ⦸			
C Pudendal Nerve ⦸			
D Femoral Nerve ⦸			
F Sciatic Nerve ⦸			
G Tibial Nerve ⦸			
H Peroneal Nerve ⦸			
K Head and Neck Sympathetic Nerve			
L Thoracic Sympathetic Nerve CC			
M Abdominal Sympathetic Nerve			
N Lumbar Sympathetic Nerve			
P Sacral Sympathetic Nerve			
Q Sacral Plexus ⦸			
R Sacral Nerve ⦸			

CC 01B30ZZ 01BL0ZZ
⦸ 01B03ZX 01B04ZX 01B13ZX 01B14ZX 01B23ZX 01B24ZX 01B33ZX 01B34ZX 01B43ZX 01B44ZX 01B53ZX 01B54ZX 01B63ZX 01B64ZX 01B83ZX 01B84ZX 01B93ZX 01B94ZX 01BA3ZX 01BA4ZX 01BB3ZX 01BB4ZX 01BC3ZX 01BC4ZX 01BD3ZX 01BD4ZX 01BF3ZX 01BF4ZX 01BG3ZX 01BG4ZX 01BH3ZX 01BH4ZX 01BQ3ZX 01BQ4ZX 01BR3ZX 01BR4ZX

0 Medical and Surgical
1 Peripheral Nervous System
C Extirpation: Taking or cutting out solid matter from a body part

Body Part Character 4	Approach Character 5	Device Character 6	Qualifier Character 7
0 Cervical Plexus	0 Open	Z No Device	Z No Qualifier
1 Cervical Nerve	3 Percutaneous		
2 Phrenic Nerve	4 Percutaneous Endoscopic		
3 Brachial Plexus			
4 Ulnar Nerve			
5 Median Nerve			
6 Radial Nerve			
8 Thoracic Nerve			
9 Lumbar Plexus			
A Lumbosacral Plexus			
B Lumbar Nerve			
C Pudendal Nerve			
D Femoral Nerve			
F Sciatic Nerve			
G Tibial Nerve			
H Peroneal Nerve			
K Head and Neck Sympathetic Nerve			
L Thoracic Sympathetic Nerve			
M Abdominal Sympathetic Nerve			
N Lumbar Sympathetic Nerve			
P Sacral Sympathetic Nerve			
Q Sacral Plexus			
R Sacral Nerve			

0 Medical and Surgical
1 Peripheral Nervous System
D Extraction: Pulling or stripping out or off all or a portion of a body part by the use of force

Body Part Character 4	Approach Character 5	Device Character 6	Qualifier Character 7
0 Cervical Plexus **1** Cervical Nerve **2** Phrenic Nerve **3** Brachial Plexus **4** Ulnar Nerve **5** Median Nerve **6** Radial Nerve **8** Thoracic Nerve **9** Lumbar Plexus **A** Lumbosacral Plexus **B** Lumbar Nerve **C** Pudendal Nerve **D** Femoral Nerve **F** Sciatic Nerve **G** Tibial Nerve **H** Peroneal Nerve **K** Head and Neck Sympathetic Nerve **L** Thoracic Sympathetic Nerve **M** Abdominal Sympathetic Nerve **N** Lumbar Sympathetic Nerve **P** Sacral Sympathetic Nerve **Q** Sacral Plexus **R** Sacral Nerve	**0** Open **3** Percutaneous **4** Percutaneous Endoscopic	**Z** No Device	**Z** No Qualifier

0 Medical and Surgical
1 Peripheral Nervous System
H Insertion: Putting in a nonbiological appliance that monitors, assists, performs, or prevents a physiological function but does not physically take the place of a body part

Body Part Character 4	Approach Character 5	Device Character 6	Qualifier Character 7
Y Peripheral Nerve CC	**0** Open **3** Percutaneous **4** Percutaneous Endoscopic	**2** Monitoring Device **M** Neurostimulator Lead	**Z** No Qualifier

CC 01HY0MZ 01HY3MZ 01HY4MZ

0 Medical and Surgical
1 Peripheral Nervous System
J Inspection: Visually and/or manually exploring a body part

Body Part Character 4	Approach Character 5	Device Character 6	Qualifier Character 7
Y Peripheral Nerve ⃠	**0** Open **3** Percutaneous **4** Percutaneous Endoscopic	**Z** No Device	**Z** No Qualifier

⃠ 01JY3ZZ

0 Medical and Surgical
1 Peripheral Nervous System
N Release: Freeing a body part from an abnormal physical constraint by cutting or by the use of force

Body Part Character 4	Approach Character 5	Device Character 6	Qualifier Character 7
0 Cervical Plexus **1** Cervical Nerve **2** Phrenic Nerve **3** Brachial Plexus **4** Ulnar Nerve **5** Median Nerve **6** Radial Nerve **8** Thoracic Nerve **9** Lumbar Plexus **A** Lumbosacral Plexus **B** Lumbar Nerve **C** Pudendal Nerve **D** Femoral Nerve **F** Sciatic Nerve **G** Tibial Nerve **H** Peroneal Nerve **K** Head and Neck Sympathetic Nerve **L** Thoracic Sympathetic Nerve **M** Abdominal Sympathetic Nerve **N** Lumbar Sympathetic Nerve **P** Sacral Sympathetic Nerve **Q** Sacral Plexus **R** Sacral Nerve	**0** Open **3** Percutaneous **4** Percutaneous Endoscopic	**Z** No Device	**Z** No Qualifier

0 Medical and Surgical
1 Peripheral Nervous System
P Removal: Taking out or off a device from a body part

Body Part Character 4	Approach Character 5	Device Character 6	Qualifier Character 7
Y Peripheral Nerve	**0** Open **3** Percutaneous **4** Percutaneous Endoscopic	**0** Drainage Device **2** Monitoring Device **7** Autologous Tissue Substitute **M** Neurostimulator Lead	**Z** No Qualifier
Y Peripheral Nerve ⃠	**X** External	**0** Drainage Device **2** Monitoring Device **M** Neurostimulator Lead	**Z** No Qualifier

⃠ 01PYX0Z 01PYX2Z

0 Medical and Surgical
1 Peripheral Nervous System
Q Repair: Restoring, to the extent possible, a body part to its normal anatomic structure and function

Body Part Character 4	Approach Character 5	Device Character 6	Qualifier Character 7
0 Cervical Plexus **1** Cervical Nerve **2** Phrenic Nerve **3** Brachial Plexus **4** Ulnar Nerve **5** Median Nerve **6** Radial Nerve **8** Thoracic Nerve **9** Lumbar Plexus **A** Lumbosacral Plexus **B** Lumbar Nerve **C** Pudendal Nerve **D** Femoral Nerve **F** Sciatic Nerve **G** Tibial Nerve **H** Peroneal Nerve **K** Head and Neck Sympathetic Nerve **L** Thoracic Sympathetic Nerve **M** Abdominal Sympathetic Nerve **N** Lumbar Sympathetic Nerve **P** Sacral Sympathetic Nerve **Q** Sacral Plexus **R** Sacral Nerve	**0** Open **3** Percutaneous **4** Percutaneous Endoscopic	**Z** No Device	**Z** No Qualifier

0 Medical and Surgical
1 Peripheral Nervous System
S Reposition: Moving to its normal location, or other suitable location, all or a portion of a body part

Body Part Character 4	Approach Character 5	Device Character 6	Qualifier Character 7
0 Cervical Plexus **1** Cervical Nerve **2** Phrenic Nerve **3** Brachial Plexus **4** Ulnar Nerve **5** Median Nerve **6** Radial Nerve **8** Thoracic Nerve **9** Lumbar Plexus **A** Lumbosacral Plexus **B** Lumbar Nerve **C** Pudendal Nerve **D** Femoral Nerve **F** Sciatic Nerve **G** Tibial Nerve **H** Peroneal Nerve **Q** Sacral Plexus **R** Sacral Nerve	**0** Open **3** Percutaneous **4** Percutaneous Endoscopic	**Z** No Device	**Z** No Qualifier

0 Medical and Surgical
1 Peripheral Nervous System
U Supplement: Putting in or on biological or synthetic material that physically reinforces and/or augments the function of a portion of a body part

Body Part Character 4	Approach Character 5	Device Character 6	Qualifier Character 7
1 Cervical Nerve 2 Phrenic Nerve 4 Ulnar Nerve 5 Median Nerve 6 Radial Nerve 8 Thoracic Nerve B Lumbar Nerve C Pudendal Nerve D Femoral Nerve F Sciatic Nerve G Tibial Nerve H Peroneal Nerve R Sacral Nerve	0 Open 3 Percutaneous 4 Percutaneous Endoscopic	7 Autologous Tissue Substitute	Z No Qualifier

0 Medical and Surgical
1 Peripheral Nervous System
W Revision: Correcting, to the extent possible, a portion of a malfunctioning device or the position of a displaced device

Body Part Character 4	Approach Character 5	Device Character 6	Qualifier Character 7
Y Peripheral Nerve ⊘	0 Open 3 Percutaneous 4 Percutaneous Endoscopic X External	0 Drainage Device 2 Monitoring Device 7 Autologous Tissue Substitute M Neurostimulator Lead	Z No Qualifier

⊘ 01WYX0Z 01WYX2Z 01WYX7Z 01WYXMZ

0 Medical and Surgical
1 Peripheral Nervous System
X Transfer: Moving, without taking out, all or a portion of a body part to another location to take over the function of all or a portion of a body part

Body Part Character 4	Approach Character 5	Device Character 6	Qualifier Character 7
1 Cervical Nerve 2 Phrenic Nerve	0 Open 4 Percutaneous Endoscopic	Z No Device	1 Cervical Nerve 2 Phrenic Nerve
4 Ulnar Nerve 5 Median Nerve 6 Radial Nerve	0 Open 4 Percutaneous Endoscopic	Z No Device	4 Ulnar Nerve 5 Median Nerve 6 Radial Nerve
8 Thoracic Nerve	0 Open 4 Percutaneous Endoscopic	Z No Device	8 Thoracic Nerve
B Lumbar Nerve C Pudendal Nerve	0 Open 4 Percutaneous Endoscopic	Z No Device	B Lumbar Nerve C Perineal Nerve
D Femoral Nerve F Sciatic Nerve G Tibial Nerve H Peroneal Nerve	0 Open 4 Percutaneous Endoscopic	Z No Device	D Femoral Nerve F Sciatic Nerve G Tibial Nerve H Peroneal Nerve

Heart and Great Vessels 021-02Y

0 Medical and Surgical
2 Heart and Great Vessels
1 Bypass: Altering the route of passage of the contents of a tubular body part

Body Part Character 4	Approach Character 5	Device Character 6	Qualifier Character 7
0 Coronary Artery, One Artery HAC ⊘ **1** Coronary Artery, Two Arteries HAC ⊘ **2** Coronary Artery, Three Arteries HAC ⊘ **3** Coronary Artery, Four or More Arteries HAC ⊘	**0** Open	**8** Zooplastic Tissue **9** Autologous Venous Tissue **A** Autologous Arterial Tissue **J** Synthetic Substitute **K** Nonautologous Tissue Substitute	**3** Coronary Artery **8** Internal Mammary, Right **9** Internal Mammary, Left **C** Thoracic Artery **F** Abdominal Artery **W** Aorta
0 Coronary Artery, One Artery HAC **1** Coronary Artery, Two Arteries HAC **2** Coronary Artery, Three Arteries HAC **3** Coronary Artery, Four or More Arteries HAC	**0** Open	**Z** No Device	**3** Coronary Artery **8** Internal Mammary, Right **9** Internal Mammary, Left **C** Thoracic Artery **F** Abdominal Artery
0 Coronary Artery, One Artery ⊘ **1** Coronary Artery, Two Arteries ⊘ **2** Coronary Artery, Three Arteries ⊘ **3** Coronary Artery, Four or More Arteries ⊘	**3** Percutaneous	**4** Intraluminal Device, Drug-eluting **D** Intraluminal Device	**4** Coronary Vein
0 Coronary Artery, One Artery ⊘ **1** Coronary Artery, Two Arteries ⊘ **2** Coronary Artery, Three Arteries ⊘ **3** Coronary Artery, Four or More Arteries ⊘	**4** Percutaneous Endoscopic	**4** Intraluminal Device, Drug-eluting **D** Intraluminal Device	**4** Coronary Vein
0 Coronary Artery, One Artery HAC ⊘ **1** Coronary Artery, Two Arteries HAC ⊘ **2** Coronary Artery, Three Arteries HAC ⊘ **3** Coronary Artery, Four or More Arteries HAC ⊘	**4** Percutaneous Endoscopic	**8** Zooplastic Tissue **9** Autologous Venous Tissue **A** Autologous Arterial Tissue **J** Synthetic Substitute **K** Nonautologous Tissue Substitute	**3** Coronary Artery **8** Internal Mammary, Right **9** Internal Mammary, Left **C** Thoracic Artery **F** Abdominal Artery **W** Aorta
0 Coronary Artery, One Artery HAC **1** Coronary Artery, Two Arteries HAC **2** Coronary Artery, Three Arteries HAC **3** Coronary Artery, Four or More Arteries HAC	**4** Percutaneous Endoscopic	**Z** No Device	**3** Coronary Artery **8** Internal Mammary, Right **9** Internal Mammary, Left **C** Thoracic Artery **F** Abdominal Artery
6 Atrium, Right ⊘	**0** Open **4** Percutaneous Endoscopic	**8** Zooplastic Tissue **9** Autologous Venous Tissue **A** Autologous Arterial Tissue **J** Synthetic Substitute **K** Nonautologous Tissue Substitute	**P** Pulmonary Trunk **Q** Pulmonary Artery, Right **R** Pulmonary Artery, Left
6 Atrium, Right	**0** Open **4** Percutaneous Endoscopic	**Z** No Device	**7** Atrium, Left **P** Pulmonary Trunk **Q** Pulmonary Artery, Right **R** Pulmonary Artery, Left

021 continued on next page

021 continued from previous page

0 Medical and Surgical
2 Heart and Great Vessels
1 Bypass: Altering the route of passage of the contents of a tubular body part

Body Part Character 4	Approach Character 5	Device Character 6	Qualifier Character 7
7 Atrium, Left LC ⦸ **V** Superior Vena Cava ⦸	**0** Open **4** Percutaneous Endoscopic	**8** Zooplastic Tissue **9** Autologous Venous Tissue **A** Autologous Arterial Tissue **J** Synthetic Substitute **K** Nonautologous Tissue Substitute **Z** No Device	**P** Pulmonary Trunk **Q** Pulmonary Artery, Right **R** Pulmonary Artery, Left **S** Pulmonary Vein, Right **T** Pulmonary Vein, Left **U** Pulmonary Vein, Confluence
K Ventricle, Right ⦸ **L** Ventricle, Left ⦸	**0** Open **4** Percutaneous Endoscopic	**8** Zooplastic Tissue **9** Autologous Venous Tissue **A** Autologous Arterial Tissue **J** Synthetic Substitute **K** Nonautologous Tissue Substitute	**P** Pulmonary Trunk **Q** Pulmonary Artery, Right **R** Pulmonary Artery, Left
K Ventricle, Right **L** Ventricle, Left	**0** Open **4** Percutaneous Endoscopic	**Z** No Device	**5** Coronary Circulation **8** Internal Mammary, Right **9** Internal Mammary, Left **C** Thoracic Artery **F** Abdominal Artery **P** Pulmonary Trunk **Q** Pulmonary Artery, Right **R** Pulmonary Artery, Left **W** Aorta
P Pulmonary Trunk ⦸ **Q** Pulmonary Artery, Right ⦸ **R** Pulmonary Artery, Left ⦸	**0** Open **4** Percutaneous Endoscopic	**8** Zooplastic Tissue **9** Autologous Venous Tissue **A** Autologous Arterial Tissue **J** Synthetic Substitute **K** Nonautologous Tissue Substitute **Z** No Device	**A** Innominate Artery **B** Subclavian **D** Carotid
W Thoracic Aorta, Descending ⦸ **X** Thoracic Aorta, Ascending/Arch ⦸	**0** Open **4** Percutaneous Endoscopic	**8** Zooplastic Tissue **9** Autologous Venous Tissue **A** Autologous Arterial Tissue **J** Synthetic Substitute **K** Nonautologous Tissue Substitute **Z** No Device	**B** Subclavian **D** Carotid **P** Pulmonary Trunk **Q** Pulmonary Artery, Right **R** Pulmonary Artery, Left

⦸ 0210083 0210088 0210089 021008C 021008F 021008W 0210344 02103D4 0210444 0210483 0210488 0210489 021048C 021048F 021048W 02104D4 0211083 0211088 0211089 021108C 021108F 021108W 0211344 02113D4 0211444 0211483 0211488 0211489 021148C 021148F 021148W 02114D4 0212083 0212088 0212089 021208C 021208F 021208W 0212344 02123D4 0212444 0212483 0212488 0212489 021248C 021248F 021248W 02124D4 0213083 0213088 0213089 021308C 021308F 021308W 0213344 02133D4 0213444 0213483 0213488 0213489 021348C 021348F 021348W 02134D4 021608P 021608Q 021608R 021648P 021648Q 021648R 021708P 021708Q 021708R 021708S 021708T 021708U 021709S 021709T 021709U 02170AS 02170AT 02170AU 02170JS 02170JT 02170JU 02170KS 02170KT 02170KU 02170ZS 02170ZT 02170ZU 021748P 021748Q 021748R 021748S 021748T 021748U 021749S 021749T 021749U 02174AS 02174AT 02174AU 02174JS 02174JT 02174JU 02174KS 02174KT 02174KU 02174ZS 02174ZT 02174ZU 021K08P 021K08Q 021K08R 021K48P 021K48Q 021K48R 021L08P 021L08Q 021L08R 021L48P 021L48Q 021L48R 021P08A 021P08B 021P08D 021P09A 021P09B 021P09D 021P0AA 021P0AB 021P0AD 021P0JA 021P0JB 021P0JD 021P0KA 021P0KB 021P0KD 021P0ZA 021P0ZB 021P0ZD 021P48A 021P48B 021P48D 021P49A 021P49B 021P49D 021P4AA 021P4AB 021P4AD 021P4JA 021P4JB 021P4JD 021P4KA 021P4KB 021P4KD 021P4ZA 021P4ZB 021P4ZD 021Q08A 021Q08B 021Q08D 021Q09A 021Q09B 021Q09D 021Q0AA 021Q0AB 021Q0AD 021Q0JA 021Q0JB 021Q0JD 021Q0KA 021Q0KB 021Q0KD 021Q0ZA 021Q0ZB 021Q0ZD 021Q48A 021Q48B 021Q48D 021Q49A 021Q49B 021Q49D 021Q4AA 021Q4AB 021Q4AD 021Q4JA 021Q4JB 021Q4JD 021Q4KA 021Q4KB 021Q4KD 021Q4ZA 021Q4ZB 021Q4ZD 021R08A 021R08B 021R08D 021R09A 021R09B 021R09D 021R0AA 021R0AB 021R0AD 021R0JA 021R0JB 021R0JD 021R0KA 021R0KB 021R0KD 021R0ZA 021R0ZB 021R0ZD 021R48A 021R48B 021R48D 021R49A 021R49B 021R49D 021R4AA 021R4AB 021R4AD 021R4JA 021R4JB 021R4JD 021R4KA 021R4KB 021R4KD 021R4ZA 021R4ZB 021R4ZD 021V08P 021V08Q 021V08R 021V08S 021V08T 021V08U 021V09S 021V09T 021V09U 021V0AS 021V0AT 021V0AU 021V0JS 021V0JT 021V0JU 021V0KS 021V0KT 021V0KU 021V0ZS 021V0ZT 021V0ZU 021V48P 021V48Q 021V48R 021V48S 021V48T 021V48U 021V49S 021V49T 021V49U 021V4AS 021V4AT 021V4AU 021V4JS 021V4JT 021V4JU 021V4KS 021V4KT 021V4KU 021V4ZS 021V4ZT 021V4ZU 021W08B 021W08D 021W08P 021W08Q 021W08R 021W48B 021W48D 021W48P 021W48Q 021W48R 021X08B 021X08D 021X08P 021X08Q 021X08R 021X09B 021X09D 021X09P 021X09Q 021X09R 021X0AB 021X0AD 021X0AP 021X0AQ 021X0AR 021X0JB 021X0JD 021X0JP 021X0JQ 021X0JR 021X0KB 021X0KD 021X0KP 021X0KQ 021X0KR 021X0ZB 021X0ZD 021X0ZP 021X0ZQ 021X0ZR 021X48B 021X48D 021X48P 021X48Q 021X48R 021X49B 021X49D 021X49P 021X49Q 021X49R 021X4AB 021X4AD 021X4AP 021X4AQ 021X4AR 021X4JB 021X4JD 021X4JP 021X4JQ 021X4JR 021X4KB 021X4KD 021X4KP 021X4KQ 021X4KR 021X4ZB 021X4ZD 021X4ZP 021X4ZQ 021X4ZR

CC 02170ZP 02170ZQ 02170ZR

021 continued on next page

021 continued from previous page

HAC 0210093 0210098 0210099 0210493 0210498 0210499 0211093 0211098 0211099 0211493 0211498 0211499 0212093 0212098 0212099 0212493 0212498 0212499 0213093 0213098 0213099 0213493 0213498 0213499 021009C 021009F 021009W 02100A3 02100A8 02100A9 02100AC 02100AF 02100AW 02100J3 02100J8 02100J9 02100JC 02100JF 02100JW 02100K3 02100K8 02100K9 02100KC 02100KF 02100KW 02100Z3 02100Z8 02100Z9 02100ZC 02100ZF 021049C 021049F 021049W 02104A3 02104A8 02104A9 02104AC 02104AF 02104AW 02104J3 02104J8 02104J9 02104JC 02104JF 02104JW 02104K3 02104K8 02104K9 02104KC 02104KF 02104KW 02104Z3 02104Z8 02104Z9 02104ZC 02104ZF 021109C 021109F 021109W 02110A3 02110A8 02110A9 02110AC 02110AF 02110AW 02110J3 02110J8 02110J9 02110JC 02110JF 02110JW 02110K3 02110K8 02110K9 02110KC 02110KF 02110KW 02110Z3 02110Z8 02110Z9 02110ZC 02110ZF 021149C 021149F 021149W 02114A3 02114A8 02114A9 02114AC 02114AF 02114AW 02114J3 02114J8 02114J9 02114JC 02114JF 02114JW 02114K3 02114K8 02114K9 02114KC 02114KF 02114KW 02114Z3 02114Z8 02114Z9 02114ZC 02114ZF 021209C 021209F 021209W 02120A3 02120A8 02120A9 02120AC 02120AF 02120AW 02120J3 02120J8 02120J9 02120JC 02120JF 02120JW 02120K3 02120K8 02120K9 02120KC 02120KF 02120KW 02120Z3 02120Z8 02120Z9 02120ZC 02120ZF 021249C 021249F 021249W 02124A3 02124A8 02124A9 02124AC 02124AF 02124AW 02124J3 02124J8 02124J9 02124JC 02124JF 02124JW 02124K3 02124K8 02124K9 02124KC 02124KF 02124KW 02124Z3 02124Z8 02124Z9 02124ZC 02124ZF 021309C 021309F 021309W 02130A3 02130A8 02130A9 02130AC 02130AF 02130AW 02130J3 02130J8 02130J9 02130JC 02130JF 02130JW 02130K3 02130K8 02130K9 02130KC 02130KF 02130KW 02130Z3 02130Z8 02130Z9 02130ZC 02130ZF 021349C 021349F 021349W 02134A3 02134A8 02134A9 02134AC 02134AF 02134AW 02134J3 02134J8 02134J9 02134JC 02134JF 02134JW 02134K3 02134K8 02134K9 02134KC 02134KF 02134KW 02134Z3 02134Z8 02134Z9 02134ZC or 02134ZF All preceding codes with the HAC symbol are classified as hospital-acquired conditions when reported with secondary diagnosis J98.5.

0 Medical and Surgical
2 Heart and Great Vessels
4 Creation: Putting in or on biological or synthetic material to form a new body part that to the extent possible replicates the anatomic structure or function of an absent body part

Body Part Character 4	Approach Character 5	Device Character 6	Qualifier Character 7
F Aortic Valve ⃠	0 Open	7 Autologous Tissue Substitute 8 Zooplastic Tissue J Synthetic Substitute K Nonautologous Tissue Substitute	J Truncal Valve
G Mitral Valve ⃠ J Tricuspid Valve ⃠	0 Open	7 Autologous Tissue Substitute 8 Zooplastic Tissue J Synthetic Substitute K Nonautologous Tissue Substitute	2 Common Atrioventricular Valve

⃠ 024F07J 024F08J 024F0JJ 024F0KJ 024G072 024G082 024G0J2 024G0K2 024J072 024J082 024J0J2 024J0K2

0 **Medical and Surgical**
2 **Heart and Great Vessels**
5 **Destruction:** Physical eradication of all or a portion of a body part by the direct use of energy, force, or a destructive agent

Body Part Character 4	Approach Character 5	Device Character 6	Qualifier Character 7
4 Coronary Vein **5** Atrial Septum **6** Atrium, Right **8** Conduction Mechanism **9** Chordae Tendineae **D** Papillary Muscle **F** Aortic Valve **G** Mitral Valve **H** Pulmonary Valve **J** Tricuspid Valve **K** Ventricle, Right **L** Ventricle, Left **M** Ventricular Septum **N** Pericardium **P** Pulmonary Trunk **Q** Pulmonary Artery, Right **R** Pulmonary Artery, Left **S** Pulmonary Vein, Right **T** Pulmonary Vein, Left **V** Superior Vena Cava **W** Thoracic Aorta, Descending **X** Thoracic Aorta, Ascending/Arch ⦸	**0** Open **3** Percutaneous **4** Percutaneous Endoscopic	**Z** No Device	**Z** No Qualifier
7 Atrium, Left DRG	**0** Open **3** Percutaneous **4** Percutaneous Endoscopic	**Z** No Device	**K** Left Atrial Appendage **Z** No Qualifier

⦸ 025X0ZZ 025X3ZZ 025X4ZZ
DRG 02570ZK 02573ZK 02574ZK

0 Medical and Surgical
2 Heart and Great Vessels
7 Dilation: Expanding an orifice or the lumen of a tubular body part

Body Part Character 4	Approach Character 5	Device Character 6	Qualifier Character 7
0 Coronary Artery, One Artery ⃠ **1** Coronary Artery, Two Arteries ⃠ **2** Coronary Artery, Three Arteries ⃠ **3** Coronary Artery, Four or More Arteries ⃠	**0** Open **3** Percutaneous **4** Percutaneous Endoscopic	**4** Intraluminal Device, Drug-eluting **5** Intraluminal Device, Drug-eluting, Two **6** Intraluminal Device, Drug-eluting, Three **7** Intraluminal Device, Drug-eluting, Four or More **D** Intraluminal Device **E** Intraluminal Device, Two **F** Intraluminal Device, Three **G** Intraluminal Device, Four or More **T** Intraluminal Device, Radioactive **Z** No Device	**6** Bifurcation **Z** No Qualifier
F Aortic Valve **G** Mitral Valve **H** Pulmonary Valve **J** Tricuspid Valve **K** Ventricle, Right **P** Pulmonary Trunk **Q** Pulmonary Artery, Right **S** Pulmonary Vein, Right **T** Pulmonary Vein, Left **V** Superior Vena Cava **W** Thoracic Aorta, Descending **X** Thoracic Aorta, Ascending/Arch ⃠	**0** Open **3** Percutaneous **4** Percutaneous Endoscopic	**4** Intraluminal Device, Drug-eluting **D** Intraluminal Device **Z** No Device	**Z** No Qualifier
R Pulmonary Artery, Left	**0** Open **3** Percutaneous **4** Percutaneous Endoscopic	**4** Intraluminal Device, Drug-eluting **D** Intraluminal Device **Z** No Device	**T** Ductus Arteriosus **Z** No Qualifier

⃠ 0270056 027005Z 0270066 027006Z 0270076 027007Z 02700E6 02700EZ 02700F6 02700FZ 02700G6 02700GZ 0270356 027035Z 0270366 027036Z 0270376 027037Z 02703E6 02703EZ 02703F6 02703FZ 02703G6 02703GZ 0270456 027045Z 0270466 027046Z 0270476 027047Z 02704E6 02704EZ 02704F6 02704FZ 02704G6 02704GZ 0271056 027105Z 0271066 027106Z 0271076 027107Z 02710E6 02710EZ 02710F6 02710FZ 02710G6 02710GZ 0271356 027135Z 0271366 027136Z 0271376 027137Z 02713E6 02713EZ 02713F6 02713FZ 02713G6 02713GZ 0271456 027145Z 0271466 027146Z 0271476 027147Z 02714E6 02714EZ 02714F6 02714FZ 02714G6 02714GZ 0272056 027205Z 0272066 027206Z 0272076 027207Z 02720E6 02720EZ 02720F6 02720FZ 02720G6 02720GZ 0272356 027235Z 0272366 027236Z 0272376 027237Z 02723E6 02723EZ 02723F6 02723FZ 02723G6 02723GZ 0272456 027245Z 0272466 027246Z 0272476 027247Z 02724E6 02724EZ 02724F6 02724FZ 02724G6 02724GZ 0273056 027305Z 0273066 027306Z 0273076 027307Z 02730E6 02730EZ 02730F6 02730FZ 02730G6 02730GZ 0273356 027335Z 0273366 027336Z 0273376 027337Z 02733E6 02733EZ 02733F6 02733FZ 02733G6 02733GZ 0273456 027345Z 0273466 027346Z 0273476 027347Z 02734E6 02734EZ 02734F6 02734FZ 02734G6 02734GZ 027X04Z 027X0DZ 027X0ZZ 027X34Z 027X3DZ 027X3ZZ 027X44Z 027X4DZ 027X4ZZ

0 Medical and Surgical
2 Heart and Great Vessels
8 Division: Cutting into a body part, without draining fluids and/or gases from the body part, in order to separate or transect a body part

Body Part Character 4	Approach Character 5	Device Character 6	Qualifier Character 7
8 Conduction Mechanism 9 Chordae Tendineae D Papillary Muscle	0 Open 3 Percutaneous 4 Percutaneous Endoscopic	Z No Device	Z No Qualifier

0 Medical and Surgical
2 Heart and Great Vessels
B Excision: Cutting out or off, without replacement, a portion of a body part

Body Part Character 4	Approach Character 5	Device Character 6	Qualifier Character 7
4 Coronary Vein ⊘ 5 Atrial Septum ⊘ 6 Atrium, Right ⊘ 8 Conduction Mechanism ⊘ 9 Chordae Tendineae ⊘ D Papillary Muscle ⊘ F Aortic Valve ⊘ G Mitral Valve ⊘ H Pulmonary Valve ⊘ J Tricuspid Valve ⊘ K Ventricle, Right NC ⊘ CC L Ventricle, Left NC ⊘ M Ventricular Septum ⊘ N Pericardium P Pulmonary Trunk Q Pulmonary Artery, Right R Pulmonary Artery, Left S Pulmonary Vein, Right T Pulmonary Vein, Left V Superior Vena Cava W Thoracic Aorta, Descending X Thoracic Aorta, Ascending/Arch ⊘	0 Open 3 Percutaneous 4 Percutaneous Endoscopic	Z No Device	X Diagnostic Z No Qualifier
7 Atrium, Left ⊘ DRG	0 Open 3 Percutaneous 4 Percutaneous Endoscopic	Z No Device	K Left Atrial Appendage X Diagnostic Z No Qualifier

⊘ 02B40ZX 02B43ZX 02B44ZX 02B50ZX 02B53ZX 02B54ZX 02B60ZX 02B63ZX 02B64ZX 02B70ZX 02B73ZX 02B74ZX 02B80ZX 02B83ZX 02B84ZX 02B90ZX 02B93ZX 02B94ZX 02BD0ZX 02BD3ZX 02BD4ZX 02BF0ZX 02BF3ZX 02BF4ZX 02BG0ZX 02BG3ZX 02BG4ZX 02BH0ZX 02BH3ZX 02BH4ZX 02BJ0ZX 02BJ3ZX 02BJ4ZX 02BK0ZX 02BK3ZX 02BK4ZX 02BL0ZX 02BL3ZX 02BL4ZX 02BM0ZX 02BM3ZX 02BM4ZX 02BX0ZX 02BX0ZZ 02BX3ZX 02BX3ZZ 02BX4ZX 02BX4ZZ

NC 02BK0ZZ 02BK3ZZ 02BK4ZZ 02BL0ZZ 02BL3ZZ 02BL4ZZ

CC 02BK0ZZ

DRG 02B70ZK 02B73ZK 02B74ZK

0 Medical and Surgical
2 Heart and Great Vessels
C Extirpation: Taking or cutting out solid matter from a body part

Body Part Character 4	Approach Character 5	Device Character 6	Qualifier Character 7
0 Coronary Artery, One Artery ⃠ **1** Coronary Artery, Two Arteries ⃠ **2** Coronary Artery, Three Arteries ⃠ **3** Coronary Artery, Four or More Arteries ⃠	**0** Open **3** Percutaneous **4** Percutaneous Endoscopic	**Z** No Device	**6** Bifurcation **Z** No Qualifier
4 Coronary Vein **5** Atrial Septum **6** Atrium, Right **7** Atrium, Left **8** Conduction Mechanism **9** Chordae Tendineae **D** Papillary Muscle **F** Aortic Valve **G** Mitral Valve **H** Pulmonary Valve **J** Tricuspid Valve **K** Ventricle, Right **L** Ventricle, Left **M** Ventricular Septum **N** Pericardium **P** Pulmonary Trunk **Q** Pulmonary Artery, Right **R** Pulmonary Artery, Left **S** Pulmonary Vein, Right **T** Pulmonary Vein, Left **V** Superior Vena Cava **W** Thoracic Aorta, Descending **X** Thoracic Aorta, Ascending/Arch ⃠	**0** Open **3** Percutaneous **4** Percutaneous Endoscopic	**Z** No Device	**Z** No Qualifier

⃠ 02C00Z6 02C03Z6 02C04Z6 02C10Z6 02C13Z6 02C14Z6 02C20Z6 02C23Z6 02C24Z6 02C30Z6 02C33Z6 02C34Z6 02CX0ZZ 02CX3ZZ 02CX4ZZ

0 Medical and Surgical
2 Heart and Great Vessels
F Fragmentation: Breaking solid matter in a body part into pieces

Body Part Character 4	Approach Character 5	Device Character 6	Qualifier Character 7
N Pericardium NC ⃠	**0** Open **3** Percutaneous **4** Percutaneous Endoscopic **X** External	**Z** No Device	**Z** No Qualifier

NC 02FNXZZ
⃠ 02FNXZZ

0 Medical and Surgical
2 Heart and Great Vessels
H Insertion: Putting in a nonbiological appliance that monitors, assists, performs, or prevents a physiological function but does not physically take the place of a body part

Body Part Character 4	Approach Character 5	Device Character 6	Qualifier Character 7
4 Coronary Vein CC DRG HAC ⊘ **6** Atrium, Right CC DRG HAC ⊘ **7** Atrium, Left CC DRG HAC ⊘ **K** Ventricle, Right CC DRG HAC ⊘ **L** Ventricle, Left CC DRG HAC ⊘	**0** Open **3** Percutaneous **4** Percutaneous Endoscopic	**0** Monitoring Device, Pressure Sensor **2** Monitoring Device **3** Infusion Device **D** Intraluminal Device **J** Cardiac Lead, Pacemaker **K** Cardiac Lead, Defibrillator **M** Cardiac Lead **N** Intracardiac Pacemaker	**Z** No Qualifier
A Heart NC LC	**0** Open **3** Percutaneous **4** Percutaneous Endoscopic	**Q** Implantable Heart Assist System	**Z** No Qualifier
A Heart CC	**0** Open **3** Percutaneous **4** Percutaneous Endoscopic	**R** External Heart Assist System	**S** Biventricular **Z** No Qualifier
N Pericardium CC HAC ⊘	**0** Open **3** Percutaneous **4** Percutaneous Endoscopic	**0** Monitoring Device, Pressure Sensor **2** Monitoring Device **J** Cardiac Lead, Pacemaker **K** Cardiac Lead, Defibrillator **M** Cardiac Lead	**Z** No Qualifier
P Pulmonary Trunk ⊘ **Q** Pulmonary Artery, Right ⊘ **R** Pulmonary Artery, Left ⊘ **S** Pulmonary Vein, Right ⊘ **T** Pulmonary Vein, Left ⊘ **V** Superior Vena Cava ⊘ **W** Thoracic Aorta, Descending ⊘ **X** Thoracic Aorta, Ascending/Arch ⊘	**0** Open **3** Percutaneous **4** Percutaneous Endoscopic	**0** Monitoring Device, Pressure Sensor **2** Monitoring Device **3** Infusion Device **D** Intraluminal Device	**Z** No Qualifier

⊘ 02H40NZ 02H432Z 02H433Z 02H43NZ 02H44NZ 02H60NZ 02H632Z 02H633Z 02H63NZ 02H64NZ 02H70NZ 02H732Z 02H733Z 02H73NZ 02H74NZ 02HK0NZ 02HK32Z 02HK33Z 02HK3NZ 02HK4NZ 02HL0NZ 02HL32Z 02HL33Z 02HL3NZ 02HL4NZ 02HN32Z 02HP00Z 02HP02Z 02HP03Z 02HP30Z 02HP32Z 02HP33Z 02HP40Z 02HP42Z 02HP43Z 02HQ02Z 02HQ03Z 02HQ32Z 02HQ33Z 02HQ42Z 02HQ43Z 02HR02Z 02HR03Z 02HR32Z 02HR33Z 02HR42Z 02HR43Z 02HS03Z 02HS32Z 02HS33Z 02HS43Z 02HT03Z 02HT32Z 02HT33Z 02HT43Z 02HV03Z 02HV32Z 02HV33Z 02HV43Z 02HW00Z 02HW03Z 02HW30Z 02HW32Z 02HW33Z 02HW40Z 02HW43Z 02HX00Z 02HX02Z 02HX03Z 02HX0DZ 02HX30Z 02HX32Z 02HX33Z 02HX3DZ 02HX40Z 02HX42Z 02HX43Z 02HX4DZ

LC 02HA0QZ

NC 02HA3QZ 02HA4QZ

HAC 02H43JZ 02H43KZ 02H43MZ 02H63JZ 02H63MZ 02H73JZ 02H73MZ 02HK3JZ 02HL3JZ 02HN0JZ 02HN0MZ 02HN3JZ 02HN3MZ 02HN4JZ or 02HN4MZ All preceding codes with the HAC symbol are classified as hospital-acquired conditions when reported with secondary diagnosis K68.11, T81.4XXA, T82.6XXA, or T82.7XXA.

CC 02H40JZ 02H40KZ 02H40MZ 02H43JZ 02H43KZ 02H43MZ 02H44JZ 02H44KZ 02H44MZ 02H60JZ 02H60KZ 02H60MZ 02H63JZ 02H63KZ 02H63MZ 02H64JZ 02H64KZ 02H64MZ 02H70JZ 02H70KZ 02H70MZ 02H73JZ 02H73KZ 02H73MZ 02H74JZ 02H74KZ 02H74MZ 02HA0RS 02HA0RZ 02HA3RS 02HA4RS 02HA4RZ 02HK00Z 02HK02Z 02HK0JZ 02HK0KZ 02HK0MZ 02HK30Z 02HK32Z 02HK3JZ 02HK3KZ 02HK3MZ 02HK40Z 02HK42Z 02HK4JZ 02HK4KZ 02HK4MZ 02HL0JZ 02HL0KZ 02HL0MZ 02HL3JZ 02HL3KZ 02HL3MZ 02HL4JZ 02HL4KZ 02HL4MZ 02HN0JZ 02HN0KZ 02HN0MZ 02HN3JZ 02HN3KZ 02HN3MZ 02HN4JZ 02HN4KZ 02HN4MZ

DRG 02H40JZ 02H40MZ 02H44JZ 02H44MZ 02H60JZ 02H60MZ 02H63JZ 02H64JZ 02H64MZ 02H70JZ 02H70MZ 02H73JZ 02H74JZ 02H74MZ 02HK0JZ 02HK0MZ 02HK3JZ 02HK3MZ 02HK4JZ 02HK4MZ 02HL0JZ 02HL0MZ 02HL3JZ 02HL3MZ 02HL4JZ 02HL4MZ

0 Medical and Surgical
2 Heart and Great Vessels
J Inspection: Visually and/or manually exploring a body part

Body Part Character 4	Approach Character 5	Device Character 6	Qualifier Character 7
A Heart ⃠ **Y** Great Vessel ⃠	**0** Open **3** Percutaneous **4** Percutaneous Endoscopic	**Z** No Device	**Z** No Qualifier

⃠ 02JA3ZZ 02JY3ZZ

0 Medical and Surgical
2 Heart and Great Vessels
K Map: Locating the route of passage of electrical impulses and/or locating functional areas in a body part

Body Part Character 4	Approach Character 5	Device Character 6	Qualifier Character 7
8 Conduction Mechanism DRG	**0** Open **3** Percutaneous **4** Percutaneous Endoscopic	**Z** No Device	**Z** No Qualifier

DRG 02K80ZZ 02K83ZZ 02K84ZZ

0 Medical and Surgical
2 Heart and Great Vessels
L Occlusion: Completely closing an orifice or the lumen of a tubular body part

Body Part Character 4	Approach Character 5	Device Character 6	Qualifier Character 7
7 Atrium, Left DRG	**0** Open **3** Percutaneous **4** Percutaneous Endoscopic	**C** Extraluminal Device **D** Intraluminal Device **Z** No Device	**K** Left Atrial Appendage
H Pulmonary Valve ⃠ **S** Pulmonary Vein, Right CC **T** Pulmonary Vein, Left CC **V** Superior Vena Cava	**0** Open **3** Percutaneous **4** Percutaneous Endoscopic	**C** Extraluminal Device **D** Intraluminal Device **Z** No Device	**Z** No Qualifier
R Pulmonary Artery, Left CC	**0** Open **3** Percutaneous **4** Percutaneous Endoscopic	**C** Extraluminal Device **D** Intraluminal Device **Z** No Device	**T** Ductus Arteriosus

CC 02LR0ZT 02LS0ZZ 02LT0ZZ
DRG 02L70CK 02L70DK 02L70ZK 02L73CK 02L73DK 02L73ZK 02L74CK 02L74DK 02L74ZK
⃠ 02LH0CZ 02LH0DZ 02LH0ZZ 02LH3CZ 02LH3DZ 02LH3ZZ 02LH4CZ 02LH4DZ 02LH4ZZ

0 Medical and Surgical
2 Heart and Great Vessels
N Release: Freeing a body part from an abnormal physical constraint by cutting or by the use of force

Body Part Character 4	Approach Character 5	Device Character 6	Qualifier Character 7
4 Coronary Vein **5** Atrial Septum **6** Atrium, Right **7** Atrium, Left **8** Conduction Mechanism **9** Chordae Tendineae **D** Papillary Muscle **F** Aortic Valve **G** Mitral Valve **H** Pulmonary Valve CC **J** Tricuspid Valve **K** Ventricle, Right **L** Ventricle, Left **M** Ventricular Septum **N** Pericardium **P** Pulmonary Trunk **Q** Pulmonary Artery, Right **R** Pulmonary Artery, Left **S** Pulmonary Vein, Right **T** Pulmonary Vein, Left **V** Superior Vena Cava **W** Thoracic Aorta, Descending **X** Thoracic Aorta, Ascending/Arch ⊘	**0** Open **3** Percutaneous **4** Percutaneous Endoscopic	**Z** No Device	**Z** No Qualifier

⊘ 02NX0ZZ 02NX3ZZ 02NX4ZZ
CC 02NH0ZZ

0 Medical and Surgical
2 Heart and Great Vessels
P Removal: Taking out or off a device from a body part

Body Part Character 4	Approach Character 5	Device Character 6	Qualifier Character 7
A Heart ⦸ CC HAC	0 Open 3 Percutaneous 4 Percutaneous Endoscopic	2 Monitoring Device 3 Infusion Device 7 Autologous Tissue Substitute 8 Zooplastic Tissue C Extraluminal Device D Intraluminal Device J Synthetic Substitute K Nonautologous Tissue Substitute M Cardiac Lead N Intracardiac Pacemaker Q Implantable Heart Assist System R External Heart Assist System	Z No Qualifier
A Heart ⦸ CC HAC	X External	2 Monitoring Device 3 Infusion Device D Intraluminal Device M Cardiac Lead	Z No Qualifier
Y Great Vessel ⦸	0 Open 3 Percutaneous 4 Percutaneous Endoscopic	2 Monitoring Device 3 Infusion Device 7 Autologous Tissue Substitute 8 Zooplastic Tissue C Extraluminal Device D Intraluminal Device J Synthetic Substitute K Nonautologous Tissue Substitute	Z No Qualifier
Y Great Vessel ⦸	X External	2 Monitoring Device 3 Infusion Device D Intraluminal Device	Z No Qualifier

⦸ 02PA0NZ 02PA32Z 02PA33Z 02PA3NZ 02PA4NZ 02PAX2Z 02PAX3Z 02PAXDZ 02PY32Z 02PY33Z 02PYX2Z 02PYX3Z 02PYXDZ
HAC 02PA0MZ 02PA3MZ 02PA4MZ or 02PAXMZ when reported with secondary diagnosis K68.11, T81.4XXA, T82.6XXA, T82.7XXA
CC 02PA0MZ 02PA0RZ 02PA3MZ 02PA3RZ 02PA4MZ 02PA4RZ 02PAXMZ

0 Medical and Surgical
2 Heart and Great Vessels
Q Repair: Restoring, to the extent possible, a body part to its normal anatomic structure and function

Body Part Character 4	Approach Character 5	Device Character 6	Qualifier Character 7
0 Coronary Artery, One Artery **1** Coronary Artery, Two Arteries **2** Coronary Artery, Three Arteries **3** Coronary Artery, Four or More Arteries **4** Coronary Vein **5** Atrial Septum **6** Atrium, Right **7** Atrium, Left **8** Conduction Mechanism **9** Chordae Tendineae **A** Heart **B** Heart, Right **C** Heart, Left **D** Papillary Muscle **H** Pulmonary Valve **K** Ventricle, Right **L** Ventricle, Left **M** Ventricular Septum **N** Pericardium **P** Pulmonary Trunk **Q** Pulmonary Artery, Right **R** Pulmonary Artery, Left **S** Pulmonary Vein, Right **T** Pulmonary Vein, Left **V** Superior Vena Cava **W** Thoracic Aorta, Descending **X** Thoracic Aorta, Ascending/Arch ⦸	**0** Open **3** Percutaneous **4** Percutaneous Endoscopic	**Z** No Device	**Z** No Qualifier
F Aortic Valve ⦸	**0** Open **3** Percutaneous **4** Percutaneous Endoscopic	**Z** No Device	**J** Truncal Valve **Z** No Qualifier
G Mitral Valve ⦸	**0** Open **3** Percutaneous **4** Percutaneous Endoscopic	**Z** No Device	**E** Atrioventricular Valve, Left **Z** No Qualifier
J Tricuspid Valve ⦸	**0** Open **3** Percutaneous **4** Percutaneous Endoscopic	**Z** No Device	**G** Atrioventricular Valve, Right **Z** No Qualifier

⦸ 02QF0ZJ 02QF3ZJ 02QF4ZJ 02QG0ZE 02QG3ZE 02QG4ZE 02QJ0ZG 02QJ3ZG 02QJ4ZG 02QX0ZZ 02QX3ZZ 02QX4ZZ

0 Medical and Surgical
2 Heart and Great Vessels
R Replacement: Putting in or on biological or synthetic material that physically takes the place and/or function of all or a portion of a body part

Body Part Character 4	Approach Character 5	Device Character 6	Qualifier Character 7
5 Atrial Septum 6 Atrium, Right 7 Atrium, Left 9 Chordae Tendineae D Papillary Muscle J Tricuspid Valve K Ventricle, Right NC LC CC L Ventricle, Left NC LC CC M Ventricular Septum CC N Pericardium P Pulmonary Trunk CC Q Pulmonary Artery, Right CC R Pulmonary Artery, Left CC S Pulmonary Vein, Right T Pulmonary Vein, Left V Superior Vena Cava W Thoracic Aorta, Descending X Thoracic Aorta, Ascending/Arch ⦸	0 Open 4 Percutaneous Endoscopic	7 Autologous Tissue Substitute 8 Zooplastic Tissue J Synthetic Substitute K Nonautologous Tissue Substitute	Z No Qualifier
F Aortic Valve G Mitral Valve H Pulmonary Valve	0 Open 4 Percutaneous Endoscopic	7 Autologous Tissue Substitute 8 Zooplastic Tissue J Synthetic Substitute K Nonautologous Tissue Substitute	Z No Qualifier
F Aortic Valve G Mitral Valve H Pulmonary Valve	3 Percutaneous	7 Autologous Tissue Substitute 8 Zooplastic Tissue J Synthetic Substitute K Nonautologous Tissue Substitute	H Transapical Z No Qualifier

⦸ 02RX07Z 02RX08Z 02RX0JZ 02RX0KZ 02RX47Z 02RX48Z 02RX4JZ 02RX4KZ
LC 02RK0JZ with 02RL0JZ limited coverage when combined with diagnosis code Z00.6
NC 02RK0JZ with 02RL0JZ noncovered except when combined with diagnosis code Z00.6
CC 02RK0JZ 02RL0JZ 02RM0JZ 02RP0JZ 02RQ07Z 02RQ0JZ 02RR07Z 02RR0JZ

0 Medical and Surgical
2 Heart and Great Vessels
S Reposition: Moving to its normal location, or other suitable location, all or a portion of a body part

Body Part Character 4	Approach Character 5	Device Character 6	Qualifier Character 7
0 Coronary Artery, One Artery ⦸ 1 Coronary Artery, Two Arteries ⦸ P Pulmonary Trunk CC Q Pulmonary Artery, Right R Pulmonary Artery, Left S Pulmonary Vein, Right T Pulmonary Vein, Left V Superior Vena Cava W Thoracic Aorta, Descending CC X Thoracic Aorta, Ascending/Arch ⦸	0 Open	Z No Device	Z No Qualifier

⦸ 02S00ZZ 02S10ZZ 02SX0ZZ
CC 02SP0ZZ 02SW0ZZ

0 Medical and Surgical
2 Heart and Great Vessels
T Resection: Cutting out or off, without replacement, all of a body part

Body Part Character 4	Approach Character 5	Device Character 6	Qualifier Character 7
5 Atrial Septum 8 Conduction Mechanism 9 Chordae Tendineae D Papillary Muscle H Pulmonary Valve M Ventricular Septum N Pericardium	0 Open 3 Percutaneous 4 Percutaneous Endoscopic	Z No Device	Z No Qualifier

0 Medical and Surgical
2 Heart and Great Vessels
U Supplement: Putting in or on biological or synthetic material that physically reinforces and/or augments the function of a portion of a body part

Body Part Character 4	Approach Character 5	Device Character 6	Qualifier Character 7
5 Atrial Septum 6 Atrium, Right 7 Atrium, Left CC DRG 9 Chordae Tendineae A Heart D Papillary Muscle H Pulmonary Valve K Ventricle, Right L Ventricle, Left M Ventricular Septum N Pericardium P Pulmonary Trunk Q Pulmonary Artery, Right R Pulmonary Artery, Left S Pulmonary Vein, Right T Pulmonary Vein, Left V Superior Vena Cava W Thoracic Aorta, Descending X Thoracic Aorta, Ascending/Arch ⊘	0 Open 3 Percutaneous 4 Percutaneous Endoscopic	7 Autologous Tissue Substitute 8 Zooplastic Tissue J Synthetic Substitute K Nonautologous Tissue Substitute	Z No Qualifier
F Aortic Valve ⊘	0 Open 3 Percutaneous 4 Percutaneous Endoscopic	7 Autologous Tissue Substitute 8 Zooplastic Tissue J Synthetic Substitute K Nonautologous Tissue Substitute	J Truncal Valve Z No Qualifier
G Mitral Valve ⊘	0 Open 3 Percutaneous 4 Percutaneous Endoscopic	7 Autologous Tissue Substitute 8 Zooplastic Tissue J Synthetic Substitute K Nonautologous Tissue Substitute	E Atrioventricular Valve, Left Z No Qualifier
J Tricuspid Valve ⊘	0 Open 3 Percutaneous 4 Percutaneous Endoscopic	7 Autologous Tissue Substitute 8 Zooplastic Tissue J Synthetic Substitute K Nonautologous Tissue Substitute	G Atrioventricular Valve, Right Z No Qualifier

⊘ 02UF07J 02UF08J 02UF0JJ 02UF0KJ 02UF37J 02UF38J 02UF3JJ 02UF3KJ 02UF47J 02UF48J 02UF4JJ 02UF4KJ 02UG07E 02UG08E 02UG0JE 02UG0KE 02UG37E 02UG38E 02UG3JE 02UG3KE 02UG47E 02UG48E 02UG4JE 02UG4KE 02UJ07G 02UJ08G 02UJ0JG 02UJ0KG 02UJ37G 02UJ38G 02UJ3JG 02UJ3KG 02UJ47G 02UJ48G 02UJ4JG 02UJ4KG 02UX07Z 02UX08Z 02UX0JZ 02UX0KZ 02UX37Z 02UX38Z 02UX3JZ 02UX3KZ 02UX47Z 02UX48Z 02UX4JZ 02UX4KZ

CC 02U70JZ

DRG 02U73JZ 02U74JZ

LC Limited Coverage NC Noncovered HAC HAC Associated Procedure CC Combination Cluster - See Appendix G for code lists
DRG Non-OR-Affecting MS-DRG Assignment ⊘ Non-OR-Not Affecting MS-DRG Assignment New/Revised Text in **Orange** ♂ Male ♀ Female

0 Medical and Surgical
2 Heart and Great Vessels
V Restriction: Partially closing an orifice or the lumen of a tubular body part

Body Part Character 4	Approach Character 5	Device Character 6	Qualifier Character 7
A Heart	**0** Open **3** Percutaneous **4** Percutaneous Endoscopic	**C** Extraluminal Device **Z** No Device	**Z** No Qualifier
P Pulmonary Trunk **Q** Pulmonary Artery, Right **S** Pulmonary Vein, Right **T** Pulmonary Vein, Left **V** Superior Vena Cava	**0** Open **3** Percutaneous **4** Percutaneous Endoscopic	**C** Extraluminal Device **D** Intraluminal Device **Z** No Device	**Z** No Qualifier
R Pulmonary Artery, Left CC	**0** Open **3** Percutaneous **4** Percutaneous Endoscopic	**C** Extraluminal Device **D** Intraluminal Device **Z** No Device	**T** Ductus Arteriosus **Z** No Qualifier
W Thoracic Aorta, Descending ⃠ **X** Thoracic Aorta, Ascending/Arch ⃠	**0** Open **3** Percutaneous **4** Percutaneous Endoscopic	**C** Extraluminal Device **D** Intraluminal Device **E** Intraluminal Device, Branched or Fenestrated, One or Two Arteries **F** Intraluminal Device, Branched or Fenestrated, Three or More Arteries **Z** No Device	**Z** No Qualifier

⃠ 02VW0EZ 02VW0FZ 02VW3EZ 02VW3FZ 02VW4EZ 02VW4FZ 02VX0CZ 02VX0DZ 02VX0EZ 02VX0FZ 02VX0ZZ 02VX3CZ 02VX3DZ 02VX3EZ 02VX3FZ 02VX3ZZ 02VX4CZ 02VX4DZ 02VX4EZ 02VX4FZ 02VX4ZZ

CC 02VR0ZT

0 Medical and Surgical
2 Heart and Great Vessels
W Revision: Correcting, to the extent possible, a portion of a malfunctioning device or the position of a displaced device

Body Part Character 4	Approach Character 5	Device Character 6	Qualifier Character 7
5 Atrial Septum **M** Ventricular Septum	**0** Open **4** Percutaneous Endoscopic	**J** Synthetic Substitute	**Z** No Qualifier
A Heart NC ⊘ CC HAC LC	**0** Open **3** Percutaneous **4** Percutaneous Endoscopic **X** External	**2** Monitoring Device **3** Infusion Device **7** Autologous Tissue Substitute **8** Zooplastic Tissue **C** Extraluminal Device **D** Intraluminal Device **J** Synthetic Substitute **K** Nonautologous Tissue Substitute **M** Cardiac Lead **N** Intracardiac Pacemaker **Q** Implantable Heart Assist System **R** External Heart Assist System	**Z** No Qualifier
F Aortic Valve **G** Mitral Valve **H** Pulmonary Valve **J** Tricuspid Valve	**0** Open **4** Percutaneous Endoscopic	**7** Autologous Tissue Substitute **8** Zooplastic Tissue **J** Synthetic Substitute **K** Nonautologous Tissue Substitute	**Z** No Qualifier
Y Great Vessel ⊘	**0** Open **3** Percutaneous **4** Percutaneous Endoscopic **X** External	**2** Monitoring Device **3** Infusion Device **7** Autologous Tissue Substitute **8** Zooplastic Tissue **C** Extraluminal Device **D** Intraluminal Device **J** Synthetic Substitute **K** Nonautologous Tissue Substitute	**Z** No Qualifier

⊘ 02WA0NZ 02WA3NZ 02WA4NZ 02WAX2Z 02WAX3Z 02WAX7Z 02WAX8Z 02WAXCZ 02WAXDZ 02WAXJZ 02WAXKZ 02WAXMZ 02WAXNZ 02WAXQZ 02WAXRZ 02WYX2Z 02WYX3Z 02WYX7Z 02WYX8Z 02WYXCZ 02WYXDZ 02WYXJZ 02WYXKZ
LC 02WA0JZ 02WA0QZ
NC 02WA3QZ 02WA4QZ
HAC 02WA0MZ 02WA3MZ or 02WA4MZ when reported with secondary diagnosis K68.11, T81.4XXA, T82.6XXA, or T82.7XXA.
CC 02WA0QZ 02WA0RZ 02WA3QZ 02WA3RZ 02WA4QZ 02WA4RZ

0 Medical and Surgical
2 Heart and Great Vessels
Y Transplantation: Putting in or on all or a portion of a living body part taken from another individual or animal to physically take the place and/or function of all or a portion of a similar body part

Body Part Character 4	Approach Character 5	Device Character 6	Qualifier Character 7
A Heart LC	**0** Open	**Z** No Device	**0** Allogeneic **1** Syngeneic **2** Zooplastic

LC 02YA0Z0 02YA0Z1 02YA0Z2

Upper Arteries 031-03W

0 Medical and Surgical
3 Upper Arteries
1 Bypass: Altering the route of passage of the contents of a tubular body part

Body Part Character 4	Approach Character 5	Device Character 6	Qualifier Character 7
2 Innominate Artery 5 Axillary Artery, Right 6 Axillary Artery, Left	0 Open	9 Autologous Venous Tissue A Autologous Arterial Tissue J Synthetic Substitute K Nonautologous Tissue Substitute Z No Device	0 Upper Arm Artery, Right 1 Upper Arm Artery, Left 2 Upper Arm Artery, Bilateral 3 Lower Arm Artery, Right 4 Lower Arm Artery, Left 5 Lower Arm Artery, Bilateral 6 Upper Leg Artery, Right 7 Upper Leg Artery, Left 8 Upper Leg Artery, Bilateral 9 Lower Leg Artery, Right B Lower Leg Artery, Left C Lower Leg Artery, Bilateral D Upper Arm Vein F Lower Arm Vein J Extracranial Artery, Right K Extracranial Artery, Left
3 Subclavian Artery, Right 4 Subclavian Artery, Left	0 Open	9 Autologous Venous Tissue A Autologous Arterial Tissue J Synthetic Substitute K Nonautologous Tissue Substitute Z No Device	0 Upper Arm Artery, Right 1 Upper Arm Artery, Left 2 Upper Arm Artery, Bilateral 3 Lower Arm Artery, Right 4 Lower Arm Artery, Left 5 Lower Arm Artery, Bilateral 6 Upper Leg Artery, Right 7 Upper Leg Artery, Left 8 Upper Leg Artery, Bilateral 9 Lower Leg Artery, Right B Lower Leg Artery, Left C Lower Leg Artery, Bilateral D Upper Arm Vein F Lower Arm Vein J Extracranial Artery, Right K Extracranial Artery, Left M Pulmonary Artery, Right N Pulmonary Artery, Left
7 Brachial Artery, Right	0 Open	9 Autologous Venous Tissue A Autologous Arterial Tissue J Synthetic Substitute K Nonautologous Tissue Substitute Z No Device	0 Upper Arm Artery, Right 3 Lower Arm Artery, Right D Upper Arm Vein F Lower Arm Vein
8 Brachial Artery, Left	0 Open	9 Autologous Venous Tissue A Autologous Arterial Tissue J Synthetic Substitute K Nonautologous Tissue Substitute Z No Device	1 Upper Arm Artery, Left 4 Lower Arm Artery, Left D Upper Arm Vein F Lower Arm Vein
9 Ulnar Artery, Right B Radial Artery, Right CC	0 Open	9 Autologous Venous Tissue A Autologous Arterial Tissue J Synthetic Substitute K Nonautologous Tissue Substitute Z No Device	3 Lower Arm Artery, Right F Lower Arm Vein
A Ulnar Artery, Left C Radial Artery, Left CC	0 Open	9 Autologous Venous Tissue A Autologous Arterial Tissue J Synthetic Substitute K Nonautologous Tissue Substitute Z No Device	4 Lower Arm Artery, Left F Lower Arm Vein

031 continued on next page

031 continued from previous page

0 Medical and Surgical
3 Upper Arteries
1 Bypass: Altering the route of passage of the contents of a tubular body part

Body Part Character 4	Approach Character 5	Device Character 6	Qualifier Character 7
G Intracranial Artery **S** Temporal Artery, Right NC **T** Temporal Artery, Left NC	**0** Open	**9** Autologous Venous Tissue **A** Autologous Arterial Tissue **J** Synthetic Substitute **K** Nonautologous Tissue Substitute **Z** No Device	**G** Intracranial Artery
H Common Carotid Artery, Right NC	**0** Open	**9** Autologous Venous Tissue **A** Autologous Arterial Tissue **J** Synthetic Substitute **K** Nonautologous Tissue Substitute **Z** No Device	**G** Intracranial Artery **J** Extracranial Artery, Right
J Common Carotid Artery, Left NC	**0** Open	**9** Autologous Venous Tissue **A** Autologous Arterial Tissue **J** Synthetic Substitute **K** Nonautologous Tissue Substitute **Z** No Device	**G** Intracranial Artery **K** Extracranial Artery, Left
K Internal Carotid Artery, Right **M** External Carotid Artery, Right	**0** Open	**9** Autologous Venous Tissue **A** Autologous Arterial Tissue **J** Synthetic Substitute **K** Nonautologous Tissue Substitute **Z** No Device	**J** Extracranial Artery, Right
L Internal Carotid Artery, Left **N** External Carotid Artery, Left	**0** Open	**9** Autologous Venous Tissue **A** Autologous Arterial Tissue **J** Synthetic Substitute **K** Nonautologous Tissue Substitute **Z** No Device	**K** Extracranial Artery, Left

NC 031H09G 031H0AG 031H0JG 031H0KG 031H0ZG 031J09G 031J0AG 031J0JG 031J0KG 031J0ZG 031S09G 031S0AG 031S0JG 031S0KG 031S0ZG 031T09G 031T0AG 031T0JG 031T0KG 031T0ZG
CC 031B0JF 031C0JF

LC Limited Coverage NC Noncovered HAC HAC Associated Procedure CC Combination Cluster - See Appendix G for code lists
DRG Non-OR-Affecting MS-DRG Assignment ⦸ Non-OR-Not Affecting MS-DRG Assignment New/Revised Text in **Orange** ♂ Male ♀ Female

0 Medical and Surgical
3 Upper Arteries
5 Destruction: Physical eradication of all or a portion of a body part by the direct use of energy, force, or a destructive agent

Body Part Character 4	Approach Character 5	Device Character 6	Qualifier Character 7
0 Internal Mammary Artery, Right **1** Internal Mammary Artery, Left **2** Innominate Artery **3** Subclavian Artery, Right **4** Subclavian Artery, Left **5** Axillary Artery, Right **6** Axillary Artery, Left **7** Brachial Artery, Right **8** Brachial Artery, Left **9** Ulnar Artery, Right **A** Ulnar Artery, Left **B** Radial Artery, Right **C** Radial Artery, Left **D** Hand Artery, Right **F** Hand Artery, Left **G** Intracranial Artery **H** Common Carotid Artery, Right **J** Common Carotid Artery, Left **K** Internal Carotid Artery, Right **L** Internal Carotid Artery, Left **M** External Carotid Artery, Right **N** External Carotid Artery, Left **P** Vertebral Artery, Right **Q** Vertebral Artery, Left **R** Face Artery **S** Temporal Artery, Right **T** Temporal Artery, Left **U** Thyroid Artery, Right **V** Thyroid Artery, Left **Y** Upper Artery	**0** Open **3** Percutaneous **4** Percutaneous Endoscopic	**Z** No Device	**Z** No Qualifier

0 Medical and Surgical
3 Upper Arteries
7 Dilation: Expanding an orifice or the lumen of a tubular body part

Body Part Character 4	Approach Character 5	Device Character 6	Qualifier Character 7
0 Internal Mammary Artery, Right ⊘	**0** Open	**4** Intraluminal Device, Drug-eluting	**6** Bifurcation
1 Internal Mammary Artery, Left ⊘	**3** Percutaneous	**5** Intraluminal Device, Drug-eluting, Two	**Z** No Qualifier
2 Innominate Artery ⊘	**4** Percutaneous Endoscopic	**6** Intraluminal Device, Drug-eluting, Three	
3 Subclavian Artery, Right ⊘		**7** Intraluminal Device, Drug-eluting, Four or More	
4 Subclavian Artery, Left ⊘		**D** Intraluminal Device	
5 Axillary Artery, Right ⊘		**E** Intraluminal Device, Two	
6 Axillary Artery, Left ⊘		**F** Intraluminal Device, Three	
7 Brachial Artery, Right ⊘		**G** Intraluminal Device, Four or More	
8 Brachial Artery, Left ⊘		**Z** No Device	
9 Ulnar Artery, Right ⊘			
A Ulnar Artery, Left ⊘			
B Radial Artery, Right ⊘			
C Radial Artery, Left ⊘			
D Hand Artery, Right ⊘			
F Hand Artery, Left ⊘			
G Intracranial Artery NC ⊘			
H Common Carotid Artery, Right ⊘			
J Common Carotid Artery, Left ⊘			
K Internal Carotid Artery, Right ⊘			
L Internal Carotid Artery, Left ⊘			
M External Carotid Artery, Right ⊘			
N External Carotid Artery, Left ⊘			
P Vertebral Artery, Right ⊘			
Q Vertebral Artery, Left ⊘			
R Face Artery ⊘			
S Temporal Artery, Right ⊘			
T Temporal Artery, Left ⊘			
U Thyroid Artery, Right ⊘			
V Thyroid Artery, Left ⊘			
Y Upper Artery ⊘			

⊘

0370046	0370056	037005Z	0370066	037006Z	0370076	037007Z	03700D6	03700E6	03700EZ	03700F6	03700FZ	03700G6
03700GZ	03700Z6	0370346	0370356	037035Z	0370366	037036Z	0370376	037037Z	03703D6	03703E6	03703EZ	03703F6
03703FZ	03703G6	03703GZ	03703Z6	0370446	0370456	037045Z	0370466	037046Z	0370476	037047Z	03704D6	03704E6
03704EZ	03704F6	03704FZ	03704G6	03704GZ	03704Z6	0371046	0371056	037105Z	0371066	037106Z	0371076	037107Z
03710D6	03710E6	03710EZ	03710F6	03710FZ	03710G6	03710GZ	03710Z6	0371346	0371356	037135Z	0371366	037136Z
0371376	037137Z	03713D6	03713E6	03713EZ	03713F6	03713FZ	03713G6	03713GZ	03713Z6	0371446	0371456	037145Z
0371466	037146Z	0371476	037147Z	03714D6	03714E6	03714EZ	03714F6	03714FZ	03714G6	03714GZ	03714Z6	0372046
0372056	037205Z	0372066	037206Z	0372076	037207Z	03720D6	03720E6	03720EZ	03720F6	03720FZ	03720G6	03720GZ
03720Z6	0372346	0372356	037235Z	0372366	037236Z	0372376	037237Z	03723D6	03723E6	03723EZ	03723F6	03723FZ
03723G6	03723GZ	03723Z6	0372446	0372456	037245Z	0372466	037246Z	0372476	037247Z	03724D6	03724E6	03724EZ
03724F6	03724FZ	03724G6	03724GZ	03724Z6	0373046	0373056	037305Z	0373066	037306Z	0373076	037307Z	03730D6
03730E6	03730EZ	03730F6	03730FZ	03730G6	03730GZ	03730Z6	0373346	0373356	037335Z	0373366	037336Z	0373376
037337Z	03733D6	03733E6	03733EZ	03733F6	03733FZ	03733G6	03733GZ	03733Z6	0373446	0373456	037345Z	0373466
037346Z	0373476	037347Z	03734D6	03734E6	03734EZ	03734F6	03734FZ	03734G6	03734GZ	03734Z6	0374046	0374056
037405Z	0374066	037406Z	0374076	037407Z	03740D6	03740E6	03740EZ	03740F6	03740FZ	03740G6	03740GZ	03740Z6
0374346	0374356	037435Z	0374366	037436Z	0374376	037437Z	03743D6	03743E6	03743EZ	03743F6	03743FZ	03743G6
03743GZ	03743Z6	0374446	0374456	037445Z	0374466	037446Z	0374476	037447Z	03744D6	03744E6	03744EZ	03744F6
03744FZ	03744G6	03744GZ	03744Z6	0375046	0375056	037505Z	0375066	037506Z	0375076	037507Z	03750D6	03750E6
03750EZ	03750F6	03750FZ	03750G6	03750GZ	03750Z6	0375346	0375356	037535Z	0375366	037536Z	0375376	037537Z
03753D6	03753E6	03753EZ	03753F6	03753FZ	03753G6	03753GZ	03753Z6	0375446	0375456	037545Z	0375466	037546Z
0375476	037547Z	03754D6	03754E6	03754EZ	03754F6	03754FZ	03754G6	03754GZ	03754Z6	0376046	0376056	037605Z
0376066	037606Z	0376076	037607Z	03760D6	03760E6	03760EZ	03760F6	03760FZ	03760G6	03760GZ	03760Z6	0376346
0376356	037635Z	0376366	037636Z	0376376	037637Z	03763D6	03763E6	03763EZ	03763F6	03763FZ	03763G6	03763GZ
03763Z6	0376446	0376456	037645Z	0376466	037646Z	0376476	037647Z	03764D6	03764E6	03764EZ	03764F6	03764FZ
03764G6	03764GZ	03764Z6	0377046	0377056	037705Z	0377066	037706Z	0377076	037707Z	03770D6	03770E6	03770EZ
03770F6	03770FZ	03770G6	03770GZ	03770Z6	0377346	0377356	037735Z	0377366	037736Z	0377376	037737Z	03773D6
03773E6	03773EZ	03773F6	03773FZ	03773G6	03773GZ	03773Z6	0377446	0377456	037745Z	0377466	037746Z	0377476
037747Z	03774D6	03774E6	03774EZ	03774F6	03774FZ	03774G6	03774GZ	03774Z6	0378046	0378056	037805Z	0378066
037806Z	0378076	037807Z	03780D6	03780E6	03780EZ	03780F6	03780FZ	03780G6	03780GZ	03780Z6	0378346	0378356
037835Z	0378366	037836Z	0378376	037837Z	03783D6	03783E6	03783EZ	03783F6	03783FZ	03783G6	03783GZ	03783Z6

037 continued on next page

037 continued from previous page

0378446 0378456 037845Z 0378466 037846Z 0378476 037847Z 03784D6 03784E6 03784EZ 03784F6 03784FZ 03784G6
03784GZ 03784Z6 0379046 0379056 037905Z 0379066 037906Z 0379076 037907Z 03790D6 03790E6 03790EZ 03790F6
03790FZ 03790G6 03790GZ 03790Z6 0379346 0379356 037935Z 0379366 037936Z 0379376 037937Z 03793D6 03793E6
03793EZ 03793F6 03793FZ 03793G6 03793GZ 03793Z6 0379446 0379456 037945Z 0379466 037946Z 0379476 037947Z
03794D6 03794E6 03794EZ 03794F6 03794FZ 03794G6 03794GZ 03794Z6 037A046 037A056 037A05Z 037A066 037A06Z
037A076 037A07Z 037A0D6 037A0E6 037A0EZ 037A0F6 037A0FZ 037A0G6 037A0GZ 037A0Z6 037A346 037A356 037A35Z
037A366 037A36Z 037A376 037A37Z 037A3D6 037A3E6 037A3EZ 037A3F6 037A3FZ 037A3G6 037A3GZ 037A3Z6 037A446
037A456 037A45Z 037A466 037A46Z 037A476 037A47Z 037A4D6 037A4E6 037A4EZ 037A4F6 037A4FZ 037A4G6 037A4GZ
037A4Z6 037B046 037B056 037B05Z 037B066 037B06Z 037B076 037B07Z 037B0D6 037B0E6 037B0EZ 037B0F6 037B0FZ
037B0G6 037B0GZ 037B0Z6 037B346 037B356 037B35Z 037B366 037B36Z 037B376 037B37Z 037B3D6 037B3E6 037B3EZ
037B3F6 037B3FZ 037B3G6 037B3GZ 037B3Z6 037B446 037B456 037B45Z 037B466 037B46Z 037B476 037B47Z 037B4D6
037B4E6 037B4EZ 037B4F6 037B4FZ 037B4G6 037B4GZ 037B4Z6 037C046 037C056 037C05Z 037C066 037C06Z 037C076
037C07Z 037C0D6 037C0E6 037C0EZ 037C0F6 037C0FZ 037C0G6 037C0GZ 037C0Z6 037C346 037C356 037C35Z 037C366
037C36Z 037C376 037C37Z 037C3D6 037C3E6 037C3EZ 037C3F6 037C3FZ 037C3G6 037C3GZ 037C3Z6 037C446 037C456
037C45Z 037C466 037C46Z 037C476 037C47Z 037C4D6 037C4E6 037C4EZ 037C4F6 037C4FZ 037C4G6 037C4GZ 037C4Z6
037D046 037D056 037D05Z 037D066 037D06Z 037D076 037D07Z 037D0D6 037D0E6 037D0EZ 037D0F6 037D0FZ 037D0G6
037D0GZ 037D0Z6 037D346 037D356 037D35Z 037D366 037D36Z 037D376 037D37Z 037D3D6 037D3E6 037D3EZ 037D3F6
037D3FZ 037D3G6 037D3GZ 037D3Z6 037D446 037D456 037D45Z 037D466 037D46Z 037D476 037D47Z 037D4D6 037D4E6
037D4EZ 037D4F6 037D4FZ 037D4G6 037D4GZ 037D4Z6 037F046 037F056 037F05Z 037F066 037F06Z 037F076 037F07Z
037F0D6 037F0E6 037F0EZ 037F0F6 037F0FZ 037F0G6 037F0GZ 037F0Z6 037F346 037F356 037F35Z 037F366 037F36Z
037F376 037F37Z 037F3D6 037F3E6 037F3EZ 037F3F6 037F3FZ 037F3G6 037F3GZ 037F3Z6 037F446 037F456 037F45Z
037F466 037F46Z 037F476 037F47Z 037F4D6 037F4E6 037F4EZ 037F4F6 037F4FZ 037F4G6 037F4GZ 037F4Z6 037G046
037G056 037G05Z 037G066 037G06Z 037G076 037G07Z 037G0D6 037G0E6 037G0EZ 037G0F6 037G0FZ 037G0G6 037G0GZ
037G0Z6 037G346 037G356 037G35Z 037G366 037G36Z 037G376 037G37Z 037G3D6 037G3E6 037G3EZ 037G3F6 037G3FZ
037G3G6 037G3GZ 037G3Z6 037G446 037G456 037G45Z 037G466 037G46Z 037G476 037G47Z 037G4D6 037G4E6 037G4EZ
037G4F6 037G4FZ 037G4G6 037G4GZ 037G4Z6 037H046 037H056 037H05Z 037H066 037H06Z 037H076 037H07Z 037H0D6
037H0E6 037H0EZ 037H0F6 037H0FZ 037H0G6 037H0GZ 037H0Z6 037H346 037H356 037H35Z 037H366 037H36Z 037H376
037H37Z 037H3D6 037H3E6 037H3EZ 037H3F6 037H3FZ 037H3G6 037H3GZ 037H3Z6 037H446 037H456 037H45Z 037H466
037H46Z 037H476 037H47Z 037H4D6 037H4E6 037H4EZ 037H4F6 037H4FZ 037H4G6 037H4GZ 037H4Z6 037J046 037J056
037J05Z 037J066 037J06Z 037J076 037J07Z 037J0D6 037J0E6 037J0EZ 037J0F6 037J0FZ 037J0G6 037J0GZ 037J0Z6
037J346 037J356 037J35Z 037J366 037J36Z 037J376 037J37Z 037J3D6 037J3E6 037J3EZ 037J3F6 037J3FZ 037J3G6
037J3GZ 037J3Z6 037J446 037J456 037J45Z 037J466 037J46Z 037J476 037J47Z 037J4D6 037J4E6 037J4EZ 037J4F6
037J4FZ 037J4G6 037J4GZ 037J4Z6 037K046 037K056 037K05Z 037K066 037K06Z 037K076 037K07Z 037K0D6 037K0E6
037K0EZ 037K0F6 037K0FZ 037K0G6 037K0GZ 037K0Z6 037K346 037K356 037K35Z 037K366 037K36Z 037K376 037K37Z
037K3D6 037K3E6 037K3EZ 037K3F6 037K3FZ 037K3G6 037K3GZ 037K3Z6 037K446 037K456 037K45Z 037K466 037K46Z
037K476 037K47Z 037K4D6 037K4E6 037K4EZ 037K4F6 037K4FZ 037K4G6 037K4GZ 037K4Z6 037L046 037L056 037L05Z
037L066 037L06Z 037L076 037L07Z 037L0D6 037L0E6 037L0EZ 037L0F6 037L0FZ 037L0G6 037L0GZ 037L0Z6 037L346
037L356 037L35Z 037L366 037L36Z 037L376 037L37Z 037L3D6 037L3E6 037L3EZ 037L3F6 037L3FZ 037L3G6 037L3GZ
037L3Z6 037L446 037L456 037L45Z 037L466 037L46Z 037L476 037L47Z 037L4D6 037L4E6 037L4EZ 037L4F6 037L4FZ
037L4G6 037L4GZ 037L4Z6 037M046 037M056 037M05Z 037M066 037M06Z 037M076 037M07Z 037M0D6 037M0E6 037M0EZ
037M0F6 037M0FZ 037M0G6 037M0GZ 037M0Z6 037M346 037M356 037M35Z 037M366 037M36Z 037M376 037M37Z 037M3D6
037M3E6 037M3EZ 037M3F6 037M3FZ 037M3G6 037M3GZ 037M3Z6 037M446 037M456 037M45Z 037M466 037M46Z 037M476
037M47Z 037M4D6 037M4E6 037M4EZ 037M4F6 037M4FZ 037M4G6 037M4GZ 037M4Z6 037N046 037N056 037N05Z 037N066
037N06Z 037N076 037N07Z 037N0D6 037N0E6 037N0EZ 037N0F6 037N0FZ 037N0G6 037N0GZ 037N0Z6 037N346 037N356
037N35Z 037N366 037N36Z 037N376 037N37Z 037N3D6 037N3E6 037N3EZ 037N3F6 037N3FZ 037N3G6 037N3GZ 037N3Z6
037N446 037N456 037N45Z 037N466 037N46Z 037N476 037N47Z 037N4D6 037N4E6 037N4EZ 037N4F6 037N4FZ 037N4G6
037N4GZ 037N4Z6 037P046 037P056 037P05Z 037P066 037P06Z 037P076 037P07Z 037P0D6 037P0E6 037P0EZ 037P0F6
037P0FZ 037P0G6 037P0GZ 037P0Z6 037P346 037P356 037P35Z 037P366 037P36Z 037P376 037P37Z 037P3D6 037P3E6
037P3EZ 037P3F6 037P3FZ 037P3G6 037P3GZ 037P3Z6 037P446 037P456 037P45Z 037P466 037P46Z 037P476 037P47Z
037P4D6 037P4E6 037P4EZ 037P4F6 037P4FZ 037P4G6 037P4GZ 037P4Z6 037Q046 037Q056 037Q05Z 037Q066 037Q06Z
037Q076 037Q07Z 037Q0D6 037Q0E6 037Q0EZ 037Q0F6 037Q0FZ 037Q0G6 037Q0GZ 037Q0Z6 037Q346 037Q356 037Q35Z
037Q366 037Q36Z 037Q376 037Q37Z 037Q3D6 037Q3E6 037Q3EZ 037Q3F6 037Q3FZ 037Q3G6 037Q3GZ 037Q3Z6 037Q446
037Q456 037Q45Z 037Q466 037Q46Z 037Q476 037Q47Z 037Q4D6 037Q4E6 037Q4EZ 037Q4F6 037Q4FZ 037Q4G6 037Q4GZ
037Q4Z6 037R046 037R056 037R05Z 037R066 037R06Z 037R076 037R07Z 037R0D6 037R0E6 037R0EZ 037R0F6 037R0FZ
037R0G6 037R0GZ 037R0Z6 037R346 037R356 037R35Z 037R366 037R36Z 037R376 037R37Z 037R3D6 037R3E6 037R3EZ
037R3F6 037R3FZ 037R3G6 037R3GZ 037R3Z6 037R446 037R456 037R45Z 037R466 037R46Z 037R476 037R47Z 037R4D6
037R4E6 037R4EZ 037R4F6 037R4FZ 037R4G6 037R4GZ 037R4Z6 037S046 037S056 037S05Z 037S066 037S06Z 037S076
037S07Z 037S0D6 037S0E6 037S0EZ 037S0F6 037S0FZ 037S0G6 037S0GZ 037S0Z6 037S346 037S356 037S35Z 037S366
037S36Z 037S376 037S37Z 037S3D6 037S3E6 037S3EZ 037S3F6 037S3FZ 037S3G6 037S3GZ 037S3Z6 037S446 037S456
037S45Z 037S466 037S46Z 037S476 037S47Z 037S4D6 037S4E6 037S4EZ 037S4F6 037S4FZ 037S4G6 037S4GZ 037S4Z6
037T046 037T056 037T05Z 037T066 037T06Z 037T076 037T07Z 037T0D6 037T0E6 037T0EZ 037T0F6 037T0FZ 037T0G6
037T0GZ 037T0Z6 037T346 037T356 037T35Z 037T366 037T36Z 037T376 037T37Z 037T3D6 037T3E6 037T3EZ 037T3F6
037T3FZ 037T3G6 037T3GZ 037T3Z6 037T446 037T456 037T45Z 037T466 037T46Z 037T476 037T47Z 037T4D6 037T4E6
037T4EZ 037T4F6 037T4FZ 037T4G6 037T4GZ 037T4Z6 037U046 037U056 037U05Z 037U066 037U06Z 037U076 037U07Z
037U0D6 037U0E6 037U0EZ 037U0F6 037U0FZ 037U0G6 037U0GZ 037U0Z6 037U346 037U356 037U35Z 037U366 037U36Z
037U376 037U37Z 037U3D6 037U3E6 037U3EZ 037U3F6 037U3FZ 037U3G6 037U3GZ 037U3Z6 037U446 037U456 037U45Z
037U466 037U46Z 037U476 037U47Z 037U4D6 037U4E6 037U4EZ 037U4F6 037U4FZ 037U4G6 037U4GZ 037U4Z6 037V046
037V056 037V05Z 037V066 037V06Z 037V076 037V07Z 037V0D6 037V0E6 037V0EZ 037V0F6 037V0FZ 037V0G6 037V0GZ
037V0Z6 037V346 037V356 037V35Z 037V366 037V36Z 037V376 037V37Z 037V3D6 037V3E6 037V3EZ 037V3F6 037V3FZ
037V3G6 037V3GZ 037V3Z6 037V446 037V456 037V45Z 037V466 037V46Z 037V476 037V47Z 037V4D6 037V4E6 037V4EZ
037V4F6 037V4FZ 037V4G6 037V4GZ 037V4Z6 037Y046 037Y056 037Y05Z 037Y066 037Y06Z 037Y076 037Y07Z 037Y0D6
037Y0E6 037Y0EZ 037Y0F6 037Y0FZ 037Y0G6 037Y0GZ 037Y0Z6 037Y346 037Y356 037Y35Z 037Y366 037Y36Z 037Y376
037Y37Z 037Y3D6 037Y3E6 037Y3EZ 037Y3F6 037Y3FZ 037Y3G6 037Y3GZ 037Y3Z6 037Y446 037Y456 037Y45Z 037Y466
037Y46Z 037Y476 037Y47Z 037Y4D6 037Y4E6 037Y4EZ 037Y4F6 037Y4FZ 037Y4G6 037Y4GZ 037Y4Z6

NC 037G3ZZ 037G4ZZ

LC Limited Coverage NC Noncovered HAC HAC Associated Procedure CC Combination Cluster - See Appendix G for code lists
DRG Non-OR-Affecting MS-DRG Assignment Non-OR-Not Affecting MS-DRG Assignment New/Revised Text in **Orange** ♂ Male ♀ Female

0 Medical and Surgical
3 Upper Arteries
9 Drainage: Taking or letting out fluids and/or gases from a body part

Body Part Character 4	Approach Character 5	Device Character 6	Qualifier Character 7
0 Internal Mammary Artery, Right ⊘ **1** Internal Mammary Artery, Left ⊘ **2** Innominate Artery ⊘ **3** Subclavian Artery, Right ⊘ **4** Subclavian Artery, Left ⊘ **5** Axillary Artery, Right ⊘ **6** Axillary Artery, Left ⊘ **7** Brachial Artery, Right ⊘ **8** Brachial Artery, Left ⊘ **9** Ulnar Artery, Right ⊘ **A** Ulnar Artery, Left ⊘ **B** Radial Artery, Right ⊘ **C** Radial Artery, Left ⊘ **D** Hand Artery, Right ⊘ **F** Hand Artery, Left ⊘ **G** Intracranial Artery ⊘ **H** Common Carotid Artery, Right ⊘ **J** Common Carotid Artery, Left ⊘ **K** Internal Carotid Artery, Right ⊘ **L** Internal Carotid Artery, Left ⊘ **M** External Carotid Artery, Right ⊘ **N** External Carotid Artery, Left ⊘ **P** Vertebral Artery, Right ⊘ **Q** Vertebral Artery, Left ⊘ **R** Face Artery ⊘ **S** Temporal Artery, Right ⊘ **T** Temporal Artery, Left ⊘ **U** Thyroid Artery, Right ⊘ **V** Thyroid Artery, Left ⊘ **Y** Upper Artery ⊘	**0** Open **3** Percutaneous **4** Percutaneous Endoscopic	**0** Drainage Device	**Z** No Qualifier
0 Internal Mammary Artery, Right ⊘ **1** Internal Mammary Artery, Left ⊘ **2** Innominate Artery ⊘ **3** Subclavian Artery, Right ⊘ **4** Subclavian Artery, Left ⊘ **5** Axillary Artery, Right ⊘ **6** Axillary Artery, Left ⊘ **7** Brachial Artery, Right ⊘ **8** Brachial Artery, Left ⊘ **9** Ulnar Artery, Right ⊘ **A** Ulnar Artery, Left ⊘ **B** Radial Artery, Right ⊘ **C** Radial Artery, Left ⊘ **D** Hand Artery, Right ⊘ **F** Hand Artery, Left ⊘ **G** Intracranial Artery ⊘ **H** Common Carotid Artery, Right ⊘ **J** Common Carotid Artery, Left ⊘ **K** Internal Carotid Artery, Right ⊘ **L** Internal Carotid Artery, Left ⊘ **M** External Carotid Artery, Right ⊘ **N** External Carotid Artery, Left ⊘ **P** Vertebral Artery, Right ⊘ **Q** Vertebral Artery, Left ⊘ **R** Face Artery ⊘ **S** Temporal Artery, Right ⊘ **T** Temporal Artery, Left ⊘ **U** Thyroid Artery, Right ⊘ **V** Thyroid Artery, Left ⊘ **Y** Upper Artery ⊘	**0** Open **3** Percutaneous **4** Percutaneous Endoscopic	**Z** No Device	**X** Diagnostic **Z** No Qualifier

⊘ 039000Z 03900ZZ 039030Z 03903ZZ 039040Z 03904ZZ 039100Z 03910ZZ 039130Z 03913ZZ 039140Z 03914ZZ 039200Z

039 continued on next page

039 continued from previous page

03920ZZ	039230Z	03923ZZ	039240Z	03924ZZ	039300Z	03930ZZ	039330Z	03933ZZ	039340Z	03934ZZ	039400Z	03940ZZ
039430Z	03943ZZ	039440Z	03944ZZ	039500Z	03950ZZ	039530Z	03953ZZ	039540Z	03954ZZ	039600Z	03960ZZ	039630Z
03963ZZ	039640Z	03964ZZ	039700Z	03970ZZ	039730Z	03973ZZ	039740Z	03974ZZ	039800Z	03980ZZ	039830Z	03983ZZ
039840Z	03984ZZ	039900Z	03990ZZ	039930Z	03993ZZ	039940Z	03994ZZ	039A00Z	039A0ZZ	039A30Z	039A3ZZ	039A40Z
039A4ZZ	039B00Z	039B0ZZ	039B30Z	039B3ZZ	039B40Z	039B4ZZ	039C00Z	039C0ZZ	039C30Z	039C3ZZ	039C40Z	039C4ZZ
039D00Z	039D0ZZ	039D30Z	039D3ZZ	039D40Z	039D4ZZ	039F00Z	039F0ZZ	039F30Z	039F3ZZ	039F40Z	039F4ZZ	039G00Z
039G0ZZ	039G30Z	039G3ZZ	039G40Z	039G4ZZ	039H00Z	039H0ZZ	039H30Z	039H3ZZ	039H40Z	039H4ZZ	039J00Z	039J0ZZ
039J30Z	039J3ZZ	039J40Z	039J4ZZ	039K00Z	039K0ZZ	039K30Z	039K3ZZ	039K40Z	039K4ZZ	039L00Z	039L0ZZ	039L30Z
039L3ZZ	039L40Z	039L4ZZ	039M00Z	039M0ZZ	039M30Z	039M3ZZ	039M40Z	039M4ZZ	039N00Z	039N0ZZ	039N30Z	039N3ZZ
039N40Z	039N4ZZ	039P00Z	039P0ZZ	039P30Z	039P3ZZ	039P40Z	039P4ZZ	039Q00Z	039Q0ZZ	039Q30Z	039Q3ZZ	039Q40Z
039Q4ZZ	039R00Z	039R0ZZ	039R30Z	039R3ZZ	039R40Z	039R4ZZ	039S00Z	039S0ZZ	039S30Z	039S3ZZ	039S40Z	039S4ZZ
039T00Z	039T0ZZ	039T30Z	039T3ZZ	039T40Z	039T4ZZ	039U00Z	039U0ZZ	039U30Z	039U3ZZ	039U40Z	039U4ZZ	039V00Z
039V0ZZ	039V30Z	039V3ZZ	039V40Z	039V4ZZ	039Y00Z	039Y0ZZ	039Y30Z	039Y3ZZ	039Y40Z	039Y4ZZ		

0 Medical and Surgical
3 Upper Arteries
B Excision: Cutting out or off, without replacement, a portion of a body part

Body Part Character 4	Approach Character 5	Device Character 6	Qualifier Character 7
0 Internal Mammary Artery, Right **1** Internal Mammary Artery, Left **2** Innominate Artery **3** Subclavian Artery, Right **4** Subclavian Artery, Left **5** Axillary Artery, Right **6** Axillary Artery, Left **7** Brachial Artery, Right **8** Brachial Artery, Left **9** Ulnar Artery, Right **A** Ulnar Artery, Left **B** Radial Artery, Right **C** Radial Artery, Left **D** Hand Artery, Right **F** Hand Artery, Left **G** Intracranial Artery **H** Common Carotid Artery, Right **J** Common Carotid Artery, Left **K** Internal Carotid Artery, Right **L** Internal Carotid Artery, Left **M** External Carotid Artery, Right **N** External Carotid Artery, Left **P** Vertebral Artery, Right **Q** Vertebral Artery, Left **R** Face Artery **S** Temporal Artery, Right **T** Temporal Artery, Left **U** Thyroid Artery, Right **V** Thyroid Artery, Left **Y** Upper Artery	**0** Open **3** Percutaneous **4** Percutaneous Endoscopic	**Z** No Device	**X** Diagnostic **Z** No Qualifier

0 Medical and Surgical
3 Upper Arteries
C Extirpation: Taking or cutting out solid matter from a body part

Body Part Character 4	Approach Character 5	Device Character 6	Qualifier Character 7
0 Internal Mammary Artery, Right ⦸ **1** Internal Mammary Artery, Left ⦸ **2** Innominate Artery ⦸ **3** Subclavian Artery, Right ⦸ **4** Subclavian Artery, Left ⦸ **5** Axillary Artery, Right ⦸ **6** Axillary Artery, Left ⦸ **7** Brachial Artery, Right ⦸ **8** Brachial Artery, Left ⦸ **9** Ulnar Artery, Right ⦸ **A** Ulnar Artery, Left ⦸ **B** Radial Artery, Right ⦸ **C** Radial Artery, Left ⦸ **D** Hand Artery, Right ⦸ **F** Hand Artery, Left ⦸ **G** Intracranial Artery ⦸ **H** Common Carotid Artery, Right ⦸ **J** Common Carotid Artery, Left ⦸ **K** Internal Carotid Artery, Right ⦸ **L** Internal Carotid Artery, Left ⦸ **M** External Carotid Artery, Right ⦸ **N** External Carotid Artery, Left ⦸ **P** Vertebral Artery, Right ⦸ **Q** Vertebral Artery, Left ⦸ **R** Face Artery ⦸ **S** Temporal Artery, Right ⦸ **T** Temporal Artery, Left ⦸ **U** Thyroid Artery, Right ⦸ **V** Thyroid Artery, Left ⦸ **Y** Upper Artery ⦸	**0** Open **3** Percutaneous **4** Percutaneous Endoscopic	**Z** No Device	**6** Bifurcation **Z** No Qualifier

⦸ 03C00Z6 03C03Z6 03C04Z6 03C10Z6 03C13Z6 03C14Z6 03C20Z6 03C23Z6 03C24Z6 03C30Z6 03C33Z6 03C34Z6 03C40Z6 03C43Z6 03C44Z6 03C50Z6 03C53Z6 03C54Z6 03C60Z6 03C63Z6 03C64Z6 03C70Z6 03C73Z6 03C74Z6 03C80Z6 03C83Z6 03C84Z6 03C90Z6 03C93Z6 03C94Z6 03CA0Z6 03CA3Z6 03CA4Z6 03CB0Z6 03CB3Z6 03CB4Z6 03CC0Z6 03CC3Z6 03CC4Z6 03CD0Z6 03CD3Z6 03CD4Z6 03CF0Z6 03CF3Z6 03CF4Z6 03CG0Z6 03CG3Z6 03CG4Z6 03CH0Z6 03CH3Z6 03CH4Z6 03CJ0Z6 03CJ3Z6 03CJ4Z6 03CK0Z6 03CK3Z6 03CK4Z6 03CL0Z6 03CL3Z6 03CL4Z6 03CM0Z6 03CM3Z6 03CM4Z6 03CN0Z6 03CN3Z6 03CN4Z6 03CP0Z6 03CP3Z6 03CP4Z6 03CQ0Z6 03CQ3Z6 03CQ4Z6 03CR0Z6 03CR3Z6 03CR4Z6 03CS0Z6 03CS3Z6 03CS4Z6 03CT0Z6 03CT3Z6 03CT4Z6 03CU0Z6 03CU3Z6 03CU4Z6 03CV0Z6 03CV3Z6 03CV4Z6 03CY0Z6 03CY3Z6 03CY4Z6

0 Medical and Surgical
3 Upper Arteries
H Insertion: Putting in a nonbiological appliance that monitors, assists, performs, or prevents a physiological function but does not physically take the place of a body part

Body Part Character 4	Approach Character 5	Device Character 6	Qualifier Character 7
0 Internal Mammary Artery, Right ⊘ **1** Internal Mammary Artery, Left ⊘ **2** Innominate Artery ⊘ **3** Subclavian Artery, Right ⊘ **4** Subclavian Artery, Left ⊘ **5** Axillary Artery, Right ⊘ **6** Axillary Artery, Left ⊘ **7** Brachial Artery, Right ⊘ **8** Brachial Artery, Left ⊘ **9** Ulnar Artery, Right ⊘ **A** Ulnar Artery, Left ⊘ **B** Radial Artery, Right ⊘ **C** Radial Artery, Left ⊘ **D** Hand Artery, Right ⊘ **F** Hand Artery, Left ⊘ **G** Intracranial Artery ⊘ **H** Common Carotid Artery, Right ⊘ **J** Common Carotid Artery, Left ⊘ **M** External Carotid Artery, Right ⊘ **N** External Carotid Artery, Left ⊘ **P** Vertebral Artery, Right ⊘ **Q** Vertebral Artery, Left ⊘ **R** Face Artery ⊘ **S** Temporal Artery, Right ⊘ **T** Temporal Artery, Left ⊘ **U** Thyroid Artery, Right ⊘ **V** Thyroid Artery, Left ⊘	**0** Open **3** Percutaneous **4** Percutaneous Endoscopic	**3** Infusion Device **D** Intraluminal Device	**Z** No Qualifier
K Internal Carotid Artery, Right ⊘ CC **L** Internal Carotid Artery, Left ⊘ CC	**0** Open **3** Percutaneous **4** Percutaneous Endoscopic	**3** Infusion Device **D** Intraluminal Device **M** Stimulator Lead	**Z** No Qualifier
Y Upper Artery ⊘	**0** Open **3** Percutaneous **4** Percutaneous Endoscopic	**2** Monitoring Device **3** Infusion Device **D** Intraluminal Device	**Z** No Qualifier

⊘ 03H003Z 03H033Z 03H043Z 03H103Z 03H133Z 03H143Z 03H203Z 03H233Z 03H243Z 03H303Z 03H333Z 03H343Z 03H403Z 03H433Z 03H443Z 03H503Z 03H533Z 03H543Z 03H603Z 03H633Z 03H643Z 03H703Z 03H733Z 03H743Z 03H803Z 03H833Z 03H843Z 03H903Z 03H933Z 03H943Z 03HA03Z 03HA33Z 03HA43Z 03HB03Z 03HB33Z 03HB43Z 03HC03Z 03HC33Z 03HC43Z 03HD03Z 03HD33Z 03HD43Z 03HF03Z 03HF33Z 03HF43Z 03HG03Z 03HG33Z 03HG43Z 03HH03Z 03HH33Z 03HH43Z 03HJ03Z 03HJ33Z 03HJ43Z 03HK03Z 03HK33Z 03HK43Z 03HL03Z 03HL33Z 03HL43Z 03HM03Z 03HM33Z 03HM43Z 03HN03Z 03HN33Z 03HN43Z 03HP03Z 03HP33Z 03HP43Z 03HQ03Z 03HQ33Z 03HQ43Z 03HR03Z 03HR33Z 03HR43Z 03HS03Z 03HS33Z 03HS43Z 03HT03Z 03HT33Z 03HT43Z 03HU03Z 03HU33Z 03HU43Z 03HV03Z 03HV33Z 03HV43Z 03HY03Z 03HY32Z 03HY33Z 03HY43Z

CC 03HK0MZ 03HK3MZ 03HK4MZ 03HL0MZ 03HL3MZ 03HL4MZ

0 Medical and Surgical
3 Upper Arteries
J Inspection: Visually and/or manually exploring a body part

Body Part Character 4	Approach Character 5	Device Character 6	Qualifier Character 7
Y Upper Artery ⊘	**0** Open **3** Percutaneous **4** Percutaneous Endoscopic **X** External	**Z** No Device	**Z** No Qualifier

⊘ 03JY3ZZ 03JY4ZZ 03JYXZZ

LC Limited Coverage NC Noncovered HAC HAC Associated Procedure CC Combination Cluster - See Appendix G for code lists
DRG Non-OR-Affecting MS-DRG Assignment ⊘ Non-OR-Not Affecting MS-DRG Assignment New/Revised Text in **Orange** ♂ Male ♀ Female

0 Medical and Surgical
3 Upper Arteries
L Occlusion: Completely closing an orifice or the lumen of a tubular body part

Body Part Character 4	Approach Character 5	Device Character 6	Qualifier Character 7
0 Internal Mammary Artery, Right **1** Internal Mammary Artery, Left **2** Innominate Artery **3** Subclavian Artery, Right **4** Subclavian Artery, Left **5** Axillary Artery, Right **6** Axillary Artery, Left **7** Brachial Artery, Right **8** Brachial Artery, Left **9** Ulnar Artery, Right **A** Ulnar Artery, Left **B** Radial Artery, Right **C** Radial Artery, Left **D** Hand Artery, Right **F** Hand Artery, Left **R** Face Artery **S** Temporal Artery, Right **T** Temporal Artery, Left **U** Thyroid Artery, Right **V** Thyroid Artery, Left **Y** Upper Artery	**0** Open **3** Percutaneous **4** Percutaneous Endoscopic	**C** Extraluminal Device **D** Intraluminal Device **Z** No Device	**Z** No Qualifier
G Intracranial Artery **H** Common Carotid Artery, Right **J** Common Carotid Artery, Left **K** Internal Carotid Artery, Right **L** Internal Carotid Artery, Left **M** External Carotid Artery, Right **N** External Carotid Artery, Left **P** Vertebral Artery, Right **Q** Vertebral Artery, Left	**0** Open **3** Percutaneous **4** Percutaneous Endoscopic	**B** Intraluminal Device, Bioactive **C** Extraluminal Device **D** Intraluminal Device **Z** No Device	**Z** No Qualifier

0 Medical and Surgical
3 Upper Arteries
N Release: Freeing a body part from an abnormal physical constraint by cutting or by the use of force

Body Part Character 4	Approach Character 5	Device Character 6	Qualifier Character 7
0 Internal Mammary Artery, Right	**0** Open	**Z** No Device	**Z** No Qualifier
1 Internal Mammary Artery, Left	**3** Percutaneous		
2 Innominate Artery	**4** Percutaneous Endoscopic		
3 Subclavian Artery, Right			
4 Subclavian Artery, Left			
5 Axillary Artery, Right			
6 Axillary Artery, Left			
7 Brachial Artery, Right			
8 Brachial Artery, Left			
9 Ulnar Artery, Right			
A Ulnar Artery, Left			
B Radial Artery, Right			
C Radial Artery, Left			
D Hand Artery, Right			
F Hand Artery, Left			
G Intracranial Artery			
H Common Carotid Artery, Right			
J Common Carotid Artery, Left			
K Internal Carotid Artery, Right			
L Internal Carotid Artery, Left			
M External Carotid Artery, Right			
N External Carotid Artery, Left			
P Vertebral Artery, Right			
Q Vertebral Artery, Left			
R Face Artery			
S Temporal Artery, Right			
T Temporal Artery, Left			
U Thyroid Artery, Right			
V Thyroid Artery, Left			
Y Upper Artery			

0 Medical and Surgical
3 Upper Arteries
P Removal: Taking out or off a device from a body part

Body Part Character 4	Approach Character 5	Device Character 6	Qualifier Character 7
Y Upper Artery ⊘ CC	**0** Open **3** Percutaneous **4** Percutaneous Endoscopic	**0** Drainage Device **2** Monitoring Device **3** Infusion Device **7** Autologous Tissue Substitute **C** Extraluminal Device **D** Intraluminal Device **J** Synthetic Substitute **K** Nonautologous Tissue Substitute **M** Stimulator Lead	**Z** No Qualifier
Y Upper Artery ⊘	**X** External	**0** Drainage Device **2** Monitoring Device **3** Infusion Device **D** Intraluminal Device **M** Stimulator Lead	**Z** No Qualifier

⊘ 03PY30Z 03PY32Z 03PY33Z 03PYX0Z 03PYX2Z 03PYX3Z 03PYXDZ 03PYXMZ
CC 03PY0JZ 03PY0MZ 03PY3JZ 03PY3MZ 03PY4JZ 03PY4MZ

0 Medical and Surgical
3 Upper Arteries
Q Repair: Restoring, to the extent possible, a body part to its normal anatomic structure and function

Body Part Character 4	Approach Character 5	Device Character 6	Qualifier Character 7
0 Internal Mammary Artery, Right **1** Internal Mammary Artery, Left **2** Innominate Artery **3** Subclavian Artery, Right **4** Subclavian Artery, Left **5** Axillary Artery, Right **6** Axillary Artery, Left **7** Brachial Artery, Right **8** Brachial Artery, Left **9** Ulnar Artery, Right **A** Ulnar Artery, Left **B** Radial Artery, Right **C** Radial Artery, Left **D** Hand Artery, Right **F** Hand Artery, Left **G** Intracranial Artery **H** Common Carotid Artery, Right **J** Common Carotid Artery, Left **K** Internal Carotid Artery, Right **L** Internal Carotid Artery, Left **M** External Carotid Artery, Right **N** External Carotid Artery, Left **P** Vertebral Artery, Right **Q** Vertebral Artery, Left **R** Face Artery **S** Temporal Artery, Right **T** Temporal Artery, Left **U** Thyroid Artery, Right **V** Thyroid Artery, Left **Y** Upper Artery	**0** Open **3** Percutaneous **4** Percutaneous Endoscopic	**Z** No Device	**Z** No Qualifier

0 Medical and Surgical
3 Upper Arteries
R Replacement: Putting in or on biological or synthetic material that physically takes the place and/or function of all or a portion of a body part

Body Part Character 4	Approach Character 5	Device Character 6	Qualifier Character 7
0 Internal Mammary Artery, Right **1** Internal Mammary Artery, Left **2** Innominate Artery **3** Subclavian Artery, Right **4** Subclavian Artery, Left **5** Axillary Artery, Right **6** Axillary Artery, Left **7** Brachial Artery, Right **8** Brachial Artery, Left **9** Ulnar Artery, Right **A** Ulnar Artery, Left **B** Radial Artery, Right **C** Radial Artery, Left **D** Hand Artery, Right **F** Hand Artery, Left **G** Intracranial Artery **H** Common Carotid Artery, Right **J** Common Carotid Artery, Left **K** Internal Carotid Artery, Right **L** Internal Carotid Artery, Left **M** External Carotid Artery, Right **N** External Carotid Artery, Left **P** Vertebral Artery, Right **Q** Vertebral Artery, Left **R** Face Artery **S** Temporal Artery, Right **T** Temporal Artery, Left **U** Thyroid Artery, Right **V** Thyroid Artery, Left **Y** Upper Artery	**0** Open **4** Percutaneous Endoscopic	**7** Autologous Tissue Substitute **J** Synthetic Substitute **K** Nonautologous Tissue Substitute	**Z** No Qualifier

0 Medical and Surgical
3 Upper Arteries
S Reposition: Moving to its normal location, or other suitable location, all or a portion of a body part

Body Part Character 4	Approach Character 5	Device Character 6	Qualifier Character 7
0 Internal Mammary Artery, Right **1** Internal Mammary Artery, Left **2** Innominate Artery **3** Subclavian Artery, Right **4** Subclavian Artery, Left **5** Axillary Artery, Right **6** Axillary Artery, Left **7** Brachial Artery, Right **8** Brachial Artery, Left **9** Ulnar Artery, Right **A** Ulnar Artery, Left **B** Radial Artery, Right **C** Radial Artery, Left **D** Hand Artery, Right **F** Hand Artery, Left **G** Intracranial Artery **H** Common Carotid Artery, Right **J** Common Carotid Artery, Left **K** Internal Carotid Artery, Right **L** Internal Carotid Artery, Left **M** External Carotid Artery, Right **N** External Carotid Artery, Left **P** Vertebral Artery, Right **Q** Vertebral Artery, Left **R** Face Artery **S** Temporal Artery, Right **T** Temporal Artery, Left **U** Thyroid Artery, Right **V** Thyroid Artery, Left **Y** Upper Artery	**0** Open **3** Percutaneous **4** Percutaneous Endoscopic	**Z** No Device	**Z** No Qualifier

0 Medical and Surgical
3 Upper Arteries
U Supplement: Putting in or on biological or synthetic material that physically reinforces and/or augments the function of a portion of a body part

Body Part Character 4	Approach Character 5	Device Character 6	Qualifier Character 7
0 Internal Mammary Artery, Right **1** Internal Mammary Artery, Left **2** Innominate Artery **3** Subclavian Artery, Right **4** Subclavian Artery, Left **5** Axillary Artery, Right **6** Axillary Artery, Left **7** Brachial Artery, Right **8** Brachial Artery, Left **9** Ulnar Artery, Right **A** Ulnar Artery, Left **B** Radial Artery, Right **C** Radial Artery, Left **D** Hand Artery, Right **F** Hand Artery, Left **G** Intracranial Artery **H** Common Carotid Artery, Right **J** Common Carotid Artery, Left **K** Internal Carotid Artery, Right **L** Internal Carotid Artery, Left **M** External Carotid Artery, Right **N** External Carotid Artery, Left **P** Vertebral Artery, Right **Q** Vertebral Artery, Left **R** Face Artery **S** Temporal Artery, Right **T** Temporal Artery, Left **U** Thyroid Artery, Right **V** Thyroid Artery, Left **Y** Upper Artery	**0** Open **3** Percutaneous **4** Percutaneous Endoscopic	**7** Autologous Tissue Substitute **J** Synthetic Substitute **K** Nonautologous Tissue Substitute	**Z** No Qualifier

0 Medical and Surgical
3 Upper Arteries
V Restriction: Partially closing an orifice or the lumen of a tubular body part

Body Part Character 4	Approach Character 5	Device Character 6	Qualifier Character 7
0 Internal Mammary Artery, Right **1** Internal Mammary Artery, Left **2** Innominate Artery **3** Subclavian Artery, Right **4** Subclavian Artery, Left **5** Axillary Artery, Right **6** Axillary Artery, Left **7** Brachial Artery, Right **8** Brachial Artery, Left **9** Ulnar Artery, Right **A** Ulnar Artery, Left **B** Radial Artery, Right **C** Radial Artery, Left **D** Hand Artery, Right **F** Hand Artery, Left **R** Face Artery **S** Temporal Artery, Right **T** Temporal Artery, Left **U** Thyroid Artery, Right **V** Thyroid Artery, Left **Y** Upper Artery	**0** Open **3** Percutaneous **4** Percutaneous Endoscopic	**C** Extraluminal Device **D** Intraluminal Device **Z** No Device	**Z** No Qualifier
G Intracranial Artery **H** Common Carotid Artery, Right **J** Common Carotid Artery, Left **K** Internal Carotid Artery, Right **L** Internal Carotid Artery, Left **M** External Carotid Artery, Right **N** External Carotid Artery, Left **P** Vertebral Artery, Right **Q** Vertebral Artery, Left	**0** Open **3** Percutaneous **4** Percutaneous Endoscopic	**B** Intraluminal Device, Bioactive **C** Extraluminal Device **D** Intraluminal Device **Z** No Device	**Z** No Qualifier

0 Medical and Surgical
3 Upper Arteries
W Revision: Correcting, to the extent possible, a portion of a malfunctioning device or the position of a displaced device

Body Part Character 4	Approach Character 5	Device Character 6	Qualifier Character 7
Y Upper Artery ⃠	**0** Open **3** Percutaneous **4** Percutaneous Endoscopic **X** External	**0** Drainage Device **2** Monitoring Device **3** Infusion Device **7** Autologous Tissue Substitute **C** Extraluminal Device **D** Intraluminal Device **J** Synthetic Substitute **K** Nonautologous Tissue Substitute **M** Stimulator Lead	**Z** No Qualifier

⃠ 03WYX0Z 03WYX2Z 03WYX3Z 03WYX7Z 03WYXCZ 03WYXDZ 03WYXJZ 03WYXKZ 03WYXMZ

Lower Arteries 041-04W

0 Medical and Surgical
4 Lower Arteries
1 Bypass: Altering the route of passage of the contents of a tubular body part

Body Part Character 4	Approach Character 5	Device Character 6	Qualifier Character 7
0 Abdominal Aorta **C** Common Iliac Artery, Right **D** Common Iliac Artery, Left	**0** Open **4** Percutaneous Endoscopic	**9** Autologous Venous Tissue **A** Autologous Arterial Tissue **J** Synthetic Substitute **K** Nonautologous Tissue Substitute **Z** No Device	**0** Abdominal Aorta **1** Celiac Artery **2** Mesenteric Artery **3** Renal Artery, Right **4** Renal Artery, Left **5** Renal Artery, Bilateral **6** Common Iliac Artery, Right **7** Common Iliac Artery, Left **8** Common Iliac Arteries, Bilateral **9** Internal Iliac Artery, Right **B** Internal Iliac Artery, Left **C** Internal Iliac Arteries, Bilateral **D** External Iliac Artery, Right **F** External Iliac Artery, Left **G** External Iliac Arteries, Bilateral **H** Femoral Artery, Right **J** Femoral Artery, Left **K** Femoral Arteries, Bilateral **Q** Lower Extremity Artery **R** Lower Artery
4 Splenic Artery	**0** Open **4** Percutaneous Endoscopic	**9** Autologous Venous Tissue **A** Autologous Arterial Tissue **J** Synthetic Substitute **K** Nonautologous Tissue Substitute **Z** No Device	**3** Renal Artery, Right **4** Renal Artery, Left **5** Renal Artery, Bilateral
E Internal Iliac Artery, Right **F** Internal Iliac Artery, Left **H** External Iliac Artery, Right **J** External Iliac Artery, Left	**0** Open **4** Percutaneous Endoscopic	**9** Autologous Venous Tissue **A** Autologous Arterial Tissue **J** Synthetic Substitute **K** Nonautologous Tissue Substitute **Z** No Device	**9** Internal Iliac Artery, Right **B** Internal Iliac Artery, Left **C** Internal Iliac Arteries, Bilateral **D** External Iliac Artery, Right **F** External Iliac Artery, Left **G** External Iliac Arteries, Bilateral **H** Femoral Artery, Right **J** Femoral Artery, Left **K** Femoral Arteries, Bilateral **P** Foot Artery **Q** Lower Extremity Artery
K Femoral Artery, Right **L** Femoral Artery, Left	**0** Open **4** Percutaneous Endoscopic	**9** Autologous Venous Tissue **A** Autologous Arterial Tissue **J** Synthetic Substitute **K** Nonautologous Tissue Substitute **Z** No Device	**H** Femoral Artery, Right **J** Femoral Artery, Left **K** Femoral Arteries, Bilateral **L** Popliteal Artery **M** Peroneal Artery **N** Posterior Tibial Artery **P** Foot Artery **Q** Lower Extremity Artery **S** Lower Extremity Vein
M Popliteal Artery, Right **N** Popliteal Artery, Left	**0** Open **4** Percutaneous Endoscopic	**9** Autologous Venous Tissue **A** Autologous Arterial Tissue **J** Synthetic Substitute **K** Nonautologous Tissue Substitute **Z** No Device	**L** Popliteal Artery **M** Peroneal Artery **P** Foot Artery **Q** Lower Extremity Artery **S** Lower Extremity Vein

0 Medical and Surgical
4 Lower Arteries
5 Destruction: Physical eradication of all or a portion of a body part by the direct use of energy, force, or a destructive agent

Body Part Character 4	Approach Character 5	Device Character 6	Qualifier Character 7
0 Abdominal Aorta **1** Celiac Artery **2** Gastric Artery **3** Hepatic Artery **4** Splenic Artery **5** Superior Mesenteric Artery **6** Colic Artery, Right **7** Colic Artery, Left **8** Colic Artery, Middle **9** Renal Artery, Right **A** Renal Artery, Left **B** Inferior Mesenteric Artery **C** Common Iliac Artery, Right **D** Common Iliac Artery, Left **E** Internal Iliac Artery, Right **F** Internal Iliac Artery, Left **H** External Iliac Artery, Right **J** External Iliac Artery, Left **K** Femoral Artery, Right **L** Femoral Artery, Left **M** Popliteal Artery, Right **N** Popliteal Artery, Left **P** Anterior Tibial Artery, Right **Q** Anterior Tibial Artery, Left **R** Posterior Tibial Artery, Right **S** Posterior Tibial Artery, Left **T** Peroneal Artery, Right **U** Peroneal Artery, Left **V** Foot Artery, Right **W** Foot Artery, Left **Y** Lower Artery	**0** Open **3** Percutaneous **4** Percutaneous Endoscopic	**Z** No Device	**Z** No Qualifier

0 Medical and Surgical
4 Lower Arteries
7 Dilation: Expanding an orifice or the lumen of a tubular body part

Body Part Character 4	Approach Character 5	Device Character 6	Qualifier Character 7
0 Abdominal Aorta ⦸ **1** Celiac Artery ⦸ **2** Gastric Artery ⦸ **3** Hepatic Artery ⦸ **4** Splenic Artery ⦸ **5** Superior Mesenteric Artery ⦸ **6** Colic Artery, Right ⦸ **7** Colic Artery, Left ⦸ **8** Colic Artery, Middle ⦸ **9** Renal Artery, Right ⦸ **A** Renal Artery, Left ⦸ **B** Inferior Mesenteric Artery ⦸ **C** Common Iliac Artery, Right ⦸ **D** Common Iliac Artery, Left ⦸ **E** Internal Iliac Artery, Right ⦸ **F** Internal Iliac Artery, Left ⦸ **H** External Iliac Artery, Right ⦸ **J** External Iliac Artery, Left ⦸ **P** Anterior Tibial Artery, Right ⦸ **Q** Anterior Tibial Artery, Left ⦸ **R** Posterior Tibial Artery, Right ⦸ **S** Posterior Tibial Artery, Left ⦸ **T** Peroneal Artery, Right ⦸ **U** Peroneal Artery, Left ⦸ **V** Foot Artery, Right ⦸ **W** Foot Artery, Left ⦸ **Y** Lower Artery ⦸	**0** Open **3** Percutaneous **4** Percutaneous Endoscopic	**4** Intraluminal Device, Drug-eluting **5** Intraluminal Device, Drug-eluting, Two **6** Intraluminal Device, Drug-eluting, Three **7** Intraluminal Device, Drug-eluting, Four or More **D** Intraluminal Device **E** Intraluminal Device, Two **F** Intraluminal Device, Three **G** Intraluminal Device, Four or More **Z** No Device	**6** Bifurcation **Z** No Qualifier
K Femoral Artery, Right ⦸ **L** Femoral Artery, Left ⦸ **M** Popliteal Artery, Right ⦸ **N** Popliteal Artery, Left ⦸	**0** Open **3** Percutaneous **4** Percutaneous Endoscopic	**4** Intraluminal Device, Drug-eluting **D** Intraluminal Device **Z** No Device	**1** Drug-Coated Balloon **6** Bifurcation **Z** No Qualifier
K Femoral Artery, Right ⦸ **L** Femoral Artery, Left ⦸ **M** Popliteal Artery, Right ⦸ **N** Popliteal Artery, Left ⦸	**0** Open **3** Percutaneous **4** Percutaneous Endoscopic	**5** Intraluminal Device, Drug-eluting, Two **6** Intraluminal Device, Drug-eluting, Three **7** Intraluminal Device, Drug-eluting, Four or More **E** Intraluminal Device, Two **F** Intraluminal Device, Three **G** Intraluminal Device, Four or More	**6** Bifurcation **Z** No Qualifier

⦸ 0470046	0470056	047005Z	0470066	047006Z	0470076	047007Z	04700D6	04700E6	04700EZ	04700F6	04700FZ	04700G6
04700GZ	04700Z6	0470346	0470356	047035Z	0470366	047036Z	0470376	047037Z	04703D6	04703E6	04703EZ	04703F6
04703FZ	04703G6	04703GZ	04703Z6	0470446	0470456	047045Z	0470466	047046Z	0470476	047047Z	04704D6	04704E6
04704EZ	04704F6	04704FZ	04704G6	04704GZ	04704Z6	0471046	0471056	047105Z	0471066	047106Z	0471076	047107Z
04710D6	04710E6	04710EZ	04710F6	04710FZ	04710G6	04710GZ	04710Z6	0471346	0471356	047135Z	0471366	047136Z
0471376	047137Z	04713D6	04713E6	04713EZ	04713F6	04713FZ	04713G6	04713GZ	04713Z6	0471446	0471456	047145Z
0471466	047146Z	0471476	047147Z	04714D6	04714E6	04714EZ	04714F6	04714FZ	04714G6	04714GZ	04714Z6	0472046
0472056	047205Z	0472066	047206Z	0472076	047207Z	04720D6	04720E6	04720EZ	04720F6	04720FZ	04720G6	04720GZ
04720Z6	0472346	0472356	047235Z	0472366	047236Z	0472376	047237Z	04723D6	04723E6	04723EZ	04723F6	04723FZ
04723G6	04723GZ	04723Z6	0472446	0472456	047245Z	0472466	047246Z	0472476	047247Z	04724D6	04724E6	04724EZ
04724F6	04724FZ	04724G6	04724GZ	04724Z6	0473046	0473056	047305Z	0473066	047306Z	0473076	047307Z	04730D6
04730E6	04730EZ	04730F6	04730FZ	04730G6	04730GZ	04730Z6	0473346	0473356	047335Z	0473366	047336Z	0473376
047337Z	04733D6	04733E6	04733EZ	04733F6	04733FZ	04733G6	04733GZ	04733Z6	0473446	0473456	047345Z	0473466
047346Z	0473476	047347Z	04734D6	04734E6	04734EZ	04734F6	04734FZ	04734G6	04734GZ	04734Z6	0474046	0474056
047405Z	0474066	047406Z	0474076	047407Z	04740D6	04740E6	04740EZ	04740F6	04740FZ	04740G6	04740GZ	04740Z6
0474346	0474356	047435Z	0474366	047436Z	0474376	047437Z	04743D6	04743E6	04743EZ	04743F6	04743FZ	04743G6
04743GZ	04743Z6	0474446	0474456	047445Z	0474466	047446Z	0474476	047447Z	04744D6	04744E6	04744EZ	04744F6
04744FZ	04744G6	04744GZ	04744Z6	0475046	0475056	047505Z	0475066	047506Z	0475076	047507Z	04750D6	04750E6
04750EZ	04750F6	04750FZ	04750G6	04750GZ	04750Z6	0475346	0475356	047535Z	0475366	047536Z	0475376	047537Z

047 continued on next page

047 continued from previous page

04753D6	04753E6	04753EZ	04753F6	04753FZ	04753G6	04753GZ	04753Z6	0475446	0475456	047545Z	0475466	047546Z
0475476	047547Z	04754D6	04754DZ	04754E6	04754EZ	04754F6	04754FZ	04754G6	04754GZ	04754Z6	0476046	0476056
047605Z	0476066	047606Z	0476076	047607Z	04760D6	04760E6	04760EZ	04760F6	04760FZ	04760G6	04760GZ	04760Z6
0476346	0476356	047635Z	0476366	047636Z	0476376	047637Z	04763D6	04763E6	04763EZ	04763F6	04763FZ	04763G6
04763GZ	04763Z6	0476446	0476456	047645Z	0476466	047646Z	0476476	047647Z	04764D6	04764E6	04764EZ	04764F6
04764FZ	04764G6	04764GZ	04764Z6	0477046	0477056	047705Z	0477066	047706Z	0477076	047707Z	04770D6	04770E6
04770EZ	04770F6	04770FZ	04770G6	04770GZ	04770Z6	0477346	0477356	047735Z	0477366	047736Z	0477376	047737Z
04773D6	04773E6	04773EZ	04773F6	04773FZ	04773G6	04773GZ	04773Z6	0477446	0477456	047745Z	0477466	047746Z
0477476	047747Z	04774D6	04774E6	04774EZ	04774F6	04774FZ	04774G6	04774GZ	04774Z6	0478046	0478056	047805Z
0478066	047806Z	0478076	047807Z	04780D6	04780E6	04780EZ	04780F6	04780FZ	04780G6	04780GZ	04780Z6	0478346
0478356	047835Z	0478366	047836Z	0478376	047837Z	04783D6	04783E6	04783EZ	04783F6	04783FZ	04783G6	04783GZ
04783Z6	0478446	0478456	047845Z	0478466	047846Z	0478476	047847Z	04784D6	04784E6	04784EZ	04784F6	04784FZ
04784G6	04784GZ	04784Z6	0479046	0479056	047905Z	0479066	047906Z	0479076	047907Z	04790D6	04790E6	04790EZ
04790F6	04790FZ	04790G6	04790GZ	04790Z6	0479346	0479356	047935Z	0479366	047936Z	0479376	047937Z	04793D6
04793E6	04793EZ	04793F6	04793FZ	04793G6	04793GZ	04793Z6	0479446	0479456	047945Z	0479466	047946Z	0479476
047947Z	04794D6	04794DZ	04794E6	04794EZ	04794F6	04794FZ	04794G6	04794GZ	04794Z6	047A046	047A056	047A05Z
047A066	047A06Z	047A076	047A07Z	047A0D6	047A0E6	047A0EZ	047A0F6	047A0FZ	047A0G6	047A0GZ	047A0Z6	047A346
047A356	047A35Z	047A366	047A36Z	047A376	047A37Z	047A3D6	047A3E6	047A3EZ	047A3F6	047A3FZ	047A3G6	047A3GZ
047A3Z6	047A446	047A456	047A45Z	047A466	047A46Z	047A476	047A47Z	047A4D6	047A4DZ	047A4E6	047A4EZ	047A4F6
047A4FZ	047A4G6	047A4GZ	047A4Z6	047B046	047B056	047B05Z	047B066	047B06Z	047B076	047B07Z	047B0D6	047B0E6
047B0EZ	047B0F6	047B0FZ	047B0G6	047B0GZ	047B0Z6	047B346	047B356	047B35Z	047B366	047B36Z	047B376	047B37Z
047B3D6	047B3E6	047B3EZ	047B3F6	047B3FZ	047B3G6	047B3GZ	047B3Z6	047B446	047B456	047B45Z	047B466	047B46Z
047B476	047B47Z	047B4D6	047B4E6	047B4EZ	047B4F6	047B4FZ	047B4G6	047B4GZ	047B4Z6	047C046	047C056	047C05Z
047C066	047C06Z	047C076	047C07Z	047C0D6	047C0E6	047C0EZ	047C0F6	047C0FZ	047C0G6	047C0GZ	047C0Z6	047C346
047C356	047C35Z	047C366	047C36Z	047C376	047C37Z	047C3D6	047C3E6	047C3EZ	047C3F6	047C3FZ	047C3G6	047C3GZ
047C3Z6	047C446	047C456	047C45Z	047C466	047C46Z	047C476	047C47Z	047C4D6	047C4E6	047C4EZ	047C4F6	047C4FZ
047C4G6	047C4GZ	047C4Z6	047D046	047D056	047D05Z	047D066	047D06Z	047D076	047D07Z	047D0D6	047D0E6	047D0EZ
047D0F6	047D0FZ	047D0G6	047D0GZ	047D0Z6	047D346	047D356	047D35Z	047D366	047D36Z	047D376	047D37Z	047D3D6
047D3E6	047D3EZ	047D3F6	047D3FZ	047D3G6	047D3GZ	047D3Z6	047D446	047D456	047D45Z	047D466	047D46Z	047D476
047D47Z	047D4D6	047D4E6	047D4EZ	047D4F6	047D4FZ	047D4G6	047D4GZ	047D4Z6	047E046	047E056	047E05Z	047E066
047E06Z	047E076	047E07Z	047E0D6	047E0E6	047E0EZ	047E0F6	047E0FZ	047E0G6	047E0GZ	047E0Z6	047E346	047E356
047E35Z	047E366	047E36Z	047E376	047E37Z	047E3D6	047E3E6	047E3EZ	047E3F6	047E3FZ	047E3G6	047E3GZ	047E3Z6
047E446	047E456	047E45Z	047E466	047E46Z	047E476	047E47Z	047E4D6	047E4E6	047E4EZ	047E4F6	047E4FZ	047E4G6
047E4GZ	047E4Z6	047F046	047F056	047F05Z	047F066	047F06Z	047F076	047F07Z	047F0D6	047F0E6	047F0EZ	047F0F6
047F0FZ	047F0G6	047F0GZ	047F0Z6	047F346	047F356	047F35Z	047F366	047F36Z	047F376	047F37Z	047F3D6	047F3E6
047F3EZ	047F3F6	047F3FZ	047F3G6	047F3GZ	047F3Z6	047F446	047F456	047F45Z	047F466	047F46Z	047F476	047F47Z
047F4D6	047F4E6	047F4EZ	047F4F6	047F4FZ	047F4G6	047F4GZ	047F4Z6	047H046	047H056	047H05Z	047H066	047H06Z
047H076	047H07Z	047H0D6	047H0E6	047H0EZ	047H0F6	047H0FZ	047H0G6	047H0GZ	047H0Z6	047H346	047H356	047H35Z
047H366	047H36Z	047H376	047H37Z	047H3D6	047H3E6	047H3EZ	047H3F6	047H3FZ	047H3G6	047H3GZ	047H3Z6	047H446
047H456	047H45Z	047H466	047H46Z	047H476	047H47Z	047H4D6	047H4E6	047H4EZ	047H4F6	047H4FZ	047H4G6	047H4GZ
047H4Z6	047J046	047J056	047J05Z	047J066	047J06Z	047J076	047J07Z	047J0D6	047J0E6	047J0EZ	047J0F6	047J0FZ
047J0G6	047J0GZ	047J0Z6	047J346	047J356	047J35Z	047J366	047J36Z	047J376	047J37Z	047J3D6	047J3E6	047J3EZ
047J3F6	047J3FZ	047J3G6	047J3GZ	047J3Z6	047J446	047J456	047J45Z	047J466	047J46Z	047J476	047J47Z	047J4D6
047J4E6	047J4EZ	047J4F6	047J4FZ	047J4G6	047J4GZ	047J4Z6	047K046	047K056	047K05Z	047K066	047K06Z	047K076
047K07Z	047K0D6	047K0E6	047K0EZ	047K0F6	047K0FZ	047K0G6	047K0GZ	047K0Z6	047K346	047K356	047K35Z	047K366
047K36Z	047K376	047K37Z	047K3D6	047K3E6	047K3EZ	047K3F6	047K3FZ	047K3G6	047K3GZ	047K3Z6	047K446	047K456
047K45Z	047K466	047K46Z	047K476	047K47Z	047K4D6	047K4E6	047K4EZ	047K4F6	047K4FZ	047K4G6	047K4GZ	047K4Z6
047L046	047L056	047L05Z	047L066	047L06Z	047L076	047L07Z	047L0D6	047L0E6	047L0EZ	047L0F6	047L0FZ	047L0G6
047L0GZ	047L0Z6	047L346	047L356	047L35Z	047L366	047L36Z	047L376	047L37Z	047L3D6	047L3E6	047L3EZ	047L3F6
047L3FZ	047L3G6	047L3GZ	047L3Z6	047L446	047L456	047L45Z	047L466	047L46Z	047L476	047L47Z	047L4D6	047L4E6
047L4EZ	047L4F6	047L4FZ	047L4G6	047L4GZ	047L4Z6	047M046	047M056	047M05Z	047M066	047M06Z	047M076	047M07Z
047M0D6	047M0E6	047M0EZ	047M0F6	047M0FZ	047M0G6	047M0GZ	047M0Z6	047M346	047M356	047M35Z	047M366	047M36Z
047M376	047M37Z	047M3D6	047M3E6	047M3EZ	047M3F6	047M3FZ	047M3G6	047M3GZ	047M3Z6	047M446	047M456	047M45Z
047M466	047M46Z	047M476	047M47Z	047M4D6	047M4E6	047M4EZ	047M4F6	047M4FZ	047M4G6	047M4GZ	047M4Z6	047N046
047N056	047N05Z	047N066	047N06Z	047N076	047N07Z	047N0D6	047N0E6	047N0EZ	047N0F6	047N0FZ	047N0G6	047N0GZ
047N0Z6	047N346	047N356	047N35Z	047N366	047N36Z	047N376	047N37Z	047N3D6	047N3E6	047N3EZ	047N3F6	047N3FZ
047N3G6	047N3GZ	047N3Z6	047N446	047N456	047N45Z	047N466	047N46Z	047N476	047N47Z	047N4D6	047N4E6	047N4EZ
047N4F6	047N4FZ	047N4G6	047N4GZ	047N4Z6	047P046	047P056	047P05Z	047P066	047P06Z	047P076	047P07Z	047P0D6
047P0E6	047P0EZ	047P0F6	047P0FZ	047P0G6	047P0GZ	047P0Z6	047P346	047P356	047P35Z	047P366	047P36Z	047P376
047P37Z	047P3D6	047P3E6	047P3EZ	047P3F6	047P3FZ	047P3G6	047P3GZ	047P3Z6	047P446	047P456	047P45Z	047P466
047P46Z	047P476	047P47Z	047P4D6	047P4E6	047P4EZ	047P4F6	047P4FZ	047P4G6	047P4GZ	047P4Z6	047Q046	047Q056
047Q05Z	047Q066	047Q06Z	047Q076	047Q07Z	047Q0D6	047Q0E6	047Q0EZ	047Q0F6	047Q0FZ	047Q0G6	047Q0GZ	047Q0Z6
047Q346	047Q356	047Q35Z	047Q366	047Q36Z	047Q376	047Q37Z	047Q3D6	047Q3E6	047Q3EZ	047Q3F6	047Q3FZ	047Q3G6
047Q3GZ	047Q3Z6	047Q446	047Q456	047Q45Z	047Q466	047Q46Z	047Q476	047Q47Z	047Q4D6	047Q4E6	047Q4EZ	047Q4F6
047Q4FZ	047Q4G6	047Q4GZ	047Q4Z6	047R046	047R056	047R05Z	047R066	047R06Z	047R076	047R07Z	047R0D6	047R0E6
047R0EZ	047R0F6	047R0FZ	047R0G6	047R0GZ	047R0Z6	047R346	047R356	047R35Z	047R366	047R36Z	047R376	047R37Z
047R3D6	047R3E6	047R3EZ	047R3F6	047R3FZ	047R3G6	047R3GZ	047R3Z6	047R446	047R456	047R45Z	047R466	047R46Z
047R476	047R47Z	047R4D6	047R4E6	047R4EZ	047R4F6	047R4FZ	047R4G6	047R4GZ	047R4Z6	047S046	047S056	047S05Z
047S066	047S06Z	047S076	047S07Z	047S0D6	047S0E6	047S0EZ	047S0F6	047S0FZ	047S0G6	047S0GZ	047S0Z6	047S346
047S356	047S35Z	047S366	047S36Z	047S376	047S37Z	047S3D6	047S3E6	047S3EZ	047S3F6	047S3FZ	047S3G6	047S3GZ
047S3Z6	047S446	047S456	047S45Z	047S466	047S46Z	047S476	047S47Z	047S4D6	047S4E6	047S4EZ	047S4F6	047S4FZ

047 continued on next page

047 continued from previous page

047S4G6	047S4GZ	047S4Z6	047T046	047T056	047T05Z	047T066	047T06Z	047T076	047T07Z	047T0D6	047T0E6	047T0EZ
047T0F6	047T0FZ	047T0G6	047T0GZ	047T0Z6	047T346	047T356	047T35Z	047T366	047T36Z	047T376	047T37Z	047T3D6
047T3E6	047T3EZ	047T3F6	047T3FZ	047T3G6	047T3GZ	047T3Z6	047T446	047T456	047T45Z	047T466	047T46Z	047T476
047T47Z	047T4D6	047T4E6	047T4EZ	047T4F6	047T4FZ	047T4G6	047T4GZ	047T4Z6	047U046	047U056	047U05Z	047U066
047U06Z	047U076	047U07Z	047U0D6	047U0E6	047U0EZ	047U0F6	047U0FZ	047U0G6	047U0GZ	047U0Z6	047U346	047U356
047U35Z	047U366	047U36Z	047U376	047U37Z	047U3D6	047U3E6	047U3EZ	047U3F6	047U3FZ	047U3G6	047U3GZ	047U3Z6
047U446	047U456	047U45Z	047U466	047U46Z	047U476	047U47Z	047U4D6	047U4E6	047U4EZ	047U4F6	047U4FZ	047U4G6
047U4GZ	047U4Z6	047V046	047V056	047V05Z	047V066	047V06Z	047V076	047V07Z	047V0D6	047V0E6	047V0EZ	047V0F6
047V0FZ	047V0G6	047V0GZ	047V0Z6	047V346	047V356	047V35Z	047V366	047V36Z	047V376	047V37Z	047V3D6	047V3E6
047V3EZ	047V3F6	047V3FZ	047V3G6	047V3GZ	047V3Z6	047V446	047V456	047V45Z	047V466	047V46Z	047V476	047V47Z
047V4D6	047V4E6	047V4EZ	047V4F6	047V4FZ	047V4G6	047V4GZ	047V4Z6	047W046	047W056	047W05Z	047W066	047W06Z
047W076	047W07Z	047W0D6	047W0E6	047W0EZ	047W0F6	047W0FZ	047W0G6	047W0GZ	047W0Z6	047W346	047W356	047W35Z
047W366	047W36Z	047W376	047W37Z	047W3D6	047W3E6	047W3EZ	047W3F6	047W3FZ	047W3G6	047W3GZ	047W3Z6	047W446
047W456	047W45Z	047W466	047W46Z	047W476	047W47Z	047W4D6	047W4E6	047W4EZ	047W4F6	047W4FZ	047W4G6	047W4GZ
047W4Z6	047Y046	047Y056	047Y05Z	047Y066	047Y06Z	047Y076	047Y07Z	047Y0D6	047Y0E6	047Y0EZ	047Y0F6	047Y0FZ
047Y0G6	047Y0GZ	047Y0Z6	047Y346	047Y356	047Y35Z	047Y366	047Y36Z	047Y376	047Y37Z	047Y3D6	047Y3E6	047Y3EZ
047Y3F6	047Y3FZ	047Y3G6	047Y3GZ	047Y3Z6	047Y446	047Y456	047Y45Z	047Y466	047Y46Z	047Y476	047Y47Z	047Y4D6
047Y4E6	047Y4EZ	047Y4F6	047Y4FZ	047Y4G6	047Y4GZ	047Y4Z6						

0 Medical and Surgical
4 Lower Arteries
9 Drainage: Taking or letting out fluids and/or gases from a body part

Body Part Character 4	Approach Character 5	Device Character 6	Qualifier Character 7
0 Abdominal Aorta ⦸ 1 Celiac Artery ⦸ 2 Gastric Artery ⦸ 3 Hepatic Artery ⦸ 4 Splenic Artery ⦸ 5 Superior Mesenteric Artery ⦸ 6 Colic Artery, Right ⦸ 7 Colic Artery, Left ⦸ 8 Colic Artery, Middle ⦸ 9 Renal Artery, Right ⦸ A Renal Artery, Left ⦸ B Inferior Mesenteric Artery ⦸ C Common Iliac Artery, Right ⦸ D Common Iliac Artery, Left ⦸ E Internal Iliac Artery, Right ⦸ F Internal Iliac Artery, Left ⦸ H External Iliac Artery, Right ⦸ J External Iliac Artery, Left ⦸ K Femoral Artery, Right ⦸ L Femoral Artery, Left ⦸ M Popliteal Artery, Right ⦸ N Popliteal Artery, Left ⦸ P Anterior Tibial Artery, Right ⦸ Q Anterior Tibial Artery, Left ⦸ R Posterior Tibial Artery, Right ⦸ S Posterior Tibial Artery, Left ⦸ T Peroneal Artery, Right ⦸ U Peroneal Artery, Left ⦸ V Foot Artery, Right ⦸ W Foot Artery, Left ⦸ Y Lower Artery ⦸	0 Open 3 Percutaneous 4 Percutaneous Endoscopic	0 Drainage Device	Z No Qualifier

049 continued on next page

049 continued from previous page

0 Medical and Surgical
4 Lower Arteries
9 Drainage: Taking or letting out fluids and/or gases from a body part

Body Part Character 4	Approach Character 5	Device Character 6	Qualifier Character 7
0 Abdominal Aorta ⃠ **1** Celiac Artery ⃠ **2** Gastric Artery ⃠ **3** Hepatic Artery ⃠ **4** Splenic Artery ⃠ **5** Superior Mesenteric Artery ⃠ **6** Colic Artery, Right ⃠ **7** Colic Artery, Left ⃠ **8** Colic Artery, Middle ⃠ **9** Renal Artery, Right ⃠ **A** Renal Artery, Left ⃠ **B** Inferior Mesenteric Artery ⃠ **C** Common Iliac Artery, Right ⃠ **D** Common Iliac Artery, Left ⃠ **E** Internal Iliac Artery, Right ⃠ **F** Internal Iliac Artery, Left ⃠ **H** External Iliac Artery, Right ⃠ **J** External Iliac Artery, Left ⃠ **K** Femoral Artery, Right ⃠ **L** Femoral Artery, Left ⃠ **M** Popliteal Artery, Right ⃠ **N** Popliteal Artery, Left ⃠ **P** Anterior Tibial Artery, Right ⃠ **Q** Anterior Tibial Artery, Left ⃠ **R** Posterior Tibial Artery, Right ⃠ **S** Posterior Tibial Artery, Left ⃠ **T** Peroneal Artery, Right ⃠ **U** Peroneal Artery, Left ⃠ **V** Foot Artery, Right ⃠ **W** Foot Artery, Left ⃠ **Y** Lower Artery ⃠	**0** Open **3** Percutaneous **4** Percutaneous Endoscopic	**Z** No Device	**X** Diagnostic **Z** No Qualifier

⃠ 049000Z 04900ZZ 049030Z 04903ZZ 049040Z 04904ZZ 049100Z 04910ZZ 049130Z 04913ZZ 049140Z 04914ZZ 049200Z 04920ZZ 049230Z 04923ZZ 049240Z 04924ZZ 049300Z 04930ZZ 049330Z 04933ZZ 049340Z 04934ZZ 049400Z 04940ZZ 049430Z 04943ZZ 049440Z 04944ZZ 049500Z 04950ZZ 049530Z 04953ZZ 049540Z 04954ZZ 049600Z 04960ZZ 049630Z 04963ZZ 049640Z 04964ZZ 049700Z 04970ZZ 049730Z 04973ZZ 049740Z 04974ZZ 049800Z 04980ZZ 049830Z 04983ZZ 049840Z 04984ZZ 049900Z 04990ZZ 049930Z 04993ZZ 049940Z 04994ZZ 049A00Z 049A0ZZ 049A30Z 049A3ZZ 049A40Z 049A4ZZ 049B00Z 049B0ZZ 049B30Z 049B3ZZ 049B40Z 049B4ZZ 049C00Z 049C0ZZ 049C30Z 049C3ZZ 049C40Z 049C4ZZ 049D00Z 049D0ZZ 049D30Z 049D3ZZ 049D40Z 049D4ZZ 049E00Z 049E0ZZ 049E30Z 049E3ZZ 049E40Z 049E4ZZ 049F00Z 049F0ZZ 049F30Z 049F3ZZ 049F40Z 049F4ZZ 049H00Z 049H0ZZ 049H30Z 049H3ZZ 049H40Z 049H4ZZ 049J00Z 049J0ZZ 049J30Z 049J3ZZ 049J40Z 049J4ZZ 049K00Z 049K0ZZ 049K30Z 049K3ZZ 049K40Z 049K4ZZ 049L00Z 049L0ZZ 049L30Z 049L3ZZ 049L40Z 049L4ZZ 049M00Z 049M0ZZ 049M30Z 049M3ZZ 049M40Z 049M4ZZ 049N00Z 049N0ZZ 049N30Z 049N3ZZ 049N40Z 049N4ZZ 049P00Z 049P0ZZ 049P30Z 049P3ZZ 049P40Z 049P4ZZ 049Q00Z 049Q0ZZ 049Q30Z 049Q3ZZ 049Q40Z 049Q4ZZ 049R00Z 049R0ZZ 049R30Z 049R3ZZ 049R40Z 049R4ZZ 049S00Z 049S0ZZ 049S30Z 049S3ZZ 049S40Z 049S4ZZ 049T00Z 049T0ZZ 049T30Z 049T3ZZ 049T40Z 049T4ZZ 049U00Z 049U0ZZ 049U30Z 049U3ZZ 049U40Z 049U4ZZ 049V00Z 049V0ZZ 049V30Z 049V3ZZ 049V40Z 049V4ZZ 049W00Z 049W0ZZ 049W30Z 049W3ZZ 049W40Z 049W4ZZ 049Y00Z 049Y0ZZ 049Y30Z 049Y3ZZ 049Y40Z 049Y4ZZ

0 Medical and Surgical
4 Lower Arteries
B Excision: Cutting out or off, without replacement, a portion of a body part

Body Part Character 4	Approach Character 5	Device Character 6	Qualifier Character 7
0 Abdominal Aorta **1** Celiac Artery **2** Gastric Artery **3** Hepatic Artery **4** Splenic Artery **5** Superior Mesenteric Artery **6** Colic Artery, Right **7** Colic Artery, Left **8** Colic Artery, Middle **9** Renal Artery, Right **A** Renal Artery, Left **B** Inferior Mesenteric Artery **C** Common Iliac Artery, Right **D** Common Iliac Artery, Left **E** Internal Iliac Artery, Right **F** Internal Iliac Artery, Left **H** External Iliac Artery, Right **J** External Iliac Artery, Left **K** Femoral Artery, Right **L** Femoral Artery, Left **M** Popliteal Artery, Right **N** Popliteal Artery, Left **P** Anterior Tibial Artery, Right **Q** Anterior Tibial Artery, Left **R** Posterior Tibial Artery, Right **S** Posterior Tibial Artery, Left **T** Peroneal Artery, Right **U** Peroneal Artery, Left **V** Foot Artery, Right **W** Foot Artery, Left **Y** Lower Artery	**0** Open **3** Percutaneous **4** Percutaneous Endoscopic	**Z** No Device	**X** Diagnostic **Z** No Qualifier

0 Medical and Surgical
4 Lower Arteries
C Extirpation: Taking or cutting out solid matter from a body part

Body Part Character 4	Approach Character 5	Device Character 6	Qualifier Character 7
0 Abdominal Aorta ⊘	**0** Open	**Z** No Device	**6** Bifurcation
1 Celiac Artery ⊘	**3** Percutaneous		**Z** No Qualifier
2 Gastric Artery ⊘	**4** Percutaneous Endoscopic		
3 Hepatic Artery ⊘			
4 Splenic Artery ⊘			
5 Superior Mesenteric Artery ⊘			
6 Colic Artery, Right ⊘			
7 Colic Artery, Left ⊘			
8 Colic Artery, Middle ⊘			
9 Renal Artery, Right ⊘			
A Renal Artery, Left ⊘			
B Inferior Mesenteric Artery ⊘			
C Common Iliac Artery, Right ⊘			
D Common Iliac Artery, Left ⊘			
E Internal Iliac Artery, Right ⊘			
F Internal Iliac Artery, Left ⊘			
H External Iliac Artery, Right ⊘			
J External Iliac Artery, Left ⊘			
K Femoral Artery, Right ⊘			
L Femoral Artery, Left ⊘			
M Popliteal Artery, Right ⊘			
N Popliteal Artery, Left ⊘			
P Anterior Tibial Artery, Right ⊘			
Q Anterior Tibial Artery, Left ⊘			
R Posterior Tibial Artery, Right ⊘			
S Posterior Tibial Artery, Left ⊘			
T Peroneal Artery, Right ⊘			
U Peroneal Artery, Left ⊘			
V Foot Artery, Right ⊘			
W Foot Artery, Left ⊘			
Y Lower Artery ⊘			

⊘ 04C00Z6 04C03Z6 04C04Z6 04C10Z6 04C13Z6 04C14Z6 04C20Z6 04C23Z6 04C24Z6 04C30Z6 04C33Z6 04C34Z6 04C40Z6 04C43Z6 04C44Z6 04C50Z6 04C53Z6 04C54Z6 04C60Z6 04C63Z6 04C64Z6 04C70Z6 04C73Z6 04C74Z6 04C80Z6 04C83Z6 04C84Z6 04C90Z6 04C93Z6 04C94Z6 04CA0Z6 04CA3Z6 04CA4Z6 04CB0Z6 04CB3Z6 04CB4Z6 04CC0Z6 04CC3Z6 04CC4Z6 04CD0Z6 04CD3Z6 04CD4Z6 04CE0Z6 04CE3Z6 04CE4Z6 04CF0Z6 04CF3Z6 04CF4Z6 04CH0Z6 04CH3Z6 04CH4Z6 04CJ0Z6 04CJ3Z6 04CJ4Z6 04CK0Z6 04CK3Z6 04CK4Z6 04CL0Z6 04CL3Z6 04CL4Z6 04CM0Z6 04CM3Z6 04CM4Z6 04CN0Z6 04CN3Z6 04CN4Z6 04CP0Z6 04CP3Z6 04CP4Z6 04CQ0Z6 04CQ3Z6 04CQ4Z6 04CR0Z6 04CR3Z6 04CR4Z6 04CS0Z6 04CS3Z6 04CS4Z6 04CT0Z6 04CT3Z6 04CT4Z6 04CU0Z6 04CU3Z6 04CU4Z6 04CV0Z6 04CV3Z6 04CV4Z6 04CW0Z6 04CW3Z6 04CW4Z6 04CY0Z6 04CY3Z6 04CY4Z6

0 Medical and Surgical
4 Lower Arteries
H Insertion: Putting in a nonbiological appliance that monitors, assists, performs, or prevents a physiological function but does not physically take the place of a body part

Body Part Character 4	Approach Character 5	Device Character 6	Qualifier Character 7
0 Abdominal Aorta ⊘ **Y** Lower Artery ⊘	**0** Open **3** Percutaneous **4** Percutaneous Endoscopic	**2** Monitoring Device **3** Infusion Device **D** Intraluminal Device	**Z** No Qualifier
1 Celiac Artery ⊘ **2** Gastric Artery ⊘ **3** Hepatic Artery ⊘ **4** Splenic Artery ⊘ **5** Superior Mesenteric Artery ⊘ **6** Colic Artery, Right ⊘ **7** Colic Artery, Left ⊘ **8** Colic Artery, Middle ⊘ **9** Renal Artery, Right ⊘ **A** Renal Artery, Left ⊘ **B** Inferior Mesenteric Artery ⊘ **C** Common Iliac Artery, Right ⊘ **D** Common Iliac Artery, Left ⊘ **E** Internal Iliac Artery, Right ⊘ **F** Internal Iliac Artery, Left ⊘ **H** External Iliac Artery, Right ⊘ **J** External Iliac Artery, Left ⊘ **K** Femoral Artery, Right ⊘ **L** Femoral Artery, Left ⊘ **M** Popliteal Artery, Right ⊘ **N** Popliteal Artery, Left ⊘ **P** Anterior Tibial Artery, Right ⊘ **Q** Anterior Tibial Artery, Left ⊘ **R** Posterior Tibial Artery, Right ⊘ **S** Posterior Tibial Artery, Left ⊘ **T** Peroneal Artery, Right ⊘ **U** Peroneal Artery, Left ⊘ **V** Foot Artery, Right ⊘ **W** Foot Artery, Left ⊘	**0** Open **3** Percutaneous **4** Percutaneous Endoscopic	**3** Infusion Device **D** Intraluminal Device	**Z** No Qualifier

⊘ 04H002Z 04H003Z 04H032Z 04H033Z 04H042Z 04H043Z 04H103Z 04H133Z 04H143Z 04H203Z 04H233Z 04H243Z 04H303Z 04H333Z 04H343Z 04H403Z 04H433Z 04H443Z 04H503Z 04H533Z 04H543Z 04H603Z 04H633Z 04H643Z 04H703Z 04H733Z 04H743Z 04H803Z 04H833Z 04H843Z 04H903Z 04H933Z 04H943Z 04HA03Z 04HA33Z 04HA43Z 04HB03Z 04HB33Z 04HB43Z 04HC03Z 04HC33Z 04HC43Z 04HD03Z 04HD33Z 04HD43Z 04HE03Z 04HE33Z 04HE43Z 04HF03Z 04HF33Z 04HF43Z 04HH03Z 04HH33Z 04HH43Z 04HJ03Z 04HJ33Z 04HJ43Z 04HK03Z 04HK33Z 04HK43Z 04HL03Z 04HL33Z 04HL43Z 04HM03Z 04HM33Z 04HM43Z 04HN03Z 04HN33Z 04HN43Z 04HP03Z 04HP33Z 04HP43Z 04HQ03Z 04HQ33Z 04HQ43Z 04HR03Z 04HR33Z 04HR43Z 04HS03Z 04HS33Z 04HS43Z 04HT03Z 04HT33Z 04HT43Z 04HU03Z 04HU33Z 04HU43Z 04HV03Z 04HV33Z 04HV43Z 04HW03Z 04HW33Z 04HW43Z 04HY03Z 04HY32Z 04HY33Z 04HY43Z

0 Medical and Surgical
4 Lower Arteries
J Inspection: Visually and/or manually exploring a body part

Body Part Character 4	Approach Character 5	Device Character 6	Qualifier Character 7
Y Lower Artery ⊘	**0** Open **3** Percutaneous **4** Percutaneous Endoscopic **X** External	**Z** No Device	**Z** No Qualifier

⊘ 04JY3ZZ 04JY4ZZ 04JYXZZ

0 Medical and Surgical
4 Lower Arteries
L Occlusion: Completely closing an orifice or the lumen of a tubular body part

Body Part Character 4	Approach Character 5	Device Character 6	Qualifier Character 7
0 Abdominal Aorta **1** Celiac Artery **2** Gastric Artery ⃠ **3** Hepatic Artery **4** Splenic Artery **5** Superior Mesenteric Artery **6** Colic Artery, Right **7** Colic Artery, Left **8** Colic Artery, Middle **9** Renal Artery, Right **A** Renal Artery, Left **B** Inferior Mesenteric Artery **C** Common Iliac Artery, Right **D** Common Iliac Artery, Left **H** External Iliac Artery, Right **J** External Iliac Artery, Left **K** Femoral Artery, Right **L** Femoral Artery, Left **M** Popliteal Artery, Right **N** Popliteal Artery, Left **P** Anterior Tibial Artery, Right **Q** Anterior Tibial Artery, Left **R** Posterior Tibial Artery, Right **S** Posterior Tibial Artery, Left **T** Peroneal Artery, Right **U** Peroneal Artery, Left **V** Foot Artery, Right **W** Foot Artery, Left **Y** Lower Artery	**0** Open **3** Percutaneous **4** Percutaneous Endoscopic	**C** Extraluminal Device **D** Intraluminal Device **Z** No Device	**Z** No Qualifier
E Internal Iliac Artery, Right ♀	**0** Open **3** Percutaneous **4** Percutaneous Endoscopic	**C** Extraluminal Device **D** Intraluminal Device **Z** No Device	**T** Uterine Artery, Right **Z** No Qualifier
F Internal Iliac Artery, Left ♀	**0** Open **3** Percutaneous **4** Percutaneous Endoscopic	**C** Extraluminal Device **D** Intraluminal Device **Z** No Device	**U** Uterine Artery, Left **Z** No Qualifier

⃠ 04L23DZ

♀ 04LE0CT 04LE0DT 04LE0ZT 04LE3CT 04LE3DT 04LE3ZT 04LE4CT 04LE4DT 04LE4ZT 04LF0CU 04LF0DU 04LF0ZU 04LF3CU 04LF3DU 04LF3ZU 04LF4CU 04LF4DU 04LF4ZU

0 Medical and Surgical
4 Lower Arteries
N Release: Freeing a body part from an abnormal physical constraint by cutting or by the use of force

Body Part Character 4	Approach Character 5	Device Character 6	Qualifier Character 7
0 Abdominal Aorta **1** Celiac Artery **2** Gastric Artery **3** Hepatic Artery **4** Splenic Artery **5** Superior Mesenteric Artery **6** Colic Artery, Right **7** Colic Artery, Left **8** Colic Artery, Middle **9** Renal Artery, Right **A** Renal Artery, Left **B** Inferior Mesenteric Artery **C** Common Iliac Artery, Right **D** Common Iliac Artery, Left **E** Internal Iliac Artery, Right **F** Internal Iliac Artery, Left **H** External Iliac Artery, Right **J** External Iliac Artery, Left **K** Femoral Artery, Right **L** Femoral Artery, Left **M** Popliteal Artery, Right **N** Popliteal Artery, Left **P** Anterior Tibial Artery, Right **Q** Anterior Tibial Artery, Left **R** Posterior Tibial Artery, Right **S** Posterior Tibial Artery, Left **T** Peroneal Artery, Right **U** Peroneal Artery, Left **V** Foot Artery, Right **W** Foot Artery, Left **Y** Lower Artery	**0** Open **3** Percutaneous **4** Percutaneous Endoscopic	**Z** No Device	**Z** No Qualifier

0 Medical and Surgical
4 Lower Arteries
P Removal: Taking out or off a device from a body part

Body Part Character 4	Approach Character 5	Device Character 6	Qualifier Character 7
Y Lower Artery ⃠	**0** Open **3** Percutaneous **4** Percutaneous Endoscopic	**0** Drainage Device **2** Monitoring Device **3** Infusion Device **7** Autologous Tissue Substitute **C** Extraluminal Device **D** Intraluminal Device **J** Synthetic Substitute **K** Nonautologous Tissue Substitute	**Z** No Qualifier
Y Lower Artery ⃠	**X** External	**0** Drainage Device **1** Radioactive Element **2** Monitoring Device **3** Infusion Device **D** Intraluminal Device	**Z** No Qualifier

⃠ 04PY30Z 04PY32Z 04PY33Z 04PYX0Z 04PYX1Z 04PYX2Z 04PYX3Z 04PYXDZ

0 **Medical and Surgical**
4 **Lower Arteries**
Q **Repair:** Restoring, to the extent possible, a body part to its normal anatomic structure and function

Body Part Character 4	Approach Character 5	Device Character 6	Qualifier Character 7
0 Abdominal Aorta **1** Celiac Artery **2** Gastric Artery **3** Hepatic Artery **4** Splenic Artery **5** Superior Mesenteric Artery **6** Colic Artery, Right **7** Colic Artery, Left **8** Colic Artery, Middle **9** Renal Artery, Right **A** Renal Artery, Left **B** Inferior Mesenteric Artery **C** Common Iliac Artery, Right **D** Common Iliac Artery, Left **E** Internal Iliac Artery, Right **F** Internal Iliac Artery, Left **H** External Iliac Artery, Right **J** External Iliac Artery, Left **K** Femoral Artery, Right **L** Femoral Artery, Left **M** Popliteal Artery, Right **N** Popliteal Artery, Left **P** Anterior Tibial Artery, Right **Q** Anterior Tibial Artery, Left **R** Posterior Tibial Artery, Right **S** Posterior Tibial Artery, Left **T** Peroneal Artery, Right **U** Peroneal Artery, Left **V** Foot Artery, Right **W** Foot Artery, Left **Y** Lower Artery	**0** Open **3** Percutaneous **4** Percutaneous Endoscopic	**Z** No Device	**Z** No Qualifier

0 Medical and Surgical
4 Lower Arteries
R Replacement: Putting in or on biological or synthetic material that physically takes the place and/or function of all or a portion of a body part

Body Part Character 4	Approach Character 5	Device Character 6	Qualifier Character 7
0 Abdominal Aorta **1** Celiac Artery **2** Gastric Artery **3** Hepatic Artery **4** Splenic Artery **5** Superior Mesenteric Artery **6** Colic Artery, Right **7** Colic Artery, Left **8** Colic Artery, Middle **9** Renal Artery, Right **A** Renal Artery, Left **B** Inferior Mesenteric Artery **C** Common Iliac Artery, Right **D** Common Iliac Artery, Left **E** Internal Iliac Artery, Right **F** Internal Iliac Artery, Left **H** External Iliac Artery, Right **J** External Iliac Artery, Left **K** Femoral Artery, Right **L** Femoral Artery, Left **M** Popliteal Artery, Right **N** Popliteal Artery, Left **P** Anterior Tibial Artery, Right **Q** Anterior Tibial Artery, Left **R** Posterior Tibial Artery, Right **S** Posterior Tibial Artery, Left **T** Peroneal Artery, Right **U** Peroneal Artery, Left **V** Foot Artery, Right **W** Foot Artery, Left **Y** Lower Artery	**0** Open **4** Percutaneous Endoscopic	**7** Autologous Tissue Substitute **J** Synthetic Substitute **K** Nonautologous Tissue Substitute	**Z** No Qualifier

0 Medical and Surgical
4 Lower Arteries
S Reposition: Moving to its normal location, or other suitable location, all or a portion of a body part

Body Part Character 4	Approach Character 5	Device Character 6	Qualifier Character 7
0 Abdominal Aorta **1** Celiac Artery **2** Gastric Artery **3** Hepatic Artery **4** Splenic Artery **5** Superior Mesenteric Artery **6** Colic Artery, Right **7** Colic Artery, Left **8** Colic Artery, Middle **9** Renal Artery, Right **A** Renal Artery, Left **B** Inferior Mesenteric Artery **C** Common Iliac Artery, Right **D** Common Iliac Artery, Left **E** Internal Iliac Artery, Right **F** Internal Iliac Artery, Left **H** External Iliac Artery, Right **J** External Iliac Artery, Left **K** Femoral Artery, Right **L** Femoral Artery, Left **M** Popliteal Artery, Right **N** Popliteal Artery, Left **P** Anterior Tibial Artery, Right **Q** Anterior Tibial Artery, Left **R** Posterior Tibial Artery, Right **S** Posterior Tibial Artery, Left **T** Peroneal Artery, Right **U** Peroneal Artery, Left **V** Foot Artery, Right **W** Foot Artery, Left **Y** Lower Artery	**0** Open **3** Percutaneous **4** Percutaneous Endoscopic	**Z** No Device	**Z** No Qualifier

LC Limited Coverage NC Noncovered HAC HAC Associated Procedure CC Combination Cluster - See Appendix G for code lists
DRG Non-OR-Affecting MS-DRG Assignment ⊘ Non-OR-Not Affecting MS-DRG Assignment New/Revised Text in **Orange** ♂ Male ♀ Female

0 Medical and Surgical
4 Lower Arteries
U Supplement: Putting in or on biological or synthetic material that physically reinforces and/or augments the function of a portion of a body part

Body Part Character 4	Approach Character 5	Device Character 6	Qualifier Character 7
0 Abdominal Aorta **1** Celiac Artery **2** Gastric Artery **3** Hepatic Artery **4** Splenic Artery **5** Superior Mesenteric Artery **6** Colic Artery, Right **7** Colic Artery, Left **8** Colic Artery, Middle **9** Renal Artery, Right **A** Renal Artery, Left **B** Inferior Mesenteric Artery **C** Common Iliac Artery, Right **D** Common Iliac Artery, Left **E** Internal Iliac Artery, Right **F** Internal Iliac Artery, Left **H** External Iliac Artery, Right **J** External Iliac Artery, Left **K** Femoral Artery, Right **L** Femoral Artery, Left **M** Popliteal Artery, Right **N** Popliteal Artery, Left **P** Anterior Tibial Artery, Right **Q** Anterior Tibial Artery, Left **R** Posterior Tibial Artery, Right **S** Posterior Tibial Artery, Left **T** Peroneal Artery, Right **U** Peroneal Artery, Left **V** Foot Artery, Right **W** Foot Artery, Left **Y** Lower Artery	**0** Open **3** Percutaneous **4** Percutaneous Endoscopic	**7** Autologous Tissue Substitute **J** Synthetic Substitute **K** Nonautologous Tissue Substitute	**Z** No Qualifier

0 Medical and Surgical
4 Lower Arteries
V Restriction: Partially closing an orifice or the lumen of a tubular body part

Body Part Character 4	Approach Character 5	Device Character 6	Qualifier Character 7
0 Abdominal Aorta ⊘	**0** Open **3** Percutaneous **4** Percutaneous Endoscopic	**C** Extraluminal Device **E** Intraluminal Device, Branched or Fenestrated, One or Two Arteries **F** Intraluminal Device, Branched or Fenestrated, Three or More Arteries **Z** No Device	**6** Bifurcation **Z** No Qualifier
0 Abdominal Aorta ⊘	**0** Open **3** Percutaneous **4** Percutaneous Endoscopic	**D** Intraluminal Device	**6** Bifurcation **J** Temporary **Z** No Qualifier
1 Celiac Artery **2** Gastric Artery **3** Hepatic Artery **4** Splenic Artery **5** Superior Mesenteric Artery **6** Colic Artery, Right **7** Colic Artery, Left **8** Colic Artery, Middle **9** Renal Artery, Right **A** Renal Artery, Left **B** Inferior Mesenteric Artery **E** Internal Iliac Artery, Right **F** Internal Iliac Artery, Left **H** External Iliac Artery, Right **J** External Iliac Artery, Left **K** Femoral Artery, Right **L** Femoral Artery, Left **M** Popliteal Artery, Right **N** Popliteal Artery, Left **P** Anterior Tibial Artery, Right **Q** Anterior Tibial Artery, Left **R** Posterior Tibial Artery, Right **S** Posterior Tibial Artery, Left **T** Peroneal Artery, Right **U** Peroneal Artery, Left **V** Foot Artery, Right **W** Foot Artery, Left **Y** Lower Artery	**0** Open **3** Percutaneous **4** Percutaneous Endoscopic	**C** Extraluminal Device **D** Intraluminal Device **Z** No Device	**Z** No Qualifier
C Common Iliac Artery, Right ⊘ **D** Common Iliac Artery, Left ⊘	**0** Open **3** Percutaneous **4** Percutaneous Endoscopic	**C** Extraluminal Device **D** Intraluminal Device **E** Intraluminal Device, Branched or Fenestrated, One or Two Arteries **F** Intraluminal Device, Branched or Fenestrated, Three or More Arteries **Z** No Device	**Z** No Qualifier

⊘ 04V00C6 04V00D6 04V00E6 04V00EZ 04V00F6 04V00FZ 04V00Z6 04V03C6 04V03D6 04V03E6 04V03EZ 04V03F6 04V03FZ 04V03Z6 04V04C6 04V04D6 04V04E6 04V04EZ 04V04F6 04V04FZ 04V04Z6 04VC0EZ 04VC0FZ 04VC3EZ 04VC3FZ 04VC4EZ 04VC4FZ 04VD0EZ 04VD0FZ 04VD3EZ 04VD3FZ 04VD4EZ 04VD4FZ

0 Medical and Surgical
4 Lower Arteries
W Revision: Correcting, to the extent possible, a portion of a malfunctioning device or the position of a displaced device

Body Part Character 4	Approach Character 5	Device Character 6	Qualifier Character 7
Y Lower Artery ⃠	**0** Open **3** Percutaneous **4** Percutaneous Endoscopic **X** External	**0** Drainage Device **2** Monitoring Device **3** Infusion Device **7** Autologous Tissue Substitute **C** Extraluminal Device **D** Intraluminal Device **J** Synthetic Substitute **K** Nonautologous Tissue Substitute	**Z** No Qualifier

⃠ 04WYX0Z 04WYX2Z 04WYX3Z 04WYX7Z 04WYXCZ 04WYXDZ 04WYXJZ 04WYXKZ

Upper Veins 051-05W

0 Medical and Surgical
5 Upper Veins
1 Bypass: Altering the route of passage of the contents of a tubular body part

Body Part Character 4	Approach Character 5	Device Character 6	Qualifier Character 7
0 Azygos Vein **1** Hemiazygos Vein **3** Innominate Vein, Right **4** Innominate Vein, Left **5** Subclavian Vein, Right **6** Subclavian Vein, Left **7** Axillary Vein, Right **8** Axillary Vein, Left **9** Brachial Vein, Right **A** Brachial Vein, Left **B** Basilic Vein, Right **C** Basilic Vein, Left **D** Cephalic Vein, Right **F** Cephalic Vein, Left **G** Hand Vein, Right **H** Hand Vein, Left **L** Intracranial Vein **M** Internal Jugular Vein, Right **N** Internal Jugular Vein, Left **P** External Jugular Vein, Right **Q** External Jugular Vein, Left **R** Vertebral Vein, Right **S** Vertebral Vein, Left **T** Face Vein, Right **V** Face Vein, Left	**0** Open **4** Percutaneous Endoscopic	**7** Autologous Tissue Substitute **9** Autologous Venous Tissue **A** Autologous Arterial Tissue **J** Synthetic Substitute **K** Nonautologous Tissue Substitute **Z** No Device	**Y** Upper Vein

0 Medical and Surgical
5 Upper Veins
5 Destruction: Physical eradication of all or a portion of a body part by the direct use of energy, force, or a destructive agent

Body Part Character 4	Approach Character 5	Device Character 6	Qualifier Character 7
0 Azygos Vein **1** Hemiazygos Vein **3** Innominate Vein, Right **4** Innominate Vein, Left **5** Subclavian Vein, Right **6** Subclavian Vein, Left **7** Axillary Vein, Right **8** Axillary Vein, Left **9** Brachial Vein, Right **A** Brachial Vein, Left **B** Basilic Vein, Right **C** Basilic Vein, Left **D** Cephalic Vein, Right **F** Cephalic Vein, Left **G** Hand Vein, Right **H** Hand Vein, Left **L** Intracranial Vein **M** Internal Jugular Vein, Right **N** Internal Jugular Vein, Left **P** External Jugular Vein, Right **Q** External Jugular Vein, Left **R** Vertebral Vein, Right **S** Vertebral Vein, Left **T** Face Vein, Right **V** Face Vein, Left **Y** Upper Vein	**0** Open **3** Percutaneous **4** Percutaneous Endoscopic	**Z** No Device	**Z** No Qualifier

0 Medical and Surgical
5 Upper Veins
7 Dilation: Expanding an orifice or the lumen of a tubular body part

Body Part Character 4	Approach Character 5	Device Character 6	Qualifier Character 7
0 Azygos Vein **1** Hemiazygos Vein **3** Innominate Vein, Right **4** Innominate Vein, Left **5** Subclavian Vein, Right **6** Subclavian Vein, Left **7** Axillary Vein, Right **8** Axillary Vein, Left **9** Brachial Vein, Right **A** Brachial Vein, Left **B** Basilic Vein, Right **C** Basilic Vein, Left **D** Cephalic Vein, Right **F** Cephalic Vein, Left **G** Hand Vein, Right **H** Hand Vein, Left **L** Intracranial Vein NC **M** Internal Jugular Vein, Right **N** Internal Jugular Vein, Left **P** External Jugular Vein, Right **Q** External Jugular Vein, Left **R** Vertebral Vein, Right **S** Vertebral Vein, Left **T** Face Vein, Right **V** Face Vein, Left **Y** Upper Vein	**0** Open **3** Percutaneous **4** Percutaneous Endoscopic	**D** Intraluminal Device **Z** No Device	**Z** No Qualifier

NC 057L3ZZ 057L4ZZ

0 Medical and Surgical
5 Upper Veins
9 Drainage: Taking or letting out fluids and/or gases from a body part

Body Part Character 4	Approach Character 5	Device Character 6	Qualifier Character 7
0 Azygos Vein ⊘ **1** Hemiazygos Vein ⊘ **3** Innominate Vein, Right ⊘ **4** Innominate Vein, Left ⊘ **5** Subclavian Vein, Right ⊘ **6** Subclavian Vein, Left ⊘ **7** Axillary Vein, Right ⊘ **8** Axillary Vein, Left ⊘ **9** Brachial Vein, Right ⊘ **A** Brachial Vein, Left ⊘ **B** Basilic Vein, Right ⊘ **C** Basilic Vein, Left ⊘ **D** Cephalic Vein, Right ⊘ **F** Cephalic Vein, Left ⊘ **G** Hand Vein, Right ⊘ **H** Hand Vein, Left ⊘ **L** Intracranial Vein ⊘ **M** Internal Jugular Vein, Right ⊘ **N** Internal Jugular Vein, Left ⊘ **P** External Jugular Vein, Right ⊘ **Q** External Jugular Vein, Left ⊘ **R** Vertebral Vein, Right ⊘ **S** Vertebral Vein, Left ⊘ **T** Face Vein, Right ⊘ **V** Face Vein, Left ⊘ **Y** Upper Vein ⊘	**0** Open **3** Percutaneous **4** Percutaneous Endoscopic	**0** Drainage Device	**Z** No Qualifier
0 Azygos Vein ⊘ **1** Hemiazygos Vein ⊘ **3** Innominate Vein, Right ⊘ **4** Innominate Vein, Left ⊘ **5** Subclavian Vein, Right ⊘ **6** Subclavian Vein, Left ⊘ **7** Axillary Vein, Right ⊘ **8** Axillary Vein, Left ⊘ **9** Brachial Vein, Right ⊘ **A** Brachial Vein, Left ⊘ **B** Basilic Vein, Right ⊘ **C** Basilic Vein, Left ⊘ **D** Cephalic Vein, Right ⊘ **F** Cephalic Vein, Left ⊘ **G** Hand Vein, Right ⊘ **H** Hand Vein, Left ⊘ **L** Intracranial Vein ⊘ **M** Internal Jugular Vein, Right ⊘ **N** Internal Jugular Vein, Left ⊘ **P** External Jugular Vein, Right ⊘ **Q** External Jugular Vein, Left ⊘ **R** Vertebral Vein, Right ⊘ **S** Vertebral Vein, Left ⊘ **T** Face Vein, Right ⊘ **V** Face Vein, Left ⊘ **Y** Upper Vein ⊘	**0** Open **3** Percutaneous **4** Percutaneous Endoscopic	**Z** No Device	**X** Diagnostic **Z** No Qualifier

⊘ 059000Z 05900ZZ 059030Z 05903ZZ 059040Z 05904ZZ 059100Z 05910ZZ 059130Z 05913ZZ 059140Z 05914ZZ 059300Z 05930ZZ 059330Z 05933ZZ 059340Z 05934ZZ 059400Z 05940ZZ 059430Z 05943ZZ 059440Z 05944ZZ 059500Z 05950ZZ 059530Z 05953ZZ 059540Z 05954ZZ 059600Z 05960ZZ 059630Z 05963ZZ 059640Z 05964ZZ 059700Z 05970ZZ 059730Z 05973ZZ 059740Z 05974ZZ 059800Z 05980ZZ 059830Z 05983ZZ 059840Z 05984ZZ 059900Z 05990ZZ 059930Z 05993ZZ 059940Z 05994ZZ 059A00Z 059A0ZZ 059A30Z 059A3ZZ 059A40Z 059A4ZZ 059B00Z 059B0ZZ 059B30Z 059B3ZZ 059B40Z 059B4ZZ 059C00Z 059C0ZZ 059C30Z 059C3ZZ 059C40Z 059C4ZZ 059D00Z 059D0ZZ 059D30Z 059D3ZZ 059D40Z 059D4ZZ 059F00Z 059F0ZZ 059F30Z 059F3ZZ 059F40Z 059F4ZZ 059G00Z 059G0ZZ 059G30Z 059G3ZZ 059G40Z 059G4ZZ 059H00Z 059H0ZZ 059H30Z 059H3ZZ 059H40Z 059H4ZZ 059L00Z 059L0ZZ 059L30Z 059L3ZZ 059L40Z 059L4ZZ 059M00Z 059M0ZZ 059M30Z 059M3ZZ 059M40Z 059M4ZZ 059N00Z 059N0ZZ 059N30Z 059N3ZZ 059N40Z 059N4ZZ 059P00Z 059P0ZZ 059P30Z 059P3ZZ 059P40Z 059P4ZZ 059Q00Z 059Q0ZZ 059Q30Z 059Q3ZZ 059Q40Z 059Q4ZZ 059R00Z 059R0ZZ 059R30Z 059R3ZZ 059R40Z 059R4ZZ 059S00Z 059S0ZZ 059S30Z 059S3ZZ 059S40Z 059S4ZZ 059T00Z 059T0ZZ 059T30Z 059T3ZZ 059T40Z 059T4ZZ 059V00Z 059V0ZZ 059V30Z 059V3ZZ 059V40Z 059V4ZZ 059Y00Z 059Y0ZZ 059Y30Z 059Y3ZZ 059Y40Z 059Y4ZZ

0 Medical and Surgical
5 Upper Veins
B Excision: Cutting out or off, without replacement, a portion of a body part

Body Part Character 4	Approach Character 5	Device Character 6	Qualifier Character 7
0 Azygos Vein **1** Hemiazygos Vein **3** Innominate Vein, Right **4** Innominate Vein, Left **5** Subclavian Vein, Right **6** Subclavian Vein, Left **7** Axillary Vein, Right **8** Axillary Vein, Left **9** Brachial Vein, Right **A** Brachial Vein, Left **B** Basilic Vein, Right **C** Basilic Vein, Left **D** Cephalic Vein, Right **F** Cephalic Vein, Left **G** Hand Vein, Right **H** Hand Vein, Left **L** Intracranial Vein **M** Internal Jugular Vein, Right **N** Internal Jugular Vein, Left **P** External Jugular Vein, Right **Q** External Jugular Vein, Left **R** Vertebral Vein, Right **S** Vertebral Vein, Left **T** Face Vein, Right **V** Face Vein, Left **Y** Upper Vein	**0** Open **3** Percutaneous **4** Percutaneous Endoscopic	**Z** No Device	**X** Diagnostic **Z** No Qualifier

0 Medical and Surgical
5 Upper Veins
C Extirpation: Taking or cutting out solid matter from a body part

Body Part Character 4	Approach Character 5	Device Character 6	Qualifier Character 7
0 Azygos Vein **1** Hemiazygos Vein **3** Innominate Vein, Right **4** Innominate Vein, Left **5** Subclavian Vein, Right **6** Subclavian Vein, Left **7** Axillary Vein, Right **8** Axillary Vein, Left **9** Brachial Vein, Right **A** Brachial Vein, Left **B** Basilic Vein, Right **C** Basilic Vein, Left **D** Cephalic Vein, Right **F** Cephalic Vein, Left **G** Hand Vein, Right **H** Hand Vein, Left **L** Intracranial Vein **M** Internal Jugular Vein, Right **N** Internal Jugular Vein, Left **P** External Jugular Vein, Right **Q** External Jugular Vein, Left **R** Vertebral Vein, Right **S** Vertebral Vein, Left **T** Face Vein, Right **V** Face Vein, Left **Y** Upper Vein	**0** Open **3** Percutaneous **4** Percutaneous Endoscopic	**Z** No Device	**Z** No Qualifier

0 Medical and Surgical
5 Upper Veins
D Extraction: Pulling or stripping out or off all or a portion of a body part by the use of force

Body Part Character 4	Approach Character 5	Device Character 6	Qualifier Character 7
9 Brachial Vein, Right **A** Brachial Vein, Left **B** Basilic Vein, Right **C** Basilic Vein, Left **D** Cephalic Vein, Right **F** Cephalic Vein, Left **G** Hand Vein, Right **H** Hand Vein, Left **Y** Upper Vein	**0** Open **3** Percutaneous	**Z** No Device	**Z** No Qualifier

0 Medical and Surgical
5 Upper Veins
H Insertion: Putting in a nonbiological appliance that monitors, assists, performs, or prevents a physiological function but does not physically take the place of a body part

Body Part Character 4	Approach Character 5	Device Character 6	Qualifier Character 7
0 Azygos Vein ⊘	**0** Open **3** Percutaneous **4** Percutaneous Endoscopic	**2** Monitoring Device **3** Infusion Device **D** Intraluminal Device **M** Neurostimulator Lead	**Z** No Qualifier
1 Hemiazygos Vein ⊘ **5** Subclavian Vein, Right ⊘ CC DRG **6** Subclavian Vein, Left ⊘ CC DRG **7** Axillary Vein, Right ⊘ **8** Axillary Vein, Left ⊘ **9** Brachial Vein, Right ⊘ **A** Brachial Vein, Left ⊘ **B** Basilic Vein, Right ⊘ **C** Basilic Vein, Left ⊘ **D** Cephalic Vein, Right ⊘ **F** Cephalic Vein, Left ⊘ **G** Hand Vein, Right ⊘ **H** Hand Vein, Left ⊘ **L** Intracranial Vein ⊘ **M** Internal Jugular Vein, Right ⊘ CC DRG HAC **N** Internal Jugular Vein, Left ⊘ CC DRG HAC **P** External Jugular Vein, Right ⊘ CC DRG HAC **Q** External Jugular Vein, Left ⊘ CC DRG HAC **R** Vertebral Vein, Right ⊘ **S** Vertebral Vein, Left ⊘ **T** Face Vein, Right ⊘ **V** Face Vein, Left ⊘	**0** Open **3** Percutaneous **4** Percutaneous Endoscopic	**3** Infusion Device **D** Intraluminal Device	**Z** No Qualifier
3 Innominate Vein, Right ⊘ **4** Innominate Vein, Left ⊘	**0** Open **3** Percutaneous **4** Percutaneous Endoscopic	**3** Infusion Device **D** Intraluminal Device **M** Neurostimulator Lead	**Z** No Qualifier
Y Upper Vein ⊘	**0** Open **3** Percutaneous **4** Percutaneous Endoscopic	**2** Monitoring Device **3** Infusion Device **D** Intraluminal Device	**Z** No Qualifier

⊘ 05H002Z 05H003Z 05H00MZ 05H032Z 05H033Z 05H03MZ 05H042Z 05H043Z 05H04MZ 05H103Z 05H133Z 05H143Z 05H303Z 05H30MZ 05H333Z 05H33MZ 05H343Z 05H34MZ 05H403Z 05H40MZ 05H433Z 05H43MZ 05H443Z 05H44MZ 05H503Z 05H543Z 05H603Z 05H643Z 05H703Z 05H733Z 05H743Z 05H803Z 05H833Z 05H843Z 05H903Z 05H933Z 05H943Z 05HA03Z 05HA33Z 05HA43Z 05HB03Z 05HB33Z 05HB43Z 05HC03Z 05HC33Z 05HC43Z 05HD03Z 05HD33Z 05HD43Z 05HF03Z 05HF33Z 05HF43Z 05HG03Z 05HG33Z 05HG43Z 05HH03Z 05HH33Z 05HH43Z 05HL03Z 05HL33Z 05HL43Z 05HM03Z 05HM43Z 05HN03Z 05HN43Z

05H continued on next page

05H continued from previous page

05HP03Z 05HP43Z 05HQ03Z 05HQ43Z 05HR03Z 05HR33Z 05HR43Z 05HS03Z 05HS33Z 05HS43Z 05HT03Z 05HT33Z 05HT43Z 05HV03Z 05HV33Z 05HV43Z 05HY03Z 05HY32Z 05HY33Z 05HY43Z

HAC 05HM33Z 05HN33Z 05HP33Z or 05HQ33Z All preceding codes with the HAC symbol are classified as hospital-acquired conditions when reported with secondary diagnosis J95.811.

CC 05H533Z 05H633Z 05HM33Z 05HN33Z 05HP33Z 05HQ33Z

DRG 05H533Z 05H633Z 05HM33Z 05HN33Z 05HP33Z 05HQ33Z

0 Medical and Surgical
5 Upper Veins
J Inspection: Visually and/or manually exploring a body part

Body Part Character 4	Approach Character 5	Device Character 6	Qualifier Character 7
Y Upper Vein ⃠	**0** Open **3** Percutaneous **4** Percutaneous Endoscopic **X** External	**Z** No Device	**Z** No Qualifier

⃠ 05JY3ZZ 05JYXZZ

0 Medical and Surgical
5 Upper Veins
L Occlusion: Completely closing an orifice or the lumen of a tubular body part

Body Part Character 4	Approach Character 5	Device Character 6	Qualifier Character 7
0 Azygos Vein **1** Hemiazygos Vein **3** Innominate Vein, Right **4** Innominate Vein, Left **5** Subclavian Vein, Right **6** Subclavian Vein, Left **7** Axillary Vein, Right **8** Axillary Vein, Left **9** Brachial Vein, Right **A** Brachial Vein, Left **B** Basilic Vein, Right **C** Basilic Vein, Left **D** Cephalic Vein, Right **F** Cephalic Vein, Left **G** Hand Vein, Right **H** Hand Vein, Left **L** Intracranial Vein **M** Internal Jugular Vein, Right **N** Internal Jugular Vein, Left **P** External Jugular Vein, Right **Q** External Jugular Vein, Left **R** Vertebral Vein, Right **S** Vertebral Vein, Left **T** Face Vein, Right **V** Face Vein, Left **Y** Upper Vein	**0** Open **3** Percutaneous **4** Percutaneous Endoscopic	**C** Extraluminal Device **D** Intraluminal Device **Z** No Device	**Z** No Qualifier

0 Medical and Surgical
5 Upper Veins
N Release: Freeing a body part from an abnormal physical constraint by cutting or by the use of force

Body Part Character 4	Approach Character 5	Device Character 6	Qualifier Character 7
0 Azygos Vein **1** Hemiazygos Vein **3** Innominate Vein, Right **4** Innominate Vein, Left **5** Subclavian Vein, Right **6** Subclavian Vein, Left **7** Axillary Vein, Right **8** Axillary Vein, Left **9** Brachial Vein, Right **A** Brachial Vein, Left **B** Basilic Vein, Right **C** Basilic Vein, Left **D** Cephalic Vein, Right **F** Cephalic Vein, Left **G** Hand Vein, Right **H** Hand Vein, Left **L** Intracranial Vein **M** Internal Jugular Vein, Right **N** Internal Jugular Vein, Left **P** External Jugular Vein, Right **Q** External Jugular Vein, Left **R** Vertebral Vein, Right **S** Vertebral Vein, Left **T** Face Vein, Right **V** Face Vein, Left **Y** Upper Vein	**0** Open **3** Percutaneous **4** Percutaneous Endoscopic	**Z** No Device	**Z** No Qualifier

0 Medical and Surgical
5 Upper Veins
P Removal: Taking out or off a device from a body part

Body Part Character 4	Approach Character 5	Device Character 6	Qualifier Character 7
0 Azygos Vein ⊘	**0** Open **3** Percutaneous **4** Percutaneous Endoscopic **X** External	**2** Monitoring Device **M** Neurostimulator Lead	**Z** No Qualifier
3 Innominate Vein, Right ⊘ **4** Innominate Vein, Left ⊘	**0** Open **3** Percutaneous **4** Percutaneous Endoscopic **X** External	**M** Neurostimulator Lead	**Z** No Qualifier
Y Upper Vein ⊘	**0** Open **3** Percutaneous **4** Percutaneous Endoscopic	**0** Drainage Device **2** Monitoring Device **3** Infusion Device **7** Autologous Tissue Substitute **C** Extraluminal Device **D** Intraluminal Device **J** Synthetic Substitute **K** Nonautologous Tissue Substitute	**Z** No Qualifier
Y Upper Vein ⊘	**X** External	**0** Drainage Device **2** Monitoring Device **3** Infusion Device **D** Intraluminal Device	**Z** No Qualifier

⊘ 05P002Z 05P00MZ 05P032Z 05P03MZ 05P042Z 05P04MZ 05P0X2Z 05P0XMZ 05P30MZ 05P33MZ 05P34MZ 05P3XMZ 05P40MZ 05P43MZ 05P44MZ 05P4XMZ 05PY30Z 05PY32Z 05PY33Z 05PYX0Z 05PYX2Z 05PYX3Z 05PYXDZ

0 Medical and Surgical
5 Upper Veins
Q Repair: Restoring, to the extent possible, a body part to its normal anatomic structure and function

Body Part Character 4	Approach Character 5	Device Character 6	Qualifier Character 7
0 Azygos Vein 1 Hemiazygos Vein 3 Innominate Vein, Right 4 Innominate Vein, Left 5 Subclavian Vein, Right 6 Subclavian Vein, Left 7 Axillary Vein, Right 8 Axillary Vein, Left 9 Brachial Vein, Right A Brachial Vein, Left B Basilic Vein, Right C Basilic Vein, Left D Cephalic Vein, Right F Cephalic Vein, Left G Hand Vein, Right H Hand Vein, Left L Intracranial Vein M Internal Jugular Vein, Right N Internal Jugular Vein, Left P External Jugular Vein, Right Q External Jugular Vein, Left R Vertebral Vein, Right S Vertebral Vein, Left T Face Vein, Right V Face Vein, Left Y Upper Vein	0 Open 3 Percutaneous 4 Percutaneous Endoscopic	Z No Device	Z No Qualifier

0 Medical and Surgical
5 Upper Veins
R Replacement: Putting in or on biological or synthetic material that physically takes the place and/or function of all or a portion of a body part

Body Part Character 4	Approach Character 5	Device Character 6	Qualifier Character 7
0 Azygos Vein 1 Hemiazygos Vein 3 Innominate Vein, Right 4 Innominate Vein, Left 5 Subclavian Vein, Right 6 Subclavian Vein, Left 7 Axillary Vein, Right 8 Axillary Vein, Left 9 Brachial Vein, Right A Brachial Vein, Left B Basilic Vein, Right C Basilic Vein, Left D Cephalic Vein, Right F Cephalic Vein, Left G Hand Vein, Right H Hand Vein, Left L Intracranial Vein M Internal Jugular Vein, Right N Internal Jugular Vein, Left P External Jugular Vein, Right Q External Jugular Vein, Left R Vertebral Vein, Right S Vertebral Vein, Left T Face Vein, Right V Face Vein, Left Y Upper Vein	0 Open 4 Percutaneous Endoscopic	7 Autologous Tissue Substitute J Synthetic Substitute K Nonautologous Tissue Substitute	Z No Qualifier

0 Medical and Surgical
5 Upper Veins
S Reposition: Moving to its normal location, or other suitable location, all or a portion of a body part

Body Part Character 4	Approach Character 5	Device Character 6	Qualifier Character 7
0 Azygos Vein **1** Hemiazygos Vein **3** Innominate Vein, Right **4** Innominate Vein, Left **5** Subclavian Vein, Right **6** Subclavian Vein, Left **7** Axillary Vein, Right **8** Axillary Vein, Left **9** Brachial Vein, Right **A** Brachial Vein, Left **B** Basilic Vein, Right **C** Basilic Vein, Left **D** Cephalic Vein, Right **F** Cephalic Vein, Left **G** Hand Vein, Right **H** Hand Vein, Left **L** Intracranial Vein **M** Internal Jugular Vein, Right **N** Internal Jugular Vein, Left **P** External Jugular Vein, Right **Q** External Jugular Vein, Left **R** Vertebral Vein, Right **S** Vertebral Vein, Left **T** Face Vein, Right **V** Face Vein, Left **Y** Upper Vein	**0** Open **3** Percutaneous **4** Percutaneous Endoscopic	**Z** No Device	**Z** No Qualifier

0 Medical and Surgical
5 Upper Veins
U Supplement: Putting in or on biological or synthetic material that physically reinforces and/or augments the function of a portion of a body part

Body Part Character 4	Approach Character 5	Device Character 6	Qualifier Character 7
0 Azygos Vein **1** Hemiazygos Vein **3** Innominate Vein, Right **4** Innominate Vein, Left **5** Subclavian Vein, Right **6** Subclavian Vein, Left **7** Axillary Vein, Right **8** Axillary Vein, Left **9** Brachial Vein, Right **A** Brachial Vein, Left **B** Basilic Vein, Right **C** Basilic Vein, Left **D** Cephalic Vein, Right **F** Cephalic Vein, Left **G** Hand Vein, Right **H** Hand Vein, Left **L** Intracranial Vein **M** Internal Jugular Vein, Right **N** Internal Jugular Vein, Left **P** External Jugular Vein, Right **Q** External Jugular Vein, Left **R** Vertebral Vein, Right **S** Vertebral Vein, Left **T** Face Vein, Right **V** Face Vein, Left **Y** Upper Vein	**0** Open **3** Percutaneous **4** Percutaneous Endoscopic	**7** Autologous Tissue Substitute **J** Synthetic Substitute **K** Nonautologous Tissue Substitute	**Z** No Qualifier

0 Medical and Surgical
5 Upper Veins
V Restriction: Partially closing an orifice or the lumen of a tubular body part

Body Part Character 4	Approach Character 5	Device Character 6	Qualifier Character 7
0 Azygos Vein **1** Hemiazygos Vein **3** Innominate Vein, Right **4** Innominate Vein, Left **5** Subclavian Vein, Right **6** Subclavian Vein, Left **7** Axillary Vein, Right **8** Axillary Vein, Left **9** Brachial Vein, Right **A** Brachial Vein, Left **B** Basilic Vein, Right **C** Basilic Vein, Left **D** Cephalic Vein, Right **F** Cephalic Vein, Left **G** Hand Vein, Right **H** Hand Vein, Left **L** Intracranial Vein **M** Internal Jugular Vein, Right **N** Internal Jugular Vein, Left **P** External Jugular Vein, Right **Q** External Jugular Vein, Left **R** Vertebral Vein, Right **S** Vertebral Vein, Left **T** Face Vein, Right **V** Face Vein, Left **Y** Upper Vein	**0** Open **3** Percutaneous **4** Percutaneous Endoscopic	**C** Extraluminal Device **D** Intraluminal Device **Z** No Device	**Z** No Qualifier

0 Medical and Surgical
5 Upper Veins
W Revision: Correcting, to the extent possible, a portion of a malfunctioning device or the position of a displaced device

Body Part Character 4	Approach Character 5	Device Character 6	Qualifier Character 7
0 Azygos Vein ⦸	**0** Open **3** Percutaneous **4** Percutaneous Endoscopic **X** External	**2** Monitoring Device **M** Neurostimulator Lead	**Z** No Qualifier
3 Innominate Vein, Right ⦸ **4** Innominate Vein, Left ⦸	**0** Open **3** Percutaneous **4** Percutaneous Endoscopic **X** External	**M** Neurostimulator Lead	**Z** No Qualifier
Y Upper Vein ⦸	**0** Open **3** Percutaneous **4** Percutaneous Endoscopic **X** External	**0** Drainage Device **2** Monitoring Device **3** Infusion Device **7** Autologous Tissue Substitute **C** Extraluminal Device **D** Intraluminal Device **J** Synthetic Substitute **K** Nonautologous Tissue Substitute	**Z** No Qualifier

⦸ 05W002Z 05W00MZ 05W032Z 05W03MZ 05W042Z 05W04MZ 05W0X2Z 05W0XMZ 05W30MZ 05W33MZ 05W34MZ 05W3XMZ 05W40MZ 05W43MZ 05W44MZ 05W4XMZ 05WYX0Z 05WYX2Z 05WYX3Z 05WYX7Z 05WYXCZ 05WYXDZ 05WYXJZ 05WYXKZ

Lower Veins 061-06W

0 Medical and Surgical
6 Lower Veins
1 Bypass: Altering the route of passage of the contents of a tubular body part

Body Part Character 4	Approach Character 5	Device Character 6	Qualifier Character 7
0 Inferior Vena Cava	0 Open 4 Percutaneous Endoscopic	7 Autologous Tissue Substitute 9 Autologous Venous Tissue A Autologous Arterial Tissue J Synthetic Substitute K Nonautologous Tissue Substitute Z No Device	5 Superior Mesenteric Vein 6 Inferior Mesenteric Vein Y Lower Vein
1 Splenic Vein	0 Open 4 Percutaneous Endoscopic	7 Autologous Tissue Substitute 9 Autologous Venous Tissue A Autologous Arterial Tissue J Synthetic Substitute K Nonautologous Tissue Substitute Z No Device	9 Renal Vein, Right B Renal Vein, Left Y Lower Vein
2 Gastric Vein 3 Esophageal Vein 4 Hepatic Vein 5 Superior Mesenteric Vein 6 Inferior Mesenteric Vein 7 Colic Vein 9 Renal Vein, Right B Renal Vein, Left C Common Iliac Vein, Right D Common Iliac Vein, Left F External Iliac Vein, Right G External Iliac Vein, Left H Hypogastric Vein, Right J Hypogastric Vein, Left M Femoral Vein, Right N Femoral Vein, Left P Greater Saphenous Vein, Right Q Greater Saphenous Vein, Left R Lesser Saphenous Vein, Right S Lesser Saphenous Vein, Left T Foot Vein, Right V Foot Vein, Left	0 Open 4 Percutaneous Endoscopic	7 Autologous Tissue Substitute 9 Autologous Venous Tissue A Autologous Arterial Tissue J Synthetic Substitute K Nonautologous Tissue Substitute Z No Device	Y Lower Vein
8 Portal Vein	0 Open	7 Autologous Tissue Substitute 9 Autologous Venous Tissue A Autologous Arterial Tissue J Synthetic Substitute K Nonautologous Tissue Substitute Z No Device	9 Renal Vein, Right B Renal Vein, Left Y Lower Vein
8 Portal Vein	3 Percutaneous	D Intraluminal Device	Y Lower Vein
8 Portal Vein	4 Percutaneous Endoscopic	7 Autologous Tissue Substitute 9 Autologous Venous Tissue A Autologous Arterial Tissue J Synthetic Substitute K Nonautologous Tissue Substitute Z No Device	9 Renal Vein, Right B Renal Vein, Left Y Lower Vein
8 Portal Vein	4 Percutaneous Endoscopic	D Intraluminal Device	Y Lower Vein

0 Medical and Surgical
6 Lower Veins
5 Destruction: Physical eradication of all or a portion of a body part by the direct use of energy, force, or a destructive agent

Body Part Character 4	Approach Character 5	Device Character 6	Qualifier Character 7
0 Inferior Vena Cava **1** Splenic Vein **2** Gastric Vein **3** Esophageal Vein **4** Hepatic Vein **5** Superior Mesenteric Vein **6** Inferior Mesenteric Vein **7** Colic Vein **8** Portal Vein **9** Renal Vein, Right **B** Renal Vein, Left **C** Common Iliac Vein, Right **D** Common Iliac Vein, Left **F** External Iliac Vein, Right **G** External Iliac Vein, Left **H** Hypogastric Vein, Right **J** Hypogastric Vein, Left **M** Femoral Vein, Right **N** Femoral Vein, Left **P** Greater Saphenous Vein, Right **Q** Greater Saphenous Vein, Left **R** Lesser Saphenous Vein, Right **S** Lesser Saphenous Vein, Left **T** Foot Vein, Right **V** Foot Vein, Left	**0** Open **3** Percutaneous **4** Percutaneous Endoscopic	**Z** No Device	**Z** No Qualifier
Y Lower Vein	**0** Open **3** Percutaneous **4** Percutaneous Endoscopic	**Z** No Device	**C** Hemorrhoidal Plexus **Z** No Qualifier

0 Medical and Surgical
6 Lower Veins
7 Dilation: Expanding an orifice or the lumen of a tubular body part

Body Part Character 4	Approach Character 5	Device Character 6	Qualifier Character 7
0 Inferior Vena Cava **1** Splenic Vein **2** Gastric Vein **3** Esophageal Vein **4** Hepatic Vein **5** Superior Mesenteric Vein **6** Inferior Mesenteric Vein **7** Colic Vein **8** Portal Vein **9** Renal Vein, Right **B** Renal Vein, Left **C** Common Iliac Vein, Right **D** Common Iliac Vein, Left **F** External Iliac Vein, Right **G** External Iliac Vein, Left **H** Hypogastric Vein, Right **J** Hypogastric Vein, Left **M** Femoral Vein, Right **N** Femoral Vein, Left **P** Greater Saphenous Vein, Right **Q** Greater Saphenous Vein, Left **R** Lesser Saphenous Vein, Right **S** Lesser Saphenous Vein, Left **T** Foot Vein, Right **V** Foot Vein, Left **Y** Lower Vein	**0** Open **3** Percutaneous **4** Percutaneous Endoscopic	**D** Intraluminal Device **Z** No Device	**Z** No Qualifier

LC Limited Coverage NC Noncovered HAC HAC Associated Procedure CC Combination Cluster - See Appendix G for code lists
DRG Non-OR-Affecting MS-DRG Assignment ⦸ Non-OR-Not Affecting MS-DRG Assignment New/Revised Text in **Orange** ♂ Male ♀ Female

0 Medical and Surgical
6 Lower Veins
9 Drainage: Taking or letting out fluids and/or gases from a body part

Body Part Character 4	Approach Character 5	Device Character 6	Qualifier Character 7
0 Inferior Vena Cava ⦸ **1** Splenic Vein ⦸ **2** Gastric Vein ⦸ **3** Esophageal Vein ⦸ **4** Hepatic Vein ⦸ **5** Superior Mesenteric Vein ⦸ **6** Inferior Mesenteric Vein ⦸ **7** Colic Vein ⦸ **8** Portal Vein ⦸ **9** Renal Vein, Right ⦸ **B** Renal Vein, Left ⦸ **C** Common Iliac Vein, Right ⦸ **D** Common Iliac Vein, Left ⦸ **F** External Iliac Vein, Right ⦸ **G** External Iliac Vein, Left ⦸ **H** Hypogastric Vein, Right ⦸ **J** Hypogastric Vein, Left ⦸ **M** Femoral Vein, Right ⦸ **N** Femoral Vein, Left ⦸ **P** Greater Saphenous Vein, Right ⦸ **Q** Greater Saphenous Vein, Left ⦸ **R** Lesser Saphenous Vein, Right ⦸ **S** Lesser Saphenous Vein, Left ⦸ **T** Foot Vein, Right ⦸ **V** Foot Vein, Left ⦸ **Y** Lower Vein ⦸	**0** Open **3** Percutaneous **4** Percutaneous Endoscopic	**0** Drainage Device	**Z** No Qualifier
0 Inferior Vena Cava ⦸ **1** Splenic Vein ⦸ **2** Gastric Vein ⦸ **3** Esophageal Vein ⦸ **4** Hepatic Vein ⦸ **5** Superior Mesenteric Vein ⦸ **6** Inferior Mesenteric Vein ⦸ **7** Colic Vein ⦸ **8** Portal Vein ⦸ **9** Renal Vein, Right ⦸ **B** Renal Vein, Left ⦸ **C** Common Iliac Vein, Right ⦸ **D** Common Iliac Vein, Left ⦸ **F** External Iliac Vein, Right ⦸ **G** External Iliac Vein, Left ⦸ **H** Hypogastric Vein, Right ⦸ **J** Hypogastric Vein, Left ⦸ **M** Femoral Vein, Right ⦸ **N** Femoral Vein, Left ⦸ **P** Greater Saphenous Vein, Right ⦸ **Q** Greater Saphenous Vein, Left ⦸ **R** Lesser Saphenous Vein, Right ⦸ **S** Lesser Saphenous Vein, Left ⦸ **T** Foot Vein, Right ⦸ **V** Foot Vein, Left ⦸ **Y** Lower Vein ⦸	**0** Open **3** Percutaneous **4** Percutaneous Endoscopic	**Z** No Device	**X** Diagnostic **Z** No Qualifier

⦸ 069000Z 06900ZZ 069030Z 06903ZZ 069040Z 06904ZZ 069100Z 06910ZZ 069130Z 06913ZZ 069140Z 06914ZZ 069200Z 06920ZZ 069230Z 06923ZZ 069240Z 06924ZZ 069330Z 06933ZZ 069400Z 06940ZZ 069430Z 06943ZZ 069440Z 06944ZZ 069500Z 06950ZZ 069530Z 06953ZZ 069540Z 06954ZZ 069600Z 06960ZZ 069630Z 06963ZZ 069640Z 06964ZZ 069700Z 06970ZZ 069730Z 06973ZZ 069740Z 06974ZZ 069800Z 06980ZZ 069830Z 06983ZZ 069840Z 06984ZZ 069900Z 06990ZZ 069930Z 06993ZZ 069940Z 06994ZZ 069B00Z 069B0ZZ 069B30Z 069B3ZZ 069B40Z 069B4ZZ 069C00Z 069C0ZZ 069C30Z

069 continued on next page

LC Limited Coverage NC Noncovered HAC HAC Associated Procedure CC Combination Cluster - See Appendix G for code lists
DRG Non-OR-Affecting MS-DRG Assignment ⦸ Non-OR-Not Affecting MS-DRG Assignment New/Revised Text in **Orange** ♂ Male ♀ Female

069 continued from previous page

069C3ZZ 069C40Z 069C4ZZ 069D00Z 069D0ZZ 069D30Z 069D3ZZ 069D40Z 069D4ZZ 069F00Z 069F0ZZ 069F30Z 069F3ZZ 069F40Z 069F4ZZ 069G00Z 069G0ZZ 069G30Z 069G3ZZ 069G40Z 069G4ZZ 069H00Z 069H0ZZ 069H30Z 069H3ZZ 069H40Z 069H4ZZ 069J00Z 069J0ZZ 069J30Z 069J3ZZ 069J40Z 069J4ZZ 069M00Z 069M0ZZ 069M30Z 069M3ZZ 069M40Z 069M4ZZ 069N00Z 069N0ZZ 069N30Z 069N3ZZ 069N40Z 069N4ZZ 069P00Z 069P0ZZ 069P30Z 069P3ZZ 069P40Z 069P4ZZ 069Q00Z 069Q0ZZ 069Q30Z 069Q3ZZ 069Q40Z 069Q4ZZ 069R00Z 069R0ZZ 069R30Z 069R3ZZ 069R40Z 069R4ZZ 069S00Z 069S0ZZ 069S30Z 069S3ZZ 069S40Z 069S4ZZ 069T00Z 069T0ZZ 069T30Z 069T3ZZ 069T40Z 069T4ZZ 069V00Z 069V0ZZ 069V30Z 069V3ZZ 069V40Z 069V4ZZ 069Y00Z 069Y0ZZ 069Y30Z 069Y3ZZ 069Y40Z 069Y4ZZ

0 Medical and Surgical
6 Lower Veins
B Excision: Cutting out or off, without replacement, a portion of a body part

Body Part Character 4	Approach Character 5	Device Character 6	Qualifier Character 7
0 Inferior Vena Cava **1** Splenic Vein **2** Gastric Vein **3** Esophageal Vein **4** Hepatic Vein **5** Superior Mesenteric Vein **6** Inferior Mesenteric Vein **7** Colic Vein **8** Portal Vein **9** Renal Vein, Right **B** Renal Vein, Left **C** Common Iliac Vein, Right **D** Common Iliac Vein, Left **F** External Iliac Vein, Right **G** External Iliac Vein, Left **H** Hypogastric Vein, Right **J** Hypogastric Vein, Left **M** Femoral Vein, Right **N** Femoral Vein, Left **P** Greater Saphenous Vein, Right **Q** Greater Saphenous Vein, Left **R** Lesser Saphenous Vein, Right **S** Lesser Saphenous Vein, Left **T** Foot Vein, Right **V** Foot Vein, Left	**0** Open **3** Percutaneous **4** Percutaneous Endoscopic	**Z** No Device	**X** Diagnostic **Z** No Qualifier
Y Lower Vein	**0** Open **3** Percutaneous **4** Percutaneous Endoscopic	**Z** No Device	**C** Hemorrhoidal Plexus **X** Diagnostic **Z** No Qualifier

0 Medical and Surgical
6 Lower Veins
C Extirpation: Taking or cutting out solid matter from a body part

Body Part Character 4	Approach Character 5	Device Character 6	Qualifier Character 7
0 Inferior Vena Cava **1** Splenic Vein **2** Gastric Vein **3** Esophageal Vein **4** Hepatic Vein **5** Superior Mesenteric Vein **6** Inferior Mesenteric Vein **7** Colic Vein **8** Portal Vein **9** Renal Vein, Right **B** Renal Vein, Left **C** Common Iliac Vein, Right **D** Common Iliac Vein, Left **F** External Iliac Vein, Right **G** External Iliac Vein, Left **H** Hypogastric Vein, Right **J** Hypogastric Vein, Left **M** Femoral Vein, Right **N** Femoral Vein, Left **P** Greater Saphenous Vein, Right **Q** Greater Saphenous Vein, Left **R** Lesser Saphenous Vein, Right **S** Lesser Saphenous Vein, Left **T** Foot Vein, Right **V** Foot Vein, Left **Y** Lower Vein	**0** Open **3** Percutaneous **4** Percutaneous Endoscopic	**Z** No Device	**Z** No Qualifier

0 Medical and Surgical
6 Lower Veins
D Extraction: Pulling or stripping out or off all or a portion of a body part by the use of force

Body Part Character 4	Approach Character 5	Device Character 6	Qualifier Character 7
M Femoral Vein, Right **N** Femoral Vein, Left **P** Greater Saphenous Vein, Right **Q** Greater Saphenous Vein, Left **R** Lesser Saphenous Vein, Right **S** Lesser Saphenous Vein, Left **T** Foot Vein, Right **V** Foot Vein, Left **Y** Lower Vein	**0** Open **3** Percutaneous **4** Percutaneous Endoscopic	**Z** No Device	**Z** No Qualifier

0 Medical and Surgical
6 Lower Veins
H Insertion: Putting in a nonbiological appliance that monitors, assists, performs, or prevents a physiological function but does not physically take the place of a body part

Body Part Character 4	Approach Character 5	Device Character 6	Qualifier Character 7
0 Inferior Vena Cava ⊘	**0** Open **3** Percutaneous	**3** Infusion Device	**T** Via Umbilical Vein **Z** No Qualifier
0 Inferior Vena Cava	**0** Open **3** Percutaneous	**D** Intraluminal Device	**Z** No Qualifier
0 Inferior Vena Cava ⊘	**4** Percutaneous Endoscopic	**3** Infusion Device **D** Intraluminal Device	**Z** No Qualifier
1 Splenic Vein ⊘ **2** Gastric Vein ⊘ **3** Esophageal Vein ⊘ **4** Hepatic Vein ⊘ **5** Superior Mesenteric Vein ⊘ **6** Inferior Mesenteric Vein ⊘ **7** Colic Vein ⊘ **8** Portal Vein ⊘ **9** Renal Vein, Right ⊘ **B** Renal Vein, Left ⊘ **C** Common Iliac Vein, Right ⊘ **D** Common Iliac Vein, Left ⊘ **F** External Iliac Vein, Right ⊘ **G** External Iliac Vein, Left ⊘ **H** Hypogastric Vein, Right ⊘ **J** Hypogastric Vein, Left ⊘ **M** Femoral Vein, Right ⊘ CC DRG **N** Femoral Vein, Left ⊘ CC DRG **P** Greater Saphenous Vein, Right ⊘ **Q** Greater Saphenous Vein, Left ⊘ **R** Lesser Saphenous Vein, Right ⊘ **S** Lesser Saphenous Vein, Left ⊘ **T** Foot Vein, Right ⊘ **V** Foot Vein, Left ⊘	**0** Open **3** Percutaneous **4** Percutaneous Endoscopic	**3** Infusion Device **D** Intraluminal Device	**Z** No Qualifier
Y Lower Vein ⊘	**0** Open **3** Percutaneous **4** Percutaneous Endoscopic	**2** Monitoring Device **3** Infusion Device **D** Intraluminal Device	**Z** No Qualifier

⊘ 06H003T 06H003Z 06H033T 06H033Z 06H043Z 06H103Z 06H133Z 06H143Z 06H203Z 06H233Z 06H243Z 06H303Z 06H333Z 06H343Z 06H403Z 06H433Z 06H443Z 06H503Z 06H533Z 06H543Z 06H603Z 06H633Z 06H643Z 06H703Z 06H733Z 06H743Z 06H803Z 06H833Z 06H843Z 06H903Z 06H933Z 06H943Z 06HB03Z 06HB33Z 06HB43Z 06HC03Z 06HC33Z 06HC43Z 06HD03Z 06HD33Z 06HD43Z 06HF03Z 06HF33Z 06HF43Z 06HG03Z 06HG33Z 06HG43Z 06HH03Z 06HH33Z 06HH43Z 06HJ03Z 06HJ33Z 06HJ43Z 06HM03Z 06HM43Z 06HN03Z 06HN43Z 06HP03Z 06HP33Z 06HP43Z 06HQ03Z 06HQ33Z 06HQ43Z 06HR03Z 06HR33Z 06HR43Z 06HS03Z 06HS33Z 06HS43Z 06HT03Z 06HT33Z 06HT43Z 06HV03Z 06HV33Z 06HV43Z 06HY03Z 06HY32Z 06HY33Z 06HY43Z

CC 06HM33Z 06HN33Z

DRG 06HM33Z 06HN33Z

0 Medical and Surgical
6 Lower Veins
J Inspection: Visually and/or manually exploring a body part

Body Part Character 4	Approach Character 5	Device Character 6	Qualifier Character 7
Y Lower Vein ⊘	**0** Open **3** Percutaneous **4** Percutaneous Endoscopic **X** External	**Z** No Device	**Z** No Qualifier

⊘ 06JY3ZZ 06JYXZZ

0 Medical and Surgical
6 Lower Veins
L Occlusion: Completely closing an orifice or the lumen of a tubular body part

Body Part Character 4	Approach Character 5	Device Character 6	Qualifier Character 7
0 Inferior Vena Cava **1** Splenic Vein **2** Gastric Vein **3** Esophageal Vein ⦸ **4** Hepatic Vein **5** Superior Mesenteric Vein **6** Inferior Mesenteric Vein **7** Colic Vein **8** Portal Vein **9** Renal Vein, Right **B** Renal Vein, Left **C** Common Iliac Vein, Right **D** Common Iliac Vein, Left **F** External Iliac Vein, Right **G** External Iliac Vein, Left **H** Hypogastric Vein, Right **J** Hypogastric Vein, Left **M** Femoral Vein, Right **N** Femoral Vein, Left **P** Greater Saphenous Vein, Right **Q** Greater Saphenous Vein, Left **R** Lesser Saphenous Vein, Right **S** Lesser Saphenous Vein, Left **T** Foot Vein, Right **V** Foot Vein, Left	**0** Open **3** Percutaneous **4** Percutaneous Endoscopic	**C** Extraluminal Device **D** Intraluminal Device **Z** No Device	**Z** No Qualifier
Y Lower Vein	**0** Open **3** Percutaneous **4** Percutaneous Endoscopic	**C** Extraluminal Device **D** Intraluminal Device **Z** No Device	**C** Hemorrhoidal Plexus **Z** No Qualifier

⦸ 06L33CZ 06L33DZ 06L33ZZ 06L34CZ 06L34DZ 06L34ZZ

0 Medical and Surgical
6 Lower Veins
N Release: Freeing a body part from an abnormal physical constraint by cutting or by the use of force

Body Part Character 4	Approach Character 5	Device Character 6	Qualifier Character 7
0 Inferior Vena Cava **1** Splenic Vein **2** Gastric Vein **3** Esophageal Vein **4** Hepatic Vein **5** Superior Mesenteric Vein **6** Inferior Mesenteric Vein **7** Colic Vein **8** Portal Vein **9** Renal Vein, Right **B** Renal Vein, Left **C** Common Iliac Vein, Right **D** Common Iliac Vein, Left **F** External Iliac Vein, Right **G** External Iliac Vein, Left **H** Hypogastric Vein, Right **J** Hypogastric Vein, Left **M** Femoral Vein, Right **N** Femoral Vein, Left **P** Greater Saphenous Vein, Right **Q** Greater Saphenous Vein, Left **R** Lesser Saphenous Vein, Right **S** Lesser Saphenous Vein, Left **T** Foot Vein, Right **V** Foot Vein, Left **Y** Lower Vein	**0** Open **3** Percutaneous **4** Percutaneous Endoscopic	**Z** No Device	**Z** No Qualifier

0 Medical and Surgical
6 Lower Veins
P Removal: Taking out or off a device from a body part

Body Part Character 4	Approach Character 5	Device Character 6	Qualifier Character 7
Y Lower Vein ⃠	**0** Open **3** Percutaneous **4** Percutaneous Endoscopic	**0** Drainage Device **2** Monitoring Device **3** Infusion Device **7** Autologous Tissue Substitute **C** Extraluminal Device **D** Intraluminal Device **J** Synthetic Substitute **K** Nonautologous Tissue Substitute	**Z** No Qualifier
Y Lower Vein ⃠	**X** External	**0** Drainage Device **2** Monitoring Device **3** Infusion Device **D** Intraluminal Device	**Z** No Qualifier

⃠ 06PY30Z 06PY32Z 06PY33Z 06PYX0Z 06PYX2Z 06PYX3Z 06PYXDZ

0 Medical and Surgical
6 Lower Veins
Q Repair: Restoring, to the extent possible, a body part to its normal anatomic structure and function

Body Part Character 4	Approach Character 5	Device Character 6	Qualifier Character 7
0 Inferior Vena Cava **1** Splenic Vein **2** Gastric Vein **3** Esophageal Vein **4** Hepatic Vein **5** Superior Mesenteric Vein **6** Inferior Mesenteric Vein **7** Colic Vein **8** Portal Vein **9** Renal Vein, Right **B** Renal Vein, Left **C** Common Iliac Vein, Right **D** Common Iliac Vein, Left **F** External Iliac Vein, Right **G** External Iliac Vein, Left **H** Hypogastric Vein, Right **J** Hypogastric Vein, Left **M** Femoral Vein, Right **N** Femoral Vein, Left **P** Greater Saphenous Vein, Right **Q** Greater Saphenous Vein, Left **R** Lesser Saphenous Vein, Right **S** Lesser Saphenous Vein, Left **T** Foot Vein, Right **V** Foot Vein, Left **Y** Lower Vein	**0** Open **3** Percutaneous **4** Percutaneous Endoscopic	**Z** No Device	**Z** No Qualifier

0 Medical and Surgical
6 Lower Veins
R Replacement: Putting in or on biological or synthetic material that physically takes the place and/or function of all or a portion of a body part

Body Part Character 4	Approach Character 5	Device Character 6	Qualifier Character 7
0 Inferior Vena Cava **1** Splenic Vein **2** Gastric Vein **3** Esophageal Vein **4** Hepatic Vein **5** Superior Mesenteric Vein **6** Inferior Mesenteric Vein **7** Colic Vein **8** Portal Vein **9** Renal Vein, Right **B** Renal Vein, Left **C** Common Iliac Vein, Right **D** Common Iliac Vein, Left **F** External Iliac Vein, Right **G** External Iliac Vein, Left **H** Hypogastric Vein, Right **J** Hypogastric Vein, Left **M** Femoral Vein, Right **N** Femoral Vein, Left **P** Greater Saphenous Vein, Right **Q** Greater Saphenous Vein, Left **R** Lesser Saphenous Vein, Right **S** Lesser Saphenous Vein, Left **T** Foot Vein, Right **V** Foot Vein, Left **Y** Lower Vein	**0** Open **4** Percutaneous Endoscopic	**7** Autologous Tissue Substitute **J** Synthetic Substitute **K** Nonautologous Tissue Substitute	**Z** No Qualifier

0 Medical and Surgical
6 Lower Veins
S Reposition: Moving to its normal location, or other suitable location, all or a portion of a body part

Body Part Character 4	Approach Character 5	Device Character 6	Qualifier Character 7
0 Inferior Vena Cava **1** Splenic Vein **2** Gastric Vein **3** Esophageal Vein **4** Hepatic Vein **5** Superior Mesenteric Vein **6** Inferior Mesenteric Vein **7** Colic Vein **8** Portal Vein **9** Renal Vein, Right **B** Renal Vein, Left **C** Common Iliac Vein, Right **D** Common Iliac Vein, Left **F** External Iliac Vein, Right **G** External Iliac Vein, Left **H** Hypogastric Vein, Right **J** Hypogastric Vein, Left **M** Femoral Vein, Right **N** Femoral Vein, Left **P** Greater Saphenous Vein, Right **Q** Greater Saphenous Vein, Left **R** Lesser Saphenous Vein, Right **S** Lesser Saphenous Vein, Left **T** Foot Vein, Right **V** Foot Vein, Left **Y** Lower Vein	**0** Open **3** Percutaneous **4** Percutaneous Endoscopic	**Z** No Device	**Z** No Qualifier

0 Medical and Surgical
6 Lower Veins
U Supplement: Putting in or on biological or synthetic material that physically reinforces and/or augments the function of a portion of a body part

Body Part Character 4	Approach Character 5	Device Character 6	Qualifier Character 7
0 Inferior Vena Cava **1** Splenic Vein **2** Gastric Vein **3** Esophageal Vein **4** Hepatic Vein **5** Superior Mesenteric Vein **6** Inferior Mesenteric Vein **7** Colic Vein **8** Portal Vein **9** Renal Vein, Right **B** Renal Vein, Left **C** Common Iliac Vein, Right **D** Common Iliac Vein, Left **F** External Iliac Vein, Right **G** External Iliac Vein, Left **H** Hypogastric Vein, Right **J** Hypogastric Vein, Left **M** Femoral Vein, Right **N** Femoral Vein, Left **P** Greater Saphenous Vein, Right **Q** Greater Saphenous Vein, Left **R** Lesser Saphenous Vein, Right **S** Lesser Saphenous Vein, Left **T** Foot Vein, Right **V** Foot Vein, Left **Y** Lower Vein	**0** Open **3** Percutaneous **4** Percutaneous Endoscopic	**7** Autologous Tissue Substitute **J** Synthetic Substitute **K** Nonautologous Tissue Substitute	**Z** No Qualifier

0 Medical and Surgical
6 Lower Veins
V Restriction: Partially closing an orifice or the lumen of a tubular body part

Body Part Character 4	Approach Character 5	Device Character 6	Qualifier Character 7
0 Inferior Vena Cava **1** Splenic Vein **2** Gastric Vein **3** Esophageal Vein **4** Hepatic Vein **5** Superior Mesenteric Vein **6** Inferior Mesenteric Vein **7** Colic Vein **8** Portal Vein **9** Renal Vein, Right **B** Renal Vein, Left **C** Common Iliac Vein, Right **D** Common Iliac Vein, Left **F** External Iliac Vein, Right **G** External Iliac Vein, Left **H** Hypogastric Vein, Right **J** Hypogastric Vein, Left **M** Femoral Vein, Right **N** Femoral Vein, Left **P** Greater Saphenous Vein, Right **Q** Greater Saphenous Vein, Left **R** Lesser Saphenous Vein, Right **S** Lesser Saphenous Vein, Left **T** Foot Vein, Right **V** Foot Vein, Left **Y** Lower Vein	**0** Open **3** Percutaneous **4** Percutaneous Endoscopic	**C** Extraluminal Device **D** Intraluminal Device **Z** No Device	**Z** No Qualifier

0 Medical and Surgical
6 Lower Veins
W Revision: Correcting, to the extent possible, a portion of a malfunctioning device or the position of a displaced device

Body Part Character 4	Approach Character 5	Device Character 6	Qualifier Character 7
Y Lower Vein ⃠	**0** Open **3** Percutaneous **4** Percutaneous Endoscopic **X** External	**0** Drainage Device **2** Monitoring Device **3** Infusion Device **7** Autologous Tissue Substitute **C** Extraluminal Device **D** Intraluminal Device **J** Synthetic Substitute **K** Nonautologous Tissue Substitute	**Z** No Qualifier

⃠ 06WYX0Z 06WYX2Z 06WYX3Z 06WYX7Z 06WYXCZ 06WYXDZ 06WYXJZ 06WYXKZ

Lymphatic and Hemic Systems 072-07Y

0 Medical and Surgical
7 Lymphatic and Hemic Systems
2 Change: Taking out or off a device from a body part and putting back an identical or similar device in or on the same body part without cutting or puncturing the skin or a mucous membrane

Body Part Character 4	Approach Character 5	Device Character 6	Qualifier Character 7
K Thoracic Duct ⊘ **L** Cisterna Chyli ⊘ **M** Thymus ⊘ **N** Lymphatic ⊘ **P** Spleen ⊘ **T** Bone Marrow ⊘	**X** External	**0** Drainage Device **Y** Other Device	**Z** No Qualifier

⊘ 072KX0Z 072KXYZ 072LX0Z 072LXYZ 072MX0Z 072MXYZ 072NX0Z 072NXYZ 072PX0Z 072PXYZ 072TX0Z 072TXYZ

0 Medical and Surgical
7 Lymphatic and Hemic Systems
5 Destruction: Physical eradication of all or a portion of a body part by the direct use of energy, force, or a destructive agent

Body Part Character 4	Approach Character 5	Device Character 6	Qualifier Character 7
0 Lymphatic, Head **1** Lymphatic, Right Neck **2** Lymphatic, Left Neck **3** Lymphatic, Right Upper Extremity **4** Lymphatic, Left Upper Extremity **5** Lymphatic, Right Axillary **6** Lymphatic, Left Axillary **7** Lymphatic, Thorax **8** Lymphatic, Internal Mammary, Right **9** Lymphatic, Internal Mammary, Left **B** Lymphatic, Mesenteric **C** Lymphatic, Pelvis **D** Lymphatic, Aortic **F** Lymphatic, Right Lower Extremity **G** Lymphatic, Left Lower Extremity **H** Lymphatic, Right Inguinal **J** Lymphatic, Left Inguinal **K** Thoracic Duct **L** Cisterna Chyli **M** Thymus **P** Spleen	**0** Open **3** Percutaneous **4** Percutaneous Endoscopic	**Z** No Device	**Z** No Qualifier

0 Medical and Surgical
7 Lymphatic and Hemic Systems
9 Drainage: Taking or letting out fluids and/or gases from a body part

Body Part Character 4	Approach Character 5	Device Character 6	Qualifier Character 7
0 Lymphatic, Head ⊘ **1** Lymphatic, Right Neck ⊘ **2** Lymphatic, Left Neck ⊘ **3** Lymphatic, Right Upper Extremity ⊘ **4** Lymphatic, Left Upper Extremity ⊘ **5** Lymphatic, Right Axillary ⊘ **6** Lymphatic, Left Axillary ⊘ **7** Lymphatic, Thorax ⊘ **8** Lymphatic, Internal Mammary, Right ⊘ **9** Lymphatic, Internal Mammary, Left ⊘ **B** Lymphatic, Mesenteric ⊘ **C** Lymphatic, Pelvis ⊘ **D** Lymphatic, Aortic ⊘ **F** Lymphatic, Right Lower Extremity ⊘ **G** Lymphatic, Left Lower Extremity ⊘ **H** Lymphatic, Right Inguinal ⊘ **J** Lymphatic, Left Inguinal ⊘ **K** Thoracic Duct ⊘ **L** Cisterna Chyli ⊘ **M** Thymus ⊘ **P** Spleen ⊘ **T** Bone Marrow ⊘	**0** Open **3** Percutaneous **4** Percutaneous Endoscopic	**0** Drainage Device	**Z** No Qualifier
0 Lymphatic, Head ⊘ **1** Lymphatic, Right Neck ⊘ **2** Lymphatic, Left Neck ⊘ **3** Lymphatic, Right Upper Extremity ⊘ **4** Lymphatic, Left Upper Extremity ⊘ **5** Lymphatic, Right Axillary ⊘ **6** Lymphatic, Left Axillary ⊘ **7** Lymphatic, Thorax ⊘ **8** Lymphatic, Internal Mammary, Right ⊘ **9** Lymphatic, Internal Mammary, Left ⊘ **B** Lymphatic, Mesenteric ⊘ **C** Lymphatic, Pelvis ⊘ **D** Lymphatic, Aortic ⊘ **F** Lymphatic, Right Lower Extremity ⊘ **G** Lymphatic, Left Lower Extremity ⊘ **H** Lymphatic, Right Inguinal ⊘ **J** Lymphatic, Left Inguinal ⊘ **K** Thoracic Duct ⊘ **L** Cisterna Chyli ⊘ **M** Thymus ⊘ **P** Spleen ⊘ **T** Bone Marrow ⊘	**0** Open **3** Percutaneous **4** Percutaneous Endoscopic	**Z** No Device	**X** Diagnostic **Z** No Qualifier

⊘ 079030Z 07903ZZ 079130Z 07913ZZ 079230Z 07923ZZ 079330Z 07933ZZ 079430Z 07943ZZ 079530Z 07953ZZ 079630Z 07963ZZ 079730Z 07973ZZ 079830Z 07983ZZ 079930Z 07993ZZ 079B30Z 079B3ZZ 079C30Z 079C3ZZ 079D30Z 079D3ZZ 079F30Z 079F3ZZ 079G30Z 079G3ZZ 079H30Z 079H3ZZ 079J30Z 079J3ZZ 079K30Z 079K3ZZ 079L30Z 079L3ZZ 079M30Z 079M3ZZ 079P30Z 079P3ZX 079P3ZZ 079P40Z 079P4ZX 079P4ZZ 079T00Z 079T0ZX 079T0ZZ 079T30Z 079T3ZX 079T3ZZ 079T40Z 079T4ZX 079T4ZZ

LC Limited Coverage NC Noncovered HAC HAC Associated Procedure CC Combination Cluster - See Appendix G for code lists
DRG Non-OR-Affecting MS-DRG Assignment ⊘ Non-OR-Not Affecting MS-DRG Assignment New/Revised Text in **Orange** ♂ Male ♀ Female

0 Medical and Surgical
7 Lymphatic and Hemic Systems
B Excision: Cutting out or off, without replacement, a portion of a body part

Body Part Character 4	Approach Character 5	Device Character 6	Qualifier Character 7
0 Lymphatic, Head **1** Lymphatic, Right Neck **2** Lymphatic, Left Neck **3** Lymphatic, Right Upper Extremity **4** Lymphatic, Left Upper Extremity **5** Lymphatic, Right Axillary **6** Lymphatic, Left Axillary **7** Lymphatic, Thorax **8** Lymphatic, Internal Mammary, Right **9** Lymphatic, Internal Mammary, Left **B** Lymphatic, Mesenteric **C** Lymphatic, Pelvis **D** Lymphatic, Aortic **F** Lymphatic, Right Lower Extremity **G** Lymphatic, Left Lower Extremity **H** Lymphatic, Right Inguinal CC **J** Lymphatic, Left Inguinal CC **K** Thoracic Duct **L** Cisterna Chyli **M** Thymus **P** Spleen ⦸	**0** Open **3** Percutaneous **4** Percutaneous Endoscopic	**Z** No Device	**X** Diagnostic **Z** No Qualifier

⦸ 07BP3ZX 07BP4ZX
CC 07BH0ZZ 07BH4ZZ 07BJ0ZZ 07BJ4ZZ

0 Medical and Surgical
7 Lymphatic and Hemic Systems
C Extirpation: Taking or cutting out solid matter from a body part

Body Part Character 4	Approach Character 5	Device Character 6	Qualifier Character 7
0 Lymphatic, Head **1** Lymphatic, Right Neck **2** Lymphatic, Left Neck **3** Lymphatic, Right Upper Extremity **4** Lymphatic, Left Upper Extremity **5** Lymphatic, Right Axillary **6** Lymphatic, Left Axillary **7** Lymphatic, Thorax **8** Lymphatic, Internal Mammary, Right **9** Lymphatic, Internal Mammary, Left **B** Lymphatic, Mesenteric **C** Lymphatic, Pelvis **D** Lymphatic, Aortic **F** Lymphatic, Right Lower Extremity **G** Lymphatic, Left Lower Extremity **H** Lymphatic, Right Inguinal **J** Lymphatic, Left Inguinal **K** Thoracic Duct **L** Cisterna Chyli **M** Thymus **P** Spleen ⃠	**0** Open **3** Percutaneous **4** Percutaneous Endoscopic	**Z** No Device	**Z** No Qualifier

⃠ 07CP3ZZ 07CP4ZZ

0 Medical and Surgical
7 Lymphatic and Hemic Systems
D Extraction: Pulling or stripping out or off all or a portion of a body part by the use of force

Body Part Character 4	Approach Character 5	Device Character 6	Qualifier Character 7
Q Bone Marrow, Sternum ⃠ **R** Bone Marrow, Iliac ⃠ **S** Bone Marrow, Vertebral ⃠	**0** Open **3** Percutaneous	**Z** No Device	**X** Diagnostic **Z** No Qualifier

⃠ 07DQ0ZX 07DQ0ZZ 07DQ3ZX 07DQ3ZZ 07DR0ZX 07DR0ZZ 07DR3ZX 07DR3ZZ 07DS0ZX 07DS0ZZ 07DS3ZX 07DS3ZZ

0 Medical and Surgical
7 Lymphatic and Hemic Systems
H Insertion: Putting in a nonbiological appliance that monitors, assists, performs, or prevents a physiological function but does not physically take the place of a body part

Body Part Character 4	Approach Character 5	Device Character 6	Qualifier Character 7
K Thoracic Duct ⃠ **L** Cisterna Chyli ⃠ **M** Thymus ⃠ **N** Lymphatic ⃠ **P** Spleen ⃠	**0** Open **3** Percutaneous **4** Percutaneous Endoscopic	**3** Infusion Device	**Z** No Qualifier

⃠ 07HK03Z 07HK33Z 07HK43Z 07HL03Z 07HL33Z 07HL43Z 07HM03Z 07HM33Z 07HM43Z 07HN03Z 07HN33Z 07HN43Z 07HP03Z 07HP33Z 07HP43Z

0 Medical and Surgical
7 Lymphatic and Hemic Systems
J Inspection: Visually and/or manually exploring a body part

Body Part Character 4	Approach Character 5	Device Character 6	Qualifier Character 7
K Thoracic Duct ⃠ **L** Cisterna Chyli ⃠ **M** Thymus ⃠ **T** Bone Marrow ⃠	**0** Open **3** Percutaneous **4** Percutaneous Endoscopic	**Z** No Device	**Z** No Qualifier
N Lymphatic ⃠ **P** Spleen ⃠	**0** Open **3** Percutaneous **4** Percutaneous Endoscopic **X** External	**Z** No Device	**Z** No Qualifier

⃠ 07JK3ZZ 07JL3ZZ 07JM3ZZ 07JN3ZZ 07JNXZZ 07JP3ZZ 07JP4ZZ 07JPXZZ 07JT0ZZ 07JT3ZZ 07JT4ZZ

0 Medical and Surgical
7 Lymphatic and Hemic Systems
L Occlusion: Completely closing an orifice or the lumen of a tubular body part

Body Part Character 4	Approach Character 5	Device Character 6	Qualifier Character 7
0 Lymphatic, Head **1** Lymphatic, Right Neck **2** Lymphatic, Left Neck **3** Lymphatic, Right Upper Extremity **4** Lymphatic, Left Upper Extremity **5** Lymphatic, Right Axillary **6** Lymphatic, Left Axillary **7** Lymphatic, Thorax **8** Lymphatic, Internal Mammary, Right **9** Lymphatic, Internal Mammary, Left **B** Lymphatic, Mesenteric **C** Lymphatic, Pelvis **D** Lymphatic, Aortic **F** Lymphatic, Right Lower Extremity **G** Lymphatic, Left Lower Extremity **H** Lymphatic, Right Inguinal **J** Lymphatic, Left Inguinal **K** Thoracic Duct **L** Cisterna Chyli	**0** Open **3** Percutaneous **4** Percutaneous Endoscopic	**C** Extraluminal Device **D** Intraluminal Device **Z** No Device	**Z** No Qualifier

0 Medical and Surgical
7 Lymphatic and Hemic Systems
N Release: Freeing a body part from an abnormal physical constraint by cutting or by the use of force

Body Part Character 4	Approach Character 5	Device Character 6	Qualifier Character 7
0 Lymphatic, Head **1** Lymphatic, Right Neck **2** Lymphatic, Left Neck **3** Lymphatic, Right Upper Extremity **4** Lymphatic, Left Upper Extremity **5** Lymphatic, Right Axillary **6** Lymphatic, Left Axillary **7** Lymphatic, Thorax **8** Lymphatic, Internal Mammary, Right **9** Lymphatic, Internal Mammary, Left **B** Lymphatic, Mesenteric **C** Lymphatic, Pelvis **D** Lymphatic, Aortic **F** Lymphatic, Right Lower Extremity **G** Lymphatic, Left Lower Extremity **H** Lymphatic, Right Inguinal **J** Lymphatic, Left Inguinal **K** Thoracic Duct **L** Cisterna Chyli **M** Thymus **P** Spleen	**0** Open **3** Percutaneous **4** Percutaneous Endoscopic	**Z** No Device	**Z** No Qualifier

0 Medical and Surgical
7 Lymphatic and Hemic Systems
P Removal: Taking out or off a device from a body part

Body Part Character 4	Approach Character 5	Device Character 6	Qualifier Character 7
K Thoracic Duct **L** Cisterna Chyli **N** Lymphatic	**0** Open **3** Percutaneous **4** Percutaneous Endoscopic	**0** Drainage Device **3** Infusion Device **7** Autologous Tissue Substitute **C** Extraluminal Device **D** Intraluminal Device **J** Synthetic Substitute **K** Nonautologous Tissue Substitute	**Z** No Qualifier
K Thoracic Duct ⦸ **L** Cisterna Chyli ⦸ **N** Lymphatic ⦸	**X** External	**0** Drainage Device **3** Infusion Device **D** Intraluminal Device	**Z** No Qualifier
M Thymus ⦸ **P** Spleen ⦸	**0** Open **3** Percutaneous **4** Percutaneous Endoscopic **X** External	**0** Drainage Device **3** Infusion Device	**Z** No Qualifier
T Bone Marrow ⦸	**0** Open **3** Percutaneous **4** Percutaneous Endoscopic **X** External	**0** Drainage Device	**Z** No Qualifier

⦸ 07PKX0Z 07PKX3Z 07PKXDZ 07PLX0Z 07PLX3Z 07PLXDZ 07PMX0Z 07PMX3Z 07PNX0Z 07PNX3Z 07PNXDZ 07PPX0Z 07PPX3Z 07PT00Z 07PT30Z 07PT40Z 07PTX0Z

0 Medical and Surgical
7 Lymphatic and Hemic Systems
Q Repair: Restoring, to the extent possible, a body part to its normal anatomic structure and function

Body Part Character 4	Approach Character 5	Device Character 6	Qualifier Character 7
0 Lymphatic, Head **1** Lymphatic, Right Neck **2** Lymphatic, Left Neck **3** Lymphatic, Right Upper Extremity **4** Lymphatic, Left Upper Extremity **5** Lymphatic, Right Axillary **6** Lymphatic, Left Axillary **7** Lymphatic, Thorax **8** Lymphatic, Internal Mammary, Right **9** Lymphatic, Internal Mammary, Left **B** Lymphatic, Mesenteric **C** Lymphatic, Pelvis **D** Lymphatic, Aortic **F** Lymphatic, Right Lower Extremity **G** Lymphatic, Left Lower Extremity **H** Lymphatic, Right Inguinal **J** Lymphatic, Left Inguinal **K** Thoracic Duct **L** Cisterna Chyli **M** Thymus **P** Spleen	**0** Open **3** Percutaneous **4** Percutaneous Endoscopic	**Z** No Device	**Z** No Qualifier

0 Medical and Surgical
7 Lymphatic and Hemic Systems
S Reposition: Moving to its normal location, or other suitable location, all or a portion of a body part

Body Part Character 4	Approach Character 5	Device Character 6	Qualifier Character 7
M Thymus **P** Spleen	**0** Open	**Z** No Device	**Z** No Qualifier

0 Medical and Surgical
7 Lymphatic and Hemic Systems
T Resection: Cutting out or off, without replacement, all of a body part

Body Part Character 4	Approach Character 5	Device Character 6	Qualifier Character 7
0 Lymphatic, Head **1** Lymphatic, Right Neck **2** Lymphatic, Left Neck **3** Lymphatic, Right Upper Extremity **4** Lymphatic, Left Upper Extremity **5** Lymphatic, Right Axillary CC **6** Lymphatic, Left Axillary CC **7** Lymphatic, Thorax CC **8** Lymphatic, Internal Mammary, Right CC **9** Lymphatic, Internal Mammary, Left CC **B** Lymphatic, Mesenteric **C** Lymphatic, Pelvis **D** Lymphatic, Aortic **F** Lymphatic, Right Lower Extremity **G** Lymphatic, Left Lower Extremity **H** Lymphatic, Right Inguinal **J** Lymphatic, Left Inguinal **K** Thoracic Duct **L** Cisterna Chyli **M** Thymus **P** Spleen	**0** Open **4** Percutaneous Endoscopic	**Z** No Device	**Z** No Qualifier

CC 07T50ZZ 07T60ZZ 07T70ZZ 07T80ZZ 07T90ZZ

0 Medical and Surgical
7 Lymphatic and Hemic Systems
U Supplement: Putting in or on biological or synthetic material that physically reinforces and/or augments the function of a portion of a body part

Body Part Character 4	Approach Character 5	Device Character 6	Qualifier Character 7
0 Lymphatic, Head **1** Lymphatic, Right Neck **2** Lymphatic, Left Neck **3** Lymphatic, Right Upper Extremity **4** Lymphatic, Left Upper Extremity **5** Lymphatic, Right Axillary **6** Lymphatic, Left Axillary **7** Lymphatic, Thorax **8** Lymphatic, Internal Mammary, Right **9** Lymphatic, Internal Mammary, Left **B** Lymphatic, Mesenteric **C** Lymphatic, Pelvis **D** Lymphatic, Aortic **F** Lymphatic, Right Lower Extremity **G** Lymphatic, Left Lower Extremity **H** Lymphatic, Right Inguinal **J** Lymphatic, Left Inguinal **K** Thoracic Duct **L** Cisterna Chyli	**0** Open **4** Percutaneous Endoscopic	**7** Autologous Tissue Substitute **J** Synthetic Substitute **K** Nonautologous Tissue Substitute	**Z** No Qualifier

0 Medical and Surgical
7 Lymphatic and Hemic Systems
V Restriction: Partially closing an orifice or the lumen of a tubular body part

Body Part Character 4	Approach Character 5	Device Character 6	Qualifier Character 7
0 Lymphatic, Head **1** Lymphatic, Right Neck **2** Lymphatic, Left Neck **3** Lymphatic, Right Upper Extremity **4** Lymphatic, Left Upper Extremity **5** Lymphatic, Right Axillary **6** Lymphatic, Left Axillary **7** Lymphatic, Thorax **8** Lymphatic, Internal Mammary, Right **9** Lymphatic, Internal Mammary, Left **B** Lymphatic, Mesenteric **C** Lymphatic, Pelvis **D** Lymphatic, Aortic **F** Lymphatic, Right Lower Extremity **G** Lymphatic, Left Lower Extremity **H** Lymphatic, Right Inguinal **J** Lymphatic, Left Inguinal **K** Thoracic Duct **L** Cisterna Chyli	**0** Open **3** Percutaneous **4** Percutaneous Endoscopic	**C** Extraluminal Device **D** Intraluminal Device **Z** No Device	**Z** No Qualifier

0 Medical and Surgical
7 Lymphatic and Hemic Systems
W Revision: Correcting, to the extent possible, a portion of a malfunctioning device or the position of a displaced device

Body Part Character 4	Approach Character 5	Device Character 6	Qualifier Character 7
K Thoracic Duct ⃠ L Cisterna Chyli ⃠ N Lymphatic ⃠	0 Open 3 Percutaneous 4 Percutaneous Endoscopic X External	0 Drainage Device 3 Infusion Device 7 Autologous Tissue Substitute C Extraluminal Device D Intraluminal Device J Synthetic Substitute K Nonautologous Tissue Substitute	Z No Qualifier
M Thymus ⃠ P Spleen ⃠	0 Open 3 Percutaneous 4 Percutaneous Endoscopic X External	0 Drainage Device 3 Infusion Device	Z No Qualifier
T Bone Marrow ⃠	0 Open 3 Percutaneous 4 Percutaneous Endoscopic X External	0 Drainage Device	Z No Qualifier

⃠ 07WKX0Z 07WKX3Z 07WKX7Z 07WKXCZ 07WKXDZ 07WKXJZ 07WKXKZ 07WLX0Z 07WLX3Z 07WLX7Z 07WLXCZ 07WLXDZ 07WLXJZ 07WLXKZ 07WMX0Z 07WMX3Z 07WNX0Z 07WNX3Z 07WNX7Z 07WNXCZ 07WNXDZ 07WNXJZ 07WNXKZ 07WPX0Z 07WPX3Z 07WT00Z 07WT30Z 07WT40Z 07WTX0Z

0 Medical and Surgical
7 Lymphatic and Hemic Systems
Y Transplantation: Putting in or on all or a portion of a living body part taken from another individual or animal to physically take the place and/or function of all or a portion of a similar body part

Body Part Character 4	Approach Character 5	Device Character 6	Qualifier Character 7
M Thymus P Spleen	0 Open	Z No Device	0 Allogeneic 1 Syngeneic 2 Zooplastic

Eye 080-08X

0 Medical and Surgical
8 Eye
0 Alteration: Modifying the anatomic structure of a body part without affecting the function of the body part

Body Part Character 4	Approach Character 5	Device Character 6	Qualifier Character 7
N Upper Eyelid, Right ⦸ **P** Upper Eyelid, Left ⦸ **Q** Lower Eyelid, Right ⦸ **R** Lower Eyelid, Left ⦸	**0** Open **3** Percutaneous **X** External	**7** Autologous Tissue Substitute **J** Synthetic Substitute **K** Nonautologous Tissue Substitute **Z** No Device	**Z** No Qualifier

⦸ 080N07Z 080N0JZ 080N0KZ 080N0ZZ 080N37Z 080N3JZ 080N3KZ 080N3ZZ 080NX7Z 080NXJZ 080NXKZ 080NXZZ 080P07Z 080P0JZ 080P0KZ 080P0ZZ 080P37Z 080P3JZ 080P3KZ 080P3ZZ 080PX7Z 080PXJZ 080PXKZ 080PXZZ 080Q07Z 080Q0JZ 080Q0KZ 080Q0ZZ 080Q37Z 080Q3JZ 080Q3KZ 080Q3ZZ 080QX7Z 080QXJZ 080QXKZ 080QXZZ 080R07Z 080R0JZ 080R0KZ 080R0ZZ 080R37Z 080R3JZ 080R3KZ 080R3ZZ 080RX7Z 080RXJZ 080RXKZ 080RXZZ

0 Medical and Surgical
8 Eye
1 Bypass: Altering the route of passage of the contents of a tubular body part

Body Part Character 4	Approach Character 5	Device Character 6	Qualifier Character 7
2 Anterior Chamber, Right **3** Anterior Chamber, Left	**3** Percutaneous	**J** Synthetic Substitute **K** Nonautologous Tissue Substitute **Z** No Device	**4** Sclera
X Lacrimal Duct, Right **Y** Lacrimal Duct, Left	**0** Open **3** Percutaneous	**J** Synthetic Substitute **K** Nonautologous Tissue Substitute **Z** No Device	**3** Nasal Cavity

0 Medical and Surgical
8 Eye
2 Change: Taking out or off a device from a body part and putting back an identical or similar device in or on the same body part without cutting or puncturing the skin or a mucous membrane

Body Part Character 4	Approach Character 5	Device Character 6	Qualifier Character 7
0 Eye, Right ⦸ **1** Eye, Left ⦸	**X** External	**0** Drainage Device **Y** Other Device	**Z** No Qualifier

⦸ 0820X0Z 0820XYZ 0821X0Z 0821XYZ

0 Medical and Surgical
8 Eye
5 Destruction: Physical eradication of all or a portion of a body part by the direct use of energy, force, or a destructive agent

Body Part Character 4	Approach Character 5	Device Character 6	Qualifier Character 7
0 Eye, Right **1** Eye, Left **6** Sclera, Right **7** Sclera, Left **8** Cornea, Right **9** Cornea, Left **S** Conjunctiva, Right **T** Conjunctiva, Left	**X** External	**Z** No Device	**Z** No Qualifier
2 Anterior Chamber, Right **3** Anterior Chamber, Left **4** Vitreous, Right **5** Vitreous, Left **C** Iris, Right **D** Iris, Left **E** Retina, Right **F** Retina, Left **G** Retinal Vessel, Right **H** Retinal Vessel, Left **J** Lens, Right **K** Lens, Left	**3** Percutaneous	**Z** No Device	**Z** No Qualifier
A Choroid, Right **B** Choroid, Left **L** Extraocular Muscle, Right **M** Extraocular Muscle, Left **V** Lacrimal Gland, Right **W** Lacrimal Gland, Left	**0** Open **3** Percutaneous	**Z** No Device	**Z** No Qualifier
N Upper Eyelid, Right **P** Upper Eyelid, Left **Q** Lower Eyelid, Right **R** Lower Eyelid, Left	**0** Open **3** Percutaneous **X** External	**Z** No Device	**Z** No Qualifier
X Lacrimal Duct, Right **Y** Lacrimal Duct, Left	**0** Open **3** Percutaneous **7** Via Natural or Artificial Opening **8** Via Natural or Artificial Opening Endoscopic	**Z** No Device	**Z** No Qualifier

0 Medical and Surgical
8 Eye
7 Dilation: Expanding an orifice or the lumen of a tubular body part

Body Part Character 4	Approach Character 5	Device Character 6	Qualifier Character 7
X Lacrimal Duct, Right **Y** Lacrimal Duct, Left	**0** Open **3** Percutaneous **7** Via Natural or Artificial Opening **8** Via Natural or Artificial Opening Endoscopic	**D** Intraluminal Device **Z** No Device	**Z** No Qualifier

0 Medical and Surgical
8 Eye
9 Drainage: Taking or letting out fluids and/or gases from a body part

Body Part Character 4	Approach Character 5	Device Character 6	Qualifier Character 7
0 Eye, Right **1** Eye, Left **6** Sclera, Right **7** Sclera, Left **8** Cornea, Right **9** Cornea, Left **S** Conjunctiva, Right **T** Conjunctiva, Left	**X** External	**0** Drainage Device	**Z** No Qualifier
0 Eye, Right **1** Eye, Left **6** Sclera, Right **7** Sclera, Left **8** Cornea, Right **9** Cornea, Left **S** Conjunctiva, Right **T** Conjunctiva, Left	**X** External	**Z** No Device	**X** Diagnostic **Z** No Qualifier
2 Anterior Chamber, Right **3** Anterior Chamber, Left **4** Vitreous, Right **5** Vitreous, Left **C** Iris, Right **D** Iris, Left **E** Retina, Right **F** Retina, Left **G** Retinal Vessel, Right **H** Retinal Vessel, Left **J** Lens, Right **K** Lens, Left	**3** Percutaneous	**0** Drainage Device	**Z** No Qualifier
2 Anterior Chamber, Right **3** Anterior Chamber, Left **4** Vitreous, Right **5** Vitreous, Left **C** Iris, Right **D** Iris, Left **E** Retina, Right **F** Retina, Left **G** Retinal Vessel, Right **H** Retinal Vessel, Left **J** Lens, Right **K** Lens, Left	**3** Percutaneous	**Z** No Device	**X** Diagnostic **Z** No Qualifier
A Choroid, Right **B** Choroid, Left **L** Extraocular Muscle, Right **M** Extraocular Muscle, Left **V** Lacrimal Gland, Right **W** Lacrimal Gland, Left	**0** Open **3** Percutaneous	**0** Drainage Device	**Z** No Qualifier
A Choroid, Right **B** Choroid, Left **L** Extraocular Muscle, Right **M** Extraocular Muscle, Left **V** Lacrimal Gland, Right **W** Lacrimal Gland, Left	**0** Open **3** Percutaneous	**Z** No Device	**X** Diagnostic **Z** No Qualifier
N Upper Eyelid, Right ⃠ **P** Upper Eyelid, Left ⃠ **Q** Lower Eyelid, Right ⃠ **R** Lower Eyelid, Left ⃠	**0** Open **3** Percutaneous **X** External	**0** Drainage Device	**Z** No Qualifier

089 continued on next page

0 Medical and Surgical
8 Eye
9 Drainage: Taking or letting out fluids and/or gases from a body part

089 continued from previous page

Body Part Character 4	Approach Character 5	Device Character 6	Qualifier Character 7
N Upper Eyelid, Right ⦸ **P** Upper Eyelid, Left ⦸ **Q** Lower Eyelid, Right ⦸ **R** Lower Eyelid, Left ⦸	**0** Open **3** Percutaneous **X** External	**Z** No Device	**X** Diagnostic **Z** No Qualifier
X Lacrimal Duct, Right **Y** Lacrimal Duct, Left	**0** Open **3** Percutaneous **7** Via Natural or Artificial Opening **8** Via Natural or Artificial Opening Endoscopic	**0** Drainage Device	**Z** No Qualifier
X Lacrimal Duct, Right **Y** Lacrimal Duct, Left	**0** Open **3** Percutaneous **7** Via Natural or Artificial Opening **8** Via Natural or Artificial Opening Endoscopic	**Z** No Device	**X** Diagnostic **Z** No Qualifier

⦸ 089N00Z 089N0ZZ 089N30Z 089N3ZZ 089NX0Z 089NXZZ 089P00Z 089P0ZZ 089P30Z 089P3ZZ 089PX0Z 089PXZZ 089Q00Z 089Q0ZZ 089Q30Z 089Q3ZZ 089QX0Z 089QXZZ 089R00Z 089R0ZZ 089R30Z 089R3ZZ 089RX0Z 089RXZZ

0 Medical and Surgical
8 Eye
B Excision: Cutting out or off, without replacement, a portion of a body part

Body Part Character 4	Approach Character 5	Device Character 6	Qualifier Character 7
0 Eye, Right **1** Eye, Left **N** Upper Eyelid, Right **P** Upper Eyelid, Left **Q** Lower Eyelid, Right **R** Lower Eyelid, Left	**0** Open **3** Percutaneous **X** External	**Z** No Device	**X** Diagnostic **Z** No Qualifier
4 Vitreous, Right **5** Vitreous, Left **C** Iris, Right CC **D** Iris, Left CC **E** Retina, Right **F** Retina, Left **J** Lens, Right **K** Lens, Left	**3** Percutaneous	**Z** No Device	**X** Diagnostic **Z** No Qualifier
6 Sclera, Right CC **7** Sclera, Left CC **8** Cornea, Right **9** Cornea, Left **S** Conjunctiva, Right **T** Conjunctiva, Left	**X** External	**Z** No Device	**X** Diagnostic **Z** No Qualifier
A Choroid, Right **B** Choroid, Left **L** Extraocular Muscle, Right **M** Extraocular Muscle, Left **V** Lacrimal Gland, Right **W** Lacrimal Gland, Left	**0** Open **3** Percutaneous	**Z** No Device	**X** Diagnostic **Z** No Qualifier
X Lacrimal Duct, Right **Y** Lacrimal Duct, Left	**0** Open **3** Percutaneous **7** Via Natural or Artificial Opening **8** Via Natural or Artificial Opening Endoscopic	**Z** No Device	**X** Diagnostic **Z** No Qualifier

CC 08B6XZZ 08B7XZZ 08BC3ZZ 08BD3ZZ

0 Medical and Surgical
8 Eye
C Extirpation: Taking or cutting out solid matter from a body part

Body Part Character 4	Approach Character 5	Device Character 6	Qualifier Character 7
0 Eye, Right **1** Eye, Left **6** Sclera, Right ⦸ **7** Sclera, Left ⦸ **8** Cornea, Right **9** Cornea, Left **S** Conjunctiva, Right **T** Conjunctiva, Left	**X** External	**Z** No Device	**Z** No Qualifier
2 Anterior Chamber, Right ⦸ **3** Anterior Chamber, Left ⦸ **4** Vitreous, Right **5** Vitreous, Left **C** Iris, Right **D** Iris, Left **E** Retina, Right **F** Retina, Left **G** Retinal Vessel, Right **H** Retinal Vessel, Left **J** Lens, Right **K** Lens, Left	**3** Percutaneous **X** External	**Z** No Device	**Z** No Qualifier
A Choroid, Right **B** Choroid, Left **L** Extraocular Muscle, Right **M** Extraocular Muscle, Left **N** Upper Eyelid, Right ⦸ **P** Upper Eyelid, Left ⦸ **Q** Lower Eyelid, Right ⦸ **R** Lower Eyelid, Left ⦸ **V** Lacrimal Gland, Right **W** Lacrimal Gland, Left	**0** Open **3** Percutaneous **X** External	**Z** No Device	**Z** No Qualifier
X Lacrimal Duct, Right **Y** Lacrimal Duct, Left	**0** Open **3** Percutaneous **7** Via Natural or Artificial Opening **8** Via Natural or Artificial Opening Endoscopic	**Z** No Device	**Z** No Qualifier

⦸ 08C2XZZ 08C3XZZ 08C6XZZ 08C7XZZ 08CN0ZZ 08CN3ZZ 08CNXZZ 08CP0ZZ 08CP3ZZ 08CPXZZ 08CQ0ZZ 08CQ3ZZ 08CQXZZ 08CR0ZZ 08CR3ZZ 08CRXZZ

0 Medical and Surgical
8 Eye
D Extraction: Pulling or stripping out or off all or a portion of a body part by the use of force

Body Part Character 4	Approach Character 5	Device Character 6	Qualifier Character 7
8 Cornea, Right **9** Cornea, Left	**X** External	**Z** No Device	**X** Diagnostic **Z** No Qualifier
J Lens, Right **K** Lens, Left	**3** Percutaneous	**Z** No Device	**Z** No Qualifier

0 Medical and Surgical
8 Eye
F Fragmentation: Breaking solid matter in a body part into pieces

Body Part Character 4	Approach Character 5	Device Character 6	Qualifier Character 7
4 Vitreous, Right NC ⦸ **5** Vitreous, Left NC ⦸	**3** Percutaneous **X** External	**Z** No Device	**Z** No Qualifier

⦸ 08F4XZZ 08F5XZZ
NC 08F4XZZ 08F5XZZ

0 Medical and Surgical
8 Eye
H Insertion: Putting in a nonbiological appliance that monitors, assists, performs, or prevents a physiological function but does not physically take the place of a body part

Body Part Character 4	Approach Character 5	Device Character 6	Qualifier Character 7
0 Eye, Right **1** Eye, Left	**0** Open	**5** Epiretinal Visual Prosthesis	**Z** No Qualifier
0 Eye, Right **1** Eye, Left	**3** Percutaneous **X** External	**1** Radioactive Element **3** Infusion Device	**Z** No Qualifier

0 Medical and Surgical
8 Eye
J Inspection: Visually and/or manually exploring a body part

Body Part Character 4	Approach Character 5	Device Character 6	Qualifier Character 7
0 Eye, Right ⦸ **1** Eye, Left ⦸ **J** Lens, Right ⦸ **K** Lens, Left ⦸	**X** External	**Z** No Device	**Z** No Qualifier
L Extraocular Muscle, Right ⦸ **M** Extraocular Muscle, Left ⦸	**0** Open **X** External	**Z** No Device	**Z** No Qualifier

⦸ 08J0XZZ 08J1XZZ 08JJXZZ 08JKXZZ 08JLXZZ 08JMXZZ

0 Medical and Surgical
8 Eye
L Occlusion: Completely closing an orifice or the lumen of a tubular body part

Body Part Character 4	Approach Character 5	Device Character 6	Qualifier Character 7
X Lacrimal Duct, Right **Y** Lacrimal Duct, Left	**0** Open **3** Percutaneous	**C** Extraluminal Device **D** Intraluminal Device **Z** No Device	**Z** No Qualifier
X Lacrimal Duct, Right **Y** Lacrimal Duct, Left	**7** Via Natural or Artificial Opening **8** Via Natural or Artificial Opening Endoscopic	**D** Intraluminal Device **Z** No Device	**Z** No Qualifier

0 Medical and Surgical
8 Eye
M Reattachment: Putting back in or on all or a portion of a separated body part to its normal location or other suitable location

Body Part Character 4	Approach Character 5	Device Character 6	Qualifier Character 7
N Upper Eyelid, Right **P** Upper Eyelid, Left **Q** Lower Eyelid, Right **R** Lower Eyelid, Left	**X** External	**Z** No Device	**Z** No Qualifier

0 Medical and Surgical
8 Eye
N Release: Freeing a body part from an abnormal physical constraint by cutting or by the use of force

Body Part Character 4	Approach Character 5	Device Character 6	Qualifier Character 7
0 Eye, Right **1** Eye, Left **6** Sclera, Right **7** Sclera, Left **8** Cornea, Right **9** Cornea, Left **S** Conjunctiva, Right **T** Conjunctiva, Left	**X** External	**Z** No Device	**Z** No Qualifier
2 Anterior Chamber, Right **3** Anterior Chamber, Left **4** Vitreous, Right **5** Vitreous, Left **C** Iris, Right **D** Iris, Left **E** Retina, Right **F** Retina, Left **G** Retinal Vessel, Right **H** Retinal Vessel, Left **J** Lens, Right **K** Lens, Left	**3** Percutaneous	**Z** No Device	**Z** No Qualifier
A Choroid, Right **B** Choroid, Left **L** Extraocular Muscle, Right **M** Extraocular Muscle, Left **V** Lacrimal Gland, Right **W** Lacrimal Gland, Left	**0** Open **3** Percutaneous	**Z** No Device	**Z** No Qualifier
N Upper Eyelid, Right **P** Upper Eyelid, Left **Q** Lower Eyelid, Right **R** Lower Eyelid, Left	**0** Open **3** Percutaneous **X** External	**Z** No Device	**Z** No Qualifier
X Lacrimal Duct, Right **Y** Lacrimal Duct, Left	**0** Open **3** Percutaneous **7** Via Natural or Artificial Opening **8** Via Natural or Artificial Opening Endoscopic	**Z** No Device	**Z** No Qualifier

0 Medical and Surgical
8 Eye
P Removal: Taking out or off a device from a body part

Body Part Character 4	Approach Character 5	Device Character 6	Qualifier Character 7
0 Eye, Right ⃠ **1** Eye, Left ⃠	**0** Open **3** Percutaneous **7** Via Natural or Artificial Opening **8** Via Natural or Artificial Opening Endoscopic **X** External	**0** Drainage Device **1** Radioactive Element **3** Infusion Device **7** Autologous Tissue Substitute **C** Extraluminal Device **D** Intraluminal Device **J** Synthetic Substitute **K** Nonautologous Tissue Substitute	**Z** No Qualifier
J Lens, Right **K** Lens, Left	**3** Percutaneous	**J** Synthetic Substitute	**Z** No Qualifier
L Extraocular Muscle, Right **M** Extraocular Muscle, Left	**0** Open **3** Percutaneous	**0** Drainage Device **7** Autologous Tissue Substitute **J** Synthetic Substitute **K** Nonautologous Tissue Substitute	**Z** No Qualifier

⃠ 08P070Z 08P073Z 08P07DZ 08P080Z 08P083Z 08P08DZ 08P0X0Z 08P0X3Z 08P0XCZ 08P0XDZ 08P170Z 08P173Z 08P17DZ 08P180Z 08P183Z 08P18DZ 08P1X0Z 08P1X1Z 08P1X3Z 08P1XCZ 08P1XDZ

LC Limited Coverage NC Noncovered HAC HAC Associated Procedure CC Combination Cluster - See Appendix G for code lists
DRG Non-OR-Affecting MS-DRG Assignment ⃠ Non-OR-Not Affecting MS-DRG Assignment New/Revised Text in **Orange** ♂ Male ♀ Female

0 Medical and Surgical
8 Eye
Q Repair: Restoring, to the extent possible, a body part to its normal anatomic structure and function

Body Part Character 4	Approach Character 5	Device Character 6	Qualifier Character 7
0 Eye, Right **1** Eye, Left **6** Sclera, Right **7** Sclera, Left **8** Cornea, Right NC **9** Cornea, Left NC **S** Conjunctiva, Right **T** Conjunctiva, Left	**X** External	**Z** No Device	**Z** No Qualifier
2 Anterior Chamber, Right **3** Anterior Chamber, Left **4** Vitreous, Right **5** Vitreous, Left **C** Iris, Right **D** Iris, Left **E** Retina, Right **F** Retina, Left **G** Retinal Vessel, Right **H** Retinal Vessel, Left **J** Lens, Right **K** Lens, Left	**3** Percutaneous	**Z** No Device	**Z** No Qualifier
A Choroid, Right **B** Choroid, Left **L** Extraocular Muscle, Right **M** Extraocular Muscle, Left **V** Lacrimal Gland, Right **W** Lacrimal Gland, Left	**0** Open **3** Percutaneous	**Z** No Device	**Z** No Qualifier
N Upper Eyelid, Right ⦸ **P** Upper Eyelid, Left ⦸ **Q** Lower Eyelid, Right ⦸ **R** Lower Eyelid, Left ⦸	**0** Open **3** Percutaneous **X** External	**Z** No Device	**Z** No Qualifier
X Lacrimal Duct, Right **Y** Lacrimal Duct, Left	**0** Open **3** Percutaneous **7** Via Natural or Artificial Opening **8** Via Natural or Artificial Opening Endoscopic	**Z** No Device	**Z** No Qualifier

⦸ 08QN0ZZ 08QN3ZZ 08QNXZZ 08QP0ZZ 08QP3ZZ 08QPXZZ 08QQ0ZZ 08QQ3ZZ 08QQXZZ 08QR0ZZ 08QR3ZZ 08QRXZZ
NC 08Q8XZZ 08Q9XZZ

0 Medical and Surgical
8 Eye
R Replacement: Putting in or on biological or synthetic material that physically takes the place and/or function of all or a portion of a body part

Body Part Character 4	Approach Character 5	Device Character 6	Qualifier Character 7
0 Eye, Right **1** Eye, Left **A** Choroid, Right **B** Choroid, Left	**0** Open **3** Percutaneous	**7** Autologous Tissue Substitute **J** Synthetic Substitute **K** Nonautologous Tissue Substitute	**Z** No Qualifier
4 Vitreous, Right **5** Vitreous, Left **C** Iris, Right **D** Iris, Left **G** Retinal Vessel, Right **H** Retinal Vessel, Left	**3** Percutaneous	**7** Autologous Tissue Substitute **J** Synthetic Substitute **K** Nonautologous Tissue Substitute	**Z** No Qualifier
6 Sclera, Right **7** Sclera, Left **S** Conjunctiva, Right **T** Conjunctiva, Left	**X** External	**7** Autologous Tissue Substitute **J** Synthetic Substitute **K** Nonautologous Tissue Substitute	**Z** No Qualifier
8 Cornea, Right **9** Cornea, Left	**3** Percutaneous **X** External	**7** Autologous Tissue Substitute **J** Synthetic Substitute **K** Nonautologous Tissue Substitute	**Z** No Qualifier
J Lens, Right **K** Lens, Left	**3** Percutaneous	**0** Synthetic Substitute, Intraocular Telescope **7** Autologous Tissue Substitute **J** Synthetic Substitute **K** Nonautologous Tissue Substitute	**Z** No Qualifier
N Upper Eyelid, Right **P** Upper Eyelid, Left **Q** Lower Eyelid, Right **R** Lower Eyelid, Left	**0** Open **3** Percutaneous **X** External	**7** Autologous Tissue Substitute **J** Synthetic Substitute **K** Nonautologous Tissue Substitute	**Z** No Qualifier
X Lacrimal Duct, Right **Y** Lacrimal Duct, Left	**0** Open **3** Percutaneous **7** Via Natural or Artificial Opening **8** Via Natural or Artificial Opening Endoscopic	**7** Autologous Tissue Substitute **J** Synthetic Substitute **K** Nonautologous Tissue Substitute	**Z** No Qualifier

0 Medical and Surgical
8 Eye
S Reposition: Moving to its normal location, or other suitable location, all or a portion of a body part

Body Part Character 4	Approach Character 5	Device Character 6	Qualifier Character 7
C Iris, Right **D** Iris, Left **G** Retinal Vessel, Right **H** Retinal Vessel, Left **J** Lens, Right **K** Lens, Left	**3** Percutaneous	**Z** No Device	**Z** No Qualifier
L Extraocular Muscle, Right **M** Extraocular Muscle, Left **V** Lacrimal Gland, Right **W** Lacrimal Gland, Left	**0** Open **3** Percutaneous	**Z** No Device	**Z** No Qualifier
N Upper Eyelid, Right CC **P** Upper Eyelid, Left CC **Q** Lower Eyelid, Right CC **R** Lower Eyelid, Left CC	**0** Open **3** Percutaneous **X** External	**Z** No Device	**Z** No Qualifier
X Lacrimal Duct, Right **Y** Lacrimal Duct, Left	**0** Open **3** Percutaneous **7** Via Natural or Artificial Opening **8** Via Natural or Artificial Opening Endoscopic	**Z** No Device	**Z** No Qualifier

CC 08SN0ZZ 08SN3ZZ 08SNXZZ 08SP0ZZ 08SP3ZZ 08SPXZZ 08SQ0ZZ 08SQ3ZZ 08SQXZZ 08SR0ZZ 08SR3ZZ 08SRXZZ

0 Medical and Surgical
8 Eye
T Resection: Cutting out or off, without replacement, all of a body part

Body Part Character 4	Approach Character 5	Device Character 6	Qualifier Character 7
0 Eye, Right CC **1** Eye, Left CC **8** Cornea, Right **9** Cornea, Left	**X** External	**Z** No Device	**Z** No Qualifier
4 Vitreous, Right **5** Vitreous, Left **C** Iris, Right **D** Iris, Left **J** Lens, Right **K** Lens, Left	**3** Percutaneous	**Z** No Device	**Z** No Qualifier
L Extraocular Muscle, Right **M** Extraocular Muscle, Left **V** Lacrimal Gland, Right **W** Lacrimal Gland, Left	**0** Open **3** Percutaneous	**Z** No Device	**Z** No Qualifier
N Upper Eyelid, Right **P** Upper Eyelid, Left **Q** Lower Eyelid, Right **R** Lower Eyelid, Left	**0** Open **X** External	**Z** No Device	**Z** No Qualifier
X Lacrimal Duct, Right **Y** Lacrimal Duct, Left	**0** Open **3** Percutaneous **7** Via Natural or Artificial Opening **8** Via Natural or Artificial Opening Endoscopic	**Z** No Device	**Z** No Qualifier

CC 08T0XZZ 08T1XZZ

0 Medical and Surgical
8 Eye
U Supplement: Putting in or on biological or synthetic material that physically reinforces and/or augments the function of a portion of a body part

Body Part Character 4	Approach Character 5	Device Character 6	Qualifier Character 7
0 Eye, Right **1** Eye, Left **C** Iris, Right **D** Iris, Left **E** Retina, Right **F** Retina, Left **G** Retinal Vessel, Right **H** Retinal Vessel, Left **L** Extraocular Muscle, Right **M** Extraocular Muscle, Left	**0** Open **3** Percutaneous	**7** Autologous Tissue Substitute **J** Synthetic Substitute **K** Nonautologous Tissue Substitute	**Z** No Qualifier
8 Cornea, Right NC **9** Cornea, Left NC **N** Upper Eyelid, Right **P** Upper Eyelid, Left **Q** Lower Eyelid, Right **R** Lower Eyelid, Left	**0** Open **3** Percutaneous **X** External	**7** Autologous Tissue Substitute **J** Synthetic Substitute **K** Nonautologous Tissue Substitute	**Z** No Qualifier
X Lacrimal Duct, Right **Y** Lacrimal Duct, Left	**0** Open **3** Percutaneous **7** Via Natural or Artificial Opening **8** Via Natural or Artificial Opening Endoscopic	**7** Autologous Tissue Substitute **J** Synthetic Substitute **K** Nonautologous Tissue Substitute	**Z** No Qualifier

NC 08U80KZ 08U83KZ 08U8XKZ 08U90KZ 08U93KZ 08U9XKZ

0 Medical and Surgical
8 Eye
V Restriction: Partially closing an orifice or the lumen of a tubular body part

Body Part Character 4	Approach Character 5	Device Character 6	Qualifier Character 7
X Lacrimal Duct, Right **Y** Lacrimal Duct, Left	**0** Open **3** Percutaneous	**C** Extraluminal Device **D** Intraluminal Device **Z** No Device	**Z** No Qualifier
X Lacrimal Duct, Right **Y** Lacrimal Duct, Left	**7** Via Natural or Artificial Opening **8** Via Natural or Artificial Opening Endoscopic	**D** Intraluminal Device **Z** No Device	**Z** No Qualifier

0 Medical and Surgical
8 Eye
W Revision: Correcting, to the extent possible, a portion of a malfunctioning device or the position of a displaced device

Body Part Character 4	Approach Character 5	Device Character 6	Qualifier Character 7
0 Eye, Right ⊘ **1** Eye, Left ⊘	**0** Open **3** Percutaneous **7** Via Natural or Artificial Opening **8** Via Natural or Artificial Opening Endoscopic **X** External	**0** Drainage Device **3** Infusion Device **7** Autologous Tissue Substitute **C** Extraluminal Device **D** Intraluminal Device **J** Synthetic Substitute **K** Nonautologous Tissue Substitute	**Z** No Qualifier
J Lens, Right ⊘ **K** Lens, Left ⊘	**3** Percutaneous **X** External	**J** Synthetic Substitute	**Z** No Qualifier
L Extraocular Muscle, Right **M** Extraocular Muscle, Left	**0** Open **3** Percutaneous	**0** Drainage Device **7** Autologous Tissue Substitute **J** Synthetic Substitute **K** Nonautologous Tissue Substitute	**Z** No Qualifier

⊘ 08W0X0Z 08W0X3Z 08W0X7Z 08W0XCZ 08W0XDZ 08W0XJZ 08W0XKZ 08W1X0Z 08W1X3Z 08W1X7Z 08W1XCZ 08W1XDZ 08W1XJZ 08W1XKZ 08WJXJZ 08WKXJZ

LC Limited Coverage NC Noncovered HAC HAC Associated Procedure CC Combination Cluster - See Appendix G for code lists
DRG Non-OR-Affecting MS-DRG Assignment ⊘ Non-OR-Not Affecting MS-DRG Assignment New/Revised Text in **Orange** ♂ Male ♀ Female

0 Medical and Surgical
8 Eye
X Transfer: Moving, without taking out, all or a portion of a body part to another location to take over the function of all or a portion of a body part

Body Part Character 4	Approach Character 5	Device Character 6	Qualifier Character 7
L Extraocular Muscle, Right **M** Extraocular Muscle, Left	**0** Open **3** Percutaneous	**Z** No Device	**Z** No Qualifier

Ear, Nose, Sinus 090-09W

0 Medical and Surgical
9 Ear, Nose, Sinus
0 Alteration: Modifying the anatomic structure of a body part without affecting the function of the body part

Body Part Character 4	Approach Character 5	Device Character 6	Qualifier Character 7
0 External Ear, Right **1** External Ear, Left **2** External Ear, Bilateral **K** Nose	**0** Open **3** Percutaneous **4** Percutaneous Endoscopic **X** External	**7** Autologous Tissue Substitute **J** Synthetic Substitute **K** Nonautologous Tissue Substitute **Z** No Device	**Z** No Qualifier

0 Medical and Surgical
9 Ear, Nose, Sinus
1 Bypass: Altering the route of passage of the contents of a tubular body part

Body Part Character 4	Approach Character 5	Device Character 6	Qualifier Character 7
D Inner Ear, Right **E** Inner Ear, Left	**0** Open	**7** Autologous Tissue Substitute **J** Synthetic Substitute **K** Nonautologous Tissue Substitute **Z** No Device	**0** Endolymphatic

0 Medical and Surgical
9 Ear, Nose, Sinus
2 Change: Taking out or off a device from a body part and putting back an identical or similar device in or on the same body part without cutting or puncturing the skin or a mucous membrane

Body Part Character 4	Approach Character 5	Device Character 6	Qualifier Character 7
H Ear, Right ⊘ **J** Ear, Left ⊘ **K** Nose ⊘ **Y** Sinus ⊘	**X** External	**0** Drainage Device **Y** Other Device	**Z** No Qualifier

⊘ 092HX0Z 092HXYZ 092JX0Z 092JXYZ 092KX0Z 092KXYZ 092YX0Z 092YXYZ

0 Medical and Surgical
9 Ear, Nose, Sinus
5 Destruction: Physical eradication of all or a portion of a body part by the direct use of energy, force, or a destructive agent

Body Part Character 4	Approach Character 5	Device Character 6	Qualifier Character 7
0 External Ear, Right ⊘ **1** External Ear, Left ⊘ **K** Nose ⊘	**0** Open **3** Percutaneous **4** Percutaneous Endoscopic **X** External	**Z** No Device	**Z** No Qualifier
3 External Auditory Canal, Right ⊘ **4** External Auditory Canal, Left ⊘	**0** Open **3** Percutaneous **4** Percutaneous Endoscopic **7** Via Natural or Artificial Opening **8** Via Natural or Artificial Opening Endoscopic **X** External	**Z** No Device	**Z** No Qualifier
5 Middle Ear, Right **6** Middle Ear, Left **9** Auditory Ossicle, Right **A** Auditory Ossicle, Left **D** Inner Ear, Right **E** Inner Ear, Left	**0** Open	**Z** No Device	**Z** No Qualifier
7 Tympanic Membrane, Right **8** Tympanic Membrane, Left **F** Eustachian Tube, Right ⊘ **G** Eustachian Tube, Left ⊘ **L** Nasal Turbinate **N** Nasopharynx	**0** Open **3** Percutaneous **4** Percutaneous Endoscopic **7** Via Natural or Artificial Opening **8** Via Natural or Artificial Opening Endoscopic	**Z** No Device	**Z** No Qualifier
B Mastoid Sinus, Right **C** Mastoid Sinus, Left **M** Nasal Septum ⊘ **P** Accessory Sinus **Q** Maxillary Sinus, Right **R** Maxillary Sinus, Left **S** Frontal Sinus, Right **T** Frontal Sinus, Left **U** Ethmoid Sinus, Right **V** Ethmoid Sinus, Left **W** Sphenoid Sinus, Right **X** Sphenoid Sinus, Left	**0** Open **3** Percutaneous **4** Percutaneous Endoscopic	**Z** No Device	**Z** No Qualifier

⊘ 09500ZZ 09503ZZ 09504ZZ 0950XZZ 09510ZZ 09513ZZ 09514ZZ 0951XZZ 09530ZZ 09533ZZ 09534ZZ 09537ZZ 09538ZZ 0953XZZ 09540ZZ 09543ZZ 09544ZZ 09547ZZ 09548ZZ 0954XZZ 095F0ZZ 095F3ZZ 095F4ZZ 095F7ZZ 095F8ZZ 095G0ZZ 095G3ZZ 095G4ZZ 095G7ZZ 095G8ZZ 095K0ZZ 095K3ZZ 095K4ZZ 095KXZZ 095M0ZZ 095M3ZZ 095M4ZZ

0 Medical and Surgical
9 Ear, Nose, Sinus
7 Dilation: Expanding an orifice or the lumen of a tubular body part

Body Part Character 4	Approach Character 5	Device Character 6	Qualifier Character 7
F Eustachian Tube, Right ⊘ **G** Eustachian Tube, Left ⊘	**0** Open **7** Via Natural or Artificial Opening **8** Via Natural or Artificial Opening Endoscopic	**D** Intraluminal Device **Z** No Device	**Z** No Qualifier
F Eustachian Tube, Right ⊘ **G** Eustachian Tube, Left ⊘	**3** Percutaneous **4** Percutaneous Endoscopic	**Z** No Device	**Z** No Qualifier

⊘ 097F0DZ 097F0ZZ 097F3ZZ 097F4ZZ 097F7DZ 097F7ZZ 097F8DZ 097F8ZZ 097G0DZ 097G0ZZ 097G3ZZ 097G4ZZ 097G7DZ 097G7ZZ 097G8DZ 097G8ZZ

0 Medical and Surgical
9 Ear, Nose, Sinus
8 Division: Cutting into a body part, without draining fluids and/or gases from the body part, in order to separate or transect a body part

Body Part Character 4	Approach Character 5	Device Character 6	Qualifier Character 7
L Nasal Turbinate	0 Open 3 Percutaneous 4 Percutaneous Endoscopic 7 Via Natural or Artificial Opening 8 Via Natural or Artificial Opening Endoscopic	Z No Device	Z No Qualifier

0 Medical and Surgical
9 Ear, Nose, Sinus
9 Drainage: Taking or letting out fluids and/or gases from a body part

Body Part Character 4	Approach Character 5	Device Character 6	Qualifier Character 7
0 External Ear, Right ⊘ 1 External Ear, Left ⊘ K Nose ⊘	0 Open 3 Percutaneous 4 Percutaneous Endoscopic X External	0 Drainage Device	Z No Qualifier
0 External Ear, Right ⊘ 1 External Ear, Left ⊘ K Nose ⊘	0 Open 3 Percutaneous 4 Percutaneous Endoscopic X External	Z No Device	X Diagnostic Z No Qualifier
3 External Auditory Canal, Right ⊘ 4 External Auditory Canal, Left ⊘	0 Open 3 Percutaneous 4 Percutaneous Endoscopic 7 Via Natural or Artificial Opening 8 Via Natural or Artificial Opening Endoscopic X External	0 Drainage Device	Z No Qualifier
3 External Auditory Canal, Right ⊘ 4 External Auditory Canal, Left ⊘	0 Open 3 Percutaneous 4 Percutaneous Endoscopic 7 Via Natural or Artificial Opening 8 Via Natural or Artificial Opening Endoscopic X External	Z No Device	X Diagnostic Z No Qualifier
5 Middle Ear, Right 6 Middle Ear, Left 9 Auditory Ossicle, Right A Auditory Ossicle, Left D Inner Ear, Right E Inner Ear, Left	0 Open	0 Drainage Device	Z No Qualifier
5 Middle Ear, Right ⊘ 6 Middle Ear, Left ⊘ 9 Auditory Ossicle, Right A Auditory Ossicle, Left D Inner Ear, Right E Inner Ear, Left	0 Open	Z No Device	X Diagnostic Z No Qualifier
7 Tympanic Membrane, Right 8 Tympanic Membrane, Left F Eustachian Tube, Right ⊘ G Eustachian Tube, Left ⊘ L Nasal Turbinate ⊘ N Nasopharynx ⊘	0 Open 3 Percutaneous 4 Percutaneous Endoscopic 7 Via Natural or Artificial Opening 8 Via Natural or Artificial Opening Endoscopic	0 Drainage Device	Z No Qualifier
7 Tympanic Membrane, Right ⊘ 8 Tympanic Membrane, Left ⊘ F Eustachian Tube, Right ⊘ G Eustachian Tube, Left ⊘ L Nasal Turbinate ⊘ N Nasopharynx ⊘	0 Open 3 Percutaneous 4 Percutaneous Endoscopic 7 Via Natural or Artificial Opening 8 Via Natural or Artificial Opening Endoscopic	Z No Device	X Diagnostic Z No Qualifier

099 continued on next page

0 Medical and Surgical
9 Ear, Nose, Sinus
9 Drainage: Taking or letting out fluids and/or gases from a body part

099 continued from previous page

Body Part Character 4	Approach Character 5	Device Character 6	Qualifier Character 7
B Mastoid Sinus, Right ⃠ **C** Mastoid Sinus, Left ⃠ **M** Nasal Septum ⃠ **P** Accessory Sinus ⃠ **Q** Maxillary Sinus, Right ⃠ **R** Maxillary Sinus, Left ⃠ **S** Frontal Sinus, Right ⃠ **T** Frontal Sinus, Left ⃠ **U** Ethmoid Sinus, Right ⃠ **V** Ethmoid Sinus, Left ⃠ **W** Sphenoid Sinus, Right ⃠ **X** Sphenoid Sinus, Left ⃠	**0** Open **3** Percutaneous **4** Percutaneous Endoscopic	**0** Drainage Device	**Z** No Qualifier
B Mastoid Sinus, Right ⃠ **C** Mastoid Sinus, Left ⃠ **M** Nasal Septum ⃠ **P** Accessory Sinus ⃠ **Q** Maxillary Sinus, Right ⃠ **R** Maxillary Sinus, Left ⃠ **S** Frontal Sinus, Right ⃠ **T** Frontal Sinus, Left ⃠ **U** Ethmoid Sinus, Right ⃠ **V** Ethmoid Sinus, Left ⃠ **W** Sphenoid Sinus, Right ⃠ **X** Sphenoid Sinus, Left ⃠	**0** Open **3** Percutaneous **4** Percutaneous Endoscopic	**Z** No Device	**X** Diagnostic **Z** No Qualifier

⃠ 099000Z 09900ZX 09900ZZ 099030Z 09903ZX 09903ZZ 099040Z 09904ZX 09904ZZ 0990X0Z 0990XZX 0990XZZ 099100Z 09910ZX 09910ZZ 099130Z 09913ZX 09913ZZ 099140Z 09914ZX 09914ZZ 0991X0Z 0991XZX 0991XZZ 099300Z 09930ZX 09930ZZ 099330Z 09933ZX 09933ZZ 099340Z 09934ZX 09934ZZ 099370Z 09937ZX 09937ZZ 099380Z 09938ZX 09938ZZ 0993X0Z 0993XZX 0993XZZ 099400Z 09940ZX 09940ZZ 099430Z 09943ZX 09943ZZ 099440Z 09944ZX 09944ZZ 099470Z 09947ZX 09947ZZ 099480Z 09948ZX 09948ZZ 0994X0Z 0994XZX 0994XZZ 09950ZZ 09960ZZ 09970ZZ 09973ZZ 09974ZZ 09977ZZ 09978ZZ 09980ZZ 09983ZZ 09984ZZ 09987ZZ 09988ZZ 099B30Z 099B3ZZ 099C30Z 099C3ZZ 099F00Z 099F0ZZ 099F30Z 099F3ZZ 099F40Z 099F4ZZ 099F70Z 099F7ZZ 099F80Z 099F8ZZ 099G00Z 099G0ZZ 099G30Z 099G3ZZ 099G40Z 099G4ZZ 099G70Z 099G7ZZ 099G80Z 099G8ZZ 099K00Z 099K0ZX 099K0ZZ 099K30Z 099K3ZX 099K3ZZ 099K40Z 099K4ZX 099K4ZZ 099KX0Z 099KXZX 099KXZZ 099L00Z 099L0ZX 099L0ZZ 099L30Z 099L3ZX 099L3ZZ 099L40Z 099L4ZX 099L4ZZ 099L70Z 099L7ZX 099L7ZZ 099L80Z 099L8ZX 099L8ZZ 099M00Z 099M0ZX 099M0ZZ 099M30Z 099M3ZX 099M3ZZ 099M40Z 099M4ZX 099M4ZZ 099N0ZX 099N30Z 099N3ZX 099N3ZZ 099N4ZX 099N7ZX 099N8ZX 099P30Z 099P3ZX 099P3ZZ 099P40Z 099P4ZX 099P4ZZ 099Q30Z 099Q3ZX 099Q3ZZ 099Q40Z 099Q4ZX 099Q4ZZ 099R30Z 099R3ZX 099R3ZZ 099R40Z 099R4ZX 099R4ZZ 099S30Z 099S3ZX 099S3ZZ 099S40Z 099S4ZX 099S4ZZ 099T30Z 099T3ZX 099T3ZZ 099T40Z 099T4ZX 099T4ZZ 099U30Z 099U3ZX 099U3ZZ 099U40Z 099U4ZX 099U4ZZ 099V30Z 099V3ZX 099V3ZZ 099V40Z 099V4ZX 099V4ZZ 099W30Z 099W3ZX 099W3ZZ 099W40Z 099W4ZX 099W4ZZ 099X30Z 099X3ZX 099X3ZZ 099X40Z 099X4ZX 099X4ZZ

0 Medical and Surgical
9 Ear, Nose, Sinus
B Excision: Cutting out or off, without replacement, a portion of a body part

Body Part Character 4	Approach Character 5	Device Character 6	Qualifier Character 7
0 External Ear, Right ⊘ **1** External Ear, Left ⊘ **K** Nose ⊘	**0** Open **3** Percutaneous **4** Percutaneous Endoscopic **X** External	**Z** No Device	**X** Diagnostic **Z** No Qualifier
3 External Auditory Canal, Right ⊘ **4** External Auditory Canal, Left ⊘	**0** Open **3** Percutaneous **4** Percutaneous Endoscopic **7** Via Natural or Artificial Opening **8** Via Natural or Artificial Opening Endoscopic **X** External	**Z** No Device	**X** Diagnostic **Z** No Qualifier
5 Middle Ear, Right **6** Middle Ear, Left **9** Auditory Ossicle, Right **A** Auditory Ossicle, Left **D** Inner Ear, Right **E** Inner Ear, Left	**0** Open	**Z** No Device	**X** Diagnostic **Z** No Qualifier
7 Tympanic Membrane, Right **8** Tympanic Membrane, Left **F** Eustachian Tube, Right ⊘ **G** Eustachian Tube, Left ⊘ **L** Nasal Turbinate ⊘ **N** Nasopharynx ⊘	**0** Open **3** Percutaneous **4** Percutaneous Endoscopic **7** Via Natural or Artificial Opening **8** Via Natural or Artificial Opening Endoscopic	**Z** No Device	**X** Diagnostic **Z** No Qualifier
B Mastoid Sinus, Right **C** Mastoid Sinus, Left **M** Nasal Septum ⊘ **P** Accessory Sinus ⊘ **Q** Maxillary Sinus, Right ⊘ **R** Maxillary Sinus, Left ⊘ **S** Frontal Sinus, Right ⊘ **T** Frontal Sinus, Left ⊘ **U** Ethmoid Sinus, Right ⊘ **V** Ethmoid Sinus, Left ⊘ **W** Sphenoid Sinus, Right ⊘ **X** Sphenoid Sinus, Left ⊘	**0** Open **3** Percutaneous **4** Percutaneous Endoscopic	**Z** No Device	**X** Diagnostic **Z** No Qualifier

⊘ 09B00ZX 09B00ZZ 09B03ZX 09B03ZZ 09B04ZX 09B04ZZ 09B0XZX 09B0XZZ 09B10ZX 09B10ZZ 09B13ZX 09B13ZZ 09B14ZX
09B14ZZ 09B1XZX 09B1XZZ 09B30ZX 09B30ZZ 09B33ZX 09B33ZZ 09B34ZX 09B34ZZ 09B37ZX 09B37ZZ 09B38ZX 09B38ZZ
09B3XZX 09B3XZZ 09B40ZX 09B40ZZ 09B43ZX 09B43ZZ 09B44ZX 09B44ZZ 09B47ZX 09B47ZZ 09B48ZX 09B48ZZ 09B4XZX
09B4XZZ 09BF0ZX 09BF0ZZ 09BF3ZX 09BF3ZZ 09BF4ZX 09BF4ZZ 09BF7ZX 09BF7ZZ 09BF8ZX 09BF8ZZ 09BG0ZX 09BG0ZZ
09BG3ZX 09BG3ZZ 09BG4ZX 09BG4ZZ 09BG7ZX 09BG7ZZ 09BG8ZX 09BG8ZZ 09BK0ZX 09BK0ZZ 09BK3ZX 09BK3ZZ 09BK4ZX
09BK4ZZ 09BKXZX 09BKXZZ 09BL0ZX 09BL3ZX 09BL4ZX 09BL7ZX 09BL8ZX 09BM0ZX 09BM3ZX 09BM4ZX 09BN0ZX 09BN3ZX
09BN4ZX 09BN7ZX 09BN8ZX 09BP3ZX 09BP4ZX 09BQ3ZX 09BQ4ZX 09BR3ZX 09BR4ZX 09BS3ZX 09BS4ZX 09BT3ZX 09BT4ZX
09BU3ZX 09BU4ZX 09BV3ZX 09BV4ZX 09BW3ZX 09BW4ZX 09BX3ZX 09BX4ZX

0 Medical and Surgical
9 Ear, Nose, Sinus
C Extirpation: Taking or cutting out solid matter from a body part

Body Part Character 4	Approach Character 5	Device Character 6	Qualifier Character 7
0 External Ear, Right ⊘ **1** External Ear, Left ⊘ **K** Nose ⊘	**0** Open **3** Percutaneous **4** Percutaneous Endoscopic **X** External	**Z** No Device	**Z** No Qualifier
3 External Auditory Canal, Right ⊘ **4** External Auditory Canal, Left ⊘	**0** Open **3** Percutaneous **4** Percutaneous Endoscopic **7** Via Natural or Artificial Opening **8** Via Natural or Artificial Opening Endoscopic **X** External	**Z** No Device	**Z** No Qualifier
5 Middle Ear, Right **6** Middle Ear, Left **9** Auditory Ossicle, Right **A** Auditory Ossicle, Left **D** Inner Ear, Right **E** Inner Ear, Left	**0** Open	**Z** No Device	**Z** No Qualifier
7 Tympanic Membrane, Right ⊘ **8** Tympanic Membrane, Left ⊘ **F** Eustachian Tube, Right ⊘ **G** Eustachian Tube, Left ⊘ **L** Nasal Turbinate ⊘ **N** Nasopharynx	**0** Open **3** Percutaneous **4** Percutaneous Endoscopic **7** Via Natural or Artificial Opening **8** Via Natural or Artificial Opening Endoscopic	**Z** No Device	**Z** No Qualifier
B Mastoid Sinus, Right **C** Mastoid Sinus, Left **M** Nasal Septum ⊘ **P** Accessory Sinus **Q** Maxillary Sinus, Right **R** Maxillary Sinus, Left **S** Frontal Sinus, Right **T** Frontal Sinus, Left **U** Ethmoid Sinus, Right **V** Ethmoid Sinus, Left **W** Sphenoid Sinus, Right **X** Sphenoid Sinus, Left	**0** Open **3** Percutaneous **4** Percutaneous Endoscopic	**Z** No Device	**Z** No Qualifier

⊘ 09C00ZZ 09C03ZZ 09C04ZZ 09C0XZZ 09C10ZZ 09C13ZZ 09C14ZZ 09C1XZZ 09C30ZZ 09C33ZZ 09C34ZZ 09C37ZZ 09C38ZZ 09C3XZZ 09C40ZZ 09C43ZZ 09C44ZZ 09C47ZZ 09C48ZZ 09C4XZZ 09C70ZZ 09C73ZZ 09C74ZZ 09C77ZZ 09C78ZZ 09C80ZZ 09C83ZZ 09C84ZZ 09C87ZZ 09C88ZZ 09CF0ZZ 09CF3ZZ 09CF4ZZ 09CF7ZZ 09CF8ZZ 09CG0ZZ 09CG3ZZ 09CG4ZZ 09CG7ZZ 09CG8ZZ 09CK0ZZ 09CK3ZZ 09CK4ZZ 09CKXZZ 09CL0ZZ 09CL3ZZ 09CL4ZZ 09CL7ZZ 09CL8ZZ 09CM0ZZ 09CM3ZZ 09CM4ZZ

0 Medical and Surgical
9 Ear, Nose, Sinus
D Extraction: Pulling or stripping out or off all or a portion of a body part by the use of force

Body Part Character 4	Approach Character 5	Device Character 6	Qualifier Character 7
7 Tympanic Membrane, Right 8 Tympanic Membrane, Left L Nasal Turbinate	0 Open 3 Percutaneous 4 Percutaneous Endoscopic 7 Via Natural or Artificial Opening 8 Via Natural or Artificial Opening Endoscopic	Z No Device	Z No Qualifier
9 Auditory Ossicle, Right A Auditory Ossicle, Left	0 Open	Z No Device	Z No Qualifier
B Mastoid Sinus, Right C Mastoid Sinus, Left M Nasal Septum P Accessory Sinus Q Maxillary Sinus, Right R Maxillary Sinus, Left S Frontal Sinus, Right T Frontal Sinus, Left U Ethmoid Sinus, Right V Ethmoid Sinus, Left W Sphenoid Sinus, Right X Sphenoid Sinus, Left	0 Open 3 Percutaneous 4 Percutaneous Endoscopic	Z No Device	Z No Qualifier

0 Medical and Surgical
9 Ear, Nose, Sinus
H Insertion: Putting in a nonbiological appliance that monitors, assists, performs, or prevents a physiological function but does not physically take the place of a body part

Body Part Character 4	Approach Character 5	Device Character 6	Qualifier Character 7
D Inner Ear, Right E Inner Ear, Left	0 Open 3 Percutaneous 4 Percutaneous Endoscopic	4 Hearing Device, Bone Conduction 5 Hearing Device, Single Channel Cochlear Prosthesis 6 Hearing Device, Multiple Channel Cochlear Prosthesis S Hearing Device	Z No Qualifier
N Nasopharynx ⃠	7 Via Natural or Artificial Opening 8 Via Natural or Artificial Opening Endoscopic	B Intraluminal Device, Airway	Z No Qualifier

⃠ 09HN7BZ 09HN8BZ

0 Medical and Surgical
9 Ear, Nose, Sinus
J Inspection: Visually and/or manually exploring a body part

Body Part Character 4	Approach Character 5	Device Character 6	Qualifier Character 7
7 Tympanic Membrane, Right ⃠ 8 Tympanic Membrane, Left ⃠ H Ear, Right ⃠ J Ear, Left ⃠	0 Open 3 Percutaneous 4 Percutaneous Endoscopic 7 Via Natural or Artificial Opening 8 Via Natural or Artificial Opening Endoscopic X External	Z No Device	Z No Qualifier
D Inner Ear, Right ⃠ E Inner Ear, Left ⃠ K Nose ⃠ Y Sinus ⃠	0 Open 3 Percutaneous 4 Percutaneous Endoscopic X External	Z No Device	Z No Qualifier

⃠ 09J73ZZ 09J77ZZ 09J78ZZ 09J7XZZ 09J83ZZ 09J87ZZ 09J88ZZ 09J8XZZ 09JD3ZZ 09JDXZZ 09JE3ZZ 09JEXZZ 09JH0ZZ 09JH3ZZ 09JH4ZZ 09JH7ZZ 09JH8ZZ 09JHXZZ 09JJ0ZZ 09JJ3ZZ 09JJ4ZZ 09JJ7ZZ 09JJ8ZZ 09JJXZZ 09JK0ZZ 09JK3ZZ 09JK4ZZ 09JKXZZ 09JY0ZZ 09JY3ZZ 09JY4ZZ 09JYXZZ

0 Medical and Surgical
9 Ear, Nose, Sinus
M Reattachment: Putting back in or on all or a portion of a separated body part to its normal location or other suitable location

Body Part Character 4	Approach Character 5	Device Character 6	Qualifier Character 7
0 External Ear, Right **1** External Ear, Left **K** Nose	**X** External	**Z** No Device	**Z** No Qualifier

0 Medical and Surgical
9 Ear, Nose, Sinus
N Release: Freeing a body part from an abnormal physical constraint by cutting or by the use of force

Body Part Character 4	Approach Character 5	Device Character 6	Qualifier Character 7
0 External Ear, Right **1** External Ear, Left **K** Nose ⃠	**0** Open **3** Percutaneous **4** Percutaneous Endoscopic **X** External	**Z** No Device	**Z** No Qualifier
3 External Auditory Canal, Right **4** External Auditory Canal, Left	**0** Open **3** Percutaneous **4** Percutaneous Endoscopic **7** Via Natural or Artificial Opening **8** Via Natural or Artificial Opening Endoscopic **X** External	**Z** No Device	**Z** No Qualifier
5 Middle Ear, Right **6** Middle Ear, Left **9** Auditory Ossicle, Right **A** Auditory Ossicle, Left **D** Inner Ear, Right **E** Inner Ear, Left	**0** Open	**Z** No Device	**Z** No Qualifier
7 Tympanic Membrane, Right **8** Tympanic Membrane, Left **F** Eustachian Tube, Right ⃠ **G** Eustachian Tube, Left ⃠ **L** Nasal Turbinate ⃠ **N** Nasopharynx	**0** Open **3** Percutaneous **4** Percutaneous Endoscopic **7** Via Natural or Artificial Opening **8** Via Natural or Artificial Opening Endoscopic	**Z** No Device	**Z** No Qualifier
B Mastoid Sinus, Right **C** Mastoid Sinus, Left **M** Nasal Septum ⃠ **P** Accessory Sinus **Q** Maxillary Sinus, Right **R** Maxillary Sinus, Left **S** Frontal Sinus, Right **T** Frontal Sinus, Left **U** Ethmoid Sinus, Right **V** Ethmoid Sinus, Left **W** Sphenoid Sinus, Right **X** Sphenoid Sinus, Left	**0** Open **3** Percutaneous **4** Percutaneous Endoscopic	**Z** No Device	**Z** No Qualifier

⃠ 09NF0ZZ 09NF3ZZ 09NF4ZZ 09NF7ZZ 09NF8ZZ 09NG0ZZ 09NG3ZZ 09NG4ZZ 09NG7ZZ 09NG8ZZ 09NK0ZZ 09NK3ZZ 09NK4ZZ 09NKXZZ 09NL0ZZ 09NL3ZZ 09NL4ZZ 09NL7ZZ 09NL8ZZ 09NM0ZZ 09NM3ZZ 09NM4ZZ

0 Medical and Surgical
9 Ear, Nose, Sinus
P Removal: Taking out or off a device from a body part

Body Part Character 4	Approach Character 5	Device Character 6	Qualifier Character 7
7 Tympanic Membrane, Right ⃠ **8** Tympanic Membrane, Left ⃠	**0** Open **7** Via Natural or Artificial Opening **8** Via Natural or Artificial Opening Endoscopic **X** External	**0** Drainage Device	**Z** No Qualifier
D Inner Ear, Right **E** Inner Ear, Left	**0** Open **7** Via Natural or Artificial Opening **8** Via Natural or Artificial Opening Endoscopic	**S** Hearing Device	**Z** No Qualifier
H Ear, Right ⃠ **J** Ear, Left ⃠ **K** Nose ⃠	**0** Open **3** Percutaneous **4** Percutaneous Endoscopic **7** Via Natural or Artificial Opening **8** Via Natural or Artificial Opening Endoscopic **X** External	**0** Drainage Device **7** Autologous Tissue Substitute **D** Intraluminal Device **J** Synthetic Substitute **K** Nonautologous Tissue Substitute	**Z** No Qualifier
Y Sinus ⃠	**0** Open **3** Percutaneous **4** Percutaneous Endoscopic **X** External	**0** Drainage Device	**Z** No Qualifier

⃠ 09P700Z 09P770Z 09P780Z 09P7X0Z 09P800Z 09P870Z 09P880Z 09P8X0Z 09PH30Z 09PH3JZ 09PH3KZ 09PH40Z 09PH4JZ 09PH4KZ 09PH70Z 09PH7DZ 09PH80Z 09PH8DZ 09PHX0Z 09PHX7Z 09PHXDZ 09PHXJZ 09PHXKZ 09PJ30Z 09PJ3JZ 09PJ3KZ 09PJ40Z 09PJ4JZ 09PJ4KZ 09PJ70Z 09PJ7DZ 09PJ80Z 09PJ8DZ 09PJX0Z 09PJX7Z 09PJXDZ 09PJXJZ 09PJXKZ 09PK00Z 09PK07Z 09PK0DZ 09PK0JZ 09PK0KZ 09PK30Z 09PK37Z 09PK3DZ 09PK3JZ 09PK3KZ 09PK40Z 09PK47Z 09PK4DZ 09PK4JZ 09PK4KZ 09PK70Z 09PK77Z 09PK7DZ 09PK7JZ 09PK7KZ 09PK80Z 09PK87Z 09PK8DZ 09PK8JZ 09PK8KZ 09PKX0Z 09PKX7Z 09PKXDZ 09PKXJZ 09PKXKZ 09PYX0Z

0 Medical and Surgical
9 Ear, Nose, Sinus
Q Repair: Restoring, to the extent possible, a body part to its normal anatomic structure and function

Body Part Character 4	Approach Character 5	Device Character 6	Qualifier Character 7
0 External Ear, Right ⃠ **1** External Ear, Left ⃠ **2** External Ear, Bilateral ⃠ **K** Nose CC	**0** Open **3** Percutaneous **4** Percutaneous Endoscopic **X** External	**Z** No Device	**Z** No Qualifier
3 External Auditory Canal, Right ⃠ **4** External Auditory Canal, Left ⃠ **F** Eustachian Tube, Right ⃠ **G** Eustachian Tube, Left ⃠	**0** Open **3** Percutaneous **4** Percutaneous Endoscopic **7** Via Natural or Artificial Opening **8** Via Natural or Artificial Opening Endoscopic **X** External	**Z** No Device	**Z** No Qualifier
5 Middle Ear, Right **6** Middle Ear, Left **9** Auditory Ossicle, Right **A** Auditory Ossicle, Left **D** Inner Ear, Right **E** Inner Ear, Left	**0** Open	**Z** No Device	**Z** No Qualifier
7 Tympanic Membrane, Right **8** Tympanic Membrane, Left **L** Nasal Turbinate **N** Nasopharynx	**0** Open **3** Percutaneous **4** Percutaneous Endoscopic **7** Via Natural or Artificial Opening **8** Via Natural or Artificial Opening Endoscopic	**Z** No Device	**Z** No Qualifier

09Q continued on next page

0 Medical and Surgical
9 Ear, Nose, Sinus
Q Repair: Restoring, to the extent possible, a body part to its normal anatomic structure and function

09Q continued from previous page

Body Part Character 4	Approach Character 5	Device Character 6	Qualifier Character 7
B Mastoid Sinus, Right **C** Mastoid Sinus, Left **M** Nasal Septum **P** Accessory Sinus **Q** Maxillary Sinus, Right CC **R** Maxillary Sinus, Left **S** Frontal Sinus, Right **T** Frontal Sinus, Left **U** Ethmoid Sinus, Right **V** Ethmoid Sinus, Left **W** Sphenoid Sinus, Right **X** Sphenoid Sinus, Left	**0** Open **3** Percutaneous **4** Percutaneous Endoscopic	**Z** No Device	**Z** No Qualifier

⦸ 09Q0XZZ 09Q1XZZ 09Q2XZZ 09Q3XZZ 09Q4XZZ 09QF0ZZ 09QF3ZZ 09QF4ZZ 09QF7ZZ 09QF8ZZ 09QFXZZ 09QG0ZZ 09QG3ZZ 09QG4ZZ 09QG7ZZ 09QG8ZZ 09QGXZZ

CC 09QK0ZZ 09QK3ZZ 09QK4ZZ 09QQ0ZZ 09QQ3ZZ 09QQ4ZZ

0 Medical and Surgical
9 Ear, Nose, Sinus
R Replacement: Putting in or on biological or synthetic material that physically takes the place and/or function of all or a portion of a body part

Body Part Character 4	Approach Character 5	Device Character 6	Qualifier Character 7
0 External Ear, Right **1** External Ear, Left **2** External Ear, Bilateral **K** Nose	**0** Open **X** External	**7** Autologous Tissue Substitute **J** Synthetic Substitute **K** Nonautologous Tissue Substitute	**Z** No Qualifier
5 Middle Ear, Right **6** Middle Ear, Left **9** Auditory Ossicle, Right **A** Auditory Ossicle, Left **D** Inner Ear, Right **E** Inner Ear, Left	**0** Open	**7** Autologous Tissue Substitute **J** Synthetic Substitute **K** Nonautologous Tissue Substitute	**Z** No Qualifier
7 Tympanic Membrane, Right **8** Tympanic Membrane, Left **N** Nasopharynx	**0** Open **7** Via Natural or Artificial Opening **8** Via Natural or Artificial Opening Endoscopic	**7** Autologous Tissue Substitute **J** Synthetic Substitute **K** Nonautologous Tissue Substitute	**Z** No Qualifier
L Nasal Turbinate	**0** Open **3** Percutaneous **4** Percutaneous Endoscopic **7** Via Natural or Artificial Opening **8** Via Natural or Artificial Opening Endoscopic	**7** Autologous Tissue Substitute **J** Synthetic Substitute **K** Nonautologous Tissue Substitute	**Z** No Qualifier
M Nasal Septum	**0** Open **3** Percutaneous **4** Percutaneous Endoscopic	**7** Autologous Tissue Substitute **J** Synthetic Substitute **K** Nonautologous Tissue Substitute	**Z** No Qualifier

0 Medical and Surgical
9 Ear, Nose, Sinus
S Reposition: Moving to its normal location, or other suitable location, all or a portion of a body part

Body Part Character 4	Approach Character 5	Device Character 6	Qualifier Character 7
0 External Ear, Right **1** External Ear, Left **2** External Ear, Bilateral **K** Nose	**0** Open **4** Percutaneous Endoscopic **X** External	**Z** No Device	**Z** No Qualifier
7 Tympanic Membrane, Right **8** Tympanic Membrane, Left **F** Eustachian Tube, Right ⃠ **G** Eustachian Tube, Left ⃠ **L** Nasal Turbinate	**0** Open **4** Percutaneous Endoscopic **7** Via Natural or Artificial Opening **8** Via Natural or Artificial Opening Endoscopic	**Z** No Device	**Z** No Qualifier
9 Auditory Ossicle, Right **A** Auditory Ossicle, Left **M** Nasal Septum	**0** Open **4** Percutaneous Endoscopic	**Z** No Device	**Z** No Qualifier

⃠ 09SF0ZZ 09SF4ZZ 09SF7ZZ 09SF8ZZ 09SG0ZZ 09SG4ZZ 09SG7ZZ 09SG8ZZ

0 Medical and Surgical
9 Ear, Nose, Sinus
T Resection: Cutting out or off, without replacement, all of a body part

Body Part Character 4	Approach Character 5	Device Character 6	Qualifier Character 7
0 External Ear, Right **1** External Ear, Left **K** Nose	**0** Open **4** Percutaneous Endoscopic **X** External	**Z** No Device	**Z** No Qualifier
5 Middle Ear, Right **6** Middle Ear, Left **9** Auditory Ossicle, Right **A** Auditory Ossicle, Left **D** Inner Ear, Right **E** Inner Ear, Left	**0** Open	**Z** No Device	**Z** No Qualifier
7 Tympanic Membrane, Right **8** Tympanic Membrane, Left **F** Eustachian Tube, Right ⃠ **G** Eustachian Tube, Left ⃠ **L** Nasal Turbinate **N** Nasopharynx	**0** Open **4** Percutaneous Endoscopic **7** Via Natural or Artificial Opening **8** Via Natural or Artificial Opening Endoscopic	**Z** No Device	**Z** No Qualifier
B Mastoid Sinus, Right **C** Mastoid Sinus, Left **M** Nasal Septum **P** Accessory Sinus **Q** Maxillary Sinus, Right **R** Maxillary Sinus, Left **S** Frontal Sinus, Right **T** Frontal Sinus, Left **U** Ethmoid Sinus, Right **V** Ethmoid Sinus, Left **W** Sphenoid Sinus, Right **X** Sphenoid Sinus, Left	**0** Open **4** Percutaneous Endoscopic	**Z** No Device	**Z** No Qualifier

⃠ 09TF0ZZ 09TF4ZZ 09TF7ZZ 09TF8ZZ 09TG0ZZ 09TG4ZZ 09TG7ZZ 09TG8ZZ

0 Medical and Surgical
9 Ear, Nose, Sinus
U Supplement: Putting in or on biological or synthetic material that physically reinforces and/or augments the function of a portion of a body part

Body Part Character 4	Approach Character 5	Device Character 6	Qualifier Character 7
0 External Ear, Right **1** External Ear, Left **2** External Ear, Bilateral **K** Nose	**0** Open **X** External	**7** Autologous Tissue Substitute **J** Synthetic Substitute **K** Nonautologous Tissue Substitute	**Z** No Qualifier
5 Middle Ear, Right **6** Middle Ear, Left **9** Auditory Ossicle, Right **A** Auditory Ossicle, Left **D** Inner Ear, Right **E** Inner Ear, Left	**0** Open	**7** Autologous Tissue Substitute **J** Synthetic Substitute **K** Nonautologous Tissue Substitute	**Z** No Qualifier
7 Tympanic Membrane, Right **8** Tympanic Membrane, Left **N** Nasopharynx	**0** Open **7** Via Natural or Artificial Opening **8** Via Natural or Artificial Opening Endoscopic	**7** Autologous Tissue Substitute **J** Synthetic Substitute **K** Nonautologous Tissue Substitute	**Z** No Qualifier
L Nasal Turbinate	**0** Open **3** Percutaneous **4** Percutaneous Endoscopic **7** Via Natural or Artificial Opening **8** Via Natural or Artificial Opening Endoscopic	**7** Autologous Tissue Substitute **J** Synthetic Substitute **K** Nonautologous Tissue Substitute	**Z** No Qualifier
M Nasal Septum	**0** Open **3** Percutaneous **4** Percutaneous Endoscopic	**7** Autologous Tissue Substitute **J** Synthetic Substitute **K** Nonautologous Tissue Substitute	**Z** No Qualifier

0 Medical and Surgical
9 Ear, Nose, Sinus
W Revision: Correcting, to the extent possible, a portion of a malfunctioning device or the position of a displaced device

Body Part Character 4	Approach Character 5	Device Character 6	Qualifier Character 7
7 Tympanic Membrane, Right **8** Tympanic Membrane, Left **9** Auditory Ossicle, Right **A** Auditory Ossicle, Left	**0** Open **7** Via Natural or Artificial Opening **8** Via Natural or Artificial Opening Endoscopic	**7** Autologous Tissue Substitute **J** Synthetic Substitute **K** Nonautologous Tissue Substitute	**Z** No Qualifier
D Inner Ear, Right **E** Inner Ear, Left	**0** Open **7** Via Natural or Artificial Opening **8** Via Natural or Artificial Opening Endoscopic	**S** Hearing Device	**Z** No Qualifier
H Ear, Right ⃠ **J** Ear, Left ⃠ **K** Nose ⃠	**0** Open **3** Percutaneous **4** Percutaneous Endoscopic **7** Via Natural or Artificial Opening **8** Via Natural or Artificial Opening Endoscopic **X** External	**0** Drainage Device **7** Autologous Tissue Substitute **D** Intraluminal Device **J** Synthetic Substitute **K** Nonautologous Tissue Substitute	**Z** No Qualifier
Y Sinus ⃠	**0** Open **3** Percutaneous **4** Percutaneous Endoscopic **X** External	**0** Drainage Device	**Z** No Qualifier

⃠ 09WH3JZ 09WH3KZ 09WH4JZ 09WH4KZ 09WH7DZ 09WH8DZ 09WHX0Z 09WHX7Z 09WHXDZ 09WHXJZ 09WHXKZ 09WJ3JZ 09WJ3KZ 09WJ4JZ 09WJ4KZ 09WJ7DZ 09WJ8DZ 09WJX0Z 09WJX7Z 09WJXDZ 09WJXJZ 09WJXKZ 09WK00Z 09WK07Z 09WK0DZ 09WK0JZ 09WK0KZ 09WK30Z 09WK37Z 09WK3DZ 09WK3JZ 09WK3KZ 09WK40Z 09WK47Z 09WK4DZ 09WK4JZ 09WK4KZ 09WK70Z 09WK77Z 09WK7DZ 09WK7JZ 09WK7KZ 09WK80Z 09WK87Z 09WK8DZ 09WK8JZ 09WK8KZ 09WKX0Z 09WKX7Z 09WKXDZ 09WKXJZ 09WKXKZ 09WYX0Z

Respiratory System 0B1-0BY

0 Medical and Surgical
B Respiratory System
1 Bypass: Altering the route of passage of the contents of a tubular body part

Body Part Character 4	Approach Character 5	Device Character 6	Qualifier Character 7
1 Trachea ⊘	0 Open	D Intraluminal Device	6 Esophagus
1 Trachea	0 Open	F Tracheostomy Device Z No Device	4 Cutaneous
1 Trachea DRG	3 Percutaneous 4 Percutaneous Endoscopic	F Tracheostomy Device Z No Device	4 Cutaneous

DRG 0B113F4 0B113Z4
⊘ 0B110D6

0 Medical and Surgical
B Respiratory System
2 Change: Taking out or off a device from a body part and putting back an identical or similar device in or on the same body part without cutting or puncturing the skin or a mucous membrane

Body Part Character 4	Approach Character 5	Device Character 6	Qualifier Character 7
0 Tracheobronchial Tree ⊘ K Lung, Right ⊘ L Lung, Left ⊘ Q Pleura ⊘ T Diaphragm ⊘	X External	0 Drainage Device Y Other Device	Z No Qualifier
1 Trachea ⊘	X External	0 Drainage Device E Intraluminal Device, Endotracheal Airway F Tracheostomy Device Y Other Device	Z No Qualifier

⊘ 0B20X0Z 0B20XYZ 0B21X0Z 0B21XEZ 0B21XFZ 0B21XYZ 0B2KX0Z 0B2KXYZ 0B2LX0Z 0B2LXYZ 0B2QX0Z 0B2QXYZ 0B2TX0Z 0B2TXYZ

0 Medical and Surgical
B Respiratory System
5 Destruction: Physical eradication of all or a portion of a body part by the direct use of energy, force, or a destructive agent

Body Part Character 4	Approach Character 5	Device Character 6	Qualifier Character 7
1 Trachea 2 Carina 3 Main Bronchus, Right ⊘ 4 Upper Lobe Bronchus, Right ⊘ 5 Middle Lobe Bronchus, Right ⊘ 6 Lower Lobe Bronchus, Right ⊘ 7 Main Bronchus, Left ⊘ 8 Upper Lobe Bronchus, Left ⊘ 9 Lingula Bronchus ⊘ B Lower Lobe Bronchus, Left ⊘ C Upper Lung Lobe, Right ⊘ D Middle Lung Lobe, Right ⊘ F Lower Lung Lobe, Right ⊘ G Upper Lung Lobe, Left ⊘ H Lung Lingula ⊘ J Lower Lung Lobe, Left ⊘ K Lung, Right ⊘ L Lung, Left ⊘ M Lungs, Bilateral ⊘	0 Open 3 Percutaneous 4 Percutaneous Endoscopic 7 Via Natural or Artificial Opening 8 Via Natural or Artificial Opening Endoscopic	Z No Device	Z No Qualifier
N Pleura, Right P Pleura, Left R Diaphragm, Right S Diaphragm, Left	0 Open 3 Percutaneous 4 Percutaneous Endoscopic	Z No Device	Z No Qualifier

⊘ 0B534ZZ 0B544ZZ 0B554ZZ 0B564ZZ 0B574ZZ 0B584ZZ 0B594ZZ 0B5B4ZZ 0B5C8ZZ 0B5D8ZZ 0B5F8ZZ 0B5G8ZZ 0B5H8ZZ 0B5J8ZZ 0B5K8ZZ 0B5L8ZZ 0B5M8ZZ

LC Limited Coverage NC Noncovered HAC HAC Associated Procedure CC Combination Cluster - See Appendix G for code lists
DRG Non-OR-Affecting MS-DRG Assignment ⊘ Non-OR-Not Affecting MS-DRG Assignment New/Revised Text in **Orange** ♂ Male ♀ Female

0 Medical and Surgical
B Respiratory System
7 Dilation: Expanding an orifice or the lumen of a tubular body part

Body Part Character 4	Approach Character 5	Device Character 6	Qualifier Character 7
1 Trachea **2** Carina **3** Main Bronchus, Right ⦸ **4** Upper Lobe Bronchus, Right ⦸ **5** Middle Lobe Bronchus, Right ⦸ **6** Lower Lobe Bronchus, Right ⦸ **7** Main Bronchus, Left ⦸ **8** Upper Lobe Bronchus, Left ⦸ **9** Lingula Bronchus ⦸ **B** Lower Lobe Bronchus, Left ⦸	**0** Open **3** Percutaneous **4** Percutaneous Endoscopic **7** Via Natural or Artificial Opening **8** Via Natural or Artificial Opening Endoscopic	**D** Intraluminal Device **Z** No Device	**Z** No Qualifier

⦸ 0B730DZ 0B730ZZ 0B733DZ 0B733ZZ 0B734DZ 0B734ZZ 0B737DZ 0B737ZZ 0B738DZ 0B738ZZ 0B740DZ 0B740ZZ 0B743DZ
0B743ZZ 0B744DZ 0B744ZZ 0B747DZ 0B747ZZ 0B748DZ 0B748ZZ 0B750DZ 0B750ZZ 0B753DZ 0B753ZZ 0B754DZ 0B754ZZ
0B757DZ 0B757ZZ 0B758DZ 0B758ZZ 0B760DZ 0B760ZZ 0B763DZ 0B763ZZ 0B764DZ 0B764ZZ 0B767DZ 0B767ZZ 0B768DZ
0B768ZZ 0B770DZ 0B770ZZ 0B773DZ 0B773ZZ 0B774DZ 0B774ZZ 0B777DZ 0B777ZZ 0B778DZ 0B778ZZ 0B780DZ 0B780ZZ
0B783DZ 0B783ZZ 0B784DZ 0B784ZZ 0B787DZ 0B787ZZ 0B788DZ 0B788ZZ 0B790DZ 0B790ZZ 0B793DZ 0B793ZZ 0B794DZ
0B794ZZ 0B797DZ 0B797ZZ 0B798DZ 0B798ZZ 0B7B0DZ 0B7B0ZZ 0B7B3DZ 0B7B3ZZ 0B7B4DZ 0B7B4ZZ 0B7B7DZ 0B7B7ZZ
0B7B8DZ 0B7B8ZZ

0 Medical and Surgical
B Respiratory System
9 Drainage: Taking or letting out fluids and/or gases from a body part

Body Part Character 4	Approach Character 5	Device Character 6	Qualifier Character 7
1 Trachea **2** Carina **3** Main Bronchus, Right **4** Upper Lobe Bronchus, Right **5** Middle Lobe Bronchus, Right **6** Lower Lobe Bronchus, Right **7** Main Bronchus, Left **8** Upper Lobe Bronchus, Left **9** Lingula Bronchus **B** Lower Lobe Bronchus, Left **C** Upper Lung Lobe, Right **D** Middle Lung Lobe, Right **F** Lower Lung Lobe, Right **G** Upper Lung Lobe, Left **H** Lung Lingula **J** Lower Lung Lobe, Left **K** Lung, Right **L** Lung, Left **M** Lungs, Bilateral	**0** Open **3** Percutaneous **4** Percutaneous Endoscopic **7** Via Natural or Artificial Opening **8** Via Natural or Artificial Opening Endoscopic	**0** Drainage Device	**Z** No Qualifier

0B9 continued on next page

0B9 continued from previous page

0 Medical and Surgical
B Respiratory System
9 Drainage: Taking or letting out fluids and/or gases from a body part

Body Part Character 4	Approach Character 5	Device Character 6	Qualifier Character 7
1 Trachea ⦸ **2** Carina ⦸ **3** Main Bronchus, Right ⦸ **4** Upper Lobe Bronchus, Right ⦸ **5** Middle Lobe Bronchus, Right ⦸ **6** Lower Lobe Bronchus, Right ⦸ **7** Main Bronchus, Left ⦸ **8** Upper Lobe Bronchus, Left ⦸ **9** Lingula Bronchus ⦸ **B** Lower Lobe Bronchus, Left ⦸ **C** Upper Lung Lobe, Right ⦸ **D** Middle Lung Lobe, Right ⦸ **F** Lower Lung Lobe, Right ⦸ **G** Upper Lung Lobe, Left ⦸ **H** Lung Lingula ⦸ **J** Lower Lung Lobe, Left ⦸ **K** Lung, Right ⦸ **L** Lung, Left ⦸ **M** Lungs, Bilateral ⦸	**0** Open **3** Percutaneous **4** Percutaneous Endoscopic **7** Via Natural or Artificial Opening **8** Via Natural or Artificial Opening Endoscopic	**Z** No Device	**X** Diagnostic **Z** No Qualifier
N Pleura, Right ⦸ **P** Pleura, Left ⦸ **R** Diaphragm, Right ⦸ **S** Diaphragm, Left ⦸	**0** Open **3** Percutaneous **4** Percutaneous Endoscopic	**0** Drainage Device	**Z** No Qualifier
N Pleura, Right ⦸ **P** Pleura, Left ⦸ **R** Diaphragm, Right ⦸ **S** Diaphragm, Left ⦸	**0** Open **3** Percutaneous **4** Percutaneous Endoscopic	**Z** No Device	**X** Diagnostic **Z** No Qualifier

⦸ 0B913ZX 0B914ZX 0B917ZX 0B918ZX 0B923ZX 0B924ZX 0B927ZX 0B928ZX 0B933ZX 0B934ZX 0B937ZX 0B938ZX 0B943ZX 0B944ZX 0B947ZX 0B948ZX 0B953ZX 0B954ZX 0B957ZX 0B958ZX 0B963ZX 0B964ZX 0B967ZX 0B968ZX 0B973ZX 0B974ZX 0B977ZX 0B978ZX 0B983ZX 0B984ZX 0B987ZX 0B988ZX 0B993ZX 0B994ZX 0B997ZX 0B998ZX 0B9B3ZX 0B9B4ZX 0B9B7ZX 0B9B8ZX 0B9C3ZX 0B9C4ZX 0B9C7ZX 0B9D3ZX 0B9D4ZX 0B9D7ZX 0B9F3ZX 0B9F4ZX 0B9F7ZX 0B9G3ZX 0B9G4ZX 0B9G7ZX 0B9H3ZX 0B9H4ZX 0B9H7ZX 0B9J3ZX 0B9J4ZX 0B9J7ZX 0B9K3ZX 0B9K4ZX 0B9K7ZX 0B9L3ZX 0B9L4ZX 0B9L7ZX 0B9M3ZX 0B9M4ZX 0B9M7ZX 0B9N00Z 0B9N0ZX 0B9N0ZZ 0B9N30Z 0B9N3ZX 0B9N3ZZ 0B9N4ZX 0B9P00Z 0B9P0ZX 0B9P0ZZ 0B9P30Z 0B9P3ZX 0B9P3ZZ 0B9P4ZX 0B9R30Z 0B9R3ZZ 0B9S30Z 0B9S3ZZ

0 Medical and Surgical
B Respiratory System
B Excision: Cutting out or off, without replacement, a portion of a body part

Body Part Character 4	Approach Character 5	Device Character 6	Qualifier Character 7
1 Trachea ⦸ **2** Carina ⦸ **3** Main Bronchus, Right ⦸ **4** Upper Lobe Bronchus, Right ⦸ **5** Middle Lobe Bronchus, Right ⦸ **6** Lower Lobe Bronchus, Right ⦸ **7** Main Bronchus, Left ⦸ **8** Upper Lobe Bronchus, Left ⦸ **9** Lingula Bronchus ⦸ **B** Lower Lobe Bronchus, Left ⦸ **C** Upper Lung Lobe, Right ⦸ **D** Middle Lung Lobe, Right ⦸ **F** Lower Lung Lobe, Right ⦸ **G** Upper Lung Lobe, Left ⦸ **H** Lung Lingula ⦸ **J** Lower Lung Lobe, Left ⦸ **K** Lung, Right ⦸ **L** Lung, Left ⦸ **M** Lungs, Bilateral ⦸	**0** Open **3** Percutaneous **4** Percutaneous Endoscopic **7** Via Natural or Artificial Opening **8** Via Natural or Artificial Opening Endoscopic	**Z** No Device	**X** Diagnostic **Z** No Qualifier
N Pleura, Right ⦸ **P** Pleura, Left ⦸ **R** Diaphragm, Right **S** Diaphragm, Left	**0** Open **3** Percutaneous **4** Percutaneous Endoscopic	**Z** No Device	**X** Diagnostic **Z** No Qualifier

⦸ 0BB13ZX 0BB14ZX 0BB17ZX 0BB18ZX 0BB23ZX 0BB24ZX 0BB27ZX 0BB28ZX 0BB33ZX 0BB34ZX 0BB34ZZ 0BB37ZX 0BB38ZX
0BB38ZZ 0BB43ZX 0BB44ZX 0BB44ZZ 0BB47ZX 0BB48ZX 0BB48ZZ 0BB53ZX 0BB54ZX 0BB54ZZ 0BB57ZX 0BB58ZX 0BB58ZZ
0BB63ZX 0BB64ZX 0BB64ZZ 0BB67ZX 0BB68ZX 0BB68ZZ 0BB73ZX 0BB74ZX 0BB74ZZ 0BB77ZX 0BB78ZX 0BB78ZZ 0BB83ZX
0BB84ZX 0BB84ZZ 0BB87ZX 0BB88ZX 0BB88ZZ 0BB93ZX 0BB94ZX 0BB94ZZ 0BB97ZX 0BB98ZX 0BB98ZZ 0BBB3ZX 0BBB4ZX
0BBB4ZZ 0BBB7ZX 0BBB8ZX 0BBB8ZZ 0BBC3ZX 0BBC8ZZ 0BBD3ZX 0BBD8ZZ 0BBF3ZX 0BBF8ZZ 0BBG3ZX 0BBG8ZZ 0BBH3ZX
0BBH8ZZ 0BBJ3ZX 0BBJ8ZZ 0BBK3ZX 0BBK8ZZ 0BBL3ZX 0BBL8ZZ 0BBM3ZX 0BBM4ZZ 0BBM8ZZ 0BBN0ZX 0BBN3ZX 0BBP0ZX
0BBP3ZX

0 Medical and Surgical
B Respiratory System
C Extirpation: Taking or cutting out solid matter from a body part

Body Part Character 4	Approach Character 5	Device Character 6	Qualifier Character 7
1 Trachea ⊘ 2 Carina ⊘ 3 Main Bronchus, Right ⊘ 4 Upper Lobe Bronchus, Right ⊘ 5 Middle Lobe Bronchus, Right ⊘ 6 Lower Lobe Bronchus, Right ⊘ 7 Main Bronchus, Left ⊘ 8 Upper Lobe Bronchus, Left ⊘ 9 Lingula Bronchus ⊘ B Lower Lobe Bronchus, Left ⊘ C Upper Lung Lobe, Right D Middle Lung Lobe, Right F Lower Lung Lobe, Right G Upper Lung Lobe, Left H Lung Lingula J Lower Lung Lobe, Left K Lung, Right L Lung, Left M Lungs, Bilateral	0 Open 3 Percutaneous 4 Percutaneous Endoscopic 7 Via Natural or Artificial Opening 8 Via Natural or Artificial Opening Endoscopic	Z No Device	Z No Qualifier
N Pleura, Right ⊘ P Pleura, Left ⊘ R Diaphragm, Right S Diaphragm, Left	0 Open 3 Percutaneous 4 Percutaneous Endoscopic	Z No Device	Z No Qualifier

⊘ 0BC17ZZ 0BC18ZZ 0BC27ZZ 0BC28ZZ 0BC37ZZ 0BC38ZZ 0BC47ZZ 0BC48ZZ 0BC57ZZ 0BC58ZZ 0BC67ZZ 0BC68ZZ 0BC77ZZ 0BC78ZZ 0BC87ZZ 0BC88ZZ 0BC97ZZ 0BC98ZZ 0BCB7ZZ 0BCB8ZZ 0BCN0ZZ 0BCN3ZZ 0BCN4ZZ 0BCP0ZZ 0BCP3ZZ 0BCP4ZZ

0 Medical and Surgical
B Respiratory System
D Extraction: Pulling or stripping out or off all or a portion of a body part by the use of force

Body Part Character 4	Approach Character 5	Device Character 6	Qualifier Character 7
N Pleura, Right P Pleura, Left	0 Open 3 Percutaneous 4 Percutaneous Endoscopic	Z No Device	X Diagnostic Z No Qualifier

0 Medical and Surgical
B Respiratory System
F Fragmentation: Breaking solid matter in a body part into pieces

Body Part Character 4	Approach Character 5	Device Character 6	Qualifier Character 7
1 Trachea NC ⊘ **2** Carina NC ⊘ **3** Main Bronchus, Right NC ⊘ **4** Upper Lobe Bronchus, Right NC ⊘ **5** Middle Lobe Bronchus, Right NC ⊘ **6** Lower Lobe Bronchus, Right NC ⊘ **7** Main Bronchus, Left NC ⊘ **8** Upper Lobe Bronchus, Left NC ⊘ **9** Lingula Bronchus NC ⊘ **B** Lower Lobe Bronchus, Left NC ⊘	**0** Open **3** Percutaneous **4** Percutaneous Endoscopic **7** Via Natural or Artificial Opening **8** Via Natural or Artificial Opening Endoscopic **X** External	**Z** No Device	**Z** No Qualifier

NC 0BF1XZZ 0BF2XZZ 0BF3XZZ 0BF4XZZ 0BF5XZZ 0BF6XZZ 0BF7XZZ 0BF8XZZ 0BF9XZZ 0BFBXZZ
⊘ 0BF1XZZ 0BF2XZZ 0BF3XZZ 0BF4XZZ 0BF5XZZ 0BF6XZZ 0BF7XZZ 0BF8XZZ 0BF9XZZ 0BFBXZZ

0 Medical and Surgical
B Respiratory System
H Insertion: Putting in a nonbiological appliance that monitors, assists, performs, or prevents a physiological function but does not physically take the place of a body part

Body Part Character 4	Approach Character 5	Device Character 6	Qualifier Character 7
0 Tracheobronchial Tree ⊘	**0** Open **3** Percutaneous **4** Percutaneous Endoscopic **7** Via Natural or Artificial Opening **8** Via Natural or Artificial Opening Endoscopic	**1** Radioactive Element **2** Monitoring Device **3** Infusion Device **D** Intraluminal Device	**Z** No Qualifier
1 Trachea	**0** Open	**2** Monitoring Device **D** Intraluminal Device	**Z** No Qualifier
1 Trachea ⊘	**3** Percutaneous	**D** Intraluminal Device **E** Intraluminal Device, Endotracheal Airway	**Z** No Qualifier
1 Trachea	**4** Percutaneous Endoscopic	**D** Intraluminal Device	**Z** No Qualifier
1 Trachea ⊘	**7** Via Natural or Artificial Opening **8** Via Natural or Artificial Opening Endoscopic	**2** Monitoring Device **D** Intraluminal Device **E** Intraluminal Device, Endotracheal Airway	**Z** No Qualifier
3 Main Bronchus, Right ⊘ **4** Upper Lobe Bronchus, Right ⊘ **5** Middle Lobe Bronchus, Right ⊘ **6** Lower Lobe Bronchus, Right ⊘ **7** Main Bronchus, Left ⊘ **8** Upper Lobe Bronchus, Left ⊘ **9** Lingula Bronchus ⊘ **B** Lower Lobe Bronchus, Left ⊘	**0** Open **3** Percutaneous **4** Percutaneous Endoscopic **7** Via Natural or Artificial Opening **8** Via Natural or Artificial Opening Endoscopic	**G** Intraluminal Device, Endobronchial Valve	**Z** No Qualifier
K Lung, Right ⊘ **L** Lung, Left ⊘	**0** Open **3** Percutaneous **4** Percutaneous Endoscopic **7** Via Natural or Artificial Opening **8** Via Natural or Artificial Opening Endoscopic	**1** Radioactive Element **2** Monitoring Device **3** Infusion Device	**Z** No Qualifier
R Diaphragm, Right **S** Diaphragm, Left	**0** Open **3** Percutaneous **4** Percutaneous Endoscopic	**2** Monitoring Device **M** Diaphragmatic Pacemaker Lead	**Z** No Qualifier

⊘ 0BH072Z 0BH073Z 0BH07DZ 0BH082Z 0BH083Z 0BH08DZ 0BH13EZ 0BH172Z 0BH17EZ 0BH182Z 0BH18EZ 0BH38GZ 0BH48GZ 0BH58GZ 0BH68GZ 0BH78GZ 0BH88GZ 0BH98GZ 0BHB8GZ 0BHK72Z 0BHK73Z 0BHK82Z 0BHK83Z 0BHL72Z 0BHL73Z 0BHL82Z 0BHL83Z

LC Limited Coverage NC Noncovered HAC HAC Associated Procedure CC Combination Cluster - See Appendix G for code lists
DRG Non-OR-Affecting MS-DRG Assignment ⊘ Non-OR-Not Affecting MS-DRG Assignment New/Revised Text in **Orange** ♂ Male ♀ Female

0 Medical and Surgical
B Respiratory System
J Inspection: Visually and/or manually exploring a body part

Body Part Character 4	Approach Character 5	Device Character 6	Qualifier Character 7
0 Tracheobronchial Tree ⦸ **1** Trachea ⦸ **K** Lung, Right ⦸ **L** Lung, Left ⦸ **Q** Pleura ⦸ **T** Diaphragm ⦸	**0** Open **3** Percutaneous **4** Percutaneous Endoscopic **7** Via Natural or Artificial Opening **8** Via Natural or Artificial Opening Endoscopic **X** External	**Z** No Device	**Z** No Qualifier

⦸ 0BJ03ZZ 0BJ07ZZ 0BJ08ZZ 0BJ0XZZ 0BJ13ZZ 0BJ14ZZ 0BJ17ZZ 0BJ18ZZ 0BJ1XZZ 0BJK3ZZ 0BJK7ZZ 0BJK8ZZ 0BJKXZZ 0BJL3ZZ 0BJL7ZZ 0BJL8ZZ 0BJLXZZ 0BJQ3ZZ 0BJQ7ZZ 0BJQ8ZZ 0BJQXZZ 0BJT3ZZ 0BJT7ZZ 0BJT8ZZ 0BJTXZZ

0 Medical and Surgical
B Respiratory System
L Occlusion: Completely closing an orifice or the lumen of a tubular body part

Body Part Character 4	Approach Character 5	Device Character 6	Qualifier Character 7
1 Trachea **2** Carina **3** Main Bronchus, Right **4** Upper Lobe Bronchus, Right **5** Middle Lobe Bronchus, Right **6** Lower Lobe Bronchus, Right **7** Main Bronchus, Left **8** Upper Lobe Bronchus, Left **9** Lingula Bronchus **B** Lower Lobe Bronchus, Left	**0** Open **3** Percutaneous **4** Percutaneous Endoscopic	**C** Extraluminal Device **D** Intraluminal Device **Z** No Device	**Z** No Qualifier
1 Trachea **2** Carina **3** Main Bronchus, Right **4** Upper Lobe Bronchus, Right **5** Middle Lobe Bronchus, Right **6** Lower Lobe Bronchus, Right **7** Main Bronchus, Left **8** Upper Lobe Bronchus, Left **9** Lingula Bronchus **B** Lower Lobe Bronchus, Left	**7** Via Natural or Artificial Opening **8** Via Natural or Artificial Opening Endoscopic	**D** Intraluminal Device **Z** No Device	**Z** No Qualifier

0 Medical and Surgical
B Respiratory System
M Reattachment: Putting back in or on all or a portion of a separated body part to its normal location or other suitable location

Body Part Character 4	Approach Character 5	Device Character 6	Qualifier Character 7
1 Trachea **2** Carina **3** Main Bronchus, Right **4** Upper Lobe Bronchus, Right **5** Middle Lobe Bronchus, Right **6** Lower Lobe Bronchus, Right **7** Main Bronchus, Left **8** Upper Lobe Bronchus, Left **9** Lingula Bronchus **B** Lower Lobe Bronchus, Left **C** Upper Lung Lobe, Right **D** Middle Lung Lobe, Right **F** Lower Lung Lobe, Right **G** Upper Lung Lobe, Left **H** Lung Lingula **J** Lower Lung Lobe, Left **K** Lung, Right **L** Lung, Left **R** Diaphragm, Right **S** Diaphragm, Left	**0** Open	**Z** No Device	**Z** No Qualifier

0 Medical and Surgical
B Respiratory System
N Release: Freeing a body part from an abnormal physical constraint by cutting or by the use of force

Body Part Character 4	Approach Character 5	Device Character 6	Qualifier Character 7
1 Trachea **2** Carina **3** Main Bronchus, Right **4** Upper Lobe Bronchus, Right **5** Middle Lobe Bronchus, Right **6** Lower Lobe Bronchus, Right **7** Main Bronchus, Left **8** Upper Lobe Bronchus, Left **9** Lingula Bronchus **B** Lower Lobe Bronchus, Left **C** Upper Lung Lobe, Right **D** Middle Lung Lobe, Right **F** Lower Lung Lobe, Right **G** Upper Lung Lobe, Left **H** Lung Lingula **J** Lower Lung Lobe, Left **K** Lung, Right **L** Lung, Left **M** Lungs, Bilateral	**0** Open **3** Percutaneous **4** Percutaneous Endoscopic **7** Via Natural or Artificial Opening **8** Via Natural or Artificial Opening Endoscopic	**Z** No Device	**Z** No Qualifier
N Pleura, Right **P** Pleura, Left **R** Diaphragm, Right **S** Diaphragm, Left	**0** Open **3** Percutaneous **4** Percutaneous Endoscopic	**Z** No Device	**Z** No Qualifier

0 Medical and Surgical
B Respiratory System
P Removal: Taking out or off a device from a body part

Body Part Character 4	Approach Character 5	Device Character 6	Qualifier Character 7
0 Tracheobronchial Tree ⦸	0 Open 3 Percutaneous 4 Percutaneous Endoscopic 7 Via Natural or Artificial Opening 8 Via Natural or Artificial Opening Endoscopic	0 Drainage Device 1 Radioactive Element 2 Monitoring Device 3 Infusion Device 7 Autologous Tissue Substitute C Extraluminal Device D Intraluminal Device J Synthetic Substitute K Nonautologous Tissue Substitute	Z No Qualifier
0 Tracheobronchial Tree ⦸	X External	0 Drainage Device 1 Radioactive Element 2 Monitoring Device 3 Infusion Device D Intraluminal Device	Z No Qualifier
1 Trachea ⦸	0 Open 3 Percutaneous 4 Percutaneous Endoscopic 7 Via Natural or Artificial Opening 8 Via Natural or Artificial Opening Endoscopic	0 Drainage Device 2 Monitoring Device 7 Autologous Tissue Substitute C Extraluminal Device D Intraluminal Device F Tracheostomy Device J Synthetic Substitute K Nonautologous Tissue Substitute	Z No Qualifier
1 Trachea ⦸	X External	0 Drainage Device 2 Monitoring Device D Intraluminal Device F Tracheostomy Device	Z No Qualifier
K Lung, Right ⦸ L Lung, Left ⦸	0 Open 3 Percutaneous 4 Percutaneous Endoscopic 7 Via Natural or Artificial Opening 8 Via Natural or Artificial Opening Endoscopic X External	0 Drainage Device 1 Radioactive Element 2 Monitoring Device 3 Infusion Device	Z No Qualifier
Q Pleura ⦸	0 Open 3 Percutaneous 4 Percutaneous Endoscopic 7 Via Natural or Artificial Opening 8 Via Natural or Artificial Opening Endoscopic X External	0 Drainage Device 1 Radioactive Element 2 Monitoring Device	Z No Qualifier
T Diaphragm ⦸	0 Open 3 Percutaneous 4 Percutaneous Endoscopic 7 Via Natural or Artificial Opening 8 Via Natural or Artificial Opening Endoscopic	0 Drainage Device 2 Monitoring Device 7 Autologous Tissue Substitute J Synthetic Substitute K Nonautologous Tissue Substitute M Diaphragmatic Pacemaker Lead	Z No Qualifier
T Diaphragm ⦸	X External	0 Drainage Device 2 Monitoring Device M Diaphragmatic Pacemaker Lead	Z No Qualifier

⦸ 0BP070Z 0BP072Z 0BP073Z 0BP07DZ 0BP080Z 0BP082Z 0BP083Z 0BP08DZ 0BP0X0Z 0BP0X1Z 0BP0X2Z 0BP0X3Z 0BP0XDZ 0BP10FZ 0BP13FZ 0BP14FZ 0BP170Z 0BP172Z 0BP17DZ 0BP17FZ 0BP180Z 0BP182Z 0BP18DZ 0BP18FZ 0BP1X0Z 0BP1X2Z 0BP1XDZ 0BP1XFZ 0BPK70Z 0BPK72Z 0BPK73Z 0BPK80Z 0BPK82Z 0BPK83Z 0BPKX0Z 0BPKX1Z 0BPKX2Z 0BPKX3Z 0BPL70Z 0BPL72Z 0BPL73Z 0BPL80Z 0BPL82Z 0BPL83Z 0BPLX0Z 0BPLX1Z 0BPLX2Z 0BPLX3Z 0BPQ00Z 0BPQ01Z 0BPQ02Z 0BPQ30Z 0BPQ31Z 0BPQ32Z 0BPQ40Z 0BPQ41Z 0BPQ42Z 0BPQ70Z 0BPQ71Z 0BPQ72Z 0BPQ80Z 0BPQ81Z 0BPQ82Z 0BPQX0Z 0BPQX1Z 0BPQX2Z 0BPT70Z 0BPT72Z 0BPT80Z 0BPT82Z 0BPTX0Z 0BPTX2Z 0BPTXMZ

0 Medical and Surgical
B Respiratory System
Q Repair: Restoring, to the extent possible, a body part to its normal anatomic structure and function

Body Part Character 4	Approach Character 5	Device Character 6	Qualifier Character 7
1 Trachea CC 2 Carina 3 Main Bronchus, Right CC 4 Upper Lobe Bronchus, Right CC 5 Middle Lobe Bronchus, Right CC 6 Lower Lobe Bronchus, Right CC 7 Main Bronchus, Left CC 8 Upper Lobe Bronchus, Left CC 9 Lingula Bronchus CC B Lower Lobe Bronchus, Left CC C Upper Lung Lobe, Right D Middle Lung Lobe, Right F Lower Lung Lobe, Right G Upper Lung Lobe, Left H Lung Lingula J Lower Lung Lobe, Left K Lung, Right CC L Lung, Left CC M Lungs, Bilateral CC	0 Open 3 Percutaneous 4 Percutaneous Endoscopic 7 Via Natural or Artificial Opening 8 Via Natural or Artificial Opening Endoscopic	Z No Device	Z No Qualifier
N Pleura, Right CC P Pleura, Left CC R Diaphragm, Right S Diaphragm, Left	0 Open 3 Percutaneous 4 Percutaneous Endoscopic	Z No Device	Z No Qualifier

CC 0BQ10ZZ 0BQ13ZZ 0BQ14ZZ 0BQ17ZZ 0BQ18ZZ 0BQ30ZZ 0BQ33ZZ 0BQ34ZZ 0BQ37ZZ 0BQ38ZZ 0BQ40ZZ 0BQ43ZZ 0BQ44ZZ 0BQ47ZZ 0BQ48ZZ 0BQ50ZZ 0BQ53ZZ 0BQ54ZZ 0BQ57ZZ 0BQ58ZZ 0BQ60ZZ 0BQ63ZZ 0BQ64ZZ 0BQ67ZZ 0BQ68ZZ 0BQ70ZZ 0BQ73ZZ 0BQ74ZZ 0BQ77ZZ 0BQ78ZZ 0BQ80ZZ 0BQ83ZZ 0BQ84ZZ 0BQ87ZZ 0BQ88ZZ 0BQ90ZZ 0BQ93ZZ 0BQ94ZZ 0BQ97ZZ 0BQ98ZZ 0BQB0ZZ 0BQB3ZZ 0BQB4ZZ 0BQB7ZZ 0BQB8ZZ 0BQK0ZZ 0BQK3ZZ 0BQK4ZZ 0BQK7ZZ 0BQK8ZZ 0BQL0ZZ 0BQL3ZZ 0BQL4ZZ 0BQL7ZZ 0BQL8ZZ 0BQM0ZZ 0BQM3ZZ 0BQM4ZZ 0BQM7ZZ 0BQM8ZZ 0BQN0ZZ 0BQN3ZZ 0BQN4ZZ 0BQP0ZZ 0BQP3ZZ 0BQP4ZZ

0 Medical and Surgical
B Respiratory System
S Reposition: Moving to its normal location, or other suitable location, all or a portion of a body part

Body Part Character 4	Approach Character 5	Device Character 6	Qualifier Character 7
1 Trachea 2 Carina 3 Main Bronchus, Right 4 Upper Lobe Bronchus, Right 5 Middle Lobe Bronchus, Right 6 Lower Lobe Bronchus, Right 7 Main Bronchus, Left 8 Upper Lobe Bronchus, Left 9 Lingula Bronchus B Lower Lobe Bronchus, Left C Upper Lung Lobe, Right D Middle Lung Lobe, Right F Lower Lung Lobe, Right G Upper Lung Lobe, Left H Lung Lingula J Lower Lung Lobe, Left K Lung, Right L Lung, Left R Diaphragm, Right S Diaphragm, Left	0 Open	Z No Device	Z No Qualifier

LC Limited Coverage NC Noncovered HAC HAC Associated Procedure CC Combination Cluster - See Appendix G for code lists
DRG Non-OR-Affecting MS-DRG Assignment Non-OR-Not Affecting MS-DRG Assignment New/Revised Text in Orange ♂ Male ♀ Female

0 Medical and Surgical
B Respiratory System
T Resection: Cutting out or off, without replacement, all of a body part

Body Part Character 4	Approach Character 5	Device Character 6	Qualifier Character 7
1 Trachea **2** Carina **3** Main Bronchus, Right **4** Upper Lobe Bronchus, Right **5** Middle Lobe Bronchus, Right **6** Lower Lobe Bronchus, Right **7** Main Bronchus, Left **8** Upper Lobe Bronchus, Left **9** Lingula Bronchus **B** Lower Lobe Bronchus, Left **C** Upper Lung Lobe, Right **D** Middle Lung Lobe, Right **F** Lower Lung Lobe, Right **G** Upper Lung Lobe, Left **H** Lung Lingula **J** Lower Lung Lobe, Left **K** Lung, Right CC **L** Lung, Left CC **M** Lungs, Bilateral CC **R** Diaphragm, Right **S** Diaphragm, Left	**0** Open **4** Percutaneous Endoscopic	**Z** No Device	**Z** No Qualifier

CC 0BTK0ZZ 0BTL0ZZ 0BTM0ZZ

0 Medical and Surgical
B Respiratory System
U Supplement: Putting in or on biological or synthetic material that physically reinforces and/or augments the function of a portion of a body part

Body Part Character 4	Approach Character 5	Device Character 6	Qualifier Character 7
1 Trachea **2** Carina **3** Main Bronchus, Right **4** Upper Lobe Bronchus, Right **5** Middle Lobe Bronchus, Right **6** Lower Lobe Bronchus, Right **7** Main Bronchus, Left **8** Upper Lobe Bronchus, Left **9** Lingula Bronchus **B** Lower Lobe Bronchus, Left **R** Diaphragm, Right **S** Diaphragm, Left	**0** Open **4** Percutaneous Endoscopic	**7** Autologous Tissue Substitute **J** Synthetic Substitute **K** Nonautologous Tissue Substitute	**Z** No Qualifier

0 Medical and Surgical
B Respiratory System
V Restriction: Partially closing an orifice or the lumen of a tubular body part

Body Part Character 4	Approach Character 5	Device Character 6	Qualifier Character 7
1 Trachea **2** Carina **3** Main Bronchus, Right **4** Upper Lobe Bronchus, Right **5** Middle Lobe Bronchus, Right **6** Lower Lobe Bronchus, Right **7** Main Bronchus, Left **8** Upper Lobe Bronchus, Left **9** Lingula Bronchus **B** Lower Lobe Bronchus, Left	**0** Open **3** Percutaneous **4** Percutaneous Endoscopic	**C** Extraluminal Device **D** Intraluminal Device **Z** No Device	**Z** No Qualifier
1 Trachea **2** Carina **3** Main Bronchus, Right **4** Upper Lobe Bronchus, Right **5** Middle Lobe Bronchus, Right **6** Lower Lobe Bronchus, Right **7** Main Bronchus, Left **8** Upper Lobe Bronchus, Left **9** Lingula Bronchus **B** Lower Lobe Bronchus, Left	**7** Via Natural or Artificial Opening **8** Via Natural or Artificial Opening Endoscopic	**D** Intraluminal Device **Z** No Device	**Z** No Qualifier

0 Medical and Surgical
B Respiratory System
W Revision: Correcting, to the extent possible, a portion of a malfunctioning device or the position of a displaced device

Body Part Character 4	Approach Character 5	Device Character 6	Qualifier Character 7
0 Tracheobronchial Tree ⊘	**0** Open **3** Percutaneous **4** Percutaneous Endoscopic **7** Via Natural or Artificial Opening **8** Via Natural or Artificial Opening Endoscopic **X** External	**0** Drainage Device **2** Monitoring Device **3** Infusion Device **7** Autologous Tissue Substitute **C** Extraluminal Device **D** Intraluminal Device **J** Synthetic Substitute **K** Nonautologous Tissue Substitute	**Z** No Qualifier
1 Trachea ⊘	**0** Open **3** Percutaneous **4** Percutaneous Endoscopic **7** Via Natural or Artificial Opening **8** Via Natural or Artificial Opening Endoscopic **X** External	**0** Drainage Device **2** Monitoring Device **7** Autologous Tissue Substitute **C** Extraluminal Device **D** Intraluminal Device **F** Tracheostomy Device **J** Synthetic Substitute **K** Nonautologous Tissue Substitute	**Z** No Qualifier
K Lung, Right ⊘ **L** Lung, Left ⊘	**0** Open **3** Percutaneous **4** Percutaneous Endoscopic **7** Via Natural or Artificial Opening **8** Via Natural or Artificial Opening Endoscopic **X** External	**0** Drainage Device **2** Monitoring Device **3** Infusion Device	**Z** No Qualifier
Q Pleura ⊘	**0** Open **3** Percutaneous **4** Percutaneous Endoscopic **7** Via Natural or Artificial Opening **8** Via Natural or Artificial Opening Endoscopic **X** External	**0** Drainage Device **2** Monitoring Device	**Z** No Qualifier

0BW continued on next page

0BW continued from previous page

0 Medical and Surgical
B Respiratory System
W Revision: Correcting, to the extent possible, a portion of a malfunctioning device or the position of a displaced device

Body Part Character 4	Approach Character 5	Device Character 6	Qualifier Character 7
T Diaphragm ⦸	**0** Open **3** Percutaneous **4** Percutaneous Endoscopic **7** Via Natural or Artificial Opening **8** Via Natural or Artificial Opening Endoscopic **X** External	**0** Drainage Device **2** Monitoring Device **7** Autologous Tissue Substitute **J** Synthetic Substitute **K** Nonautologous Tissue Substitute **M** Diaphragmatic Pacemaker Lead	**Z** No Qualifier

⦸ 0BW0X0Z 0BW0X2Z 0BW0X3Z 0BW0X7Z 0BW0XCZ 0BW0XDZ 0BW0XJZ 0BW0XKZ 0BW1X0Z 0BW1X2Z 0BW1X7Z 0BW1XCZ 0BW1XDZ 0BW1XFZ 0BW1XJZ 0BW1XKZ 0BWKX0Z 0BWKX2Z 0BWKX3Z 0BWLX0Z 0BWLX2Z 0BWLX3Z 0BWQ00Z 0BWQ02Z 0BWQ30Z 0BWQ32Z 0BWQ40Z 0BWQ42Z 0BWQ70Z 0BWQ72Z 0BWQ80Z 0BWQ82Z 0BWQX0Z 0BWQX2Z 0BWTX0Z 0BWTX2Z 0BWTX7Z 0BWTXJZ 0BWTXKZ 0BWTXMZ

0 Medical and Surgical
B Respiratory System
Y Transplantation: Putting in or on all or a portion of a living body part taken from another individual or animal to physically take the place and/or function of all or a portion of a similar body part

Body Part Character 4	Approach Character 5	Device Character 6	Qualifier Character 7
C Upper Lung Lobe, Right LC **D** Middle Lung Lobe, Right LC **F** Lower Lung Lobe, Right LC **G** Upper Lung Lobe, Left LC **H** Lung Lingula LC **J** Lower Lung Lobe, Left LC **K** Lung, Right LC **L** Lung, Left LC **M** Lungs, Bilateral LC	**0** Open	**Z** No Device	**0** Allogeneic **1** Syngeneic **2** Zooplastic

LC 0BYC0Z0 0BYC0Z1 0BYC0Z2 0BYD0Z0 0BYD0Z1 0BYD0Z2 0BYF0Z0 0BYF0Z1 0BYF0Z2 0BYG0Z0 0BYG0Z1 0BYG0Z2 0BYH0Z0 0BYH0Z1 0BYH0Z2 0BYJ0Z0 0BYJ0Z1 0BYJ0Z2 0BYK0Z0 0BYK0Z1 0BYK0Z2 0BYL0Z0 0BYL0Z1 0BYL0Z2 0BYM0Z0 0BYM0Z1 0BYM0Z2

Mouth and Throat 0C0-0CX

0 Medical and Surgical
C Mouth and Throat
0 Alteration: Modifying the anatomic structure of a body part without affecting the function of the body part

Body Part Character 4	Approach Character 5	Device Character 6	Qualifier Character 7
0 Upper Lip **1** Lower Lip	**X** External	**7** Autologous Tissue Substitute **J** Synthetic Substitute **K** Nonautologous Tissue Substitute **Z** No Device	**Z** No Qualifier

0 Medical and Surgical
C Mouth and Throat
2 Change: Taking out or off a device from a body part and putting back an identical or similar device in or on the same body part without cutting or puncturing the skin or a mucous membrane

Body Part Character 4	Approach Character 5	Device Character 6	Qualifier Character 7
A Salivary Gland ⊘ **S** Larynx ⊘ **Y** Mouth and Throat ⊘	**X** External	**0** Drainage Device **Y** Other Device	**Z** No Qualifier

⊘ 0C2AX0Z 0C2AXYZ 0C2SX0Z 0C2SXYZ 0C2YX0Z 0C2YXYZ

0 Medical and Surgical
C Mouth and Throat
5 Destruction: Physical eradication of all or a portion of a body part by the direct use of energy, force, or a destructive agent

Body Part Character 4	Approach Character 5	Device Character 6	Qualifier Character 7
0 Upper Lip **1** Lower Lip **2** Hard Palate **3** Soft Palate **4** Buccal Mucosa **5** Upper Gingiva ⊘ **6** Lower Gingiva ⊘ **7** Tongue **N** Uvula **P** Tonsils **Q** Adenoids	**0** Open **3** Percutaneous **X** External	**Z** No Device	**Z** No Qualifier
8 Parotid Gland, Right **9** Parotid Gland, Left **B** Parotid Duct, Right **C** Parotid Duct, Left **D** Sublingual Gland, Right **F** Sublingual Gland, Left **G** Submaxillary Gland, Right **H** Submaxillary Gland, Left **J** Minor Salivary Gland	**0** Open **3** Percutaneous	**Z** No Device	**Z** No Qualifier
M Pharynx **R** Epiglottis **S** Larynx **T** Vocal Cord, Right **V** Vocal Cord, Left	**0** Open **3** Percutaneous **4** Percutaneous Endoscopic **7** Via Natural or Artificial Opening **8** Via Natural or Artificial Opening Endoscopic	**Z** No Device	**Z** No Qualifier
W Upper Tooth ⊘ **X** Lower Tooth ⊘	**0** Open **X** External	**Z** No Device	**0** Single **1** Multiple **2** All

⊘ 0C550ZZ 0C553ZZ 0C55XZZ 0C560ZZ 0C563ZZ 0C56XZZ 0C5W0Z0 0C5W0Z1 0C5W0Z2 0C5WXZ0 0C5WXZ1 0C5WXZ2 0C5X0Z0 0C5X0Z1 0C5X0Z2 0C5XXZ0 0C5XXZ1 0C5XXZ2

0 Medical and Surgical
C Mouth and Throat
7 Dilation: Expanding an orifice or the lumen of a tubular body part

Body Part Character 4	Approach Character 5	Device Character 6	Qualifier Character 7
B Parotid Duct, Right ⊘ **C** Parotid Duct, Left ⊘	**0** Open **3** Percutaneous **7** Via Natural or Artificial Opening	**D** Intraluminal Device **Z** No Device	**Z** No Qualifier
M Pharynx ⊘	**7** Via Natural or Artificial Opening **8** Via Natural or Artificial Opening Endoscopic	**D** Intraluminal Device **Z** No Device	**Z** No Qualifier
S Larynx CC	**0** Open **3** Percutaneous **4** Percutaneous Endoscopic **7** Via Natural or Artificial Opening **8** Via Natural or Artificial Opening Endoscopic	**D** Intraluminal Device **Z** No Device	**Z** No Qualifier

CC 0C7S0DZ 0C7S3DZ 0C7S4DZ 0C7S7DZ 0C7S8DZ
⊘ 0C7B0DZ 0C7B0ZZ 0C7B3DZ 0C7B3ZZ 0C7B7DZ 0C7B7ZZ 0C7C0DZ 0C7C0ZZ 0C7C3DZ 0C7C3ZZ 0C7C7DZ 0C7C7ZZ 0C7M7DZ 0C7M7ZZ 0C7M8DZ 0C7M8ZZ

0 Medical and Surgical
C Mouth and Throat
9 Drainage: Taking or letting out fluids and/or gases from a body part

Body Part Character 4	Approach Character 5	Device Character 6	Qualifier Character 7
0 Upper Lip ⊘ **1** Lower Lip ⊘ **2** Hard Palate ⊘ **3** Soft Palate ⊘ **4** Buccal Mucosa **5** Upper Gingiva ⊘ **6** Lower Gingiva ⊘ **7** Tongue ⊘ **N** Uvula ⊘ **P** Tonsils ⊘ **Q** Adenoids ⊘	**0** Open **3** Percutaneous **X** External	**0** Drainage Device	**Z** No Qualifier
0 Upper Lip ⊘ **1** Lower Lip ⊘ **2** Hard Palate ⊘ **3** Soft Palate ⊘ **4** Buccal Mucosa ⊘ **5** Upper Gingiva ⊘ **6** Lower Gingiva ⊘ **7** Tongue ⊘ **N** Uvula ⊘ **P** Tonsils ⊘ **Q** Adenoids ⊘	**0** Open **3** Percutaneous **X** External	**Z** No Device	**X** Diagnostic **Z** No Qualifier
8 Parotid Gland, Right ⊘ **9** Parotid Gland, Left ⊘ **B** Parotid Duct, Right ⊘ **C** Parotid Duct, Left ⊘ **D** Sublingual Gland, Right ⊘ **F** Sublingual Gland, Left ⊘ **G** Submaxillary Gland, Right ⊘ **H** Submaxillary Gland, Left ⊘ **J** Minor Salivary Gland ⊘	**0** Open **3** Percutaneous	**0** Drainage Device	**Z** No Qualifier

0C9 continued on next page

0 Medical and Surgical
C Mouth and Throat
9 Drainage: Taking or letting out fluids and/or gases from a body part

0C9 continued from previous page

Body Part Character 4	Approach Character 5	Device Character 6	Qualifier Character 7
8 Parotid Gland, Right ⦸ **9** Parotid Gland, Left ⦸ **B** Parotid Duct, Right ⦸ **C** Parotid Duct, Left ⦸ **D** Sublingual Gland, Right ⦸ **F** Sublingual Gland, Left ⦸ **G** Submaxillary Gland, Right ⦸ **H** Submaxillary Gland, Left ⦸ **J** Minor Salivary Gland ⦸	**0** Open **3** Percutaneous	**Z** No Device	**X** Diagnostic **Z** No Qualifier
M Pharynx ⦸ **R** Epiglottis ⦸ **S** Larynx ⦸ **T** Vocal Cord, Right ⦸ **V** Vocal Cord, Left ⦸	**0** Open **3** Percutaneous **4** Percutaneous Endoscopic **7** Via Natural or Artificial Opening **8** Via Natural or Artificial Opening Endoscopic	**0** Drainage Device	**Z** No Qualifier
M Pharynx ⦸ **R** Epiglottis ⦸ **S** Larynx ⦸ **T** Vocal Cord, Right ⦸ **V** Vocal Cord, Left ⦸	**0** Open **3** Percutaneous **4** Percutaneous Endoscopic **7** Via Natural or Artificial Opening **8** Via Natural or Artificial Opening Endoscopic	**Z** No Device	**X** Diagnostic **Z** No Qualifier
W Upper Tooth ⦸ **X** Lower Tooth ⦸	**0** Open **X** External	**0** Drainage Device **Z** No Device	**0** Single **1** Multiple **2** All

⦸	0C900ZX	0C9030Z	0C903ZX	0C903ZZ	0C90XZX	0C910ZX	0C9130Z	0C913ZX	0C913ZZ	0C91XZX	0C9230Z	0C923ZZ	0C9330Z
	0C933ZZ	0C940ZX	0C9430Z	0C943ZX	0C943ZZ	0C94XZX	0C9500Z	0C950ZX	0C950ZZ	0C9530Z	0C953ZX	0C953ZZ	0C95X0Z
	0C95XZX	0C95XZZ	0C9600Z	0C960ZX	0C960ZZ	0C9630Z	0C963ZX	0C963ZZ	0C96X0Z	0C96XZX	0C96XZZ	0C9730Z	0C973ZX
	0C973ZZ	0C97XZX	0C9800Z	0C980ZZ	0C9830Z	0C983ZX	0C983ZZ	0C9900Z	0C990ZZ	0C9930Z	0C993ZX	0C993ZZ	0C9B00Z
	0C9B0ZZ	0C9B30Z	0C9B3ZX	0C9B3ZZ	0C9C00Z	0C9C0ZZ	0C9C30Z	0C9C3ZX	0C9C3ZZ	0C9D00Z	0C9D0ZZ	0C9D30Z	0C9D3ZX
	0C9D3ZZ	0C9F00Z	0C9F0ZZ	0C9F30Z	0C9F3ZX	0C9F3ZZ	0C9G00Z	0C9G0ZZ	0C9G30Z	0C9G3ZX	0C9G3ZZ	0C9H00Z	0C9H0ZZ
	0C9H30Z	0C9H3ZX	0C9H3ZZ	0C9J00Z	0C9J0ZZ	0C9J30Z	0C9J3ZX	0C9J3ZZ	0C9M0ZX	0C9M30Z	0C9M3ZX	0C9M3ZZ	0C9M4ZX
	0C9M7ZX	0C9M8ZX	0C9N30Z	0C9N3ZZ	0C9P30Z	0C9P3ZZ	0C9Q30Z	0C9Q3ZZ	0C9R30Z	0C9R3ZX	0C9R3ZZ	0C9R4ZX	0C9R7ZX
	0C9R8ZX	0C9S30Z	0C9S3ZX	0C9S3ZZ	0C9S4ZX	0C9S7ZX	0C9S8ZX	0C9T30Z	0C9T3ZX	0C9T3ZZ	0C9T4ZX	0C9T7ZX	0C9T8ZX
	0C9V30Z	0C9V3ZX	0C9V3ZZ	0C9V4ZX	0C9V7ZX	0C9V8ZX	0C9W000	0C9W001	0C9W002	0C9W0Z0	0C9W0Z1	0C9W0Z2	0C9WX00
	0C9WX01	0C9WX02	0C9WXZ0	0C9WXZ1	0C9WXZ2	0C9X000	0C9X001	0C9X002	0C9X0Z0	0C9X0Z1	0C9X0Z2	0C9XX00	0C9XX01
	0C9XX02	0C9XXZ0	0C9XXZ1	0C9XXZ2									

0 Medical and Surgical
C Mouth and Throat
B Excision: Cutting out or off, without replacement, a portion of a body part

Body Part Character 4	Approach Character 5	Device Character 6	Qualifier Character 7
0 Upper Lip ⦸ **1** Lower Lip ⦸ **2** Hard Palate **3** Soft Palate **4** Buccal Mucosa ⦸ **5** Upper Gingiva ⦸ **6** Lower Gingiva ⦸ **7** Tongue ⦸ **N** Uvula **P** Tonsils **Q** Adenoids	**0** Open **3** Percutaneous **X** External	**Z** No Device	**X** Diagnostic **Z** No Qualifier
8 Parotid Gland, Right ⦸ **9** Parotid Gland, Left ⦸ **B** Parotid Duct, Right ⦸ **C** Parotid Duct, Left ⦸ **D** Sublingual Gland, Right ⦸ **F** Sublingual Gland, Left ⦸ **G** Submaxillary Gland, Right ⦸ **H** Submaxillary Gland, Left ⦸ **J** Minor Salivary Gland ⦸	**0** Open **3** Percutaneous	**Z** No Device	**X** Diagnostic **Z** No Qualifier
M Pharynx ⦸ **R** Epiglottis ⦸ **S** Larynx ⦸ **T** Vocal Cord, Right ⦸ **V** Vocal Cord, Left ⦸	**0** Open **3** Percutaneous **4** Percutaneous Endoscopic **7** Via Natural or Artificial Opening **8** Via Natural or Artificial Opening Endoscopic	**Z** No Device	**X** Diagnostic **Z** No Qualifier
W Upper Tooth ⦸ **X** Lower Tooth ⦸	**0** Open **X** External	**Z** No Device	**0** Single **1** Multiple **2** All

⦸ 0CB00ZX 0CB03ZX 0CB0XZX 0CB10ZX 0CB13ZX 0CB1XZX 0CB40ZX 0CB43ZX 0CB4XZX 0CB50ZX 0CB50ZZ 0CB53ZX 0CB53ZZ 0CB5XZX 0CB5XZZ 0CB60ZX 0CB60ZZ 0CB63ZX 0CB63ZZ 0CB6XZX 0CB6XZZ 0CB73ZX 0CB7XZX 0CB83ZX 0CB93ZX 0CBB3ZX 0CBC3ZX 0CBD3ZX 0CBF3ZX 0CBG3ZX 0CBH3ZX 0CBJ3ZX 0CBM0ZX 0CBM3ZX 0CBM4ZX 0CBM7ZX 0CBM8ZX 0CBR3ZX 0CBR4ZX 0CBR7ZX 0CBR8ZX 0CBS3ZX 0CBS4ZX 0CBS7ZX 0CBS8ZX 0CBT3ZX 0CBT4ZX 0CBT7ZX 0CBT8ZX 0CBV3ZX 0CBV4ZX 0CBV7ZX 0CBV8ZX 0CBW0Z0 0CBW0Z1 0CBW0Z2 0CBWXZ0 0CBWXZ1 0CBWXZ2 0CBX0Z0 0CBX0Z1 0CBX0Z2 0CBXXZ0 0CBXXZ1 0CBXXZ2

0 Medical and Surgical
C Mouth and Throat
C Extirpation: Taking or cutting out solid matter from a body part

Body Part Character 4	Approach Character 5	Device Character 6	Qualifier Character 7
0 Upper Lip ⊘ **1** Lower Lip ⊘ **2** Hard Palate ⊘ **3** Soft Palate ⊘ **4** Buccal Mucosa ⊘ **5** Upper Gingiva ⊘ **6** Lower Gingiva ⊘ **7** Tongue ⊘ **N** Uvula ⊘ **P** Tonsils ⊘ **Q** Adenoids ⊘	**0** Open **3** Percutaneous **X** External	**Z** No Device	**Z** No Qualifier
8 Parotid Gland, Right ⊘ **9** Parotid Gland, Left ⊘ **B** Parotid Duct, Right ⊘ **C** Parotid Duct, Left ⊘ **D** Sublingual Gland, Right ⊘ **F** Sublingual Gland, Left ⊘ **G** Submaxillary Gland, Right ⊘ **H** Submaxillary Gland, Left ⊘ **J** Minor Salivary Gland ⊘	**0** Open **3** Percutaneous	**Z** No Device	**Z** No Qualifier
M Pharynx ⊘ **R** Epiglottis **S** Larynx ⊘ **T** Vocal Cord, Right **V** Vocal Cord, Left	**0** Open **3** Percutaneous **4** Percutaneous Endoscopic **7** Via Natural or Artificial Opening **8** Via Natural or Artificial Opening Endoscopic	**Z** No Device	**Z** No Qualifier
W Upper Tooth ⊘ **X** Lower Tooth ⊘	**0** Open **X** External	**Z** No Device	**0** Single **1** Multiple **2** All

⊘ 0CC0XZZ 0CC1XZZ 0CC2XZZ 0CC3XZZ 0CC4XZZ 0CC50ZZ 0CC53ZZ 0CC5XZZ 0CC60ZZ 0CC63ZZ 0CC6XZZ 0CC7XZZ 0CC80ZZ 0CC83ZZ 0CC90ZZ 0CC93ZZ 0CCB0ZZ 0CCB3ZZ 0CCC0ZZ 0CCC3ZZ 0CCD0ZZ 0CCD3ZZ 0CCF0ZZ 0CCF3ZZ 0CCG0ZZ 0CCG3ZZ 0CCH0ZZ 0CCH3ZZ 0CCJ0ZZ 0CCJ3ZZ 0CCM7ZZ 0CCM8ZZ 0CCNXZZ 0CCPXZZ 0CCQXZZ 0CCS7ZZ 0CCS8ZZ 0CCW0Z0 0CCW0Z1 0CCW0Z2 0CCWXZ0 0CCWXZ1 0CCWXZ2 0CCX0Z0 0CCX0Z1 0CCX0Z2 0CCXXZ0 0CCXXZ1 0CCXXZ2

0 Medical and Surgical
C Mouth and Throat
D Extraction: Pulling or stripping out or off all or a portion of a body part by the use of force

Body Part Character 4	Approach Character 5	Device Character 6	Qualifier Character 7
T Vocal Cord, Right **V** Vocal Cord, Left	**0** Open **3** Percutaneous **4** Percutaneous Endoscopic **7** Via Natural or Artificial Opening **8** Via Natural or Artificial Opening Endoscopic	**Z** No Device	**Z** No Qualifier
W Upper Tooth ⊘ **X** Lower Tooth ⊘	**X** External	**Z** No Device	**0** Single **1** Multiple **2** All

⊘ 0CDWXZ0 0CDWXZ1 0CDWXZ2 0CDXXZ0 0CDXXZ1 0CDXXZ2

0 Medical and Surgical
C Mouth and Throat
F Fragmentation: Breaking solid matter in a body part into pieces

Body Part Character 4	Approach Character 5	Device Character 6	Qualifier Character 7
B Parotid Duct, Right NC ⃠ C Parotid Duct, Left NC ⃠	0 Open 3 Percutaneous 7 Via Natural or Artificial Opening X External	Z No Device	Z No Qualifier

NC 0CFBXZZ 0CFCXZZ
⃠ 0CFB0ZZ 0CFB3ZZ 0CFB7ZZ 0CFBXZZ 0CFC0ZZ 0CFC3ZZ 0CFC7ZZ 0CFCXZZ

0 Medical and Surgical
C Mouth and Throat
H Insertion: Putting in a nonbiological appliance that monitors, assists, performs, or prevents a physiological function but does not physically take the place of a body part

Body Part Character 4	Approach Character 5	Device Character 6	Qualifier Character 7
7 Tongue	0 Open 3 Percutaneous X External	1 Radioactive Element	Z No Qualifier
Y Mouth and Throat ⃠	7 Via Natural or Artificial Opening 8 Via Natural or Artificial Opening Endoscopic	B Intraluminal Device, Airway	Z No Qualifier

⃠ 0CHY7BZ 0CHY8BZ

0 Medical and Surgical
C Mouth and Throat
J Inspection: Visually and/or manually exploring a body part

Body Part Character 4	Approach Character 5	Device Character 6	Qualifier Character 7
A Salivary Gland ⃠	0 Open 3 Percutaneous X External	Z No Device	Z No Qualifier
S Larynx ⃠ Y Mouth and Throat ⃠	0 Open 3 Percutaneous 4 Percutaneous Endoscopic 7 Via Natural or Artificial Opening 8 Via Natural or Artificial Opening Endoscopic X External	Z No Device	Z No Qualifier

⃠ 0CJA0ZZ 0CJA3ZZ 0CJAXZZ 0CJS0ZZ 0CJS3ZZ 0CJS4ZZ 0CJS7ZZ 0CJS8ZZ 0CJSXZZ 0CJY0ZZ 0CJY3ZZ 0CJY4ZZ 0CJY7ZZ 0CJY8ZZ 0CJYXZZ

0 Medical and Surgical
C Mouth and Throat
L Occlusion: Completely closing an orifice or the lumen of a tubular body part

Body Part Character 4	Approach Character 5	Device Character 6	Qualifier Character 7
B Parotid Duct, Right C Parotid Duct, Left	0 Open 3 Percutaneous 4 Percutaneous Endoscopic	C Extraluminal Device D Intraluminal Device Z No Device	Z No Qualifier
B Parotid Duct, Right C Parotid Duct, Left	7 Via Natural or Artificial Opening 8 Via Natural or Artificial Opening Endoscopic	D Intraluminal Device Z No Device	Z No Qualifier

0 Medical and Surgical
C Mouth and Throat
M Reattachment: Putting back in or on all or a portion of a separated body part to its normal location or other suitable location

Body Part Character 4	Approach Character 5	Device Character 6	Qualifier Character 7
0 Upper Lip **1** Lower Lip **3** Soft Palate **7** Tongue **N** Uvula	**0** Open	**Z** No Device	**Z** No Qualifier
W Upper Tooth ⦸ **X** Lower Tooth ⦸	**0** Open **X** External	**Z** No Device	**0** Single **1** Multiple **2** All

⦸ 0CMW0Z0 0CMW0Z1 0CMW0Z2 0CMWXZ0 0CMWXZ1 0CMWXZ2 0CMX0Z0 0CMX0Z1 0CMX0Z2 0CMXXZ0 0CMXXZ1 0CMXXZ2

0 Medical and Surgical
C Mouth and Throat
N Release: Freeing a body part from an abnormal physical constraint by cutting or by the use of force

Body Part Character 4	Approach Character 5	Device Character 6	Qualifier Character 7
0 Upper Lip ⦸ **1** Lower Lip ⦸ **2** Hard Palate **3** Soft Palate **4** Buccal Mucosa **5** Upper Gingiva ⦸ **6** Lower Gingiva ⦸ **7** Tongue ⦸ **N** Uvula **P** Tonsils **Q** Adenoids	**0** Open **3** Percutaneous **X** External	**Z** No Device	**Z** No Qualifier
8 Parotid Gland, Right **9** Parotid Gland, Left **B** Parotid Duct, Right **C** Parotid Duct, Left **D** Sublingual Gland, Right **F** Sublingual Gland, Left **G** Submaxillary Gland, Right **H** Submaxillary Gland, Left **J** Minor Salivary Gland	**0** Open **3** Percutaneous	**Z** No Device	**Z** No Qualifier
M Pharynx **R** Epiglottis **S** Larynx **T** Vocal Cord, Right **V** Vocal Cord, Left	**0** Open **3** Percutaneous **4** Percutaneous Endoscopic **7** Via Natural or Artificial Opening **8** Via Natural or Artificial Opening Endoscopic	**Z** No Device	**Z** No Qualifier
W Upper Tooth ⦸ **X** Lower Tooth ⦸	**0** Open **X** External	**Z** No Device	**0** Single **1** Multiple **2** All

⦸ 0CN00ZZ 0CN03ZZ 0CN0XZZ 0CN10ZZ 0CN13ZZ 0CN1XZZ 0CN50ZZ 0CN53ZZ 0CN5XZZ 0CN60ZZ 0CN63ZZ 0CN6XZZ 0CN70ZZ 0CN73ZZ 0CN7XZZ 0CNW0Z0 0CNW0Z1 0CNW0Z2 0CNWXZ0 0CNWXZ1 0CNWXZ2 0CNX0Z0 0CNX0Z1 0CNX0Z2 0CNXXZ0 0CNXXZ1 0CNXXZ2

0 Medical and Surgical
C Mouth and Throat
P Removal: Taking out or off a device from a body part

Body Part Character 4	Approach Character 5	Device Character 6	Qualifier Character 7
A Salivary Gland ⊘	**0** Open **3** Percutaneous	**0** Drainage Device **C** Extraluminal Device	**Z** No Qualifier
S Larynx ⊘ CC	**0** Open **3** Percutaneous **7** Via Natural or Artificial Opening **8** Via Natural or Artificial Opening Endoscopic **X** External	**0** Drainage Device **7** Autologous Tissue Substitute **D** Intraluminal Device **J** Synthetic Substitute **K** Nonautologous Tissue Substitute	**Z** No Qualifier
Y Mouth and Throat ⊘	**0** Open **3** Percutaneous **7** Via Natural or Artificial Opening **8** Via Natural or Artificial Opening Endoscopic **X** External	**0** Drainage Device **1** Radioactive Element **7** Autologous Tissue Substitute **D** Intraluminal Device **J** Synthetic Substitute **K** Nonautologous Tissue Substitute	**Z** No Qualifier

CC 0CPS0DZ 0CPS3DZ 0CPS7DZ 0CPS8DZ
⊘ 0CPA00Z 0CPA0CZ 0CPA30Z 0CPA3CZ 0CPS70Z 0CPS7DZ 0CPS80Z 0CPS8DZ 0CPSX0Z 0CPSX7Z 0CPSXDZ 0CPSXJZ 0CPSXKZ 0CPY70Z 0CPY7DZ 0CPY80Z 0CPY8DZ 0CPYX0Z 0CPYX1Z 0CPYX7Z 0CPYXDZ 0CPYXJZ 0CPYXKZ

0 Medical and Surgical
C Mouth and Throat
Q Repair: Restoring, to the extent possible, a body part to its normal anatomic structure and function

Body Part Character 4	Approach Character 5	Device Character 6	Qualifier Character 7
0 Upper Lip ⊘ CC **1** Lower Lip ⊘ CC **2** Hard Palate **3** Soft Palate **4** Buccal Mucosa CC **5** Upper Gingiva ⊘ **6** Lower Gingiva ⊘ **7** Tongue **N** Uvula **P** Tonsils **Q** Adenoids	**0** Open **3** Percutaneous **X** External	**Z** No Device	**Z** No Qualifier
8 Parotid Gland, Right **9** Parotid Gland, Left **B** Parotid Duct, Right **C** Parotid Duct, Left **D** Sublingual Gland, Right **F** Sublingual Gland, Left **G** Submaxillary Gland, Right **H** Submaxillary Gland, Left **J** Minor Salivary Gland	**0** Open **3** Percutaneous	**Z** No Device	**Z** No Qualifier
M Pharynx CC **R** Epiglottis **S** Larynx **T** Vocal Cord, Right **V** Vocal Cord, Left	**0** Open **3** Percutaneous **4** Percutaneous Endoscopic **7** Via Natural or Artificial Opening **8** Via Natural or Artificial Opening Endoscopic	**Z** No Device	**Z** No Qualifier
W Upper Tooth ⊘ **X** Lower Tooth ⊘	**0** Open **X** External	**Z** No Device	**0** Single **1** Multiple **2** All

CC 0CQ00ZZ 0CQ03ZZ 0CQ10ZZ 0CQ13ZZ 0CQ40ZZ 0CQ43ZZ 0CQ4XZZ 0CQM0ZZ 0CQM3ZZ 0CQM4ZZ 0CQM7ZZ 0CQM8ZZ
⊘ 0CQ0XZZ 0CQ1XZZ 0CQ50ZZ 0CQ53ZZ 0CQ5XZZ 0CQ60ZZ 0CQ63ZZ 0CQ6XZZ 0CQW0Z0 0CQW0Z1 0CQW0Z2 0CQWXZ0 0CQWXZ1 0CQWXZ2 0CQX0Z0 0CQX0Z1 0CQX0Z2 0CQXXZ0 0CQXXZ1 0CQXXZ2

0 Medical and Surgical
C Mouth and Throat
R Replacement: Putting in or on biological or synthetic material that physically takes the place and/or function of all or a portion of a body part

Body Part Character 4	Approach Character 5	Device Character 6	Qualifier Character 7
0 Upper Lip **1** Lower Lip **2** Hard Palate **3** Soft Palate **4** Buccal Mucosa **5** Upper Gingiva **6** Lower Gingiva **7** Tongue **N** Uvula	**0** Open **3** Percutaneous **X** External	**7** Autologous Tissue Substitute **J** Synthetic Substitute **K** Nonautologous Tissue Substitute	**Z** No Qualifier
B Parotid Duct, Right **C** Parotid Duct, Left	**0** Open **3** Percutaneous	**7** Autologous Tissue Substitute **J** Synthetic Substitute **K** Nonautologous Tissue Substitute	**Z** No Qualifier
M Pharynx **R** Epiglottis **S** Larynx CC **T** Vocal Cord, Right **V** Vocal Cord, Left	**0** Open **7** Via Natural or Artificial Opening **8** Via Natural or Artificial Opening Endoscopic	**7** Autologous Tissue Substitute **J** Synthetic Substitute **K** Nonautologous Tissue Substitute	**Z** No Qualifier
W Upper Tooth ⊘ **X** Lower Tooth ⊘	**0** Open **X** External	**7** Autologous Tissue Substitute **J** Synthetic Substitute **K** Nonautologous Tissue Substitute	**0** Single **1** Multiple **2** All

CC 0CRS0JZ 0CRS7JZ 0CRS8JZ

⊘ 0CRW070 0CRW071 0CRW072 0CRW0J0 0CRW0J1 0CRW0J2 0CRW0K0 0CRW0K1 0CRW0K2 0CRWX70 0CRWX71 0CRWX72 0CRWXJ0 0CRWXJ1 0CRWXJ2 0CRWXK0 0CRWXK1 0CRWXK2 0CRX070 0CRX071 0CRX072 0CRX0J0 0CRX0J1 0CRX0J2 0CRX0K0 0CRX0K1 0CRX0K2 0CRXX70 0CRXX71 0CRXX72 0CRXXJ0 0CRXXJ1 0CRXXJ2 0CRXXK0 0CRXXK1 0CRXXK2

0 Medical and Surgical
C Mouth and Throat
S Reposition: Moving to its normal location, or other suitable location, all or a portion of a body part

Body Part Character 4	Approach Character 5	Device Character 6	Qualifier Character 7
0 Upper Lip **1** Lower Lip **2** Hard Palate **3** Soft Palate **7** Tongue **N** Uvula	**0** Open **X** External	**Z** No Device	**Z** No Qualifier
B Parotid Duct, Right **C** Parotid Duct, Left	**0** Open **3** Percutaneous	**Z** No Device	**Z** No Qualifier
R Epiglottis **T** Vocal Cord, Right **V** Vocal Cord, Left	**0** Open **7** Via Natural or Artificial Opening **8** Via Natural or Artificial Opening Endoscopic	**Z** No Device	**Z** No Qualifier
W Upper Tooth ⊘ **X** Lower Tooth ⊘	**0** Open **X** External	**5** External Fixation Device **Z** No Device	**0** Single **1** Multiple **2** All

⊘ 0CSW050 0CSW051 0CSW052 0CSW0Z0 0CSW0Z1 0CSW0Z2 0CSWX50 0CSWX51 0CSWX52 0CSWXZ0 0CSWXZ1 0CSWXZ2 0CSX050 0CSX051 0CSX052 0CSX0Z0 0CSX0Z1 0CSX0Z2 0CSXX50 0CSXX51 0CSXX52 0CSXXZ0 0CSXXZ1 0CSXXZ2

0 Medical and Surgical
C Mouth and Throat
T Resection: Cutting out or off, without replacement, all of a body part

Body Part Character 4	Approach Character 5	Device Character 6	Qualifier Character 7
0 Upper Lip 1 Lower Lip 2 Hard Palate 3 Soft Palate 7 Tongue N Uvula P Tonsils CC Q Adenoids CC	0 Open X External	Z No Device	Z No Qualifier
8 Parotid Gland, Right 9 Parotid Gland, Left B Parotid Duct, Right C Parotid Duct, Left D Sublingual Gland, Right F Sublingual Gland, Left G Submaxillary Gland, Right H Submaxillary Gland, Left J Minor Salivary Gland	0 Open	Z No Device	Z No Qualifier
M Pharynx R Epiglottis S Larynx T Vocal Cord, Right V Vocal Cord, Left	0 Open 4 Percutaneous Endoscopic 7 Via Natural or Artificial Opening 8 Via Natural or Artificial Opening Endoscopic	Z No Device	Z No Qualifier
W Upper Tooth ⦸ X Lower Tooth ⦸	0 Open	Z No Device	0 Single 1 Multiple 2 All

CC 0CTP0ZZ 0CTPXZZ 0CTQ0ZZ 0CTQXZZ
⦸ 0CTW0Z0 0CTW0Z1 0CTW0Z2 0CTX0Z0 0CTX0Z1 0CTX0Z2

0 Medical and Surgical
C Mouth and Throat
U Supplement: Putting in or on biological or synthetic material that physically reinforces and/or augments the function of a portion of a body part

Body Part Character 4	Approach Character 5	Device Character 6	Qualifier Character 7
0 Upper Lip 1 Lower Lip 2 Hard Palate ⦸ 3 Soft Palate 4 Buccal Mucosa 5 Upper Gingiva 6 Lower Gingiva 7 Tongue N Uvula	0 Open 3 Percutaneous X External	7 Autologous Tissue Substitute J Synthetic Substitute K Nonautologous Tissue Substitute	Z No Qualifier
M Pharynx R Epiglottis S Larynx CC T Vocal Cord, Right V Vocal Cord, Left	0 Open 7 Via Natural or Artificial Opening 8 Via Natural or Artificial Opening Endoscopic	7 Autologous Tissue Substitute J Synthetic Substitute K Nonautologous Tissue Substitute	Z No Qualifier

CC 0CUS0JZ 0CUS7JZ 0CUS8JZ
⦸ 0CU20JZ 0CU23JZ

LC Limited Coverage NC Noncovered HAC HAC Associated Procedure CC Combination Cluster - See Appendix G for code lists
DRG Non-OR-Affecting MS-DRG Assignment ⦸ Non-OR-Not Affecting MS-DRG Assignment New/Revised Text in **Orange** ♂ Male ♀ Female

0 Medical and Surgical
C Mouth and Throat
V Restriction: Partially closing an orifice or the lumen of a tubular body part

Body Part Character 4	Approach Character 5	Device Character 6	Qualifier Character 7
B Parotid Duct, Right **C** Parotid Duct, Left	**0** Open **3** Percutaneous	**C** Extraluminal Device **D** Intraluminal Device **Z** No Device	**Z** No Qualifier
B Parotid Duct, Right **C** Parotid Duct, Left	**7** Via Natural or Artificial Opening **8** Via Natural or Artificial Opening Endoscopic	**D** Intraluminal Device **Z** No Device	**Z** No Qualifier

0 Medical and Surgical
C Mouth and Throat
W Revision: Correcting, to the extent possible, a portion of a malfunctioning device or the position of a displaced device

Body Part Character 4	Approach Character 5	Device Character 6	Qualifier Character 7
A Salivary Gland ⦸	**0** Open **3** Percutaneous **X** External	**0** Drainage Device **C** Extraluminal Device	**Z** No Qualifier
S Larynx ⦸	**0** Open **3** Percutaneous **7** Via Natural or Artificial Opening **8** Via Natural or Artificial Opening Endoscopic **X** External	**0** Drainage Device **7** Autologous Tissue Substitute **D** Intraluminal Device **J** Synthetic Substitute **K** Nonautologous Tissue Substitute	**Z** No Qualifier
Y Mouth and Throat ⦸	**0** Open **3** Percutaneous **7** Via Natural or Artificial Opening **8** Via Natural or Artificial Opening Endoscopic **X** External	**0** Drainage Device **1** Radioactive Element **7** Autologous Tissue Substitute **D** Intraluminal Device **J** Synthetic Substitute **K** Nonautologous Tissue Substitute	**Z** No Qualifier

⦸ 0CWA00Z 0CWA0CZ 0CWA30Z 0CWA3CZ 0CWAX0Z 0CWAXCZ 0CWSX0Z 0CWSX7Z 0CWSXDZ 0CWSXJZ 0CWSXKZ 0CWY07Z 0CWYX0Z 0CWYX1Z 0CWYX7Z 0CWYXDZ 0CWYXJZ 0CWYXKZ

0 Medical and Surgical
C Mouth and Throat
X Transfer: Moving, without taking out, all or a portion of a body part to another location to take over the function of all or a portion of a body part

Body Part Character 4	Approach Character 5	Device Character 6	Qualifier Character 7
0 Upper Lip **1** Lower Lip **3** Soft Palate **4** Buccal Mucosa **5** Upper Gingiva **6** Lower Gingiva **7** Tongue	**0** Open **X** External	**Z** No Device	**Z** No Qualifier

Gastrointestinal System 0D1-0DY

0 Medical and Surgical
D Gastrointestinal System
1 Bypass: Altering the route of passage of the contents of a tubular body part

Body Part Character 4	Approach Character 5	Device Character 6	Qualifier Character 7
1 Esophagus, Upper **2** Esophagus, Middle **3** Esophagus, Lower **5** Esophagus	**0** Open **4** Percutaneous Endoscopic **8** Via Natural or Artificial Opening Endoscopic	**7** Autologous Tissue Substitute **J** Synthetic Substitute **K** Nonautologous Tissue Substitute **Z** No Device	**4** Cutaneous **6** Stomach **9** Duodenum **A** Jejunum **B** Ileum
1 Esophagus, Upper **2** Esophagus, Middle **3** Esophagus, Lower **5** Esophagus	**3** Percutaneous	**J** Synthetic Substitute	**4** Cutaneous
6 Stomach ⊘ CC HAC **9** Duodenum	**0** Open **4** Percutaneous Endoscopic **8** Via Natural or Artificial Opening Endoscopic	**7** Autologous Tissue Substitute **J** Synthetic Substitute **K** Nonautologous Tissue Substitute **Z** No Device	**4** Cutaneous **9** Duodenum **A** Jejunum **B** Ileum **L** Transverse Colon
6 Stomach ⊘ HAC **9** Duodenum	**3** Percutaneous	**J** Synthetic Substitute	**4** Cutaneous
A Jejunum	**0** Open **4** Percutaneous Endoscopic **8** Via Natural or Artificial Opening Endoscopic	**7** Autologous Tissue Substitute **J** Synthetic Substitute **K** Nonautologous Tissue Substitute **Z** No Device	**4** Cutaneous **A** Jejunum **B** Ileum **H** Cecum **K** Ascending Colon **L** Transverse Colon **M** Descending Colon **N** Sigmoid Colon **P** Rectum **Q** Anus
A Jejunum	**3** Percutaneous	**J** Synthetic Substitute	**4** Cutaneous
B Ileum	**0** Open **4** Percutaneous Endoscopic **8** Via Natural or Artificial Opening Endoscopic	**7** Autologous Tissue Substitute **J** Synthetic Substitute **K** Nonautologous Tissue Substitute **Z** No Device	**4** Cutaneous **B** Ileum **H** Cecum **K** Ascending Colon **L** Transverse Colon **M** Descending Colon **N** Sigmoid Colon **P** Rectum **Q** Anus
B Ileum	**3** Percutaneous	**J** Synthetic Substitute	**4** Cutaneous
H Cecum	**0** Open **4** Percutaneous Endoscopic **8** Via Natural or Artificial Opening Endoscopic	**7** Autologous Tissue Substitute **J** Synthetic Substitute **K** Nonautologous Tissue Substitute **Z** No Device	**4** Cutaneous **H** Cecum **K** Ascending Colon **L** Transverse Colon **M** Descending Colon **N** Sigmoid Colon **P** Rectum
H Cecum	**3** Percutaneous	**J** Synthetic Substitute	**4** Cutaneous
K Ascending Colon	**0** Open **4** Percutaneous Endoscopic **8** Via Natural or Artificial Opening Endoscopic	**7** Autologous Tissue Substitute **J** Synthetic Substitute **K** Nonautologous Tissue Substitute **Z** No Device	**4** Cutaneous **K** Ascending Colon **L** Transverse Colon **M** Descending Colon **N** Sigmoid Colon **P** Rectum
K Ascending Colon	**3** Percutaneous	**J** Synthetic Substitute	**4** Cutaneous

0D1 continued on next page

0 **Medical and Surgical**
D **Gastrointestinal System**
1 **Bypass:** Altering the route of passage of the contents of a tubular body part

0D1 continued from previous page

Body Part Character 4	Approach Character 5	Device Character 6	Qualifier Character 7
L Transverse Colon	**0** Open **4** Percutaneous Endoscopic **8** Via Natural or Artificial Opening Endoscopic	**7** Autologous Tissue Substitute **J** Synthetic Substitute **K** Nonautologous Tissue Substitute **Z** No Device	**4** Cutaneous **L** Transverse Colon **M** Descending Colon **N** Sigmoid Colon **P** Rectum
L Transverse Colon	**3** Percutaneous	**J** Synthetic Substitute	**4** Cutaneous
M Descending Colon	**0** Open **4** Percutaneous Endoscopic **8** Via Natural or Artificial Opening Endoscopic	**7** Autologous Tissue Substitute **J** Synthetic Substitute **K** Nonautologous Tissue Substitute **Z** No Device	**4** Cutaneous **M** Descending Colon **N** Sigmoid Colon **P** Rectum
M Descending Colon	**3** Percutaneous	**J** Synthetic Substitute	**4** Cutaneous
N Sigmoid Colon CC	**0** Open **4** Percutaneous Endoscopic **8** Via Natural or Artificial Opening Endoscopic	**7** Autologous Tissue Substitute **J** Synthetic Substitute **K** Nonautologous Tissue Substitute **Z** No Device	**4** Cutaneous **N** Sigmoid Colon **P** Rectum
N Sigmoid Colon	**3** Percutaneous	**J** Synthetic Substitute	**4** Cutaneous

CC 0D1607A 0D160JA 0D160KA 0D160ZA 0D160ZB 0D1N0Z4 0D1N4Z4

HAC 0D16079 0D1607A 0D1607B 0D1607L 0D160J9 0D160JA 0D160JB 0D160JL 0D160K9 0D160KA 0D160KB 0D160KL 0D160Z9 0D160ZA 0D160ZB 0D160ZL 0D16479 0D1647A 0D1647B 0D1647L 0D164J9 0D164JA 0D164JB 0D164JL 0D164K9 0D164KA 0D164KB 0D164KL 0D164Z9 0D164ZA 0D164ZB 0D164ZL 0D16879 0D1687A 0D1687B 0D1687L 0D168J9 0D168JA 0D168JB 0D168JL 0D168K9 0D168KA 0D168KB 0D168KL 0D168Z9 0D168ZA 0D168ZB or 0D168ZL All preceding codes with the HAC symbol are classified as hospital-acquired conditions when reported with principal diagnosis E66.01 and secondary diagnosis K68.11, K95.01, K95.81, or T81.4XXA.

⦸ 0D16074 0D160J4 0D160K4 0D160Z4 0D163J4 0D16474 0D164J4 0D164K4 0D164Z4 0D16874 0D168J4 0D168K4 0D168Z4

0 **Medical and Surgical**
D **Gastrointestinal System**
2 **Change:** Taking out or off a device from a body part and putting back an identical or similar device in or on the same body part without cutting or puncturing the skin or a mucous membrane

Body Part Character 4	Approach Character 5	Device Character 6	Qualifier Character 7
0 Upper Intestinal Tract ⦸ **D** Lower Intestinal Tract ⦸	**X** External	**0** Drainage Device **U** Feeding Device **Y** Other Device	**Z** No Qualifier
U Omentum ⦸ **V** Mesentery ⦸ **W** Peritoneum ⦸	**X** External	**0** Drainage Device **Y** Other Device	**Z** No Qualifier

⦸ 0D20X0Z 0D20XUZ 0D20XYZ 0D2DX0Z 0D2DXUZ 0D2DXYZ 0D2UX0Z 0D2UXYZ 0D2VX0Z 0D2VXYZ 0D2WX0Z 0D2WXYZ

0 Medical and Surgical
D Gastrointestinal System
5 Destruction: Physical eradication of all or a portion of a body part by the direct use of energy, force, or a destructive agent

Body Part Character 4	Approach Character 5	Device Character 6	Qualifier Character 7
1 Esophagus, Upper ⊘ **2** Esophagus, Middle ⊘ **3** Esophagus, Lower ⊘ **4** Esophagogastric Junction ⊘ **5** Esophagus ⊘ **6** Stomach ⊘ **7** Stomach, Pylorus ⊘ **8** Small Intestine **9** Duodenum ⊘ **A** Jejunum **B** Ileum **C** Ileocecal Valve **E** Large Intestine ⊘ **F** Large Intestine, Right ⊘ **G** Large Intestine, Left ⊘ **H** Cecum ⊘ **J** Appendix **K** Ascending Colon ⊘ **L** Transverse Colon ⊘ **M** Descending Colon ⊘ **N** Sigmoid Colon ⊘ **P** Rectum ⊘	**0** Open **3** Percutaneous **4** Percutaneous Endoscopic **7** Via Natural or Artificial Opening **8** Via Natural or Artificial Opening Endoscopic	**Z** No Device	**Z** No Qualifier
Q Anus ⊘	**0** Open **3** Percutaneous **4** Percutaneous Endoscopic **7** Via Natural or Artificial Opening **8** Via Natural or Artificial Opening Endoscopic **X** External	**Z** No Device	**Z** No Qualifier
R Anal Sphincter ⊘ **S** Greater Omentum **T** Lesser Omentum **V** Mesentery **W** Peritoneum	**0** Open **3** Percutaneous **4** Percutaneous Endoscopic	**Z** No Device	**Z** No Qualifier

⊘ 0D514ZZ 0D518ZZ 0D524ZZ 0D528ZZ 0D534ZZ 0D538ZZ 0D544ZZ 0D548ZZ 0D554ZZ 0D558ZZ 0D564ZZ 0D568ZZ 0D574ZZ 0D578ZZ 0D594ZZ 0D598ZZ 0D5E4ZZ 0D5E8ZZ 0D5F4ZZ 0D5F8ZZ 0D5G4ZZ 0D5G8ZZ 0D5H4ZZ 0D5H8ZZ 0D5K4ZZ 0D5K8ZZ 0D5L4ZZ 0D5L8ZZ 0D5M4ZZ 0D5M8ZZ 0D5N4ZZ 0D5N8ZZ 0D5P0ZZ 0D5P3ZZ 0D5P4ZZ 0D5P7ZZ 0D5P8ZZ 0D5Q4ZZ 0D5Q8ZZ 0D5R4ZZ

0 Medical and Surgical
D Gastrointestinal System
7 Dilation: Expanding an orifice or the lumen of a tubular body part

Body Part Character 4	Approach Character 5	Device Character 6	Qualifier Character 7
1 Esophagus, Upper ⦸ **2** Esophagus, Middle ⦸ **3** Esophagus, Lower ⦸ **4** Esophagogastric Junction ⦸ **5** Esophagus ⦸ **6** Stomach ⦸ **7** Stomach, Pylorus ⦸ **8** Small Intestine ⦸ **9** Duodenum ⦸ **A** Jejunum ⦸ **B** Ileum ⦸ **C** Ileocecal Valve ⦸ **E** Large Intestine ⦸ **F** Large Intestine, Right ⦸ **G** Large Intestine, Left ⦸ **H** Cecum ⦸ **K** Ascending Colon ⦸ **L** Transverse Colon ⦸ **M** Descending Colon ⦸ **N** Sigmoid Colon ⦸ **P** Rectum ⦸ **Q** Anus ⦸	**0** Open **3** Percutaneous **4** Percutaneous Endoscopic **7** Via Natural or Artificial Opening **8** Via Natural or Artificial Opening Endoscopic	**D** Intraluminal Device **Z** No Device	**Z** No Qualifier

⦸ 0D717DZ 0D717ZZ 0D718DZ 0D718ZZ 0D727DZ 0D727ZZ 0D728DZ 0D728ZZ 0D737DZ 0D737ZZ 0D738DZ 0D738ZZ 0D747DZ 0D747ZZ 0D748DZ 0D748ZZ 0D757DZ 0D757ZZ 0D758DZ 0D758ZZ 0D767DZ 0D767ZZ 0D768DZ 0D768ZZ 0D774DZ 0D777DZ 0D777ZZ 0D778DZ 0D778ZZ 0D780DZ 0D783DZ 0D784DZ 0D787DZ 0D787ZZ 0D788DZ 0D788ZZ 0D790DZ 0D793DZ 0D794DZ 0D797DZ 0D797ZZ 0D798DZ 0D798ZZ 0D7A0DZ 0D7A3DZ 0D7A4DZ 0D7A7DZ 0D7A7ZZ 0D7A8DZ 0D7A8ZZ 0D7B0DZ 0D7B3DZ 0D7B4DZ 0D7B7DZ 0D7B7ZZ 0D7B8DZ 0D7B8ZZ 0D7C0DZ 0D7C3DZ 0D7C4DZ 0D7C7DZ 0D7C7ZZ 0D7C8DZ 0D7C8ZZ 0D7E0DZ 0D7E3DZ 0D7E4DZ 0D7E7DZ 0D7E7ZZ 0D7E8DZ 0D7E8ZZ 0D7F0DZ 0D7F3DZ 0D7F4DZ 0D7F7DZ 0D7F7ZZ 0D7F8DZ 0D7F8ZZ 0D7G0DZ 0D7G3DZ 0D7G4DZ 0D7G7DZ 0D7G7ZZ 0D7G8DZ 0D7G8ZZ 0D7H0DZ 0D7H3DZ 0D7H4DZ 0D7H7DZ 0D7H7ZZ 0D7H8DZ 0D7H8ZZ 0D7K0DZ 0D7K3DZ 0D7K4DZ 0D7K7DZ 0D7K7ZZ 0D7K8DZ 0D7K8ZZ 0D7L0DZ 0D7L3DZ 0D7L4DZ 0D7L7DZ 0D7L7ZZ 0D7L8DZ 0D7L8ZZ 0D7M0DZ 0D7M3DZ 0D7M4DZ 0D7M7DZ 0D7M7ZZ 0D7M8DZ 0D7M8ZZ 0D7N0DZ 0D7N3DZ 0D7N4DZ 0D7N7DZ 0D7N7ZZ 0D7N8DZ 0D7N8ZZ 0D7P7DZ 0D7P7ZZ 0D7P8DZ 0D7P8ZZ 0D7Q7DZ 0D7Q7ZZ 0D7Q8DZ 0D7Q8ZZ

0 Medical and Surgical
D Gastrointestinal System
8 Division: Cutting into a body part, without draining fluids and/or gases from the body part, in order to separate or transect a body part

Body Part Character 4	Approach Character 5	Device Character 6	Qualifier Character 7
4 Esophagogastric Junction **7** Stomach, Pylorus	**0** Open **3** Percutaneous **4** Percutaneous Endoscopic **7** Via Natural or Artificial Opening **8** Via Natural or Artificial Opening Endoscopic	**Z** No Device	**Z** No Qualifier
R Anal Sphincter	**0** Open **3** Percutaneous	**Z** No Device	**Z** No Qualifier

0 Medical and Surgical
D Gastrointestinal System
9 Drainage: Taking or letting out fluids and/or gases from a body part

Body Part Character 4	Approach Character 5	Device Character 6	Qualifier Character 7
1 Esophagus, Upper ⦸ **2** Esophagus, Middle ⦸ **3** Esophagus, Lower ⦸ **4** Esophagogastric Junction ⦸ **5** Esophagus ⦸ **6** Stomach ⦸ **7** Stomach, Pylorus ⦸ **8** Small Intestine ⦸ **9** Duodenum ⦸ **A** Jejunum ⦸ **B** Ileum ⦸ **C** Ileocecal Valve ⦸ **E** Large Intestine ⦸ **F** Large Intestine, Right ⦸ **G** Large Intestine, Left ⦸ **H** Cecum ⦸ **J** Appendix ⦸ **K** Ascending Colon ⦸ **L** Transverse Colon ⦸ **M** Descending Colon ⦸ **N** Sigmoid Colon ⦸ **P** Rectum ⦸	**0** Open **3** Percutaneous **4** Percutaneous Endoscopic **7** Via Natural or Artificial Opening **8** Via Natural or Artificial Opening Endoscopic	**0** Drainage Device	**Z** No Qualifier
1 Esophagus, Upper ⦸ **2** Esophagus, Middle ⦸ **3** Esophagus, Lower ⦸ **4** Esophagogastric Junction ⦸ **5** Esophagus ⦸ **6** Stomach ⦸ **7** Stomach, Pylorus ⦸ **8** Small Intestine ⦸ **9** Duodenum ⦸ **A** Jejunum ⦸ **B** Ileum ⦸ **C** Ileocecal Valve ⦸ **E** Large Intestine ⦸ **F** Large Intestine, Right ⦸ **G** Large Intestine, Left ⦸ **H** Cecum ⦸ **J** Appendix ⦸ **K** Ascending Colon ⦸ **L** Transverse Colon ⦸ **M** Descending Colon ⦸ **N** Sigmoid Colon ⦸ **P** Rectum ⦸	**0** Open **3** Percutaneous **4** Percutaneous Endoscopic **7** Via Natural or Artificial Opening **8** Via Natural or Artificial Opening Endoscopic	**Z** No Device	**X** Diagnostic **Z** No Qualifier
Q Anus ⦸	**0** Open **3** Percutaneous **4** Percutaneous Endoscopic **7** Via Natural or Artificial Opening **8** Via Natural or Artificial Opening Endoscopic **X** External	**0** Drainage Device	**Z** No Qualifier
Q Anus ⦸	**0** Open **3** Percutaneous **4** Percutaneous Endoscopic **7** Via Natural or Artificial Opening **8** Via Natural or Artificial Opening Endoscopic **X** External	**Z** No Device	**X** Diagnostic **Z** No Qualifier

0D9 continued on next page

0D9 continued from previous page

0 Medical and Surgical
D Gastrointestinal System
9 Drainage: Taking or letting out fluids and/or gases from a body part

Body Part Character 4	Approach Character 5	Device Character 6	Qualifier Character 7
R Anal Sphincter ⃠ **S** Greater Omentum ⃠ **T** Lesser Omentum ⃠ **V** Mesentery ⃠ **W** Peritoneum ⃠	**0** Open **3** Percutaneous **4** Percutaneous Endoscopic	**0** Drainage Device	**Z** No Qualifier
R Anal Sphincter ⃠ **S** Greater Omentum ⃠ **T** Lesser Omentum ⃠ **V** Mesentery ⃠ **W** Peritoneum ⃠	**0** Open **3** Percutaneous **4** Percutaneous Endoscopic	**Z** No Device	**X** Diagnostic **Z** No Qualifier

⃠ 0D9130Z 0D913ZX 0D913ZZ 0D914ZX 0D917ZX 0D918ZX 0D9230Z 0D923ZX 0D923ZZ 0D924ZX 0D927ZX 0D928ZX 0D9330Z 0D933ZX 0D933ZZ 0D934ZX 0D937ZX 0D938ZX 0D9430Z 0D943ZX 0D943ZZ 0D944ZX 0D947ZX 0D948ZX 0D9530Z 0D953ZX 0D953ZZ 0D954ZX 0D957ZX 0D958ZX 0D9630Z 0D963ZX 0D963ZZ 0D964ZX 0D9670Z 0D967ZX 0D9680Z 0D968ZX 0D9730Z 0D973ZX 0D973ZZ 0D974ZX 0D9770Z 0D977ZX 0D9780Z 0D978ZX 0D9830Z 0D983ZX 0D983ZZ 0D984ZX 0D9870Z 0D987ZX 0D9880Z 0D988ZX 0D9930Z 0D993ZX 0D993ZZ 0D994ZX 0D9970Z 0D997ZX 0D9980Z 0D998ZX 0D9A30Z 0D9A3ZX 0D9A3ZZ 0D9A4ZX 0D9A70Z 0D9A7ZX 0D9A80Z 0D9A8ZX 0D9B30Z 0D9B3ZX 0D9B3ZZ 0D9B4ZX 0D9B70Z 0D9B7ZX 0D9B80Z 0D9B8ZX 0D9C30Z 0D9C3ZX 0D9C3ZZ 0D9C4ZX 0D9C7ZX 0D9C8ZX 0D9E30Z 0D9E3ZX 0D9E3ZZ 0D9E4ZX 0D9E70Z 0D9E7ZX 0D9E80Z 0D9E8ZX 0D9F30Z 0D9F3ZX 0D9F3ZZ 0D9F4ZX 0D9F70Z 0D9F7ZX 0D9F80Z 0D9F8ZX 0D9G30Z 0D9G3ZX 0D9G3ZZ 0D9G4ZX 0D9G70Z 0D9G7ZX 0D9G80Z 0D9G8ZX 0D9H30Z 0D9H3ZX 0D9H3ZZ 0D9H4ZX 0D9H70Z 0D9H7ZX 0D9H80Z 0D9H8ZX 0D9J30Z 0D9J3ZZ 0D9K30Z 0D9K3ZX 0D9K3ZZ 0D9K4ZX 0D9K70Z 0D9K7ZX 0D9K80Z 0D9K8ZX 0D9L30Z 0D9L3ZX 0D9L3ZZ 0D9L4ZX 0D9L70Z 0D9L7ZX 0D9L80Z 0D9L8ZX 0D9M30Z 0D9M3ZX 0D9M3ZZ 0D9M4ZX 0D9M70Z 0D9M7ZX 0D9M80Z 0D9M8ZX 0D9N30Z 0D9N3ZX 0D9N3ZZ 0D9N4ZX 0D9N70Z 0D9N7ZX 0D9N80Z 0D9N8ZX 0D9P30Z 0D9P3ZX 0D9P3ZZ 0D9P4ZX 0D9P70Z 0D9P7ZX 0D9P80Z 0D9P8ZX 0D9Q0ZX 0D9Q30Z 0D9Q3ZX 0D9Q3ZZ 0D9Q4ZX 0D9Q7ZX 0D9Q8ZX 0D9QXZX 0D9R0ZX 0D9R30Z 0D9R3ZX 0D9R3ZZ 0D9R4ZX 0D9S30Z 0D9S3ZZ 0D9S40Z 0D9S4ZZ 0D9T30Z 0D9T3ZZ 0D9T40Z 0D9T4ZZ 0D9V30Z 0D9V3ZZ 0D9V40Z 0D9V4ZZ 0D9W30Z 0D9W3ZZ 0D9W40Z 0D9W4ZZ

0 Medical and Surgical
D Gastrointestinal System
B Excision: Cutting out or off, without replacement, a portion of a body part

Body Part Character 4	Approach Character 5	Device Character 6	Qualifier Character 7
1 Esophagus, Upper ⊘ **2** Esophagus, Middle ⊘ **3** Esophagus, Lower ⊘ **4** Esophagogastric Junction ⊘ **5** Esophagus ⊘ **7** Stomach, Pylorus ⊘ **8** Small Intestine ⊘ CC **9** Duodenum ⊘ CC **A** Jejunum ⊘ **B** Ileum ⊘ CC **C** Ileocecal Valve ⊘ **E** Large Intestine ⊘ CC **F** Large Intestine, Right ⊘ **G** Large Intestine, Left ⊘ **H** Cecum ⊘ **J** Appendix **K** Ascending Colon ⊘ **L** Transverse Colon ⊘ **M** Descending Colon ⊘ **N** Sigmoid Colon ⊘ CC **P** Rectum ⊘	**0** Open **3** Percutaneous **4** Percutaneous Endoscopic **7** Via Natural or Artificial Opening **8** Via Natural or Artificial Opening Endoscopic	**Z** No Device	**X** Diagnostic **Z** No Qualifier
6 Stomach ⊘	**0** Open **3** Percutaneous **4** Percutaneous Endoscopic **7** Via Natural or Artificial Opening **8** Via Natural or Artificial Opening Endoscopic	**Z** No Device	**3** Vertical **X** Diagnostic **Z** No Qualifier
Q Anus ⊘	**0** Open **3** Percutaneous **4** Percutaneous Endoscopic **7** Via Natural or Artificial Opening **8** Via Natural or Artificial Opening Endoscopic **X** External	**Z** No Device	**X** Diagnostic **Z** No Qualifier
R Anal Sphincter ⊘ **S** Greater Omentum ⊘ **T** Lesser Omentum ⊘ **V** Mesentery ⊘ **W** Peritoneum ⊘	**0** Open **3** Percutaneous **4** Percutaneous Endoscopic	**Z** No Device	**X** Diagnostic **Z** No Qualifier

CC 0DB80ZZ 0DB90ZZ 0DBB0ZZ 0DBE0ZZ 0DBN0ZZ

⊘ 0DB13ZX 0DB14ZX 0DB14ZZ 0DB17ZX 0DB18ZX 0DB18ZZ 0DB23ZX 0DB24ZX 0DB24ZZ 0DB27ZX 0DB28ZX 0DB28ZZ 0DB33ZX 0DB34ZX 0DB34ZZ 0DB37ZX 0DB38ZX 0DB38ZZ 0DB43ZX 0DB44ZX 0DB47ZX 0DB48ZX 0DB48ZZ 0DB53ZX 0DB54ZX 0DB54ZZ 0DB57ZX 0DB58ZX 0DB58ZZ 0DB63ZX 0DB64ZX 0DB64ZZ 0DB67ZX 0DB68ZX 0DB68ZZ 0DB73ZX 0DB74ZX 0DB74ZZ 0DB77ZX 0DB78ZX 0DB78ZZ 0DB83ZX 0DB84ZX 0DB87ZX 0DB88ZX 0DB93ZX 0DB94ZX 0DB94ZZ 0DB97ZX 0DB98ZX 0DB98ZZ 0DBA3ZX 0DBA4ZX 0DBA7ZX 0DBA8ZX 0DBB3ZX 0DBB4ZX 0DBB7ZX 0DBB8ZX 0DBC3ZX 0DBC4ZX 0DBC7ZX 0DBC8ZX 0DBE3ZX 0DBE4ZX 0DBE7ZX 0DBE8ZX 0DBE8ZZ 0DBF3ZX 0DBF4ZX 0DBF7ZX 0DBF8ZX 0DBF8ZZ 0DBG3ZX 0DBG4ZX 0DBG7ZX 0DBG8ZX 0DBG8ZZ 0DBH3ZX 0DBH4ZX 0DBH7ZX 0DBH8ZX 0DBH8ZZ 0DBK3ZX 0DBK4ZX 0DBK7ZX 0DBK8ZX 0DBK8ZZ 0DBL3ZX 0DBL4ZX 0DBL7ZX 0DBL8ZX 0DBL8ZZ 0DBM3ZX 0DBM4ZX 0DBM7ZX 0DBM8ZX 0DBM8ZZ 0DBN3ZX 0DBN4ZX 0DBN7ZX 0DBN8ZX 0DBN8ZZ 0DBP3ZX 0DBP4ZX 0DBP7ZX 0DBP8ZX 0DBP8ZZ 0DBQ0ZX 0DBQ3ZX 0DBQ4ZX 0DBQ7ZX 0DBQ8ZX 0DBQXZX 0DBR0ZX 0DBR3ZX 0DBR4ZX 0DBS3ZX 0DBS4ZX 0DBT3ZX 0DBT4ZX 0DBV3ZX 0DBV4ZX 0DBW3ZX 0DBW4ZX

0 Medical and Surgical
D Gastrointestinal System
C Extirpation: Taking or cutting out solid matter from a body part

Body Part Character 4	Approach Character 5	Device Character 6	Qualifier Character 7
1 Esophagus, Upper ⦸ **2** Esophagus, Middle ⦸ **3** Esophagus, Lower ⦸ **4** Esophagogastric Junction ⦸ **5** Esophagus ⦸ **6** Stomach ⦸ **7** Stomach, Pylorus ⦸ **8** Small Intestine ⦸ **9** Duodenum ⦸ **A** Jejunum ⦸ **B** Ileum ⦸ **C** Ileocecal Valve ⦸ **E** Large Intestine ⦸ **F** Large Intestine, Right ⦸ **G** Large Intestine, Left ⦸ **H** Cecum ⦸ **J** Appendix **K** Ascending Colon ⦸ **L** Transverse Colon ⦸ **M** Descending Colon ⦸ **N** Sigmoid Colon ⦸ **P** Rectum ⦸	**0** Open **3** Percutaneous **4** Percutaneous Endoscopic **7** Via Natural or Artificial Opening **8** Via Natural or Artificial Opening Endoscopic	**Z** No Device	**Z** No Qualifier
Q Anus ⦸	**0** Open **3** Percutaneous **4** Percutaneous Endoscopic **7** Via Natural or Artificial Opening **8** Via Natural or Artificial Opening Endoscopic **X** External	**Z** No Device	**Z** No Qualifier
R Anal Sphincter **S** Greater Omentum **T** Lesser Omentum **V** Mesentery **W** Peritoneum	**0** Open **3** Percutaneous **4** Percutaneous Endoscopic	**Z** No Device	**Z** No Qualifier

⦸ 0DC17ZZ 0DC18ZZ 0DC27ZZ 0DC28ZZ 0DC37ZZ 0DC38ZZ 0DC47ZZ 0DC48ZZ 0DC57ZZ 0DC58ZZ 0DC67ZZ 0DC68ZZ 0DC77ZZ 0DC78ZZ 0DC87ZZ 0DC88ZZ 0DC97ZZ 0DC98ZZ 0DCA7ZZ 0DCA8ZZ 0DCB7ZZ 0DCB8ZZ 0DCC7ZZ 0DCC8ZZ 0DCE7ZZ 0DCE8ZZ 0DCF7ZZ 0DCF8ZZ 0DCG7ZZ 0DCG8ZZ 0DCH7ZZ 0DCH8ZZ 0DCK7ZZ 0DCK8ZZ 0DCL7ZZ 0DCL8ZZ 0DCM7ZZ 0DCM8ZZ 0DCN7ZZ 0DCN8ZZ 0DCP7ZZ 0DCP8ZZ 0DCQ7ZZ 0DCQ8ZZ 0DCQXZZ

LC Limited Coverage NC Noncovered HAC HAC Associated Procedure CC Combination Cluster - See Appendix G for code lists
DRG Non-OR-Affecting MS-DRG Assignment ⦸ Non-OR-Not Affecting MS-DRG Assignment New/Revised Text in **Orange** ♂ Male ♀ Female

0 Medical and Surgical
D Gastrointestinal System
F Fragmentation: Breaking solid matter in a body part into pieces

Body Part Character 4	Approach Character 5	Device Character 6	Qualifier Character 7
5 Esophagus NC ⊘ 6 Stomach NC ⊘ 8 Small Intestine NC ⊘ 9 Duodenum NC ⊘ A Jejunum NC ⊘ B Ileum NC ⊘ E Large Intestine NC ⊘ F Large Intestine, Right NC ⊘ G Large Intestine, Left NC ⊘ H Cecum NC ⊘ J Appendix NC ⊘ K Ascending Colon NC ⊘ L Transverse Colon NC ⊘ M Descending Colon NC ⊘ N Sigmoid Colon NC ⊘ P Rectum NC ⊘ Q Anus NC ⊘	0 Open 3 Percutaneous 4 Percutaneous Endoscopic 7 Via Natural or Artificial Opening 8 Via Natural or Artificial Opening Endoscopic X External	Z No Device	Z No Qualifier

NC 0DF5XZZ 0DF6XZZ 0DF8XZZ 0DF9XZZ 0DFAXZZ 0DFBXZZ 0DFEXZZ 0DFFXZZ 0DFGXZZ 0DFHXZZ 0DFJXZZ 0DFKXZZ 0DFLXZZ 0DFMXZZ 0DFNXZZ 0DFPXZZ 0DFQXZZ

⊘ 0DF5XZZ 0DF6XZZ 0DF8XZZ 0DF9XZZ 0DFAXZZ 0DFBXZZ 0DFEXZZ 0DFFXZZ 0DFGXZZ 0DFHXZZ 0DFJXZZ 0DFKXZZ 0DFLXZZ 0DFMXZZ 0DFNXZZ 0DFPXZZ 0DFQXZZ

0 Medical and Surgical
D Gastrointestinal System
H Insertion: Putting in a nonbiological appliance that monitors, assists, performs, or prevents a physiological function but does not physically take the place of a body part

Body Part Character 4	Approach Character 5	Device Character 6	Qualifier Character 7
5 Esophagus ⊘	0 Open 3 Percutaneous 4 Percutaneous Endoscopic	1 Radioactive Element 2 Monitoring Device 3 Infusion Device D Intraluminal Device U Feeding Device	Z No Qualifier
5 Esophagus ⊘	7 Via Natural or Artificial Opening 8 Via Natural or Artificial Opening Endoscopic	1 Radioactive Element 2 Monitoring Device 3 Infusion Device B Intraluminal Device, Airway D Intraluminal Device U Feeding Device	Z No Qualifier
6 Stomach ⊘ CC	0 Open 3 Percutaneous 4 Percutaneous Endoscopic	2 Monitoring Device 3 Infusion Device D Intraluminal Device M Stimulator Lead U Feeding Device	Z No Qualifier
6 Stomach ⊘	7 Via Natural or Artificial Opening 8 Via Natural or Artificial Opening Endoscopic	2 Monitoring Device 3 Infusion Device D Intraluminal Device U Feeding Device	Z No Qualifier
8 Small Intestine ⊘ 9 Duodenum ⊘ A Jejunum ⊘ B Ileum ⊘	0 Open 3 Percutaneous 4 Percutaneous Endoscopic 7 Via Natural or Artificial Opening 8 Via Natural or Artificial Opening Endoscopic	2 Monitoring Device 3 Infusion Device D Intraluminal Device U Feeding Device	Z No Qualifier

0DH continued on next page

LC Limited Coverage NC Noncovered HAC HAC Associated Procedure CC Combination Cluster - See Appendix G for code lists
DRG Non-OR-Affecting MS-DRG Assignment ⊘ Non-OR-Not Affecting MS-DRG Assignment New/Revised Text in **Orange** ♂ Male ♀ Female

0D9 continued from previous page

0 Medical and Surgical
D Gastrointestinal System
H Insertion: Putting in a nonbiological appliance that monitors, assists, performs, or prevents a physiological function but does not physically take the place of a body part

Body Part Character 4	Approach Character 5	Device Character 6	Qualifier Character 7
E Large Intestine ⊘	**0** Open **3** Percutaneous **4** Percutaneous Endoscopic **7** Via Natural or Artificial Opening **8** Via Natural or Artificial Opening Endoscopic	**D** Intraluminal Device	**Z** No Qualifier
P Rectum ⊘	**0** Open **3** Percutaneous **4** Percutaneous Endoscopic **7** Via Natural or Artificial Opening **8** Via Natural or Artificial Opening Endoscopic	**1** Radioactive Element **D** Intraluminal Device	**Z** No Qualifier
Q Anus	**0** Open **3** Percutaneous **4** Percutaneous Endoscopic	**D** Intraluminal Device **L** Artificial Sphincter	**Z** No Qualifier
Q Anus	**7** Via Natural or Artificial Opening **8** Via Natural or Artificial Opening Endoscopic	**D** Intraluminal Device	**Z** No Qualifier
R Anal Sphincter	**0** Open **3** Percutaneous **4** Percutaneous Endoscopic	**M** Stimulator Lead	**Z** No Qualifier

CC 0DH60MZ 0DH63MZ 0DH64MZ

⊘ 0DH50DZ 0DH50UZ 0DH53DZ 0DH53UZ 0DH54DZ 0DH54UZ 0DH572Z 0DH573Z 0DH57BZ 0DH57DZ 0DH57UZ 0DH582Z 0DH583Z 0DH58BZ 0DH58DZ 0DH58UZ 0DH63UZ 0DH64UZ 0DH672Z 0DH673Z 0DH67UZ 0DH682Z 0DH683Z 0DH68UZ 0DH80DZ 0DH80UZ 0DH83DZ 0DH83UZ 0DH84DZ 0DH84UZ 0DH872Z 0DH873Z 0DH87DZ 0DH87UZ 0DH882Z 0DH883Z 0DH88DZ 0DH88UZ 0DH90DZ 0DH90UZ 0DH93DZ 0DH93UZ 0DH94DZ 0DH94UZ 0DH972Z 0DH973Z 0DH97DZ 0DH97UZ 0DH982Z 0DH983Z 0DH98DZ 0DH98UZ 0DHA0DZ 0DHA0UZ 0DHA3DZ 0DHA3UZ 0DHA4DZ 0DHA4UZ 0DHA72Z 0DHA73Z 0DHA7DZ 0DHA7UZ 0DHA82Z 0DHA83Z 0DHA8DZ 0DHA8UZ 0DHB0DZ 0DHB0UZ 0DHB3DZ 0DHB3UZ 0DHB4DZ 0DHB4UZ 0DHB72Z 0DHB73Z 0DHB7DZ 0DHB7UZ 0DHB82Z 0DHB83Z 0DHB8DZ 0DHB8UZ 0DHE0DZ 0DHE3DZ 0DHE4DZ 0DHE7DZ 0DHE8DZ 0DHP0DZ 0DHP3DZ 0DHP4DZ 0DHP7DZ 0DHP8DZ

0 Medical and Surgical
D Gastrointestinal System
J Inspection: Visually and/or manually exploring a body part

Body Part Character 4	Approach Character 5	Device Character 6	Qualifier Character 7
0 Upper Intestinal Tract ⊘ **6** Stomach ⊘ **D** Lower Intestinal Tract ⊘	**0** Open **3** Percutaneous **4** Percutaneous Endoscopic **7** Via Natural or Artificial Opening **8** Via Natural or Artificial Opening Endoscopic **X** External	**Z** No Device	**Z** No Qualifier
U Omentum ⊘ **V** Mesentery ⊘ **W** Peritoneum ⊘	**0** Open **3** Percutaneous **4** Percutaneous Endoscopic **X** External	**Z** No Device	**Z** No Qualifier

⊘ 0DJ03ZZ 0DJ07ZZ 0DJ08ZZ 0DJ0XZZ 0DJ63ZZ 0DJ67ZZ 0DJ68ZZ 0DJ6XZZ 0DJD3ZZ 0DJD7ZZ 0DJD8ZZ 0DJDXZZ 0DJU3ZZ 0DJUXZZ 0DJV3ZZ 0DJVXZZ 0DJW3ZZ 0DJWXZZ

0 Medical and Surgical
D Gastrointestinal System
L Occlusion: Completely closing an orifice or the lumen of a tubular body part

Body Part Character 4	Approach Character 5	Device Character 6	Qualifier Character 7
1 Esophagus, Upper ⊘ 2 Esophagus, Middle ⊘ 3 Esophagus, Lower ⊘ 4 Esophagogastric Junction ⊘ 5 Esophagus ⊘ 6 Stomach 7 Stomach, Pylorus 8 Small Intestine 9 Duodenum A Jejunum B Ileum C Ileocecal Valve E Large Intestine F Large Intestine, Right G Large Intestine, Left H Cecum K Ascending Colon L Transverse Colon M Descending Colon N Sigmoid Colon P Rectum	0 Open 3 Percutaneous 4 Percutaneous Endoscopic	C Extraluminal Device D Intraluminal Device Z No Device	Z No Qualifier
1 Esophagus, Upper ⊘ 2 Esophagus, Middle ⊘ 3 Esophagus, Lower ⊘ 4 Esophagogastric Junction ⊘ 5 Esophagus ⊘ 6 Stomach 7 Stomach, Pylorus 8 Small Intestine 9 Duodenum A Jejunum B Ileum C Ileocecal Valve E Large Intestine F Large Intestine, Right G Large Intestine, Left H Cecum K Ascending Colon L Transverse Colon M Descending Colon N Sigmoid Colon P Rectum	7 Via Natural or Artificial Opening 8 Via Natural or Artificial Opening Endoscopic	D Intraluminal Device Z No Device	Z No Qualifier
Q Anus	0 Open 3 Percutaneous 4 Percutaneous Endoscopic X External	C Extraluminal Device D Intraluminal Device Z No Device	Z No Qualifier
Q Anus	7 Via Natural or Artificial Opening 8 Via Natural or Artificial Opening Endoscopic	D Intraluminal Device Z No Device	Z No Qualifier

⊘ 0DL10CZ 0DL10DZ 0DL10ZZ 0DL13CZ 0DL13DZ 0DL13ZZ 0DL14CZ 0DL14DZ 0DL14ZZ 0DL17DZ 0DL17ZZ 0DL18DZ 0DL18ZZ
0DL20CZ 0DL20DZ 0DL20ZZ 0DL23CZ 0DL23DZ 0DL23ZZ 0DL24CZ 0DL24DZ 0DL24ZZ 0DL27DZ 0DL27ZZ 0DL28DZ 0DL28ZZ
0DL30CZ 0DL30DZ 0DL30ZZ 0DL33CZ 0DL33DZ 0DL33ZZ 0DL34CZ 0DL34DZ 0DL34ZZ 0DL37DZ 0DL37ZZ 0DL38DZ 0DL38ZZ
0DL40CZ 0DL40DZ 0DL40ZZ 0DL43CZ 0DL43DZ 0DL43ZZ 0DL44CZ 0DL44DZ 0DL44ZZ 0DL47DZ 0DL47ZZ 0DL48DZ 0DL48ZZ
0DL50CZ 0DL50DZ 0DL50ZZ 0DL53CZ 0DL53DZ 0DL53ZZ 0DL54CZ 0DL54DZ 0DL54ZZ 0DL57DZ 0DL57ZZ 0DL58DZ 0DL58ZZ

0 Medical and Surgical
D Gastrointestinal System
M Reattachment: Putting back in or on all or a portion of a separated body part to its normal location or other suitable location

Body Part Character 4	Approach Character 5	Device Character 6	Qualifier Character 7
5 Esophagus **6** Stomach **8** Small Intestine **9** Duodenum **A** Jejunum **B** Ileum **E** Large Intestine **F** Large Intestine, Right **G** Large Intestine, Left **H** Cecum **K** Ascending Colon **L** Transverse Colon **M** Descending Colon **N** Sigmoid Colon **P** Rectum	**0** Open **4** Percutaneous Endoscopic	**Z** No Device	**Z** No Qualifier

0 Medical and Surgical
D Gastrointestinal System
N Release: Freeing a body part from an abnormal physical constraint by cutting or by the use of force

Body Part Character 4	Approach Character 5	Device Character 6	Qualifier Character 7
1 Esophagus, Upper **2** Esophagus, Middle **3** Esophagus, Lower **4** Esophagogastric Junction **5** Esophagus **6** Stomach **7** Stomach, Pylorus **8** Small Intestine ⊘ **9** Duodenum ⊘ **A** Jejunum ⊘ **B** Ileum ⊘ **C** Ileocecal Valve **E** Large Intestine ⊘ **F** Large Intestine, Right ⊘ **G** Large Intestine, Left ⊘ **H** Cecum ⊘ **J** Appendix **K** Ascending Colon ⊘ **L** Transverse Colon ⊘ **M** Descending Colon ⊘ **N** Sigmoid Colon ⊘ **P** Rectum	**0** Open **3** Percutaneous **4** Percutaneous Endoscopic **7** Via Natural or Artificial Opening **8** Via Natural or Artificial Opening Endoscopic	**Z** No Device	**Z** No Qualifier
Q Anus	**0** Open **3** Percutaneous **4** Percutaneous Endoscopic **7** Via Natural or Artificial Opening **8** Via Natural or Artificial Opening Endoscopic **X** External	**Z** No Device	**Z** No Qualifier
R Anal Sphincter **S** Greater Omentum **T** Lesser Omentum **V** Mesentery **W** Peritoneum	**0** Open **3** Percutaneous **4** Percutaneous Endoscopic	**Z** No Device	**Z** No Qualifier

⊘ 0DN87ZZ 0DN88ZZ 0DN97ZZ 0DN98ZZ 0DNA7ZZ 0DNA8ZZ 0DNB7ZZ 0DNB8ZZ 0DNE7ZZ 0DNE8ZZ 0DNF7ZZ 0DNF8ZZ 0DNG7ZZ 0DNG8ZZ 0DNH7ZZ 0DNH8ZZ 0DNK7ZZ 0DNK8ZZ 0DNL7ZZ 0DNL8ZZ 0DNM7ZZ 0DNM8ZZ 0DNN7ZZ 0DNN8ZZ

0 Medical and Surgical
D Gastrointestinal System
P Removal: Taking out or off a device from a body part

Body Part Character 4	Approach Character 5	Device Character 6	Qualifier Character 7
0 Upper Intestinal Tract ⃠ **D** Lower Intestinal Tract ⃠	**0** Open **3** Percutaneous **4** Percutaneous Endoscopic **7** Via Natural or Artificial Opening **8** Via Natural or Artificial Opening Endoscopic	**0** Drainage Device **2** Monitoring Device **3** Infusion Device **7** Autologous Tissue Substitute **C** Extraluminal Device **D** Intraluminal Device **J** Synthetic Substitute **K** Nonautologous Tissue Substitute **U** Feeding Device	**Z** No Qualifier
0 Upper Intestinal Tract ⃠ **D** Lower Intestinal Tract ⃠	**X** External	**0** Drainage Device **2** Monitoring Device **3** Infusion Device **D** Intraluminal Device **U** Feeding Device	**Z** No Qualifier
5 Esophagus	**0** Open **3** Percutaneous **4** Percutaneous Endoscopic	**1** Radioactive Element **2** Monitoring Device **3** Infusion Device **U** Feeding Device	**Z** No Qualifier
5 Esophagus ⃠	**7** Via Natural or Artificial Opening **8** Via Natural or Artificial Opening Endoscopic	**1** Radioactive Element **D** Intraluminal Device	**Z** No Qualifier
5 Esophagus ⃠	**X** External	**1** Radioactive Element **2** Monitoring Device **3** Infusion Device **D** Intraluminal Device **U** Feeding Device	**Z** No Qualifier
6 Stomach	**0** Open **3** Percutaneous **4** Percutaneous Endoscopic	**0** Drainage Device **2** Monitoring Device **3** Infusion Device **7** Autologous Tissue Substitute **C** Extraluminal Device **D** Intraluminal Device **J** Synthetic Substitute **K** Nonautologous Tissue Substitute **M** Stimulator Lead **U** Feeding Device	**Z** No Qualifier
6 Stomach ⃠	**7** Via Natural or Artificial Opening **8** Via Natural or Artificial Opening Endoscopic	**0** Drainage Device **2** Monitoring Device **3** Infusion Device **7** Autologous Tissue Substitute **C** Extraluminal Device **D** Intraluminal Device **J** Synthetic Substitute **K** Nonautologous Tissue Substitute **U** Feeding Device	**Z** No Qualifier
6 Stomach ⃠	**X** External	**0** Drainage Device **2** Monitoring Device **3** Infusion Device **D** Intraluminal Device **U** Feeding Device	**Z** No Qualifier

0DP continued on next page

0 Medical and Surgical
D Gastrointestinal System
P Removal: Taking out or off a device from a body part

0DP continued from previous page

Body Part Character 4	Approach Character 5	Device Character 6	Qualifier Character 7
P Rectum ⦸	**0** Open **3** Percutaneous **4** Percutaneous Endoscopic **7** Via Natural or Artificial Opening **8** Via Natural or Artificial Opening Endoscopic **X** External	**1** Radioactive Element	**Z** No Qualifier
Q Anus	**0** Open **3** Percutaneous **4** Percutaneous Endoscopic **7** Via Natural or Artificial Opening **8** Via Natural or Artificial Opening Endoscopic	**L** Artificial Sphincter	**Z** No Qualifier
R Anal Sphincter	**0** Open **3** Percutaneous **4** Percutaneous Endoscopic	**M** Stimulator Lead	**Z** No Qualifier
U Omentum **V** Mesentery **W** Peritoneum	**0** Open **3** Percutaneous **4** Percutaneous Endoscopic	**0** Drainage Device **1** Radioactive Element **7** Autologous Tissue Substitute **J** Synthetic Substitute **K** Nonautologous Tissue Substitute	**Z** No Qualifier

⦸ 0DP070Z 0DP072Z 0DP073Z 0DP07DZ 0DP080Z 0DP082Z 0DP083Z 0DP08DZ 0DP0X0Z 0DP0X2Z 0DP0X3Z 0DP0XDZ 0DP0XUZ 0DP571Z 0DP57DZ 0DP581Z 0DP58DZ 0DP5X1Z 0DP5X2Z 0DP5X3Z 0DP5XDZ 0DP5XUZ 0DP670Z 0DP672Z 0DP673Z 0DP67DZ 0DP680Z 0DP682Z 0DP683Z 0DP68DZ 0DP6X0Z 0DP6X2Z 0DP6X3Z 0DP6XDZ 0DP6XUZ 0DPD70Z 0DPD72Z 0DPD73Z 0DPD7DZ 0DPD80Z 0DPD82Z 0DPD83Z 0DPD8DZ 0DPDX0Z 0DPDX2Z 0DPDX3Z 0DPDXDZ 0DPDXUZ 0DPP71Z 0DPP81Z 0DPPX1Z

0 Medical and Surgical
D Gastrointestinal System
Q Repair: Restoring, to the extent possible, a body part to its normal anatomic structure and function

Body Part Character 4	Approach Character 5	Device Character 6	Qualifier Character 7
1 Esophagus, Upper 2 Esophagus, Middle 3 Esophagus, Lower 4 Esophagogastric Junction 5 Esophagus CC 6 Stomach CC 7 Stomach, Pylorus 8 Small Intestine CC 9 Duodenum CC A Jejunum CC B Ileum CC C Ileocecal Valve E Large Intestine CC F Large Intestine, Right CC G Large Intestine, Left CC H Cecum CC J Appendix CC K Ascending Colon CC L Transverse Colon CC M Descending Colon CC N Sigmoid Colon CC P Rectum CC	0 Open 3 Percutaneous 4 Percutaneous Endoscopic 7 Via Natural or Artificial Opening 8 Via Natural or Artificial Opening Endoscopic	Z No Device	Z No Qualifier
Q Anus CC	0 Open 3 Percutaneous 4 Percutaneous Endoscopic 7 Via Natural or Artificial Opening 8 Via Natural or Artificial Opening Endoscopic X External	Z No Device	Z No Qualifier
R Anal Sphincter S Greater Omentum T Lesser Omentum V Mesentery W Peritoneum CC	0 Open 3 Percutaneous 4 Percutaneous Endoscopic	Z No Device	Z No Qualifier

CC 0DQ50ZZ 0DQ53ZZ 0DQ54ZZ 0DQ57ZZ 0DQ58ZZ 0DQ60ZZ 0DQ63ZZ 0DQ64ZZ 0DQ67ZZ 0DQ68ZZ 0DQ80ZZ 0DQ90ZZ 0DQA0ZZ 0DQB0ZZ 0DQE0ZZ 0DQF0ZZ 0DQG0ZZ 0DQH0ZZ 0DQJ0ZZ 0DQJ3ZZ 0DQJ4ZZ 0DQJ7ZZ 0DQJ8ZZ 0DQK0ZZ 0DQL0ZZ 0DQM0ZZ 0DQN0ZZ 0DQN3ZZ 0DQN4ZZ 0DQN7ZZ 0DQN8ZZ 0DQP0ZZ 0DQP3ZZ 0DQP4ZZ 0DQP7ZZ 0DQP8ZZ 0DQQ0ZZ 0DQQ3ZZ 0DQQ4ZZ 0DQQ7ZZ 0DQQ8ZZ 0DQW0ZZ 0DQW3ZZ 0DQW4ZZ

0 Medical and Surgical
D Gastrointestinal System
R Replacement: Putting in or on biological or synthetic material that physically takes the place and/or function of all or a portion of a body part

Body Part Character 4	Approach Character 5	Device Character 6	Qualifier Character 7
5 Esophagus	0 Open 4 Percutaneous Endoscopic 7 Via Natural or Artificial Opening 8 Via Natural or Artificial Opening Endoscopic	7 Autologous Tissue Substitute J Synthetic Substitute K Nonautologous Tissue Substitute	Z No Qualifier
R Anal Sphincter S Greater Omentum T Lesser Omentum V Mesentery W Peritoneum	0 Open 4 Percutaneous Endoscopic	7 Autologous Tissue Substitute J Synthetic Substitute K Nonautologous Tissue Substitute	Z No Qualifier

0 Medical and Surgical
D Gastrointestinal System
S Reposition: Moving to its normal location, or other suitable location, all or a portion of a body part

Body Part Character 4	Approach Character 5	Device Character 6	Qualifier Character 7
5 Esophagus **6** Stomach ⦸ **9** Duodenum ⦸ **A** Jejunum ⦸ **B** Ileum ⦸ **H** Cecum ⦸ **K** Ascending Colon ⦸ **L** Transverse Colon ⦸ **M** Descending Colon ⦸ **N** Sigmoid Colon ⦸ **P** Rectum ⦸ **Q** Anus	**0** Open **4** Percutaneous Endoscopic **7** Via Natural or Artificial Opening **8** Via Natural or Artificial Opening Endoscopic **X** External	**Z** No Device	**Z** No Qualifier

⦸ 0DS6XZZ 0DS9XZZ 0DSAXZZ 0DSBXZZ 0DSHXZZ 0DSKXZZ 0DSLXZZ 0DSMXZZ 0DSNXZZ 0DSPXZZ

0 Medical and Surgical
D Gastrointestinal System
T Resection: Cutting out or off, without replacement, all of a body part

Body Part Character 4	Approach Character 5	Device Character 6	Qualifier Character 7
1 Esophagus, Upper **2** Esophagus, Middle **3** Esophagus, Lower **4** Esophagogastric Junction **5** Esophagus **6** Stomach **7** Stomach, Pylorus **8** Small Intestine **9** Duodenum CC **A** Jejunum **B** Ileum **C** Ileocecal Valve **E** Large Intestine **F** Large Intestine, Right **G** Large Intestine, Left **H** Cecum **J** Appendix **K** Ascending Colon **L** Transverse Colon **M** Descending Colon **N** Sigmoid Colon CC **P** Rectum CC **Q** Anus	**0** Open **4** Percutaneous Endoscopic **7** Via Natural or Artificial Opening **8** Via Natural or Artificial Opening Endoscopic	**Z** No Device	**Z** No Qualifier
R Anal Sphincter **S** Greater Omentum **T** Lesser Omentum	**0** Open **4** Percutaneous Endoscopic	**Z** No Device	**Z** No Qualifier

CC 0DT90ZZ 0DTN0ZZ 0DTN4ZZ 0DTP0ZZ 0DTP4ZZ 0DTP7ZZ 0DTP8ZZ

LC Limited Coverage NC Noncovered HAC HAC Associated Procedure CC Combination Cluster - See Appendix G for code lists
DRG Non-OR-Affecting MS-DRG Assignment ⦸ Non-OR-Not Affecting MS-DRG Assignment New/Revised Text in **Orange** ♂ Male ♀ Female

0 Medical and Surgical
D Gastrointestinal System
U Supplement: Putting in or on biological or synthetic material that physically reinforces and/or augments the function of a portion of a body part

Body Part Character 4	Approach Character 5	Device Character 6	Qualifier Character 7
1 Esophagus, Upper **2** Esophagus, Middle **3** Esophagus, Lower **4** Esophagogastric Junction **5** Esophagus **6** Stomach **7** Stomach, Pylorus **8** Small Intestine **9** Duodenum **A** Jejunum **B** Ileum **C** Ileocecal Valve **E** Large Intestine **F** Large Intestine, Right **G** Large Intestine, Left **H** Cecum **K** Ascending Colon **L** Transverse Colon **M** Descending Colon **N** Sigmoid Colon **P** Rectum	**0** Open **4** Percutaneous Endoscopic **7** Via Natural or Artificial Opening **8** Via Natural or Artificial Opening Endoscopic	**7** Autologous Tissue Substitute **J** Synthetic Substitute **K** Nonautologous Tissue Substitute	**Z** No Qualifier
Q Anus	**0** Open **4** Percutaneous Endoscopic **7** Via Natural or Artificial Opening **8** Via Natural or Artificial Opening Endoscopic **X** External	**7** Autologous Tissue Substitute **J** Synthetic Substitute **K** Nonautologous Tissue Substitute	**Z** No Qualifier
R Anal Sphincter **S** Greater Omentum **T** Lesser Omentum **V** Mesentery **W** Peritoneum	**0** Open **4** Percutaneous Endoscopic	**7** Autologous Tissue Substitute **J** Synthetic Substitute **K** Nonautologous Tissue Substitute	**Z** No Qualifier

0 Medical and Surgical
D Gastrointestinal System
V Restriction: Partially closing an orifice or the lumen of a tubular body part

Body Part Character 4	Approach Character 5	Device Character 6	Qualifier Character 7
1 Esophagus, Upper **2** Esophagus, Middle **3** Esophagus, Lower **4** Esophagogastric Junction **5** Esophagus **6** Stomach HAC **7** Stomach, Pylorus **8** Small Intestine **9** Duodenum **A** Jejunum **B** Ileum **C** Ileocecal Valve **E** Large Intestine **F** Large Intestine, Right **G** Large Intestine, Left **H** Cecum **K** Ascending Colon **L** Transverse Colon **M** Descending Colon **N** Sigmoid Colon **P** Rectum	**0** Open **3** Percutaneous **4** Percutaneous Endoscopic	**C** Extraluminal Device **D** Intraluminal Device **Z** No Device	**Z** No Qualifier
1 Esophagus, Upper **2** Esophagus, Middle **3** Esophagus, Lower **4** Esophagogastric Junction **5** Esophagus **6** Stomach NC ⃠ **7** Stomach, Pylorus **8** Small Intestine **9** Duodenum **A** Jejunum **B** Ileum **C** Ileocecal Valve **E** Large Intestine **F** Large Intestine, Right **G** Large Intestine, Left **H** Cecum **K** Ascending Colon **L** Transverse Colon **M** Descending Colon **N** Sigmoid Colon **P** Rectum	**7** Via Natural or Artificial Opening **8** Via Natural or Artificial Opening Endoscopic	**D** Intraluminal Device **Z** No Device	**Z** No Qualifier
Q Anus	**0** Open **3** Percutaneous **4** Percutaneous Endoscopic **X** External	**C** Extraluminal Device **D** Intraluminal Device **Z** No Device	**Z** No Qualifier
Q Anus	**7** Via Natural or Artificial Opening **8** Via Natural or Artificial Opening Endoscopic	**D** Intraluminal Device **Z** No Device	**Z** No Qualifier

NC 0DV67DZ 0DV68DZ
HAC 0DV64CZ when reported with principal diagnosis E66.01 and secondary diagnosis K68.11, K95.01, K95.81, or T81.4XXA
⃠ 0DV67DZ 0DV68DZ

0 Medical and Surgical
D Gastrointestinal System
W Revision: Correcting, to the extent possible, a portion of a malfunctioning device or the position of a displaced device

Body Part Character 4	Approach Character 5	Device Character 6	Qualifier Character 7
0 Upper Intestinal Tract ⊘ **D** Lower Intestinal Tract ⊘	**0** Open **3** Percutaneous **4** Percutaneous Endoscopic **7** Via Natural or Artificial Opening **8** Via Natural or Artificial Opening Endoscopic **X** External	**0** Drainage Device **2** Monitoring Device **3** Infusion Device **7** Autologous Tissue Substitute **C** Extraluminal Device **D** Intraluminal Device **J** Synthetic Substitute **K** Nonautologous Tissue Substitute **U** Feeding Device	**Z** No Qualifier
5 Esophagus ⊘	**7** Via Natural or Artificial Opening **8** Via Natural or Artificial Opening Endoscopic **X** External	**D** Intraluminal Device	**Z** No Qualifier
6 Stomach	**0** Open **3** Percutaneous **4** Percutaneous Endoscopic	**0** Drainage Device **2** Monitoring Device **3** Infusion Device **7** Autologous Tissue Substitute **C** Extraluminal Device **D** Intraluminal Device **J** Synthetic Substitute **K** Nonautologous Tissue Substitute **M** Stimulator Lead **U** Feeding Device	**Z** No Qualifier
6 Stomach ⊘	**7** Via Natural or Artificial Opening **8** Via Natural or Artificial Opening Endoscopic **X** External	**0** Drainage Device **2** Monitoring Device **3** Infusion Device **7** Autologous Tissue Substitute **C** Extraluminal Device **D** Intraluminal Device **J** Synthetic Substitute **K** Nonautologous Tissue Substitute **U** Feeding Device	**Z** No Qualifier
8 Small Intestine **E** Large Intestine	**0** Open **4** Percutaneous Endoscopic **7** Via Natural or Artificial Opening **8** Via Natural or Artificial Opening Endoscopic	**7** Autologous Tissue Substitute **J** Synthetic Substitute **K** Nonautologous Tissue Substitute	**Z** No Qualifier
Q Anus	**0** Open **3** Percutaneous **4** Percutaneous Endoscopic **7** Via Natural or Artificial Opening **8** Via Natural or Artificial Opening Endoscopic	**L** Artificial Sphincter	**Z** No Qualifier
R Anal Sphincter	**0** Open **3** Percutaneous **4** Percutaneous Endoscopic	**M** Stimulator Lead	**Z** No Qualifier
U Omentum ⊘ **V** Mesentery ⊘ **W** Peritoneum ⊘	**0** Open **3** Percutaneous **4** Percutaneous Endoscopic	**0** Drainage Device **7** Autologous Tissue Substitute **J** Synthetic Substitute **K** Nonautologous Tissue Substitute	**Z** No Qualifier

⊘ 0DW0X0Z 0DW0X2Z 0DW0X3Z 0DW0X7Z 0DW0XCZ 0DW0XDZ 0DW0XJZ 0DW0XKZ 0DW0XUZ 0DW5XDZ 0DW6X0Z 0DW6X2Z 0DW6X3Z 0DW6X7Z 0DW6XCZ 0DW6XDZ 0DW6XJZ 0DW6XKZ 0DW6XUZ 0DWDX0Z 0DWDX2Z 0DWDX3Z 0DWDX7Z 0DWDXCZ 0DWDXDZ 0DWDXJZ 0DWDXKZ 0DWDXUZ 0DWU00Z 0DWU30Z 0DWU40Z 0DWV00Z 0DWV30Z 0DWV40Z 0DWW00Z 0DWW30Z 0DWW40Z

0 Medical and Surgical
D Gastrointestinal System
X Transfer: Moving, without taking out, all or a portion of a body part to another location to take over the function of all or a portion of a body part

Body Part Character 4	Approach Character 5	Device Character 6	Qualifier Character 7
6 Stomach **8** Small Intestine **E** Large Intestine	**0** Open **4** Percutaneous Endoscopic	**Z** No Device	**5** Esophagus

0 Medical and Surgical
D Gastrointestinal System
Y Transplantation: Putting in or on all or a portion of a living body part taken from another individual or animal to physically take the place and/or function of all or a portion of a similar body part

Body Part Character 4	Approach Character 5	Device Character 6	Qualifier Character 7
5 Esophagus ⊘ **6** Stomach **8** Small Intestine LC **E** Large Intestine LC	**0** Open	**Z** No Device	**0** Allogeneic **1** Syngeneic **2** Zooplastic

LC 0DY80Z0 0DY80Z1 0DY80Z2 0DYE0Z0 0DYE0Z1 0DYE0Z2
⊘ 0DY50Z0 0DY50Z1 0DY50Z2

LC Limited Coverage NC Noncovered HAC HAC Associated Procedure CC Combination Cluster - See Appendix G for code lists
DRG Non-OR-Affecting MS-DRG Assignment ⊘ Non-OR-Not Affecting MS-DRG Assignment New/Revised Text in **Orange** ♂ Male ♀ Female

Hepatobiliary System and Pancreas 0F1-0FY

0 Medical and Surgical
F Hepatobiliary System and Pancreas
1 Bypass: Altering the route of passage of the contents of a tubular body part

Body Part Character 4	Approach Character 5	Device Character 6	Qualifier Character 7
4 Gallbladder 5 Hepatic Duct, Right 6 Hepatic Duct, Left 8 Cystic Duct 9 Common Bile Duct CC	0 Open 4 Percutaneous Endoscopic	D Intraluminal Device Z No Device	3 Duodenum 4 Stomach 5 Hepatic Duct, Right 6 Hepatic Duct, Left 7 Hepatic Duct, Caudate 8 Cystic Duct 9 Common Bile Duct B Small Intestine
D Pancreatic Duct F Pancreatic Duct, Accessory G Pancreas CC	0 Open 4 Percutaneous Endoscopic	D Intraluminal Device Z No Device	3 Duodenum B Small Intestine C Large Intestine

CC 0F190Z3 0F1G0ZC

0 Medical and Surgical
F Hepatobiliary System and Pancreas
2 Change: Taking out or off a device from a body part and putting back an identical or similar device in or on the same body part without cutting or puncturing the skin or a mucous membrane

Body Part Character 4	Approach Character 5	Device Character 6	Qualifier Character 7
0 Liver ⊘ 4 Gallbladder ⊘ B Hepatobiliary Duct ⊘ D Pancreatic Duct ⊘ G Pancreas ⊘	X External	0 Drainage Device Y Other Device	Z No Qualifier

⊘ 0F20X0Z 0F20XYZ 0F24X0Z 0F24XYZ 0F2BX0Z 0F2BXYZ 0F2DX0Z 0F2DXYZ 0F2GX0Z 0F2GXYZ

0 Medical and Surgical
F Hepatobiliary System and Pancreas
5 Destruction: Physical eradication of all or a portion of a body part by the direct use of energy, force, or a destructive agent

Body Part Character 4	Approach Character 5	Device Character 6	Qualifier Character 7
0 Liver 1 Liver, Right Lobe 2 Liver, Left Lobe 4 Gallbladder G Pancreas ⊘	0 Open 3 Percutaneous 4 Percutaneous Endoscopic	Z No Device	Z No Qualifier
5 Hepatic Duct, Right ⊘ 6 Hepatic Duct, Left ⊘ 8 Cystic Duct ⊘ 9 Common Bile Duct ⊘ C Ampulla of Vater ⊘ D Pancreatic Duct ⊘ F Pancreatic Duct, Accessory ⊘	0 Open 3 Percutaneous 4 Percutaneous Endoscopic 7 Via Natural or Artificial Opening 8 Via Natural or Artificial Opening Endoscopic	Z No Device	Z No Qualifier

⊘ 0F554ZZ 0F558ZZ 0F564ZZ 0F568ZZ 0F584ZZ 0F588ZZ 0F594ZZ 0F598ZZ 0F5C4ZZ 0F5C8ZZ 0F5D4ZZ 0F5D8ZZ 0F5F4ZZ 0F5F8ZZ 0F5G4ZZ

LC Limited Coverage NC Noncovered HAC HAC Associated Procedure CC Combination Cluster - See Appendix G for code lists
DRG Non-OR-Affecting MS-DRG Assignment ⊘ Non-OR-Not Affecting MS-DRG Assignment New/Revised Text in Orange ♂ Male ♀ Female

0 Medical and Surgical
F Hepatobiliary System and Pancreas
7 Dilation: Expanding an orifice or the lumen of a tubular body part

Body Part Character 4	Approach Character 5	Device Character 6	Qualifier Character 7
5 Hepatic Duct, Right ⊘ CC DRG **6** Hepatic Duct, Left ⊘ CC DRG **8** Cystic Duct ⊘ CC DRG **9** Common Bile Duct ⊘ CC DRG **C** Ampulla of Vater ⊘ **D** Pancreatic Duct ⊘ CC DRG **F** Pancreatic Duct, Accessory ⊘	**0** Open **3** Percutaneous **4** Percutaneous Endoscopic **7** Via Natural or Artificial Opening **8** Via Natural or Artificial Opening Endoscopic	**D** Intraluminal Device **Z** No Device	**Z** No Qualifier

CC 0F757DZ 0F758DZ 0F767DZ 0F768DZ 0F787DZ 0F788DZ 0F797DZ 0F798DZ 0F7D7DZ 0F7D8DZ
DRG 0F757DZ 0F758DZ 0F767DZ 0F768DZ 0F787DZ 0F788DZ 0F797DZ 0F798DZ 0F7D7DZ 0F7D8DZ
⊘ 0F753DZ 0F753ZZ 0F754DZ 0F754ZZ 0F758ZZ 0F763DZ 0F763ZZ 0F764DZ 0F764ZZ 0F768ZZ 0F783DZ 0F783ZZ 0F784DZ 0F784ZZ 0F788ZZ 0F793DZ 0F793ZZ 0F794DZ 0F794ZZ 0F798ZZ 0F7C8DZ 0F7C8ZZ 0F7D4DZ 0F7D4ZZ 0F7D8ZZ 0F7F4DZ 0F7F4ZZ 0F7F8DZ 0F7F8ZZ

0 Medical and Surgical
F Hepatobiliary System and Pancreas
8 Division: Cutting into a body part, without draining fluids and/or gases from the body part, in order to separate or transect a body part

Body Part Character 4	Approach Character 5	Device Character 6	Qualifier Character 7
G Pancreas	**0** Open **3** Percutaneous **4** Percutaneous Endoscopic	**Z** No Device	**Z** No Qualifier

0 Medical and Surgical
F Hepatobiliary System and Pancreas
9 Drainage: Taking or letting out fluids and/or gases from a body part

Body Part Character 4	Approach Character 5	Device Character 6	Qualifier Character 7
0 Liver ⊘ **1** Liver, Right Lobe ⊘ **2** Liver, Left Lobe ⊘ **4** Gallbladder ⊘ **G** Pancreas	**0** Open **3** Percutaneous **4** Percutaneous Endoscopic	**0** Drainage Device	**Z** No Qualifier
0 Liver ⊘ **1** Liver, Right Lobe ⊘ **2** Liver, Left Lobe ⊘ **4** Gallbladder ⊘ **G** Pancreas ⊘	**0** Open **3** Percutaneous **4** Percutaneous Endoscopic	**Z** No Device	**X** Diagnostic **Z** No Qualifier
5 Hepatic Duct, Right ⊘ **6** Hepatic Duct, Left ⊘ **8** Cystic Duct ⊘ **9** Common Bile Duct ⊘ **C** Ampulla of Vater ⊘ **D** Pancreatic Duct ⊘ **F** Pancreatic Duct, Accessory ⊘	**0** Open **3** Percutaneous **4** Percutaneous Endoscopic **7** Via Natural or Artificial Opening **8** Via Natural or Artificial Opening Endoscopic	**0** Drainage Device	**Z** No Qualifier
5 Hepatic Duct, Right ⊘ **6** Hepatic Duct, Left ⊘ **8** Cystic Duct ⊘ **9** Common Bile Duct ⊘ **C** Ampulla of Vater ⊘ **D** Pancreatic Duct ⊘ **F** Pancreatic Duct, Accessory ⊘	**0** Open **3** Percutaneous **4** Percutaneous Endoscopic **7** Via Natural or Artificial Opening **8** Via Natural or Artificial Opening Endoscopic	**Z** No Device	**X** Diagnostic **Z** No Qualifier

⊘ 0F9030Z 0F903ZX 0F903ZZ 0F9040Z 0F904ZX 0F904ZZ 0F9130Z 0F913ZX 0F913ZZ 0F9140Z 0F914ZX 0F914ZZ 0F9230Z 0F923ZX 0F923ZZ 0F9240Z 0F924ZX 0F924ZZ 0F9430Z 0F943ZX 0F943ZZ 0F9440Z 0F944ZX 0F944ZZ 0F9530Z 0F953ZX 0F953ZZ 0F954ZX 0F957ZX 0F958ZX 0F9630Z 0F963ZX 0F963ZZ 0F964ZX 0F967ZX 0F968ZX 0F9830Z 0F983ZX 0F983ZZ 0F984ZX 0F987ZX 0F988ZX 0F9930Z 0F993ZX 0F993ZZ 0F994ZX 0F994ZZ 0F997ZX 0F997ZZ 0F9980Z 0F998ZX 0F998ZZ 0F9C30Z 0F9C3ZX 0F9C3ZZ 0F9C40Z 0F9C4ZX 0F9C4ZZ 0F9C7ZX 0F9C80Z 0F9C8ZX 0F9C8ZZ 0F9D30Z 0F9D3ZX 0F9D3ZZ 0F9D4ZX 0F9D7ZX 0F9D80Z 0F9D8ZX 0F9F30Z 0F9F3ZX 0F9F3ZZ 0F9F4ZX 0F9F7ZX 0F9F80Z 0F9F8ZX 0F9G30Z 0F9G3ZX 0F9G3ZZ 0F9G4ZX

0 Medical and Surgical
F Hepatobiliary System and Pancreas
B Excision: Cutting out or off, without replacement, a portion of a body part

Body Part Character 4	Approach Character 5	Device Character 6	Qualifier Character 7
0 Liver ⊘ **1** Liver, Right Lobe ⊘ **2** Liver, Left Lobe ⊘ **4** Gallbladder ⊘ **G** Pancreas ⊘	**0** Open **3** Percutaneous **4** Percutaneous Endoscopic	**Z** No Device	**X** Diagnostic **Z** No Qualifier
5 Hepatic Duct, Right ⊘ **6** Hepatic Duct, Left ⊘ **8** Cystic Duct ⊘ **9** Common Bile Duct ⊘ **C** Ampulla of Vater ⊘ **D** Pancreatic Duct ⊘ **F** Pancreatic Duct, Accessory ⊘	**0** Open **3** Percutaneous **4** Percutaneous Endoscopic **7** Via Natural or Artificial Opening **8** Via Natural or Artificial Opening Endoscopic	**Z** No Device	**X** Diagnostic **Z** No Qualifier

⊘ 0FB03ZX 0FB13ZX 0FB23ZX 0FB43ZX 0FB44ZX 0FB53ZX 0FB54ZX 0FB54ZZ 0FB57ZX 0FB58ZX 0FB58ZZ 0FB63ZX 0FB64ZX 0FB64ZZ 0FB67ZX 0FB68ZX 0FB68ZZ 0FB83ZX 0FB84ZX 0FB84ZZ 0FB87ZX 0FB88ZX 0FB88ZZ 0FB93ZX 0FB94ZX 0FB94ZZ 0FB97ZX 0FB98ZX 0FB98ZZ 0FBC3ZX 0FBC4ZX 0FBC4ZZ 0FBC7ZX 0FBC8ZX 0FBC8ZZ 0FBD3ZX 0FBD4ZX 0FBD4ZZ 0FBD7ZX 0FBD8ZX 0FBD8ZZ 0FBF3ZX 0FBF4ZX 0FBF4ZZ 0FBF7ZX 0FBF8ZX 0FBF8ZZ 0FBG3ZX 0FBG4ZX

0 Medical and Surgical
F Hepatobiliary System and Pancreas
C Extirpation: Taking or cutting out solid matter from a body part

Body Part Character 4	Approach Character 5	Device Character 6	Qualifier Character 7
0 Liver **1** Liver, Right Lobe **2** Liver, Left Lobe **4** Gallbladder **G** Pancreas	**0** Open **3** Percutaneous **4** Percutaneous Endoscopic	**Z** No Device	**Z** No Qualifier
5 Hepatic Duct, Right ⊘ **6** Hepatic Duct, Left ⊘ **8** Cystic Duct ⊘ **9** Common Bile Duct ⊘ **C** Ampulla of Vater ⊘ **D** Pancreatic Duct ⊘ **F** Pancreatic Duct, Accessory ⊘	**0** Open **3** Percutaneous **4** Percutaneous Endoscopic **7** Via Natural or Artificial Opening **8** Via Natural or Artificial Opening Endoscopic	**Z** No Device	**Z** No Qualifier

⊘ 0FC53ZZ 0FC54ZZ 0FC57ZZ 0FC58ZZ 0FC63ZZ 0FC64ZZ 0FC67ZZ 0FC68ZZ 0FC83ZZ 0FC84ZZ 0FC87ZZ 0FC88ZZ 0FC93ZZ 0FC94ZZ 0FC97ZZ 0FC98ZZ 0FCC4ZZ 0FCC8ZZ 0FCD3ZZ 0FCD4ZZ 0FCD8ZZ 0FCF3ZZ 0FCF4ZZ 0FCF8ZZ

0 Medical and Surgical
F Hepatobiliary System and Pancreas
F Fragmentation: Breaking solid matter in a body part into pieces

Body Part Character 4	Approach Character 5	Device Character 6	Qualifier Character 7
4 Gallbladder NC ⊘ **5** Hepatic Duct, Right NC ⊘ **6** Hepatic Duct, Left NC ⊘ **8** Cystic Duct NC ⊘ **9** Common Bile Duct NC ⊘ **C** Ampulla of Vater NC ⊘ **D** Pancreatic Duct NC ⊘ **F** Pancreatic Duct, Accessory NC ⊘	**0** Open **3** Percutaneous **4** Percutaneous Endoscopic **7** Via Natural or Artificial Opening **8** Via Natural or Artificial Opening Endoscopic **X** External	**Z** No Device	**Z** No Qualifier

NC 0FF4XZZ 0FF5XZZ 0FF6XZZ 0FF8XZZ 0FF9XZZ 0FFCXZZ 0FFDXZZ 0FFFXZZ
⊘ 0FF48ZZ 0FF4XZZ 0FF58ZZ 0FF5XZZ 0FF68ZZ 0FF6XZZ 0FF88ZZ 0FF8XZZ 0FF98ZZ 0FF9XZZ 0FFC8ZZ 0FFCXZZ 0FFDXZZ 0FFFXZZ

0 Medical and Surgical
F Hepatobiliary System and Pancreas
H Insertion: Putting in a nonbiological appliance that monitors, assists, performs, or prevents a physiological function but does not physically take the place of a body part

Body Part Character 4	Approach Character 5	Device Character 6	Qualifier Character 7
0 Liver ⊘ 1 Liver, Right Lobe ⊘ 2 Liver, Left Lobe ⊘ 4 Gallbladder ⊘ G Pancreas ⊘	0 Open 3 Percutaneous 4 Percutaneous Endoscopic	2 Monitoring Device 3 Infusion Device	Z No Qualifier
B Hepatobiliary Duct ⊘ CC DRG D Pancreatic Duct ⊘	0 Open 3 Percutaneous 4 Percutaneous Endoscopic 7 Via Natural or Artificial Opening 8 Via Natural or Artificial Opening Endoscopic	1 Radioactive Element 2 Monitoring Device 3 Infusion Device D Intraluminal Device	Z No Qualifier

DRG 0FHB8DZ
CC 0FHB7DZ 0FHB8DZ
⊘ 0FH003Z 0FH033Z 0FH043Z 0FH103Z 0FH133Z 0FH143Z 0FH203Z 0FH233Z 0FH243Z 0FH403Z 0FH433Z 0FH443Z 0FHB03Z 0FHB33Z 0FHB43Z 0FHB4DZ 0FHB72Z 0FHB73Z 0FHB82Z 0FHB83Z 0FHD03Z 0FHD33Z 0FHD43Z 0FHD4DZ 0FHD72Z 0FHD73Z 0FHD82Z 0FHD83Z 0FHD8DZ 0FHG03Z 0FHG33Z 0FHG43Z

0 Medical and Surgical
F Hepatobiliary System and Pancreas
J Inspection: Visually and/or manually exploring a body part

Body Part Character 4	Approach Character 5	Device Character 6	Qualifier Character 7
0 Liver ⊘ 4 Gallbladder ⊘ G Pancreas ⊘	0 Open 3 Percutaneous 4 Percutaneous Endoscopic X External	Z No Device	Z No Qualifier
B Hepatobiliary Duct ⊘ D Pancreatic Duct ⊘	0 Open 3 Percutaneous 4 Percutaneous Endoscopic 7 Via Natural or Artificial Opening 8 Via Natural or Artificial Opening Endoscopic	Z No Device	Z No Qualifier

⊘ 0FJ03ZZ 0FJ0XZZ 0FJ43ZZ 0FJ4XZZ 0FJB3ZZ 0FJB7ZZ 0FJB8ZZ 0FJD3ZZ 0FJD7ZZ 0FJD8ZZ 0FJG3ZZ 0FJGXZZ

0 Medical and Surgical
F Hepatobiliary System and Pancreas
L Occlusion: Completely closing an orifice or the lumen of a tubular body part

Body Part Character 4	Approach Character 5	Device Character 6	Qualifier Character 7
5 Hepatic Duct, Right ⊘ 6 Hepatic Duct, Left ⊘ 8 Cystic Duct ⊘ 9 Common Bile Duct ⊘ C Ampulla of Vater D Pancreatic Duct F Pancreatic Duct, Accessory	0 Open 3 Percutaneous 4 Percutaneous Endoscopic	C Extraluminal Device D Intraluminal Device Z No Device	Z No Qualifier
5 Hepatic Duct, Right ⊘ 6 Hepatic Duct, Left ⊘ 8 Cystic Duct ⊘ 9 Common Bile Duct ⊘ C Ampulla of Vater D Pancreatic Duct F Pancreatic Duct, Accessory	7 Via Natural or Artificial Opening 8 Via Natural or Artificial Opening Endoscopic	D Intraluminal Device Z No Device	Z No Qualifier

⊘ 0FL53CZ 0FL53DZ 0FL53ZZ 0FL54CZ 0FL54DZ 0FL54ZZ 0FL57DZ 0FL57ZZ 0FL58DZ 0FL58ZZ 0FL63CZ 0FL63DZ 0FL63ZZ 0FL64CZ 0FL64DZ 0FL64ZZ 0FL67DZ 0FL67ZZ 0FL68DZ 0FL68ZZ 0FL83CZ 0FL83DZ 0FL83ZZ 0FL84CZ 0FL84DZ 0FL84ZZ 0FL87DZ 0FL87ZZ 0FL88DZ 0FL88ZZ 0FL93CZ 0FL93DZ 0FL93ZZ 0FL94CZ 0FL94DZ 0FL94ZZ 0FL97DZ 0FL97ZZ 0FL98DZ 0FL98ZZ

LC Limited Coverage NC Noncovered HAC HAC Associated Procedure CC Combination Cluster - See Appendix G for code lists
DRG Non-OR-Affecting MS-DRG Assignment ⊘ Non-OR-Not Affecting MS-DRG Assignment New/Revised Text in **Orange** ♂ Male ♀ Female

0 Medical and Surgical
F Hepatobiliary System and Pancreas
M Reattachment: Putting back in or on all or a portion of a separated body part to its normal location or other suitable location

Body Part Character 4	Approach Character 5	Device Character 6	Qualifier Character 7
0 Liver **1** Liver, Right Lobe **2** Liver, Left Lobe **4** Gallbladder ⊘ **5** Hepatic Duct, Right ⊘ **6** Hepatic Duct, Left ⊘ **8** Cystic Duct ⊘ **9** Common Bile Duct ⊘ **C** Ampulla of Vater **D** Pancreatic Duct **F** Pancreatic Duct, Accessory **G** Pancreas	**0** Open **4** Percutaneous Endoscopic	**Z** No Device	**Z** No Qualifier

⊘ 0FM44ZZ 0FM54ZZ 0FM64ZZ 0FM84ZZ 0FM94ZZ

0 Medical and Surgical
F Hepatobiliary System and Pancreas
N Release: Freeing a body part from an abnormal physical constraint by cutting or by the use of force

Body Part Character 4	Approach Character 5	Device Character 6	Qualifier Character 7
0 Liver **1** Liver, Right Lobe **2** Liver, Left Lobe **4** Gallbladder **G** Pancreas	**0** Open **3** Percutaneous **4** Percutaneous Endoscopic	**Z** No Device	**Z** No Qualifier
5 Hepatic Duct, Right **6** Hepatic Duct, Left **8** Cystic Duct **9** Common Bile Duct **C** Ampulla of Vater **D** Pancreatic Duct **F** Pancreatic Duct, Accessory	**0** Open **3** Percutaneous **4** Percutaneous Endoscopic **7** Via Natural or Artificial Opening **8** Via Natural or Artificial Opening Endoscopic	**Z** No Device	**Z** No Qualifier

0 Medical and Surgical
F Hepatobiliary System and Pancreas
P Removal: Taking out or off a device from a body part

Body Part Character 4	Approach Character 5	Device Character 6	Qualifier Character 7
0 Liver ⊘	**0** Open **3** Percutaneous **4** Percutaneous Endoscopic **X** External	**0** Drainage Device **2** Monitoring Device **3** Infusion Device	**Z** No Qualifier
4 Gallbladder ⊘ **G** Pancreas ⊘	**0** Open **3** Percutaneous **4** Percutaneous Endoscopic **X** External	**0** Drainage Device **2** Monitoring Device **3** Infusion Device **D** Intraluminal Device	**Z** No Qualifier
B Hepatobiliary Duct ⊘ CC **D** Pancreatic Duct ⊘ CC	**0** Open **3** Percutaneous **4** Percutaneous Endoscopic **7** Via Natural or Artificial Opening **8** Via Natural or Artificial Opening Endoscopic	**0** Drainage Device **1** Radioactive Element **2** Monitoring Device **3** Infusion Device **7** Autologous Tissue Substitute **C** Extraluminal Device **D** Intraluminal Device **J** Synthetic Substitute **K** Nonautologous Tissue Substitute	**Z** No Qualifier
B Hepatobiliary Duct ⊘ CC DRG **D** Pancreatic Duct ⊘ CC DRG	**X** External	**0** Drainage Device **1** Radioactive Element **2** Monitoring Device **3** Infusion Device **D** Intraluminal Device	**Z** No Qualifier

CC 0FPB7DZ 0FPB8DZ 0FPBXDZ 0FPD7DZ 0FPD8DZ 0FPDXDZ
DRG 0FPBXDZ 0FPDXDZ
⊘ 0FP0X0Z 0FP0X2Z 0FP0X3Z 0FP4X0Z 0FP4X2Z 0FP4X3Z 0FP4XDZ 0FPB70Z 0FPB72Z 0FPB73Z 0FPB7DZ 0FPB80Z 0FPB82Z 0FPB83Z 0FPB8DZ 0FPBX0Z 0FPBX1Z 0FPBX2Z 0FPBX3Z 0FPD70Z 0FPD72Z 0FPD73Z 0FPD7DZ 0FPD80Z 0FPD82Z 0FPD83Z 0FPD8DZ 0FPDX0Z 0FPDX1Z 0FPDX2Z 0FPDX3Z 0FPGX0Z 0FPGX2Z 0FPGX3Z

0 Medical and Surgical
F Hepatobiliary System and Pancreas
Q Repair: Restoring, to the extent possible, a body part to its normal anatomic structure and function

Body Part Character 4	Approach Character 5	Device Character 6	Qualifier Character 7
0 Liver CC **1** Liver, Right Lobe **2** Liver, Left Lobe **4** Gallbladder CC **G** Pancreas	**0** Open **3** Percutaneous **4** Percutaneous Endoscopic	**Z** No Device	**Z** No Qualifier
5 Hepatic Duct, Right **6** Hepatic Duct, Left **8** Cystic Duct **9** Common Bile Duct **C** Ampulla of Vater **D** Pancreatic Duct **F** Pancreatic Duct, Accessory	**0** Open **3** Percutaneous **4** Percutaneous Endoscopic **7** Via Natural or Artificial Opening **8** Via Natural or Artificial Opening Endoscopic	**Z** No Device	**Z** No Qualifier

CC 0FQ00ZZ 0FQ03ZZ 0FQ04ZZ 0FQ40ZZ 0FQ43ZZ 0FQ44ZZ

0 Medical and Surgical
F Hepatobiliary System and Pancreas
R Replacement: Putting in or on biological or synthetic material that physically takes the place and/or function of all or a portion of a body part

Body Part Character 4	Approach Character 5	Device Character 6	Qualifier Character 7
5 Hepatic Duct, Right **6** Hepatic Duct, Left **8** Cystic Duct **9** Common Bile Duct **C** Ampulla of Vater **D** Pancreatic Duct **F** Pancreatic Duct, Accessory	**0** Open **4** Percutaneous Endoscopic	**7** Autologous Tissue Substitute **J** Synthetic Substitute **K** Nonautologous Tissue Substitute	**Z** No Qualifier

0 Medical and Surgical
F Hepatobiliary System and Pancreas
S Reposition: Moving to its normal location, or other suitable location, all or a portion of a body part

Body Part Character 4	Approach Character 5	Device Character 6	Qualifier Character 7
0 Liver **4** Gallbladder **5** Hepatic Duct, Right **6** Hepatic Duct, Left **8** Cystic Duct **9** Common Bile Duct **C** Ampulla of Vater **D** Pancreatic Duct **F** Pancreatic Duct, Accessory **G** Pancreas	**0** Open **4** Percutaneous Endoscopic	**Z** No Device	**Z** No Qualifier

0 Medical and Surgical
F Hepatobiliary System and Pancreas
T Resection: Cutting out or off, without replacement, all of a body part

Body Part Character 4	Approach Character 5	Device Character 6	Qualifier Character 7
0 Liver **1** Liver, Right Lobe **2** Liver, Left Lobe **4** Gallbladder **G** Pancreas CC	**0** Open **4** Percutaneous Endoscopic	**Z** No Device	**Z** No Qualifier
5 Hepatic Duct, Right **6** Hepatic Duct, Left **8** Cystic Duct **9** Common Bile Duct **C** Ampulla of Vater **D** Pancreatic Duct ⃠ **F** Pancreatic Duct, Accessory ⃠	**0** Open **4** Percutaneous Endoscopic **7** Via Natural or Artificial Opening **8** Via Natural or Artificial Opening Endoscopic	**Z** No Device	**Z** No Qualifier

CC 0FTG0ZZ
⃠ 0FTD4ZZ 0FTD8ZZ 0FTF4ZZ 0FTF8ZZ

0 Medical and Surgical
F Hepatobiliary System and Pancreas
U Supplement: Putting in or on biological or synthetic material that physically reinforces and/or augments the function of a portion of a body part

Body Part Character 4	Approach Character 5	Device Character 6	Qualifier Character 7
5 Hepatic Duct, Right **6** Hepatic Duct, Left **8** Cystic Duct **9** Common Bile Duct **C** Ampulla of Vater **D** Pancreatic Duct **F** Pancreatic Duct, Accessory	**0** Open **3** Percutaneous **4** Percutaneous Endoscopic	**7** Autologous Tissue Substitute **J** Synthetic Substitute **K** Nonautologous Tissue Substitute	**Z** No Qualifier

0 Medical and Surgical
F Hepatobiliary System and Pancreas
V Restriction: Partially closing an orifice or the lumen of a tubular body part

Body Part Character 4	Approach Character 5	Device Character 6	Qualifier Character 7
5 Hepatic Duct, Right ⊘ **6** Hepatic Duct, Left ⊘ **8** Cystic Duct ⊘ **9** Common Bile Duct ⊘ **C** Ampulla of Vater **D** Pancreatic Duct **F** Pancreatic Duct, Accessory	**0** Open **3** Percutaneous **4** Percutaneous Endoscopic	**C** Extraluminal Device **D** Intraluminal Device **Z** No Device	**Z** No Qualifier
5 Hepatic Duct, Right ⊘ **6** Hepatic Duct, Left ⊘ **8** Cystic Duct ⊘ **9** Common Bile Duct ⊘ **C** Ampulla of Vater **D** Pancreatic Duct **F** Pancreatic Duct, Accessory	**7** Via Natural or Artificial Opening **8** Via Natural or Artificial Opening Endoscopic	**D** Intraluminal Device **Z** No Device	**Z** No Qualifier

⊘ 0FV53CZ 0FV53DZ 0FV53ZZ 0FV54CZ 0FV54DZ 0FV54ZZ 0FV57DZ 0FV57ZZ 0FV58DZ 0FV58ZZ 0FV63CZ 0FV63DZ 0FV63ZZ 0FV64CZ 0FV64DZ 0FV64ZZ 0FV67DZ 0FV67ZZ 0FV68DZ 0FV68ZZ 0FV83CZ 0FV83DZ 0FV83ZZ 0FV84CZ 0FV84DZ 0FV84ZZ 0FV87DZ 0FV87ZZ 0FV88DZ 0FV88ZZ 0FV93CZ 0FV93DZ 0FV93ZZ 0FV94CZ 0FV94DZ 0FV94ZZ 0FV97DZ 0FV97ZZ 0FV98DZ 0FV98ZZ

0 Medical and Surgical
F Hepatobiliary System and Pancreas
W Revision: Correcting, to the extent possible, a portion of a malfunctioning device or the position of a displaced device

Body Part Character 4	Approach Character 5	Device Character 6	Qualifier Character 7
0 Liver ⊘	**0** Open **3** Percutaneous **4** Percutaneous Endoscopic **X** External	**0** Drainage Device **2** Monitoring Device **3** Infusion Device	**Z** No Qualifier
4 Gallbladder ⊘ **G** Pancreas ⊘	**0** Open **3** Percutaneous **4** Percutaneous Endoscopic **X** External	**0** Drainage Device **2** Monitoring Device **3** Infusion Device **D** Intraluminal Device	**Z** No Qualifier
B Hepatobiliary Duct ⊘ **D** Pancreatic Duct ⊘	**0** Open **3** Percutaneous **4** Percutaneous Endoscopic **7** Via Natural or Artificial Opening **8** Via Natural or Artificial Opening Endoscopic **X** External	**0** Drainage Device **2** Monitoring Device **3** Infusion Device **7** Autologous Tissue Substitute **C** Extraluminal Device **D** Intraluminal Device **J** Synthetic Substitute **K** Nonautologous Tissue Substitute	**Z** No Qualifier

⊘ 0FW0X0Z 0FW0X2Z 0FW0X3Z 0FW4X0Z 0FW4X2Z 0FW4X3Z 0FW4XDZ 0FWBX0Z 0FWBX2Z 0FWBX3Z 0FWBX7Z 0FWBXCZ 0FWBXDZ 0FWBXJZ 0FWBXKZ 0FWDX0Z 0FWDX2Z 0FWDX3Z 0FWDX7Z 0FWDXCZ 0FWDXDZ 0FWDXJZ 0FWDXKZ 0FWGX0Z 0FWGX2Z 0FWGX3Z 0FWGXDZ

0 Medical and Surgical
F Hepatobiliary System and Pancreas
Y Transplantation: Putting in or on all or a portion of a living body part taken from another individual or animal to physically take the place and/or function of all or a portion of a similar body part

Body Part Character 4	Approach Character 5	Device Character 6	Qualifier Character 7
0 Liver LC **G** Pancreas NC LC CC	**0** Open	**Z** No Device	**0** Allogeneic **1** Syngeneic **2** Zooplastic

LC 0FY00Z0 0FY00Z1 0FY00Z2 0FYG0Z0 0FYG0Z1

NC 0FYG0Z0 0FYG0Z1 or 0FYG0Z2 ICD-10-PCS procedure codes for pancreas transplants (0FYG0Z0, 0FYG0Z1) alone [without kidney transplant codes (0TY00Z0, 0TY00Z1, 0TY00Z2, 0TY10Z0, 0TY10Z1, 0TY10Z2)] are considered noncovered procedures except for the following condition: When either 0FYG0Z0 (Transplantation of Pancreas, Allogeneic, Open Approach) or 0FYG0Z1 (Transplantation of Pancreas, Syngeneic, Open Approach) is combined with at least one principal or secondary diagnosis code from the following diagnoses list: E10.10-E10.9, E89.1.

CC 0FYG0Z0 0FYG0Z1 0FYG0Z2

Endocrine System 0G2-0GW

0 Medical and Surgical
G Endocrine System
2 Change: Taking out or off a device from a body part and putting back an identical or similar device in or on the same body part without cutting or puncturing the skin or a mucous membrane

Body Part Character 4	Approach Character 5	Device Character 6	Qualifier Character 7
0 Pituitary Gland ⦸ **1** Pineal Body ⦸ **5** Adrenal Gland ⦸ **K** Thyroid Gland ⦸ **R** Parathyroid Gland ⦸ **S** Endocrine Gland ⦸	**X** External	**0** Drainage Device **Y** Other Device	**Z** No Qualifier

⦸ 0G20X0Z 0G20XYZ 0G21X0Z 0G21XYZ 0G25X0Z 0G25XYZ 0G2KX0Z 0G2KXYZ 0G2RX0Z 0G2RXYZ 0G2SX0Z 0G2SXYZ

0 Medical and Surgical
G Endocrine System
5 Destruction: Physical eradication of all or a portion of a body part by the direct use of energy, force, or a destructive agent

Body Part Character 4	Approach Character 5	Device Character 6	Qualifier Character 7
0 Pituitary Gland **1** Pineal Body **2** Adrenal Gland, Left **3** Adrenal Gland, Right **4** Adrenal Glands, Bilateral **6** Carotid Body, Left ⦸ **7** Carotid Body, Right ⦸ **8** Carotid Bodies, Bilateral ⦸ **9** Para-aortic Body ⦸ **B** Coccygeal Glomus ⦸ **C** Glomus Jugulare ⦸ **D** Aortic Body ⦸ **F** Paraganglion Extremity ⦸ **G** Thyroid Gland Lobe, Left **H** Thyroid Gland Lobe, Right **K** Thyroid Gland **L** Superior Parathyroid Gland, Right **M** Superior Parathyroid Gland, Left **N** Inferior Parathyroid Gland, Right **P** Inferior Parathyroid Gland, Left **Q** Parathyroid Glands, Multiple **R** Parathyroid Gland	**0** Open **3** Percutaneous **4** Percutaneous Endoscopic	**Z** No Device	**Z** No Qualifier

⦸ 0G560ZZ 0G563ZZ 0G564ZZ 0G570ZZ 0G573ZZ 0G574ZZ 0G580ZZ 0G583ZZ 0G584ZZ 0G590ZZ 0G593ZZ 0G594ZZ 0G5B0ZZ 0G5B3ZZ 0G5B4ZZ 0G5C0ZZ 0G5C3ZZ 0G5C4ZZ 0G5D0ZZ 0G5D3ZZ 0G5D4ZZ 0G5F0ZZ 0G5F3ZZ 0G5F4ZZ

0 Medical and Surgical
G Endocrine System
8 Division: Cutting into a body part, without draining fluids and/or gases from the body part, in order to separate or transect a body part

Body Part Character 4	Approach Character 5	Device Character 6	Qualifier Character 7
0 Pituitary Gland **J** Thyroid Gland Isthmus	**0** Open **3** Percutaneous **4** Percutaneous Endoscopic	**Z** No Device	**Z** No Qualifier

0 Medical and Surgical
G Endocrine System
9 Drainage: Taking or letting out fluids and/or gases from a body part

Body Part Character 4	Approach Character 5	Device Character 6	Qualifier Character 7
0 Pituitary Gland ⊘ **1** Pineal Body ⊘ **2** Adrenal Gland, Left ⊘ **3** Adrenal Gland, Right ⊘ **4** Adrenal Glands, Bilateral ⊘ **6** Carotid Body, Left ⊘ **7** Carotid Body, Right ⊘ **8** Carotid Bodies, Bilateral ⊘ **9** Para-aortic Body ⊘ **B** Coccygeal Glomus ⊘ **C** Glomus Jugulare ⊘ **D** Aortic Body ⊘ **F** Paraganglion Extremity ⊘ **G** Thyroid Gland Lobe, Left ⊘ **H** Thyroid Gland Lobe, Right ⊘ **K** Thyroid Gland ⊘ **L** Superior Parathyroid Gland, Right ⊘ **M** Superior Parathyroid Gland, Left ⊘ **N** Inferior Parathyroid Gland, Right ⊘ **P** Inferior Parathyroid Gland, Left ⊘ **Q** Parathyroid Glands, Multiple ⊘ **R** Parathyroid Gland ⊘	**0** Open **3** Percutaneous **4** Percutaneous Endoscopic	**0** Drainage Device	**Z** No Qualifier
0 Pituitary Gland **1** Pineal Body **2** Adrenal Gland, Left ⊘ **3** Adrenal Gland, Right ⊘ **4** Adrenal Glands, Bilateral ⊘ **6** Carotid Body, Left ⊘ **7** Carotid Body, Right ⊘ **8** Carotid Bodies, Bilateral ⊘ **9** Para-aortic Body ⊘ **B** Coccygeal Glomus ⊘ **C** Glomus Jugulare ⊘ **D** Aortic Body ⊘ **F** Paraganglion Extremity ⊘ **G** Thyroid Gland Lobe, Left ⊘ **H** Thyroid Gland Lobe, Right ⊘ **K** Thyroid Gland ⊘ **L** Superior Parathyroid Gland, Right ⊘ **M** Superior Parathyroid Gland, Left ⊘ **N** Inferior Parathyroid Gland, Right ⊘ **P** Inferior Parathyroid Gland, Left ⊘ **Q** Parathyroid Glands, Multiple ⊘ **R** Parathyroid Gland ⊘	**0** Open **3** Percutaneous **4** Percutaneous Endoscopic	**Z** No Device	**X** Diagnostic **Z** No Qualifier

⊘ 0G9030Z 0G903ZZ 0G9130Z 0G913ZZ 0G9230Z 0G923ZX 0G923ZZ 0G924ZX 0G9330Z 0G933ZX 0G933ZZ 0G934ZX 0G9430Z 0G943ZX 0G943ZZ 0G944ZX 0G9600Z 0G960ZX 0G960ZZ 0G9630Z 0G963ZX 0G963ZZ 0G9640Z 0G964ZX 0G964ZZ 0G9700Z 0G970ZX 0G970ZZ 0G9730Z 0G973ZX 0G973ZZ 0G9740Z 0G974ZX 0G974ZZ 0G9800Z 0G980ZX 0G980ZZ 0G9830Z 0G983ZX 0G983ZZ 0G9840Z 0G984ZX 0G984ZZ 0G9900Z 0G990ZX 0G990ZZ 0G9930Z 0G993ZX 0G993ZZ 0G9940Z 0G994ZX 0G994ZZ 0G9B00Z 0G9B0ZX 0G9B0ZZ 0G9B30Z 0G9B3ZX 0G9B3ZZ 0G9B40Z 0G9B4ZX 0G9B4ZZ 0G9C00Z 0G9C0ZX 0G9C0ZZ 0G9C30Z 0G9C3ZX 0G9C3ZZ 0G9C40Z 0G9C4ZX 0G9C4ZZ 0G9D00Z 0G9D0ZX 0G9D0ZZ 0G9D30Z 0G9D3ZX 0G9D3ZZ 0G9D40Z 0G9D4ZX 0G9D4ZZ 0G9F00Z 0G9F0ZX 0G9F0ZZ 0G9F30Z 0G9F3ZX 0G9F3ZZ 0G9F40Z 0G9F4ZX 0G9F4ZZ 0G9G30Z 0G9G3ZX 0G9G3ZZ 0G9G40Z 0G9G4ZX 0G9G4ZZ 0G9H30Z 0G9H3ZX 0G9H3ZZ 0G9H40Z 0G9H4ZX 0G9H4ZZ 0G9K30Z 0G9K3ZX 0G9K3ZZ 0G9K40Z 0G9K4ZX 0G9K4ZZ 0G9L30Z 0G9L3ZZ 0G9L40Z 0G9L4ZZ 0G9M30Z 0G9M3ZZ 0G9M40Z 0G9M4ZZ 0G9N30Z 0G9N3ZZ 0G9N40Z 0G9N4ZZ 0G9P30Z 0G9P3ZZ 0G9P40Z 0G9P4ZZ 0G9Q30Z 0G9Q3ZZ 0G9Q40Z 0G9Q4ZZ 0G9R30Z 0G9R3ZZ 0G9R40Z 0G9R4ZZ

LC Limited Coverage NC Noncovered HAC HAC Associated Procedure CC Combination Cluster - See Appendix G for code lists
DRG Non-OR-Affecting MS-DRG Assignment ⊘ Non-OR-Not Affecting MS-DRG Assignment New/Revised Text in **Orange** ♂ Male ♀ Female

0 Medical and Surgical
G Endocrine System
B Excision: Cutting out or off, without replacement, a portion of a body part

Body Part Character 4	Approach Character 5	Device Character 6	Qualifier Character 7
0 Pituitary Gland **1** Pineal Body **2** Adrenal Gland, Left ⃠ **3** Adrenal Gland, Right ⃠ **4** Adrenal Glands, Bilateral ⃠ **6** Carotid Body, Left ⃠ **7** Carotid Body, Right ⃠ **8** Carotid Bodies, Bilateral ⃠ **9** Para-aortic Body ⃠ **B** Coccygeal Glomus ⃠ **C** Glomus Jugulare ⃠ **D** Aortic Body ⃠ **F** Paraganglion Extremity ⃠ **G** Thyroid Gland Lobe, Left ⃠ **H** Thyroid Gland Lobe, Right ⃠ **L** Superior Parathyroid Gland, Right **M** Superior Parathyroid Gland, Left **N** Inferior Parathyroid Gland, Right **P** Inferior Parathyroid Gland, Left **Q** Parathyroid Glands, Multiple **R** Parathyroid Gland	**0** Open **3** Percutaneous **4** Percutaneous Endoscopic	**Z** No Device	**X** Diagnostic **Z** No Qualifier

⃠ 0GB23ZX 0GB24ZX 0GB33ZX 0GB34ZX 0GB43ZX 0GB44ZX 0GB60ZX 0GB60ZZ 0GB63ZX 0GB63ZZ 0GB64ZX 0GB64ZZ 0GB70ZX 0GB70ZZ 0GB73ZX 0GB73ZZ 0GB74ZX 0GB74ZZ 0GB80ZX 0GB80ZZ 0GB83ZX 0GB83ZZ 0GB84ZX 0GB84ZZ 0GB90ZX 0GB90ZZ 0GB93ZX 0GB93ZZ 0GB94ZX 0GB94ZZ 0GBB0ZX 0GBB0ZZ 0GBB3ZX 0GBB3ZZ 0GBB4ZX 0GBB4ZZ 0GBC0ZX 0GBC0ZZ 0GBC3ZX 0GBC3ZZ 0GBC4ZX 0GBC4ZZ 0GBD0ZX 0GBD0ZZ 0GBD3ZX 0GBD3ZZ 0GBD4ZX 0GBD4ZZ 0GBF0ZX 0GBF0ZZ 0GBF3ZX 0GBF3ZZ 0GBF4ZX 0GBF4ZZ 0GBG3ZX 0GBG4ZX 0GBH3ZX 0GBH4ZX

0 Medical and Surgical
G Endocrine System
C Extirpation: Taking or cutting out solid matter from a body part

Body Part Character 4	Approach Character 5	Device Character 6	Qualifier Character 7
0 Pituitary Gland **1** Pineal Body **2** Adrenal Gland, Left **3** Adrenal Gland, Right **4** Adrenal Glands, Bilateral **6** Carotid Body, Left ⃠ **7** Carotid Body, Right ⃠ **8** Carotid Bodies, Bilateral ⃠ **9** Para-aortic Body ⃠ **B** Coccygeal Glomus ⃠ **C** Glomus Jugulare ⃠ **D** Aortic Body ⃠ **F** Paraganglion Extremity ⃠ **G** Thyroid Gland Lobe, Left **H** Thyroid Gland Lobe, Right **K** Thyroid Gland **L** Superior Parathyroid Gland, Right **M** Superior Parathyroid Gland, Left **N** Inferior Parathyroid Gland, Right **P** Inferior Parathyroid Gland, Left **Q** Parathyroid Glands, Multiple **R** Parathyroid Gland	**0** Open **3** Percutaneous **4** Percutaneous Endoscopic	**Z** No Device	**Z** No Qualifier

⃠ 0GC60ZZ 0GC63ZZ 0GC64ZZ 0GC70ZZ 0GC73ZZ 0GC74ZZ 0GC80ZZ 0GC83ZZ 0GC84ZZ 0GC90ZZ 0GC93ZZ 0GC94ZZ 0GCB0ZZ 0GCB3ZZ 0GCB4ZZ 0GCC0ZZ 0GCC3ZZ 0GCC4ZZ 0GCD0ZZ 0GCD3ZZ 0GCD4ZZ 0GCF0ZZ 0GCF3ZZ 0GCF4ZZ

0 Medical and Surgical
G Endocrine System
H Insertion: Putting in a nonbiological appliance that monitors, assists, performs, or prevents a physiological function but does not physically take the place of a body part

Body Part Character 4	Approach Character 5	Device Character 6	Qualifier Character 7
S Endocrine Gland	0 Open 3 Percutaneous 4 Percutaneous Endoscopic	2 Monitoring Device 3 Infusion Device	Z No Qualifier

0 Medical and Surgical
G Endocrine System
J Inspection: Visually and/or manually exploring a body part

Body Part Character 4	Approach Character 5	Device Character 6	Qualifier Character 7
0 Pituitary Gland ⃠ 1 Pineal Body ⃠ 5 Adrenal Gland ⃠ K Thyroid Gland ⃠ R Parathyroid Gland ⃠ S Endocrine Gland ⃠	0 Open 3 Percutaneous 4 Percutaneous Endoscopic	Z No Device	Z No Qualifier

⃠ 0GJ03ZZ 0GJ13ZZ 0GJ53ZZ 0GJK3ZZ 0GJR3ZZ 0GJS3ZZ

0 Medical and Surgical
G Endocrine System
M Reattachment: Putting back in or on all or a portion of a separated body part to its normal location or other suitable location

Body Part Character 4	Approach Character 5	Device Character 6	Qualifier Character 7
2 Adrenal Gland, Left 3 Adrenal Gland, Right G Thyroid Gland Lobe, Left H Thyroid Gland Lobe, Right L Superior Parathyroid Gland, Right M Superior Parathyroid Gland, Left N Inferior Parathyroid Gland, Right P Inferior Parathyroid Gland, Left Q Parathyroid Glands, Multiple R Parathyroid Gland	0 Open 4 Percutaneous Endoscopic	Z No Device	Z No Qualifier

0 Medical and Surgical
G Endocrine System
N Release: Freeing a body part from an abnormal physical constraint by cutting or by the use of force

Body Part Character 4	Approach Character 5	Device Character 6	Qualifier Character 7
0 Pituitary Gland **1** Pineal Body **2** Adrenal Gland, Left **3** Adrenal Gland, Right **4** Adrenal Glands, Bilateral **6** Carotid Body, Left ⦸ **7** Carotid Body, Right ⦸ **8** Carotid Bodies, Bilateral ⦸ **9** Para-aortic Body ⦸ **B** Coccygeal Glomus ⦸ **C** Glomus Jugulare ⦸ **D** Aortic Body ⦸ **F** Paraganglion Extremity ⦸ **G** Thyroid Gland Lobe, Left **H** Thyroid Gland Lobe, Right **K** Thyroid Gland **L** Superior Parathyroid Gland, Right **M** Superior Parathyroid Gland, Left **N** Inferior Parathyroid Gland, Right **P** Inferior Parathyroid Gland, Left **Q** Parathyroid Glands, Multiple **R** Parathyroid Gland	**0** Open **3** Percutaneous **4** Percutaneous Endoscopic	**Z** No Device	**Z** No Qualifier

⦸ 0GN60ZZ 0GN63ZZ 0GN64ZZ 0GN70ZZ 0GN73ZZ 0GN74ZZ 0GN80ZZ 0GN83ZZ 0GN84ZZ 0GN90ZZ 0GN93ZZ 0GN94ZZ 0GNB0ZZ 0GNB3ZZ 0GNB4ZZ 0GNC0ZZ 0GNC3ZZ 0GNC4ZZ 0GND0ZZ 0GND3ZZ 0GND4ZZ 0GNF0ZZ 0GNF3ZZ 0GNF4ZZ

0 Medical and Surgical
G Endocrine System
P Removal: Taking out or off a device from a body part

Body Part Character 4	Approach Character 5	Device Character 6	Qualifier Character 7
0 Pituitary Gland ⦸ **1** Pineal Body ⦸ **5** Adrenal Gland ⦸ **K** Thyroid Gland ⦸ **R** Parathyroid Gland ⦸	**0** Open **3** Percutaneous **4** Percutaneous Endoscopic **X** External	**0** Drainage Device	**Z** No Qualifier
S Endocrine Gland ⦸	**0** Open **3** Percutaneous **4** Percutaneous Endoscopic **X** External	**0** Drainage Device **2** Monitoring Device **3** Infusion Device	**Z** No Qualifier

⦸ 0GP0X0Z 0GP1X0Z 0GP5X0Z 0GPKX0Z 0GPRX0Z 0GPS00Z 0GPS02Z 0GPS03Z 0GPS30Z 0GPS32Z 0GPS33Z 0GPS40Z 0GPS42Z 0GPS43Z 0GPSX0Z 0GPSX2Z 0GPSX3Z

0 Medical and Surgical
G Endocrine System
Q Repair: Restoring, to the extent possible, a body part to its normal anatomic structure and function

Body Part Character 4	Approach Character 5	Device Character 6	Qualifier Character 7
0 Pituitary Gland **1** Pineal Body **2** Adrenal Gland, Left **3** Adrenal Gland, Right **4** Adrenal Glands, Bilateral **6** Carotid Body, Left ⃠ **7** Carotid Body, Right ⃠ **8** Carotid Bodies, Bilateral ⃠ **9** Para-aortic Body ⃠ **B** Coccygeal Glomus ⃠ **C** Glomus Jugulare ⃠ **D** Aortic Body ⃠ **F** Paraganglion Extremity ⃠ **G** Thyroid Gland Lobe, Left **H** Thyroid Gland Lobe, Right **J** Thyroid Gland Isthmus **K** Thyroid Gland **L** Superior Parathyroid Gland, Right **M** Superior Parathyroid Gland, Left **N** Inferior Parathyroid Gland, Right **P** Inferior Parathyroid Gland, Left **Q** Parathyroid Glands, Multiple **R** Parathyroid Gland	**0** Open **3** Percutaneous **4** Percutaneous Endoscopic	**Z** No Device	**Z** No Qualifier

⃠ 0GQ60ZZ 0GQ63ZZ 0GQ64ZZ 0GQ70ZZ 0GQ73ZZ 0GQ74ZZ 0GQ80ZZ 0GQ83ZZ 0GQ84ZZ 0GQ90ZZ 0GQ93ZZ 0GQ94ZZ 0GQB0ZZ 0GQB3ZZ 0GQB4ZZ 0GQC0ZZ 0GQC3ZZ 0GQC4ZZ 0GQD0ZZ 0GQD3ZZ 0GQD4ZZ 0GQF0ZZ 0GQF3ZZ 0GQF4ZZ

0 Medical and Surgical
G Endocrine System
S Reposition: Moving to its normal location, or other suitable location, all or a portion of a body part

Body Part Character 4	Approach Character 5	Device Character 6	Qualifier Character 7
2 Adrenal Gland, Left **3** Adrenal Gland, Right **G** Thyroid Gland Lobe, Left **H** Thyroid Gland Lobe, Right **L** Superior Parathyroid Gland, Right **M** Superior Parathyroid Gland, Left **N** Inferior Parathyroid Gland, Right **P** Inferior Parathyroid Gland, Left **Q** Parathyroid Glands, Multiple **R** Parathyroid Gland	**0** Open **4** Percutaneous Endoscopic	**Z** No Device	**Z** No Qualifier

0 Medical and Surgical
G Endocrine System
T Resection: Cutting out or off, without replacement, all of a body part

Body Part Character 4	Approach Character 5	Device Character 6	Qualifier Character 7
0 Pituitary Gland 1 Pineal Body 2 Adrenal Gland, Left 3 Adrenal Gland, Right 4 Adrenal Glands, Bilateral 6 Carotid Body, Left ⊘ 7 Carotid Body, Right ⊘ 8 Carotid Bodies, Bilateral ⊘ 9 Para-aortic Body ⊘ B Coccygeal Glomus ⊘ C Glomus Jugulare ⊘ D Aortic Body ⊘ F Paraganglion Extremity ⊘ G Thyroid Gland Lobe, Left H Thyroid Gland Lobe, Right K Thyroid Gland L Superior Parathyroid Gland, Right M Superior Parathyroid Gland, Left N Inferior Parathyroid Gland, Right P Inferior Parathyroid Gland, Left Q Parathyroid Glands, Multiple R Parathyroid Gland	0 Open 4 Percutaneous Endoscopic	Z No Device	Z No Qualifier

⊘ 0GT60ZZ 0GT64ZZ 0GT70ZZ 0GT74ZZ 0GT80ZZ 0GT84ZZ 0GT90ZZ 0GT94ZZ 0GTB0ZZ 0GTB4ZZ 0GTC0ZZ 0GTC4ZZ 0GTD0ZZ 0GTD4ZZ 0GTF0ZZ 0GTF4ZZ

0 Medical and Surgical
G Endocrine System
W Revision: Correcting, to the extent possible, a portion of a malfunctioning device or the position of a displaced device

Body Part Character 4	Approach Character 5	Device Character 6	Qualifier Character 7
0 Pituitary Gland ⊘ 1 Pineal Body ⊘ 5 Adrenal Gland ⊘ K Thyroid Gland ⊘ R Parathyroid Gland ⊘	0 Open 3 Percutaneous 4 Percutaneous Endoscopic X External	0 Drainage Device	Z No Qualifier
S Endocrine Gland ⊘	0 Open 3 Percutaneous 4 Percutaneous Endoscopic X External	0 Drainage Device 2 Monitoring Device 3 Infusion Device	Z No Qualifier

⊘ 0GW0X0Z 0GW1X0Z 0GW5X0Z 0GWKX0Z 0GWRX0Z 0GWS00Z 0GWS02Z 0GWS03Z 0GWS30Z 0GWS32Z 0GWS33Z 0GWS40Z 0GWS42Z 0GWS43Z 0GWSX0Z 0GWSX2Z 0GWSX3Z

Skin and Breast 0H0-0HX

0 Medical and Surgical
H Skin and Breast
0 Alteration: Modifying the anatomic structure of a body part without affecting the function of the body part

Body Part Character 4	Approach Character 5	Device Character 6	Qualifier Character 7
T Breast, Right U Breast, Left V Breast, Bilateral	0 Open 3 Percutaneous X External	7 Autologous Tissue Substitute J Synthetic Substitute K Nonautologous Tissue Substitute Z No Device	Z No Qualifier

0 Medical and Surgical
H Skin and Breast
2 Change: Taking out or off a device from a body part and putting back an identical or similar device in or on the same body part without cutting or puncturing the skin or a mucous membrane

Body Part Character 4	Approach Character 5	Device Character 6	Qualifier Character 7
P Skin ⊘ T Breast, Right ⊘ U Breast, Left ⊘	X External	0 Drainage Device Y Other Device	Z No Qualifier

⊘ 0H2PX0Z 0H2PXYZ 0H2TX0Z 0H2TXYZ 0H2UX0Z 0H2UXYZ

0 Medical and Surgical
H Skin and Breast
5 Destruction: Physical eradication of all or a portion of a body part by the direct use of energy, force, or a destructive agent

Body Part Character 4	Approach Character 5	Device Character 6	Qualifier Character 7
0 Skin, Scalp DRG 1 Skin, Face DRG 2 Skin, Right Ear ⊘ 3 Skin, Left Ear ⊘ 4 Skin, Neck DRG 5 Skin, Chest DRG 6 Skin, Back DRG 7 Skin, Abdomen DRG 8 Skin, Buttock DRG 9 Skin, Perineum DRG A Skin, Genitalia DRG B Skin, Right Upper Arm DRG C Skin, Left Upper Arm DRG D Skin, Right Lower Arm DRG E Skin, Left Lower Arm DRG F Skin, Right Hand DRG G Skin, Left Hand DRG H Skin, Right Upper Leg DRG J Skin, Left Upper Leg DRG K Skin, Right Lower Leg DRG L Skin, Left Lower Leg DRG M Skin, Right Foot DRG N Skin, Left Foot DRG	X External	Z No Device	D Multiple Z No Qualifier
Q Finger Nail DRG R Toe Nail DRG	X External	Z No Device	Z No Qualifier
T Breast, Right U Breast, Left V Breast, Bilateral W Nipple, Right X Nipple, Left	0 Open 3 Percutaneous 7 Via Natural or Artificial Opening 8 Via Natural or Artificial Opening Endoscopic X External	Z No Device	Z No Qualifier

DRG 0H50XZD 0H50XZZ 0H51XZD 0H51XZZ 0H54XZD 0H54XZZ 0H55XZD 0H55XZZ 0H56XZD 0H56XZZ 0H57XZD 0H57XZZ 0H58XZD 0H58XZZ 0H59XZD 0H59XZZ 0H5AXZD 0H5AXZZ 0H5BXZD 0H5BXZZ 0H5CXZD 0H5CXZZ 0H5DXZD 0H5DXZZ 0H5EXZD 0H5EXZZ 0H5FXZD 0H5FXZZ 0H5GXZD 0H5GXZZ 0H5HXZD 0H5HXZZ 0H5JXZD 0H5JXZZ 0H5KXZD 0H5KXZZ 0H5LXZD 0H5LXZZ 0H5MXZD 0H5MXZZ 0H5NXZD 0H5NXZZ 0H5QXZZ 0H5RXZZ

⊘ 0H52XZD 0H52XZZ 0H53XZD 0H53XZZ

0 Medical and Surgical
H Skin and Breast
8 Division: Cutting into a body part, without draining fluids and/or gases from the body part, in order to separate or transect a body part

Body Part Character 4	Approach Character 5	Device Character 6	Qualifier Character 7
0 Skin, Scalp **1** Skin, Face **2** Skin, Right Ear ⃠ **3** Skin, Left Ear ⃠ **4** Skin, Neck **5** Skin, Chest **6** Skin, Back **7** Skin, Abdomen **8** Skin, Buttock **9** Skin, Perineum **A** Skin, Genitalia **B** Skin, Right Upper Arm **C** Skin, Left Upper Arm **D** Skin, Right Lower Arm **E** Skin, Left Lower Arm **F** Skin, Right Hand **G** Skin, Left Hand **H** Skin, Right Upper Leg **J** Skin, Left Upper Leg **K** Skin, Right Lower Leg **L** Skin, Left Lower Leg **M** Skin, Right Foot **N** Skin, Left Foot	**X** External	**Z** No Device	**Z** No Qualifier

⃠ 0H82XZZ 0H83XZZ

0 Medical and Surgical
H Skin and Breast
9 Drainage: Taking or letting out fluids and/or gases from a body part

Body Part Character 4	Approach Character 5	Device Character 6	Qualifier Character 7
0 Skin, Scalp ⃠ **1** Skin, Face ⃠ **2** Skin, Right Ear ⃠ **3** Skin, Left Ear ⃠ **4** Skin, Neck ⃠ **5** Skin, Chest ⃠ **6** Skin, Back ⃠ **7** Skin, Abdomen ⃠ **8** Skin, Buttock ⃠ **9** Skin, Perineum ⃠ **A** Skin, Genitalia ⃠ **B** Skin, Right Upper Arm ⃠ **C** Skin, Left Upper Arm ⃠ **D** Skin, Right Lower Arm ⃠ **E** Skin, Left Lower Arm ⃠ **F** Skin, Right Hand ⃠ **G** Skin, Left Hand ⃠ **H** Skin, Right Upper Leg ⃠ **J** Skin, Left Upper Leg ⃠ **K** Skin, Right Lower Leg ⃠ **L** Skin, Left Lower Leg ⃠ **M** Skin, Right Foot ⃠ **N** Skin, Left Foot ⃠ **Q** Finger Nail ⃠ **R** Toe Nail ⃠	**X** External	**0** Drainage Device	**Z** No Qualifier

0H9 continued on next page

0 Medical and Surgical
H Skin and Breast
9 Drainage: Taking or letting out fluids and/or gases from a body part

0H9 continued from previous page

Body Part Character 4	Approach Character 5	Device Character 6	Qualifier Character 7
0 Skin, Scalp ⦸ **1** Skin, Face ⦸ **2** Skin, Right Ear ⦸ **3** Skin, Left Ear ⦸ **4** Skin, Neck ⦸ **5** Skin, Chest ⦸ **6** Skin, Back ⦸ **7** Skin, Abdomen ⦸ **8** Skin, Buttock ⦸ **9** Skin, Perineum ⦸ **A** Skin, Genitalia ⦸ **B** Skin, Right Upper Arm ⦸ **C** Skin, Left Upper Arm ⦸ **D** Skin, Right Lower Arm ⦸ **E** Skin, Left Lower Arm ⦸ **F** Skin, Right Hand ⦸ **G** Skin, Left Hand ⦸ **H** Skin, Right Upper Leg ⦸ **J** Skin, Left Upper Leg ⦸ **K** Skin, Right Lower Leg ⦸ **L** Skin, Left Lower Leg ⦸ **M** Skin, Right Foot ⦸ **N** Skin, Left Foot ⦸ **Q** Finger Nail ⦸ **R** Toe Nail ⦸	**X** External	**Z** No Device	**X** Diagnostic **Z** No Qualifier
T Breast, Right ⦸ **U** Breast, Left ⦸ **V** Breast, Bilateral ⦸ **W** Nipple, Right ⦸ **X** Nipple, Left ⦸	**0** Open **3** Percutaneous **7** Via Natural or Artificial Opening **8** Via Natural or Artificial Opening Endoscopic **X** External	**0** Drainage Device	**Z** No Qualifier
T Breast, Right ⦸ **U** Breast, Left ⦸ **V** Breast, Bilateral ⦸ **W** Nipple, Right ⦸ **X** Nipple, Left ⦸	**0** Open **3** Percutaneous **7** Via Natural or Artificial Opening **8** Via Natural or Artificial Opening Endoscopic **X** External	**Z** No Device	**X** Diagnostic **Z** No Qualifier

⦸ 0H90X0Z 0H90XZX 0H90XZZ 0H91X0Z 0H91XZX 0H91XZZ 0H92X0Z 0H92XZX 0H92XZZ 0H93X0Z 0H93XZX 0H93XZZ 0H94X0Z 0H94XZX 0H94XZZ 0H95X0Z 0H95XZX 0H95XZZ 0H96X0Z 0H96XZX 0H96XZZ 0H97X0Z 0H97XZX 0H97XZZ 0H98X0Z 0H98XZX 0H98XZZ 0H99XZX 0H9AX0Z 0H9AXZX 0H9AXZZ 0H9BX0Z 0H9BXZX 0H9BXZZ 0H9CX0Z 0H9CXZX 0H9CXZZ 0H9DX0Z 0H9DXZX 0H9DXZZ 0H9EX0Z 0H9EXZX 0H9EXZZ 0H9FX0Z 0H9FXZX 0H9FXZZ 0H9GX0Z 0H9GXZX 0H9GXZZ 0H9HX0Z 0H9HXZX 0H9HXZZ 0H9JX0Z 0H9JXZX 0H9JXZZ 0H9KX0Z 0H9KXZX 0H9KXZZ 0H9LX0Z 0H9LXZX 0H9LXZZ 0H9MX0Z 0H9MXZX 0H9MXZZ 0H9NX0Z 0H9NXZX 0H9NXZZ 0H9QX0Z 0H9QXZX 0H9QXZZ 0H9RX0Z 0H9RXZX 0H9RXZZ 0H9T00Z 0H9T0ZZ 0H9T30Z 0H9T3ZX 0H9T3ZZ 0H9T70Z 0H9T7ZX 0H9T7ZZ 0H9T80Z 0H9T8ZX 0H9T8ZZ 0H9TX0Z 0H9TXZX 0H9TXZZ 0H9U00Z 0H9U0ZZ 0H9U30Z 0H9U3ZX 0H9U3ZZ 0H9U70Z 0H9U7ZX 0H9U7ZZ 0H9U80Z 0H9U8ZX 0H9U8ZZ 0H9UX0Z 0H9UXZX 0H9UXZZ 0H9V00Z 0H9V0ZZ 0H9V30Z 0H9V3ZX 0H9V3ZZ 0H9V70Z 0H9V7ZX 0H9V7ZZ 0H9V80Z 0H9V8ZX 0H9V8ZZ 0H9VX0Z 0H9VXZX 0H9VXZZ 0H9W00Z 0H9W0ZZ 0H9W30Z 0H9W3ZX 0H9W3ZZ 0H9W70Z 0H9W7ZX 0H9W7ZZ 0H9W80Z 0H9W8ZX 0H9W8ZZ 0H9WX0Z 0H9WXZX 0H9WXZZ 0H9X00Z 0H9X0ZZ 0H9X30Z 0H9X3ZX 0H9X3ZZ 0H9X70Z 0H9X7ZX 0H9X7ZZ 0H9X80Z 0H9X8ZX 0H9X8ZZ 0H9XX0Z 0H9XXZX 0H9XXZZ

0 Medical and Surgical
H Skin and Breast
B Excision: Cutting out or off, without replacement, a portion of a body part

Body Part Character 4	Approach Character 5	Device Character 6	Qualifier Character 7
0 Skin, Scalp ⊘ **1** Skin, Face ⊘ **2** Skin, Right Ear ⊘ **3** Skin, Left Ear ⊘ **4** Skin, Neck ⊘ **5** Skin, Chest ⊘ **6** Skin, Back ⊘ **7** Skin, Abdomen ⊘ **8** Skin, Buttock ⊘ **9** Skin, Perineum ⊘ DRG **A** Skin, Genitalia ⊘ **B** Skin, Right Upper Arm ⊘ **C** Skin, Left Upper Arm ⊘ **D** Skin, Right Lower Arm ⊘ **E** Skin, Left Lower Arm ⊘ **F** Skin, Right Hand ⊘ **G** Skin, Left Hand ⊘ **H** Skin, Right Upper Leg ⊘ **J** Skin, Left Upper Leg ⊘ **K** Skin, Right Lower Leg ⊘ **L** Skin, Left Lower Leg ⊘ **M** Skin, Right Foot ⊘ **N** Skin, Left Foot ⊘ **Q** Finger Nail ⊘ **R** Toe Nail ⊘	**X** External	**Z** No Device	**X** Diagnostic **Z** No Qualifier
T Breast, Right ⊘ **U** Breast, Left ⊘ **V** Breast, Bilateral ⊘ **W** Nipple, Right ⊘ **X** Nipple, Left ⊘ **Y** Supernumerary Breast ⊘	**0** Open **3** Percutaneous **7** Via Natural or Artificial Opening **8** Via Natural or Artificial Opening Endoscopic **X** External	**Z** No Device	**X** Diagnostic **Z** No Qualifier

DRG 0HB9XZZ

⊘ 0HB0XZX 0HB1XZX 0HB2XZX 0HB2XZZ 0HB3XZX 0HB3XZZ 0HB4XZX 0HB5XZX 0HB6XZX 0HB7XZX 0HB8XZX 0HB9XZX 0HBAXZX 0HBBXZX 0HBCXZX 0HBDXZX 0HBEXZX 0HBFXZX 0HBGXZX 0HBHXZX 0HBJXZX 0HBKXZX 0HBLXZX 0HBMXZX 0HBNXZX 0HBQXZX 0HBQXZZ 0HBRXZX 0HBRXZZ 0HBT3ZX 0HBT7ZX 0HBT8ZX 0HBTXZX 0HBU3ZX 0HBU7ZX 0HBU8ZX 0HBUXZX 0HBV3ZX 0HBV7ZX 0HBV8ZX 0HBVXZX 0HBW3ZX 0HBW7ZX 0HBW8ZX 0HBWXZX 0HBX3ZX 0HBX7ZX 0HBX8ZX 0HBXXZX 0HBY3ZX 0HBY7ZX 0HBY8ZX 0HBYXZX

0 Medical and Surgical
H Skin and Breast
C Extirpation: Taking or cutting out solid matter from a body part

Body Part Character 4	Approach Character 5	Device Character 6	Qualifier Character 7
0 Skin, Scalp ⦸ **1** Skin, Face ⦸ **2** Skin, Right Ear ⦸ **3** Skin, Left Ear ⦸ **4** Skin, Neck ⦸ **5** Skin, Chest ⦸ **6** Skin, Back ⦸ **7** Skin, Abdomen ⦸ **8** Skin, Buttock ⦸ **9** Skin, Perineum ⦸ **A** Skin, Genitalia ⦸ **B** Skin, Right Upper Arm ⦸ **C** Skin, Left Upper Arm ⦸ **D** Skin, Right Lower Arm ⦸ **E** Skin, Left Lower Arm ⦸ **F** Skin, Right Hand ⦸ **G** Skin, Left Hand ⦸ **H** Skin, Right Upper Leg ⦸ **J** Skin, Left Upper Leg ⦸ **K** Skin, Right Lower Leg ⦸ **L** Skin, Left Lower Leg ⦸ **M** Skin, Right Foot ⦸ **N** Skin, Left Foot ⦸ **Q** Finger Nail ⦸ **R** Toe Nail ⦸	**X** External	**Z** No Device	**Z** No Qualifier
T Breast, Right ⦸ **U** Breast, Left ⦸ **V** Breast, Bilateral ⦸ **W** Nipple, Right ⦸ **X** Nipple, Left ⦸	**0** Open **3** Percutaneous **7** Via Natural or Artificial Opening **8** Via Natural or Artificial Opening Endoscopic **X** External	**Z** No Device	**Z** No Qualifier

⦸ 0HC0XZZ 0HC1XZZ 0HC2XZZ 0HC3XZZ 0HC4XZZ 0HC5XZZ 0HC6XZZ 0HC7XZZ 0HC8XZZ 0HC9XZZ 0HCAXZZ 0HCBXZZ 0HCCXZZ 0HCDXZZ 0HCEXZZ 0HCFXZZ 0HCGXZZ 0HCHXZZ 0HCJXZZ 0HCKXZZ 0HCLXZZ 0HCMXZZ 0HCNXZZ 0HCQXZZ 0HCRXZZ 0HCT0ZZ 0HCT3ZZ 0HCT7ZZ 0HCT8ZZ 0HCTXZZ 0HCU0ZZ 0HCU3ZZ 0HCU7ZZ 0HCU8ZZ 0HCUXZZ 0HCV0ZZ 0HCV3ZZ 0HCV7ZZ 0HCV8ZZ 0HCVXZZ 0HCW0ZZ 0HCW3ZZ 0HCW7ZZ 0HCW8ZZ 0HCWXZZ 0HCX0ZZ 0HCX3ZZ 0HCX7ZZ 0HCX8ZZ 0HCXXZZ

0 Medical and Surgical
H Skin and Breast
D Extraction: Pulling or stripping out or off all or a portion of a body part by the use of force

Body Part Character 4	Approach Character 5	Device Character 6	Qualifier Character 7
0 Skin, Scalp ⊘ 1 Skin, Face ⊘ 2 Skin, Right Ear ⊘ 3 Skin, Left Ear ⊘ 4 Skin, Neck ⊘ 5 Skin, Chest ⊘ 6 Skin, Back ⊘ 7 Skin, Abdomen ⊘ 8 Skin, Buttock ⊘ 9 Skin, Perineum ⊘ A Skin, Genitalia ⊘ B Skin, Right Upper Arm ⊘ C Skin, Left Upper Arm ⊘ D Skin, Right Lower Arm ⊘ E Skin, Left Lower Arm ⊘ F Skin, Right Hand ⊘ G Skin, Left Hand ⊘ H Skin, Right Upper Leg ⊘ J Skin, Left Upper Leg ⊘ K Skin, Right Lower Leg ⊘ L Skin, Left Lower Leg ⊘ M Skin, Right Foot ⊘ N Skin, Left Foot ⊘ Q Finger Nail ⊘ R Toe Nail ⊘ S Hair ⊘	X External	Z No Device	Z No Qualifier

⊘ 0HD0XZZ 0HD1XZZ 0HD2XZZ 0HD3XZZ 0HD4XZZ 0HD5XZZ 0HD6XZZ 0HD7XZZ 0HD8XZZ 0HD9XZZ 0HDAXZZ 0HDBXZZ 0HDCXZZ 0HDDXZZ 0HDEXZZ 0HDFXZZ 0HDGXZZ 0HDHXZZ 0HDJXZZ 0HDKXZZ 0HDLXZZ 0HDMXZZ 0HDNXZZ 0HDQXZZ 0HDRXZZ 0HDSXZZ

0 Medical and Surgical
H Skin and Breast
H Insertion: Putting in a nonbiological appliance that monitors, assists, performs, or prevents a physiological function but does not physically take the place of a body part

Body Part Character 4	Approach Character 5	Device Character 6	Qualifier Character 7
T Breast, Right U Breast, Left V Breast, Bilateral W Nipple, Right X Nipple, Left	0 Open 3 Percutaneous 7 Via Natural or Artificial Opening 8 Via Natural or Artificial Opening Endoscopic	1 Radioactive Element N Tissue Expander	Z No Qualifier
T Breast, Right U Breast, Left V Breast, Bilateral W Nipple, Right X Nipple, Left	X External	1 Radioactive Element	Z No Qualifier

0 Medical and Surgical
H Skin and Breast
J Inspection: Visually and/or manually exploring a body part

Body Part Character 4	Approach Character 5	Device Character 6	Qualifier Character 7
P Skin ⦸ **Q** Finger Nail ⦸ **R** Toe Nail ⦸	**X** External	**Z** No Device	**Z** No Qualifier
T Breast, Right ⦸ **U** Breast, Left ⦸	**0** Open **3** Percutaneous **7** Via Natural or Artificial Opening **8** Via Natural or Artificial Opening Endoscopic **X** External	**Z** No Device	**Z** No Qualifier

⦸ 0HJPXZZ 0HJQXZZ 0HJRXZZ 0HJT0ZZ 0HJT3ZZ 0HJT7ZZ 0HJT8ZZ 0HJTXZZ 0HJU0ZZ 0HJU3ZZ 0HJU7ZZ 0HJU8ZZ 0HJUXZZ

0 Medical and Surgical
H Skin and Breast
M Reattachment: Putting back in or on all or a portion of a separated body part to its normal location or other suitable location

Body Part Character 4	Approach Character 5	Device Character 6	Qualifier Character 7
0 Skin, Scalp ⦸ **1** Skin, Face **2** Skin, Right Ear **3** Skin, Left Ear **4** Skin, Neck **5** Skin, Chest **6** Skin, Back **7** Skin, Abdomen **8** Skin, Buttock **9** Skin, Perineum **A** Skin, Genitalia **B** Skin, Right Upper Arm **C** Skin, Left Upper Arm **D** Skin, Right Lower Arm **E** Skin, Left Lower Arm **F** Skin, Right Hand **G** Skin, Left Hand **H** Skin, Right Upper Leg **J** Skin, Left Upper Leg **K** Skin, Right Lower Leg **L** Skin, Left Lower Leg **M** Skin, Right Foot **N** Skin, Left Foot **T** Breast, Right **U** Breast, Left **V** Breast, Bilateral **W** Nipple, Right **X** Nipple, Left	**X** External	**Z** No Device	**Z** No Qualifier

⦸ 0HM0XZZ

0 Medical and Surgical
H Skin and Breast
N Release: Freeing a body part from an abnormal physical constraint by cutting or by the use of force

Body Part Character 4	Approach Character 5	Device Character 6	Qualifier Character 7
0 Skin, Scalp **1** Skin, Face **2** Skin, Right Ear **3** Skin, Left Ear **4** Skin, Neck **5** Skin, Chest **6** Skin, Back **7** Skin, Abdomen **8** Skin, Buttock **9** Skin, Perineum **A** Skin, Genitalia **B** Skin, Right Upper Arm **C** Skin, Left Upper Arm **D** Skin, Right Lower Arm **E** Skin, Left Lower Arm **F** Skin, Right Hand **G** Skin, Left Hand **H** Skin, Right Upper Leg **J** Skin, Left Upper Leg **K** Skin, Right Lower Leg **L** Skin, Left Lower Leg **M** Skin, Right Foot **N** Skin, Left Foot **Q** Finger Nail **R** Toe Nail	**X** External	**Z** No Device	**Z** No Qualifier
T Breast, Right **U** Breast, Left **V** Breast, Bilateral **W** Nipple, Right **X** Nipple, Left	**0** Open **3** Percutaneous **7** Via Natural or Artificial Opening **8** Via Natural or Artificial Opening Endoscopic **X** External	**Z** No Device	**Z** No Qualifier

0 Medical and Surgical
H Skin and Breast
P Removal: Taking out or off a device from a body part

Body Part Character 4	Approach Character 5	Device Character 6	Qualifier Character 7
P Skin ⃠ **Q** Finger Nail ⃠ **R** Toe Nail ⃠	**X** External	**0** Drainage Device **7** Autologous Tissue Substitute **J** Synthetic Substitute **K** Nonautologous Tissue Substitute	**Z** No Qualifier
S Hair ⃠	**X** External	**7** Autologous Tissue Substitute **J** Synthetic Substitute **K** Nonautologous Tissue Substitute	**Z** No Qualifier
T Breast, Right ⃠ **U** Breast, Left ⃠	**0** Open **3** Percutaneous **7** Via Natural or Artificial Opening **8** Via Natural or Artificial Opening Endoscopic	**0** Drainage Device **1** Radioactive Element **7** Autologous Tissue Substitute **J** Synthetic Substitute **K** Nonautologous Tissue Substitute **N** Tissue Expander	**Z** No Qualifier
T Breast, Right ⃠ **U** Breast, Left ⃠	**X** External	**0** Drainage Device **1** Radioactive Element **7** Autologous Tissue Substitute **J** Synthetic Substitute **K** Nonautologous Tissue Substitute	**Z** No Qualifier

⃠ 0HPPX0Z 0HPPX7Z 0HPPXJZ 0HPPXKZ 0HPQX0Z 0HPQX7Z 0HPQXJZ 0HPQXKZ 0HPRX0Z 0HPRX7Z 0HPRXJZ 0HPRXKZ 0HPSX7Z 0HPSXJZ 0HPSXKZ 0HPT00Z 0HPT01Z 0HPT07Z 0HPT0KZ 0HPT30Z 0HPT31Z 0HPT37Z 0HPT3KZ 0HPT70Z 0HPT71Z 0HPT77Z 0HPT7JZ 0HPT7KZ 0HPT7NZ 0HPT80Z 0HPT81Z 0HPT87Z 0HPT8JZ 0HPT8KZ 0HPT8NZ 0HPTX0Z 0HPTX1Z 0HPTX7Z 0HPTXJZ 0HPTXKZ 0HPU00Z 0HPU01Z 0HPU07Z 0HPU0KZ 0HPU30Z 0HPU31Z 0HPU37Z 0HPU3KZ 0HPU70Z 0HPU71Z 0HPU77Z 0HPU7JZ 0HPU7KZ 0HPU7NZ 0HPU80Z 0HPU81Z 0HPU87Z 0HPU8JZ 0HPU8KZ 0HPU8NZ 0HPUX0Z 0HPUX1Z 0HPUX7Z 0HPUXJZ 0HPUXKZ

LC Limited Coverage NC Noncovered HAC HAC Associated Procedure CC Combination Cluster - See Appendix G for code lists
DRG Non-OR-Affecting MS-DRG Assignment ⃠ Non-OR-Not Affecting MS-DRG Assignment New/Revised Text in **Orange** ♂ Male ♀ Female

0 Medical and Surgical
H Skin and Breast
Q Repair: Restoring, to the extent possible, a body part to its normal anatomic structure and function

Body Part Character 4	Approach Character 5	Device Character 6	Qualifier Character 7
0 Skin, Scalp ⊘ **1** Skin, Face ⊘ **2** Skin, Right Ear ⊘ **3** Skin, Left Ear ⊘ **4** Skin, Neck ⊘ **5** Skin, Chest ⊘ **6** Skin, Back ⊘ **7** Skin, Abdomen ⊘ **8** Skin, Buttock ⊘ **9** Skin, Perineum CC DRG **A** Skin, Genitalia ⊘ **B** Skin, Right Upper Arm ⊘ **C** Skin, Left Upper Arm ⊘ **D** Skin, Right Lower Arm ⊘ **E** Skin, Left Lower Arm ⊘ **F** Skin, Right Hand ⊘ **G** Skin, Left Hand ⊘ **H** Skin, Right Upper Leg ⊘ **J** Skin, Left Upper Leg ⊘ **K** Skin, Right Lower Leg ⊘ **L** Skin, Left Lower Leg ⊘ **M** Skin, Right Foot ⊘ **N** Skin, Left Foot ⊘ **Q** Finger Nail **R** Toe Nail	**X** External	**Z** No Device	**Z** No Qualifier
T Breast, Right ⊘ **U** Breast, Left ⊘ **V** Breast, Bilateral ⊘ **W** Nipple, Right **X** Nipple, Left **Y** Supernumerary Breast ⊘	**0** Open **3** Percutaneous **7** Via Natural or Artificial Opening **8** Via Natural or Artificial Opening Endoscopic **X** External	**Z** No Device	**Z** No Qualifier

CC 0HQ9XZZ
DRG 0HQ9XZZ
⊘ 0HQ0XZZ 0HQ1XZZ 0HQ2XZZ 0HQ3XZZ 0HQ4XZZ 0HQ5XZZ 0HQ6XZZ 0HQ7XZZ 0HQ8XZZ 0HQAXZZ 0HQBXZZ 0HQCXZZ 0HQDXZZ 0HQEXZZ 0HQFXZZ 0HQGXZZ 0HQHXZZ 0HQJXZZ 0HQKXZZ 0HQLXZZ 0HQMXZZ 0HQNXZZ 0HQTXZZ 0HQUXZZ 0HQVXZZ 0HQYXZZ

0 Medical and Surgical
H Skin and Breast
R Replacement: Putting in or on biological or synthetic material that physically takes the place and/or function of all or a portion of a body part

Body Part Character 4	Approach Character 5	Device Character 6	Qualifier Character 7
0 Skin, Scalp **1** Skin, Face **2** Skin, Right Ear **3** Skin, Left Ear **4** Skin, Neck **5** Skin, Chest **6** Skin, Back **7** Skin, Abdomen **8** Skin, Buttock **9** Skin, Perineum **A** Skin, Genitalia **B** Skin, Right Upper Arm **C** Skin, Left Upper Arm **D** Skin, Right Lower Arm **E** Skin, Left Lower Arm **F** Skin, Right Hand **G** Skin, Left Hand **H** Skin, Right Upper Leg **J** Skin, Left Upper Leg **K** Skin, Right Lower Leg **L** Skin, Left Lower Leg **M** Skin, Right Foot **N** Skin, Left Foot	**X** External	**7** Autologous Tissue Substitute **K** Nonautologous Tissue Substitute	**3** Full Thickness **4** Partial Thickness
0 Skin, Scalp **1** Skin, Face **2** Skin, Right Ear **3** Skin, Left Ear **4** Skin, Neck **5** Skin, Chest **6** Skin, Back **7** Skin, Abdomen **8** Skin, Buttock **9** Skin, Perineum **A** Skin, Genitalia **B** Skin, Right Upper Arm **C** Skin, Left Upper Arm **D** Skin, Right Lower Arm **E** Skin, Left Lower Arm **F** Skin, Right Hand **G** Skin, Left Hand **H** Skin, Right Upper Leg **J** Skin, Left Upper Leg **K** Skin, Right Lower Leg **L** Skin, Left Lower Leg **M** Skin, Right Foot **N** Skin, Left Foot	**X** External	**J** Synthetic Substitute	**3** Full Thickness **4** Partial Thickness **Z** No Qualifier
Q Finger Nail **R** Toe Nail **S** Hair ⊘	**X** External	**7** Autologous Tissue Substitute **J** Synthetic Substitute **K** Nonautologous Tissue Substitute	**Z** No Qualifier

0HR continued on next page

0HR continued from previous page

0 Medical and Surgical
H Skin and Breast
R Replacement: Putting in or on biological or synthetic material that physically takes the place and/or function of all or a portion of a body part

Body Part Character 4	Approach Character 5	Device Character 6	Qualifier Character 7
T Breast, Right **U** Breast, Left **V** Breast, Bilateral	**0** Open	**7** Autologous Tissue Substitute	**5** Latissimus Dorsi Myocutaneous Flap **6** Transverse Rectus Abdominis Myocutaneous Flap **7** Deep Inferior Epigastric Artery Perforator Flap **8** Superficial Inferior Epigastric Artery Flap **9** Gluteal Artery Perforator Flap **Z** No Qualifier
T Breast, Right **U** Breast, Left **V** Breast, Bilateral	**0** Open	**J** Synthetic Substitute **K** Nonautologous Tissue Substitute	**Z** No Qualifier
T Breast, Right CC **U** Breast, Left CC **V** Breast, Bilateral CC	**3** Percutaneous **X** External	**7** Autologous Tissue Substitute **J** Synthetic Substitute **K** Nonautologous Tissue Substitute	**Z** No Qualifier
W Nipple, Right **X** Nipple, Left	**0** Open **3** Percutaneous **X** External	**7** Autologous Tissue Substitute **J** Synthetic Substitute **K** Nonautologous Tissue Substitute	**Z** No Qualifier

CC 0HRT37Z 0HRU37Z 0HRV37Z
⊘ 0HRSX7Z

0 Medical and Surgical
H Skin and Breast
S Reposition: Moving to its normal location, or other suitable location, all or a portion of a body part

Body Part Character 4	Approach Character 5	Device Character 6	Qualifier Character 7
S Hair ⊘ **W** Nipple, Right **X** Nipple, Left	**X** External	**Z** No Device	**Z** No Qualifier
T Breast, Right **U** Breast, Left **V** Breast, Bilateral	**0** Open	**Z** No Device	**Z** No Qualifier

⊘ 0HSSXZZ

0 Medical and Surgical
H Skin and Breast
T Resection: Cutting out or off, without replacement, all of a body part

Body Part Character 4	Approach Character 5	Device Character 6	Qualifier Character 7
Q Finger Nail ⊘ **R** Toe Nail ⊘ **W** Nipple, Right **X** Nipple, Left	**X** External	**Z** No Device	**Z** No Qualifier
T Breast, Right CC **U** Breast, Left CC **V** Breast, Bilateral CC **Y** Supernumerary Breast	**0** Open	**Z** No Device	**Z** No Qualifier

CC 0HTT0ZZ 0HTU0ZZ 0HTV0ZZ
⊘ 0HTQXZZ 0HTRXZZ

0 Medical and Surgical
H Skin and Breast
U Supplement: Putting in or on biological or synthetic material that physically reinforces and/or augments the function of a portion of a body part

Body Part Character 4	Approach Character 5	Device Character 6	Qualifier Character 7
T Breast, Right **U** Breast, Left **V** Breast, Bilateral **W** Nipple, Right **X** Nipple, Left	**0** Open **3** Percutaneous **7** Via Natural or Artificial Opening **8** Via Natural or Artificial Opening Endoscopic **X** External	**7** Autologous Tissue Substitute **J** Synthetic Substitute **K** Nonautologous Tissue Substitute	**Z** No Qualifier

0 Medical and Surgical
H Skin and Breast
W Revision: Correcting, to the extent possible, a portion of a malfunctioning device or the position of a displaced device

Body Part Character 4	Approach Character 5	Device Character 6	Qualifier Character 7
P Skin ⃠ **Q** Finger Nail ⃠ **R** Toe Nail ⃠	**X** External	**0** Drainage Device **7** Autologous Tissue Substitute **J** Synthetic Substitute **K** Nonautologous Tissue Substitute	**Z** No Qualifier
S Hair ⃠	**X** External	**7** Autologous Tissue Substitute **J** Synthetic Substitute **K** Nonautologous Tissue Substitute	**Z** No Qualifier
T Breast, Right ⃠ **U** Breast, Left ⃠	**0** Open **3** Percutaneous **7** Via Natural or Artificial Opening **8** Via Natural or Artificial Opening Endoscopic	**0** Drainage Device **7** Autologous Tissue Substitute **J** Synthetic Substitute **K** Nonautologous Tissue Substitute **N** Tissue Expander	**Z** No Qualifier
T Breast, Right ⃠ **U** Breast, Left ⃠	**X** External	**0** Drainage Device **7** Autologous Tissue Substitute **J** Synthetic Substitute **K** Nonautologous Tissue Substitute	**Z** No Qualifier

⃠ 0HWPX0Z 0HWPX7Z 0HWPXJZ 0HWPXKZ 0HWQX0Z 0HWQX7Z 0HWQXJZ 0HWQXKZ 0HWRX0Z 0HWRX7Z 0HWRXJZ 0HWRXKZ 0HWSX7Z 0HWSXJZ 0HWSXKZ 0HWT00Z 0HWT07Z 0HWT0KZ 0HWT0NZ 0HWT30Z 0HWT37Z 0HWT3KZ 0HWT3NZ 0HWT70Z 0HWT77Z 0HWT7JZ 0HWT7KZ 0HWT7NZ 0HWT80Z 0HWT87Z 0HWT8JZ 0HWT8KZ 0HWT8NZ 0HWTX0Z 0HWTX7Z 0HWTXJZ 0HWTXKZ 0HWU00Z 0HWU07Z 0HWU0KZ 0HWU0NZ 0HWU30Z 0HWU37Z 0HWU3KZ 0HWU3NZ 0HWU70Z 0HWU77Z 0HWU7JZ 0HWU7KZ 0HWU7NZ 0HWU80Z 0HWU87Z 0HWU8JZ 0HWU8KZ 0HWU8NZ 0HWUX0Z 0HWUX7Z 0HWUXJZ 0HWUXKZ

0 Medical and Surgical
H Skin and Breast
X Transfer: Moving, without taking out, all or a portion of a body part to another location to take over the function of all or a portion of a body part

Body Part Character 4	Approach Character 5	Device Character 6	Qualifier Character 7
0 Skin, Scalp **1** Skin, Face **2** Skin, Right Ear **3** Skin, Left Ear **4** Skin, Neck **5** Skin, Chest **6** Skin, Back **7** Skin, Abdomen **8** Skin, Buttock **9** Skin, Perineum **A** Skin, Genitalia **B** Skin, Right Upper Arm **C** Skin, Left Upper Arm **D** Skin, Right Lower Arm **E** Skin, Left Lower Arm **F** Skin, Right Hand **G** Skin, Left Hand **H** Skin, Right Upper Leg **J** Skin, Left Upper Leg **K** Skin, Right Lower Leg **L** Skin, Left Lower Leg **M** Skin, Right Foot **N** Skin, Left Foot	**X** External	**Z** No Device	**Z** No Qualifier

Subcutaneous Tissue and Fascia 0J0-0JX

0 Medical and Surgical
J Subcutaneous Tissue and Fascia
0 Alteration: Modifying the anatomic structure of a body part without affecting the function of the body part

Body Part Character 4	Approach Character 5	Device Character 6	Qualifier Character 7
1 Subcutaneous Tissue and Fascia, Face **4** Subcutaneous Tissue and Fascia, Anterior Neck **5** Subcutaneous Tissue and Fascia, Posterior Neck **6** Subcutaneous Tissue and Fascia, Chest **7** Subcutaneous Tissue and Fascia, Back **8** Subcutaneous Tissue and Fascia, Abdomen **9** Subcutaneous Tissue and Fascia, Buttock **D** Subcutaneous Tissue and Fascia, Right Upper Arm **F** Subcutaneous Tissue and Fascia, Left Upper Arm **G** Subcutaneous Tissue and Fascia, Right Lower Arm **H** Subcutaneous Tissue and Fascia, Left Lower Arm **L** Subcutaneous Tissue and Fascia, Right Upper Leg **M** Subcutaneous Tissue and Fascia, Left Upper Leg **N** Subcutaneous Tissue and Fascia, Right Lower Leg **P** Subcutaneous Tissue and Fascia, Left Lower Leg	**0** Open **3** Percutaneous	**Z** No Device	**Z** No Qualifier

0 Medical and Surgical
J Subcutaneous Tissue and Fascia
2 Change: Taking out or off a device from a body part and putting back an identical or similar device in or on the same body part without cutting or puncturing the skin or a mucous membrane

Body Part Character 4	Approach Character 5	Device Character 6	Qualifier Character 7
S Subcutaneous Tissue and Fascia, Head and Neck ⦸ **T** Subcutaneous Tissue and Fascia, Trunk ⦸ **V** Subcutaneous Tissue and Fascia, Upper Extremity ⦸ **W** Subcutaneous Tissue and Fascia, Lower Extremity ⦸	**X** External	**0** Drainage Device **Y** Other Device	**Z** No Qualifier

⦸ 0J2SX0Z 0J2SXYZ 0J2TX0Z 0J2TXYZ 0J2VX0Z 0J2VXYZ 0J2WX0Z 0J2WXYZ

0 Medical and Surgical
J Subcutaneous Tissue and Fascia
5 Destruction: Physical eradication of all or a portion of a body part by the direct use of energy, force, or a destructive agent

Body Part Character 4	Approach Character 5	Device Character 6	Qualifier Character 7
0 Subcutaneous Tissue and Fascia, Scalp DRG **1** Subcutaneous Tissue and Fascia, Face DRG **4** Subcutaneous Tissue and Fascia, Anterior Neck DRG **5** Subcutaneous Tissue and Fascia, Posterior Neck DRG **6** Subcutaneous Tissue and Fascia, Chest DRG **7** Subcutaneous Tissue and Fascia, Back DRG **8** Subcutaneous Tissue and Fascia, Abdomen DRG **9** Subcutaneous Tissue and Fascia, Buttock DRG **B** Subcutaneous Tissue and Fascia, Perineum DRG **C** Subcutaneous Tissue and Fascia, Pelvic Region DRG **D** Subcutaneous Tissue and Fascia, Right Upper Arm DRG **F** Subcutaneous Tissue and Fascia, Left Upper Arm DRG **G** Subcutaneous Tissue and Fascia, Right Lower Arm DRG **H** Subcutaneous Tissue and Fascia, Left Lower Arm DRG **J** Subcutaneous Tissue and Fascia, Right Hand DRG **K** Subcutaneous Tissue and Fascia, Left Hand DRG **L** Subcutaneous Tissue and Fascia, Right Upper Leg DRG **M** Subcutaneous Tissue and Fascia, Left Upper Leg DRG **N** Subcutaneous Tissue and Fascia, Right Lower Leg DRG **P** Subcutaneous Tissue and Fascia, Left Lower Leg DRG **Q** Subcutaneous Tissue and Fascia, Right Foot DRG **R** Subcutaneous Tissue and Fascia, Left Foot DRG	**0** Open **3** Percutaneous	**Z** No Device	**Z** No Qualifier

DRG 0J500ZZ 0J503ZZ 0J510ZZ 0J513ZZ 0J540ZZ 0J543ZZ 0J550ZZ 0J553ZZ 0J560ZZ 0J563ZZ 0J570ZZ 0J573ZZ 0J580ZZ 0J583ZZ 0J590ZZ 0J593ZZ 0J5B0ZZ 0J5B3ZZ 0J5C0ZZ 0J5C3ZZ 0J5D0ZZ 0J5D3ZZ 0J5F0ZZ 0J5F3ZZ 0J5G0ZZ 0J5G3ZZ 0J5H0ZZ 0J5H3ZZ 0J5J0ZZ 0J5J3ZZ 0J5K0ZZ 0J5K3ZZ 0J5L0ZZ 0J5L3ZZ 0J5M0ZZ 0J5M3ZZ 0J5N0ZZ 0J5N3ZZ 0J5P0ZZ 0J5P3ZZ 0J5Q0ZZ 0J5Q3ZZ 0J5R0ZZ 0J5R3ZZ

0 Medical and Surgical
J Subcutaneous Tissue and Fascia
8 Division: Cutting into a body part, without draining fluids and/or gases from the body part, in order to separate or transect a body part

Body Part Character 4	Approach Character 5	Device Character 6	Qualifier Character 7
0 Subcutaneous Tissue and Fascia, Scalp **1** Subcutaneous Tissue and Fascia, Face **4** Subcutaneous Tissue and Fascia, Anterior Neck **5** Subcutaneous Tissue and Fascia, Posterior Neck **6** Subcutaneous Tissue and Fascia, Chest **7** Subcutaneous Tissue and Fascia, Back **8** Subcutaneous Tissue and Fascia, Abdomen **9** Subcutaneous Tissue and Fascia, Buttock **B** Subcutaneous Tissue and Fascia, Perineum **C** Subcutaneous Tissue and Fascia, Pelvic Region **D** Subcutaneous Tissue and Fascia, Right Upper Arm **F** Subcutaneous Tissue and Fascia, Left Upper Arm **G** Subcutaneous Tissue and Fascia, Right Lower Arm **H** Subcutaneous Tissue and Fascia, Left Lower Arm **J** Subcutaneous Tissue and Fascia, Right Hand **K** Subcutaneous Tissue and Fascia, Left Hand **L** Subcutaneous Tissue and Fascia, Right Upper Leg **M** Subcutaneous Tissue and Fascia, Left Upper Leg **N** Subcutaneous Tissue and Fascia, Right Lower Leg **P** Subcutaneous Tissue and Fascia, Left Lower Leg **Q** Subcutaneous Tissue and Fascia, Right Foot **R** Subcutaneous Tissue and Fascia, Left Foot **S** Subcutaneous Tissue and Fascia, Head and Neck **T** Subcutaneous Tissue and Fascia, Trunk **V** Subcutaneous Tissue and Fascia, Upper Extremity **W** Subcutaneous Tissue and Fascia, Lower Extremity	**0** Open **3** Percutaneous	**Z** No Device	**Z** No Qualifier

0 Medical and Surgical
J Subcutaneous Tissue and Fascia
9 Drainage: Taking or letting out fluids and/or gases from a body part

Body Part Character 4	Approach Character 5	Device Character 6	Qualifier Character 7
0 Subcutaneous Tissue and Fascia, Scalp ⊘ **1** Subcutaneous Tissue and Fascia, Face ⊘ **4** Subcutaneous Tissue and Fascia, Anterior Neck ⊘ **5** Subcutaneous Tissue and Fascia, Posterior Neck ⊘ **6** Subcutaneous Tissue and Fascia, Chest ⊘ **7** Subcutaneous Tissue and Fascia, Back ⊘ **8** Subcutaneous Tissue and Fascia, Abdomen ⊘ **9** Subcutaneous Tissue and Fascia, Buttock ⊘ **B** Subcutaneous Tissue and Fascia, Perineum ⊘ **C** Subcutaneous Tissue and Fascia, Pelvic Region ⊘ **D** Subcutaneous Tissue and Fascia, Right Upper Arm ⊘ **F** Subcutaneous Tissue and Fascia, Left Upper Arm ⊘ **G** Subcutaneous Tissue and Fascia, Right Lower Arm ⊘ **H** Subcutaneous Tissue and Fascia, Left Lower Arm ⊘ **J** Subcutaneous Tissue and Fascia, Right Hand ⊘ **K** Subcutaneous Tissue and Fascia, Left Hand ⊘ **L** Subcutaneous Tissue and Fascia, Right Upper Leg ⊘ **M** Subcutaneous Tissue and Fascia, Left Upper Leg ⊘ **N** Subcutaneous Tissue and Fascia, Right Lower Leg ⊘ **P** Subcutaneous Tissue and Fascia, Left Lower Leg ⊘ **Q** Subcutaneous Tissue and Fascia, Right Foot ⊘ **R** Subcutaneous Tissue and Fascia, Left Foot ⊘	**0** Open **3** Percutaneous	**0** Drainage Device	**Z** No Qualifier

0J9 continued on next page

0 Medical and Surgical
J Subcutaneous Tissue and Fascia
9 Drainage: Taking or letting out fluids and/or gases from a body part

0J9 continued from previous page

Body Part Character 4	Approach Character 5	Device Character 6	Qualifier Character 7
0 Subcutaneous Tissue and Fascia, Scalp ⦸ **1** Subcutaneous Tissue and Fascia, Face ⦸ **4** Subcutaneous Tissue and Fascia, Anterior Neck ⦸ **5** Subcutaneous Tissue and Fascia, Posterior Neck ⦸ **6** Subcutaneous Tissue and Fascia, Chest ⦸ **7** Subcutaneous Tissue and Fascia, Back ⦸ **8** Subcutaneous Tissue and Fascia, Abdomen ⦸ **9** Subcutaneous Tissue and Fascia, Buttock ⦸ **B** Subcutaneous Tissue and Fascia, Perineum ⦸ **C** Subcutaneous Tissue and Fascia, Pelvic Region ⦸ **D** Subcutaneous Tissue and Fascia, Right Upper Arm ⦸ **F** Subcutaneous Tissue and Fascia, Left Upper Arm ⦸ **G** Subcutaneous Tissue and Fascia, Right Lower Arm ⦸ **H** Subcutaneous Tissue and Fascia, Left Lower Arm ⦸ **J** Subcutaneous Tissue and Fascia, Right Hand ⦸ **K** Subcutaneous Tissue and Fascia, Left Hand ⦸ **L** Subcutaneous Tissue and Fascia, Right Upper Leg ⦸ **M** Subcutaneous Tissue and Fascia, Left Upper Leg ⦸ **N** Subcutaneous Tissue and Fascia, Right Lower Leg ⦸ **P** Subcutaneous Tissue and Fascia, Left Lower Leg ⦸ **Q** Subcutaneous Tissue and Fascia, Right Foot ⦸ **R** Subcutaneous Tissue and Fascia, Left Foot ⦸	**0** Open **3** Percutaneous	**Z** No Device	**X** Diagnostic **Z** No Qualifier

⦸ 0J9000Z 0J900ZX 0J9030Z 0J903ZX 0J903ZZ 0J910ZX 0J9130Z 0J913ZX 0J913ZZ 0J9400Z 0J940ZX 0J9430Z 0J943ZX 0J943ZZ 0J9500Z 0J950ZX 0J9530Z 0J953ZX 0J953ZZ 0J9600Z 0J960ZX 0J9630Z 0J963ZX 0J963ZZ 0J9700Z 0J970ZX 0J9730Z 0J973ZX 0J973ZZ 0J9800Z 0J980ZX 0J9830Z 0J983ZX 0J983ZZ 0J9900Z 0J990ZX 0J9930Z 0J993ZX 0J993ZZ 0J9B00Z 0J9B0ZX 0J9B30Z 0J9B3ZX 0J9B3ZZ 0J9C00Z 0J9C0ZX 0J9C30Z 0J9C3ZX 0J9C3ZZ 0J9D00Z 0J9D0ZX 0J9D30Z 0J9D3ZX 0J9D3ZZ 0J9F00Z 0J9F0ZX 0J9F30Z 0J9F3ZX 0J9F3ZZ 0J9G00Z 0J9G0ZX 0J9G30Z 0J9G3ZX 0J9G3ZZ 0J9H00Z 0J9H0ZX 0J9H30Z 0J9H3ZX 0J9H3ZZ 0J9J0ZX 0J9J30Z 0J9J3ZX 0J9K0ZX 0J9K30Z 0J9K3ZX 0J9L00Z 0J9L0ZX 0J9L30Z 0J9L3ZX 0J9L3ZZ 0J9M00Z 0J9M0ZX 0J9M30Z 0J9M3ZX 0J9M3ZZ 0J9N00Z 0J9N0ZX 0J9N30Z 0J9N3ZX 0J9N3ZZ 0J9P00Z 0J9P0ZX 0J9P30Z 0J9P3ZX 0J9P3ZZ 0J9Q00Z 0J9Q0ZX 0J9Q30Z 0J9Q3ZX 0J9Q3ZZ 0J9R00Z 0J9R0ZX 0J9R30Z 0J9R3ZX 0J9R3ZZ

0 Medical and Surgical
J Subcutaneous Tissue and Fascia
B Excision: Cutting out or off, without replacement, a portion of a body part

Body Part Character 4	Approach Character 5	Device Character 6	Qualifier Character 7
0 Subcutaneous Tissue and Fascia, Scalp ⃠ **1** Subcutaneous Tissue and Fascia, Face ⃠ **4** Subcutaneous Tissue and Fascia, Anterior Neck ⃠ **5** Subcutaneous Tissue and Fascia, Posterior Neck ⃠ **6** Subcutaneous Tissue and Fascia, Chest ⃠ **7** Subcutaneous Tissue and Fascia, Back ⃠ **8** Subcutaneous Tissue and Fascia, Abdomen ⃠ **9** Subcutaneous Tissue and Fascia, Buttock ⃠ **B** Subcutaneous Tissue and Fascia, Perineum ⃠ **C** Subcutaneous Tissue and Fascia, Pelvic Region ⃠ **D** Subcutaneous Tissue and Fascia, Right Upper Arm ⃠ **F** Subcutaneous Tissue and Fascia, Left Upper Arm ⃠ **G** Subcutaneous Tissue and Fascia, Right Lower Arm ⃠ **H** Subcutaneous Tissue and Fascia, Left Lower Arm ⃠ **J** Subcutaneous Tissue and Fascia, Right Hand ⃠ **K** Subcutaneous Tissue and Fascia, Left Hand ⃠ **L** Subcutaneous Tissue and Fascia, Right Upper Leg ⃠ CC **M** Subcutaneous Tissue and Fascia, Left Upper Leg ⃠ CC **N** Subcutaneous Tissue and Fascia, Right Lower Leg ⃠ **P** Subcutaneous Tissue and Fascia, Left Lower Leg ⃠ **Q** Subcutaneous Tissue and Fascia, Right Foot ⃠ **R** Subcutaneous Tissue and Fascia, Left Foot ⃠	**0** Open **3** Percutaneous	**Z** No Device	**X** Diagnostic **Z** No Qualifier

CC 0JBL0ZZ 0JBM0ZZ

⃠ 0JB00ZX 0JB03ZX 0JB03ZZ 0JB10ZX 0JB13ZX 0JB40ZX 0JB43ZX 0JB43ZZ 0JB50ZX 0JB53ZX 0JB53ZZ 0JB60ZX 0JB63ZX 0JB63ZZ 0JB70ZX 0JB73ZX 0JB73ZZ 0JB80ZX 0JB83ZX 0JB83ZZ 0JB90ZX 0JB93ZX 0JB93ZZ 0JBB0ZX 0JBB3ZX 0JBB3ZZ 0JBC0ZX 0JBC3ZX 0JBC3ZZ 0JBD0ZX 0JBD3ZX 0JBD3ZZ 0JBF0ZX 0JBF3ZX 0JBF3ZZ 0JBG0ZX 0JBG3ZX 0JBG3ZZ 0JBH0ZX 0JBH3ZX 0JBH3ZZ 0JBJ0ZX 0JBJ3ZX 0JBK0ZX 0JBK3ZX 0JBL0ZX 0JBL3ZX 0JBL3ZZ 0JBM0ZX 0JBM3ZX 0JBM3ZZ 0JBN0ZX 0JBN3ZX 0JBN3ZZ 0JBP0ZX 0JBP3ZX 0JBP3ZZ 0JBQ0ZX 0JBQ3ZX 0JBQ3ZZ 0JBR0ZX 0JBR3ZX 0JBR3ZZ

0 Medical and Surgical
J Subcutaneous Tissue and Fascia
C Extirpation: Taking or cutting out solid matter from a body part

Body Part Character 4	Approach Character 5	Device Character 6	Qualifier Character 7
0 Subcutaneous Tissue and Fascia, Scalp ⊘ **1** Subcutaneous Tissue and Fascia, Face ⊘ **4** Subcutaneous Tissue and Fascia, Anterior Neck ⊘ **5** Subcutaneous Tissue and Fascia, Posterior Neck ⊘ **6** Subcutaneous Tissue and Fascia, Chest ⊘ **7** Subcutaneous Tissue and Fascia, Back ⊘ **8** Subcutaneous Tissue and Fascia, Abdomen ⊘ **9** Subcutaneous Tissue and Fascia, Buttock ⊘ **B** Subcutaneous Tissue and Fascia, Perineum ⊘ **C** Subcutaneous Tissue and Fascia, Pelvic Region ⊘ **D** Subcutaneous Tissue and Fascia, Right Upper Arm ⊘ **F** Subcutaneous Tissue and Fascia, Left Upper Arm ⊘ **G** Subcutaneous Tissue and Fascia, Right Lower Arm ⊘ **H** Subcutaneous Tissue and Fascia, Left Lower Arm ⊘ **J** Subcutaneous Tissue and Fascia, Right Hand ⊘ **K** Subcutaneous Tissue and Fascia, Left Hand ⊘ **L** Subcutaneous Tissue and Fascia, Right Upper Leg ⊘ **M** Subcutaneous Tissue and Fascia, Left Upper Leg ⊘ **N** Subcutaneous Tissue and Fascia, Right Lower Leg ⊘ **P** Subcutaneous Tissue and Fascia, Left Lower Leg ⊘ **Q** Subcutaneous Tissue and Fascia, Right Foot ⊘ **R** Subcutaneous Tissue and Fascia, Left Foot ⊘	**0** Open **3** Percutaneous	**Z** No Device	**Z** No Qualifier

⊘ 0JC00ZZ 0JC03ZZ 0JC10ZZ 0JC13ZZ 0JC40ZZ 0JC43ZZ 0JC50ZZ 0JC53ZZ 0JC60ZZ 0JC63ZZ 0JC70ZZ 0JC73ZZ 0JC80ZZ 0JC83ZZ 0JC90ZZ 0JC93ZZ 0JCB0ZZ 0JCB3ZZ 0JCC0ZZ 0JCC3ZZ 0JCD0ZZ 0JCD3ZZ 0JCF0ZZ 0JCF3ZZ 0JCG0ZZ 0JCG3ZZ 0JCH0ZZ 0JCH3ZZ 0JCJ0ZZ 0JCJ3ZZ 0JCK0ZZ 0JCK3ZZ 0JCL0ZZ 0JCL3ZZ 0JCM0ZZ 0JCM3ZZ 0JCN0ZZ 0JCN3ZZ 0JCP0ZZ 0JCP3ZZ 0JCQ0ZZ 0JCQ3ZZ 0JCR0ZZ 0JCR3ZZ

0 Medical and Surgical
J Subcutaneous Tissue and Fascia
D Extraction: Pulling or stripping out or off all or a portion of a body part by the use of force

Body Part Character 4	Approach Character 5	Device Character 6	Qualifier Character 7
0 Subcutaneous Tissue and Fascia, Scalp **1** Subcutaneous Tissue and Fascia, Face **4** Subcutaneous Tissue and Fascia, Anterior Neck **5** Subcutaneous Tissue and Fascia, Posterior Neck **6** Subcutaneous Tissue and Fascia, Chest CC **7** Subcutaneous Tissue and Fascia, Back CC **8** Subcutaneous Tissue and Fascia, Abdomen CC **9** Subcutaneous Tissue and Fascia, Buttock CC **B** Subcutaneous Tissue and Fascia, Perineum **C** Subcutaneous Tissue and Fascia, Pelvic Region **D** Subcutaneous Tissue and Fascia, Right Upper Arm **F** Subcutaneous Tissue and Fascia, Left Upper Arm **G** Subcutaneous Tissue and Fascia, Right Lower Arm **H** Subcutaneous Tissue and Fascia, Left Lower Arm **J** Subcutaneous Tissue and Fascia, Right Hand **K** Subcutaneous Tissue and Fascia, Left Hand **L** Subcutaneous Tissue and Fascia, Right Upper Leg CC **M** Subcutaneous Tissue and Fascia, Left Upper Leg CC **N** Subcutaneous Tissue and Fascia, Right Lower Leg **P** Subcutaneous Tissue and Fascia, Left Lower Leg **Q** Subcutaneous Tissue and Fascia, Right Foot **R** Subcutaneous Tissue and Fascia, Left Foot	**0** Open **3** Percutaneous	**Z** No Device	**Z** No Qualifier

CC 0JD63ZZ 0JD73ZZ 0JD83ZZ 0JD93ZZ 0JDL3ZZ 0JDM3ZZ

0 Medical and Surgical
J Subcutaneous Tissue and Fascia
H Insertion: Putting in a nonbiological appliance that monitors, assists, performs, or prevents a physiological function but does not physically take the place of a body part

Body Part Character 4	Approach Character 5	Device Character 6	Qualifier Character 7
0 Subcutaneous Tissue and Fascia, Scalp **1** Subcutaneous Tissue and Fascia, Face **4** Subcutaneous Tissue and Fascia, Anterior Neck **5** Subcutaneous Tissue and Fascia, Posterior Neck **9** Subcutaneous Tissue and Fascia, Buttock **B** Subcutaneous Tissue and Fascia, Perineum **C** Subcutaneous Tissue and Fascia, Pelvic Region **J** Subcutaneous Tissue and Fascia, Right Hand **K** Subcutaneous Tissue and Fascia, Left Hand **Q** Subcutaneous Tissue and Fascia, Right Foot **R** Subcutaneous Tissue and Fascia, Left Foot	**0** Open **3** Percutaneous	**N** Tissue Expander	**Z** No Qualifier
6 Subcutaneous Tissue and Fascia, Chest CC DRG HAC **8** Subcutaneous Tissue and Fascia, Abdomen NC CC DRG HAC	**0** Open **3** Percutaneous	**0** Monitoring Device, Hemodynamic **2** Monitoring Device **4** Pacemaker, Single Chamber **5** Pacemaker, Single Chamber Rate Responsive **6** Pacemaker, Dual Chamber **7** Cardiac Resynchronization Pacemaker Pulse Generator **8** Defibrillator Generator **9** Cardiac Resynchronization Defibrillator Pulse Generator **A** Contractility Modulation Device **B** Stimulator Generator, Single Array **C** Stimulator Generator, Single Array Rechargeable **D** Stimulator Generator, Multiple Array **E** Stimulator Generator, Multiple Array Rechargeable **H** Contraceptive Device **M** Stimulator Generator **N** Tissue Expander **P** Cardiac Rhythm Related Device **V** Infusion Device, Pump **W** Vascular Access Device, Reservoir **X** Vascular Access Device	**Z** No Qualifier

0JH continued on next page

0JH continued from previous page

0 Medical and Surgical
J Subcutaneous Tissue and Fascia
H Insertion: Putting in a nonbiological appliance that monitors, assists, performs, or prevents a physiological function but does not physically take the place of a body part

Body Part Character 4	Approach Character 5	Device Character 6	Qualifier Character 7
7 Subcutaneous Tissue and Fascia, Back NC CC	**0** Open **3** Percutaneous	**B** Stimulator Generator, Single Array **C** Stimulator Generator, Single Array Rechargeable **D** Stimulator Generator, Multiple Array **E** Stimulator Generator, Multiple Array Rechargeable **M** Stimulator Generator **N** Tissue Expander **V** Infusion Device, Pump	**Z** No Qualifier
D Subcutaneous Tissue and Fascia, Right Upper Arm ⃠ DRG **F** Subcutaneous Tissue and Fascia, Left Upper Arm ⃠ DRG **G** Subcutaneous Tissue and Fascia, Right Lower Arm ⃠ DRG **H** Subcutaneous Tissue and Fascia, Left Lower Arm ⃠ DRG **L** Subcutaneous Tissue and Fascia, Right Upper Leg ⃠ DRG **M** Subcutaneous Tissue and Fascia, Left Upper Leg ⃠ DRG **N** Subcutaneous Tissue and Fascia, Right Lower Leg ⃠ DRG **P** Subcutaneous Tissue and Fascia, Left Lower Leg ⃠ DRG	**0** Open **3** Percutaneous	**H** Contraceptive Device **N** Tissue Expander **V** Infusion Device, Pump **W** Vascular Access Device, Reservoir **X** Vascular Access Device	**Z** No Qualifier
S Subcutaneous Tissue and Fascia, Head and Neck ⃠ **V** Subcutaneous Tissue and Fascia, Upper Extremity ⃠ **W** Subcutaneous Tissue and Fascia, Lower Extremity ⃠	**0** Open **3** Percutaneous	**1** Radioactive Element **3** Infusion Device	**Z** No Qualifier
T Subcutaneous Tissue and Fascia, Trunk ⃠	**0** Open **3** Percutaneous	**1** Radioactive Element **3** Infusion Device **V** Infusion Device, Pump	**Z** No Qualifier

NC 0JH70MZ 0JH73MZ 0JH80MZ 0JH83MZ

CC 0JH600Z 0JH604Z 0JH605Z 0JH606Z 0JH607Z 0JH608Z 0JH609Z 0JH60AZ 0JH60BZ 0JH60CZ 0JH60DZ 0JH60EZ 0JH60MZ 0JH60PZ 0JH630Z 0JH634Z 0JH635Z 0JH636Z 0JH637Z 0JH638Z 0JH639Z 0JH63AZ 0JH63BZ 0JH63CZ 0JH63DZ 0JH63EZ 0JH63MZ 0JH63PZ 0JH70BZ 0JH70CZ 0JH70DZ 0JH70EZ 0JH70MZ 0JH73BZ 0JH73CZ 0JH73DZ 0JH73EZ 0JH73MZ 0JH800Z 0JH804Z 0JH805Z 0JH806Z 0JH807Z 0JH808Z 0JH809Z 0JH80AZ 0JH80BZ 0JH80CZ 0JH80DZ 0JH80EZ 0JH80MZ 0JH80PZ 0JH830Z 0JH834Z 0JH835Z 0JH836Z 0JH837Z 0JH838Z 0JH839Z 0JH83AZ 0JH83BZ 0JH83CZ 0JH83DZ 0JH83EZ 0JH83MZ 0JH83PZ

HAC 0JH604Z 0JH605Z 0JH606Z 0JH607Z 0JH608Z 0JH609Z 0JH60PZ 0JH634Z 0JH635Z 0JH636Z 0JH637Z 0JH638Z 0JH639Z 0JH63PZ 0JH804Z 0JH805Z 0JH806Z 0JH807Z 0JH808Z 0JH809Z 0JH80PZ 0JH834Z 0JH835Z 0JH836Z 0JH837Z 0JH838Z 0JH839Z or 0JH83PZ All preceding codes with the HAC symbol are classified as hospital-acquired conditions when reported with secondary diagnosis K68.11, T81.4XXA, T82.6XXA, or T82.7XXA.

HAC 0JH63XZ when reported with secondary diagnosis J95.811

DRG 0JH604Z 0JH605Z 0JH606Z 0JH60HZ 0JH60WZ 0JH60XZ 0JH634Z 0JH635Z 0JH636Z 0JH63HZ 0JH63WZ 0JH63XZ 0JH802Z 0JH804Z 0JH805Z 0JH806Z 0JH80HZ 0JH80WZ 0JH80XZ 0JH832Z 0JH834Z 0JH835Z 0JH836Z 0JH83HZ 0JH83WZ 0JH83XZ 0JHD0WZ 0JHD0XZ 0JHD3WZ 0JHD3XZ 0JHF0WZ 0JHF0XZ 0JHF3WZ 0JHF3XZ 0JHG0WZ 0JHG0XZ 0JHG3WZ 0JHG3XZ 0JHH0WZ 0JHH0XZ 0JHH3WZ 0JHH3XZ 0JHL0WZ 0JHL0XZ 0JHL3WZ 0JHL3XZ 0JHM0WZ 0JHM0XZ 0JHM3WZ 0JHM3XZ 0JHN0WZ 0JHN0XZ 0JHN3HZ 0JHN3WZ 0JHN3XZ 0JHP0HZ 0JHP0WZ 0JHP0XZ 0JHP3HZ 0JHP3WZ 0JHP3XZ

⃠ 0JHD0HZ 0JHD0VZ 0JHD3HZ 0JHD3VZ 0JHF0HZ 0JHF0VZ 0JHF3HZ 0JHF3VZ 0JHG0HZ 0JHG0VZ 0JHG3HZ 0JHG3VZ 0JHH0HZ 0JHH0VZ 0JHH3HZ 0JHH3VZ 0JHL0HZ 0JHL0VZ 0JHL3HZ 0JHL3VZ 0JHM0HZ 0JHM0VZ 0JHM3HZ 0JHM3VZ 0JHN0HZ 0JHN0VZ 0JHN3VZ 0JHP0VZ 0JHP3VZ 0JHS03Z 0JHS33Z 0JHT03Z 0JHT33Z 0JHV03Z 0JHV33Z 0JHW03Z 0JHW33Z

0 Medical and Surgical
J Subcutaneous Tissue and Fascia
J Inspection: Visually and/or manually exploring a body part

Body Part Character 4	Approach Character 5	Device Character 6	Qualifier Character 7
S Subcutaneous Tissue and Fascia, Head and Neck ⦸ **T** Subcutaneous Tissue and Fascia, Trunk ⦸ **V** Subcutaneous Tissue and Fascia, Upper Extremity ⦸ **W** Subcutaneous Tissue and Fascia, Lower Extremity ⦸	**0** Open **3** Percutaneous **X** External	**Z** No Device	**Z** No Qualifier

⦸ 0JJS0ZZ 0JJS3ZZ 0JJSXZZ 0JJT0ZZ 0JJT3ZZ 0JJTXZZ 0JJV0ZZ 0JJV3ZZ 0JJVXZZ 0JJW0ZZ 0JJW3ZZ 0JJWXZZ

0 Medical and Surgical
J Subcutaneous Tissue and Fascia
N Release: Freeing a body part from an abnormal physical constraint by cutting or by the use of force

Body Part Character 4	Approach Character 5	Device Character 6	Qualifier Character 7
0 Subcutaneous Tissue and Fascia, Scalp ⦸ **1** Subcutaneous Tissue and Fascia, Face ⦸ **4** Subcutaneous Tissue and Fascia, Anterior Neck ⦸ **5** Subcutaneous Tissue and Fascia, Posterior Neck ⦸ **6** Subcutaneous Tissue and Fascia, Chest ⦸ **7** Subcutaneous Tissue and Fascia, Back ⦸ **8** Subcutaneous Tissue and Fascia, Abdomen ⦸ **9** Subcutaneous Tissue and Fascia, Buttock ⦸ **B** Subcutaneous Tissue and Fascia, Perineum ⦸ **C** Subcutaneous Tissue and Fascia, Pelvic Region ⦸ **D** Subcutaneous Tissue and Fascia, Right Upper Arm ⦸ **F** Subcutaneous Tissue and Fascia, Left Upper Arm ⦸ **G** Subcutaneous Tissue and Fascia, Right Lower Arm ⦸ **H** Subcutaneous Tissue and Fascia, Left Lower Arm ⦸ **J** Subcutaneous Tissue and Fascia, Right Hand ⦸ **K** Subcutaneous Tissue and Fascia, Left Hand ⦸ **L** Subcutaneous Tissue and Fascia, Right Upper Leg ⦸ **M** Subcutaneous Tissue and Fascia, Left Upper Leg ⦸ **N** Subcutaneous Tissue and Fascia, Right Lower Leg ⦸ **P** Subcutaneous Tissue and Fascia, Left Lower Leg ⦸ **Q** Subcutaneous Tissue and Fascia, Right Foot ⦸ **R** Subcutaneous Tissue and Fascia, Left Foot ⦸	**0** Open **3** Percutaneous **X** External	**Z** No Device	**Z** No Qualifier

⦸ 0JN0XZZ 0JN1XZZ 0JN4XZZ 0JN5XZZ 0JN6XZZ 0JN7XZZ 0JN8XZZ 0JN9XZZ 0JNBXZZ 0JNCXZZ 0JNDXZZ 0JNFXZZ 0JNGXZZ 0JNHXZZ 0JNJXZZ 0JNKXZZ 0JNLXZZ 0JNMXZZ 0JNNXZZ 0JNPXZZ 0JNQXZZ 0JNRXZZ

LC Limited Coverage NC Noncovered HAC HAC Associated Procedure CC Combination Cluster - See Appendix G for code lists
DRG Non-OR-Affecting MS-DRG Assignment ⦸ Non-OR-Not Affecting MS-DRG Assignment New/Revised Text in Orange ♂ Male ♀ Female

0 Medical and Surgical
J Subcutaneous Tissue and Fascia
P Removal: Taking out or off a device from a body part

Body Part Character 4	Approach Character 5	Device Character 6	Qualifier Character 7
S Subcutaneous Tissue and Fascia, Head and Neck ⃠	**0** Open **3** Percutaneous	**0** Drainage Device **1** Radioactive Element **3** Infusion Device **7** Autologous Tissue Substitute **J** Synthetic Substitute **K** Nonautologous Tissue Substitute **N** Tissue Expander	**Z** No Qualifier
S Subcutaneous Tissue and Fascia, Head and Neck ⃠	**X** External	**0** Drainage Device **1** Radioactive Element **3** Infusion Device	**Z** No Qualifier
T Subcutaneous Tissue and Fascia, Trunk ⃠ CC HAC	**0** Open **3** Percutaneous	**0** Drainage Device **1** Radioactive Element **2** Monitoring Device **3** Infusion Device **7** Autologous Tissue Substitute **H** Contraceptive Device **J** Synthetic Substitute **K** Nonautologous Tissue Substitute **M** Stimulator Generator **N** Tissue Expander **P** Cardiac Rhythm Related Device **V** Infusion Device, Pump **W** Vascular Access Device, Reservoir **X** Vascular Access Device	**Z** No Qualifier
T Subcutaneous Tissue and Fascia, Trunk ⃠	**X** External	**0** Drainage Device **1** Radioactive Element **2** Monitoring Device **3** Infusion Device **H** Contraceptive Device **V** Infusion Device, Pump **X** Vascular Access Device	**Z** No Qualifier
V Subcutaneous Tissue and Fascia, Upper Extremity ⃠ **W** Subcutaneous Tissue and Fascia, Lower Extremity ⃠	**0** Open **3** Percutaneous	**0** Drainage Device **1** Radioactive Element **3** Infusion Device **7** Autologous Tissue Substitute **H** Contraceptive Device **J** Synthetic Substitute **K** Nonautologous Tissue Substitute **N** Tissue Expander **V** Infusion Device, Pump **W** Vascular Access Device, Reservoir **X** Vascular Access Device	**Z** No Qualifier
V Subcutaneous Tissue and Fascia, Upper Extremity ⃠ **W** Subcutaneous Tissue and Fascia, Lower Extremity ⃠	**X** External	**0** Drainage Device **1** Radioactive Element **3** Infusion Device **H** Contraceptive Device **V** Infusion Device, Pump **X** Vascular Access Device	**Z** No Qualifier

CC 0JPT0PZ 0JPT3PZ

HAC 0JPT0PZ or 0JPT3PZ when reported with secondary diagnosis K68.11, T81.4XXA, T82.6XXA, or T82.7XXA

⃠ 0JPS00Z 0JPS01Z 0JPS03Z 0JPS07Z 0JPS0JZ 0JPS0KZ 0JPS0NZ 0JPS30Z 0JPS31Z 0JPS33Z 0JPS37Z 0JPS3JZ 0JPS3KZ 0JPS3NZ 0JPSX0Z 0JPSX1Z 0JPSX3Z 0JPT00Z 0JPT01Z 0JPT02Z 0JPT03Z 0JPT07Z 0JPT0HZ 0JPT0JZ 0JPT0KZ 0JPT0MZ 0JPT0NZ 0JPT0VZ 0JPT0WZ 0JPT0XZ 0JPT30Z 0JPT31Z 0JPT32Z 0JPT33Z 0JPT37Z 0JPT3HZ 0JPT3JZ 0JPT3KZ 0JPT3MZ 0JPT3NZ 0JPT3VZ 0JPT3WZ 0JPT3XZ 0JPTX0Z 0JPTX1Z 0JPTX2Z 0JPTX3Z 0JPTXHZ 0JPTXVZ 0JPTXXZ 0JPV00Z 0JPV01Z 0JPV03Z 0JPV07Z 0JPV0HZ 0JPV0JZ 0JPV0KZ 0JPV0NZ 0JPV0VZ 0JPV0WZ 0JPV0XZ 0JPV30Z 0JPV31Z 0JPV33Z 0JPV37Z 0JPV3HZ 0JPV3JZ 0JPV3KZ 0JPV3NZ 0JPV3VZ 0JPV3WZ 0JPV3XZ 0JPVX0Z 0JPVX1Z 0JPVX3Z 0JPVXHZ 0JPVXVZ 0JPVXXZ 0JPW00Z 0JPW01Z 0JPW03Z 0JPW07Z 0JPW0HZ 0JPW0JZ 0JPW0KZ 0JPW0NZ 0JPW0VZ 0JPW0WZ 0JPW0XZ 0JPW30Z 0JPW31Z 0JPW33Z 0JPW37Z 0JPW3HZ 0JPW3JZ 0JPW3KZ 0JPW3NZ 0JPW3VZ 0JPW3WZ 0JPW3XZ 0JPWX0Z 0JPWX1Z 0JPWX3Z 0JPWXHZ 0JPWXVZ 0JPWXXZ

0 Medical and Surgical
J Subcutaneous Tissue and Fascia
Q Repair: Restoring, to the extent possible, a body part to its normal anatomic structure and function

Body Part Character 4	Approach Character 5	Device Character 6	Qualifier Character 7
0 Subcutaneous Tissue and Fascia, Scalp **1** Subcutaneous Tissue and Fascia, Face **4** Subcutaneous Tissue and Fascia, Anterior Neck **5** Subcutaneous Tissue and Fascia, Posterior Neck **6** Subcutaneous Tissue and Fascia, Chest **7** Subcutaneous Tissue and Fascia, Back **8** Subcutaneous Tissue and Fascia, Abdomen **9** Subcutaneous Tissue and Fascia, Buttock **B** Subcutaneous Tissue and Fascia, Perineum **C** Subcutaneous Tissue and Fascia, Pelvic Region **D** Subcutaneous Tissue and Fascia, Right Upper Arm **F** Subcutaneous Tissue and Fascia, Left Upper Arm **G** Subcutaneous Tissue and Fascia, Right Lower Arm **H** Subcutaneous Tissue and Fascia, Left Lower Arm **J** Subcutaneous Tissue and Fascia, Right Hand **K** Subcutaneous Tissue and Fascia, Left Hand **L** Subcutaneous Tissue and Fascia, Right Upper Leg **M** Subcutaneous Tissue and Fascia, Left Upper Leg **N** Subcutaneous Tissue and Fascia, Right Lower Leg **P** Subcutaneous Tissue and Fascia, Left Lower Leg **Q** Subcutaneous Tissue and Fascia, Right Foot **R** Subcutaneous Tissue and Fascia, Left Foot	**0** Open **3** Percutaneous	**Z** No Device	**Z** No Qualifier

0 Medical and Surgical
J Subcutaneous Tissue and Fascia
R Replacement: Putting in or on biological or synthetic material that physically takes the place and/or function of all or a portion of a body part

Body Part Character 4	Approach Character 5	Device Character 6	Qualifier Character 7
0 Subcutaneous Tissue and Fascia, Scalp **1** Subcutaneous Tissue and Fascia, Face **4** Subcutaneous Tissue and Fascia, Anterior Neck **5** Subcutaneous Tissue and Fascia, Posterior Neck **6** Subcutaneous Tissue and Fascia, Chest **7** Subcutaneous Tissue and Fascia, Back **8** Subcutaneous Tissue and Fascia, Abdomen **9** Subcutaneous Tissue and Fascia, Buttock **B** Subcutaneous Tissue and Fascia, Perineum **C** Subcutaneous Tissue and Fascia, Pelvic Region **D** Subcutaneous Tissue and Fascia, Right Upper Arm **F** Subcutaneous Tissue and Fascia, Left Upper Arm **G** Subcutaneous Tissue and Fascia, Right Lower Arm **H** Subcutaneous Tissue and Fascia, Left Lower Arm **J** Subcutaneous Tissue and Fascia, Right Hand **K** Subcutaneous Tissue and Fascia, Left Hand **L** Subcutaneous Tissue and Fascia, Right Upper Leg **M** Subcutaneous Tissue and Fascia, Left Upper Leg **N** Subcutaneous Tissue and Fascia, Right Lower Leg **P** Subcutaneous Tissue and Fascia, Left Lower Leg **Q** Subcutaneous Tissue and Fascia, Right Foot **R** Subcutaneous Tissue and Fascia, Left Foot	**0** Open **3** Percutaneous	**7** Autologous Tissue Substitute **J** Synthetic Substitute **K** Nonautologous Tissue Substitute	**Z** No Qualifier

0 Medical and Surgical
J Subcutaneous Tissue and Fascia
U Supplement: Putting in or on biological or synthetic material that physically reinforces and/or augments the function of a portion of a body part

Body Part Character 4	Approach Character 5	Device Character 6	Qualifier Character 7
0 Subcutaneous Tissue and Fascia, Scalp **1** Subcutaneous Tissue and Fascia, Face **4** Subcutaneous Tissue and Fascia, Anterior Neck **5** Subcutaneous Tissue and Fascia, Posterior Neck **6** Subcutaneous Tissue and Fascia, Chest **7** Subcutaneous Tissue and Fascia, Back **8** Subcutaneous Tissue and Fascia, Abdomen **9** Subcutaneous Tissue and Fascia, Buttock **B** Subcutaneous Tissue and Fascia, Perineum **C** Subcutaneous Tissue and Fascia, Pelvic Region **D** Subcutaneous Tissue and Fascia, Right Upper Arm **F** Subcutaneous Tissue and Fascia, Left Upper Arm **G** Subcutaneous Tissue and Fascia, Right Lower Arm **H** Subcutaneous Tissue and Fascia, Left Lower Arm **J** Subcutaneous Tissue and Fascia, Right Hand **K** Subcutaneous Tissue and Fascia, Left Hand **L** Subcutaneous Tissue and Fascia, Right Upper Leg **M** Subcutaneous Tissue and Fascia, Left Upper Leg **N** Subcutaneous Tissue and Fascia, Right Lower Leg **P** Subcutaneous Tissue and Fascia, Left Lower Leg **Q** Subcutaneous Tissue and Fascia, Right Foot **R** Subcutaneous Tissue and Fascia, Left Foot	**0** Open **3** Percutaneous	**7** Autologous Tissue Substitute **J** Synthetic Substitute **K** Nonautologous Tissue Substitute	**Z** No Qualifier

0 Medical and Surgical
J Subcutaneous Tissue and Fascia
W Revision: Correcting, to the extent possible, a portion of a malfunctioning device or the position of a displaced device

Body Part Character 4	Approach Character 5	Device Character 6	Qualifier Character 7
S Subcutaneous Tissue and Fascia, Head and Neck ⊘ DRG	**0** Open **3** Percutaneous **X** External	**0** Drainage Device **3** Infusion Device **7** Autologous Tissue Substitute **J** Synthetic Substitute **K** Nonautologous Tissue Substitute **N** Tissue Expander	**Z** No Qualifier
T Subcutaneous Tissue and Fascia, Trunk ⊘ HAC DRG	**0** Open **3** Percutaneous **X** External	**0** Drainage Device **2** Monitoring Device **3** Infusion Device **7** Autologous Tissue Substitute **H** Contraceptive Device **J** Synthetic Substitute **K** Nonautologous Tissue Substitute **M** Stimulator Generator **N** Tissue Expander **P** Cardiac Rhythm Related Device **V** Infusion Device, Pump **W** Vascular Access Device, Reservoir **X** Vascular Access Device	**Z** No Qualifier
V Subcutaneous Tissue and Fascia, Upper Extremity ⊘ DRG **W** Subcutaneous Tissue and Fascia, Lower Extremity ⊘ DRG	**0** Open **3** Percutaneous **X** External	**0** Drainage Device **3** Infusion Device **7** Autologous Tissue Substitute **H** Contraceptive Device **J** Synthetic Substitute **K** Nonautologous Tissue Substitute **N** Tissue Expander **V** Infusion Device, Pump **W** Vascular Access Device, Reservoir **X** Vascular Access Device	**Z** No Qualifier

HAC 0JWT0PZ or 0JWT3PZ when reported with secondary diagnosis K68.11, T81.4XXA, T82.6XXA, T82.7XXA

DRG 0JWS00Z 0JWS03Z 0JWS07Z 0JWS0JZ 0JWS0KZ 0JWS0NZ 0JWS30Z 0JWS33Z 0JWS37Z 0JWS3JZ 0JWS3KZ 0JWS3NZ 0JWT00Z 0JWT03Z 0JWT07Z 0JWT0HZ 0JWT0JZ 0JWT0KZ 0JWT0NZ 0JWT0VZ 0JWT0WZ 0JWT0XZ 0JWT30Z 0JWT33Z 0JWT37Z 0JWT3HZ 0JWT3JZ 0JWT3KZ 0JWT3NZ 0JWT3VZ 0JWT3WZ 0JWT3XZ 0JWV00Z 0JWV03Z 0JWV07Z 0JWV0HZ 0JWV0JZ 0JWV0KZ 0JWV0NZ 0JWV0VZ 0JWV0WZ 0JWV0XZ 0JWV30Z 0JWV33Z 0JWV37Z 0JWV3HZ 0JWV3JZ 0JWV3KZ 0JWV3NZ 0JWV3VZ 0JWV3WZ 0JWV3XZ 0JWW00Z 0JWW03Z 0JWW07Z 0JWW0HZ 0JWW0JZ 0JWW0KZ 0JWW0NZ 0JWW0VZ 0JWW0WZ 0JWW0XZ 0JWW30Z 0JWW33Z 0JWW37Z 0JWW3HZ 0JWW3JZ 0JWW3KZ 0JWW3NZ 0JWW3VZ 0JWW3WZ 0JWW3XZ

⊘ 0JWSX0Z 0JWSX3Z 0JWSX7Z 0JWSXJZ 0JWSXKZ 0JWSXNZ 0JWTX0Z 0JWTX2Z 0JWTX3Z 0JWTX7Z 0JWTXHZ 0JWTXJZ 0JWTXKZ 0JWTXNZ 0JWTXPZ 0JWTXVZ 0JWTXWZ 0JWTXXZ 0JWVX0Z 0JWVX3Z 0JWVX7Z 0JWVXHZ 0JWVXJZ 0JWVXKZ 0JWVXNZ 0JWVXVZ 0JWVXWZ 0JWVXXZ 0JWWX0Z 0JWWX3Z 0JWWX7Z 0JWWXHZ 0JWWXJZ 0JWWXKZ 0JWWXNZ 0JWWXVZ 0JWWXWZ 0JWWXXZ

0 Medical and Surgical
J Subcutaneous Tissue and Fascia
X Transfer: Moving, without taking out, all or a portion of a body part to another location to take over the function of all or a portion of a body part

Body Part Character 4	Approach Character 5	Device Character 6	Qualifier Character 7
0 Subcutaneous Tissue and Fascia, Scalp **1** Subcutaneous Tissue and Fascia, Face **4** Subcutaneous Tissue and Fascia, Anterior Neck **5** Subcutaneous Tissue and Fascia, Posterior Neck **6** Subcutaneous Tissue and Fascia, Chest **7** Subcutaneous Tissue and Fascia, Back **8** Subcutaneous Tissue and Fascia, Abdomen **9** Subcutaneous Tissue and Fascia, Buttock **B** Subcutaneous Tissue and Fascia, Perineum **C** Subcutaneous Tissue and Fascia, Pelvic Region **D** Subcutaneous Tissue and Fascia, Right Upper Arm **F** Subcutaneous Tissue and Fascia, Left Upper Arm **G** Subcutaneous Tissue and Fascia, Right Lower Arm **H** Subcutaneous Tissue and Fascia, Left Lower Arm **J** Subcutaneous Tissue and Fascia, Right Hand **K** Subcutaneous Tissue and Fascia, Left Hand **L** Subcutaneous Tissue and Fascia, Right Upper Leg **M** Subcutaneous Tissue and Fascia, Left Upper Leg **N** Subcutaneous Tissue and Fascia, Right Lower Leg **P** Subcutaneous Tissue and Fascia, Left Lower Leg **Q** Subcutaneous Tissue and Fascia, Right Foot **R** Subcutaneous Tissue and Fascia, Left Foot	**0** Open **3** Percutaneous	**Z** No Device	**B** Skin and Subcutaneous Tissue **C** Skin, Subcutaneous Tissue and Fascia **Z** No Qualifier

Muscles 0K2-0KX

0 Medical and Surgical
K Muscles
2 Change: Taking out or off a device from a body part and putting back an identical or similar device in or on the same body part without cutting or puncturing the skin or a mucous membrane

Body Part Character 4	Approach Character 5	Device Character 6	Qualifier Character 7
X Upper Muscle ⃠ **Y** Lower Muscle ⃠	**X** External	**0** Drainage Device **Y** Other Device	**Z** No Qualifier

⃠ 0K2XX0Z 0K2XXYZ 0K2YX0Z 0K2YXYZ

0 Medical and Surgical
K Muscles
5 Destruction: Physical eradication of all or a portion of a body part by the direct use of energy, force, or a destructive agent

Body Part Character 4	Approach Character 5	Device Character 6	Qualifier Character 7
0 Head Muscle **1** Facial Muscle **2** Neck Muscle, Right **3** Neck Muscle, Left **4** Tongue, Palate, Pharynx Muscle **5** Shoulder Muscle, Right **6** Shoulder Muscle, Left **7** Upper Arm Muscle, Right **8** Upper Arm Muscle, Left **9** Lower Arm and Wrist Muscle, Right **B** Lower Arm and Wrist Muscle, Left **C** Hand Muscle, Right **D** Hand Muscle, Left **F** Trunk Muscle, Right **G** Trunk Muscle, Left **H** Thorax Muscle, Right **J** Thorax Muscle, Left **K** Abdomen Muscle, Right **L** Abdomen Muscle, Left **M** Perineum Muscle **N** Hip Muscle, Right **P** Hip Muscle, Left **Q** Upper Leg Muscle, Right **R** Upper Leg Muscle, Left **S** Lower Leg Muscle, Right **T** Lower Leg Muscle, Left **V** Foot Muscle, Right **W** Foot Muscle, Left	**0** Open **3** Percutaneous **4** Percutaneous Endoscopic	**Z** No Device	**Z** No Qualifier

0 Medical and Surgical
K Muscles
8 Division: Cutting into a body part, without draining fluids and/or gases from the body part, in order to separate or transect a body part

Body Part Character 4	Approach Character 5	Device Character 6	Qualifier Character 7
0 Head Muscle **1** Facial Muscle **2** Neck Muscle, Right **3** Neck Muscle, Left **4** Tongue, Palate, Pharynx Muscle **5** Shoulder Muscle, Right **6** Shoulder Muscle, Left **7** Upper Arm Muscle, Right **8** Upper Arm Muscle, Left **9** Lower Arm and Wrist Muscle, Right **B** Lower Arm and Wrist Muscle, Left **C** Hand Muscle, Right **D** Hand Muscle, Left **F** Trunk Muscle, Right **G** Trunk Muscle, Left **H** Thorax Muscle, Right **J** Thorax Muscle, Left **K** Abdomen Muscle, Right **L** Abdomen Muscle, Left **M** Perineum Muscle **N** Hip Muscle, Right **P** Hip Muscle, Left **Q** Upper Leg Muscle, Right **R** Upper Leg Muscle, Left **S** Lower Leg Muscle, Right **T** Lower Leg Muscle, Left **V** Foot Muscle, Right **W** Foot Muscle, Left	**0** Open **3** Percutaneous **4** Percutaneous Endoscopic	**Z** No Device	**Z** No Qualifier

0 Medical and Surgical
K Muscles
9 Drainage: Taking or letting out fluids and/or gases from a body part

Body Part Character 4	Approach Character 5	Device Character 6	Qualifier Character 7
0 Head Muscle ⊘ **1** Facial Muscle ⊘ **2** Neck Muscle, Right ⊘ **3** Neck Muscle, Left ⊘ **4** Tongue, Palate, Pharynx Muscle ⊘ **5** Shoulder Muscle, Right ⊘ **6** Shoulder Muscle, Left ⊘ **7** Upper Arm Muscle, Right ⊘ **8** Upper Arm Muscle, Left ⊘ **9** Lower Arm and Wrist Muscle, Right ⊘ **B** Lower Arm and Wrist Muscle, Left ⊘ **C** Hand Muscle, Right ⊘ **D** Hand Muscle, Left ⊘ **F** Trunk Muscle, Right ⊘ **G** Trunk Muscle, Left ⊘ **H** Thorax Muscle, Right ⊘ **J** Thorax Muscle, Left ⊘ **K** Abdomen Muscle, Right ⊘ **L** Abdomen Muscle, Left ⊘ **M** Perineum Muscle ⊘ **N** Hip Muscle, Right ⊘ **P** Hip Muscle, Left ⊘ **Q** Upper Leg Muscle, Right ⊘ **R** Upper Leg Muscle, Left ⊘ **S** Lower Leg Muscle, Right ⊘ **T** Lower Leg Muscle, Left ⊘ **V** Foot Muscle, Right ⊘ **W** Foot Muscle, Left ⊘	**0** Open **3** Percutaneous **4** Percutaneous Endoscopic	**0** Drainage Device	**Z** No Qualifier
0 Head Muscle ⊘ **1** Facial Muscle ⊘ **2** Neck Muscle, Right ⊘ **3** Neck Muscle, Left ⊘ **4** Tongue, Palate, Pharynx Muscle ⊘ **5** Shoulder Muscle, Right ⊘ **6** Shoulder Muscle, Left ⊘ **7** Upper Arm Muscle, Right ⊘ **8** Upper Arm Muscle, Left ⊘ **9** Lower Arm and Wrist Muscle, Right ⊘ **B** Lower Arm and Wrist Muscle, Left ⊘ **C** Hand Muscle, Right ⊘ **D** Hand Muscle, Left ⊘ **F** Trunk Muscle, Right ⊘ **G** Trunk Muscle, Left ⊘ **H** Thorax Muscle, Right ⊘ **J** Thorax Muscle, Left ⊘ **K** Abdomen Muscle, Right ⊘ **L** Abdomen Muscle, Left ⊘ **M** Perineum Muscle ⊘ **N** Hip Muscle, Right ⊘ **P** Hip Muscle, Left ⊘ **Q** Upper Leg Muscle, Right ⊘ **R** Upper Leg Muscle, Left ⊘ **S** Lower Leg Muscle, Right ⊘ **T** Lower Leg Muscle, Left ⊘ **V** Foot Muscle, Right ⊘ **W** Foot Muscle, Left ⊘	**0** Open **3** Percutaneous **4** Percutaneous Endoscopic	**Z** No Device	**X** Diagnostic **Z** No Qualifier

⊘ 0K9030Z 0K903ZZ 0K9130Z 0K913ZZ 0K9230Z 0K923ZZ 0K9330Z 0K933ZZ 0K9430Z 0K943ZZ 0K9530Z 0K953ZZ 0K9630Z 0K963ZZ 0K9730Z 0K973ZZ 0K9830Z 0K983ZZ 0K9930Z 0K993ZZ 0K9B30Z 0K9B3ZZ 0K9C30Z 0K9C3ZZ 0K9C4ZZ 0K9D30Z 0K9D3ZZ 0K9D4ZZ 0K9F30Z 0K9F3ZZ 0K9G30Z 0K9G3ZZ 0K9H30Z 0K9H3ZZ 0K9J30Z 0K9J3ZZ 0K9K30Z 0K9K3ZZ 0K9L30Z 0K9L3ZZ 0K9M30Z 0K9M3ZZ 0K9N30Z 0K9N3ZZ 0K9P30Z 0K9P3ZZ 0K9Q30Z 0K9Q3ZZ 0K9R30Z 0K9R3ZZ 0K9S30Z 0K9S3ZZ 0K9T30Z 0K9T3ZZ 0K9V30Z 0K9V3ZZ 0K9W30Z 0K9W3ZZ

0 Medical and Surgical
K Muscles
B Excision: Cutting out or off, without replacement, a portion of a body part

Body Part Character 4	Approach Character 5	Device Character 6	Qualifier Character 7
0 Head Muscle **1** Facial Muscle **2** Neck Muscle, Right **3** Neck Muscle, Left **4** Tongue, Palate, Pharynx Muscle **5** Shoulder Muscle, Right **6** Shoulder Muscle, Left **7** Upper Arm Muscle, Right **8** Upper Arm Muscle, Left **9** Lower Arm and Wrist Muscle, Right **B** Lower Arm and Wrist Muscle, Left **C** Hand Muscle, Right **D** Hand Muscle, Left **F** Trunk Muscle, Right **G** Trunk Muscle, Left **H** Thorax Muscle, Right **J** Thorax Muscle, Left **K** Abdomen Muscle, Right **L** Abdomen Muscle, Left **M** Perineum Muscle **N** Hip Muscle, Right **P** Hip Muscle, Left **Q** Upper Leg Muscle, Right **R** Upper Leg Muscle, Left **S** Lower Leg Muscle, Right **T** Lower Leg Muscle, Left **V** Foot Muscle, Right **W** Foot Muscle, Left	**0** Open **3** Percutaneous **4** Percutaneous Endoscopic	**Z** No Device	**X** Diagnostic **Z** No Qualifier

0 Medical and Surgical
K Muscles
C Extirpation: Taking or cutting out solid matter from a body part

Body Part Character 4	Approach Character 5	Device Character 6	Qualifier Character 7
0 Head Muscle **1** Facial Muscle **2** Neck Muscle, Right **3** Neck Muscle, Left **4** Tongue, Palate, Pharynx Muscle **5** Shoulder Muscle, Right **6** Shoulder Muscle, Left **7** Upper Arm Muscle, Right **8** Upper Arm Muscle, Left **9** Lower Arm and Wrist Muscle, Right **B** Lower Arm and Wrist Muscle, Left **C** Hand Muscle, Right **D** Hand Muscle, Left **F** Trunk Muscle, Right **G** Trunk Muscle, Left **H** Thorax Muscle, Right **J** Thorax Muscle, Left **K** Abdomen Muscle, Right **L** Abdomen Muscle, Left **M** Perineum Muscle **N** Hip Muscle, Right **P** Hip Muscle, Left **Q** Upper Leg Muscle, Right **R** Upper Leg Muscle, Left **S** Lower Leg Muscle, Right **T** Lower Leg Muscle, Left **V** Foot Muscle, Right **W** Foot Muscle, Left	**0** Open **3** Percutaneous **4** Percutaneous Endoscopic	**Z** No Device	**Z** No Qualifier

0 **Medical and Surgical**
K **Muscles**
H **Insertion:** Putting in a nonbiological appliance that monitors, assists, performs, or prevents a physiological function but does not physically take the place of a body part

Body Part Character 4	Approach Character 5	Device Character 6	Qualifier Character 7
X Upper Muscle **Y** Lower Muscle	**0** Open **3** Percutaneous **4** Percutaneous Endoscopic	**M** Stimulator Lead	**Z** No Qualifier

0 **Medical and Surgical**
K **Muscles**
J **Inspection:** Visually and/or manually exploring a body part

Body Part Character 4	Approach Character 5	Device Character 6	Qualifier Character 7
X Upper Muscle ⃠ **Y** Lower Muscle ⃠	**0** Open **3** Percutaneous **4** Percutaneous Endoscopic **X** External	**Z** No Device	**Z** No Qualifier

⃠ 0KJX3ZZ 0KJXXZZ 0KJY3ZZ 0KJYXZZ

0 **Medical and Surgical**
K **Muscles**
M **Reattachment:** Putting back in or on all or a portion of a separated body part to its normal location or other suitable location

Body Part Character 4	Approach Character 5	Device Character 6	Qualifier Character 7
0 Head Muscle **1** Facial Muscle **2** Neck Muscle, Right **3** Neck Muscle, Left **4** Tongue, Palate, Pharynx Muscle **5** Shoulder Muscle, Right **6** Shoulder Muscle, Left **7** Upper Arm Muscle, Right **8** Upper Arm Muscle, Left **9** Lower Arm and Wrist Muscle, Right **B** Lower Arm and Wrist Muscle, Left **C** Hand Muscle, Right **D** Hand Muscle, Left **F** Trunk Muscle, Right **G** Trunk Muscle, Left **H** Thorax Muscle, Right **J** Thorax Muscle, Left **K** Abdomen Muscle, Right **L** Abdomen Muscle, Left **M** Perineum Muscle **N** Hip Muscle, Right **P** Hip Muscle, Left **Q** Upper Leg Muscle, Right **R** Upper Leg Muscle, Left **S** Lower Leg Muscle, Right **T** Lower Leg Muscle, Left **V** Foot Muscle, Right **W** Foot Muscle, Left	**0** Open **4** Percutaneous Endoscopic	**Z** No Device	**Z** No Qualifier

0 Medical and Surgical
K Muscles
N Release: Freeing a body part from an abnormal physical constraint by cutting or by the use of force

Body Part Character 4	Approach Character 5	Device Character 6	Qualifier Character 7
0 Head Muscle ⦸ **1** Facial Muscle ⦸ **2** Neck Muscle, Right ⦸ **3** Neck Muscle, Left ⦸ **4** Tongue, Palate, Pharynx Muscle ⦸ **5** Shoulder Muscle, Right ⦸ **6** Shoulder Muscle, Left ⦸ **7** Upper Arm Muscle, Right ⦸ **8** Upper Arm Muscle, Left ⦸ **9** Lower Arm and Wrist Muscle, Right ⦸ **B** Lower Arm and Wrist Muscle, Left ⦸ **C** Hand Muscle, Right ⦸ **D** Hand Muscle, Left ⦸ **F** Trunk Muscle, Right ⦸ **G** Trunk Muscle, Left ⦸ **H** Thorax Muscle, Right ⦸ **J** Thorax Muscle, Left ⦸ **K** Abdomen Muscle, Right ⦸ **L** Abdomen Muscle, Left ⦸ **M** Perineum Muscle ⦸ **N** Hip Muscle, Right ⦸ **P** Hip Muscle, Left ⦸ **Q** Upper Leg Muscle, Right ⦸ **R** Upper Leg Muscle, Left ⦸ **S** Lower Leg Muscle, Right ⦸ **T** Lower Leg Muscle, Left ⦸ **V** Foot Muscle, Right ⦸ **W** Foot Muscle, Left ⦸	**0** Open **3** Percutaneous **4** Percutaneous Endoscopic **X** External	**Z** No Device	**Z** No Qualifier

⦸ 0KN0XZZ 0KN1XZZ 0KN2XZZ 0KN3XZZ 0KN4XZZ 0KN5XZZ 0KN6XZZ 0KN7XZZ 0KN8XZZ 0KN9XZZ 0KNBXZZ 0KNCXZZ 0KNDXZZ 0KNFXZZ 0KNGXZZ 0KNHXZZ 0KNJXZZ 0KNKXZZ 0KNLXZZ 0KNMXZZ 0KNNXZZ 0KNPXZZ 0KNQXZZ 0KNRXZZ 0KNSXZZ 0KNTXZZ 0KNVXZZ 0KNWXZZ

0 Medical and Surgical
K Muscles
P Removal: Taking out or off a device from a body part

Body Part Character 4	Approach Character 5	Device Character 6	Qualifier Character 7
X Upper Muscle ⦸ **Y** Lower Muscle ⦸	**0** Open **3** Percutaneous **4** Percutaneous Endoscopic	**0** Drainage Device **7** Autologous Tissue Substitute **J** Synthetic Substitute **K** Nonautologous Tissue Substitute **M** Stimulator Lead	**Z** No Qualifier
X Upper Muscle ⦸ **Y** Lower Muscle ⦸	**X** External	**0** Drainage Device **M** Stimulator Lead	**Z** No Qualifier

⦸ 0KPXX0Z 0KPXXMZ 0KPYX0Z 0KPYXMZ

0 Medical and Surgical
K Muscles
Q Repair: Restoring, to the extent possible, a body part to its normal anatomic structure and function

Body Part Character 4	Approach Character 5	Device Character 6	Qualifier Character 7
0 Head Muscle **1** Facial Muscle **2** Neck Muscle, Right **3** Neck Muscle, Left **4** Tongue, Palate, Pharynx Muscle **5** Shoulder Muscle, Right **6** Shoulder Muscle, Left **7** Upper Arm Muscle, Right **8** Upper Arm Muscle, Left **9** Lower Arm and Wrist Muscle, Right **B** Lower Arm and Wrist Muscle, Left **C** Hand Muscle, Right **D** Hand Muscle, Left **F** Trunk Muscle, Right **G** Trunk Muscle, Left **H** Thorax Muscle, Right **J** Thorax Muscle, Left **K** Abdomen Muscle, Right **L** Abdomen Muscle, Left **M** Perineum Muscle **N** Hip Muscle, Right **P** Hip Muscle, Left **Q** Upper Leg Muscle, Right **R** Upper Leg Muscle, Left **S** Lower Leg Muscle, Right **T** Lower Leg Muscle, Left **V** Foot Muscle, Right **W** Foot Muscle, Left	**0** Open **3** Percutaneous **4** Percutaneous Endoscopic	**Z** No Device	**Z** No Qualifier

0 Medical and Surgical
K Muscles
S Reposition: Moving to its normal location, or other suitable location, all or a portion of a body part

Body Part Character 4	Approach Character 5	Device Character 6	Qualifier Character 7
0 Head Muscle **1** Facial Muscle **2** Neck Muscle, Right **3** Neck Muscle, Left **4** Tongue, Palate, Pharynx Muscle **5** Shoulder Muscle, Right **6** Shoulder Muscle, Left **7** Upper Arm Muscle, Right **8** Upper Arm Muscle, Left **9** Lower Arm and Wrist Muscle, Right **B** Lower Arm and Wrist Muscle, Left **C** Hand Muscle, Right **D** Hand Muscle, Left **F** Trunk Muscle, Right **G** Trunk Muscle, Left **H** Thorax Muscle, Right **J** Thorax Muscle, Left **K** Abdomen Muscle, Right **L** Abdomen Muscle, Left **M** Perineum Muscle **N** Hip Muscle, Right **P** Hip Muscle, Left **Q** Upper Leg Muscle, Right **R** Upper Leg Muscle, Left **S** Lower Leg Muscle, Right **T** Lower Leg Muscle, Left **V** Foot Muscle, Right **W** Foot Muscle, Left	**0** Open **4** Percutaneous Endoscopic	**Z** No Device	**Z** No Qualifier

0 Medical and Surgical
K Muscles
T Resection: Cutting out or off, without replacement, all of a body part

Body Part Character 4	Approach Character 5	Device Character 6	Qualifier Character 7
0 Head Muscle **1** Facial Muscle **2** Neck Muscle, Right **3** Neck Muscle, Left **4** Tongue, Palate, Pharynx Muscle **5** Shoulder Muscle, Right **6** Shoulder Muscle, Left **7** Upper Arm Muscle, Right **8** Upper Arm Muscle, Left **9** Lower Arm and Wrist Muscle, Right **B** Lower Arm and Wrist Muscle, Left **C** Hand Muscle, Right **D** Hand Muscle, Left **F** Trunk Muscle, Right **G** Trunk Muscle, Left **H** Thorax Muscle, Right CC **J** Thorax Muscle, Left CC **K** Abdomen Muscle, Right **L** Abdomen Muscle, Left **M** Perineum Muscle **N** Hip Muscle, Right **P** Hip Muscle, Left **Q** Upper Leg Muscle, Right **R** Upper Leg Muscle, Left **S** Lower Leg Muscle, Right **T** Lower Leg Muscle, Left **V** Foot Muscle, Right **W** Foot Muscle, Left	**0** Open **4** Percutaneous Endoscopic	**Z** No Device	**Z** No Qualifier

CC 0KTH0ZZ 0KTJ0ZZ

0 Medical and Surgical
K Muscles
U Supplement: Putting in or on biological or synthetic material that physically reinforces and/or augments the function of a portion of a body part

Body Part Character 4	Approach Character 5	Device Character 6	Qualifier Character 7
0 Head Muscle **1** Facial Muscle **2** Neck Muscle, Right **3** Neck Muscle, Left **4** Tongue, Palate, Pharynx Muscle **5** Shoulder Muscle, Right **6** Shoulder Muscle, Left **7** Upper Arm Muscle, Right **8** Upper Arm Muscle, Left **9** Lower Arm and Wrist Muscle, Right **B** Lower Arm and Wrist Muscle, Left **C** Hand Muscle, Right **D** Hand Muscle, Left **F** Trunk Muscle, Right **G** Trunk Muscle, Left **H** Thorax Muscle, Right **J** Thorax Muscle, Left **K** Abdomen Muscle, Right **L** Abdomen Muscle, Left **M** Perineum Muscle **N** Hip Muscle, Right **P** Hip Muscle, Left **Q** Upper Leg Muscle, Right **R** Upper Leg Muscle, Left **S** Lower Leg Muscle, Right **T** Lower Leg Muscle, Left **V** Foot Muscle, Right **W** Foot Muscle, Left	**0** Open **4** Percutaneous Endoscopic	**7** Autologous Tissue Substitute **J** Synthetic Substitute **K** Nonautologous Tissue Substitute	**Z** No Qualifier

0 Medical and Surgical
K Muscles
W Revision: Correcting, to the extent possible, a portion of a malfunctioning device or the position of a displaced device

Body Part Character 4	Approach Character 5	Device Character 6	Qualifier Character 7
X Upper Muscle ⊘ **Y** Lower Muscle ⊘	**0** Open **3** Percutaneous **4** Percutaneous Endoscopic **X** External	**0** Drainage Device **7** Autologous Tissue Substitute **J** Synthetic Substitute **K** Nonautologous Tissue Substitute **M** Stimulator Lead	**Z** No Qualifier

⊘ 0KWXX0Z 0KWXX7Z 0KWXXJZ 0KWXXKZ 0KWXXMZ 0KWYX0Z 0KWYX7Z 0KWYXJZ 0KWYXKZ 0KWYXMZ

0 **Medical and Surgical**
K **Muscles**
X **Transfer:** Moving, without taking out, all or a portion of a body part to another location to take over the function of all or a portion of a body part

Body Part Character 4	Approach Character 5	Device Character 6	Qualifier Character 7
0 Head Muscle 1 Facial Muscle CC 2 Neck Muscle, Right 3 Neck Muscle, Left 4 Tongue, Palate, Pharynx Muscle 5 Shoulder Muscle, Right 6 Shoulder Muscle, Left 7 Upper Arm Muscle, Right 8 Upper Arm Muscle, Left 9 Lower Arm and Wrist Muscle, Right B Lower Arm and Wrist Muscle, Left C Hand Muscle, Right D Hand Muscle, Left F Trunk Muscle, Right G Trunk Muscle, Left H Thorax Muscle, Right J Thorax Muscle, Left M Perineum Muscle N Hip Muscle, Right P Hip Muscle, Left Q Upper Leg Muscle, Right R Upper Leg Muscle, Left S Lower Leg Muscle, Right CC T Lower Leg Muscle, Left CC V Foot Muscle, Right W Foot Muscle, Left	0 Open 4 Percutaneous Endoscopic	Z No Device	0 Skin 1 Subcutaneous Tissue 2 Skin and Subcutaneous Tissue Z No Qualifier
K Abdomen Muscle, Right L Abdomen Muscle, Left	0 Open 4 Percutaneous Endoscopic	Z No Device	0 Skin 1 Subcutaneous Tissue 2 Skin and Subcutaneous Tissue 6 Transverse Rectus Abdominis Myocutaneous Flap Z No Qualifier

CC 0KX10ZZ 0KX14ZZ 0KXS0ZZ 0KXS4ZZ 0KXT0ZZ 0KXT4ZZ

Tendons 0L2-0LX

0 Medical and Surgical
L Tendons
2 Change: Taking out or off a device from a body part and putting back an identical or similar device in or on the same body part without cutting or puncturing the skin or a mucous membrane

Body Part Character 4	Approach Character 5	Device Character 6	Qualifier Character 7
X Upper Tendon ⦸ **Y** Lower Tendon ⦸	**X** External	**0** Drainage Device **Y** Other Device	**Z** No Qualifier

⦸ 0L2XX0Z 0L2XXYZ 0L2YX0Z 0L2YXYZ

0 Medical and Surgical
L Tendons
5 Destruction: Physical eradication of all or a portion of a body part by the direct use of energy, force, or a destructive agent

Body Part Character 4	Approach Character 5	Device Character 6	Qualifier Character 7
0 Head and Neck Tendon **1** Shoulder Tendon, Right **2** Shoulder Tendon, Left **3** Upper Arm Tendon, Right **4** Upper Arm Tendon, Left **5** Lower Arm and Wrist Tendon, Right **6** Lower Arm and Wrist Tendon, Left **7** Hand Tendon, Right **8** Hand Tendon, Left **9** Trunk Tendon, Right **B** Trunk Tendon, Left **C** Thorax Tendon, Right **D** Thorax Tendon, Left **F** Abdomen Tendon, Right **G** Abdomen Tendon, Left **H** Perineum Tendon **J** Hip Tendon, Right **K** Hip Tendon, Left **L** Upper Leg Tendon, Right **M** Upper Leg Tendon, Left **N** Lower Leg Tendon, Right **P** Lower Leg Tendon, Left **Q** Knee Tendon, Right **R** Knee Tendon, Left **S** Ankle Tendon, Right **T** Ankle Tendon, Left **V** Foot Tendon, Right **W** Foot Tendon, Left	**0** Open **3** Percutaneous **4** Percutaneous Endoscopic	**Z** No Device	**Z** No Qualifier

0 Medical and Surgical
L Tendons
8 Division: Cutting into a body part, without draining fluids and/or gases from the body part, in order to separate or transect a body part

Body Part Character 4	Approach Character 5	Device Character 6	Qualifier Character 7
0 Head and Neck Tendon **1** Shoulder Tendon, Right **2** Shoulder Tendon, Left **3** Upper Arm Tendon, Right **4** Upper Arm Tendon, Left **5** Lower Arm and Wrist Tendon, Right **6** Lower Arm and Wrist Tendon, Left **7** Hand Tendon, Right **8** Hand Tendon, Left **9** Trunk Tendon, Right **B** Trunk Tendon, Left **C** Thorax Tendon, Right **D** Thorax Tendon, Left **F** Abdomen Tendon, Right **G** Abdomen Tendon, Left **H** Perineum Tendon **J** Hip Tendon, Right **K** Hip Tendon, Left **L** Upper Leg Tendon, Right **M** Upper Leg Tendon, Left **N** Lower Leg Tendon, Right **P** Lower Leg Tendon, Left **Q** Knee Tendon, Right **R** Knee Tendon, Left **S** Ankle Tendon, Right **T** Ankle Tendon, Left **V** Foot Tendon, Right **W** Foot Tendon, Left	**0** Open **3** Percutaneous **4** Percutaneous Endoscopic	**Z** No Device	**Z** No Qualifier

0 Medical and Surgical
L Tendons
9 Drainage: Taking or letting out fluids and/or gases from a body part

Body Part Character 4	Approach Character 5	Device Character 6	Qualifier Character 7
0 Head and Neck Tendon ⦸ **1** Shoulder Tendon, Right ⦸ **2** Shoulder Tendon, Left ⦸ **3** Upper Arm Tendon, Right ⦸ **4** Upper Arm Tendon, Left ⦸ **5** Lower Arm and Wrist Tendon, Right ⦸ **6** Lower Arm and Wrist Tendon, Left ⦸ **7** Hand Tendon, Right ⦸ **8** Hand Tendon, Left ⦸ **9** Trunk Tendon, Right ⦸ **B** Trunk Tendon, Left ⦸ **C** Thorax Tendon, Right ⦸ **D** Thorax Tendon, Left ⦸ **F** Abdomen Tendon, Right ⦸ **G** Abdomen Tendon, Left ⦸ **H** Perineum Tendon ⦸ **J** Hip Tendon, Right ⦸ **K** Hip Tendon, Left ⦸ **L** Upper Leg Tendon, Right ⦸ **M** Upper Leg Tendon, Left ⦸ **N** Lower Leg Tendon, Right ⦸ **P** Lower Leg Tendon, Left ⦸ **Q** Knee Tendon, Right ⦸ **R** Knee Tendon, Left ⦸ **S** Ankle Tendon, Right ⦸ **T** Ankle Tendon, Left ⦸ **V** Foot Tendon, Right ⦸ **W** Foot Tendon, Left ⦸	**0** Open **3** Percutaneous **4** Percutaneous Endoscopic	**0** Drainage Device	**Z** No Qualifier
0 Head and Neck Tendon ⦸ **1** Shoulder Tendon, Right ⦸ **2** Shoulder Tendon, Left ⦸ **3** Upper Arm Tendon, Right ⦸ **4** Upper Arm Tendon, Left ⦸ **5** Lower Arm and Wrist Tendon, Right ⦸ **6** Lower Arm and Wrist Tendon, Left ⦸ **7** Hand Tendon, Right ⦸ **8** Hand Tendon, Left ⦸ **9** Trunk Tendon, Right ⦸ **B** Trunk Tendon, Left ⦸ **C** Thorax Tendon, Right ⦸ **D** Thorax Tendon, Left ⦸ **F** Abdomen Tendon, Right ⦸ **G** Abdomen Tendon, Left ⦸ **H** Perineum Tendon ⦸ **J** Hip Tendon, Right ⦸ **K** Hip Tendon, Left ⦸ **L** Upper Leg Tendon, Right ⦸ **M** Upper Leg Tendon, Left ⦸ **N** Lower Leg Tendon, Right ⦸ **P** Lower Leg Tendon, Left ⦸ **Q** Knee Tendon, Right ⦸ **R** Knee Tendon, Left ⦸ **S** Ankle Tendon, Right ⦸ **T** Ankle Tendon, Left ⦸ **V** Foot Tendon, Right ⦸ **W** Foot Tendon, Left ⦸	**0** Open **3** Percutaneous **4** Percutaneous Endoscopic	**Z** No Device	**X** Diagnostic **Z** No Qualifier

⦸ 0L9030Z 0L903ZZ 0L9130Z 0L913ZZ 0L9230Z 0L923ZZ 0L9330Z 0L933ZZ 0L9430Z 0L943ZZ 0L9530Z 0L953ZZ 0L9630Z 0L963ZZ 0L9730Z 0L973ZZ 0L974ZZ 0L9830Z 0L983ZZ 0L984ZZ 0L9930Z 0L993ZZ 0L9B30Z 0L9B3ZZ 0L9C30Z 0L9C3ZZ 0L9D30Z 0L9D3ZZ 0L9F30Z 0L9F3ZZ 0L9G30Z 0L9G3ZZ 0L9H30Z 0L9H3ZZ 0L9J30Z 0L9J3ZZ 0L9K30Z 0L9K3ZZ 0L9L30Z 0L9L3ZZ 0L9M30Z 0L9M3ZZ 0L9N30Z 0L9N3ZZ 0L9P30Z 0L9P3ZZ 0L9Q30Z 0L9Q3ZZ 0L9R30Z 0L9R3ZZ 0L9S30Z 0L9S3ZZ 0L9T30Z 0L9T3ZZ 0L9V30Z 0L9V3ZZ 0L9W30Z 0L9W3ZZ

0 Medical and Surgical
L Tendons
B Excision: Cutting out or off, without replacement, a portion of a body part

Body Part Character 4	Approach Character 5	Device Character 6	Qualifier Character 7
0 Head and Neck Tendon **1** Shoulder Tendon, Right **2** Shoulder Tendon, Left **3** Upper Arm Tendon, Right **4** Upper Arm Tendon, Left **5** Lower Arm and Wrist Tendon, Right **6** Lower Arm and Wrist Tendon, Left **7** Hand Tendon, Right **8** Hand Tendon, Left **9** Trunk Tendon, Right **B** Trunk Tendon, Left **C** Thorax Tendon, Right **D** Thorax Tendon, Left **F** Abdomen Tendon, Right **G** Abdomen Tendon, Left **H** Perineum Tendon **J** Hip Tendon, Right **K** Hip Tendon, Left **L** Upper Leg Tendon, Right **M** Upper Leg Tendon, Left **N** Lower Leg Tendon, Right **P** Lower Leg Tendon, Left **Q** Knee Tendon, Right **R** Knee Tendon, Left **S** Ankle Tendon, Right **T** Ankle Tendon, Left **V** Foot Tendon, Right **W** Foot Tendon, Left	**0** Open **3** Percutaneous **4** Percutaneous Endoscopic	**Z** No Device	**X** Diagnostic **Z** No Qualifier

0 Medical and Surgical
L Tendons
C Extirpation: Taking or cutting out solid matter from a body part

Body Part Character 4	Approach Character 5	Device Character 6	Qualifier Character 7
0 Head and Neck Tendon **1** Shoulder Tendon, Right **2** Shoulder Tendon, Left **3** Upper Arm Tendon, Right **4** Upper Arm Tendon, Left **5** Lower Arm and Wrist Tendon, Right **6** Lower Arm and Wrist Tendon, Left **7** Hand Tendon, Right **8** Hand Tendon, Left **9** Trunk Tendon, Right **B** Trunk Tendon, Left **C** Thorax Tendon, Right **D** Thorax Tendon, Left **F** Abdomen Tendon, Right **G** Abdomen Tendon, Left **H** Perineum Tendon **J** Hip Tendon, Right **K** Hip Tendon, Left **L** Upper Leg Tendon, Right **M** Upper Leg Tendon, Left **N** Lower Leg Tendon, Right **P** Lower Leg Tendon, Left **Q** Knee Tendon, Right **R** Knee Tendon, Left **S** Ankle Tendon, Right **T** Ankle Tendon, Left **V** Foot Tendon, Right **W** Foot Tendon, Left	**0** Open **3** Percutaneous **4** Percutaneous Endoscopic	**Z** No Device	**Z** No Qualifier

0 Medical and Surgical
L Tendons
J Inspection: Visually and/or manually exploring a body part

Body Part Character 4	Approach Character 5	Device Character 6	Qualifier Character 7
X Upper Tendon ⦸ **Y** Lower Tendon ⦸	**0** Open **3** Percutaneous **4** Percutaneous Endoscopic **X** External	**Z** No Device	**Z** No Qualifier

⦸ 0LJX3ZZ 0LJXXZZ 0LJY3ZZ 0LJYXZZ

0 Medical and Surgical
L Tendons
M Reattachment: Putting back in or on all or a portion of a separated body part to its normal location or other suitable location

Body Part Character 4	Approach Character 5	Device Character 6	Qualifier Character 7
0 Head and Neck Tendon **1** Shoulder Tendon, Right **2** Shoulder Tendon, Left **3** Upper Arm Tendon, Right **4** Upper Arm Tendon, Left **5** Lower Arm and Wrist Tendon, Right **6** Lower Arm and Wrist Tendon, Left **7** Hand Tendon, Right **8** Hand Tendon, Left **9** Trunk Tendon, Right **B** Trunk Tendon, Left **C** Thorax Tendon, Right **D** Thorax Tendon, Left **F** Abdomen Tendon, Right **G** Abdomen Tendon, Left **H** Perineum Tendon **J** Hip Tendon, Right **K** Hip Tendon, Left **L** Upper Leg Tendon, Right **M** Upper Leg Tendon, Left **N** Lower Leg Tendon, Right **P** Lower Leg Tendon, Left **Q** Knee Tendon, Right **R** Knee Tendon, Left **S** Ankle Tendon, Right **T** Ankle Tendon, Left **V** Foot Tendon, Right **W** Foot Tendon, Left	**0** Open **4** Percutaneous Endoscopic	**Z** No Device	**Z** No Qualifier

0 Medical and Surgical
L Tendons
N Release: Freeing a body part from an abnormal physical constraint by cutting or by the use of force

Body Part Character 4	Approach Character 5	Device Character 6	Qualifier Character 7
0 Head and Neck Tendon ⦸ **1** Shoulder Tendon, Right ⦸ **2** Shoulder Tendon, Left ⦸ **3** Upper Arm Tendon, Right ⦸ **4** Upper Arm Tendon, Left ⦸ **5** Lower Arm and Wrist Tendon, Right ⦸ **6** Lower Arm and Wrist Tendon, Left ⦸ **7** Hand Tendon, Right ⦸ **8** Hand Tendon, Left ⦸ **9** Trunk Tendon, Right ⦸ **B** Trunk Tendon, Left ⦸ **C** Thorax Tendon, Right ⦸ **D** Thorax Tendon, Left ⦸ **F** Abdomen Tendon, Right ⦸ **G** Abdomen Tendon, Left ⦸ **H** Perineum Tendon ⦸ **J** Hip Tendon, Right ⦸ **K** Hip Tendon, Left ⦸ **L** Upper Leg Tendon, Right ⦸ **M** Upper Leg Tendon, Left ⦸ **N** Lower Leg Tendon, Right ⦸ **P** Lower Leg Tendon, Left ⦸ **Q** Knee Tendon, Right ⦸ **R** Knee Tendon, Left ⦸ **S** Ankle Tendon, Right ⦸ **T** Ankle Tendon, Left ⦸ **V** Foot Tendon, Right ⦸ **W** Foot Tendon, Left ⦸	**0** Open **3** Percutaneous **4** Percutaneous Endoscopic **X** External	**Z** No Device	**Z** No Qualifier

⦸ 0LN0XZZ 0LN1XZZ 0LN2XZZ 0LN3XZZ 0LN4XZZ 0LN5XZZ 0LN6XZZ 0LN7XZZ 0LN8XZZ 0LN9XZZ 0LNBXZZ 0LNCXZZ 0LNDXZZ 0LNFXZZ 0LNGXZZ 0LNHXZZ 0LNJXZZ 0LNKXZZ 0LNLXZZ 0LNMXZZ 0LNNXZZ 0LNPXZZ 0LNQXZZ 0LNRXZZ 0LNSXZZ 0LNTXZZ 0LNVXZZ 0LNWXZZ

0 Medical and Surgical
L Tendons
P Removal: Taking out or off a device from a body part

Body Part Character 4	Approach Character 5	Device Character 6	Qualifier Character 7
X Upper Tendon ⦸ **Y** Lower Tendon ⦸	**0** Open **3** Percutaneous **4** Percutaneous Endoscopic	**0** Drainage Device **7** Autologous Tissue Substitute **J** Synthetic Substitute **K** Nonautologous Tissue Substitute	**Z** No Qualifier
X Upper Tendon ⦸ **Y** Lower Tendon ⦸	**X** External	**0** Drainage Device	**Z** No Qualifier

⦸ 0LPX30Z 0LPXX0Z 0LPY30Z 0LPYX0Z

0 Medical and Surgical
L Tendons
Q Repair: Restoring, to the extent possible, a body part to its normal anatomic structure and function

Body Part Character 4	Approach Character 5	Device Character 6	Qualifier Character 7
0 Head and Neck Tendon	**0** Open	**Z** No Device	**Z** No Qualifier
1 Shoulder Tendon, Right	**3** Percutaneous		
2 Shoulder Tendon, Left	**4** Percutaneous Endoscopic		
3 Upper Arm Tendon, Right			
4 Upper Arm Tendon, Left			
5 Lower Arm and Wrist Tendon, Right			
6 Lower Arm and Wrist Tendon, Left			
7 Hand Tendon, Right			
8 Hand Tendon, Left			
9 Trunk Tendon, Right			
B Trunk Tendon, Left			
C Thorax Tendon, Right			
D Thorax Tendon, Left			
F Abdomen Tendon, Right			
G Abdomen Tendon, Left			
H Perineum Tendon			
J Hip Tendon, Right			
K Hip Tendon, Left			
L Upper Leg Tendon, Right			
M Upper Leg Tendon, Left			
N Lower Leg Tendon, Right			
P Lower Leg Tendon, Left			
Q Knee Tendon, Right			
R Knee Tendon, Left			
S Ankle Tendon, Right			
T Ankle Tendon, Left			
V Foot Tendon, Right			
W Foot Tendon, Left			

0 Medical and Surgical
L Tendons
R Replacement: Putting in or on biological or synthetic material that physically takes the place and/or function of all or a portion of a body part

Body Part Character 4	Approach Character 5	Device Character 6	Qualifier Character 7
0 Head and Neck Tendon	**0** Open	**7** Autologous Tissue Substitute	**Z** No Qualifier
1 Shoulder Tendon, Right	**4** Percutaneous Endoscopic	**J** Synthetic Substitute	
2 Shoulder Tendon, Left		**K** Nonautologous Tissue Substitute	
3 Upper Arm Tendon, Right			
4 Upper Arm Tendon, Left			
5 Lower Arm and Wrist Tendon, Right			
6 Lower Arm and Wrist Tendon, Left			
7 Hand Tendon, Right			
8 Hand Tendon, Left			
9 Trunk Tendon, Right			
B Trunk Tendon, Left			
C Thorax Tendon, Right			
D Thorax Tendon, Left			
F Abdomen Tendon, Right			
G Abdomen Tendon, Left			
H Perineum Tendon			
J Hip Tendon, Right			
K Hip Tendon, Left			
L Upper Leg Tendon, Right			
M Upper Leg Tendon, Left			
N Lower Leg Tendon, Right			
P Lower Leg Tendon, Left			
Q Knee Tendon, Right			
R Knee Tendon, Left			
S Ankle Tendon, Right			
T Ankle Tendon, Left			
V Foot Tendon, Right			
W Foot Tendon, Left			

0 Medical and Surgical
L Tendons
S Reposition: Moving to its normal location, or other suitable location, all or a portion of a body part

Body Part Character 4	Approach Character 5	Device Character 6	Qualifier Character 7
0 Head and Neck Tendon **1** Shoulder Tendon, Right **2** Shoulder Tendon, Left **3** Upper Arm Tendon, Right **4** Upper Arm Tendon, Left **5** Lower Arm and Wrist Tendon, Right **6** Lower Arm and Wrist Tendon, Left **7** Hand Tendon, Right **8** Hand Tendon, Left **9** Trunk Tendon, Right **B** Trunk Tendon, Left **C** Thorax Tendon, Right **D** Thorax Tendon, Left **F** Abdomen Tendon, Right **G** Abdomen Tendon, Left **H** Perineum Tendon **J** Hip Tendon, Right **K** Hip Tendon, Left **L** Upper Leg Tendon, Right **M** Upper Leg Tendon, Left **N** Lower Leg Tendon, Right **P** Lower Leg Tendon, Left **Q** Knee Tendon, Right CC **R** Knee Tendon, Left CC **S** Ankle Tendon, Right **T** Ankle Tendon, Left **V** Foot Tendon, Right **W** Foot Tendon, Left	**0** Open **4** Percutaneous Endoscopic	**Z** No Device	**Z** No Qualifier

CC 0LSQ0ZZ 0LSQ4ZZ 0LSR0ZZ 0LSR4ZZ

0 Medical and Surgical
L Tendons
T Resection: Cutting out or off, without replacement, all of a body part

Body Part Character 4	Approach Character 5	Device Character 6	Qualifier Character 7
0 Head and Neck Tendon **1** Shoulder Tendon, Right **2** Shoulder Tendon, Left **3** Upper Arm Tendon, Right **4** Upper Arm Tendon, Left **5** Lower Arm and Wrist Tendon, Right **6** Lower Arm and Wrist Tendon, Left **7** Hand Tendon, Right **8** Hand Tendon, Left **9** Trunk Tendon, Right **B** Trunk Tendon, Left **C** Thorax Tendon, Right **D** Thorax Tendon, Left **F** Abdomen Tendon, Right **G** Abdomen Tendon, Left **H** Perineum Tendon **J** Hip Tendon, Right **K** Hip Tendon, Left **L** Upper Leg Tendon, Right **M** Upper Leg Tendon, Left **N** Lower Leg Tendon, Right **P** Lower Leg Tendon, Left **Q** Knee Tendon, Right **R** Knee Tendon, Left **S** Ankle Tendon, Right **T** Ankle Tendon, Left **V** Foot Tendon, Right **W** Foot Tendon, Left	**0** Open **4** Percutaneous Endoscopic	**Z** No Device	**Z** No Qualifier

0 Medical and Surgical
L Tendons
U Supplement: Putting in or on biological or synthetic material that physically reinforces and/or augments the function of a portion of a body part

Body Part Character 4	Approach Character 5	Device Character 6	Qualifier Character 7
0 Head and Neck Tendon **1** Shoulder Tendon, Right **2** Shoulder Tendon, Left **3** Upper Arm Tendon, Right **4** Upper Arm Tendon, Left **5** Lower Arm and Wrist Tendon, Right **6** Lower Arm and Wrist Tendon, Left **7** Hand Tendon, Right **8** Hand Tendon, Left **9** Trunk Tendon, Right **B** Trunk Tendon, Left **C** Thorax Tendon, Right **D** Thorax Tendon, Left **F** Abdomen Tendon, Right **G** Abdomen Tendon, Left **H** Perineum Tendon **J** Hip Tendon, Right **K** Hip Tendon, Left **L** Upper Leg Tendon, Right **M** Upper Leg Tendon, Left **N** Lower Leg Tendon, Right **P** Lower Leg Tendon, Left **Q** Knee Tendon, Right **R** Knee Tendon, Left **S** Ankle Tendon, Right **T** Ankle Tendon, Left **V** Foot Tendon, Right **W** Foot Tendon, Left	**0** Open **4** Percutaneous Endoscopic	**7** Autologous Tissue Substitute **J** Synthetic Substitute **K** Nonautologous Tissue Substitute	**Z** No Qualifier

0 Medical and Surgical
L Tendons
W Revision: Correcting, to the extent possible, a portion of a malfunctioning device or the position of a displaced device

Body Part Character 4	Approach Character 5	Device Character 6	Qualifier Character 7
X Upper Tendon ⦸ **Y** Lower Tendon ⦸	**0** Open **3** Percutaneous **4** Percutaneous Endoscopic **X** External	**0** Drainage Device **7** Autologous Tissue Substitute **J** Synthetic Substitute **K** Nonautologous Tissue Substitute	**Z** No Qualifier

⦸ 0LWXX0Z 0LWXX7Z 0LWXXJZ 0LWXXKZ 0LWYX0Z 0LWYX7Z 0LWYXJZ 0LWYXKZ

0 Medical and Surgical
L Tendons
X Transfer: Moving, without taking out, all or a portion of a body part to another location to take over the function of all or a portion of a body part

Body Part Character 4	Approach Character 5	Device Character 6	Qualifier Character 7
0 Head and Neck Tendon **1** Shoulder Tendon, Right **2** Shoulder Tendon, Left **3** Upper Arm Tendon, Right **4** Upper Arm Tendon, Left **5** Lower Arm and Wrist Tendon, Right **6** Lower Arm and Wrist Tendon, Left **7** Hand Tendon, Right **8** Hand Tendon, Left **9** Trunk Tendon, Right **B** Trunk Tendon, Left **C** Thorax Tendon, Right **D** Thorax Tendon, Left **F** Abdomen Tendon, Right **G** Abdomen Tendon, Left **H** Perineum Tendon **J** Hip Tendon, Right **K** Hip Tendon, Left **L** Upper Leg Tendon, Right **M** Upper Leg Tendon, Left **N** Lower Leg Tendon, Right **P** Lower Leg Tendon, Left **Q** Knee Tendon, Right **R** Knee Tendon, Left **S** Ankle Tendon, Right **T** Ankle Tendon, Left **V** Foot Tendon, Right **W** Foot Tendon, Left	**0** Open **4** Percutaneous Endoscopic	**Z** No Device	**Z** No Qualifier

Bursae and Ligaments 0M2-0MX

0 Medical and Surgical
M Bursae and Ligaments
2 Change: Taking out or off a device from a body part and putting back an identical or similar device in or on the same body part without cutting or puncturing the skin or a mucous membrane

Body Part Character 4	Approach Character 5	Device Character 6	Qualifier Character 7
X Upper Bursa and Ligament ⃠ **Y** Lower Bursa and Ligament ⃠	**X** External	**0** Drainage Device **Y** Other Device	**Z** No Qualifier

⃠ 0M2XX0Z 0M2XXYZ 0M2YX0Z 0M2YXYZ

0 Medical and Surgical
M Bursae and Ligaments
5 Destruction: Physical eradication of all or a portion of a body part by the direct use of energy, force, or a destructive agent

Body Part Character 4	Approach Character 5	Device Character 6	Qualifier Character 7
0 Head and Neck Bursa and Ligament **1** Shoulder Bursa and Ligament, Right **2** Shoulder Bursa and Ligament, Left **3** Elbow Bursa and Ligament, Right **4** Elbow Bursa and Ligament, Left **5** Wrist Bursa and Ligament, Right **6** Wrist Bursa and Ligament, Left **7** Hand Bursa and Ligament, Right **8** Hand Bursa and Ligament, Left **9** Upper Extremity Bursa and Ligament, Right **B** Upper Extremity Bursa and Ligament, Left **C** Trunk Bursa and Ligament, Right **D** Trunk Bursa and Ligament, Left **F** Thorax Bursa and Ligament, Right **G** Thorax Bursa and Ligament, Left **H** Abdomen Bursa and Ligament, Right **J** Abdomen Bursa and Ligament, Left **K** Perineum Bursa and Ligament **L** Hip Bursa and Ligament, Right **M** Hip Bursa and Ligament, Left **N** Knee Bursa and Ligament, Right **P** Knee Bursa and Ligament, Left **Q** Ankle Bursa and Ligament, Right **R** Ankle Bursa and Ligament, Left **S** Foot Bursa and Ligament, Right **T** Foot Bursa and Ligament, Left **V** Lower Extremity Bursa and Ligament, Right **W** Lower Extremity Bursa and Ligament, Left	**0** Open **3** Percutaneous **4** Percutaneous Endoscopic	**Z** No Device	**Z** No Qualifier

0 Medical and Surgical
M Bursae and Ligaments
8 Division: Cutting into a body part, without draining fluids and/or gases from the body part, in order to separate or transect a body part

Body Part Character 4	Approach Character 5	Device Character 6	Qualifier Character 7
0 Head and Neck Bursa and Ligament **1** Shoulder Bursa and Ligament, Right **2** Shoulder Bursa and Ligament, Left **3** Elbow Bursa and Ligament, Right **4** Elbow Bursa and Ligament, Left **5** Wrist Bursa and Ligament, Right ⦸ **6** Wrist Bursa and Ligament, Left ⦸ **7** Hand Bursa and Ligament, Right **8** Hand Bursa and Ligament, Left **9** Upper Extremity Bursa and Ligament, Right **B** Upper Extremity Bursa and Ligament, Left **C** Trunk Bursa and Ligament, Right **D** Trunk Bursa and Ligament, Left **F** Thorax Bursa and Ligament, Right **G** Thorax Bursa and Ligament, Left **H** Abdomen Bursa and Ligament, Right **J** Abdomen Bursa and Ligament, Left **K** Perineum Bursa and Ligament **L** Hip Bursa and Ligament, Right **M** Hip Bursa and Ligament, Left **N** Knee Bursa and Ligament, Right **P** Knee Bursa and Ligament, Left **Q** Ankle Bursa and Ligament, Right **R** Ankle Bursa and Ligament, Left **S** Foot Bursa and Ligament, Right **T** Foot Bursa and Ligament, Left **V** Lower Extremity Bursa and Ligament, Right **W** Lower Extremity Bursa and Ligament, Left	**0** Open **3** Percutaneous **4** Percutaneous Endoscopic	**Z** No Device	**Z** No Qualifier

⦸ 0M850ZZ 0M853ZZ 0M854ZZ 0M860ZZ 0M863ZZ 0M864ZZ

0 Medical and Surgical
M Bursae and Ligaments
9 Drainage: Taking or letting out fluids and/or gases from a body part

Body Part Character 4	Approach Character 5	Device Character 6	Qualifier Character 7
0 Head and Neck Bursa and Ligament ⊘	**0** Open	**0** Drainage Device	**Z** No Qualifier
1 Shoulder Bursa and Ligament, Right ⊘	**3** Percutaneous		
2 Shoulder Bursa and Ligament, Left ⊘	**4** Percutaneous Endoscopic		
3 Elbow Bursa and Ligament, Right ⊘			
4 Elbow Bursa and Ligament, Left ⊘			
5 Wrist Bursa and Ligament, Right			
6 Wrist Bursa and Ligament, Left			
7 Hand Bursa and Ligament, Right ⊘			
8 Hand Bursa and Ligament, Left ⊘			
9 Upper Extremity Bursa and Ligament, Right ⊘			
B Upper Extremity Bursa and Ligament, Left ⊘			
C Trunk Bursa and Ligament, Right ⊘			
D Trunk Bursa and Ligament, Left ⊘			
F Thorax Bursa and Ligament, Right ⊘			
G Thorax Bursa and Ligament, Left ⊘			
H Abdomen Bursa and Ligament, Right ⊘			
J Abdomen Bursa and Ligament, Left ⊘			
K Perineum Bursa and Ligament ⊘			
L Hip Bursa and Ligament, Right ⊘			
M Hip Bursa and Ligament, Left ⊘			
N Knee Bursa and Ligament, Right			
P Knee Bursa and Ligament, Left			
Q Ankle Bursa and Ligament, Right			
R Ankle Bursa and Ligament, Left ⊘			
S Foot Bursa and Ligament, Right ⊘			
T Foot Bursa and Ligament, Left ⊘			
V Lower Extremity Bursa and ⊘ Ligament, Right ⊘			
W Lower Extremity Bursa and Ligament, Left ⊘			

0M9 continued on next page

0 Medical and Surgical
M Bursae and Ligaments
9 Drainage: Taking or letting out fluids and/or gases from a body part

0M9 continued from previous page

Body Part Character 4	Approach Character 5	Device Character 6	Qualifier Character 7
0 Head and Neck Bursa and Ligament ⃠ **1** Shoulder Bursa and Ligament, Right ⃠ **2** Shoulder Bursa and Ligament, Left ⃠ **3** Elbow Bursa and Ligament, Right ⃠ **4** Elbow Bursa and Ligament, Left ⃠ **5** Wrist Bursa and Ligament, Right ⃠ **6** Wrist Bursa and Ligament, Left ⃠ **7** Hand Bursa and Ligament, Right ⃠ **8** Hand Bursa and Ligament, Left ⃠ **9** Upper Extremity Bursa and Ligament, Right ⃠ **B** Upper Extremity Bursa and Ligament, Left ⃠ **C** Trunk Bursa and Ligament, Right ⃠ **D** Trunk Bursa and Ligament, Left ⃠ **F** Thorax Bursa and Ligament, Right ⃠ **G** Thorax Bursa and Ligament, Left ⃠ **H** Abdomen Bursa and Ligament, Right ⃠ **J** Abdomen Bursa and Ligament, Left ⃠ **K** Perineum Bursa and Ligament ⃠ **L** Hip Bursa and Ligament, Right ⃠ **M** Hip Bursa and Ligament, Left ⃠ **N** Knee Bursa and Ligament, Right ⃠ **P** Knee Bursa and Ligament, Left ⃠ **Q** Ankle Bursa and Ligament, Right ⃠ **R** Ankle Bursa and Ligament, Left ⃠ **S** Foot Bursa and Ligament, Right ⃠ **T** Foot Bursa and Ligament, Left ⃠ **V** Lower Extremity Bursa and Ligament, Right ⃠ **W** Lower Extremity Bursa and Ligament, Left ⃠	**0** Open **3** Percutaneous **4** Percutaneous Endoscopic	**Z** No Device	**X** Diagnostic **Z** No Qualifier

⃠ 0M900ZX 0M9030Z 0M903ZX 0M903ZZ 0M904ZX 0M904ZZ 0M910ZX 0M9130Z 0M913ZX 0M913ZZ 0M9140Z 0M914ZX 0M920ZX 0M9230Z 0M923ZX 0M923ZZ 0M9240Z 0M924ZX 0M930ZX 0M9330Z 0M933ZX 0M933ZZ 0M9340Z 0M934ZX 0M940ZX 0M9430Z 0M943ZX 0M943ZZ 0M9440Z 0M944ZX 0M950ZX 0M9530Z 0M953ZX 0M953ZZ 0M954ZX 0M954ZZ 0M960ZX 0M9630Z 0M963ZX 0M963ZZ 0M964ZX 0M964ZZ 0M970ZX 0M9730Z 0M973ZX 0M973ZZ 0M9740Z 0M974ZX 0M974ZZ 0M980ZX 0M9830Z 0M983ZX 0M983ZZ 0M9840Z 0M984ZX 0M984ZZ 0M9930Z 0M993ZZ 0M9940Z 0M994ZZ 0M9B30Z 0M9B3ZZ 0M9B40Z 0M9B4ZZ 0M9C0ZX 0M9C30Z 0M9C3ZX 0M9C3ZZ 0M9C40Z 0M9C4ZX 0M9C4ZZ 0M9D0ZX 0M9D30Z 0M9D3ZX 0M9D3ZZ 0M9D40Z 0M9D4ZX 0M9D4ZZ 0M9F0ZX 0M9F30Z 0M9F3ZX 0M9F3ZZ 0M9F40Z 0M9F4ZX 0M9F4ZZ 0M9G0ZX 0M9G30Z 0M9G3ZX 0M9G3ZZ 0M9G40Z 0M9G4ZX

0M9 continued on next page

0M9 continued from previous page

0M9G4ZZ	0M9H30Z	0M9H3ZZ	0M9H40Z	0M9H4ZZ	0M9J30Z	0M9J3ZZ	0M9J40Z	0M9J4ZZ	0M9K30Z	0M9K3ZZ	0M9K40Z	0M9K4ZZ
0M9L0ZX	0M9L30Z	0M9L3ZX	0M9L3ZZ	0M9L40Z	0M9L4ZX	0M9M0ZX	0M9M30Z	0M9M3ZX	0M9M3ZZ	0M9M40Z	0M9M4ZX	0M9N0ZX
0M9N30Z	0M9N3ZX	0M9N3ZZ	0M9N4ZX	0M9N4ZZ	0M9P0ZX	0M9P30Z	0M9P3ZX	0M9P3ZZ	0M9P4ZX	0M9P4ZZ	0M9Q0ZX	0M9Q30Z
0M9Q3ZX	0M9Q3ZZ	0M9Q4ZX	0M9Q4ZZ	0M9R0ZX	0M9R30Z	0M9R3ZX	0M9R3ZZ	0M9R4ZX	0M9R4ZZ	0M9S0ZX	0M9S30Z	0M9S3ZX
0M9S3ZZ	0M9S4ZX	0M9S4ZZ	0M9T0ZX	0M9T30Z	0M9T3ZX	0M9T3ZZ	0M9T4ZX	0M9T4ZZ	0M9V30Z	0M9V3ZZ	0M9V40Z	0M9V4ZZ
0M9W30Z	0M9W3ZZ	0M9W40Z	0M9W4ZZ									

0 Medical and Surgical
M Bursae and Ligaments
B Excision: Cutting out or off, without replacement, a portion of a body part

Body Part Character 4	Approach Character 5	Device Character 6	Qualifier Character 7
0 Head and Neck Bursa and Ligament ⊘ **1** Shoulder Bursa and Ligament, Right ⊘ **2** Shoulder Bursa and Ligament, Left ⊘ **3** Elbow Bursa and Ligament, Right ⊘ **4** Elbow Bursa and Ligament, Left ⊘ **5** Wrist Bursa and Ligament, Right ⊘ **6** Wrist Bursa and Ligament, Left ⊘ **7** Hand Bursa and Ligament, Right ⊘ **8** Hand Bursa and Ligament, Left ⊘ **9** Upper Extremity Bursa and Ligament, Right ⊘ **B** Upper Extremity Bursa and Ligament, Left ⊘ **C** Trunk Bursa and Ligament, Right ⊘ **D** Trunk Bursa and Ligament, Left ⊘ **F** Thorax Bursa and Ligament, Right ⊘ **G** Thorax Bursa and Ligament, Left ⊘ **H** Abdomen Bursa and Ligament, Right **J** Abdomen Bursa and Ligament, Left **K** Perineum Bursa and Ligament **L** Hip Bursa and Ligament, Right ⊘ **M** Hip Bursa and Ligament, Left ⊘ **N** Knee Bursa and Ligament, Right ⊘ **P** Knee Bursa and Ligament, Left ⊘ **Q** Ankle Bursa and Ligament, Right ⊘ **R** Ankle Bursa and Ligament, Left ⊘ **S** Foot Bursa and Ligament, Right ⊘ **T** Foot Bursa and Ligament, Left ⊘ **V** Lower Extremity Bursa and Ligament, Right **W** Lower Extremity Bursa and Ligament, Left	**0** Open **3** Percutaneous **4** Percutaneous Endoscopic	**Z** No Device	**X** Diagnostic **Z** No Qualifier

0MB continued on next page

0MB continued from previous page

⊘ 0MB00ZX 0MB03ZX 0MB04ZX 0MB10ZX 0MB13ZX 0MB14ZX 0MB20ZX 0MB23ZX 0MB24ZX 0MB30ZX 0MB33ZX 0MB34ZX 0MB40ZX 0MB43ZX 0MB44ZX 0MB50ZX 0MB53ZX 0MB54ZX 0MB60ZX 0MB63ZX 0MB64ZX 0MB70ZX 0MB73ZX 0MB74ZX 0MB80ZX 0MB83ZX 0MB84ZX 0MB94ZX 0MBB0ZX 0MBB3ZX 0MBB4ZX 0MBC0ZX 0MBC3ZX 0MBC4ZX 0MBD0ZX 0MBD3ZX 0MBD4ZX 0MBF0ZX 0MBF3ZX 0MBF4ZX 0MBG0ZX 0MBG3ZX 0MBG4ZX 0MBL0ZX 0MBL3ZX 0MBL4ZX 0MBM0ZX 0MBM3ZX 0MBM4ZX 0MBN0ZX 0MBN3ZX 0MBN4ZX 0MBP0ZX 0MBP3ZX 0MBP4ZX 0MBQ0ZX 0MBQ3ZX 0MBQ4ZX 0MBR0ZX 0MBR3ZX 0MBR4ZX 0MBS0ZX 0MBS3ZX 0MBS4ZX 0MBT0ZX 0MBT3ZX 0MBT4ZX

0 Medical and Surgical
M Bursae and Ligaments
C Extirpation: Taking or cutting out solid matter from a body part

Body Part Character 4	Approach Character 5	Device Character 6	Qualifier Character 7
0 Head and Neck Bursa and Ligament **1** Shoulder Bursa and Ligament, Right **2** Shoulder Bursa and Ligament, Left **3** Elbow Bursa and Ligament, Right **4** Elbow Bursa and Ligament, Left **5** Wrist Bursa and Ligament, Right **6** Wrist Bursa and Ligament, Left **7** Hand Bursa and Ligament, Right **8** Hand Bursa and Ligament, Left **9** Upper Extremity Bursa and Ligament, Right **B** Upper Extremity Bursa and Ligament, Left **C** Trunk Bursa and Ligament, Right **D** Trunk Bursa and Ligament, Left **F** Thorax Bursa and Ligament, Right **G** Thorax Bursa and Ligament, Left **H** Abdomen Bursa and Ligament, Right **J** Abdomen Bursa and Ligament, Left **K** Perineum Bursa and Ligament **L** Hip Bursa and Ligament, Right **M** Hip Bursa and Ligament, Left **N** Knee Bursa and Ligament, Right **P** Knee Bursa and Ligament, Left **Q** Ankle Bursa and Ligament, Right **R** Ankle Bursa and Ligament, Left **S** Foot Bursa and Ligament, Right **T** Foot Bursa and Ligament, Left **V** Lower Extremity Bursa and Ligament, Right **W** Lower Extremity Bursa and Ligament, Left	**0** Open **3** Percutaneous **4** Percutaneous Endoscopic	**Z** No Device	**Z** No Qualifier

0 Medical and Surgical
M Bursae and Ligaments
D Extraction: Pulling or stripping out or off all or a portion of a body part by the use of force

Body Part Character 4	Approach Character 5	Device Character 6	Qualifier Character 7
0 Head and Neck Bursa and Ligament **1** Shoulder Bursa and Ligament, Right **2** Shoulder Bursa and Ligament, Left **3** Elbow Bursa and Ligament, Right **4** Elbow Bursa and Ligament, Left **5** Wrist Bursa and Ligament, Right **6** Wrist Bursa and Ligament, Left **7** Hand Bursa and Ligament, Right **8** Hand Bursa and Ligament, Left **9** Upper Extremity Bursa and Ligament, Right **B** Upper Extremity Bursa and Ligament, Left **C** Trunk Bursa and Ligament, Right **D** Trunk Bursa and Ligament, Left **F** Thorax Bursa and Ligament, Right **G** Thorax Bursa and Ligament, Left **H** Abdomen Bursa and Ligament, Right **J** Abdomen Bursa and Ligament, Left **K** Perineum Bursa and Ligament **L** Hip Bursa and Ligament, Right **M** Hip Bursa and Ligament, Left **N** Knee Bursa and Ligament, Right **P** Knee Bursa and Ligament, Left **Q** Ankle Bursa and Ligament, Right **R** Ankle Bursa and Ligament, Left **S** Foot Bursa and Ligament, Right **T** Foot Bursa and Ligament, Left **V** Lower Extremity Bursa and Ligament, Right **W** Lower Extremity Bursa and Ligament, Left	**0** Open **3** Percutaneous **4** Percutaneous Endoscopic	**Z** No Device	**Z** No Qualifier

0 Medical and Surgical
M Bursae and Ligaments
J Inspection: Visually and/or manually exploring a body part

Body Part Character 4	Approach Character 5	Device Character 6	Qualifier Character 7
X Upper Bursa and Ligament ⃠ **Y** Lower Bursa and Ligament ⃠	**0** Open **3** Percutaneous **4** Percutaneous Endoscopic **X** External	**Z** No Device	**Z** No Qualifier

⃠ 0MJX3ZZ 0MJXXZZ 0MJY3ZZ 0MJYXZZ

0 Medical and Surgical
M Bursae and Ligaments
M Reattachment: Putting back in or on all or a portion of a separated body part to its normal location or other suitable location

Body Part Character 4	Approach Character 5	Device Character 6	Qualifier Character 7
0 Head and Neck Bursa and Ligament **1** Shoulder Bursa and Ligament, Right **2** Shoulder Bursa and Ligament, Left **3** Elbow Bursa and Ligament, Right **4** Elbow Bursa and Ligament, Left **5** Wrist Bursa and Ligament, Right **6** Wrist Bursa and Ligament, Left **7** Hand Bursa and Ligament, Right **8** Hand Bursa and Ligament, Left **9** Upper Extremity Bursa and Ligament, Right **B** Upper Extremity Bursa and Ligament, Left **C** Trunk Bursa and Ligament, Right **D** Trunk Bursa and Ligament, Left **F** Thorax Bursa and Ligament, Right **G** Thorax Bursa and Ligament, Left **H** Abdomen Bursa and Ligament, Right **J** Abdomen Bursa and Ligament, Left **K** Perineum Bursa and Ligament **L** Hip Bursa and Ligament, Right **M** Hip Bursa and Ligament, Left **N** Knee Bursa and Ligament, Right **P** Knee Bursa and Ligament, Left **Q** Ankle Bursa and Ligament, Right **R** Ankle Bursa and Ligament, Left **S** Foot Bursa and Ligament, Right **T** Foot Bursa and Ligament, Left **V** Lower Extremity Bursa and Ligament, Right **W** Lower Extremity Bursa and Ligament, Left	**0** Open **4** Percutaneous Endoscopic	**Z** No Device	**Z** No Qualifier

0 Medical and Surgical
M Bursae and Ligaments
N Release: Freeing a body part from an abnormal physical constraint by cutting or by the use of force

Body Part Character 4	Approach Character 5	Device Character 6	Qualifier Character 7
0 Head and Neck Bursa and Ligament **1** Shoulder Bursa and Ligament, Right **2** Shoulder Bursa and Ligament, Left **3** Elbow Bursa and Ligament, Right **4** Elbow Bursa and Ligament, Left **5** Wrist Bursa and Ligament, Right **6** Wrist Bursa and Ligament, Left **7** Hand Bursa and Ligament, Right **8** Hand Bursa and Ligament, Left **9** Upper Extremity Bursa and Ligament, Right **B** Upper Extremity Bursa and Ligament, Left **C** Trunk Bursa and Ligament, Right **D** Trunk Bursa and Ligament, Left **F** Thorax Bursa and Ligament, Right **G** Thorax Bursa and Ligament, Left **H** Abdomen Bursa and Ligament, Right **J** Abdomen Bursa and Ligament, Left **K** Perineum Bursa and Ligament **L** Hip Bursa and Ligament, Right **M** Hip Bursa and Ligament, Left **N** Knee Bursa and Ligament, Right **P** Knee Bursa and Ligament, Left **Q** Ankle Bursa and Ligament, Right **R** Ankle Bursa and Ligament, Left **S** Foot Bursa and Ligament, Right **T** Foot Bursa and Ligament, Left **V** Lower Extremity Bursa and Ligament, Right **W** Lower Extremity Bursa and Ligament, Left	**0** Open **3** Percutaneous **4** Percutaneous Endoscopic **X** External	**Z** No Device	**Z** No Qualifier

0 Medical and Surgical
M Bursae and Ligaments
P Removal: Taking out or off a device from a body part

Body Part Character 4	Approach Character 5	Device Character 6	Qualifier Character 7
X Upper Bursa and Ligament ⊘ **Y** Lower Bursa and Ligament ⊘	**0** Open **3** Percutaneous **4** Percutaneous Endoscopic	**0** Drainage Device **7** Autologous Tissue Substitute **J** Synthetic Substitute **K** Nonautologous Tissue Substitute	**Z** No Qualifier
X Upper Bursa and Ligament ⊘ **Y** Lower Bursa and Ligament ⊘	**X** External	**0** Drainage Device	**Z** No Qualifier

⊘ 0MPX30Z 0MPXX0Z 0MPY30Z 0MPYX0Z

0 Medical and Surgical
M Bursae and Ligaments
Q Repair: Restoring, to the extent possible, a body part to its normal anatomic structure and function

Body Part Character 4	Approach Character 5	Device Character 6	Qualifier Character 7
0 Head and Neck Bursa and Ligament **1** Shoulder Bursa and Ligament, Right **2** Shoulder Bursa and Ligament, Left **3** Elbow Bursa and Ligament, Right **4** Elbow Bursa and Ligament, Left **5** Wrist Bursa and Ligament, Right **6** Wrist Bursa and Ligament, Left **7** Hand Bursa and Ligament, Right **8** Hand Bursa and Ligament, Left **9** Upper Extremity Bursa and Ligament, Right **B** Upper Extremity Bursa and Ligament, Left **C** Trunk Bursa and Ligament, Right **D** Trunk Bursa and Ligament, Left **F** Thorax Bursa and Ligament, Right **G** Thorax Bursa and Ligament, Left **H** Abdomen Bursa and Ligament, Right **J** Abdomen Bursa and Ligament, Left **K** Perineum Bursa and Ligament **L** Hip Bursa and Ligament, Right **M** Hip Bursa and Ligament, Left **N** Knee Bursa and Ligament, Right CC **P** Knee Bursa and Ligament, Left CC **Q** Ankle Bursa and Ligament, Right **R** Ankle Bursa and Ligament, Left **S** Foot Bursa and Ligament, Right CC **T** Foot Bursa and Ligament, Left CC **V** Lower Extremity Bursa and Ligament, Right **W** Lower Extremity Bursa and Ligament, Left	**0** Open **3** Percutaneous **4** Percutaneous Endoscopic	**Z** No Device	**Z** No Qualifier

CC 0MQN0ZZ 0MQN3ZZ 0MQN4ZZ 0MQP0ZZ 0MQP3ZZ 0MQP4ZZ 0MQS0ZZ 0MQS3ZZ 0MQS4ZZ 0MQT0ZZ 0MQT3ZZ 0MQT4ZZ

0 Medical and Surgical
M Bursae and Ligaments
S Reposition: Moving to its normal location, or other suitable location, all or a portion of a body part

Body Part Character 4	Approach Character 5	Device Character 6	Qualifier Character 7
0 Head and Neck Bursa and Ligament **1** Shoulder Bursa and Ligament, Right **2** Shoulder Bursa and Ligament, Left **3** Elbow Bursa and Ligament, Right **4** Elbow Bursa and Ligament, Left **5** Wrist Bursa and Ligament, Right **6** Wrist Bursa and Ligament, Left **7** Hand Bursa and Ligament, Right **8** Hand Bursa and Ligament, Left **9** Upper Extremity Bursa and Ligament, Right **B** Upper Extremity Bursa and Ligament, Left **C** Trunk Bursa and Ligament, Right **D** Trunk Bursa and Ligament, Left **F** Thorax Bursa and Ligament, Right **G** Thorax Bursa and Ligament, Left **H** Abdomen Bursa and Ligament, Right **J** Abdomen Bursa and Ligament, Left **K** Perineum Bursa and Ligament **L** Hip Bursa and Ligament, Right **M** Hip Bursa and Ligament, Left **N** Knee Bursa and Ligament, Right **P** Knee Bursa and Ligament, Left **Q** Ankle Bursa and Ligament, Right **R** Ankle Bursa and Ligament, Left **S** Foot Bursa and Ligament, Right **T** Foot Bursa and Ligament, Left **V** Lower Extremity Bursa and Ligament, Right **W** Lower Extremity Bursa and Ligament, Left	**0** Open **4** Percutaneous Endoscopic	**Z** No Device	**Z** No Qualifier

0 Medical and Surgical
M Bursae and Ligaments
T Resection: Cutting out or off, without replacement, all of a body part

Body Part Character 4	Approach Character 5	Device Character 6	Qualifier Character 7
0 Head and Neck Bursa and Ligament **1** Shoulder Bursa and Ligament, Right **2** Shoulder Bursa and Ligament, Left **3** Elbow Bursa and Ligament, Right **4** Elbow Bursa and Ligament, Left **5** Wrist Bursa and Ligament, Right **6** Wrist Bursa and Ligament, Left **7** Hand Bursa and Ligament, Right **8** Hand Bursa and Ligament, Left **9** Upper Extremity Bursa and Ligament, Right **B** Upper Extremity Bursa and Ligament, Left **C** Trunk Bursa and Ligament, Right **D** Trunk Bursa and Ligament, Left **F** Thorax Bursa and Ligament, Right **G** Thorax Bursa and Ligament, Left **H** Abdomen Bursa and Ligament, Right **J** Abdomen Bursa and Ligament, Left **K** Perineum Bursa and Ligament **L** Hip Bursa and Ligament, Right **M** Hip Bursa and Ligament, Left **N** Knee Bursa and Ligament, Right **P** Knee Bursa and Ligament, Left **Q** Ankle Bursa and Ligament, Right **R** Ankle Bursa and Ligament, Left **S** Foot Bursa and Ligament, Right **T** Foot Bursa and Ligament, Left **V** Lower Extremity Bursa and Ligament, Right **W** Lower Extremity Bursa and Ligament, Left	**0** Open **4** Percutaneous Endoscopic	**Z** No Device	**Z** No Qualifier

0 Medical and Surgical
M Bursae and Ligaments
U Supplement: Putting in or on biological or synthetic material that physically reinforces and/or augments the function of a portion of a body part

Body Part Character 4	Approach Character 5	Device Character 6	Qualifier Character 7
0 Head and Neck Bursa and Ligament **1** Shoulder Bursa and Ligament, Right **2** Shoulder Bursa and Ligament, Left **3** Elbow Bursa and Ligament, Right **4** Elbow Bursa and Ligament, Left **5** Wrist Bursa and Ligament, Right **6** Wrist Bursa and Ligament, Left **7** Hand Bursa and Ligament, Right **8** Hand Bursa and Ligament, Left **9** Upper Extremity Bursa and Ligament, Right **B** Upper Extremity Bursa and Ligament, Left **C** Trunk Bursa and Ligament, Right **D** Trunk Bursa and Ligament, Left **F** Thorax Bursa and Ligament, Right **G** Thorax Bursa and Ligament, Left **H** Abdomen Bursa and Ligament, Right **J** Abdomen Bursa and Ligament, Left **K** Perineum Bursa and Ligament **L** Hip Bursa and Ligament, Right **M** Hip Bursa and Ligament, Left **N** Knee Bursa and Ligament, Right **P** Knee Bursa and Ligament, Left **Q** Ankle Bursa and Ligament, Right **R** Ankle Bursa and Ligament, Left **S** Foot Bursa and Ligament, Right **T** Foot Bursa and Ligament, Left **V** Lower Extremity Bursa and Ligament, Right **W** Lower Extremity Bursa and Ligament, Left	**0** Open **4** Percutaneous Endoscopic	**7** Autologous Tissue Substitute **J** Synthetic Substitute **K** Nonautologous Tissue Substitute	**Z** No Qualifier

0 Medical and Surgical
M Bursae and Ligaments
W Revision: Correcting, to the extent possible, a portion of a malfunctioning device or the position of a displaced device

Body Part Character 4	Approach Character 5	Device Character 6	Qualifier Character 7
X Upper Bursa and Ligament ⃠ **Y** Lower Bursa and Ligament ⃠	**0** Open **3** Percutaneous **4** Percutaneous Endoscopic **X** External	**0** Drainage Device **7** Autologous Tissue Substitute **J** Synthetic Substitute **K** Nonautologous Tissue Substitute	**Z** No Qualifier

⃠ 0MWXX0Z 0MWXX7Z 0MWXXJZ 0MWXXKZ 0MWYX0Z 0MWYX7Z 0MWYXJZ 0MWYXKZ

0 Medical and Surgical
M Bursae and Ligaments
X Transfer: Moving, without taking out, all or a portion of a body part to another location to take over the function of all or a portion of a body part

Body Part Character 4	Approach Character 5	Device Character 6	Qualifier Character 7
0 Head and Neck Bursa and Ligament **1** Shoulder Bursa and Ligament, Right **2** Shoulder Bursa and Ligament, Left **3** Elbow Bursa and Ligament, Right **4** Elbow Bursa and Ligament, Left **5** Wrist Bursa and Ligament, Right **6** Wrist Bursa and Ligament, Left **7** Hand Bursa and Ligament, Right **8** Hand Bursa and Ligament, Left **9** Upper Extremity Bursa and Ligament, Right **B** Upper Extremity Bursa and Ligament, Left **C** Trunk Bursa and Ligament, Right **D** Trunk Bursa and Ligament, Left **F** Thorax Bursa and Ligament, Right **G** Thorax Bursa and Ligament, Left **H** Abdomen Bursa and Ligament, Right **J** Abdomen Bursa and Ligament, Left **K** Perineum Bursa and Ligament **L** Hip Bursa and Ligament, Right **M** Hip Bursa and Ligament, Left **N** Knee Bursa and Ligament, Right **P** Knee Bursa and Ligament, Left **Q** Ankle Bursa and Ligament, Right **R** Ankle Bursa and Ligament, Left **S** Foot Bursa and Ligament, Right **T** Foot Bursa and Ligament, Left **V** Lower Extremity Bursa and Ligament, Right **W** Lower Extremity Bursa and Ligament, Left	**0** Open **4** Percutaneous Endoscopic	**Z** No Device	**Z** No Qualifier

Head and Facial Bones 0N2-0NW

0 Medical and Surgical
N Head and Facial Bones
2 Change: Taking out or off a device from a body part and putting back an identical or similar device in or on the same body part without cutting or puncturing the skin or a mucous membrane

Body Part Character 4	Approach Character 5	Device Character 6	Qualifier Character 7
0 Skull ⃠ B Nasal Bone ⃠ W Facial Bone ⃠	X External	0 Drainage Device Y Other Device	Z No Qualifier

⃠ 0N20X0Z 0N20XYZ 0N2BX0Z 0N2BXYZ 0N2WX0Z 0N2WXYZ

0 Medical and Surgical
N Head and Facial Bones
5 Destruction: Physical eradication of all or a portion of a body part by the direct use of energy, force, or a destructive agent

Body Part Character 4	Approach Character 5	Device Character 6	Qualifier Character 7
0 Skull 1 Frontal Bone, Right 2 Frontal Bone, Left 3 Parietal Bone, Right 4 Parietal Bone, Left 5 Temporal Bone, Right 6 Temporal Bone, Left 7 Occipital Bone, Right 8 Occipital Bone, Left B Nasal Bone C Sphenoid Bone, Right D Sphenoid Bone, Left F Ethmoid Bone, Right G Ethmoid Bone, Left H Lacrimal Bone, Right J Lacrimal Bone, Left K Palatine Bone, Right L Palatine Bone, Left M Zygomatic Bone, Right N Zygomatic Bone, Left P Orbit, Right Q Orbit, Left R Maxilla, Right S Maxilla, Left T Mandible, Right V Mandible, Left X Hyoid Bone	0 Open 3 Percutaneous 4 Percutaneous Endoscopic	Z No Device	Z No Qualifier

0 Medical and Surgical
N Head and Facial Bones
8 Division: Cutting into a body part, without draining fluids and/or gases from the body part, in order to separate or transect a body part

Body Part Character 4	Approach Character 5	Device Character 6	Qualifier Character 7
0 Skull **1** Frontal Bone, Right **2** Frontal Bone, Left **3** Parietal Bone, Right **4** Parietal Bone, Left **5** Temporal Bone, Right **6** Temporal Bone, Left **7** Occipital Bone, Right **8** Occipital Bone, Left **B** Nasal Bone ⃠ **C** Sphenoid Bone, Right **D** Sphenoid Bone, Left **F** Ethmoid Bone, Right **G** Ethmoid Bone, Left **H** Lacrimal Bone, Right **J** Lacrimal Bone, Left **K** Palatine Bone, Right **L** Palatine Bone, Left **M** Zygomatic Bone, Right **N** Zygomatic Bone, Left **P** Orbit, Right **Q** Orbit, Left **R** Maxilla, Right **S** Maxilla, Left **T** Mandible, Right **V** Mandible, Left **X** Hyoid Bone	**0** Open **3** Percutaneous **4** Percutaneous Endoscopic	**Z** No Device	**Z** No Qualifier

⃠ 0N8B0ZZ 0N8B3ZZ 0N8B4ZZ

0 Medical and Surgical
N Head and Facial Bones
9 Drainage: Taking or letting out fluids and/or gases from a body part

Body Part Character 4	Approach Character 5	Device Character 6	Qualifier Character 7
0 Skull ⊘ **1** Frontal Bone, Right ⊘ **2** Frontal Bone, Left ⊘ **3** Parietal Bone, Right ⊘ **4** Parietal Bone, Left ⊘ **5** Temporal Bone, Right ⊘ **6** Temporal Bone, Left ⊘ **7** Occipital Bone, Right ⊘ **8** Occipital Bone, Left ⊘ **B** Nasal Bone ⊘ **C** Sphenoid Bone, Right ⊘ **D** Sphenoid Bone, Left ⊘ **F** Ethmoid Bone, Right ⊘ **G** Ethmoid Bone, Left ⊘ **H** Lacrimal Bone, Right ⊘ **J** Lacrimal Bone, Left ⊘ **K** Palatine Bone, Right ⊘ **L** Palatine Bone, Left ⊘ **M** Zygomatic Bone, Right ⊘ **N** Zygomatic Bone, Left ⊘ **P** Orbit, Right ⊘ **Q** Orbit, Left **R** Maxilla, Right ⊘ **S** Maxilla, Left ⊘ **T** Mandible, Right ⊘ **V** Mandible, Left ⊘ **X** Hyoid Bone ⊘	**0** Open **3** Percutaneous **4** Percutaneous Endoscopic	**0** Drainage Device	**Z** No Qualifier
0 Skull ⊘ **1** Frontal Bone, Right ⊘ **2** Frontal Bone, Left ⊘ **3** Parietal Bone, Right ⊘ **4** Parietal Bone, Left ⊘ **5** Temporal Bone, Right ⊘ **6** Temporal Bone, Left ⊘ **7** Occipital Bone, Right ⊘ **8** Occipital Bone, Left ⊘ **B** Nasal Bone ⊘ **C** Sphenoid Bone, Right ⊘ **D** Sphenoid Bone, Left ⊘ **F** Ethmoid Bone, Right ⊘ **G** Ethmoid Bone, Left ⊘ **H** Lacrimal Bone, Right ⊘ **J** Lacrimal Bone, Left ⊘ **K** Palatine Bone, Right ⊘ **L** Palatine Bone, Left ⊘ **M** Zygomatic Bone, Right ⊘ **N** Zygomatic Bone, Left **P** Orbit, Right ⊘ **Q** Orbit, Left ⊘ **R** Maxilla, Right ⊘ **S** Maxilla, Left ⊘ **T** Mandible, Right ⊘ **V** Mandible, Left ⊘ **X** Hyoid Bone ⊘	**0** Open **3** Percutaneous **4** Percutaneous Endoscopic	**Z** No Device	**X** Diagnostic **Z** No Qualifier

⊘ 0N9030Z 0N903ZZ 0N9130Z 0N913ZZ 0N9230Z 0N923ZZ 0N9330Z 0N933ZZ 0N9430Z 0N943ZZ 0N9530Z 0N953ZZ 0N9630Z 0N963ZZ 0N9730Z 0N973ZZ 0N9830Z 0N983ZZ 0N9B00Z 0N9B0ZX 0N9B0ZZ 0N9B30Z 0N9B3ZX 0N9B3ZZ 0N9B40Z 0N9B4ZX 0N9B4ZZ 0N9C30Z 0N9C3ZZ 0N9D30Z 0N9D3ZZ 0N9F30Z 0N9F3ZZ 0N9G30Z 0N9G3ZZ 0N9H30Z 0N9H3ZZ 0N9J30Z 0N9J3ZZ 0N9K30Z 0N9K3ZZ 0N9L30Z 0N9L3ZZ 0N9M30Z 0N9M3ZZ 0N9N30Z 0N9N3ZZ 0N9P30Z 0N9P3ZZ 0N9Q30Z 0N9Q3ZZ 0N9R00Z 0N9R0ZZ 0N9R30Z 0N9R3ZZ 0N9R40Z 0N9R4ZZ 0N9S00Z 0N9S0ZZ 0N9S30Z 0N9S3ZZ 0N9S40Z 0N9S4ZZ 0N9T00Z 0N9T0ZZ 0N9T30Z 0N9T3ZZ 0N9T40Z 0N9T4ZZ 0N9V00Z 0N9V0ZZ 0N9V30Z 0N9V3ZZ 0N9V40Z 0N9V4ZZ 0N9X30Z 0N9X3ZZ

LC Limited Coverage NC Noncovered HAC HAC Associated Procedure CC Combination Cluster - See Appendix G for code lists
DRG Non-OR-Affecting MS-DRG Assignment ⊘ Non-OR-Not Affecting MS-DRG Assignment New/Revised Text in **Orange** ♂ Male ♀ Female

0 Medical and Surgical
N Head and Facial Bones
B Excision: Cutting out or off, without replacement, a portion of a body part

Body Part Character 4	Approach Character 5	Device Character 6	Qualifier Character 7
0 Skull **1** Frontal Bone, Right **2** Frontal Bone, Left **3** Parietal Bone, Right **4** Parietal Bone, Left **5** Temporal Bone, Right **6** Temporal Bone, Left **7** Occipital Bone, Right **8** Occipital Bone, Left **B** Nasal Bone ⦸ **C** Sphenoid Bone, Right **D** Sphenoid Bone, Left **F** Ethmoid Bone, Right **G** Ethmoid Bone, Left **H** Lacrimal Bone, Right **J** Lacrimal Bone, Left **K** Palatine Bone, Right **L** Palatine Bone, Left **M** Zygomatic Bone, Right **N** Zygomatic Bone, Left **P** Orbit, Right CC **Q** Orbit, Left CC **R** Maxilla, Right ⦸ CC **S** Maxilla, Left ⦸ CC **T** Mandible, Right ⦸ **V** Mandible, Left ⦸ **X** Hyoid Bone	**0** Open **3** Percutaneous **4** Percutaneous Endoscopic	**Z** No Device	**X** Diagnostic **Z** No Qualifier

⦸ 0NBB0ZX 0NBB3ZX 0NBB4ZX 0NBR0ZX 0NBR3ZX 0NBR4ZX 0NBS0ZX 0NBS3ZX 0NBS4ZX 0NBT0ZX 0NBT3ZX 0NBT4ZX 0NBV0ZX 0NBV3ZX 0NBV4ZX

CC 0NBP0ZZ 0NBP3ZZ 0NBP4ZZ 0NBQ0ZZ 0NBQ3ZZ 0NBQ4ZZ 0NBR0ZZ 0NBR4ZZ 0NBS0ZZ 0NBS4ZZ

0 Medical and Surgical
N Head and Facial Bones
C Extirpation: Taking or cutting out solid matter from a body part

Body Part Character 4	Approach Character 5	Device Character 6	Qualifier Character 7
1 Frontal Bone, Right **2** Frontal Bone, Left **3** Parietal Bone, Right **4** Parietal Bone, Left **5** Temporal Bone, Right **6** Temporal Bone, Left **7** Occipital Bone, Right **8** Occipital Bone, Left **B** Nasal Bone ⃠ **C** Sphenoid Bone, Right **D** Sphenoid Bone, Left **F** Ethmoid Bone, Right **G** Ethmoid Bone, Left **H** Lacrimal Bone, Right **J** Lacrimal Bone, Left **K** Palatine Bone, Right **L** Palatine Bone, Left **M** Zygomatic Bone, Right **N** Zygomatic Bone, Left **P** Orbit, Right **Q** Orbit, Left **R** Maxilla, Right ⃠ **S** Maxilla, Left ⃠ **T** Mandible, Right ⃠ **V** Mandible, Left ⃠ **X** Hyoid Bone	**0** Open **3** Percutaneous **4** Percutaneous Endoscopic	**Z** No Device	**Z** No Qualifier

⃠ 0NCB0ZZ 0NCB3ZZ 0NCB4ZZ 0NCR0ZZ 0NCR3ZZ 0NCR4ZZ 0NCS0ZZ 0NCS3ZZ 0NCS4ZZ 0NCT0ZZ 0NCT3ZZ 0NCT4ZZ 0NCV0ZZ 0NCV3ZZ 0NCV4ZZ

0 Medical and Surgical
N Head and Facial Bones
H Insertion: Putting in a nonbiological appliance that monitors, assists, performs, or prevents a physiological function but does not physically take the place of a body part

Body Part Character 4	Approach Character 5	Device Character 6	Qualifier Character 7
0 Skull ⊘ CC	0 Open	4 Internal Fixation Device 5 External Fixation Device M Bone Growth Stimulator N Neurostimulator Generator	Z No Qualifier
0 Skull ⊘	3 Percutaneous 4 Percutaneous Endoscopic	4 Internal Fixation Device 5 External Fixation Device M Bone Growth Stimulator	Z No Qualifier
1 Frontal Bone, Right 2 Frontal Bone, Left 3 Parietal Bone, Right 4 Parietal Bone, Left 7 Occipital Bone, Right 8 Occipital Bone, Left C Sphenoid Bone, Right D Sphenoid Bone, Left F Ethmoid Bone, Right G Ethmoid Bone, Left H Lacrimal Bone, Right J Lacrimal Bone, Left K Palatine Bone, Right L Palatine Bone, Left M Zygomatic Bone, Right N Zygomatic Bone, Left P Orbit, Right Q Orbit, Left X Hyoid Bone	0 Open 3 Percutaneous 4 Percutaneous Endoscopic	4 Internal Fixation Device	Z No Qualifier
5 Temporal Bone, Right 6 Temporal Bone, Left	0 Open 3 Percutaneous 4 Percutaneous Endoscopic	4 Internal Fixation Device S Hearing Device	Z No Qualifier
B Nasal Bone ⊘	0 Open 3 Percutaneous 4 Percutaneous Endoscopic	4 Internal Fixation Device M Bone Growth Stimulator	Z No Qualifier
R Maxilla, Right S Maxilla, Left T Mandible, Right V Mandible, Left	0 Open 3 Percutaneous 4 Percutaneous Endoscopic	4 Internal Fixation Device 5 External Fixation Device	Z No Qualifier
W Facial Bone	0 Open 3 Percutaneous 4 Percutaneous Endoscopic	M Bone Growth Stimulator	Z No Qualifier

⊘ 0NH005Z 0NH035Z 0NH045Z 0NHB04Z 0NHB0MZ 0NHB34Z 0NHB3MZ 0NHB44Z 0NHB4MZ
CC 0NH00NZ

0 Medical and Surgical
N Head and Facial Bones
J Inspection: Visually and/or manually exploring a body part

Body Part Character 4	Approach Character 5	Device Character 6	Qualifier Character 7
0 Skull ⊘ B Nasal Bone ⊘ W Facial Bone ⊘	0 Open 3 Percutaneous 4 Percutaneous Endoscopic X External	Z No Device	Z No Qualifier

⊘ 0NJ03ZZ 0NJ0XZZ 0NJB3ZZ 0NJBXZZ 0NJW3ZZ 0NJWXZZ

0 Medical and Surgical
N Head and Facial Bones
N Release: Freeing a body part from an abnormal physical constraint by cutting or by the use of force

Body Part Character 4	Approach Character 5	Device Character 6	Qualifier Character 7
1 Frontal Bone, Right **2** Frontal Bone, Left **3** Parietal Bone, Right **4** Parietal Bone, Left **5** Temporal Bone, Right **6** Temporal Bone, Left **7** Occipital Bone, Right **8** Occipital Bone, Left **B** Nasal Bone ⃠ **C** Sphenoid Bone, Right **D** Sphenoid Bone, Left **F** Ethmoid Bone, Right **G** Ethmoid Bone, Left **H** Lacrimal Bone, Right **J** Lacrimal Bone, Left **K** Palatine Bone, Right **L** Palatine Bone, Left **M** Zygomatic Bone, Right **N** Zygomatic Bone, Left **P** Orbit, Right **Q** Orbit, Left **R** Maxilla, Right **S** Maxilla, Left **T** Mandible, Right **V** Mandible, Left **X** Hyoid Bone	**0** Open **3** Percutaneous **4** Percutaneous Endoscopic	**Z** No Device	**Z** No Qualifier

⃠ 0NNB0ZZ 0NNB3ZZ 0NNB4ZZ

0 Medical and Surgical
N Head and Facial Bones
P Removal: Taking out or off a device from a body part

Body Part Character 4	Approach Character 5	Device Character 6	Qualifier Character 7
0 Skull	**0** Open	**0** Drainage Device **4** Internal Fixation Device **5** External Fixation Device **7** Autologous Tissue Substitute **J** Synthetic Substitute **K** Nonautologous Tissue Substitute **M** Bone Growth Stimulator **N** Neurostimulator Generator **S** Hearing Device	**Z** No Qualifier
0 Skull ⊘	**3** Percutaneous **4** Percutaneous Endoscopic	**0** Drainage Device **4** Internal Fixation Device **5** External Fixation Device **7** Autologous Tissue Substitute **J** Synthetic Substitute **K** Nonautologous Tissue Substitute **M** Bone Growth Stimulator **S** Hearing Device	**Z** No Qualifier
0 Skull ⊘	**X** External	**0** Drainage Device **4** Internal Fixation Device **5** External Fixation Device **M** Bone Growth Stimulator **S** Hearing Device	**Z** No Qualifier
B Nasal Bone ⊘ **W** Facial Bone	**0** Open **3** Percutaneous **4** Percutaneous Endoscopic	**0** Drainage Device **4** Internal Fixation Device **7** Autologous Tissue Substitute **J** Synthetic Substitute **K** Nonautologous Tissue Substitute **M** Bone Growth Stimulator	**Z** No Qualifier
B Nasal Bone ⊘ **W** Facial Bone ⊘	**X** External	**0** Drainage Device **4** Internal Fixation Device **M** Bone Growth Stimulator	**Z** No Qualifier

⊘ 0NP035Z 0NP045Z 0NP0X0Z 0NP0X5Z 0NPB00Z 0NPB04Z 0NPB07Z 0NPB0JZ 0NPB0KZ 0NPB0MZ 0NPB30Z 0NPB34Z 0NPB37Z 0NPB3JZ 0NPB3KZ 0NPB3MZ 0NPB40Z 0NPB44Z 0NPB47Z 0NPB4JZ 0NPB4KZ 0NPB4MZ 0NPBX0Z 0NPBX4Z 0NPBXMZ 0NPWX0Z 0NPWXMZ

0 Medical and Surgical
N Head and Facial Bones
Q Repair: Restoring, to the extent possible, a body part to its normal anatomic structure and function

Body Part Character 4	Approach Character 5	Device Character 6	Qualifier Character 7
0 Skull 1 Frontal Bone, Right 2 Frontal Bone, Left 3 Parietal Bone, Right 4 Parietal Bone, Left 5 Temporal Bone, Right 6 Temporal Bone, Left 7 Occipital Bone, Right 8 Occipital Bone, Left B Nasal Bone C Sphenoid Bone, Right D Sphenoid Bone, Left F Ethmoid Bone, Right G Ethmoid Bone, Left H Lacrimal Bone, Right J Lacrimal Bone, Left K Palatine Bone, Right L Palatine Bone, Left M Zygomatic Bone, Right N Zygomatic Bone, Left P Orbit, Right Q Orbit, Left R Maxilla, Right S Maxilla, Left T Mandible, Right V Mandible, Left X Hyoid Bone	0 Open 3 Percutaneous 4 Percutaneous Endoscopic X External	Z No Device	Z No Qualifier

0 Medical and Surgical
N Head and Facial Bones
R Replacement: Putting in or on biological or synthetic material that physically takes the place and/or function of all or a portion of a body part

Body Part Character 4	Approach Character 5	Device Character 6	Qualifier Character 7
0 Skull 1 Frontal Bone, Right 2 Frontal Bone, Left 3 Parietal Bone, Right 4 Parietal Bone, Left 5 Temporal Bone, Right 6 Temporal Bone, Left 7 Occipital Bone, Right 8 Occipital Bone, Left B Nasal Bone C Sphenoid Bone, Right D Sphenoid Bone, Left F Ethmoid Bone, Right G Ethmoid Bone, Left H Lacrimal Bone, Right J Lacrimal Bone, Left K Palatine Bone, Right L Palatine Bone, Left M Zygomatic Bone, Right N Zygomatic Bone, Left P Orbit, Right Q Orbit, Left R Maxilla, Right S Maxilla, Left T Mandible, Right V Mandible, Left X Hyoid Bone	0 Open 3 Percutaneous 4 Percutaneous Endoscopic	7 Autologous Tissue Substitute J Synthetic Substitute K Nonautologous Tissue Substitute	Z No Qualifier

0 Medical and Surgical
N Head and Facial Bones
S Reposition: Moving to its normal location, or other suitable location, all or a portion of a body part

Body Part Character 4	Approach Character 5	Device Character 6	Qualifier Character 7
0 Skull **R** Maxilla, Right ⦸ **S** Maxilla, Left ⦸ **T** Mandible, Right ⦸ **V** Mandible, Left ⦸	**0** Open **3** Percutaneous **4** Percutaneous Endoscopic	**4** Internal Fixation Device **5** External Fixation Device **Z** No Device	**Z** No Qualifier
0 Skull **R** Maxilla, Right ⦸ **S** Maxilla, Left ⦸ **T** Mandible, Right ⦸ **V** Mandible, Left ⦸	**X** External	**Z** No Device	**Z** No Qualifier
1 Frontal Bone, Right **2** Frontal Bone, Left **3** Parietal Bone, Right **4** Parietal Bone, Left **5** Temporal Bone, Right **6** Temporal Bone, Left **7** Occipital Bone, Right **8** Occipital Bone, Left **B** Nasal Bone ⦸ **C** Sphenoid Bone, Right ⦸ **D** Sphenoid Bone, Left ⦸ **F** Ethmoid Bone, Right ⦸ **G** Ethmoid Bone, Left ⦸ **H** Lacrimal Bone, Right ⦸ **J** Lacrimal Bone, Left ⦸ **K** Palatine Bone, Right ⦸ **L** Palatine Bone, Left ⦸ **M** Zygomatic Bone, Right ⦸ **N** Zygomatic Bone, Left ⦸ **P** Orbit, Right ⦸ **Q** Orbit, Left ⦸ **X** Hyoid Bone ⦸	**0** Open **3** Percutaneous **4** Percutaneous Endoscopic	**4** Internal Fixation Device **Z** No Device	**Z** No Qualifier
1 Frontal Bone, Right **2** Frontal Bone, Left **3** Parietal Bone, Right **4** Parietal Bone, Left **5** Temporal Bone, Right **6** Temporal Bone, Left **7** Occipital Bone, Right **8** Occipital Bone, Left **B** Nasal Bone ⦸ **C** Sphenoid Bone, Right ⦸ **D** Sphenoid Bone, Left ⦸ **F** Ethmoid Bone, Right ⦸ **G** Ethmoid Bone, Left ⦸ **H** Lacrimal Bone, Right ⦸ **J** Lacrimal Bone, Left ⦸ **K** Palatine Bone, Right ⦸ **L** Palatine Bone, Left ⦸ **M** Zygomatic Bone, Right ⦸ **N** Zygomatic Bone, Left ⦸ **P** Orbit, Right ⦸ **Q** Orbit, Left ⦸ **X** Hyoid Bone ⦸	**X** External	**Z** No Device	**Z** No Qualifier

⦸ 0NSB34Z 0NSB3ZZ 0NSB44Z 0NSB4ZZ 0NSBXZZ 0NSC34Z 0NSC3ZZ 0NSC44Z 0NSC4ZZ 0NSCXZZ 0NSD34Z 0NSD3ZZ 0NSD44Z 0NSD4ZZ 0NSDXZZ 0NSF34Z 0NSF3ZZ 0NSF44Z 0NSF4ZZ 0NSFXZZ 0NSG34Z 0NSG3ZZ 0NSG44Z 0NSG4ZZ 0NSGXZZ 0NSH34Z 0NSH3ZZ 0NSH44Z 0NSH4ZZ 0NSHXZZ 0NSJ34Z 0NSJ3ZZ 0NSJ44Z 0NSJ4ZZ 0NSJXZZ 0NSK34Z 0NSK3ZZ 0NSK44Z 0NSK4ZZ 0NSKXZZ 0NSL34Z 0NSL3ZZ 0NSL44Z 0NSL4ZZ 0NSLXZZ 0NSM34Z 0NSM3ZZ 0NSM44Z 0NSM4ZZ 0NSMXZZ 0NSN34Z 0NSN3ZZ 0NSN44Z 0NSN4ZZ 0NSNXZZ 0NSP34Z 0NSP3ZZ 0NSP44Z 0NSP4ZZ 0NSPXZZ 0NSQ34Z 0NSQ3ZZ 0NSQ44Z 0NSQ4ZZ 0NSQXZZ 0NSR34Z 0NSR35Z 0NSR3ZZ 0NSR44Z 0NSR45Z 0NSR4ZZ 0NSRXZZ 0NSS34Z 0NSS35Z 0NSS3ZZ 0NSS44Z 0NSS45Z 0NSS4ZZ 0NSSXZZ 0NST34Z 0NST35Z 0NST3ZZ 0NST44Z 0NST45Z 0NST4ZZ 0NSTXZZ 0NSV34Z 0NSV35Z 0NSV3ZZ 0NSV44Z 0NSV45Z 0NSV4ZZ 0NSVXZZ 0NSX34Z 0NSX3ZZ 0NSX44Z 0NSX4ZZ 0NSXXZZ

0 Medical and Surgical
N Head and Facial Bones
T Resection: Cutting out or off, without replacement, all of a body part

Body Part Character 4	Approach Character 5	Device Character 6	Qualifier Character 7
1 Frontal Bone, Right **2** Frontal Bone, Left **3** Parietal Bone, Right **4** Parietal Bone, Left **5** Temporal Bone, Right **6** Temporal Bone, Left **7** Occipital Bone, Right **8** Occipital Bone, Left **B** Nasal Bone **C** Sphenoid Bone, Right **D** Sphenoid Bone, Left **F** Ethmoid Bone, Right **G** Ethmoid Bone, Left **H** Lacrimal Bone, Right **J** Lacrimal Bone, Left **K** Palatine Bone, Right **L** Palatine Bone, Left **M** Zygomatic Bone, Right **N** Zygomatic Bone, Left **P** Orbit, Right **Q** Orbit, Left **R** Maxilla, Right **S** Maxilla, Left **T** Mandible, Right **V** Mandible, Left **X** Hyoid Bone	**0** Open	**Z** No Device	**Z** No Qualifier

0 Medical and Surgical
N Head and Facial Bones
U Supplement: Putting in or on biological or synthetic material that physically reinforces and/or augments the function of a portion of a body part

Body Part Character 4	Approach Character 5	Device Character 6	Qualifier Character 7
0 Skull **1** Frontal Bone, Right **2** Frontal Bone, Left **3** Parietal Bone, Right **4** Parietal Bone, Left **5** Temporal Bone, Right **6** Temporal Bone, Left **7** Occipital Bone, Right **8** Occipital Bone, Left **B** Nasal Bone **C** Sphenoid Bone, Right **D** Sphenoid Bone, Left **F** Ethmoid Bone, Right **G** Ethmoid Bone, Left **H** Lacrimal Bone, Right **J** Lacrimal Bone, Left **K** Palatine Bone, Right **L** Palatine Bone, Left **M** Zygomatic Bone, Right **N** Zygomatic Bone, Left **P** Orbit, Right **Q** Orbit, Left **R** Maxilla, Right **S** Maxilla, Left **T** Mandible, Right **V** Mandible, Left **X** Hyoid Bone	**0** Open **3** Percutaneous **4** Percutaneous Endoscopic	**7** Autologous Tissue Substitute **J** Synthetic Substitute **K** Nonautologous Tissue Substitute	**Z** No Qualifier

0 Medical and Surgical
N Head and Facial Bones
W Revision: Correcting, to the extent possible, a portion of a malfunctioning device or the position of a displaced device

Body Part Character 4	Approach Character 5	Device Character 6	Qualifier Character 7
0 Skull	**0** Open	**0** Drainage Device **4** Internal Fixation Device **5** External Fixation Device **7** Autologous Tissue Substitute **J** Synthetic Substitute **K** Nonautologous Tissue Substitute **M** Bone Growth Stimulator **N** Neurostimulator Generator **S** Hearing Device	**Z** No Qualifier
0 Skull ⃠	**3** Percutaneous **4** Percutaneous Endoscopic **X** External	**0** Drainage Device **4** Internal Fixation Device **5** External Fixation Device **7** Autologous Tissue Substitute **J** Synthetic Substitute **K** Nonautologous Tissue Substitute **M** Bone Growth Stimulator **S** Hearing Device	**Z** No Qualifier
B Nasal Bone ⃠ **W** Facial Bone ⃠	**0** Open **3** Percutaneous **4** Percutaneous Endoscopic **X** External	**0** Drainage Device **4** Internal Fixation Device **7** Autologous Tissue Substitute **J** Synthetic Substitute **K** Nonautologous Tissue Substitute **M** Bone Growth Stimulator	**Z** No Qualifier

⃠ 0NW0X0Z 0NW0X4Z 0NW0X5Z 0NW0X7Z 0NW0XJZ 0NW0XKZ 0NW0XMZ 0NW0XSZ 0NWB00Z 0NWB04Z 0NWB07Z 0NWB0JZ 0NWB0KZ 0NWB0MZ 0NWB30Z 0NWB34Z 0NWB37Z 0NWB3JZ 0NWB3KZ 0NWB3MZ 0NWB40Z 0NWB44Z 0NWB47Z 0NWB4JZ 0NWB4KZ 0NWB4MZ 0NWBX0Z 0NWBX4Z 0NWBX7Z 0NWBXJZ 0NWBXKZ 0NWBXMZ 0NWWX0Z 0NWWX4Z 0NWWX7Z 0NWWXJZ 0NWWXKZ 0NWWXMZ

Upper Bones 0P2-0PW

0 Medical and Surgical
P Upper Bones
2 Change: Taking out or off a device from a body part and putting back an identical or similar device in or on the same body part without cutting or puncturing the skin or a mucous membrane

Body Part Character 4	Approach Character 5	Device Character 6	Qualifier Character 7
Y Upper Bone ⊘	**X** External	**0** Drainage Device **Y** Other Device	**Z** No Qualifier

⊘ 0P2YX0Z 0P2YXYZ

0 Medical and Surgical
P Upper Bones
5 Destruction: Physical eradication of all or a portion of a body part by the direct use of energy, force, or a destructive agent

Body Part Character 4	Approach Character 5	Device Character 6	Qualifier Character 7
0 Sternum **1** Rib, Right **2** Rib, Left **3** Cervical Vertebra **4** Thoracic Vertebra **5** Scapula, Right **6** Scapula, Left **7** Glenoid Cavity, Right **8** Glenoid Cavity, Left **9** Clavicle, Right **B** Clavicle, Left **C** Humeral Head, Right **D** Humeral Head, Left **F** Humeral Shaft, Right **G** Humeral Shaft, Left **H** Radius, Right **J** Radius, Left **K** Ulna, Right **L** Ulna, Left **M** Carpal, Right **N** Carpal, Left **P** Metacarpal, Right **Q** Metacarpal, Left **R** Thumb Phalanx, Right **S** Thumb Phalanx, Left **T** Finger Phalanx, Right **V** Finger Phalanx, Left	**0** Open **3** Percutaneous **4** Percutaneous Endoscopic	**Z** No Device	**Z** No Qualifier

0 Medical and Surgical
P Upper Bones
8 Division: Cutting into a body part, without draining fluids and/or gases from the body part, in order to separate or transect a body part

Body Part Character 4	Approach Character 5	Device Character 6	Qualifier Character 7
0 Sternum	**0** Open	**Z** No Device	**Z** No Qualifier
1 Rib, Right	**3** Percutaneous		
2 Rib, Left	**4** Percutaneous Endoscopic		
3 Cervical Vertebra			
4 Thoracic Vertebra			
5 Scapula, Right			
6 Scapula, Left			
7 Glenoid Cavity, Right			
8 Glenoid Cavity, Left			
9 Clavicle, Right			
B Clavicle, Left			
C Humeral Head, Right			
D Humeral Head, Left			
F Humeral Shaft, Right CC			
G Humeral Shaft, Left CC			
H Radius, Right CC			
J Radius, Left CC			
K Ulna, Right CC			
L Ulna, Left CC			
M Carpal, Right CC			
N Carpal, Left CC			
P Metacarpal, Right CC			
Q Metacarpal, Left CC			
R Thumb Phalanx, Right			
S Thumb Phalanx, Left			
T Finger Phalanx, Right CC			
V Finger Phalanx, Left CC			

CC 0P8F0ZZ 0P8F3ZZ 0P8F4ZZ 0P8G0ZZ 0P8G3ZZ 0P8G4ZZ 0P8H0ZZ 0P8H3ZZ 0P8H4ZZ 0P8J0ZZ 0P8J3ZZ 0P8J4ZZ 0P8K0ZZ 0P8K3ZZ 0P8K4ZZ 0P8L0ZZ 0P8L3ZZ 0P8L4ZZ 0P8M0ZZ 0P8M3ZZ 0P8M4ZZ 0P8N0ZZ 0P8N3ZZ 0P8N4ZZ 0P8P0ZZ 0P8P3ZZ 0P8P4ZZ 0P8Q0ZZ 0P8Q3ZZ 0P8Q4ZZ 0P8T0ZZ 0P8T3ZZ 0P8T4ZZ 0P8V0ZZ 0P8V3ZZ 0P8V4ZZ

0 Medical and Surgical
P Upper Bones
9 Drainage: Taking or letting out fluids and/or gases from a body part

Body Part Character 4	Approach Character 5	Device Character 6	Qualifier Character 7
0 Sternum ⦸ **1** Rib, Right ⦸ **2** Rib, Left ⦸ **3** Cervical Vertebra ⦸ **4** Thoracic Vertebra ⦸ **5** Scapula, Right ⦸ **6** Scapula, Left ⦸ **7** Glenoid Cavity, Right ⦸ **8** Glenoid Cavity, Left ⦸ **9** Clavicle, Right ⦸ **B** Clavicle, Left ⦸ **C** Humeral Head, Right ⦸ **D** Humeral Head, Left ⦸ **F** Humeral Shaft, Right ⦸ **G** Humeral Shaft, Left ⦸ **H** Radius, Right ⦸ **J** Radius, Left ⦸ **K** Ulna, Right ⦸ **L** Ulna, Left ⦸ **M** Carpal, Right ⦸ **N** Carpal, Left ⦸ **P** Metacarpal, Right ⦸ **Q** Metacarpal, Left ⦸ **R** Thumb Phalanx, Right ⦸ **S** Thumb Phalanx, Left ⦸ **T** Finger Phalanx, Right ⦸ **V** Finger Phalanx, Left ⦸	**0** Open **3** Percutaneous **4** Percutaneous Endoscopic	**0** Drainage Device	**Z** No Qualifier
0 Sternum ⦸ **1** Rib, Right ⦸ **2** Rib, Left ⦸ **3** Cervical Vertebra ⦸ **4** Thoracic Vertebra ⦸ **5** Scapula, Right ⦸ **6** Scapula, Left ⦸ **7** Glenoid Cavity, Right ⦸ **8** Glenoid Cavity, Left ⦸ **9** Clavicle, Right ⦸ **B** Clavicle, Left ⦸ **C** Humeral Head, Right ⦸ **D** Humeral Head, Left ⦸ **F** Humeral Shaft, Right ⦸ **G** Humeral Shaft, Left ⦸ **H** Radius, Right ⦸ **J** Radius, Left ⦸ **K** Ulna, Right ⦸ **L** Ulna, Left ⦸ **M** Carpal, Right ⦸ **N** Carpal, Left ⦸ **P** Metacarpal, Right ⦸ **Q** Metacarpal, Left ⦸ **R** Thumb Phalanx, Right ⦸ **S** Thumb Phalanx, Left ⦸ **T** Finger Phalanx, Right ⦸ **V** Finger Phalanx, Left ⦸	**0** Open **3** Percutaneous **4** Percutaneous Endoscopic	**Z** No Device	**X** Diagnostic **Z** No Qualifier

⦸ 0P9030Z 0P903ZZ 0P9130Z 0P913ZZ 0P9230Z 0P923ZZ 0P9330Z 0P933ZZ 0P9430Z 0P943ZZ 0P9530Z 0P953ZZ 0P9630Z 0P963ZZ 0P9730Z 0P973ZZ 0P9830Z 0P983ZZ 0P9930Z 0P993ZZ 0P9B30Z 0P9B3ZZ 0P9C30Z 0P9C3ZZ 0P9D30Z 0P9D3ZZ 0P9F30Z 0P9F3ZZ 0P9G30Z 0P9G3ZZ 0P9H30Z 0P9H3ZZ 0P9J30Z 0P9J3ZZ 0P9K30Z 0P9K3ZZ 0P9L30Z 0P9L3ZZ 0P9M30Z 0P9M3ZZ 0P9N30Z 0P9N3ZZ 0P9P30Z 0P9P3ZZ 0P9Q30Z 0P9Q3ZZ 0P9R30Z 0P9R3ZZ 0P9S30Z 0P9S3ZZ 0P9T30Z 0P9T3ZZ 0P9V30Z 0P9V3ZZ

0 Medical and Surgical
P Upper Bones
B Excision: Cutting out or off, without replacement, a portion of a body part

Body Part Character 4	Approach Character 5	Device Character 6	Qualifier Character 7
0 Sternum **1** Rib, Right CC **2** Rib, Left CC **3** Cervical Vertebra **4** Thoracic Vertebra **5** Scapula, Right **6** Scapula, Left **7** Glenoid Cavity, Right **8** Glenoid Cavity, Left **9** Clavicle, Right **B** Clavicle, Left **C** Humeral Head, Right **D** Humeral Head, Left **F** Humeral Shaft, Right **G** Humeral Shaft, Left **H** Radius, Right **J** Radius, Left **K** Ulna, Right **L** Ulna, Left **M** Carpal, Right **N** Carpal, Left **P** Metacarpal, Right **Q** Metacarpal, Left **R** Thumb Phalanx, Right **S** Thumb Phalanx, Left **T** Finger Phalanx, Right **V** Finger Phalanx, Left	**0** Open **3** Percutaneous **4** Percutaneous Endoscopic	**Z** No Device	**X** Diagnostic **Z** No Qualifier

CC 0PB10ZZ 0PB20ZZ

0 Medical and Surgical
P Upper Bones
C Extirpation: Taking or cutting out solid matter from a body part

Body Part Character 4	Approach Character 5	Device Character 6	Qualifier Character 7
0 Sternum **1** Rib, Right **2** Rib, Left **3** Cervical Vertebra **4** Thoracic Vertebra **5** Scapula, Right **6** Scapula, Left **7** Glenoid Cavity, Right **8** Glenoid Cavity, Left **9** Clavicle, Right **B** Clavicle, Left **C** Humeral Head, Right **D** Humeral Head, Left **F** Humeral Shaft, Right **G** Humeral Shaft, Left **H** Radius, Right **J** Radius, Left **K** Ulna, Right **L** Ulna, Left **M** Carpal, Right **N** Carpal, Left **P** Metacarpal, Right **Q** Metacarpal, Left **R** Thumb Phalanx, Right **S** Thumb Phalanx, Left **T** Finger Phalanx, Right **V** Finger Phalanx, Left	**0** Open **3** Percutaneous **4** Percutaneous Endoscopic	**Z** No Device	**Z** No Qualifier

0 Medical and Surgical
P Upper Bones
H Insertion: Putting in a nonbiological appliance that monitors, assists, performs, or prevents a physiological function but does not physically take the place of a body part

Body Part Character 4	Approach Character 5	Device Character 6	Qualifier Character 7
0 Sternum	0 Open 3 Percutaneous 4 Percutaneous Endoscopic	0 Internal Fixation Device, Rigid Plate 4 Internal Fixation Device	Z No Qualifier
1 Rib, Right 2 Rib, Left 3 Cervical Vertebra 4 Thoracic Vertebra 5 Scapula, Right 6 Scapula, Left 7 Glenoid Cavity, Right 8 Glenoid Cavity, Left 9 Clavicle, Right B Clavicle, Left	0 Open 3 Percutaneous 4 Percutaneous Endoscopic	4 Internal Fixation Device	Z No Qualifier
C Humeral Head, Right ⊘ D Humeral Head, Left ⊘ F Humeral Shaft, Right ⊘ G Humeral Shaft, Left ⊘ H Radius, Right ⊘ J Radius, Left ⊘ K Ulna, Right ⊘ L Ulna, Left ⊘	0 Open 3 Percutaneous 4 Percutaneous Endoscopic	4 Internal Fixation Device 5 External Fixation Device 6 Internal Fixation Device, Intramedullary 8 External Fixation Device, Limb Lengthening B External Fixation Device, Monoplanar C External Fixation Device, Ring D External Fixation Device, Hybrid	Z No Qualifier
M Carpal, Right N Carpal, Left P Metacarpal, Right Q Metacarpal, Left R Thumb Phalanx, Right S Thumb Phalanx, Left T Finger Phalanx, Right V Finger Phalanx, Left	0 Open 3 Percutaneous 4 Percutaneous Endoscopic	4 Internal Fixation Device 5 External Fixation Device	Z No Qualifier
Y Upper Bone	0 Open 3 Percutaneous 4 Percutaneous Endoscopic	M Bone Growth Stimulator	Z No Qualifier

⊘ 0PHC08Z 0PHC38Z 0PHC48Z 0PHD08Z 0PHD38Z 0PHD48Z 0PHF08Z 0PHF38Z 0PHF48Z 0PHG08Z 0PHG38Z 0PHG48Z 0PHH08Z 0PHH38Z 0PHH48Z 0PHJ08Z 0PHJ38Z 0PHJ48Z 0PHK08Z 0PHK38Z 0PHK48Z 0PHL08Z 0PHL38Z 0PHL48Z

0 Medical and Surgical
P Upper Bones
J Inspection: Visually and/or manually exploring a body part

Body Part Character 4	Approach Character 5	Device Character 6	Qualifier Character 7
Y Upper Bone ⊘	0 Open 3 Percutaneous 4 Percutaneous Endoscopic X External	Z No Device	Z No Qualifier

⊘ 0PJY3ZZ 0PJYXZZ

0 Medical and Surgical
P Upper Bones
N Release: Freeing a body part from an abnormal physical constraint by cutting or by the use of force

Body Part Character 4	Approach Character 5	Device Character 6	Qualifier Character 7
0 Sternum **1** Rib, Right **2** Rib, Left **3** Cervical Vertebra **4** Thoracic Vertebra **5** Scapula, Right **6** Scapula, Left **7** Glenoid Cavity, Right **8** Glenoid Cavity, Left **9** Clavicle, Right **B** Clavicle, Left **C** Humeral Head, Right **D** Humeral Head, Left **F** Humeral Shaft, Right **G** Humeral Shaft, Left **H** Radius, Right **J** Radius, Left **K** Ulna, Right **L** Ulna, Left **M** Carpal, Right **N** Carpal, Left **P** Metacarpal, Right **Q** Metacarpal, Left **R** Thumb Phalanx, Right **S** Thumb Phalanx, Left **T** Finger Phalanx, Right **V** Finger Phalanx, Left	**0** Open **3** Percutaneous **4** Percutaneous Endoscopic	**Z** No Device	**Z** No Qualifier

0 Medical and Surgical
P Upper Bones
P Removal: Taking out or off a device from a body part

Body Part Character 4	Approach Character 5	Device Character 6	Qualifier Character 7
0 Sternum **1** Rib, Right **2** Rib, Left **3** Cervical Vertebra **4** Thoracic Vertebra **5** Scapula, Right **6** Scapula, Left **7** Glenoid Cavity, Right **8** Glenoid Cavity, Left **9** Clavicle, Right **B** Clavicle, Left	**0** Open **3** Percutaneous **4** Percutaneous Endoscopic	**4** Internal Fixation Device **7** Autologous Tissue Substitute **J** Synthetic Substitute **K** Nonautologous Tissue Substitute	**Z** No Qualifier
0 Sternum ⦸ **1** Rib, Right ⦸ **2** Rib, Left ⦸ **3** Cervical Vertebra ⦸ **4** Thoracic Vertebra ⦸ **5** Scapula, Right ⦸ **6** Scapula, Left ⦸ **7** Glenoid Cavity, Right ⦸ **8** Glenoid Cavity, Left ⦸ **9** Clavicle, Right ⦸ **B** Clavicle, Left ⦸	**X** External	**4** Internal Fixation Device	**Z** No Qualifier

0PP continued on next page

0 Medical and Surgical
P Upper Bones
P Removal: Taking out or off a device from a body part

0PP continued from previous page

Body Part Character 4	Approach Character 5	Device Character 6	Qualifier Character 7
C Humeral Head, Right **D** Humeral Head, Left **F** Humeral Shaft, Right **G** Humeral Shaft, Left **H** Radius, Right **J** Radius, Left **K** Ulna, Right **L** Ulna, Left **M** Carpal, Right **N** Carpal, Left **P** Metacarpal, Right **Q** Metacarpal, Left **R** Thumb Phalanx, Right **S** Thumb Phalanx, Left **T** Finger Phalanx, Right **V** Finger Phalanx, Left	**0** Open **3** Percutaneous **4** Percutaneous Endoscopic	**4** Internal Fixation Device **5** External Fixation Device **7** Autologous Tissue Substitute **J** Synthetic Substitute **K** Nonautologous Tissue Substitute	**Z** No Qualifier
C Humeral Head, Right ⊘ **D** Humeral Head, Left ⊘ **F** Humeral Shaft, Right ⊘ **G** Humeral Shaft, Left ⊘ **H** Radius, Right ⊘ **J** Radius, Left ⊘ **K** Ulna, Right ⊘ **L** Ulna, Left ⊘ **M** Carpal, Right ⊘ **N** Carpal, Left ⊘ **P** Metacarpal, Right ⊘ **Q** Metacarpal, Left ⊘ **R** Thumb Phalanx, Right ⊘ **S** Thumb Phalanx, Left ⊘ **T** Finger Phalanx, Right ⊘ **V** Finger Phalanx, Left ⊘	**X** External	**4** Internal Fixation Device **5** External Fixation Device	**Z** No Qualifier
Y Upper Bone ⊘	**0** Open **3** Percutaneous **4** Percutaneous Endoscopic **X** External	**0** Drainage Device **M** Bone Growth Stimulator	**Z** No Qualifier

⊘ 0PP0X4Z 0PP1X4Z 0PP2X4Z 0PP3X4Z 0PP4X4Z 0PP5X4Z 0PP6X4Z 0PP7X4Z 0PP8X4Z 0PP9X4Z 0PPBX4Z 0PPCX4Z 0PPCX5Z 0PPDX4Z 0PPDX5Z 0PPFX4Z 0PPFX5Z 0PPGX4Z 0PPGX5Z 0PPHX4Z 0PPHX5Z 0PPJX4Z 0PPJX5Z 0PPKX4Z 0PPKX5Z 0PPLX4Z 0PPLX5Z 0PPMX4Z 0PPMX5Z 0PPNX4Z 0PPNX5Z 0PPPX4Z 0PPPX5Z 0PPQX4Z 0PPQX5Z 0PPRX4Z 0PPRX5Z 0PPSX4Z 0PPSX5Z 0PPTX4Z 0PPTX5Z 0PPVX4Z 0PPVX5Z 0PPY30Z 0PPYX0Z 0PPYXMZ

0 Medical and Surgical
P Upper Bones
Q Repair: Restoring, to the extent possible, a body part to its normal anatomic structure and function

Body Part Character 4	Approach Character 5	Device Character 6	Qualifier Character 7
0 Sternum **1** Rib, Right **2** Rib, Left **3** Cervical Vertebra **4** Thoracic Vertebra **5** Scapula, Right **6** Scapula, Left **7** Glenoid Cavity, Right **8** Glenoid Cavity, Left **9** Clavicle, Right **B** Clavicle, Left **C** Humeral Head, Right **D** Humeral Head, Left **F** Humeral Shaft, Right **G** Humeral Shaft, Left **H** Radius, Right **J** Radius, Left **K** Ulna, Right **L** Ulna, Left **M** Carpal, Right **N** Carpal, Left **P** Metacarpal, Right **Q** Metacarpal, Left **R** Thumb Phalanx, Right **S** Thumb Phalanx, Left **T** Finger Phalanx, Right **V** Finger Phalanx, Left	**0** Open **3** Percutaneous **4** Percutaneous Endoscopic **X** External	**Z** No Device	**Z** No Qualifier

0 Medical and Surgical
P Upper Bones
R Replacement: Putting in or on biological or synthetic material that physically takes the place and/or function of all or a portion of a body part

Body Part Character 4	Approach Character 5	Device Character 6	Qualifier Character 7
0 Sternum **1** Rib, Right **2** Rib, Left **3** Cervical Vertebra **4** Thoracic Vertebra **5** Scapula, Right **6** Scapula, Left **7** Glenoid Cavity, Right **8** Glenoid Cavity, Left **9** Clavicle, Right **B** Clavicle, Left **C** Humeral Head, Right ⃠ **D** Humeral Head, Left ⃠ **F** Humeral Shaft, Right **G** Humeral Shaft, Left **H** Radius, Right **J** Radius, Left **K** Ulna, Right **L** Ulna, Left **M** Carpal, Right **N** Carpal, Left **P** Metacarpal, Right **Q** Metacarpal, Left **R** Thumb Phalanx, Right **S** Thumb Phalanx, Left **T** Finger Phalanx, Right **V** Finger Phalanx, Left	**0** Open **3** Percutaneous **4** Percutaneous Endoscopic	**7** Autologous Tissue Substitute **J** Synthetic Substitute **K** Nonautologous Tissue Substitute	**Z** No Qualifier

⃠ 0PRC0JZ 0PRD0JZ

0 Medical and Surgical
P Upper Bones
S Reposition: Moving to its normal location, or other suitable location, all or a portion of a body part

Body Part Character 4	Approach Character 5	Device Character 6	Qualifier Character 7
0 Sternum ⊘	**0** Open **3** Percutaneous **4** Percutaneous Endoscopic	**0** Internal Fixation Device, Rigid Plate **4** Internal Fixation Device **Z** No Device	**Z** No Qualifier
0 Sternum ⊘	**X** External	**Z** No Device	**Z** No Qualifier
1 Rib, Right ⊘ **2** Rib, Left ⊘ **3** Cervical Vertebra CC **4** Thoracic Vertebra CC **5** Scapula, Right ⊘ **6** Scapula, Left ⊘ **7** Glenoid Cavity, Right ⊘ **8** Glenoid Cavity, Left ⊘ **9** Clavicle, Right ⊘ **B** Clavicle, Left ⊘	**0** Open **3** Percutaneous **4** Percutaneous Endoscopic	**4** Internal Fixation Device **Z** No Device	**Z** No Qualifier
1 Rib, Right ⊘ **2** Rib, Left ⊘ **3** Cervical Vertebra **4** Thoracic Vertebra **5** Scapula, Right ⊘ **6** Scapula, Left ⊘ **7** Glenoid Cavity, Right ⊘ **8** Glenoid Cavity, Left ⊘ **9** Clavicle, Right ⊘ **B** Clavicle, Left ⊘	**X** External	**Z** No Device	**Z** No Qualifier
C Humeral Head, Right ⊘ **D** Humeral Head, Left ⊘ **F** Humeral Shaft, Right ⊘ **G** Humeral Shaft, Left ⊘ **H** Radius, Right ⊘ **J** Radius, Left ⊘ **K** Ulna, Right ⊘ **L** Ulna, Left ⊘	**0** Open **3** Percutaneous **4** Percutaneous Endoscopic	**4** Internal Fixation Device **5** External Fixation Device **6** Internal Fixation Device, Intramedullary **B** External Fixation Device, Monoplanar **C** External Fixation Device, Ring **D** External Fixation Device, Hybrid **Z** No Device	**Z** No Qualifier
C Humeral Head, Right ⊘ **D** Humeral Head, Left ⊘ **F** Humeral Shaft, Right ⊘ **G** Humeral Shaft, Left ⊘ **H** Radius, Right ⊘ **J** Radius, Left ⊘ **K** Ulna, Right ⊘ **L** Ulna, Left ⊘	**X** External	**Z** No Device	**Z** No Qualifier
M Carpal, Right ⊘ **N** Carpal, Left ⊘ **P** Metacarpal, Right ⊘ **Q** Metacarpal, Left ⊘ **R** Thumb Phalanx, Right ⊘ **S** Thumb Phalanx, Left ⊘ **T** Finger Phalanx, Right ⊘ **V** Finger Phalanx, Left ⊘	**0** Open **3** Percutaneous **4** Percutaneous Endoscopic	**4** Internal Fixation Device **5** External Fixation Device **Z** No Device	**Z** No Qualifier
M Carpal, Right ⊘ **N** Carpal, Left ⊘ **P** Metacarpal, Right ⊘ **Q** Metacarpal, Left ⊘ **R** Thumb Phalanx, Right ⊘ **S** Thumb Phalanx, Left ⊘ **T** Finger Phalanx, Right ⊘ **V** Finger Phalanx, Left ⊘	**X** External	**Z** No Device	**Z** No Qualifier

⊘ 0PS03ZZ 0PS04ZZ 0PS0XZZ 0PS13ZZ 0PS14ZZ 0PS1XZZ 0PS23ZZ 0PS24ZZ 0PS2XZZ 0PS53ZZ 0PS54ZZ 0PS5XZZ 0PS63ZZ 0PS64ZZ 0PS6XZZ 0PS73ZZ 0PS74ZZ 0PS7XZZ 0PS83ZZ 0PS84ZZ 0PS8XZZ 0PS93ZZ 0PS94ZZ 0PS9XZZ 0PSB3ZZ 0PSB4ZZ 0PSBXZZ 0PSC3ZZ 0PSC4ZZ 0PSCXZZ 0PSD3ZZ 0PSD4ZZ 0PSDXZZ 0PSF3ZZ 0PSF4ZZ 0PSFXZZ 0PSG3ZZ 0PSG4ZZ 0PSGXZZ 0PSH3ZZ 0PSH4ZZ 0PSHXZZ 0PSJ3ZZ 0PSJ4ZZ 0PSJXZZ 0PSK3ZZ 0PSK4ZZ 0PSKXZZ 0PSL3ZZ 0PSL4ZZ 0PSLXZZ 0PSM3ZZ 0PSM4ZZ 0PSMXZZ 0PSN3ZZ 0PSN4ZZ 0PSNXZZ 0PSP3ZZ 0PSP4ZZ 0PSPXZZ 0PSQ3ZZ 0PSQ4ZZ 0PSQXZZ 0PSR3ZZ 0PSR4ZZ 0PSRXZZ 0PSS3ZZ 0PSS4ZZ 0PSSXZZ 0PST3ZZ 0PST4ZZ 0PSTXZZ 0PSV3ZZ 0PSV4ZZ 0PSVXZZ

CC 0PS33ZZ 0PS43ZZ

LC Limited Coverage NC Noncovered HAC HAC Associated Procedure CC Combination Cluster - See Appendix G for code lists
DRG Non-OR-Affecting MS-DRG Assignment ⊘ Non-OR-Not Affecting MS-DRG Assignment New/Revised Text in **Orange** ♂ Male ♀ Female

0 Medical and Surgical
P Upper Bones
T Resection: Cutting out or off, without replacement, all of a body part

Body Part Character 4	Approach Character 5	Device Character 6	Qualifier Character 7
0 Sternum	**0** Open	**Z** No Device	**Z** No Qualifier
1 Rib, Right			
2 Rib, Left			
5 Scapula, Right			
6 Scapula, Left			
7 Glenoid Cavity, Right			
8 Glenoid Cavity, Left			
9 Clavicle, Right			
B Clavicle, Left			
C Humeral Head, Right CC			
D Humeral Head, Left CC			
F Humeral Shaft, Right CC			
G Humeral Shaft, Left CC			
H Radius, Right			
J Radius, Left			
K Ulna, Right			
L Ulna, Left			
M Carpal, Right			
N Carpal, Left			
P Metacarpal, Right			
Q Metacarpal, Left			
R Thumb Phalanx, Right			
S Thumb Phalanx, Left			
T Finger Phalanx, Right			
V Finger Phalanx, Left			

CC 0PTC0ZZ 0PTD0ZZ 0PTF0ZZ 0PTG0ZZ

0 Medical and Surgical
P Upper Bones
U Supplement: Putting in or on biological or synthetic material that physically reinforces and/or augments the function of a portion of a body part

Body Part Character 4	Approach Character 5	Device Character 6	Qualifier Character 7
0 Sternum	**0** Open	**7** Autologous Tissue Substitute	**Z** No Qualifier
1 Rib, Right	**3** Percutaneous	**J** Synthetic Substitute	
2 Rib, Left	**4** Percutaneous Endoscopic	**K** Nonautologous Tissue Substitute	
3 Cervical Vertebra CC			
4 Thoracic Vertebra CC			
5 Scapula, Right			
6 Scapula, Left			
7 Glenoid Cavity, Right			
8 Glenoid Cavity, Left			
9 Clavicle, Right			
B Clavicle, Left			
C Humeral Head, Right			
D Humeral Head, Left			
F Humeral Shaft, Right CC			
G Humeral Shaft, Left CC			
H Radius, Right CC			
J Radius, Left CC			
K Ulna, Right CC			
L Ulna, Left CC			
M Carpal, Right CC			
N Carpal, Left CC			
P Metacarpal, Right CC			
Q Metacarpal, Left CC			
R Thumb Phalanx, Right			
S Thumb Phalanx, Left			
T Finger Phalanx, Right CC			
V Finger Phalanx, Left CC			

CC 0PU33JZ 0PU43JZ 0PUF07Z 0PUF0KZ 0PUF37Z 0PUF3KZ 0PUF47Z 0PUF4KZ 0PUG07Z 0PUG0KZ 0PUG37Z 0PUG3KZ 0PUG47Z 0PUG4KZ 0PUH07Z 0PUH0KZ 0PUH37Z 0PUH3KZ 0PUH47Z 0PUH4KZ 0PUJ07Z 0PUJ0KZ 0PUJ37Z 0PUJ3KZ 0PUJ47Z 0PUJ4KZ

0PU continued on next page

0PU continued from previous page

0PUK07Z 0PUK0KZ 0PUK37Z 0PUK3KZ 0PUK47Z 0PUK4KZ 0PUL07Z 0PUL0KZ 0PUL37Z 0PUL3KZ 0PUL47Z 0PUL4KZ 0PUM07Z 0PUM0KZ 0PUM37Z 0PUM3KZ 0PUM47Z 0PUM4KZ 0PUN07Z 0PUN0KZ 0PUN37Z 0PUN3KZ 0PUN47Z 0PUN4KZ 0PUP07Z 0PUP0KZ 0PUP37Z 0PUP3KZ 0PUP47Z 0PUP4KZ 0PUQ07Z 0PUQ0KZ 0PUQ37Z 0PUQ3KZ 0PUQ47Z 0PUQ4KZ 0PUT07Z 0PUT0KZ 0PUT37Z 0PUT3KZ 0PUT47Z 0PUT4KZ 0PUV07Z 0PUV0KZ 0PUV37Z 0PUV3KZ 0PUV47Z 0PUV4KZ

0 Medical and Surgical
P Upper Bones
W Revision: Correcting, to the extent possible, a portion of a malfunctioning device or the position of a displaced device

Body Part Character 4	Approach Character 5	Device Character 6	Qualifier Character 7
0 Sternum ⊘ 1 Rib, Right ⊘ 2 Rib, Left ⊘ 3 Cervical Vertebra ⊘ 4 Thoracic Vertebra ⊘ 5 Scapula, Right ⊘ 6 Scapula, Left ⊘ 7 Glenoid Cavity, Right ⊘ 8 Glenoid Cavity, Left ⊘ 9 Clavicle, Right ⊘ B Clavicle, Left ⊘	0 Open 3 Percutaneous 4 Percutaneous Endoscopic X External	4 Internal Fixation Device 7 Autologous Tissue Substitute J Synthetic Substitute K Nonautologous Tissue Substitute	Z No Qualifier
C Humeral Head, Right ⊘ D Humeral Head, Left ⊘ F Humeral Shaft, Right ⊘ G Humeral Shaft, Left ⊘ H Radius, Right ⊘ J Radius, Left ⊘ K Ulna, Right ⊘ L Ulna, Left ⊘ M Carpal, Right ⊘ N Carpal, Left ⊘ P Metacarpal, Right ⊘ Q Metacarpal, Left ⊘ R Thumb Phalanx, Right ⊘ S Thumb Phalanx, Left ⊘ T Finger Phalanx, Right ⊘ V Finger Phalanx, Left ⊘	0 Open 3 Percutaneous 4 Percutaneous Endoscopic X External	4 Internal Fixation Device 5 External Fixation Device 7 Autologous Tissue Substitute J Synthetic Substitute K Nonautologous Tissue Substitute	Z No Qualifier
Y Upper Bone ⊘	0 Open 3 Percutaneous 4 Percutaneous Endoscopic X External	0 Drainage Device M Bone Growth Stimulator	Z No Qualifier

⊘ 0PW0X4Z 0PW0X7Z 0PW0XJZ 0PW0XKZ 0PW1X4Z 0PW1X7Z 0PW1XJZ 0PW1XKZ 0PW2X4Z 0PW2X7Z 0PW2XJZ 0PW2XKZ 0PW3X4Z 0PW3X7Z 0PW3XJZ 0PW3XKZ 0PW4X4Z 0PW4X7Z 0PW4XJZ 0PW4XKZ 0PW5X4Z 0PW5X7Z 0PW5XJZ 0PW5XKZ 0PW6X4Z 0PW6X7Z 0PW6XJZ 0PW6XKZ 0PW7X4Z 0PW7X7Z 0PW7XJZ 0PW7XKZ 0PW8X4Z 0PW8X7Z 0PW8XJZ 0PW8XKZ 0PW9X4Z 0PW9X7Z 0PW9XJZ 0PW9XKZ 0PWBX4Z 0PWBX7Z 0PWBXJZ 0PWBXKZ 0PWCX4Z 0PWCX5Z 0PWCX7Z 0PWCXJZ 0PWCXKZ 0PWDX4Z 0PWDX5Z 0PWDX7Z 0PWDXJZ 0PWDXKZ 0PWFX4Z 0PWFX5Z 0PWFX7Z 0PWFXJZ 0PWFXKZ 0PWGX4Z 0PWGX5Z 0PWGX7Z 0PWGXJZ 0PWGXKZ 0PWHX4Z 0PWHX5Z 0PWHX7Z 0PWHXJZ 0PWHXKZ 0PWJX4Z 0PWJX5Z 0PWJX7Z 0PWJXJZ 0PWJXKZ 0PWKX4Z 0PWKX5Z 0PWKX7Z 0PWKXJZ 0PWKXKZ 0PWLX4Z 0PWLX5Z 0PWLX7Z 0PWLXJZ 0PWLXKZ 0PWMX4Z 0PWMX5Z 0PWMX7Z 0PWMXJZ 0PWMXKZ 0PWNX4Z 0PWNX5Z 0PWNX7Z 0PWNXJZ 0PWNXKZ 0PWPX4Z 0PWPX5Z 0PWPX7Z 0PWPXJZ 0PWPXKZ 0PWQX4Z 0PWQX5Z 0PWQX7Z 0PWQXJZ 0PWQXKZ 0PWRX4Z 0PWRX5Z 0PWRX7Z 0PWRXJZ 0PWRXKZ 0PWSX4Z 0PWSX5Z 0PWSX7Z 0PWSXJZ 0PWSXKZ 0PWTX4Z 0PWTX5Z 0PWTX7Z 0PWTXJZ 0PWTXKZ 0PWVX4Z 0PWVX5Z 0PWVX7Z 0PWVXJZ 0PWVXKZ 0PWYX0Z 0PWYXMZ

Lower Bones 0Q2-0QW

0 Medical and Surgical
Q Lower Bones
2 Change: Taking out or off a device from a body part and putting back an identical or similar device in or on the same body part without cutting or puncturing the skin or a mucous membrane

Body Part Character 4	Approach Character 5	Device Character 6	Qualifier Character 7
Y Lower Bone ⃠	X External	0 Drainage Device Y Other Device	Z No Qualifier

⃠ 0Q2YX0Z 0Q2YXYZ

0 Medical and Surgical
Q Lower Bones
5 Destruction: Physical eradication of all or a portion of a body part by the direct use of energy, force, or a destructive agent

Body Part Character 4	Approach Character 5	Device Character 6	Qualifier Character 7
0 Lumbar Vertebra 1 Sacrum 2 Pelvic Bone, Right 3 Pelvic Bone, Left 4 Acetabulum, Right 5 Acetabulum, Left 6 Upper Femur, Right 7 Upper Femur, Left 8 Femoral Shaft, Right 9 Femoral Shaft, Left B Lower Femur, Right C Lower Femur, Left D Patella, Right F Patella, Left G Tibia, Right H Tibia, Left J Fibula, Right K Fibula, Left L Tarsal, Right M Tarsal, Left N Metatarsal, Right P Metatarsal, Left Q Toe Phalanx, Right R Toe Phalanx, Left S Coccyx	0 Open 3 Percutaneous 4 Percutaneous Endoscopic	Z No Device	Z No Qualifier

0 Medical and Surgical
Q Lower Bones
8 Division: Cutting into a body part, without draining fluids and/or gases from the body part, in order to separate or transect a body part

Body Part Character 4	Approach Character 5	Device Character 6	Qualifier Character 7
0 Lumbar Vertebra **1** Sacrum **2** Pelvic Bone, Right **3** Pelvic Bone, Left **4** Acetabulum, Right **5** Acetabulum, Left **6** Upper Femur, Right **7** Upper Femur, Left **8** Femoral Shaft, Right CC **9** Femoral Shaft, Left CC **B** Lower Femur, Right **C** Lower Femur, Left **D** Patella, Right **F** Patella, Left **G** Tibia, Right CC **H** Tibia, Left CC **J** Fibula, Right CC **K** Fibula, Left CC **L** Tarsal, Right CC **M** Tarsal, Left CC **N** Metatarsal, Right CC **P** Metatarsal, Left CC **Q** Toe Phalanx, Right CC **R** Toe Phalanx, Left CC **S** Coccyx	**0** Open **3** Percutaneous **4** Percutaneous Endoscopic	**Z** No Device	**Z** No Qualifier

CC 0Q880ZZ 0Q883ZZ 0Q884ZZ 0Q890ZZ 0Q893ZZ 0Q894ZZ 0Q8G0ZZ 0Q8G3ZZ 0Q8G4ZZ 0Q8H0ZZ 0Q8H3ZZ 0Q8H4ZZ 0Q8J0ZZ 0Q8J3ZZ 0Q8J4ZZ 0Q8K0ZZ 0Q8K3ZZ 0Q8K4ZZ 0Q8L0ZZ 0Q8L3ZZ 0Q8L4ZZ 0Q8M0ZZ 0Q8M3ZZ 0Q8M4ZZ 0Q8N0ZZ 0Q8N3ZZ 0Q8N4ZZ 0Q8P0ZZ 0Q8P3ZZ 0Q8P4ZZ 0Q8Q0ZZ 0Q8Q3ZZ 0Q8Q4ZZ 0Q8R0ZZ 0Q8R3ZZ 0Q8R4ZZ

0 Medical and Surgical
Q Lower Bones
9 Drainage: Taking or letting out fluids and/or gases from a body part

Body Part Character 4	Approach Character 5	Device Character 6	Qualifier Character 7
0 Lumbar Vertebra ⊘ **1** Sacrum ⊘ **2** Pelvic Bone, Right ⊘ **3** Pelvic Bone, Left ⊘ **4** Acetabulum, Right ⊘ **5** Acetabulum, Left ⊘ **6** Upper Femur, Right ⊘ **7** Upper Femur, Left ⊘ **8** Femoral Shaft, Right ⊘ **9** Femoral Shaft, Left ⊘ **B** Lower Femur, Right ⊘ **C** Lower Femur, Left ⊘ **D** Patella, Right ⊘ **F** Patella, Left ⊘ **G** Tibia, Right ⊘ **H** Tibia, Left ⊘ **J** Fibula, Right ⊘ **K** Fibula, Left ⊘ **L** Tarsal, Right ⊘ **M** Tarsal, Left ⊘ **N** Metatarsal, Right ⊘ **P** Metatarsal, Left ⊘ **Q** Toe Phalanx, Right ⊘ **R** Toe Phalanx, Left ⊘ **S** Coccyx ⊘	**0** Open **3** Percutaneous **4** Percutaneous Endoscopic	**0** Drainage Device	**Z** No Qualifier
0 Lumbar Vertebra ⊘ **1** Sacrum ⊘ **2** Pelvic Bone, Right ⊘ **3** Pelvic Bone, Left ⊘ **4** Acetabulum, Right ⊘ **5** Acetabulum, Left ⊘ **6** Upper Femur, Right ⊘ **7** Upper Femur, Left ⊘ **8** Femoral Shaft, Right ⊘ **9** Femoral Shaft, Left ⊘ **B** Lower Femur, Right ⊘ **C** Lower Femur, Left ⊘ **D** Patella, Right ⊘ **F** Patella, Left ⊘ **G** Tibia, Right ⊘ **H** Tibia, Left ⊘ **J** Fibula, Right ⊘ **K** Fibula, Left ⊘ **L** Tarsal, Right ⊘ **M** Tarsal, Left ⊘ **N** Metatarsal, Right ⊘ **P** Metatarsal, Left ⊘ **Q** Toe Phalanx, Right ⊘ **R** Toe Phalanx, Left ⊘ **S** Coccyx ⊘	**0** Open **3** Percutaneous **4** Percutaneous Endoscopic	**Z** No Device	**X** Diagnostic **Z** No Qualifier

⊘ 0Q9030Z 0Q903ZZ 0Q9130Z 0Q913ZZ 0Q9230Z 0Q923ZZ 0Q9330Z 0Q933ZZ 0Q9430Z 0Q943ZZ 0Q9530Z 0Q953ZZ 0Q9630Z 0Q963ZZ 0Q9730Z 0Q973ZZ 0Q9830Z 0Q983ZZ 0Q9930Z 0Q993ZZ 0Q9B30Z 0Q9B3ZZ 0Q9C30Z 0Q9C3ZZ 0Q9D30Z 0Q9D3ZZ 0Q9F30Z 0Q9F3ZZ 0Q9G30Z 0Q9G3ZZ 0Q9H30Z 0Q9H3ZZ 0Q9J30Z 0Q9J3ZZ 0Q9K30Z 0Q9K3ZZ 0Q9L30Z 0Q9L3ZZ 0Q9M30Z 0Q9M3ZZ 0Q9N30Z 0Q9N3ZZ 0Q9P30Z 0Q9P3ZZ 0Q9Q30Z 0Q9Q3ZZ 0Q9R30Z 0Q9R3ZZ 0Q9S30Z 0Q9S3ZZ

0 Medical and Surgical
Q Lower Bones
B Excision: Cutting out or off, without replacement, a portion of a body part

Body Part Character 4	Approach Character 5	Device Character 6	Qualifier Character 7
0 Lumbar Vertebra 1 Sacrum 2 Pelvic Bone, Right 3 Pelvic Bone, Left 4 Acetabulum, Right 5 Acetabulum, Left 6 Upper Femur, Right 7 Upper Femur, Left 8 Femoral Shaft, Right 9 Femoral Shaft, Left B Lower Femur, Right C Lower Femur, Left D Patella, Right F Patella, Left G Tibia, Right H Tibia, Left J Fibula, Right K Fibula, Left L Tarsal, Right M Tarsal, Left N Metatarsal, Right CC P Metatarsal, Left CC Q Toe Phalanx, Right R Toe Phalanx, Left S Coccyx	0 Open 3 Percutaneous 4 Percutaneous Endoscopic	Z No Device	X Diagnostic Z No Qualifier

CC 0QBN0ZZ 0QBN3ZZ 0QBN4ZZ 0QBP0ZZ 0QBP3ZZ 0QBP4ZZ

0 Medical and Surgical
Q Lower Bones
C Extirpation: Taking or cutting out solid matter from a body part

Body Part Character 4	Approach Character 5	Device Character 6	Qualifier Character 7
0 Lumbar Vertebra 1 Sacrum 2 Pelvic Bone, Right 3 Pelvic Bone, Left 4 Acetabulum, Right 5 Acetabulum, Left 6 Upper Femur, Right 7 Upper Femur, Left 8 Femoral Shaft, Right 9 Femoral Shaft, Left B Lower Femur, Right C Lower Femur, Left D Patella, Right F Patella, Left G Tibia, Right H Tibia, Left J Fibula, Right K Fibula, Left L Tarsal, Right M Tarsal, Left N Metatarsal, Right P Metatarsal, Left Q Toe Phalanx, Right R Toe Phalanx, Left S Coccyx	0 Open 3 Percutaneous 4 Percutaneous Endoscopic	Z No Device	Z No Qualifier

LC Limited Coverage NC Noncovered HAC HAC Associated Procedure CC Combination Cluster - See Appendix G for code lists
DRG Non-OR-Affecting MS-DRG Assignment ⊘ Non-OR-Not Affecting MS-DRG Assignment New/Revised Text in **Orange** ♂ Male ♀ Female

0 Medical and Surgical
Q Lower Bones
H Insertion: Putting in a nonbiological appliance that monitors, assists, performs, or prevents a physiological function but does not physically take the place of a body part

Body Part Character 4	Approach Character 5	Device Character 6	Qualifier Character 7
0 Lumbar Vertebra **1** Sacrum **2** Pelvic Bone, Right **3** Pelvic Bone, Left **4** Acetabulum, Right **5** Acetabulum, Left **D** Patella, Right **F** Patella, Left **L** Tarsal, Right **M** Tarsal, Left **N** Metatarsal, Right **P** Metatarsal, Left **Q** Toe Phalanx, Right **R** Toe Phalanx, Left **S** Coccyx	**0** Open **3** Percutaneous **4** Percutaneous Endoscopic	**4** Internal Fixation Device **5** External Fixation Device	**Z** No Qualifier
6 Upper Femur, Right ⦸ **7** Upper Femur, Left ⦸ **8** Femoral Shaft, Right ⦸ **9** Femoral Shaft, Left ⦸ **B** Lower Femur, Right ⦸ **C** Lower Femur, Left ⦸ **G** Tibia, Right ⦸ **H** Tibia, Left ⦸ **J** Fibula, Right ⦸ **K** Fibula, Left ⦸	**0** Open **3** Percutaneous **4** Percutaneous Endoscopic	**4** Internal Fixation Device **5** External Fixation Device **6** Internal Fixation Device, Intramedullary **8** External Fixation Device, Limb Lengthening **B** External Fixation Device, Monoplanar **C** External Fixation Device, Ring **D** External Fixation Device, Hybrid	**Z** No Qualifier
Y Lower Bone	**0** Open **3** Percutaneous **4** Percutaneous Endoscopic	**M** Bone Growth Stimulator	**Z** No Qualifier

⦸ 0QH608Z 0QH638Z 0QH648Z 0QH708Z 0QH738Z 0QH748Z 0QH808Z 0QH838Z 0QH848Z 0QH908Z 0QH938Z 0QH948Z 0QHB08Z 0QHB38Z 0QHB48Z 0QHC08Z 0QHC38Z 0QHC48Z 0QHG08Z 0QHG38Z 0QHG48Z 0QHH08Z 0QHH38Z 0QHH48Z 0QHJ08Z 0QHJ38Z 0QHJ48Z 0QHK08Z 0QHK38Z 0QHK48Z

0 Medical and Surgical
Q Lower Bones
J Inspection: Visually and/or manually exploring a body part

Body Part Character 4	Approach Character 5	Device Character 6	Qualifier Character 7
Y Lower Bone ⦸	**0** Open **3** Percutaneous **4** Percutaneous Endoscopic **X** External	**Z** No Device	**Z** No Qualifier

⦸ 0QJY3ZZ 0QJYXZZ

0 Medical and Surgical
Q Lower Bones
N Release: Freeing a body part from an abnormal physical constraint by cutting or by the use of force

Body Part Character 4	Approach Character 5	Device Character 6	Qualifier Character 7
0 Lumbar Vertebra **1** Sacrum **2** Pelvic Bone, Right **3** Pelvic Bone, Left **4** Acetabulum, Right **5** Acetabulum, Left **6** Upper Femur, Right **7** Upper Femur, Left **8** Femoral Shaft, Right **9** Femoral Shaft, Left **B** Lower Femur, Right **C** Lower Femur, Left **D** Patella, Right **F** Patella, Left **G** Tibia, Right **H** Tibia, Left **J** Fibula, Right **K** Fibula, Left **L** Tarsal, Right **M** Tarsal, Left **N** Metatarsal, Right **P** Metatarsal, Left **Q** Toe Phalanx, Right **R** Toe Phalanx, Left **S** Coccyx	**0** Open **3** Percutaneous **4** Percutaneous Endoscopic	**Z** No Device	**Z** No Qualifier

0 Medical and Surgical
Q Lower Bones
P Removal: Taking out or off a device from a body part

Body Part Character 4	Approach Character 5	Device Character 6	Qualifier Character 7
0 Lumbar Vertebra **1** Sacrum **4** Acetabulum, Right **5** Acetabulum, Left **S** Coccyx	**0** Open **3** Percutaneous **4** Percutaneous Endoscopic	**4** Internal Fixation Device **7** Autologous Tissue Substitute **J** Synthetic Substitute **K** Nonautologous Tissue Substitute	**Z** No Qualifier
0 Lumbar Vertebra ⊘ **1** Sacrum ⊘ **4** Acetabulum, Right ⊘ **5** Acetabulum, Left ⊘ **S** Coccyx ⊘	**X** External	**4** Internal Fixation Device	**Z** No Qualifier
2 Pelvic Bone, Right **3** Pelvic Bone, Left **6** Upper Femur, Right **7** Upper Femur, Left **8** Femoral Shaft, Right **9** Femoral Shaft, Left **B** Lower Femur, Right **C** Lower Femur, Left **D** Patella, Right CC **F** Patella, Left CC **G** Tibia, Right **H** Tibia, Left **J** Fibula, Right **K** Fibula, Left **L** Tarsal, Right **M** Tarsal, Left **N** Metatarsal, Right **P** Metatarsal, Left **Q** Toe Phalanx, Right **R** Toe Phalanx, Left	**0** Open **3** Percutaneous **4** Percutaneous Endoscopic	**4** Internal Fixation Device **5** External Fixation Device **7** Autologous Tissue Substitute **J** Synthetic Substitute **K** Nonautologous Tissue Substitute	**Z** No Qualifier
2 Pelvic Bone, Right ⊘ **3** Pelvic Bone, Left ⊘ **6** Upper Femur, Right ⊘ **7** Upper Femur, Left ⊘ **8** Femoral Shaft, Right ⊘ **9** Femoral Shaft, Left ⊘ **B** Lower Femur, Right ⊘ **C** Lower Femur, Left ⊘ **D** Patella, Right ⊘ **F** Patella, Left ⊘ **G** Tibia, Right ⊘ **H** Tibia, Left ⊘ **J** Fibula, Right ⊘ **K** Fibula, Left ⊘ **L** Tarsal, Right ⊘ **M** Tarsal, Left ⊘ **N** Metatarsal, Right ⊘ **P** Metatarsal, Left ⊘ **Q** Toe Phalanx, Right ⊘ **R** Toe Phalanx, Left ⊘	**X** External	**4** Internal Fixation Device **5** External Fixation Device	**Z** No Qualifier
Y Lower Bone ⊘	**0** Open **3** Percutaneous **4** Percutaneous Endoscopic **X** External	**0** Drainage Device **M** Bone Growth Stimulator	**Z** No Qualifier

⊘ 0QP0X4Z 0QP1X4Z 0QP2X4Z 0QP2X5Z 0QP3X4Z 0QP3X5Z 0QP4X4Z 0QP5X4Z 0QP6X4Z 0QP6X5Z 0QP7X4Z 0QP7X5Z 0QP8X4Z 0QP8X5Z 0QP9X4Z 0QP9X5Z 0QPBX4Z 0QPBX5Z 0QPCX4Z 0QPCX5Z 0QPDX4Z 0QPDX5Z 0QPFX4Z 0QPFX5Z 0QPGX4Z 0QPGX5Z 0QPHX4Z 0QPHX5Z 0QPJX4Z 0QPJX5Z 0QPKX4Z 0QPKX5Z 0QPLX4Z 0QPLX5Z 0QPMX4Z 0QPMX5Z 0QPNX4Z 0QPNX5Z 0QPPX4Z 0QPPX5Z 0QPQX4Z 0QPQX5Z 0QPRX4Z 0QPRX5Z 0QPSX4Z 0QPY30Z 0QPYX0Z 0QPYXMZ

CC 0QPD0JZ 0QPD3JZ 0QPD4JZ 0QPF0JZ 0QPF3JZ 0QPF4JZ

LC Limited Coverage NC Noncovered HAC HAC Associated Procedure CC Combination Cluster - See Appendix G for code lists
DRG Non-OR-Affecting MS-DRG Assignment ⊘ Non-OR-Not Affecting MS-DRG Assignment New/Revised Text in **Orange** ♂ Male ♀ Female

0 Medical and Surgical
Q Lower Bones
Q Repair: Restoring, to the extent possible, a body part to its normal anatomic structure and function

Body Part Character 4	Approach Character 5	Device Character 6	Qualifier Character 7
0 Lumbar Vertebra **1** Sacrum **2** Pelvic Bone, Right **3** Pelvic Bone, Left **4** Acetabulum, Right **5** Acetabulum, Left **6** Upper Femur, Right **7** Upper Femur, Left **8** Femoral Shaft, Right **9** Femoral Shaft, Left **B** Lower Femur, Right **C** Lower Femur, Left **D** Patella, Right **F** Patella, Left **G** Tibia, Right **H** Tibia, Left **J** Fibula, Right **K** Fibula, Left **L** Tarsal, Right **M** Tarsal, Left **N** Metatarsal, Right **P** Metatarsal, Left **Q** Toe Phalanx, Right **R** Toe Phalanx, Left **S** Coccyx	**0** Open **3** Percutaneous **4** Percutaneous Endoscopic **X** External	**Z** No Device	**Z** No Qualifier

0 Medical and Surgical
Q Lower Bones
R Replacement: Putting in or on biological or synthetic material that physically takes the place and/or function of all or a portion of a body part

Body Part Character 4	Approach Character 5	Device Character 6	Qualifier Character 7
0 Lumbar Vertebra **1** Sacrum **2** Pelvic Bone, Right **3** Pelvic Bone, Left **4** Acetabulum, Right **5** Acetabulum, Left **6** Upper Femur, Right **7** Upper Femur, Left **8** Femoral Shaft, Right CC **9** Femoral Shaft, Left CC **B** Lower Femur, Right **C** Lower Femur, Left **D** Patella, Right CC **F** Patella, Left CC **G** Tibia, Right CC **H** Tibia, Left CC **J** Fibula, Right CC **K** Fibula, Left CC **L** Tarsal, Right CC **M** Tarsal, Left CC **N** Metatarsal, Right CC **P** Metatarsal, Left CC **Q** Toe Phalanx, Right CC **R** Toe Phalanx, Left CC **S** Coccyx	**0** Open **3** Percutaneous **4** Percutaneous Endoscopic	**7** Autologous Tissue Substitute **J** Synthetic Substitute **K** Nonautologous Tissue Substitute	**Z** No Qualifier

CC 0QR807Z 0QR80KZ 0QR837Z 0QR83KZ 0QR847Z 0QR84KZ 0QR907Z 0QR90KZ 0QR937Z 0QR93KZ 0QR947Z 0QR94KZ 0QRD0JZ 0QRD3JZ 0QRD4JZ 0QRF0JZ 0QRF3JZ 0QRF4JZ 0QRG07Z 0QRG0KZ 0QRG37Z 0QRG3KZ 0QRG47Z 0QRG4KZ 0QRH07Z 0QRH0KZ 0QRH37Z 0QRH3KZ 0QRH47Z 0QRH4KZ 0QRJ07Z 0QRJ0KZ 0QRJ37Z 0QRJ3KZ 0QRJ47Z 0QRJ4KZ 0QRK07Z 0QRK0KZ 0QRK37Z 0QRK3KZ 0QRK47Z 0QRK4KZ 0QRL07Z 0QRL0KZ 0QRL37Z 0QRL3KZ 0QRL47Z 0QRL4KZ 0QRM07Z 0QRM0KZ 0QRM37Z 0QRM3KZ 0QRM47Z 0QRM4KZ 0QRN07Z 0QRN0KZ 0QRN37Z 0QRN3KZ 0QRN47Z 0QRN4KZ 0QRP07Z 0QRP0KZ 0QRP37Z 0QRP3KZ 0QRP47Z 0QRP4KZ 0QRQ07Z 0QRQ0KZ 0QRQ37Z 0QRQ3KZ 0QRQ47Z 0QRQ4KZ 0QRR07Z 0QRR0KZ 0QRR37Z 0QRR3KZ 0QRR47Z 0QRR4KZ

LC Limited Coverage NC Noncovered HAC HAC Associated Procedure CC Combination Cluster - See Appendix G for code lists
DRG Non-OR-Affecting MS-DRG Assignment ⊘ Non-OR-Not Affecting MS-DRG Assignment New/Revised Text in **Orange** ♂ Male ♀ Female

0 Medical and Surgical
Q Lower Bones
S Reposition: Moving to its normal location, or other suitable location, all or a portion of a body part

Body Part Character 4	Approach Character 5	Device Character 6	Qualifier Character 7
0 Lumbar Vertebra CC **1** Sacrum CC **4** Acetabulum, Right ⊘ **5** Acetabulum, Left ⊘ **S** Coccyx CC	**0** Open **3** Percutaneous **4** Percutaneous Endoscopic	**4** Internal Fixation Device **Z** No Device	**Z** No Qualifier
0 Lumbar Vertebra **1** Sacrum **4** Acetabulum, Right ⊘ **5** Acetabulum, Left ⊘ **S** Coccyx	**X** External	**Z** No Device	**Z** No Qualifier
2 Pelvic Bone, Right ⊘ **3** Pelvic Bone, Left ⊘ **D** Patella, Right ⊘ **F** Patella, Left ⊘ **L** Tarsal, Right ⊘ **M** Tarsal, Left ⊘ **N** Metatarsal, Right ⊘ **P** Metatarsal, Left ⊘ **Q** Toe Phalanx, Right ⊘ **R** Toe Phalanx, Left ⊘	**0** Open **3** Percutaneous **4** Percutaneous Endoscopic	**4** Internal Fixation Device **5** External Fixation Device **Z** No Device	**Z** No Qualifier
2 Pelvic Bone, Right ⊘ **3** Pelvic Bone, Left ⊘ **D** Patella, Right ⊘ **F** Patella, Left ⊘ **L** Tarsal, Right ⊘ **M** Tarsal, Left ⊘ **N** Metatarsal, Right ⊘ **P** Metatarsal, Left ⊘ **Q** Toe Phalanx, Right ⊘ **R** Toe Phalanx, Left ⊘	**X** External	**Z** No Device	**Z** No Qualifier
6 Upper Femur, Right ⊘ **7** Upper Femur, Left ⊘ **8** Femoral Shaft, Right ⊘ **9** Femoral Shaft, Left ⊘ **B** Lower Femur, Right ⊘ **C** Lower Femur, Left ⊘ **G** Tibia, Right ⊘ **H** Tibia, Left ⊘ **J** Fibula, Right ⊘ **K** Fibula, Left ⊘	**0** Open **3** Percutaneous **4** Percutaneous Endoscopic	**4** Internal Fixation Device **5** External Fixation Device **6** Internal Fixation Device, Intramedullary **B** External Fixation Device, Monoplanar **C** External Fixation Device, Ring **D** External Fixation Device, Hybrid **Z** No Device	**Z** No Qualifier
6 Upper Femur, Right ⊘ **7** Upper Femur, Left ⊘ **8** Femoral Shaft, Right ⊘ **9** Femoral Shaft, Left ⊘ **B** Lower Femur, Right ⊘ **C** Lower Femur, Left ⊘ **G** Tibia, Right ⊘ **H** Tibia, Left ⊘ **J** Fibula, Right ⊘ **K** Fibula, Left ⊘	**X** External	**Z** No Device	**Z** No Qualifier

⊘ 0QS23ZZ 0QS24ZZ 0QS2XZZ 0QS33ZZ 0QS34ZZ 0QS3XZZ 0QS43ZZ 0QS44ZZ 0QS4XZZ 0QS53ZZ 0QS54ZZ 0QS5XZZ 0QS63ZZ 0QS64ZZ 0QS6XZZ 0QS73ZZ 0QS74ZZ 0QS7XZZ 0QS83ZZ 0QS84ZZ 0QS8XZZ 0QS93ZZ 0QS94ZZ 0QS9XZZ 0QSB3ZZ 0QSB4ZZ 0QSBXZZ 0QSC3ZZ 0QSC4ZZ 0QSCXZZ 0QSD3ZZ 0QSD4ZZ 0QSDXZZ 0QSF3ZZ 0QSF4ZZ 0QSFXZZ 0QSG3ZZ 0QSG4ZZ 0QSGXZZ 0QSH3ZZ 0QSH4ZZ 0QSHXZZ 0QSJ3ZZ 0QSJ4ZZ 0QSJXZZ 0QSK3ZZ 0QSK4ZZ 0QSKXZZ 0QSL3ZZ 0QSL4ZZ 0QSLXZZ 0QSM3ZZ 0QSM4ZZ 0QSMXZZ 0QSN3ZZ 0QSN4ZZ 0QSNXZZ 0QSP3ZZ 0QSP4ZZ 0QSPXZZ 0QSQ3ZZ 0QSQ4ZZ 0QSQXZZ 0QSR3ZZ 0QSR4ZZ 0QSRXZZ

CC 0QS03ZZ 0QS13ZZ 0QSS3ZZ

0 Medical and Surgical
Q Lower Bones
T Resection: Cutting out or off, without replacement, all of a body part

Body Part Character 4	Approach Character 5	Device Character 6	Qualifier Character 7
2 Pelvic Bone, Right **3** Pelvic Bone, Left **4** Acetabulum, Right **5** Acetabulum, Left **6** Upper Femur, Right CC **7** Upper Femur, Left CC **8** Femoral Shaft, Right CC **9** Femoral Shaft, Left CC **B** Lower Femur, Right CC **C** Lower Femur, Left CC **D** Patella, Right **F** Patella, Left **G** Tibia, Right **H** Tibia, Left **J** Fibula, Right **K** Fibula, Left **L** Tarsal, Right **M** Tarsal, Left **N** Metatarsal, Right **P** Metatarsal, Left **Q** Toe Phalanx, Right **R** Toe Phalanx, Left **S** Coccyx	**0** Open	**Z** No Device	**Z** No Qualifier

CC 0QT60ZZ 0QT70ZZ 0QT80ZZ 0QT90ZZ 0QTB0ZZ 0QTC0ZZ

0 Medical and Surgical
Q Lower Bones
U Supplement: Putting in or on biological or synthetic material that physically reinforces and/or augments the function of a portion of a body part

Body Part Character 4	Approach Character 5	Device Character 6	Qualifier Character 7
0 Lumbar Vertebra CC **1** Sacrum CC **2** Pelvic Bone, Right **3** Pelvic Bone, Left **4** Acetabulum, Right **5** Acetabulum, Left **6** Upper Femur, Right **7** Upper Femur, Left **8** Femoral Shaft, Right CC **9** Femoral Shaft, Left CC **B** Lower Femur, Right **C** Lower Femur, Left **D** Patella, Right CC **F** Patella, Left CC **G** Tibia, Right CC **H** Tibia, Left CC **J** Fibula, Right CC **K** Fibula, Left CC **L** Tarsal, Right CC **M** Tarsal, Left CC **N** Metatarsal, Right CC **P** Metatarsal, Left CC **Q** Toe Phalanx, Right CC **R** Toe Phalanx, Left CC **S** Coccyx CC	**0** Open **3** Percutaneous **4** Percutaneous Endoscopic	**7** Autologous Tissue Substitute **J** Synthetic Substitute **K** Nonautologous Tissue Substitute	**Z** No Qualifier

CC 0QU03JZ 0QU13JZ 0QU807Z 0QU80KZ 0QU837Z 0QU83KZ 0QU847Z 0QU84KZ 0QU907Z 0QU90KZ 0QU937Z 0QU93KZ 0QU947Z 0QU94KZ 0QUD0JZ 0QUD3JZ 0QUD4JZ 0QUF0JZ 0QUF3JZ 0QUF4JZ 0QUG07Z 0QUG0KZ 0QUG37Z 0QUG3KZ 0QUG47Z 0QUG4KZ 0QUH07Z 0QUH0KZ 0QUH37Z 0QUH3KZ 0QUH47Z 0QUH4KZ 0QUJ07Z 0QUJ0KZ 0QUJ37Z 0QUJ3KZ 0QUJ47Z 0QUJ4KZ 0QUK07Z 0QUK0KZ 0QUK37Z 0QUK3KZ 0QUK47Z 0QUK4KZ 0QUL07Z 0QUL0KZ 0QUL37Z 0QUL3KZ 0QUL47Z 0QUL4KZ 0QUM07Z 0QUM0KZ 0QUM37Z 0QUM3KZ 0QUM47Z 0QUM4KZ 0QUN07Z 0QUN0KZ 0QUN37Z 0QUN3KZ 0QUN47Z 0QUN4KZ 0QUP07Z 0QUP0KZ 0QUP37Z 0QUP3KZ 0QUP47Z 0QUP4KZ 0QUQ07Z 0QUQ0KZ 0QUQ37Z 0QUQ3KZ 0QUQ47Z 0QUQ4KZ 0QUR07Z 0QUR0KZ 0QUR37Z 0QUR3KZ 0QUR47Z 0QUR4KZ 0QUS3JZ

0 Medical and Surgical
Q Lower Bones
W Revision: Correcting, to the extent possible, a portion of a malfunctioning device or the position of a displaced device

Body Part Character 4	Approach Character 5	Device Character 6	Qualifier Character 7
0 Lumbar Vertebra ⦸ **1** Sacrum ⦸ **4** Acetabulum, Right ⦸ **5** Acetabulum, Left ⦸ **S** Coccyx ⦸	**0** Open **3** Percutaneous **4** Percutaneous Endoscopic **X** External	**4** Internal Fixation Device **7** Autologous Tissue Substitute **J** Synthetic Substitute **K** Nonautologous Tissue Substitute	**Z** No Qualifier
2 Pelvic Bone, Right ⦸ **3** Pelvic Bone, Left ⦸ **6** Upper Femur, Right ⦸ **7** Upper Femur, Left ⦸ **8** Femoral Shaft, Right ⦸ **9** Femoral Shaft, Left ⦸ **B** Lower Femur, Right ⦸ **C** Lower Femur, Left ⦸ **D** Patella, Right ⦸ **F** Patella, Left ⦸ **G** Tibia, Right ⦸ **H** Tibia, Left ⦸ **J** Fibula, Right ⦸ **K** Fibula, Left ⦸ **L** Tarsal, Right ⦸ **M** Tarsal, Left ⦸ **N** Metatarsal, Right ⦸ **P** Metatarsal, Left ⦸ **Q** Toe Phalanx, Right ⦸ **R** Toe Phalanx, Left ⦸	**0** Open **3** Percutaneous **4** Percutaneous Endoscopic **X** External	**4** Internal Fixation Device **5** External Fixation Device **7** Autologous Tissue Substitute **J** Synthetic Substitute **K** Nonautologous Tissue Substitute	**Z** No Qualifier
Y Lower Bone ⦸	**0** Open **3** Percutaneous **4** Percutaneous Endoscopic **X** External	**0** Drainage Device **M** Bone Growth Stimulator	**Z** No Qualifier

⦸ 0QW0X4Z 0QW0X7Z 0QW0XJZ 0QW0XKZ 0QW1X4Z 0QW1X7Z 0QW1XJZ 0QW1XKZ 0QW2X4Z 0QW2X5Z 0QW2X7Z 0QW2XJZ 0QW2XKZ 0QW3X4Z 0QW3X5Z 0QW3X7Z 0QW3XJZ 0QW3XKZ 0QW4X4Z 0QW4X7Z 0QW4XJZ 0QW4XKZ 0QW5X4Z 0QW5X7Z 0QW5XJZ 0QW5XKZ 0QW6X4Z 0QW6X5Z 0QW6X7Z 0QW6XJZ 0QW6XKZ 0QW7X4Z 0QW7X5Z 0QW7X7Z 0QW7XJZ 0QW7XKZ 0QW8X4Z 0QW8X5Z 0QW8X7Z 0QW8XJZ 0QW8XKZ 0QW9X4Z 0QW9X5Z 0QW9X7Z 0QW9XJZ 0QW9XKZ 0QWBX4Z 0QWBX5Z 0QWBX7Z 0QWBXJZ 0QWBXKZ 0QWCX4Z 0QWCX5Z 0QWCX7Z 0QWCXJZ 0QWCXKZ 0QWDX4Z 0QWDX5Z 0QWDX7Z 0QWDXJZ 0QWDXKZ 0QWFX4Z 0QWFX5Z 0QWFX7Z 0QWFXJZ 0QWFXKZ 0QWGX4Z 0QWGX5Z 0QWGX7Z 0QWGXJZ 0QWGXKZ 0QWHX4Z 0QWHX5Z 0QWHX7Z 0QWHXJZ 0QWHXKZ 0QWJX4Z 0QWJX5Z 0QWJX7Z 0QWJXJZ 0QWJXKZ 0QWKX4Z 0QWKX5Z 0QWKX7Z 0QWKXJZ 0QWKXKZ 0QWLX4Z 0QWLX5Z 0QWLX7Z 0QWLXJZ 0QWLXKZ 0QWMX4Z 0QWMX5Z 0QWMX7Z 0QWMXJZ 0QWMXKZ 0QWNX4Z 0QWNX5Z 0QWNX7Z 0QWNXJZ 0QWNXKZ 0QWPX4Z 0QWPX5Z 0QWPX7Z 0QWPXJZ 0QWPXKZ 0QWQX4Z 0QWQX5Z 0QWQX7Z 0QWQXJZ 0QWQXKZ 0QWRX4Z 0QWRX5Z 0QWRX7Z 0QWRXJZ 0QWRXKZ 0QWSX4Z 0QWSX7Z 0QWSXJZ 0QWSXKZ 0QWYX0Z 0QWYXMZ

Upper Joints 0R2-0RW

0 Medical and Surgical
R Upper Joints
2 Change: Taking out or off a device from a body part and putting back an identical or similar device in or on the same body part without cutting or puncturing the skin or a mucous membrane

Body Part Character 4	Approach Character 5	Device Character 6	Qualifier Character 7
Y Upper Joint ⃠	X External	0 Drainage Device Y Other Device	Z No Qualifier

⃠ 0R2YX0Z 0R2YXYZ

0 Medical and Surgical
R Upper Joints
5 Destruction: Physical eradication of all or a portion of a body part by the direct use of energy, force, or a destructive agent

Body Part Character 4	Approach Character 5	Device Character 6	Qualifier Character 7
0 Occipital-cervical Joint 1 Cervical Vertebral Joint 3 Cervical Vertebral Disc ⃠ 4 Cervicothoracic Vertebral Joint 5 Cervicothoracic Vertebral Disc ⃠ 6 Thoracic Vertebral Joint 9 Thoracic Vertebral Disc ⃠ A Thoracolumbar Vertebral Joint B Thoracolumbar Vertebral Disc ⃠ C Temporomandibular Joint, Right D Temporomandibular Joint, Left E Sternoclavicular Joint, Right F Sternoclavicular Joint, Left G Acromioclavicular Joint, Right H Acromioclavicular Joint, Left J Shoulder Joint, Right K Shoulder Joint, Left L Elbow Joint, Right M Elbow Joint, Left N Wrist Joint, Right P Wrist Joint, Left Q Carpal Joint, Right R Carpal Joint, Left S Metacarpocarpal Joint, Right T Metacarpocarpal Joint, Left U Metacarpophalangeal Joint, Right V Metacarpophalangeal Joint, Left W Finger Phalangeal Joint, Right X Finger Phalangeal Joint, Left	0 Open 3 Percutaneous 4 Percutaneous Endoscopic	Z No Device	Z No Qualifier

⃠ 0R533ZZ 0R534ZZ 0R553ZZ 0R554ZZ 0R593ZZ 0R594ZZ 0R5B3ZZ 0R5B4ZZ

0 Medical and Surgical
R Upper Joints
9 Drainage: Taking or letting out fluids and/or gases from a body part

Body Part Character 4	Approach Character 5	Device Character 6	Qualifier Character 7
0 Occipital-cervical Joint ⃠ **1** Cervical Vertebral Joint ⃠ **3** Cervical Vertebral Disc ⃠ **4** Cervicothoracic Vertebral Joint ⃠ **5** Cervicothoracic Vertebral Disc ⃠ **6** Thoracic Vertebral Joint ⃠ **9** Thoracic Vertebral Disc ⃠ **A** Thoracolumbar Vertebral Joint ⃠ **B** Thoracolumbar Vertebral Disc ⃠ **C** Temporomandibular Joint, Right **D** Temporomandibular Joint, Left **E** Sternoclavicular Joint, Right ⃠ **F** Sternoclavicular Joint, Left ⃠ **G** Acromioclavicular Joint, Right ⃠ **H** Acromioclavicular Joint, Left ⃠ **J** Shoulder Joint, Right ⃠ **K** Shoulder Joint, Left ⃠ **L** Elbow Joint, Right ⃠ **M** Elbow Joint, Left ⃠ **N** Wrist Joint, Right ⃠ **P** Wrist Joint, Left ⃠ **Q** Carpal Joint, Right ⃠ **R** Carpal Joint, Left ⃠ **S** Metacarpocarpal Joint, Right ⃠ **T** Metacarpocarpal Joint, Left ⃠ **U** Metacarpophalangeal Joint, Right ⃠ **V** Metacarpophalangeal Joint, Left ⃠ **W** Finger Phalangeal Joint, Right ⃠ **X** Finger Phalangeal Joint, Left ⃠	**0** Open **3** Percutaneous **4** Percutaneous Endoscopic	**0** Drainage Device	**Z** No Qualifier

0R9 continued on next page

0R9 continued from previous page

0 Medical and Surgical
R Upper Joints
9 Drainage: Taking or letting out fluids and/or gases from a body part

Body Part Character 4	Approach Character 5	Device Character 6	Qualifier Character 7
0 Occipital-cervical Joint ⊘ **1** Cervical Vertebral Joint ⊘ **3** Cervical Vertebral Disc ⊘ **4** Cervicothoracic Vertebral Joint ⊘ **5** Cervicothoracic Vertebral Disc ⊘ **6** Thoracic Vertebral Joint ⊘ **9** Thoracic Vertebral Disc ⊘ **A** Thoracolumbar Vertebral Joint ⊘ **B** Thoracolumbar Vertebral Disc ⊘ **C** Temporomandibular Joint, Right ⊘ **D** Temporomandibular Joint, Left ⊘ **E** Sternoclavicular Joint, Right ⊘ **F** Sternoclavicular Joint, Left ⊘ **G** Acromioclavicular Joint, Right ⊘ **H** Acromioclavicular Joint, Left ⊘ **J** Shoulder Joint, Right ⊘ **K** Shoulder Joint, Left ⊘ **L** Elbow Joint, Right ⊘ **M** Elbow Joint, Left ⊘ **N** Wrist Joint, Right ⊘ **P** Wrist Joint, Left ⊘ **Q** Carpal Joint, Right ⊘ **R** Carpal Joint, Left ⊘ **S** Metacarpocarpal Joint, Right ⊘ **T** Metacarpocarpal Joint, Left ⊘ **U** Metacarpophalangeal Joint, Right ⊘ **V** Metacarpophalangeal Joint, Left ⊘ **W** Finger Phalangeal Joint, Right ⊘ **X** Finger Phalangeal Joint, Left ⊘	**0** Open **3** Percutaneous **4** Percutaneous Endoscopic	**Z** No Device	**X** Diagnostic **Z** No Qualifier

⊘ 0R900ZX	0R9030Z	0R903ZX	0R903ZZ	0R9040Z	0R904ZX	0R904ZZ	0R910ZX	0R9130Z	0R913ZX	0R913ZZ	0R9140Z	0R914ZX
0R914ZZ	0R930ZX	0R9330Z	0R933ZX	0R933ZZ	0R9340Z	0R934ZX	0R934ZZ	0R940ZX	0R9430Z	0R943ZX	0R943ZZ	0R9440Z
0R944ZX	0R944ZZ	0R950ZX	0R9530Z	0R953ZX	0R953ZZ	0R9540Z	0R954ZX	0R954ZZ	0R960ZX	0R9630Z	0R963ZX	0R963ZZ
0R9640Z	0R964ZX	0R964ZZ	0R990ZX	0R9930Z	0R993ZX	0R993ZZ	0R9940Z	0R994ZX	0R994ZZ	0R9A0ZX	0R9A30Z	0R9A3ZX
0R9A3ZZ	0R9A40Z	0R9A4ZX	0R9A4ZZ	0R9B0ZX	0R9B30Z	0R9B3ZX	0R9B3ZZ	0R9B40Z	0R9B4ZX	0R9B4ZZ	0R9C30Z	0R9C3ZZ
0R9D30Z	0R9D3ZZ	0R9E0ZX	0R9E30Z	0R9E3ZX	0R9E3ZZ	0R9E40Z	0R9E4ZX	0R9E4ZZ	0R9F0ZX	0R9F30Z	0R9F3ZX	0R9F3ZZ
0R9F40Z	0R9F4ZX	0R9F4ZZ	0R9G0ZX	0R9G30Z	0R9G3ZX	0R9G3ZZ	0R9G40Z	0R9G4ZX	0R9G4ZZ	0R9H0ZX	0R9H30Z	0R9H3ZX
0R9H3ZZ	0R9H40Z	0R9H4ZX	0R9H4ZZ	0R9J0ZX	0R9J30Z	0R9J3ZX	0R9J3ZZ	0R9J40Z	0R9J4ZX	0R9J4ZZ	0R9K0ZX	0R9K30Z
0R9K3ZX	0R9K3ZZ	0R9K40Z	0R9K4ZX	0R9K4ZZ	0R9L0ZX	0R9L30Z	0R9L3ZX	0R9L3ZZ	0R9L40Z	0R9L4ZX	0R9L4ZZ	0R9M0ZX
0R9M30Z	0R9M3ZX	0R9M3ZZ	0R9M40Z	0R9M4ZX	0R9M4ZZ	0R9N0ZX	0R9N30Z	0R9N3ZX	0R9N3ZZ	0R9N40Z	0R9N4ZX	0R9N4ZZ
0R9P0ZX	0R9P30Z	0R9P3ZX	0R9P3ZZ	0R9P40Z	0R9P4ZX	0R9P4ZZ	0R9Q0ZX	0R9Q30Z	0R9Q3ZX	0R9Q3ZZ	0R9Q40Z	0R9Q4ZX
0R9Q4ZZ	0R9R0ZX	0R9R30Z	0R9R3ZX	0R9R3ZZ	0R9R40Z	0R9R4ZX	0R9R4ZZ	0R9S0ZX	0R9S30Z	0R9S3ZX	0R9S3ZZ	0R9S40Z
0R9S4ZX	0R9S4ZZ	0R9T0ZX	0R9T30Z	0R9T3ZX	0R9T3ZZ	0R9T40Z	0R9T4ZX	0R9T4ZZ	0R9U0ZX	0R9U30Z	0R9U3ZX	0R9U3ZZ
0R9U40Z	0R9U4ZX	0R9U4ZZ	0R9V0ZX	0R9V30Z	0R9V3ZX	0R9V3ZZ	0R9V40Z	0R9V4ZX	0R9V4ZZ	0R9W0ZX	0R9W30Z	0R9W3ZX
0R9W3ZZ	0R9W40Z	0R9W4ZX	0R9W4ZZ	0R9X0ZX	0R9X30Z	0R9X3ZX	0R9X3ZZ	0R9X40Z	0R9X4ZX	0R9X4ZZ		

0 Medical and Surgical
R Upper Joints
B Excision: Cutting out or off, without replacement, a portion of a body part

Body Part Character 4	Approach Character 5	Device Character 6	Qualifier Character 7
0 Occipital-cervical Joint ⃠ **1** Cervical Vertebral Joint ⃠ **3** Cervical Vertebral Disc ⃠ **4** Cervicothoracic Vertebral Joint ⃠ **5** Cervicothoracic Vertebral Disc ⃠ **6** Thoracic Vertebral Joint ⃠ **9** Thoracic Vertebral Disc ⃠ **A** Thoracolumbar Vertebral Joint ⃠ **B** Thoracolumbar Vertebral Disc ⃠ **C** Temporomandibular Joint, Right **D** Temporomandibular Joint, Left **E** Sternoclavicular Joint, Right ⃠ **F** Sternoclavicular Joint, Left ⃠ **G** Acromioclavicular Joint, Right ⃠ **H** Acromioclavicular Joint, Left ⃠ **J** Shoulder Joint, Right ⃠ **K** Shoulder Joint, Left ⃠ **L** Elbow Joint, Right ⃠ **M** Elbow Joint, Left ⃠ **N** Wrist Joint, Right ⃠ **P** Wrist Joint, Left ⃠ **Q** Carpal Joint, Right ⃠ **R** Carpal Joint, Left ⃠ **S** Metacarpocarpal Joint, Right ⃠ **T** Metacarpocarpal Joint, Left ⃠ **U** Metacarpophalangeal Joint, Right ⃠ **V** Metacarpophalangeal Joint, Left ⃠ **W** Finger Phalangeal Joint, Right ⃠ **X** Finger Phalangeal Joint, Left ⃠	**0** Open **3** Percutaneous **4** Percutaneous Endoscopic	**Z** No Device	**X** Diagnostic **Z** No Qualifier

⃠ 0RB00ZX 0RB03ZX 0RB04ZX 0RB10ZX 0RB13ZX 0RB14ZX 0RB30ZX 0RB33ZX 0RB34ZX 0RB40ZX 0RB43ZX 0RB44ZX 0RB50ZX 0RB53ZX 0RB54ZX 0RB60ZX 0RB63ZX 0RB64ZX 0RB90ZX 0RB93ZX 0RB94ZX 0RBA0ZX 0RBA3ZX 0RBA4ZX 0RBB0ZX 0RBB3ZX 0RBB4ZX 0RBE0ZX 0RBE3ZX 0RBE4ZX 0RBF0ZX 0RBF3ZX 0RBF4ZX 0RBG0ZX 0RBG3ZX 0RBG4ZX 0RBH0ZX 0RBH3ZX 0RBH4ZX 0RBJ0ZX 0RBJ3ZX 0RBJ4ZX 0RBK0ZX 0RBK3ZX 0RBK4ZX 0RBL0ZX 0RBL3ZX 0RBL4ZX 0RBM0ZX 0RBM3ZX 0RBM4ZX 0RBN0ZX 0RBN3ZX 0RBN4ZX 0RBP0ZX 0RBP3ZX 0RBP4ZX 0RBQ0ZX 0RBQ3ZX 0RBQ4ZX 0RBR0ZX 0RBR3ZX 0RBR4ZX 0RBS0ZX 0RBS3ZX 0RBS4ZX 0RBT0ZX 0RBT3ZX 0RBT4ZX 0RBU0ZX 0RBU3ZX 0RBU4ZX 0RBV0ZX 0RBV3ZX 0RBV4ZX 0RBW0ZX 0RBW3ZX 0RBW4ZX 0RBX0ZX 0RBX3ZX 0RBX4ZX

0 Medical and Surgical
R Upper Joints
C Extirpation: Taking or cutting out solid matter from a body part

Body Part Character 4	Approach Character 5	Device Character 6	Qualifier Character 7
0 Occipital-cervical Joint **1** Cervical Vertebral Joint **3** Cervical Vertebral Disc **4** Cervicothoracic Vertebral Joint **5** Cervicothoracic Vertebral Disc **6** Thoracic Vertebral Joint **9** Thoracic Vertebral Disc **A** Thoracolumbar Vertebral Joint **B** Thoracolumbar Vertebral Disc **C** Temporomandibular Joint, Right **D** Temporomandibular Joint, Left **E** Sternoclavicular Joint, Right **F** Sternoclavicular Joint, Left **G** Acromioclavicular Joint, Right **H** Acromioclavicular Joint, Left **J** Shoulder Joint, Right **K** Shoulder Joint, Left **L** Elbow Joint, Right **M** Elbow Joint, Left **N** Wrist Joint, Right **P** Wrist Joint, Left **Q** Carpal Joint, Right **R** Carpal Joint, Left **S** Metacarpocarpal Joint, Right **T** Metacarpocarpal Joint, Left **U** Metacarpophalangeal Joint, Right **V** Metacarpophalangeal Joint, Left **W** Finger Phalangeal Joint, Right **X** Finger Phalangeal Joint, Left	**0** Open **3** Percutaneous **4** Percutaneous Endoscopic	**Z** No Device	**Z** No Qualifier

0 Medical and Surgical
R Upper Joints
G Fusion: Joining together portions of an articular body part rendering the articular body part immobile

Body Part Character 4	Approach Character 5	Device Character 6	Qualifier Character 7
0 Occipital-cervical Joint HAC **1** Cervical Vertebral Joint HAC **2** Cervical Vertebral Joints, 2 or more HAC **4** Cervicothoracic Vertebral Joint HAC **6** Thoracic Vertebral Joint HAC **7** Thoracic Vertebral Joints, 2 to 7 CC HAC **8** Thoracic Vertebral Joints, 8 or more HAC **A** Thoracolumbar Vertebral Joint HAC	**0** Open **3** Percutaneous **4** Percutaneous Endoscopic	**7** Autologous Tissue Substitute **A** Interbody Fusion Device **J** Synthetic Substitute **K** Nonautologous Tissue Substitute **Z** No Device	**0** Anterior Approach, Anterior Column **1** Posterior Approach, Posterior Column **J** Posterior Approach, Anterior Column
C Temporomandibular Joint, Right **D** Temporomandibular Joint, Left **E** Sternoclavicular Joint, Right HAC **F** Sternoclavicular Joint, Left HAC **G** Acromioclavicular Joint, Right HAC **H** Acromioclavicular Joint, Left HAC **J** Shoulder Joint, Right HAC **K** Shoulder Joint, Left HAC	**0** Open **3** Percutaneous **4** Percutaneous Endoscopic	**4** Internal Fixation Device **7** Autologous Tissue Substitute **J** Synthetic Substitute **K** Nonautologous Tissue Substitute **Z** No Device	**Z** No Qualifier
L Elbow Joint, Right HAC **M** Elbow Joint, Left HAC **N** Wrist Joint, Right **P** Wrist Joint, Left **Q** Carpal Joint, Right **R** Carpal Joint, Left **S** Metacarpocarpal Joint, Right **T** Metacarpocarpal Joint, Left **U** Metacarpophalangeal Joint, Right **V** Metacarpophalangeal Joint, Left **W** Finger Phalangeal Joint, Right **X** Finger Phalangeal Joint, Left	**0** Open **3** Percutaneous **4** Percutaneous Endoscopic	**4** Internal Fixation Device **5** External Fixation Device **7** Autologous Tissue Substitute **J** Synthetic Substitute **K** Nonautologous Tissue Substitute **Z** No Device	**Z** No Qualifier

CC 0RG7070 0RG7071 0RG707J 0RG70A0 0RG70A1 0RG70AJ 0RG70J0 0RG70J1 0RG70JJ 0RG70K0 0RG70K1 0RG70KJ 0RG70Z0 0RG70Z1 0RG70ZJ 0RG7370 0RG7371 0RG737J 0RG73A0 0RG73A1 0RG73AJ 0RG73J0 0RG73J1 0RG73JJ 0RG73K0 0RG73K1 0RG73KJ 0RG73Z0 0RG73Z1 0RG73ZJ 0RG7470 0RG7471 0RG747J 0RG74A0 0RG74A1 0RG74AJ 0RG74J0 0RG74J1 0RG74JJ 0RG74K0 0RG74K1 0RG74KJ 0RG74Z0 0RG74Z1 0RG74ZJ

HAC 0RG0070 0RG0071 0RG007J 0RG00A0 0RG00A1 0RG00AJ 0RG00J0 0RG00J1 0RG00JJ 0RG00K0 0RG00K1 0RG00KJ 0RG00Z0 0RG00Z1 0RG00ZJ 0RG0370 0RG0371 0RG037J 0RG03A0 0RG03A1 0RG03AJ 0RG03J0 0RG03J1 0RG03JJ 0RG03K0 0RG03K1 0RG03KJ 0RG03Z0 0RG03Z1 0RG03ZJ 0RG0470 0RG0471 0RG047J 0RG04A0 0RG04A1 0RG04AJ 0RG04J0 0RG04J1 0RG04JJ 0RG04K0 0RG04K1 0RG04KJ 0RG04Z0 0RG04Z1 0RG04ZJ 0RG1070 0RG1071 0RG107J 0RG10A0 0RG10A1 0RG10AJ 0RG10J0 0RG10J1 0RG10JJ 0RG10K0 0RG10K1 0RG10KJ 0RG10Z0 0RG10Z1 0RG10ZJ 0RG1370 0RG1371 0RG137J 0RG13A0 0RG13A1 0RG13AJ 0RG13J0 0RG13J1 0RG13JJ 0RG13K0 0RG13K1 0RG13KJ 0RG13Z0 0RG13Z1 0RG13ZJ 0RG1470 0RG1471 0RG147J 0RG14A0 0RG14A1 0RG14AJ 0RG14J0 0RG14J1 0RG14JJ 0RG14K0 0RG14K1 0RG14KJ 0RG14Z0 0RG14Z1 0RG14ZJ 0RG2070 0RG2071 0RG207J 0RG20A0 0RG20A1 0RG20AJ 0RG20J0 0RG20J1 0RG20JJ 0RG20K0 0RG20K1 0RG20KJ 0RG20Z0 0RG20Z1 0RG20ZJ 0RG2370 0RG2371 0RG237J 0RG23A0 0RG23A1 0RG23AJ 0RG23J0 0RG23J1 0RG23JJ 0RG23K0 0RG23K1 0RG23KJ 0RG23Z0 0RG23Z1 0RG23ZJ 0RG2470 0RG2471 0RG247J 0RG24A0 0RG24A1 0RG24AJ 0RG24J0 0RG24J1 0RG24JJ 0RG24K0 0RG24K1 0RG24KJ 0RG24Z0 0RG24Z1 0RG24ZJ 0RG4070 0RG4071 0RG407J 0RG40A0 0RG40A1 0RG40AJ 0RG40J0 0RG40J1 0RG40JJ 0RG40K0 0RG40K1 0RG40KJ 0RG40Z0 0RG40Z1 0RG40ZJ 0RG4370 0RG4371 0RG437J 0RG43A0 0RG43A1 0RG43AJ 0RG43J0 0RG43J1 0RG43JJ 0RG43K0 0RG43K1 0RG43KJ 0RG43Z0 0RG43Z1 0RG43ZJ 0RG4470 0RG4471 0RG447J 0RG44A0 0RG44A1 0RG44AJ 0RG44J0 0RG44J1 0RG44JJ 0RG44K0 0RG44K1 0RG44KJ 0RG44Z0 0RG44Z1 0RG44ZJ 0RG6070 0RG6071 0RG607J 0RG60A0 0RG60A1 0RG60AJ 0RG60J0 0RG60J1 0RG60JJ 0RG60K0 0RG60K1 0RG60KJ 0RG60Z0 0RG60Z1 0RG60ZJ 0RG6370 0RG6371 0RG637J 0RG63A0 0RG63A1 0RG63AJ 0RG63J0 0RG63J1 0RG63JJ 0RG63K0 0RG63K1 0RG63KJ 0RG63Z0 0RG63Z1 0RG63ZJ 0RG6470 0RG6471 0RG647J 0RG64A0 0RG64A1 0RG64AJ 0RG64J0 0RG64J1 0RG64JJ 0RG64K0 0RG64K1 0RG64KJ 0RG64Z0 0RG64Z1 0RG64ZJ 0RG7070 0RG7071 0RG707J 0RG70A0 0RG70A1 0RG70AJ 0RG70J0 0RG70J1 0RG70JJ 0RG70K0 0RG70K1 0RG70KJ 0RG70Z0 0RG70Z1 0RG70ZJ 0RG7370 0RG7371 0RG737J 0RG73A0 0RG73A1 0RG73AJ 0RG73J0 0RG73J1 0RG73JJ 0RG73K0 0RG73K1 0RG73KJ 0RG73Z0 0RG73Z1 0RG73ZJ 0RG7470 0RG7471 0RG747J 0RG74A0 0RG74A1 0RG74AJ 0RG74J0 0RG74J1 0RG74JJ 0RG74K0 0RG74K1 0RG74KJ 0RG74Z0 0RG74Z1 0RG74ZJ 0RG8070 0RG8071 0RG807J 0RG80A0 0RG80A1 0RG80AJ 0RG80J0 0RG80J1 0RG80JJ 0RG80K0 0RG80K1 0RG80KJ 0RG80Z0 0RG80Z1 0RG80ZJ 0RG8370

0RG continued on next page

LC Limited Coverage NC Noncovered HAC HAC Associated Procedure CC Combination Cluster - See Appendix G for code lists
0RG Non-OR-Affecting MS-DRG Assignment ⊘ Non-OR-Not Affecting MS-DRG Assignment New/Revised Text in **Orange** ♂ Male ♀ Female

0RG continued from previous page

0RG8371 0RG837J 0RG83A0 0RG83A1 0RG83AJ 0RG83J0 0RG83J1 0RG83JJ 0RG83K0 0RG83K1 0RG83KJ 0RG83Z0 0RG83Z1 0RG83ZJ 0RG8470 0RG8471 0RG847J 0RG84A0 0RG84A1 0RG84AJ 0RG84J0 0RG84J1 0RG84JJ 0RG84K0 0RG84K1 0RG84KJ 0RG84Z0 0RG84Z1 0RG84ZJ 0RGA070 0RGA071 0RGA07J 0RGA0A0 0RGA0A1 0RGA0AJ 0RGA0J0 0RGA0J1 0RGA0JJ 0RGA0K0 0RGA0K1 0RGA0KJ 0RGA0Z0 0RGA0Z1 0RGA0ZJ 0RGA370 0RGA371 0RGA37J 0RGA3A0 0RGA3A1 0RGA3AJ 0RGA3J0 0RGA3J1 0RGA3JJ 0RGA3K0 0RGA3K1 0RGA3KJ 0RGA3Z0 0RGA3Z1 0RGA3ZJ 0RGA470 0RGA471 0RGA47J 0RGA4A0 0RGA4A1 0RGA4AJ 0RGA4J0 0RGA4J1 0RGA4JJ 0RGA4K0 0RGA4K1 0RGA4KJ 0RGA4Z0 0RGA4Z1 0RGA4ZJ 0RGE04Z 0RGE07Z 0RGE0JZ 0RGE0KZ 0RGE0ZZ 0RGE34Z 0RGE37Z 0RGE3JZ 0RGE3KZ 0RGE3ZZ 0RGE44Z 0RGE47Z 0RGE4JZ 0RGE4KZ 0RGE4ZZ 0RGF04Z 0RGF07Z 0RGF0JZ 0RGF0KZ 0RGF0ZZ 0RGF34Z 0RGF37Z 0RGF3JZ 0RGF3KZ 0RGF3ZZ 0RGF44Z 0RGF47Z 0RGF4JZ 0RGF4KZ 0RGF4ZZ 0RGG04Z 0RGG07Z 0RGG0JZ 0RGG0KZ 0RGG0ZZ 0RGG34Z 0RGG37Z 0RGG3JZ 0RGG3KZ 0RGG3ZZ 0RGG44Z 0RGG47Z 0RGG4JZ 0RGG4KZ 0RGG4ZZ 0RGH04Z 0RGH07Z 0RGH0JZ 0RGH0KZ 0RGH0ZZ 0RGH34Z 0RGH37Z 0RGH3JZ 0RGH3KZ 0RGH3ZZ 0RGH44Z 0RGH47Z 0RGH4JZ 0RGH4KZ 0RGH4ZZ 0RGJ04Z 0RGJ07Z 0RGJ0JZ 0RGJ0KZ 0RGJ0ZZ 0RGJ34Z 0RGJ37Z 0RGJ3JZ 0RGJ3KZ 0RGJ3ZZ 0RGJ44Z 0RGJ47Z 0RGJ4JZ 0RGJ4KZ 0RGJ4ZZ 0RGK04Z 0RGK07Z 0RGK0JZ 0RGK0KZ 0RGK0ZZ 0RGK34Z 0RGK37Z 0RGK3JZ 0RGK3KZ 0RGK3ZZ 0RGK44Z 0RGK47Z 0RGK4JZ 0RGK4KZ 0RGK4ZZ 0RGL04Z 0RGL05Z 0RGL07Z 0RGL0JZ 0RGL0KZ 0RGL0ZZ 0RGL34Z 0RGL35Z 0RGL37Z 0RGL3JZ 0RGL3KZ 0RGL3ZZ 0RGL44Z 0RGL45Z 0RGL47Z 0RGL4JZ 0RGL4KZ 0RGL4ZZ 0RGM04Z 0RGM05Z 0RGM07Z 0RGM0JZ 0RGM0KZ 0RGM0ZZ 0RGM34Z 0RGM35Z 0RGM37Z 0RGM3JZ 0RGM3KZ 0RGM3ZZ 0RGM44Z 0RGM45Z 0RGM47Z 0RGM4JZ 0RGM4KZ or 0RGM4ZZ All preceding codes with the HAC symbol are classified as hospital-acquired conditions when reported with secondary diagnosis K68.11, T81.4XXA, T84.60XA, T84.610A, T84.611A, T84.612A, T84.613A, T84.614A, T84.615A, T84.619A, T84.63XA, T84.69XA, or T84.7XXA.

0 Medical and Surgical
R Upper Joints
H Insertion: Putting in a nonbiological appliance that monitors, assists, performs, or prevents a physiological function but does not physically take the place of a body part

Body Part Character 4	Approach Character 5	Device Character 6	Qualifier Character 7
0 Occipital-cervical Joint ⊘ **1** Cervical Vertebral Joint ⊘ **4** Cervicothoracic Vertebral Joint ⊘ **6** Thoracic Vertebral Joint ⊘ **A** Thoracolumbar Vertebral Joint ⊘	**0** Open **3** Percutaneous **4** Percutaneous Endoscopic	**3** Infusion Device **4** Internal Fixation Device **8** Spacer **B** Spinal Stabilization Device, Interspinous Process **C** Spinal Stabilization Device, Pedicle-Based **D** Spinal Stabilization Device, Facet Replacement	**Z** No Qualifier
3 Cervical Vertebral Disc ⊘ **5** Cervicothoracic Vertebral Disc ⊘ **9** Thoracic Vertebral Disc ⊘ **B** Thoracolumbar Vertebral Disc ⊘	**0** Open **3** Percutaneous **4** Percutaneous Endoscopic	**3** Infusion Device	**Z** No Qualifier
C Temporomandibular Joint, Right ⊘ **D** Temporomandibular Joint, Left ⊘ **E** Sternoclavicular Joint, Right ⊘ **F** Sternoclavicular Joint, Left ⊘ **G** Acromioclavicular Joint, Right ⊘ **H** Acromioclavicular Joint, Left ⊘ **J** Shoulder Joint, Right ⊘ **K** Shoulder Joint, Left ⊘	**0** Open **3** Percutaneous **4** Percutaneous Endoscopic	**3** Infusion Device **4** Internal Fixation Device **8** Spacer	**Z** No Qualifier
L Elbow Joint, Right ⊘ **M** Elbow Joint, Left ⊘ **N** Wrist Joint, Right ⊘ **P** Wrist Joint, Left ⊘ **Q** Carpal Joint, Right ⊘ **R** Carpal Joint, Left ⊘ **S** Metacarpocarpal Joint, Right ⊘ **T** Metacarpocarpal Joint, Left ⊘ **U** Metacarpophalangeal Joint, Right ⊘ **V** Metacarpophalangeal Joint, Left ⊘ **W** Finger Phalangeal Joint, Right ⊘ **X** Finger Phalangeal Joint, Left ⊘	**0** Open **3** Percutaneous **4** Percutaneous Endoscopic	**3** Infusion Device **4** Internal Fixation Device **5** External Fixation Device **8** Spacer	**Z** No Qualifier

⊘ 0RH003Z 0RH008Z 0RH033Z 0RH038Z 0RH043Z 0RH048Z 0RH103Z 0RH108Z 0RH133Z 0RH138Z 0RH143Z 0RH148Z 0RH303Z 0RH333Z 0RH343Z 0RH403Z 0RH408Z 0RH433Z 0RH438Z 0RH443Z 0RH448Z 0RH503Z 0RH533Z 0RH543Z 0RH603Z 0RH608Z

0RH continued on next page

0RH continued from previous page

0RH633Z 0RH638Z 0RH643Z 0RH648Z 0RH903Z 0RH933Z 0RH943Z 0RHA03Z 0RHA08Z 0RHA33Z 0RHA38Z 0RHA43Z 0RHA48Z
0RHB03Z 0RHB33Z 0RHB43Z 0RHC08Z 0RHC33Z 0RHC38Z 0RHC48Z 0RHD08Z 0RHD33Z 0RHD38Z 0RHD48Z 0RHE03Z 0RHE08Z
0RHE33Z 0RHE38Z 0RHE43Z 0RHE48Z 0RHF03Z 0RHF08Z 0RHF33Z 0RHF38Z 0RHF43Z 0RHF48Z 0RHG03Z 0RHG08Z 0RHG33Z
0RHG38Z 0RHG43Z 0RHG48Z 0RHH03Z 0RHH08Z 0RHH33Z 0RHH38Z 0RHH43Z 0RHH48Z 0RHJ03Z 0RHJ08Z 0RHJ33Z 0RHJ38Z
0RHJ43Z 0RHJ48Z 0RHK03Z 0RHK08Z 0RHK33Z 0RHK38Z 0RHK43Z 0RHK48Z 0RHL03Z 0RHL08Z 0RHL33Z 0RHL38Z 0RHL43Z
0RHL48Z 0RHM03Z 0RHM08Z 0RHM33Z 0RHM38Z 0RHM43Z 0RHM48Z 0RHN03Z 0RHN08Z 0RHN33Z 0RHN38Z 0RHN43Z 0RHN48Z
0RHP03Z 0RHP08Z 0RHP33Z 0RHP38Z 0RHP43Z 0RHP48Z 0RHQ03Z 0RHQ08Z 0RHQ33Z 0RHQ38Z 0RHQ43Z 0RHQ48Z 0RHR03Z
0RHR08Z 0RHR33Z 0RHR38Z 0RHR43Z 0RHR48Z 0RHS03Z 0RHS08Z 0RHS33Z 0RHS38Z 0RHS43Z 0RHS48Z 0RHT03Z 0RHT08Z
0RHT33Z 0RHT38Z 0RHT43Z 0RHT48Z 0RHU03Z 0RHU08Z 0RHU33Z 0RHU38Z 0RHU43Z 0RHU48Z 0RHV03Z 0RHV08Z 0RHV33Z
0RHV38Z 0RHV43Z 0RHV48Z 0RHW03Z 0RHW08Z 0RHW33Z 0RHW38Z 0RHW43Z 0RHW48Z 0RHX03Z 0RHX08Z 0RHX33Z 0RHX38Z
0RHX43Z 0RHX48Z

0 Medical and Surgical
R Upper Joints
J Inspection: Visually and/or manually exploring a body part

Body Part Character 4	Approach Character 5	Device Character 6	Qualifier Character 7
0 Occipital-cervical Joint ⃠ **1** Cervical Vertebral Joint ⃠ **3** Cervical Vertebral Disc ⃠ **4** Cervicothoracic Vertebral Joint ⃠ **5** Cervicothoracic Vertebral Disc ⃠ **6** Thoracic Vertebral Joint ⃠ **9** Thoracic Vertebral Disc ⃠ **A** Thoracolumbar Vertebral Joint ⃠ **B** Thoracolumbar Vertebral Disc ⃠ **C** Temporomandibular Joint, Right ⃠ **D** Temporomandibular Joint, Left ⃠ **E** Sternoclavicular Joint, Right ⃠ **F** Sternoclavicular Joint, Left ⃠ **G** Acromioclavicular Joint, Right ⃠ **H** Acromioclavicular Joint, Left ⃠ **J** Shoulder Joint, Right ⃠ **K** Shoulder Joint, Left ⃠ **L** Elbow Joint, Right ⃠ **M** Elbow Joint, Left ⃠ **N** Wrist Joint, Right ⃠ **P** Wrist Joint, Left ⃠ **Q** Carpal Joint, Right ⃠ **R** Carpal Joint, Left ⃠ **S** Metacarpocarpal Joint, Right ⃠ **T** Metacarpocarpal Joint, Left ⃠ **U** Metacarpophalangeal Joint, Right ⃠ **V** Metacarpophalangeal Joint, Left ⃠ **W** Finger Phalangeal Joint, Right ⃠ **X** Finger Phalangeal Joint, Left ⃠	**0** Open **3** Percutaneous **4** Percutaneous Endoscopic **X** External	**Z** No Device	**Z** No Qualifier

⃠ 0RJ03ZZ 0RJ0XZZ 0RJ13ZZ 0RJ1XZZ 0RJ33ZZ 0RJ3XZZ 0RJ43ZZ 0RJ4XZZ 0RJ53ZZ 0RJ5XZZ 0RJ63ZZ 0RJ6XZZ 0RJ93ZZ
0RJ9XZZ 0RJA3ZZ 0RJAXZZ 0RJB3ZZ 0RJBXZZ 0RJC3ZZ 0RJCXZZ 0RJD3ZZ 0RJDXZZ 0RJE3ZZ 0RJEXZZ 0RJF3ZZ 0RJFXZZ
0RJG3ZZ 0RJGXZZ 0RJH3ZZ 0RJHXZZ 0RJJ3ZZ 0RJJXZZ 0RJK3ZZ 0RJKXZZ 0RJL3ZZ 0RJLXZZ 0RJM3ZZ 0RJMXZZ 0RJN3ZZ
0RJNXZZ 0RJP3ZZ 0RJPXZZ 0RJQ3ZZ 0RJQXZZ 0RJR3ZZ 0RJRXZZ 0RJS3ZZ 0RJSXZZ 0RJT3ZZ 0RJTXZZ 0RJU3ZZ 0RJUXZZ
0RJV3ZZ 0RJVXZZ 0RJW3ZZ 0RJWXZZ 0RJX3ZZ 0RJXXZZ

LC Limited Coverage NC Noncovered HAC HAC Associated Procedure CC Combination Cluster - See Appendix G for code lists
DRG Non-OR-Affecting MS-DRG Assignment ⃠ Non-OR-Not Affecting MS-DRG Assignment New/Revised Text in **Orange** ♂ Male ♀ Female

0 Medical and Surgical
R Upper Joints
N Release: Freeing a body part from an abnormal physical constraint by cutting or by the use of force

Body Part Character 4	Approach Character 5	Device Character 6	Qualifier Character 7
0 Occipital-cervical Joint ⦸ 1 Cervical Vertebral Joint ⦸ 3 Cervical Vertebral Disc ⦸ 4 Cervicothoracic Vertebral Joint ⦸ 5 Cervicothoracic Vertebral Disc ⦸ 6 Thoracic Vertebral Joint ⦸ 9 Thoracic Vertebral Disc ⦸ A Thoracolumbar Vertebral Joint ⦸ B Thoracolumbar Vertebral Disc ⦸ C Temporomandibular Joint, Right ⦸ D Temporomandibular Joint, Left ⦸ E Sternoclavicular Joint, Right ⦸ F Sternoclavicular Joint, Left ⦸ G Acromioclavicular Joint, Right ⦸ H Acromioclavicular Joint, Left ⦸ J Shoulder Joint, Right ⦸ K Shoulder Joint, Left ⦸ L Elbow Joint, Right ⦸ M Elbow Joint, Left ⦸ N Wrist Joint, Right ⦸ P Wrist Joint, Left ⦸ Q Carpal Joint, Right ⦸ R Carpal Joint, Left ⦸ S Metacarpocarpal Joint, Right ⦸ T Metacarpocarpal Joint, Left ⦸ U Metacarpophalangeal Joint, Right ⦸ V Metacarpophalangeal Joint, Left ⦸ W Finger Phalangeal Joint, Right ⦸ X Finger Phalangeal Joint, Left ⦸	0 Open 3 Percutaneous 4 Percutaneous Endoscopic X External	Z No Device	Z No Qualifier

⦸ 0RN0XZZ 0RN1XZZ 0RN3XZZ 0RN4XZZ 0RN5XZZ 0RN6XZZ 0RN9XZZ 0RNAXZZ 0RNBXZZ 0RNCXZZ 0RNDXZZ 0RNEXZZ 0RNFXZZ 0RNGXZZ 0RNHXZZ 0RNJXZZ 0RNKXZZ 0RNLXZZ 0RNMXZZ 0RNNXZZ 0RNPXZZ 0RNQXZZ 0RNRXZZ 0RNSXZZ 0RNTXZZ 0RNUXZZ 0RNVXZZ 0RNWXZZ 0RNXXZZ

0 Medical and Surgical
R Upper Joints
P Removal: Taking out or off a device from a body part

Body Part Character 4	Approach Character 5	Device Character 6	Qualifier Character 7
0 Occipital-cervical Joint ⦸ 1 Cervical Vertebral Joint ⦸ 4 Cervicothoracic Vertebral Joint ⦸ 6 Thoracic Vertebral Joint ⦸ A Thoracolumbar Vertebral Joint ⦸	0 Open 3 Percutaneous 4 Percutaneous Endoscopic	0 Drainage Device 3 Infusion Device 4 Internal Fixation Device 7 Autologous Tissue Substitute 8 Spacer A Interbody Fusion Device J Synthetic Substitute K Nonautologous Tissue Substitute	Z No Qualifier
0 Occipital-cervical Joint ⦸ 1 Cervical Vertebral Joint ⦸ 4 Cervicothoracic Vertebral Joint ⦸ 6 Thoracic Vertebral Joint ⦸ A Thoracolumbar Vertebral Joint ⦸	X External	0 Drainage Device 3 Infusion Device 4 Internal Fixation Device	Z No Qualifier

0RP continued on next page

0 Medical and Surgical
R Upper Joints
P Removal: Taking out or off a device from a body part

0RP continued from previous page

Body Part Character 4	Approach Character 5	Device Character 6	Qualifier Character 7
3 Cervical Vertebral Disc ⦸ **5** Cervicothoracic Vertebral Disc ⦸ **9** Thoracic Vertebral Disc ⦸ **B** Thoracolumbar Vertebral Disc ⦸	**0** Open **3** Percutaneous **4** Percutaneous Endoscopic	**0** Drainage Device **3** Infusion Device **7** Autologous Tissue Substitute **J** Synthetic Substitute **K** Nonautologous Tissue Substitute	**Z** No Qualifier
3 Cervical Vertebral Disc ⦸ **5** Cervicothoracic Vertebral Disc ⦸ **9** Thoracic Vertebral Disc ⦸ **B** Thoracolumbar Vertebral Disc ⦸	**X** External	**0** Drainage Device **3** Infusion Device	**Z** No Qualifier
C Temporomandibular Joint, Right ⦸ **D** Temporomandibular Joint, Left ⦸ **E** Sternoclavicular Joint, Right ⦸ **F** Sternoclavicular Joint, Left ⦸ **G** Acromioclavicular Joint, Right ⦸ **H** Acromioclavicular Joint, Left ⦸ **J** Shoulder Joint, Right ⦸ **K** Shoulder Joint, Left ⦸	**0** Open **3** Percutaneous **4** Percutaneous Endoscopic	**0** Drainage Device **3** Infusion Device **4** Internal Fixation Device **7** Autologous Tissue Substitute **8** Spacer **J** Synthetic Substitute **K** Nonautologous Tissue Substitute	**Z** No Qualifier
C Temporomandibular Joint, Right ⦸ **D** Temporomandibular Joint, Left ⦸ **E** Sternoclavicular Joint, Right ⦸ **F** Sternoclavicular Joint, Left ⦸ **G** Acromioclavicular Joint, Right ⦸ **H** Acromioclavicular Joint, Left ⦸ **J** Shoulder Joint, Right ⦸ **K** Shoulder Joint, Left ⦸	**X** External	**0** Drainage Device **3** Infusion Device **4** Internal Fixation Device	**Z** No Qualifier
L Elbow Joint, Right ⦸ **M** Elbow Joint, Left ⦸ **N** Wrist Joint, Right ⦸ **P** Wrist Joint, Left ⦸ **Q** Carpal Joint, Right ⦸ **R** Carpal Joint, Left ⦸ **S** Metacarpocarpal Joint, Right ⦸ **T** Metacarpocarpal Joint, Left ⦸ **U** Metacarpophalangeal Joint, Right ⦸ **V** Metacarpophalangeal Joint, Left ⦸ **W** Finger Phalangeal Joint, Right ⦸ **X** Finger Phalangeal Joint, Left ⦸	**0** Open **3** Percutaneous **4** Percutaneous Endoscopic	**0** Drainage Device **3** Infusion Device **4** Internal Fixation Device **5** External Fixation Device **7** Autologous Tissue Substitute **8** Spacer **J** Synthetic Substitute **K** Nonautologous Tissue Substitute	**Z** No Qualifier
L Elbow Joint, Right ⦸ **M** Elbow Joint, Left ⦸ **N** Wrist Joint, Right ⦸ **P** Wrist Joint, Left ⦸ **Q** Carpal Joint, Right ⦸ **R** Carpal Joint, Left ⦸ **S** Metacarpocarpal Joint, Right ⦸ **T** Metacarpocarpal Joint, Left ⦸ **U** Metacarpophalangeal Joint, Right ⦸ **V** Metacarpophalangeal Joint, Left ⦸ **W** Finger Phalangeal Joint, Right ⦸ **X** Finger Phalangeal Joint, Left ⦸	**X** External	**0** Drainage Device **3** Infusion Device **4** Internal Fixation Device **5** External Fixation Device	**Z** No Qualifier

⦸ 0RP008Z 0RP030Z 0RP033Z 0RP038Z 0RP048Z 0RP0X0Z 0RP0X3Z 0RP0X4Z 0RP108Z 0RP130Z 0RP133Z 0RP138Z 0RP148Z 0RP1X0Z 0RP1X3Z 0RP1X4Z 0RP330Z 0RP333Z 0RP3X0Z 0RP3X3Z 0RP408Z 0RP430Z 0RP433Z 0RP438Z 0RP448Z 0RP4X0Z 0RP4X3Z 0RP4X4Z 0RP530Z 0RP533Z 0RP5X0Z 0RP5X3Z 0RP608Z 0RP630Z 0RP633Z 0RP638Z 0RP648Z 0RP6X0Z 0RP6X3Z

0RP continued on next page

0RP continued from previous page

0RP6X4Z 0RP930Z 0RP933Z 0RP9X0Z 0RP9X3Z 0RPA08Z 0RPA30Z 0RPA33Z 0RPA38Z 0RPA48Z 0RPAX0Z 0RPAX3Z 0RPAX4Z
0RPB30Z 0RPB33Z 0RPBX0Z 0RPBX3Z 0RPC08Z 0RPC30Z 0RPC33Z 0RPC38Z 0RPC48Z 0RPCX0Z 0RPCX3Z 0RPD08Z 0RPD30Z
0RPD33Z 0RPD38Z 0RPD48Z 0RPDX0Z 0RPDX3Z 0RPE08Z 0RPE30Z 0RPE33Z 0RPE38Z 0RPE48Z 0RPEX0Z 0RPEX3Z 0RPEX4Z
0RPF08Z 0RPF30Z 0RPF33Z 0RPF38Z 0RPF48Z 0RPFX0Z 0RPFX3Z 0RPFX4Z 0RPG08Z 0RPG30Z 0RPG33Z 0RPG38Z 0RPG48Z
0RPGX0Z 0RPGX3Z 0RPGX4Z 0RPH08Z 0RPH30Z 0RPH33Z 0RPH38Z 0RPH48Z 0RPHX0Z 0RPHX3Z 0RPHX4Z 0RPJ08Z 0RPJ30Z
0RPJ33Z 0RPJ38Z 0RPJ48Z 0RPJX0Z 0RPJX3Z 0RPJX4Z 0RPK08Z 0RPK30Z 0RPK33Z 0RPK38Z 0RPK48Z 0RPKX0Z 0RPKX3Z
0RPKX4Z 0RPL08Z 0RPL30Z 0RPL33Z 0RPL38Z 0RPL48Z 0RPLX0Z 0RPLX3Z 0RPLX4Z 0RPLX5Z 0RPM08Z 0RPM30Z 0RPM33Z
0RPM38Z 0RPM48Z 0RPMX0Z 0RPMX3Z 0RPMX4Z 0RPMX5Z 0RPN08Z 0RPN30Z 0RPN33Z 0RPN38Z 0RPN48Z 0RPNX0Z 0RPNX3Z
0RPNX4Z 0RPNX5Z 0RPP08Z 0RPP30Z 0RPP33Z 0RPP38Z 0RPP48Z 0RPPX0Z 0RPPX3Z 0RPPX4Z 0RPPX5Z 0RPQ08Z 0RPQ30Z
0RPQ33Z 0RPQ38Z 0RPQ48Z 0RPQX0Z 0RPQX3Z 0RPQX4Z 0RPQX5Z 0RPR08Z 0RPR30Z 0RPR33Z 0RPR38Z 0RPR48Z 0RPRX0Z
0RPRX3Z 0RPRX4Z 0RPRX5Z 0RPS08Z 0RPS30Z 0RPS33Z 0RPS38Z 0RPS48Z 0RPSX0Z 0RPSX3Z 0RPSX4Z 0RPSX5Z 0RPT08Z
0RPT30Z 0RPT33Z 0RPT38Z 0RPT48Z 0RPTX0Z 0RPTX3Z 0RPTX4Z 0RPTX5Z 0RPU08Z 0RPU30Z 0RPU33Z 0RPU38Z 0RPU48Z
0RPUX0Z 0RPUX3Z 0RPUX4Z 0RPUX5Z 0RPV08Z 0RPV30Z 0RPV33Z 0RPV38Z 0RPV48Z 0RPVX0Z 0RPVX3Z 0RPVX4Z 0RPVX5Z
0RPW08Z 0RPW30Z 0RPW33Z 0RPW38Z 0RPW48Z 0RPWX0Z 0RPWX3Z 0RPWX4Z 0RPWX5Z 0RPX08Z 0RPX30Z 0RPX33Z 0RPX38Z
0RPX48Z 0RPXX0Z 0RPXX3Z 0RPXX4Z 0RPXX5Z

0 Medical and Surgical
R Upper Joints
Q Repair: Restoring, to the extent possible, a body part to its normal anatomic structure and function

Body Part Character 4	Approach Character 5	Device Character 6	Qualifier Character 7
0 Occipital-cervical Joint **1** Cervical Vertebral Joint **3** Cervical Vertebral Disc **4** Cervicothoracic Vertebral Joint **5** Cervicothoracic Vertebral Disc **6** Thoracic Vertebral Joint **9** Thoracic Vertebral Disc **A** Thoracolumbar Vertebral Joint **B** Thoracolumbar Vertebral Disc **C** Temporomandibular Joint, Right ⦸ **D** Temporomandibular Joint, Left ⦸ **E** Sternoclavicular Joint, Right HAC **F** Sternoclavicular Joint, Left HAC **G** Acromioclavicular Joint, Right HAC **H** Acromioclavicular Joint, Left HAC **J** Shoulder Joint, Right HAC **K** Shoulder Joint, Left HAC **L** Elbow Joint, Right HAC **M** Elbow Joint, Left HAC **N** Wrist Joint, Right **P** Wrist Joint, Left **Q** Carpal Joint, Right **R** Carpal Joint, Left **S** Metacarpocarpal Joint, Right **T** Metacarpocarpal Joint, Left **U** Metacarpophalangeal Joint, Right **V** Metacarpophalangeal Joint, Left **W** Finger Phalangeal Joint, Right **X** Finger Phalangeal Joint, Left	**0** Open **3** Percutaneous **4** Percutaneous Endoscopic **X** External	**Z** No Device	**Z** No Qualifier

⦸ 0RQCXZZ 0RQDXZZ

HAC 0RQE0ZZ 0RQE3ZZ 0RQE4ZZ 0RQEXZZ 0RQF0ZZ 0RQF3ZZ 0RQF4ZZ 0RQFXZZ 0RQG0ZZ 0RQG3ZZ 0RQG4ZZ 0RQGXZZ 0RQH0ZZ 0RQH3ZZ 0RQH4ZZ 0RQHXZZ 0RQJ0ZZ 0RQJ3ZZ 0RQJ4ZZ 0RQJXZZ 0RQK0ZZ 0RQK3ZZ 0RQK4ZZ 0RQKXZZ 0RQL0ZZ 0RQL3ZZ 0RQL4ZZ 0RQLXZZ 0RQM0ZZ 0RQM3ZZ 0RQM4ZZ or 0RQMXZZ All preceding codes with the HAC symbol are classified as hospital-acquired conditions when reported with secondary diagnosis K68.11, T81.4XXA, T84.60XA, T84.610A, T84.611A, T84.612A, T84.613A, T84.614A, T84.615A, T84.619A, T84.63XA, T84.69XA, or T84.7XXA.

0 Medical and Surgical
R Upper Joints
R Replacement: Putting in or on biological or synthetic material that physically takes the place and/or function of all or a portion of a body part

Body Part Character 4	Approach Character 5	Device Character 6	Qualifier Character 7
0 Occipital-cervical Joint **1** Cervical Vertebral Joint **3** Cervical Vertebral Disc **4** Cervicothoracic Vertebral Joint **5** Cervicothoracic Vertebral Disc **6** Thoracic Vertebral Joint **9** Thoracic Vertebral Disc **A** Thoracolumbar Vertebral Joint **B** Thoracolumbar Vertebral Disc **C** Temporomandibular Joint, Right **D** Temporomandibular Joint, Left **E** Sternoclavicular Joint, Right **F** Sternoclavicular Joint, Left **G** Acromioclavicular Joint, Right **H** Acromioclavicular Joint, Left **L** Elbow Joint, Right **M** Elbow Joint, Left **N** Wrist Joint, Right **P** Wrist Joint, Left **Q** Carpal Joint, Right **R** Carpal Joint, Left **S** Metacarpocarpal Joint, Right **T** Metacarpocarpal Joint, Left **U** Metacarpophalangeal Joint, Right **V** Metacarpophalangeal Joint, Left **W** Finger Phalangeal Joint, Right **X** Finger Phalangeal Joint, Left	**0** Open	**7** Autologous Tissue Substitute **J** Synthetic Substitute **K** Nonautologous Tissue Substitute	**Z** No Qualifier
J Shoulder Joint, Right **K** Shoulder Joint, Left	**0** Open	**0** Synthetic Substitute, Reverse Ball and Socket **7** Autologous Tissue Substitute **K** Nonautologous Tissue Substitute	**Z** No Qualifier
J Shoulder Joint, Right **K** Shoulder Joint, Left	**0** Open	**J** Synthetic Substitute	**6** Humeral Surface **7** Glenoid Surface **Z** No Qualifier

0 Medical and Surgical
R Upper Joints
S Reposition: Moving to its normal location, or other suitable location, all or a portion of a body part

Body Part Character 4	Approach Character 5	Device Character 6	Qualifier Character 7
0 Occipital-cervical Joint ⊘ **1** Cervical Vertebral Joint ⊘ **4** Cervicothoracic Vertebral Joint ⊘ **6** Thoracic Vertebral Joint ⊘ **A** Thoracolumbar Vertebral Joint ⊘ **C** Temporomandibular Joint, Right ⊘ **D** Temporomandibular Joint, Left ⊘ **E** Sternoclavicular Joint, Right ⊘ **F** Sternoclavicular Joint, Left ⊘ **G** Acromioclavicular Joint, Right ⊘ **H** Acromioclavicular Joint, Left ⊘ **J** Shoulder Joint, Right ⊘ **K** Shoulder Joint, Left ⊘	**0** Open **3** Percutaneous **4** Percutaneous Endoscopic **X** External	**4** Internal Fixation Device **Z** No Device	**Z** No Qualifier
L Elbow Joint, Right ⊘ **M** Elbow Joint, Left ⊘ **N** Wrist Joint, Right ⊘ **P** Wrist Joint, Left ⊘ **Q** Carpal Joint, Right ⊘ **R** Carpal Joint, Left ⊘ **S** Metacarpocarpal Joint, Right ⊘ **T** Metacarpocarpal Joint, Left ⊘ **U** Metacarpophalangeal Joint, Right ⊘ **V** Metacarpophalangeal Joint, Left ⊘ **W** Finger Phalangeal Joint, Right ⊘ **X** Finger Phalangeal Joint, Left ⊘	**0** Open **3** Percutaneous **4** Percutaneous Endoscopic **X** External	**4** Internal Fixation Device **5** External Fixation Device **Z** No Device	**Z** No Qualifier

⊘ 0RS034Z 0RS03ZZ 0RS044Z 0RS04ZZ 0RS0X4Z 0RS0XZZ 0RS134Z 0RS13ZZ 0RS144Z 0RS14ZZ 0RS1X4Z 0RS1XZZ 0RS434Z 0RS43ZZ 0RS444Z 0RS44ZZ 0RS4X4Z 0RS4XZZ 0RS634Z 0RS63ZZ 0RS644Z 0RS64ZZ 0RS6X4Z 0RS6XZZ 0RSA34Z 0RSA3ZZ 0RSA44Z 0RSA4ZZ 0RSAX4Z 0RSAXZZ 0RSC34Z 0RSC3ZZ 0RSC44Z 0RSC4ZZ 0RSCX4Z 0RSCXZZ 0RSD34Z 0RSD3ZZ 0RSD44Z 0RSD4ZZ 0RSDX4Z 0RSDXZZ 0RSE34Z 0RSE3ZZ 0RSE44Z 0RSE4ZZ 0RSEX4Z 0RSEXZZ 0RSF34Z 0RSF3ZZ 0RSF44Z 0RSF4ZZ 0RSFX4Z 0RSFXZZ 0RSG34Z 0RSG3ZZ 0RSG44Z 0RSG4ZZ 0RSGX4Z 0RSGXZZ 0RSH34Z 0RSH3ZZ 0RSH44Z 0RSH4ZZ 0RSHX4Z 0RSHXZZ 0RSJ34Z 0RSJ3ZZ 0RSJ44Z 0RSJ4ZZ 0RSJX4Z 0RSJXZZ 0RSK34Z 0RSK3ZZ 0RSK44Z 0RSK4ZZ 0RSKX4Z 0RSKXZZ 0RSL34Z 0RSL35Z 0RSL3ZZ 0RSL44Z 0RSL45Z 0RSL4ZZ 0RSLX4Z 0RSLX5Z 0RSLXZZ 0RSM34Z 0RSM35Z 0RSM3ZZ 0RSM44Z 0RSM45Z 0RSM4ZZ 0RSMX4Z 0RSMX5Z 0RSMXZZ 0RSN34Z 0RSN35Z 0RSN3ZZ 0RSN44Z 0RSN45Z 0RSN4ZZ 0RSNX4Z 0RSNX5Z 0RSNXZZ 0RSP34Z 0RSP35Z 0RSP3ZZ 0RSP44Z 0RSP45Z 0RSP4ZZ 0RSPX4Z 0RSPX5Z 0RSPXZZ 0RSQ34Z 0RSQ35Z 0RSQ3ZZ 0RSQ44Z 0RSQ45Z 0RSQ4ZZ 0RSQX4Z 0RSQX5Z 0RSQXZZ 0RSR34Z 0RSR35Z 0RSR3ZZ 0RSR44Z 0RSR45Z 0RSR4ZZ 0RSRX4Z 0RSRX5Z 0RSRXZZ 0RSS34Z 0RSS35Z 0RSS3ZZ 0RSS44Z 0RSS45Z 0RSS4ZZ 0RSSX4Z 0RSSX5Z 0RSSXZZ 0RST34Z 0RST35Z 0RST3ZZ 0RST44Z 0RST45Z 0RST4ZZ 0RSTX4Z 0RSTX5Z 0RSTXZZ 0RSU34Z 0RSU35Z 0RSU3ZZ 0RSU44Z 0RSU45Z 0RSU4ZZ 0RSUX4Z 0RSUX5Z 0RSUXZZ 0RSV34Z 0RSV35Z 0RSV3ZZ 0RSV44Z 0RSV45Z 0RSV4ZZ 0RSVX4Z 0RSVX5Z 0RSVXZZ 0RSW34Z 0RSW35Z 0RSW3ZZ 0RSW44Z 0RSW45Z 0RSW4ZZ 0RSWX4Z 0RSWX5Z 0RSWXZZ 0RSX34Z 0RSX35Z 0RSX3ZZ 0RSX44Z 0RSX45Z 0RSX4ZZ 0RSXX4Z 0RSXX5Z 0RSXXZZ

0 Medical and Surgical
R Upper Joints
T Resection: Cutting out or off, without replacement, all of a body part

Body Part Character 4	Approach Character 5	Device Character 6	Qualifier Character 7
3 Cervical Vertebral Disc **4** Cervicothoracic Vertebral Joint **5** Cervicothoracic Vertebral Disc **9** Thoracic Vertebral Disc **B** Thoracolumbar Vertebral Disc **C** Temporomandibular Joint, Right **D** Temporomandibular Joint, Left **E** Sternoclavicular Joint, Right **F** Sternoclavicular Joint, Left **G** Acromioclavicular Joint, Right **H** Acromioclavicular Joint, Left **J** Shoulder Joint, Right **K** Shoulder Joint, Left **L** Elbow Joint, Right **M** Elbow Joint, Left **N** Wrist Joint, Right **P** Wrist Joint, Left **Q** Carpal Joint, Right **R** Carpal Joint, Left **S** Metacarpocarpal Joint, Right **T** Metacarpocarpal Joint, Left **U** Metacarpophalangeal Joint, Right **V** Metacarpophalangeal Joint, Left **W** Finger Phalangeal Joint, Right **X** Finger Phalangeal Joint, Left	**0** Open	**Z** No Device	**Z** No Qualifier

0 Medical and Surgical
R Upper Joints
U Supplement: Putting in or on biological or synthetic material that physically reinforces and/or augments the function of a portion of a body part

Body Part Character 4	Approach Character 5	Device Character 6	Qualifier Character 7
0 Occipital-cervical Joint **1** Cervical Vertebral Joint **3** Cervical Vertebral Disc **4** Cervicothoracic Vertebral Joint **5** Cervicothoracic Vertebral Disc **6** Thoracic Vertebral Joint **9** Thoracic Vertebral Disc **A** Thoracolumbar Vertebral Joint **B** Thoracolumbar Vertebral Disc **C** Temporomandibular Joint, Right **D** Temporomandibular Joint, Left **E** Sternoclavicular Joint, Right HAC **F** Sternoclavicular Joint, Left HAC **G** Acromioclavicular Joint, Right HAC **H** Acromioclavicular Joint, Left HAC **J** Shoulder Joint, Right HAC **K** Shoulder Joint, Left HAC **L** Elbow Joint, Right HAC **M** Elbow Joint, Left HAC **N** Wrist Joint, Right **P** Wrist Joint, Left **Q** Carpal Joint, Right **R** Carpal Joint, Left **S** Metacarpocarpal Joint, Right **T** Metacarpocarpal Joint, Left **U** Metacarpophalangeal Joint, Right **V** Metacarpophalangeal Joint, Left **W** Finger Phalangeal Joint, Right **X** Finger Phalangeal Joint, Left	**0** Open **3** Percutaneous **4** Percutaneous Endoscopic	**7** Autologous Tissue Substitute **J** Synthetic Substitute **K** Nonautologous Tissue Substitute	**Z** No Qualifier

HAC 0RUE07Z 0RUE0JZ 0RUE0KZ 0RUE37Z 0RUE3JZ 0RUE3KZ 0RUE47Z 0RUE4JZ 0RUE4KZ 0RUF07Z 0RUF0JZ 0RUF0KZ 0RUF37Z 0RUF3JZ 0RUF3KZ 0RUF47Z 0RUF4JZ 0RUF4KZ 0RUG07Z 0RUG0JZ 0RUG0KZ 0RUG37Z 0RUG3JZ 0RUG3KZ 0RUG47Z 0RUG4JZ 0RUG4KZ 0RUH07Z 0RUH0JZ 0RUH0KZ 0RUH37Z 0RUH3JZ 0RUH3KZ 0RUH4JZ 0RUH4KZ 0RUJ07Z 0RUJ0JZ 0RUJ0KZ 0RUJ37Z 0RUJ3JZ 0RUJ3KZ 0RUJ47Z 0RUJ4JZ 0RUJ4KZ 0RUK07Z 0RUK0JZ 0RUK0KZ 0RUK37Z 0RUK3JZ 0RUK3KZ 0RUK47Z 0RUK4JZ 0RUK4KZ 0RUL07Z 0RUL0JZ 0RUL0KZ 0RUL37Z 0RUL3JZ 0RUL3KZ 0RUL47Z 0RUL4JZ 0RUL4KZ 0RUM07Z 0RUM0JZ 0RUM0KZ 0RUM37Z 0RUM3JZ 0RUM3KZ 0RUM47Z 0RUM4JZ or 0RUM4KZ All preceding codes with the HAC symbol are classified as hospital-acquired conditions when reported with secondary diagnosis K68.11, T81.4XXA, T84.60XA, T84.610A, T84.611A, T84.612A, T84.613A, T84.614A, T84.615A, T84.619A, T84.63XA, T84.69XA, or T84.7XXA.

0 Medical and Surgical
R Upper Joints
W Revision: Correcting, to the extent possible, a portion of a malfunctioning device or the position of a displaced device

Body Part Character 4	Approach Character 5	Device Character 6	Qualifier Character 7
0 Occipital-cervical Joint ⦸ **1** Cervical Vertebral Joint ⦸ **4** Cervicothoracic Vertebral Joint ⦸ **6** Thoracic Vertebral Joint ⦸ **A** Thoracolumbar Vertebral Joint ⦸	**0** Open **3** Percutaneous **4** Percutaneous Endoscopic **X** External	**0** Drainage Device **3** Infusion Device **4** Internal Fixation Device **7** Autologous Tissue Substitute **8** Spacer **A** Interbody Fusion Device **J** Synthetic Substitute **K** Nonautologous Tissue Substitute	**Z** No Qualifier
3 Cervical Vertebral Disc ⦸ **5** Cervicothoracic Vertebral Disc ⦸ **9** Thoracic Vertebral Disc ⦸ **B** Thoracolumbar Vertebral Disc ⦸	**0** Open **3** Percutaneous **4** Percutaneous Endoscopic **X** External	**0** Drainage Device **3** Infusion Device **7** Autologous Tissue Substitute **J** Synthetic Substitute **K** Nonautologous Tissue Substitute	**Z** No Qualifier
C Temporomandibular Joint, Right ⦸ **D** Temporomandibular Joint, Left ⦸ **E** Sternoclavicular Joint, Right ⦸ **F** Sternoclavicular Joint, Left ⦸ **G** Acromioclavicular Joint, Right ⦸ **H** Acromioclavicular Joint, Left ⦸ **J** Shoulder Joint, Right ⦸ **K** Shoulder Joint, Left ⦸	**0** Open **3** Percutaneous **4** Percutaneous Endoscopic **X** External	**0** Drainage Device **3** Infusion Device **4** Internal Fixation Device **7** Autologous Tissue Substitute **8** Spacer **J** Synthetic Substitute **K** Nonautologous Tissue Substitute	**Z** No Qualifier
L Elbow Joint, Right ⦸ **M** Elbow Joint, Left ⦸ **N** Wrist Joint, Right ⦸ **P** Wrist Joint, Left ⦸ **Q** Carpal Joint, Right ⦸ **R** Carpal Joint, Left ⦸ **S** Metacarpocarpal Joint, Right ⦸ **T** Metacarpocarpal Joint, Left ⦸ **U** Metacarpophalangeal Joint, Right ⦸ **V** Metacarpophalangeal Joint, Left ⦸ **W** Finger Phalangeal Joint, Right ⦸ **X** Finger Phalangeal Joint, Left ⦸	**0** Open **3** Percutaneous **4** Percutaneous Endoscopic **X** External	**0** Drainage Device **3** Infusion Device **4** Internal Fixation Device **5** External Fixation Device **7** Autologous Tissue Substitute **8** Spacer **J** Synthetic Substitute **K** Nonautologous Tissue Substitute	**Z** No Qualifier

⦸ 0RW0X0Z 0RW0X3Z 0RW0X4Z 0RW0X7Z 0RW0X8Z 0RW0XAZ 0RW0XJZ 0RW0XKZ 0RW1X0Z 0RW1X3Z 0RW1X4Z 0RW1X7Z 0RW1X8Z 0RW1XAZ 0RW1XJZ 0RW1XKZ 0RW3X0Z 0RW3X3Z 0RW3X7Z 0RW3XJZ 0RW3XKZ 0RW4X0Z 0RW4X3Z 0RW4X4Z 0RW4X7Z 0RW4X8Z 0RW4XAZ 0RW4XJZ 0RW4XKZ 0RW5X0Z 0RW5X3Z 0RW5X7Z 0RW5XJZ 0RW5XKZ 0RW6X0Z 0RW6X3Z 0RW6X4Z 0RW6X7Z 0RW6X8Z 0RW6XAZ 0RW6XJZ 0RW6XKZ 0RW9X0Z 0RW9X3Z 0RW9X7Z 0RW9XJZ 0RW9XKZ 0RWAX0Z 0RWAX3Z 0RWAX4Z 0RWAX7Z 0RWAX8Z 0RWAXAZ 0RWAXJZ 0RWAXKZ 0RWBX0Z 0RWBX3Z 0RWBX7Z 0RWBXJZ 0RWBXKZ 0RWCX0Z 0RWCX3Z 0RWCX4Z 0RWCX7Z 0RWCX8Z 0RWCXJZ 0RWCXKZ 0RWDX0Z 0RWDX3Z 0RWDX4Z 0RWDX7Z 0RWDX8Z 0RWDXJZ 0RWDXKZ 0RWEX0Z 0RWEX3Z 0RWEX4Z 0RWEX7Z 0RWEX8Z 0RWEXJZ 0RWEXKZ 0RWFX0Z 0RWFX3Z 0RWFX4Z 0RWFX7Z 0RWFX8Z 0RWFXJZ 0RWFXKZ 0RWGX0Z 0RWGX3Z 0RWGX4Z 0RWGX7Z 0RWGX8Z 0RWGXJZ 0RWGXKZ 0RWHX0Z 0RWHX3Z 0RWHX4Z 0RWHX7Z 0RWHX8Z 0RWHXJZ 0RWHXKZ 0RWJX0Z 0RWJX3Z 0RWJX4Z 0RWJX7Z 0RWJX8Z 0RWJXJZ 0RWJXKZ 0RWKX0Z 0RWKX3Z 0RWKX4Z 0RWKX7Z 0RWKX8Z 0RWKXJZ 0RWKXKZ 0RWLX0Z 0RWLX3Z 0RWLX4Z 0RWLX5Z 0RWLX7Z 0RWLX8Z 0RWLXJZ 0RWLXKZ 0RWMX0Z 0RWMX3Z 0RWMX4Z 0RWMX5Z 0RWMX7Z 0RWMX8Z 0RWMXJZ 0RWMXKZ 0RWNX0Z 0RWNX3Z 0RWNX4Z 0RWNX5Z 0RWNX7Z 0RWNX8Z 0RWNXJZ 0RWNXKZ 0RWPX0Z 0RWPX3Z 0RWPX4Z 0RWPX5Z 0RWPX7Z 0RWPX8Z 0RWPXJZ 0RWPXKZ 0RWQX0Z 0RWQX3Z 0RWQX4Z 0RWQX5Z 0RWQX7Z 0RWQX8Z 0RWQXJZ 0RWQXKZ 0RWRX0Z 0RWRX3Z 0RWRX4Z 0RWRX5Z 0RWRX7Z 0RWRX8Z 0RWRXJZ 0RWRXKZ 0RWSX0Z 0RWSX3Z 0RWSX4Z 0RWSX5Z 0RWSX7Z 0RWSX8Z 0RWSXJZ 0RWSXKZ 0RWTX0Z 0RWTX3Z 0RWTX4Z 0RWTX5Z 0RWTX7Z 0RWTX8Z 0RWTXJZ 0RWTXKZ 0RWUX0Z 0RWUX3Z 0RWUX4Z 0RWUX5Z 0RWUX7Z 0RWUX8Z 0RWUXJZ 0RWUXKZ 0RWVX0Z 0RWVX3Z 0RWVX4Z 0RWVX5Z 0RWVX7Z 0RWVX8Z 0RWVXJZ 0RWVXKZ 0RWWX0Z 0RWWX3Z 0RWWX4Z 0RWWX5Z 0RWWX7Z 0RWWX8Z 0RWWXJZ 0RWWXKZ 0RWXX0Z 0RWXX3Z 0RWXX4Z 0RWXX5Z 0RWXX7Z 0RWXX8Z 0RWXXJZ 0RWXXKZ

Lower Joints 0S2-0SW

0 Medical and Surgical
S Lower Joints
2 Change: Taking out or off a device from a body part and putting back an identical or similar device in or on the same body part without cutting or puncturing the skin or a mucous membrane

Body Part Character 4	Approach Character 5	Device Character 6	Qualifier Character 7
Y Lower Joint ⊘	**X** External	**0** Drainage Device **Y** Other Device	**Z** No Qualifier

⊘ 0S2YX0Z 0S2YXYZ

0 Medical and Surgical
S Lower Joints
5 Destruction: Physical eradication of all or a portion of a body part by the direct use of energy, force, or a destructive agent

Body Part Character 4	Approach Character 5	Device Character 6	Qualifier Character 7
0 Lumbar Vertebral Joint **2** Lumbar Vertebral Disc **3** Lumbosacral Joint **4** Lumbosacral Disc **5** Sacrococcygeal Joint **6** Coccygeal Joint **7** Sacroiliac Joint, Right **8** Sacroiliac Joint, Left **9** Hip Joint, Right **B** Hip Joint, Left **C** Knee Joint, Right **D** Knee Joint, Left **F** Ankle Joint, Right **G** Ankle Joint, Left **H** Tarsal Joint, Right **J** Tarsal Joint, Left **K** Metatarsal-Tarsal Joint, Right **L** Metatarsal-Tarsal Joint, Left **M** Metatarsal-Phalangeal Joint, Right **N** Metatarsal-Phalangeal Joint, Left **P** Toe Phalangeal Joint, Right **Q** Toe Phalangeal Joint, Left	**0** Open **3** Percutaneous **4** Percutaneous Endoscopic	**Z** No Device	**Z** No Qualifier

0 Medical and Surgical
S Lower Joints
9 Drainage: Taking or letting out fluids and/or gases from a body part

Body Part Character 4	Approach Character 5	Device Character 6	Qualifier Character 7
0 Lumbar Vertebral Joint ⊘ **2** Lumbar Vertebral Disc ⊘ **3** Lumbosacral Joint ⊘ **4** Lumbosacral Disc ⊘ **5** Sacrococcygeal Joint ⊘ **6** Coccygeal Joint ⊘ **7** Sacroiliac Joint, Right ⊘ **8** Sacroiliac Joint, Left ⊘ **9** Hip Joint, Right ⊘ **B** Hip Joint, Left ⊘ **C** Knee Joint, Right ⊘ **D** Knee Joint, Left ⊘ **F** Ankle Joint, Right ⊘ **G** Ankle Joint, Left ⊘ **H** Tarsal Joint, Right ⊘ **J** Tarsal Joint, Left ⊘ **K** Metatarsal-Tarsal Joint, Right ⊘ **L** Metatarsal-Tarsal Joint, Left ⊘ **M** Metatarsal-Phalangeal Joint, Right ⊘ **N** Metatarsal-Phalangeal Joint, Left ⊘ **P** Toe Phalangeal Joint, Right ⊘ **Q** Toe Phalangeal Joint, Left ⊘	**0** Open **3** Percutaneous **4** Percutaneous Endoscopic	**0** Drainage Device	**Z** No Qualifier
0 Lumbar Vertebral Joint ⊘ **2** Lumbar Vertebral Disc ⊘ **3** Lumbosacral Joint ⊘ **4** Lumbosacral Disc ⊘ **5** Sacrococcygeal Joint ⊘ **6** Coccygeal Joint ⊘ **7** Sacroiliac Joint, Right ⊘ **8** Sacroiliac Joint, Left ⊘ **9** Hip Joint, Right ⊘ **B** Hip Joint, Left ⊘ **C** Knee Joint, Right ⊘ **D** Knee Joint, Left ⊘ **F** Ankle Joint, Right ⊘ **G** Ankle Joint, Left ⊘ **H** Tarsal Joint, Right ⊘ **J** Tarsal Joint, Left ⊘ **K** Metatarsal-Tarsal Joint, Right ⊘ **L** Metatarsal-Tarsal Joint, Left ⊘ **M** Metatarsal-Phalangeal Joint, Right ⊘ **N** Metatarsal-Phalangeal Joint, Left ⊘ **P** Toe Phalangeal Joint, Right ⊘ **Q** Toe Phalangeal Joint, Left ⊘	**0** Open **3** Percutaneous **4** Percutaneous Endoscopic	**Z** No Device	**X** Diagnostic **Z** No Qualifier

⊘ 0S900ZX 0S9030Z 0S903ZX 0S903ZZ 0S9040Z 0S904ZX 0S904ZZ 0S920ZX 0S9230Z 0S923ZX 0S923ZZ 0S9240Z 0S924ZX
0S924ZZ 0S930ZX 0S9330Z 0S933ZX 0S933ZZ 0S9340Z 0S934ZX 0S934ZZ 0S940ZX 0S9430Z 0S943ZX 0S943ZZ 0S9440Z
0S944ZX 0S944ZZ 0S950ZX 0S9530Z 0S953ZX 0S953ZZ 0S9540Z 0S954ZX 0S954ZZ 0S960ZX 0S9630Z 0S963ZX 0S963ZZ
0S9640Z 0S964ZX 0S964ZZ 0S970ZX 0S9730Z 0S973ZX 0S973ZZ 0S9740Z 0S974ZX 0S974ZZ 0S980ZX 0S9830Z 0S983ZX
0S983ZZ 0S9840Z 0S984ZX 0S984ZZ 0S990ZX 0S9930Z 0S993ZX 0S993ZZ 0S9940Z 0S994ZX 0S994ZZ 0S9B0ZX 0S9B30Z
0S9B3ZX 0S9B3ZZ 0S9B40Z 0S9B4ZX 0S9B4ZZ 0S9C0ZX 0S9C30Z 0S9C3ZX 0S9C3ZZ 0S9C40Z 0S9C4ZX 0S9C4ZZ 0S9D0ZX
0S9D30Z 0S9D3ZX 0S9D3ZZ 0S9D40Z 0S9D4ZX 0S9D4ZZ 0S9F0ZX 0S9F30Z 0S9F3ZX 0S9F3ZZ 0S9F40Z 0S9F4ZX 0S9F4ZZ
0S9G0ZX 0S9G30Z 0S9G3ZX 0S9G3ZZ 0S9G40Z 0S9G4ZX 0S9G4ZZ 0S9H0ZX 0S9H30Z 0S9H3ZX 0S9H3ZZ 0S9H40Z 0S9H4ZX
0S9H4ZZ 0S9J0ZX 0S9J30Z 0S9J3ZX 0S9J3ZZ 0S9J40Z 0S9J4ZX 0S9J4ZZ 0S9K0ZX 0S9K30Z 0S9K3ZX 0S9K3ZZ 0S9K40Z
0S9K4ZX 0S9K4ZZ 0S9L0ZX 0S9L30Z 0S9L3ZX 0S9L3ZZ 0S9L40Z 0S9L4ZX 0S9L4ZZ 0S9M0ZX 0S9M30Z 0S9M3ZX 0S9M3ZZ
0S9M40Z 0S9M4ZX 0S9M4ZZ 0S9N0ZX 0S9N30Z 0S9N3ZX 0S9N3ZZ 0S9N40Z 0S9N4ZX 0S9N4ZZ 0S9P0ZX 0S9P30Z 0S9P3ZX
0S9P3ZZ 0S9P40Z 0S9P4ZX 0S9P4ZZ 0S9Q0ZX 0S9Q30Z 0S9Q3ZX 0S9Q3ZZ 0S9Q40Z 0S9Q4ZX 0S9Q4ZZ

LC Limited Coverage NC Noncovered HAC HAC Associated Procedure CC Combination Cluster - See Appendix G for code lists
DRG Non-OR-Affecting MS-DRG Assignment ⊘ Non-OR-Not Affecting MS-DRG Assignment New/Revised Text in **Orange** ♂ Male ♀ Female

0 Medical and Surgical
S Lower Joints
B Excision: Cutting out or off, without replacement, a portion of a body part

Body Part Character 4	Approach Character 5	Device Character 6	Qualifier Character 7
0 Lumbar Vertebral Joint ⃠ **2** Lumbar Vertebral Disc ⃠ **3** Lumbosacral Joint ⃠ **4** Lumbosacral Disc ⃠ **5** Sacrococcygeal Joint ⃠ **6** Coccygeal Joint ⃠ **7** Sacroiliac Joint, Right ⃠ **8** Sacroiliac Joint, Left ⃠ **9** Hip Joint, Right ⃠ **B** Hip Joint, Left ⃠ **C** Knee Joint, Right ⃠ CC **D** Knee Joint, Left ⃠ CC **F** Ankle Joint, Right ⃠ **G** Ankle Joint, Left ⃠ **H** Tarsal Joint, Right ⃠ **J** Tarsal Joint, Left ⃠ **K** Metatarsal-Tarsal Joint, Right ⃠ **L** Metatarsal-Tarsal Joint, Left ⃠ **M** Metatarsal-Phalangeal Joint, Right ⃠ **N** Metatarsal-Phalangeal Joint, Left ⃠ **P** Toe Phalangeal Joint, Right ⃠ **Q** Toe Phalangeal Joint, Left ⃠	**0** Open **3** Percutaneous **4** Percutaneous Endoscopic	**Z** No Device	**X** Diagnostic **Z** No Qualifier

⃠ 0SB00ZX 0SB03ZX 0SB04ZX 0SB20ZX 0SB23ZX 0SB24ZX 0SB30ZX 0SB33ZX 0SB34ZX 0SB40ZX 0SB43ZX 0SB44ZX 0SB50ZX 0SB53ZX 0SB54ZX 0SB60ZX 0SB63ZX 0SB64ZX 0SB70ZX 0SB73ZX 0SB74ZX 0SB80ZX 0SB83ZX 0SB84ZX 0SB90ZX 0SB93ZX 0SB94ZX 0SBB0ZX 0SBB3ZX 0SBB4ZX 0SBC0ZX 0SBC3ZX 0SBC4ZX 0SBD0ZX 0SBD3ZX 0SBD4ZX 0SBF0ZX 0SBF3ZX 0SBF4ZX 0SBG0ZX 0SBG3ZX 0SBG4ZX 0SBH0ZX 0SBH3ZX 0SBH4ZX 0SBJ0ZX 0SBJ3ZX 0SBJ4ZX 0SBK0ZX 0SBK3ZX 0SBK4ZX 0SBL0ZX 0SBL3ZX 0SBL4ZX 0SBM0ZX 0SBM3ZX 0SBM4ZX 0SBN0ZX 0SBN3ZX 0SBN4ZX 0SBP0ZX 0SBP3ZX 0SBP4ZX 0SBQ0ZX 0SBQ3ZX 0SBQ4ZX

CC 0SBC0ZZ 0SBC3ZZ 0SBC4ZZ 0SBD0ZZ 0SBD3ZZ 0SBD4ZZ

0 Medical and Surgical
S Lower Joints
C Extirpation: Taking or cutting out solid matter from a body part

Body Part Character 4	Approach Character 5	Device Character 6	Qualifier Character 7
0 Lumbar Vertebral Joint **2** Lumbar Vertebral Disc **3** Lumbosacral Joint **4** Lumbosacral Disc **5** Sacrococcygeal Joint **6** Coccygeal Joint **7** Sacroiliac Joint, Right **8** Sacroiliac Joint, Left **9** Hip Joint, Right **B** Hip Joint, Left **C** Knee Joint, Right **D** Knee Joint, Left **F** Ankle Joint, Right **G** Ankle Joint, Left **H** Tarsal Joint, Right **J** Tarsal Joint, Left **K** Metatarsal-Tarsal Joint, Right **L** Metatarsal-Tarsal Joint, Left **M** Metatarsal-Phalangeal Joint, Right **N** Metatarsal-Phalangeal Joint, Left **P** Toe Phalangeal Joint, Right **Q** Toe Phalangeal Joint, Left	**0** Open **3** Percutaneous **4** Percutaneous Endoscopic	**Z** No Device	**Z** No Qualifier

0 Medical and Surgical
S Lower Joints
G Fusion: Joining together portions of an articular body part rendering the articular body part immobile

Body Part Character 4	Approach Character 5	Device Character 6	Qualifier Character 7
0 Lumbar Vertebral Joint HAC **1** Lumbar Vertebral Joints, 2 or more CC HAC **3** Lumbosacral Joint HAC	**0** Open **3** Percutaneous **4** Percutaneous Endoscopic	**7** Autologous Tissue Substitute **A** Interbody Fusion Device **J** Synthetic Substitute **K** Nonautologous Tissue Substitute **Z** No Device	**0** Anterior Approach, Anterior Column **1** Posterior Approach, Posterior Column **J** Posterior Approach, Anterior Column
5 Sacrococcygeal Joint **6** Coccygeal Joint **7** Sacroiliac Joint, Right HAC **8** Sacroiliac Joint, Left HAC	**0** Open **3** Percutaneous **4** Percutaneous Endoscopic	**4** Internal Fixation Device **7** Autologous Tissue Substitute **J** Synthetic Substitute **K** Nonautologous Tissue Substitute **Z** No Device	**Z** No Qualifier
9 Hip Joint, Right **B** Hip Joint, Left **C** Knee Joint, Right **D** Knee Joint, Left **F** Ankle Joint, Right **G** Ankle Joint, Left **H** Tarsal Joint, Right **J** Tarsal Joint, Left **K** Metatarsal-Tarsal Joint, Right **L** Metatarsal-Tarsal Joint, Left **M** Metatarsal-Phalangeal Joint, Right CC **N** Metatarsal-Phalangeal Joint, Left CC **P** Toe Phalangeal Joint, Right **Q** Toe Phalangeal Joint, Left	**0** Open **3** Percutaneous **4** Percutaneous Endoscopic	**4** Internal Fixation Device **5** External Fixation Device **7** Autologous Tissue Substitute **J** Synthetic Substitute **K** Nonautologous Tissue Substitute **Z** No Device	**Z** No Qualifier

CC	0SG1070	0SG1071	0SG107J	0SG10A0	0SG10A1	0SG10AJ	0SG10J0	0SG10J1	0SG10JJ	0SG10K0	0SG10K1	0SG10KJ	0SG10Z0
	0SG10Z1	0SG10ZJ	0SG1370	0SG1371	0SG137J	0SG13A0	0SG13A1	0SG13AJ	0SG13J0	0SG13J1	0SG13JJ	0SG13K0	0SG13K1

0SG continued on next page

0SG continued from previous page

0SG13KJ 0SG13Z0 0SG13Z1 0SG13ZJ 0SG1470 0SG1471 0SG147J 0SG14A0 0SG14A1 0SG14AJ 0SG14J0 0SG14J1 0SG14JJ 0SG14K0 0SG14K1 0SG14KJ 0SG14Z0 0SG14Z1 0SG14ZJ 0SGM0ZZ 0SGM3ZZ 0SGM4ZZ 0SGN0ZZ 0SGN3ZZ 0SGN4ZZ

HAC 0SG0070 0SG0071 0SG007J 0SG00A0 0SG00A1 0SG00AJ 0SG00J0 0SG00J1 0SG00JJ 0SG00K0 0SG00K1 0SG00KJ 0SG00Z0 0SG00Z1 0SG00ZJ 0SG0370 0SG0371 0SG037J 0SG03A0 0SG03A1 0SG03AJ 0SG03J0 0SG03J1 0SG03JJ 0SG03K0 0SG03K1 0SG03KJ 0SG03Z0 0SG03Z1 0SG03ZJ 0SG0470 0SG0471 0SG047J 0SG04A0 0SG04A1 0SG04AJ 0SG04J0 0SG04J1 0SG04JJ 0SG04K0 0SG04K1 0SG04KJ 0SG04Z0 0SG04Z1 0SG04ZJ 0SG1070 0SG1071 0SG107J 0SG10A0 0SG10A1 0SG10AJ 0SG10J0 0SG10J1 0SG10JJ 0SG10K0 0SG10K1 0SG10KJ 0SG10Z0 0SG10Z1 0SG10ZJ 0SG1370 0SG1371 0SG137J 0SG13A0 0SG13A1 0SG13AJ 0SG13J0 0SG13J1 0SG13JJ 0SG13K0 0SG13K1 0SG13KJ 0SG13Z0 0SG13Z1 0SG13ZJ 0SG1470 0SG1471 0SG147J 0SG14A0 0SG14A1 0SG14AJ 0SG14J0 0SG14J1 0SG14JJ 0SG14K0 0SG14K1 0SG14KJ 0SG14Z0 0SG14Z1 0SG14ZJ 0SG3070 0SG3071 0SG307J 0SG30A0 0SG30A1 0SG30AJ 0SG30J0 0SG30J1 0SG30JJ 0SG30K0 0SG30K1 0SG30KJ 0SG30Z0 0SG30Z1 0SG30ZJ 0SG3370 0SG3371 0SG337J 0SG33A0 0SG33A1 0SG33AJ 0SG33J0 0SG33J1 0SG33JJ 0SG33K0 0SG33K1 0SG33KJ 0SG33Z0 0SG33Z1 0SG33ZJ 0SG3470 0SG3471 0SG347J 0SG34A0 0SG34A1 0SG34AJ 0SG34J0 0SG34J1 0SG34JJ 0SG34K0 0SG34K1 0SG34KJ 0SG34Z0 0SG34Z1 0SG34ZJ 0SG704Z 0SG707Z 0SG70JZ 0SG70KZ 0SG70ZZ 0SG734Z 0SG737Z 0SG73JZ 0SG73KZ 0SG73ZZ 0SG744Z 0SG747Z 0SG74JZ 0SG74KZ 0SG74ZZ 0SG804Z 0SG807Z 0SG80JZ 0SG80KZ 0SG80ZZ 0SG834Z 0SG837Z 0SG83JZ 0SG83KZ 0SG83ZZ 0SG844Z 0SG847Z 0SG84JZ 0SG84KZ or 0SG84ZZ All preceding codes with the HAC symbol are classified as hospital-acquired conditions when reported with secondary diagnosis K68.11, T81.4XXA, T84.60XA, T84.610A, T84.611A, T84.612A, T84.613A, T84.614A, T84.615A, T84.619A, T84.63XA, T84.69XA, or T84.7XXA.

0 Medical and Surgical
S Lower Joints
H Insertion: Putting in a nonbiological appliance that monitors, assists, performs, or prevents a physiological function but does not physically take the place of a body part

Body Part Character 4	Approach Character 5	Device Character 6	Qualifier Character 7
0 Lumbar Vertebral Joint ⃠ **3** Lumbosacral Joint ⃠	**0** Open **3** Percutaneous **4** Percutaneous Endoscopic	**3** Infusion Device **4** Internal Fixation Device **8** Spacer **B** Spinal Stabilization Device, Interspinous Process **C** Spinal Stabilization Device, Pedicle-Based **D** Spinal Stabilization Device, Facet Replacement	**Z** No Qualifier
2 Lumbar Vertebral Disc ⃠ **4** Lumbosacral Disc ⃠	**0** Open **3** Percutaneous **4** Percutaneous Endoscopic	**3** Infusion Device **8** Spacer	**Z** No Qualifier
5 Sacrococcygeal Joint ⃠ **6** Coccygeal Joint ⃠ **7** Sacroiliac Joint, Right ⃠ **8** Sacroiliac Joint, Left ⃠	**0** Open **3** Percutaneous **4** Percutaneous Endoscopic	**3** Infusion Device **4** Internal Fixation Device **8** Spacer	**Z** No Qualifier
9 Hip Joint, Right ⃠ **B** Hip Joint, Left ⃠ **C** Knee Joint, Right ⃠ **D** Knee Joint, Left ⃠ **F** Ankle Joint, Right ⃠ **G** Ankle Joint, Left ⃠ **H** Tarsal Joint, Right ⃠ **J** Tarsal Joint, Left ⃠ **K** Metatarsal-Tarsal Joint, Right ⃠ **L** Metatarsal-Tarsal Joint, Left ⃠ **M** Metatarsal-Phalangeal Joint, Right ⃠ **N** Metatarsal-Phalangeal Joint, Left ⃠ **P** Toe Phalangeal Joint, Right ⃠ **Q** Toe Phalangeal Joint, Left ⃠	**0** Open **3** Percutaneous **4** Percutaneous Endoscopic	**3** Infusion Device **4** Internal Fixation Device **5** External Fixation Device **8** Spacer	**Z** No Qualifier

⃠ 0SH003Z 0SH008Z 0SH033Z 0SH038Z 0SH043Z 0SH048Z 0SH203Z 0SH208Z 0SH233Z 0SH238Z 0SH243Z 0SH248Z 0SH303Z 0SH308Z 0SH333Z 0SH338Z 0SH343Z 0SH348Z 0SH403Z 0SH408Z 0SH433Z 0SH438Z 0SH443Z 0SH448Z 0SH503Z 0SH508Z 0SH533Z 0SH538Z 0SH543Z 0SH548Z 0SH603Z 0SH608Z 0SH633Z 0SH638Z 0SH643Z 0SH648Z 0SH703Z 0SH708Z 0SH733Z 0SH738Z 0SH743Z 0SH748Z 0SH803Z 0SH808Z 0SH833Z 0SH838Z 0SH843Z 0SH848Z 0SH903Z 0SH908Z 0SH933Z 0SH938Z 0SH943Z 0SH948Z 0SHB03Z 0SHB08Z 0SHB33Z 0SHB38Z 0SHB43Z 0SHB48Z 0SHC03Z 0SHC08Z 0SHC33Z 0SHC38Z 0SHC43Z 0SHC48Z 0SHD03Z 0SHD08Z 0SHD33Z 0SHD38Z 0SHD43Z 0SHD48Z 0SHF03Z 0SHF08Z 0SHF33Z 0SHF38Z 0SHF43Z 0SHF48Z 0SHG03Z 0SHG08Z 0SHG33Z 0SHG38Z 0SHG43Z 0SHG48Z 0SHH03Z 0SHH08Z 0SHH33Z 0SHH38Z 0SHH43Z 0SHH48Z 0SHJ03Z 0SHJ08Z 0SHJ33Z 0SHJ38Z 0SHJ43Z 0SHJ48Z 0SHK03Z 0SHK08Z 0SHK33Z 0SHK38Z 0SHK43Z 0SHK48Z 0SHL03Z 0SHL08Z 0SHL33Z 0SHL38Z 0SHL43Z 0SHL48Z 0SHM03Z 0SHM08Z 0SHM33Z 0SHM38Z 0SHM43Z 0SHM48Z 0SHN03Z 0SHN08Z 0SHN33Z 0SHN38Z 0SHN43Z 0SHN48Z 0SHP03Z 0SHP08Z 0SHP33Z 0SHP38Z 0SHP43Z 0SHP48Z 0SHQ03Z 0SHQ08Z 0SHQ33Z 0SHQ38Z 0SHQ43Z 0SHQ48Z

LC Limited Coverage NC Noncovered HAC HAC Associated Procedure CC Combination Cluster - See Appendix G for code lists
DRG Non-OR-Affecting MS-DRG Assignment ⃠ Non-OR-Not Affecting MS-DRG Assignment New/Revised Text in **Orange** ♂ Male ♀ Female

0 Medical and Surgical
S Lower Joints
J Inspection: Visually and/or manually exploring a body part

Body Part Character 4	Approach Character 5	Device Character 6	Qualifier Character 7
0 Lumbar Vertebral Joint ⦸	**0** Open	**Z** No Device	**Z** No Qualifier
2 Lumbar Vertebral Disc ⦸	**3** Percutaneous		
3 Lumbosacral Joint ⦸	**4** Percutaneous Endoscopic		
4 Lumbosacral Disc ⦸	**X** External		
5 Sacrococcygeal Joint ⦸			
6 Coccygeal Joint ⦸			
7 Sacroiliac Joint, Right ⦸			
8 Sacroiliac Joint, Left ⦸			
9 Hip Joint, Right ⦸			
B Hip Joint, Left ⦸			
C Knee Joint, Right ⦸			
D Knee Joint, Left ⦸			
F Ankle Joint, Right ⦸			
G Ankle Joint, Left ⦸			
H Tarsal Joint, Right ⦸			
J Tarsal Joint, Left ⦸			
K Metatarsal-Tarsal Joint, Right ⦸			
L Metatarsal-Tarsal Joint, Left ⦸			
M Metatarsal-Phalangeal Joint, Right ⦸			
N Metatarsal-Phalangeal Joint, Left ⦸			
P Toe Phalangeal Joint, Right ⦸			
Q Toe Phalangeal Joint, Left ⦸			

⦸ 0SJ03ZZ 0SJ0XZZ 0SJ23ZZ 0SJ2XZZ 0SJ33ZZ 0SJ3XZZ 0SJ43ZZ 0SJ4XZZ 0SJ53ZZ 0SJ5XZZ 0SJ63ZZ 0SJ6XZZ 0SJ73ZZ
0SJ7XZZ 0SJ83ZZ 0SJ8XZZ 0SJ93ZZ 0SJ9XZZ 0SJB3ZZ 0SJBXZZ 0SJC3ZZ 0SJCXZZ 0SJD3ZZ 0SJDXZZ 0SJF3ZZ 0SJFXZZ
0SJG3ZZ 0SJGXZZ 0SJH3ZZ 0SJHXZZ 0SJJ3ZZ 0SJJXZZ 0SJK3ZZ 0SJKXZZ 0SJL3ZZ 0SJLXZZ 0SJM3ZZ 0SJMXZZ 0SJN3ZZ
0SJNXZZ 0SJP3ZZ 0SJPXZZ 0SJQ3ZZ 0SJQXZZ

0 Medical and Surgical
S Lower Joints
N Release: Freeing a body part from an abnormal physical constraint by cutting or by the use of force

Body Part Character 4	Approach Character 5	Device Character 6	Qualifier Character 7
0 Lumbar Vertebral Joint ⦸	**0** Open	**Z** No Device	**Z** No Qualifier
2 Lumbar Vertebral Disc ⦸	**3** Percutaneous		
3 Lumbosacral Joint ⦸	**4** Percutaneous Endoscopic		
4 Lumbosacral Disc ⦸	**X** External		
5 Sacrococcygeal Joint ⦸			
6 Coccygeal Joint ⦸			
7 Sacroiliac Joint, Right ⦸			
8 Sacroiliac Joint, Left ⦸			
9 Hip Joint, Right ⦸			
B Hip Joint, Left ⦸			
C Knee Joint, Right ⦸			
D Knee Joint, Left ⦸			
F Ankle Joint, Right ⦸			
G Ankle Joint, Left ⦸			
H Tarsal Joint, Right ⦸			
J Tarsal Joint, Left ⦸			
K Metatarsal-Tarsal Joint, Right ⦸			
L Metatarsal-Tarsal Joint, Left ⦸			
M Metatarsal-Phalangeal Joint, Right ⦸			
N Metatarsal-Phalangeal Joint, Left ⦸			
P Toe Phalangeal Joint, Right ⦸			
Q Toe Phalangeal Joint, Left ⦸			

⦸ 0SN0XZZ 0SN2XZZ 0SN3XZZ 0SN4XZZ 0SN5XZZ 0SN6XZZ 0SN7XZZ 0SN8XZZ 0SN9XZZ 0SNBXZZ 0SNCXZZ 0SNDXZZ 0SNFXZZ
0SNGXZZ 0SNHXZZ 0SNJXZZ 0SNKXZZ 0SNLXZZ 0SNMXZZ 0SNNXZZ 0SNPXZZ 0SNQXZZ

LC Limited Coverage NC Noncovered HAC HAC Associated Procedure CC Combination Cluster - See Appendix G for code lists
DRG Non-OR-Affecting MS-DRG Assignment ⦸ Non-OR-Not Affecting MS-DRG Assignment New/Revised Text in **Orange** ♂ Male ♀ Female

0 Medical and Surgical
S Lower Joints
P Removal: Taking out or off a device from a body part

Body Part Character 4	Approach Character 5	Device Character 6	Qualifier Character 7
0 Lumbar Vertebral Joint ⊘ **3** Lumbosacral Joint ⊘	**0** Open **3** Percutaneous **4** Percutaneous Endoscopic	**0** Drainage Device **3** Infusion Device **4** Internal Fixation Device **7** Autologous Tissue Substitute **8** Spacer **A** Interbody Fusion Device **J** Synthetic Substitute **K** Nonautologous Tissue Substitute	**Z** No Qualifier
0 Lumbar Vertebral Joint ⊘ **3** Lumbosacral Joint ⊘	**X** External	**0** Drainage Device **3** Infusion Device **4** Internal Fixation Device	**Z** No Qualifier
2 Lumbar Vertebral Disc ⊘ **4** Lumbosacral Disc ⊘	**0** Open **3** Percutaneous **4** Percutaneous Endoscopic	**0** Drainage Device **3** Infusion Device **7** Autologous Tissue Substitute **J** Synthetic Substitute **K** Nonautologous Tissue Substitute	**Z** No Qualifier
2 Lumbar Vertebral Disc ⊘ **4** Lumbosacral Disc ⊘	**X** External	**0** Drainage Device **3** Infusion Device	**Z** No Qualifier
5 Sacrococcygeal Joint ⊘ **6** Coccygeal Joint ⊘ **7** Sacroiliac Joint, Right ⊘ **8** Sacroiliac Joint, Left ⊘	**0** Open **3** Percutaneous **4** Percutaneous Endoscopic	**0** Drainage Device **3** Infusion Device **4** Internal Fixation Device **7** Autologous Tissue Substitute **8** Spacer **J** Synthetic Substitute **K** Nonautologous Tissue Substitute	**Z** No Qualifier
5 Sacrococcygeal Joint ⊘ **6** Coccygeal Joint ⊘ **7** Sacroiliac Joint, Right ⊘ **8** Sacroiliac Joint, Left ⊘	**X** External	**0** Drainage Device **3** Infusion Device **4** Internal Fixation Device	**Z** No Qualifier
9 Hip Joint, Right CC DRG **B** Hip Joint, Left CC DRG	**0** Open	**0** Drainage Device **3** Infusion Device **4** Internal Fixation Device **5** External Fixation Device **7** Autologous Tissue Substitute **8** Spacer **9** Liner **B** Resurfacing Device **J** Synthetic Substitute **K** Nonautologous Tissue Substitute	**Z** No Qualifier
9 Hip Joint, Right ⊘ CC DRG **B** Hip Joint, Left ⊘ CC DRG	**3** Percutaneous **4** Percutaneous Endoscopic	**0** Drainage Device **3** Infusion Device **4** Internal Fixation Device **5** External Fixation Device **7** Autologous Tissue Substitute **8** Spacer **J** Synthetic Substitute **K** Nonautologous Tissue Substitute	**Z** No Qualifier
9 Hip Joint, Right ⊘ **B** Hip Joint, Left ⊘	**X** External	**0** Drainage Device **3** Infusion Device **4** Internal Fixation Device **5** External Fixation Device	**Z** No Qualifier

0SP continued on next page

0 Medical and Surgical
S Lower Joints
P Removal: Taking out or off a device from a body part

0SP continued from previous page

Body Part Character 4	Approach Character 5	Device Character 6	Qualifier Character 7
A Hip Joint, Acetabular Surface, Right ⦸ E Hip Joint, Acetabular Surface, Left ⦸ R Hip Joint, Femoral Surface, Right ⦸ S Hip Joint, Femoral Surface, Left ⦸ T Knee Joint, Femoral Surface, Right ⦸ U Knee Joint, Femoral Surface, Left ⦸ V Knee Joint, Tibial Surface, Right ⦸ W Knee Joint, Tibial Surface, Left ⦸	0 Open 3 Percutaneous 4 Percutaneous Endoscopic	J Synthetic Substitute	Z No Qualifier
C Knee Joint, Right CC ⦸ **D** Knee Joint, Left CC ⦸	**0** Open	**0** Drainage Device **3** Infusion Device **4** Internal Fixation Device **5** External Fixation Device **7** Autologous Tissue Substitute **8** Spacer **9** Liner **K** Nonautologous Tissue Substitute	**Z** No Qualifier
C Knee Joint, Right CC ⦸ D Knee Joint, Left CC ⦸	0 Open	J Synthetic Substitute	C Patellar Surface Z No Qualifier
C Knee Joint, Right CC ⦸ **D** Knee Joint, Left CC ⦸	**3** Percutaneous **4** Percutaneous Endoscopic	**0** Drainage Device **3** Infusion Device **4** Internal Fixation Device **5** External Fixation Device **7** Autologous Tissue Substitute **8** Spacer **K** Nonautologous Tissue Substitute	**Z** No Qualifier
C Knee Joint, Right CC ⦸ D Knee Joint, Left CC ⦸	3 Percutaneous 4 Percutaneous Endoscopic	J Synthetic Substitute	C Patellar Surface Z No Qualifier
C Knee Joint, Right ⦸ **D** Knee Joint, Left ⦸	**X** External	**0** Drainage Device **3** Infusion Device **4** Internal Fixation Device **5** External Fixation Device	**Z** No Qualifier
F Ankle Joint, Right ⦸ **G** Ankle Joint, Left ⦸ **H** Tarsal Joint, Right ⦸ **J** Tarsal Joint, Left ⦸ **K** Metatarsal-Tarsal Joint, Right ⦸ **L** Metatarsal-Tarsal Joint, Left ⦸ **M** Metatarsal-Phalangeal Joint, Right ⦸ **N** Metatarsal-Phalangeal Joint, Left ⦸ **P** Toe Phalangeal Joint, Right ⦸ **Q** Toe Phalangeal Joint, Left ⦸	**0** Open **3** Percutaneous **4** Percutaneous Endoscopic	**0** Drainage Device **3** Infusion Device **4** Internal Fixation Device **5** External Fixation Device **7** Autologous Tissue Substitute **8** Spacer **J** Synthetic Substitute **K** Nonautologous Tissue Substitute	**Z** No Qualifier

0SP continued on next page

0 Medical and Surgical
S Lower Joints
P Removal: Taking out or off a device from a body part

0SP continued from previous page

Body Part Character 4	Approach Character 5	Device Character 6	Qualifier Character 7
F Ankle Joint, Right ⊘ **G** Ankle Joint, Left ⊘ **H** Tarsal Joint, Right ⊘ **J** Tarsal Joint, Left ⊘ **K** Metatarsal-Tarsal Joint, Right ⊘ **L** Metatarsal-Tarsal Joint, Left ⊘ **M** Metatarsal-Phalangeal Joint, Right ⊘ **N** Metatarsal-Phalangeal Joint, Left ⊘ **P** Toe Phalangeal Joint, Right ⊘ **Q** Toe Phalangeal Joint, Left ⊘	**X** External	**0** Drainage Device **3** Infusion Device **4** Internal Fixation Device **5** External Fixation Device	**Z** No Qualifier

⊘ 0SP008Z 0SP030Z 0SP033Z 0SP038Z 0SP048Z 0SP0X0Z 0SP0X3Z 0SP0X4Z 0SP230Z 0SP233Z 0SP2X0Z 0SP2X3Z 0SP308Z 0SP330Z 0SP333Z 0SP338Z 0SP348Z 0SP3X0Z 0SP3X3Z 0SP3X4Z 0SP430Z 0SP433Z 0SP4X0Z 0SP4X3Z 0SP508Z 0SP530Z 0SP533Z 0SP538Z 0SP548Z 0SP5X0Z 0SP5X3Z 0SP5X4Z 0SP608Z 0SP630Z 0SP633Z 0SP638Z 0SP648Z 0SP6X0Z 0SP6X3Z 0SP6X4Z 0SP708Z 0SP730Z 0SP733Z 0SP738Z 0SP748Z 0SP7X0Z 0SP7X3Z 0SP7X4Z 0SP808Z 0SP830Z 0SP833Z 0SP838Z 0SP848Z 0SP8X0Z 0SP8X3Z 0SP8X4Z 0SP930Z 0SP933Z 0SP938Z 0SP9X0Z 0SP9X3Z 0SP9X4Z 0SP9X5Z 0SPA0JZ 0SPA3JZ 0SPA4JZ 0SPB30Z 0SPB33Z 0SPB38Z 0SPBX0Z 0SPBX3Z 0SPBX4Z 0SPBX5Z 0SPC08Z 0SPC0JC 0SPC30Z 0SPC33Z 0SPC38Z 0SPC3JC 0SPC48Z 0SPC4JC 0SPCX0Z 0SPCX3Z 0SPCX4Z 0SPCX5Z 0SPD08Z 0SPD0JC 0SPD30Z 0SPD33Z 0SPD38Z 0SPD3JC 0SPD48Z 0SPD4JC 0SPDX0Z 0SPDX3Z 0SPDX4Z 0SPDX5Z 0SPE0JZ 0SPE3JZ 0SPE4JZ 0SPF08Z 0SPF30Z 0SPF33Z 0SPF38Z 0SPF48Z 0SPFX0Z 0SPFX3Z 0SPFX4Z 0SPFX5Z 0SPG08Z 0SPG30Z 0SPG33Z 0SPG38Z 0SPG48Z 0SPGX0Z 0SPGX3Z 0SPGX4Z 0SPGX5Z 0SPH08Z 0SPH30Z 0SPH33Z 0SPH38Z 0SPH48Z 0SPHX0Z 0SPHX3Z 0SPHX4Z 0SPHX5Z 0SPJ08Z 0SPJ30Z 0SPJ33Z 0SPJ38Z 0SPJ48Z 0SPJX0Z 0SPJX3Z 0SPJX4Z 0SPJX5Z 0SPK08Z 0SPK30Z 0SPK33Z 0SPK38Z 0SPK48Z 0SPKX0Z 0SPKX3Z 0SPKX4Z 0SPKX5Z 0SPL08Z 0SPL30Z 0SPL33Z 0SPL38Z 0SPL48Z 0SPLX0Z 0SPLX3Z 0SPLX4Z 0SPLX5Z 0SPM08Z 0SPM30Z 0SPM33Z 0SPM38Z 0SPM48Z 0SPMX0Z 0SPMX3Z 0SPMX4Z 0SPMX5Z 0SPN08Z 0SPN30Z 0SPN33Z 0SPN38Z 0SPN48Z 0SPNX0Z 0SPNX3Z 0SPNX4Z 0SPNX5Z 0SPP08Z 0SPP30Z 0SPP33Z 0SPP38Z 0SPP48Z 0SPPX0Z 0SPPX3Z 0SPPX4Z 0SPPX5Z 0SPQ08Z 0SPQ30Z 0SPQ33Z 0SPQ38Z 0SPQ48Z 0SPQX0Z 0SPQX3Z 0SPQX4Z 0SPQX5Z 0SPR0JZ 0SPR3JZ 0SPR4JZ 0SPS0JZ 0SPS3JZ 0SPS4JZ 0SPT0JZ 0SPT3JZ 0SPT4JZ 0SPU0JZ 0SPU3JZ 0SPU4JZ 0SPV0JZ 0SPV3JZ 0SPV4JZ 0SPW0JZ 0SPW3JZ 0SPW4JZ

CC 0SP908Z 0SP909Z 0SP90BZ 0SP90JZ 0SP948Z 0SP94JZ 0SPB08Z 0SPB09Z 0SPB0BZ 0SPB0JZ 0SPB48Z 0SPB4JZ 0SPC08Z 0SPC09Z 0SPC0JZ 0SPC38Z 0SPC48Z 0SPC4JZ 0SPD08Z 0SPD09Z 0SPD0JZ 0SPD38Z 0SPD48Z 0SPD4JZ

DRG 0SP908Z 0SP948Z 0SPB08Z 0SPB48Z

0 Medical and Surgical
S Lower Joints
Q Repair: Restoring, to the extent possible, a body part to its normal anatomic structure and function

Body Part Character 4	Approach Character 5	Device Character 6	Qualifier Character 7
0 Lumbar Vertebral Joint **2** Lumbar Vertebral Disc **3** Lumbosacral Joint **4** Lumbosacral Disc **5** Sacrococcygeal Joint **6** Coccygeal Joint **7** Sacroiliac Joint, Right **8** Sacroiliac Joint, Left **9** Hip Joint, Right **B** Hip Joint, Left **C** Knee Joint, Right **D** Knee Joint, Left **F** Ankle Joint, Right **G** Ankle Joint, Left **H** Tarsal Joint, Right **J** Tarsal Joint, Left **K** Metatarsal-Tarsal Joint, Right **L** Metatarsal-Tarsal Joint, Left **M** Metatarsal-Phalangeal Joint, Right **N** Metatarsal-Phalangeal Joint, Left **P** Toe Phalangeal Joint, Right **Q** Toe Phalangeal Joint, Left	**0** Open **3** Percutaneous **4** Percutaneous Endoscopic **X** External	**Z** No Device	**Z** No Qualifier

0 Medical and Surgical
S Lower Joints
R Replacement: Putting in or on biological or synthetic material that physically takes the place and/or function of all or a portion of a body part

Body Part Character 4	Approach Character 5	Device Character 6	Qualifier Character 7
0 Lumbar Vertebral Joint **2** Lumbar Vertebral Disc NC **3** Lumbosacral Joint **4** Lumbosacral Disc NC **5** Sacrococcygeal Joint **6** Coccygeal Joint **7** Sacroiliac Joint, Right **8** Sacroiliac Joint, Left **H** Tarsal Joint, Right **J** Tarsal Joint, Left **K** Metatarsal-Tarsal Joint, Right **L** Metatarsal-Tarsal Joint, Left **M** Metatarsal-Phalangeal Joint, Right **N** Metatarsal-Phalangeal Joint, Left **P** Toe Phalangeal Joint, Right **Q** Toe Phalangeal Joint, Left	**0** Open	**7** Autologous Tissue Substitute **J** Synthetic Substitute **K** Nonautologous Tissue Substitute	**Z** No Qualifier
9 Hip Joint, Right CC HAC **B** Hip Joint, Left CC HAC	**0** Open	**1** Synthetic Substitute, Metal **2** Synthetic Substitute, Metal on Polyethylene **3** Synthetic Substitute, Ceramic **4** Synthetic Substitute, Ceramic on Polyethylene **J** Synthetic Substitute	**9** Cemented **A** Uncemented **Z** No Qualifier
9 Hip Joint, Right HAC **B** Hip Joint, Left HAC	**0** Open	**7** Autologous Tissue Substitute **K** Nonautologous Tissue Substitute	**Z** No Qualifier
A Hip Joint, Acetabular Surface, Right CC HAC **E** Hip Joint, Acetabular Surface, Left CC HAC	**0** Open	**0** Synthetic Substitute, Polyethylene **1** Synthetic Substitute, Metal **3** Synthetic Substitute, Ceramic **J** Synthetic Substitute	**9** Cemented **A** Uncemented **Z** No Qualifier
A Hip Joint, Acetabular Surface, Right HAC **E** Hip Joint, Acetabular Surface, Left HAC	**0** Open	**7** Autologous Tissue Substitute **K** Nonautologous Tissue Substitute	**Z** No Qualifier
C Knee Joint, Right HAC **D** Knee Joint, Left HAC	**0** Open	**7** Autologous Tissue Substitute **K** Nonautologous Tissue Substitute	**Z** No Qualifier
C Knee Joint, Right CC HAC ⃠ **D** Knee Joint, Left CC HAC ⃠	**0** Open	**J** Synthetic Substitute **L** Synthetic Substitute, Unicondylar	**9** Cemented **A** Uncemented **Z** No Qualifier
F Ankle Joint, Right **G** Ankle Joint, Left **T** Knee Joint, Femoral Surface, Right HAC **U** Knee Joint, Femoral Surface, Left HAC **V** Knee Joint, Tibial Surface, Right HAC **W** Knee Joint, Tibial Surface, Left HAC	**0** Open	**7** Autologous Tissue Substitute **K** Nonautologous Tissue Substitute	**Z** No Qualifier

0SR continued on next page

LC Limited Coverage NC Noncovered HAC HAC Associated Procedure CC Combination Cluster - See Appendix G for code lists
DRG Non-OR-Affecting MS-DRG Assignment ⃠ Non-OR-Not Affecting MS-DRG Assignment New/Revised Text in **Orange** ♂ Male ♀ Female

0SR continued from previous page

0 Medical and Surgical
S Lower Joints
R Replacement: Putting in or on biological or synthetic material that physically takes the place and/or function of all or a portion of a body part

Body Part Character 4	Approach Character 5	Device Character 6	Qualifier Character 7
F Ankle Joint, Right **G** Ankle Joint, Left **T** Knee Joint, Femoral Surface, Right CC HAC **U** Knee Joint, Femoral Surface, Left CC HAC **V** Knee Joint, Tibial Surface, Right CC HAC **W** Knee Joint, Tibial Surface, Left CC HAC	**0** Open	**J** Synthetic Substitute	**9** Cemented **A** Uncemented **Z** No Qualifier
R Hip Joint, Femoral Surface, Right CC HAC **S** Hip Joint, Femoral Surface, Left CC HAC	**0** Open	**1** Synthetic Substitute, Metal **3** Synthetic Substitute, Ceramic **J** Synthetic Substitute	**9** Cemented **A** Uncemented **Z** No Qualifier
R Hip Joint, Femoral Surface, Right HAC **S** Hip Joint, Femoral Surface, Left HAC	**0** Open	**7** Autologous Tissue Substitute **K** Nonautologous Tissue Substitute	**Z** No Qualifier

⦸ 0SRC0L9 0SRC0LA 0SRC0LZ 0SRD0L9 0SRD0LA 0SRD0LZ

CC 0SR9019 0SR901A 0SR901Z 0SR9029 0SR902A 0SR902Z 0SR9039 0SR903A 0SR903Z 0SR9049 0SR904A 0SR904Z 0SR90J9 0SR90JA 0SR90JZ 0SRA009 0SRA00A 0SRA00Z 0SRA019 0SRA01A 0SRA01Z 0SRA039 0SRA03A 0SRA03Z 0SRA0J9 0SRA0JA 0SRA0JZ 0SRB019 0SRB01A 0SRB01Z 0SRB029 0SRB02A 0SRB02Z 0SRB039 0SRB03A 0SRB03Z 0SRB049 0SRB04A 0SRB04Z 0SRB0J9 0SRB0JA 0SRB0JZ 0SRC0J9 0SRC0JA 0SRC0JZ 0SRD0J9 0SRD0JA 0SRD0JZ 0SRE009 0SRE00A 0SRE00Z 0SRE019 0SRE01A 0SRE01Z 0SRE039 0SRE03A 0SRE03Z 0SRE0J9 0SRE0JA 0SRE0JZ 0SRR019 0SRR01A 0SRR01Z 0SRR039 0SRR03A 0SRR03Z 0SRR0J9 0SRR0JA 0SRR0JZ 0SRS019 0SRS01A 0SRS01Z 0SRS039 0SRS03A 0SRS03Z 0SRS0J9 0SRS0JA 0SRS0JZ 0SRT0J9 0SRT0JA 0SRT0JZ 0SRU0J9 0SRU0JA 0SRU0JZ 0SRV0J9 0SRV0JA 0SRV0JZ 0SRW0J9 0SRW0JA 0SRW0JZ

NC 0SR20JZ or 0SR40JZ when the beneficiary is over age 60

HAC 0SR9019 0SR901A 0SR901Z 0SR9029 0SR902A 0SR902Z 0SR9039 0SR903A 0SR903Z 0SR9049 0SR904A 0SR904Z 0SR907Z 0SR90J9 0SR90JA 0SR90JZ 0SR90KZ 0SRA009 0SRA00A 0SRA00Z 0SRA019 0SRA01A 0SRA01Z 0SRA039 0SRA03A 0SRA03Z 0SRA07Z 0SRA0J9 0SRA0JA 0SRA0JZ 0SRA0KZ 0SRB019 0SRB01A 0SRB01Z 0SRB029 0SRB02A 0SRB02Z 0SRB039 0SRB03A 0SRB03Z 0SRB049 0SRB04A 0SRB04Z 0SRB07Z 0SRB0J9 0SRB0JA 0SRB0JZ 0SRB0KZ 0SRC07Z 0SRC0J9 0SRC0JA 0SRC0JZ 0SRC0KZ 0SRD07Z 0SRD0J9 0SRD0JA 0SRD0JZ 0SRD0KZ 0SRE009 0SRE00A 0SRE00Z 0SRE019 0SRE01A 0SRE01Z 0SRE039 0SRE03A 0SRE03Z 0SRE07Z 0SRE0J9 0SRE0JA 0SRE0JZ 0SRE0KZ 0SRR019 0SRR01A 0SRR01Z 0SRR039 0SRR03A 0SRR03Z 0SRR07Z 0SRR0J9 0SRR0JA 0SRR0JZ 0SRR0KZ 0SRS019 0SRS01A 0SRS01Z 0SRS039 0SRS03A 0SRS03Z 0SRS07Z 0SRS0J9 0SRS0JA 0SRS0JZ 0SRS0KZ 0SRT07Z 0SRT0J9 0SRT0JA 0SRT0JZ 0SRT0KZ 0SRU07Z 0SRU0J9 0SRU0JA 0SRU0JZ 0SRU0KZ 0SRV07Z 0SRV0J9 0SRV0JA 0SRV0JZ 0SRV0KZ 0SRW07Z 0SRW0J9 0SRW0JA 0SRW0JZ or 0SRW0KZ All preceding codes with the HAC symbol are classified as hospital-acquired conditions when reported with secondary diagnosis I26.02-I26.09, I26.92-I26.99, or I82.401-I82.4Z9.

0 Medical and Surgical
S Lower Joints
S Reposition: Moving to its normal location, or other suitable location, all or a portion of a body part

Body Part Character 4	Approach Character 5	Device Character 6	Qualifier Character 7
0 Lumbar Vertebral Joint ⦸ **3** Lumbosacral Joint ⦸ **5** Sacrococcygeal Joint ⦸ **6** Coccygeal Joint ⦸ **7** Sacroiliac Joint, Right ⦸ **8** Sacroiliac Joint, Left ⦸	**0** Open **3** Percutaneous **4** Percutaneous Endoscopic **X** External	**4** Internal Fixation Device **Z** No Device	**Z** No Qualifier
9 Hip Joint, Right ⦸ **B** Hip Joint, Left ⦸ **C** Knee Joint, Right ⦸ **D** Knee Joint, Left ⦸ **F** Ankle Joint, Right ⦸ **G** Ankle Joint, Left ⦸ **H** Tarsal Joint, Right ⦸ **J** Tarsal Joint, Left ⦸ **K** Metatarsal-Tarsal Joint, Right ⦸ **L** Metatarsal-Tarsal Joint, Left ⦸ **M** Metatarsal-Phalangeal Joint, Right ⦸ **N** Metatarsal-Phalangeal Joint, Left ⦸ **P** Toe Phalangeal Joint, Right ⦸ **Q** Toe Phalangeal Joint, Left ⦸	**0** Open **3** Percutaneous **4** Percutaneous Endoscopic **X** External	**4** Internal Fixation Device **5** External Fixation Device **Z** No Device	**Z** No Qualifier

⦸ 0SS034Z 0SS03ZZ 0SS044Z 0SS04ZZ 0SS0X4Z 0SS0XZZ 0SS334Z 0SS33ZZ 0SS344Z 0SS34ZZ 0SS3X4Z 0SS3XZZ 0SS534Z 0SS53ZZ 0SS544Z 0SS54ZZ 0SS5X4Z 0SS5XZZ 0SS634Z 0SS63ZZ 0SS644Z 0SS64ZZ 0SS6X4Z 0SS6XZZ 0SS734Z 0SS73ZZ 0SS744Z 0SS74ZZ 0SS7X4Z 0SS7XZZ 0SS834Z 0SS83ZZ 0SS844Z 0SS84ZZ 0SS8X4Z 0SS8XZZ 0SS934Z 0SS935Z 0SS93ZZ 0SS944Z 0SS945Z 0SS94ZZ 0SS9X4Z 0SS9X5Z 0SS9XZZ 0SSB34Z 0SSB35Z 0SSB3ZZ 0SSB44Z 0SSB45Z 0SSB4ZZ 0SSBX4Z 0SSBX5Z 0SSBXZZ 0SSC34Z 0SSC35Z 0SSC3ZZ 0SSC44Z 0SSC45Z 0SSC4ZZ 0SSCX4Z 0SSCX5Z 0SSCXZZ 0SSD34Z 0SSD35Z 0SSD3ZZ 0SSD44Z 0SSD45Z 0SSD4ZZ 0SSDX4Z 0SSDX5Z 0SSDXZZ 0SSF34Z 0SSF35Z 0SSF3ZZ 0SSF44Z 0SSF45Z 0SSF4ZZ 0SSFX4Z 0SSFX5Z 0SSFXZZ 0SSG34Z 0SSG35Z 0SSG3ZZ 0SSG44Z 0SSG45Z 0SSG4ZZ 0SSGX4Z 0SSGX5Z 0SSGXZZ 0SSH34Z 0SSH35Z 0SSH3ZZ 0SSH44Z 0SSH45Z 0SSH4ZZ 0SSHX4Z 0SSHX5Z 0SSHXZZ 0SSJ34Z 0SSJ35Z 0SSJ3ZZ 0SSJ44Z 0SSJ45Z 0SSJ4ZZ 0SSJX4Z 0SSJX5Z 0SSJXZZ 0SSK34Z 0SSK35Z 0SSK3ZZ 0SSK44Z 0SSK45Z 0SSK4ZZ 0SSKX4Z 0SSKX5Z 0SSKXZZ 0SSL34Z 0SSL35Z 0SSL3ZZ 0SSL44Z 0SSL45Z 0SSL4ZZ 0SSLX4Z 0SSLX5Z 0SSLXZZ 0SSM34Z 0SSM35Z 0SSM3ZZ 0SSM44Z 0SSM45Z 0SSM4ZZ 0SSMX4Z 0SSMX5Z 0SSMXZZ 0SSN34Z 0SSN35Z 0SSN3ZZ 0SSN44Z 0SSN45Z 0SSN4ZZ 0SSNX4Z 0SSNX5Z 0SSNXZZ 0SSP34Z 0SSP35Z 0SSP3ZZ 0SSP44Z 0SSP45Z 0SSP4ZZ 0SSPX4Z 0SSPX5Z 0SSPXZZ 0SSQ34Z 0SSQ35Z 0SSQ3ZZ 0SSQ44Z 0SSQ45Z 0SSQ4ZZ 0SSQX4Z 0SSQX5Z 0SSQXZZ

0 Medical and Surgical
S Lower Joints
T Resection: Cutting out or off, without replacement, all of a body part

Body Part Character 4	Approach Character 5	Device Character 6	Qualifier Character 7
2 Lumbar Vertebral Disc **4** Lumbosacral Disc **5** Sacrococcygeal Joint **6** Coccygeal Joint **7** Sacroiliac Joint, Right **8** Sacroiliac Joint, Left **9** Hip Joint, Right **B** Hip Joint, Left **C** Knee Joint, Right **D** Knee Joint, Left **F** Ankle Joint, Right **G** Ankle Joint, Left **H** Tarsal Joint, Right **J** Tarsal Joint, Left **K** Metatarsal-Tarsal Joint, Right **L** Metatarsal-Tarsal Joint, Left **M** Metatarsal-Phalangeal Joint, Right **N** Metatarsal-Phalangeal Joint, Left **P** Toe Phalangeal Joint, Right **Q** Toe Phalangeal Joint, Left	**0** Open	**Z** No Device	**Z** No Qualifier

LC Limited Coverage NC Noncovered HAC HAC Associated Procedure CC Combination Cluster - See Appendix G for code lists
DRG Non-OR-Affecting MS-DRG Assignment ⦸ Non-OR-Not Affecting MS-DRG Assignment New/Revised Text in **Orange** ♂ Male ♀ Female

0 Medical and Surgical
S Lower Joints
U Supplement: Putting in or on biological or synthetic material that physically reinforces and/or augments the function of a portion of a body part

Body Part Character 4	Approach Character 5	Device Character 6	Qualifier Character 7
0 Lumbar Vertebral Joint **2** Lumbar Vertebral Disc **3** Lumbosacral Joint **4** Lumbosacral Disc **5** Sacrococcygeal Joint **6** Coccygeal Joint **7** Sacroiliac Joint, Right **8** Sacroiliac Joint, Left **F** Ankle Joint, Right **G** Ankle Joint, Left **H** Tarsal Joint, Right **J** Tarsal Joint, Left **K** Metatarsal-Tarsal Joint, Right **L** Metatarsal-Tarsal Joint, Left **M** Metatarsal-Phalangeal Joint, Right **N** Metatarsal-Phalangeal Joint, Left **P** Toe Phalangeal Joint, Right **Q** Toe Phalangeal Joint, Left	**0** Open **3** Percutaneous **4** Percutaneous Endoscopic	**7** Autologous Tissue Substitute **J** Synthetic Substitute **K** Nonautologous Tissue Substitute	**Z** No Qualifier
9 Hip Joint, Right CC HAC **B** Hip Joint, Left CC HAC	**0** Open	**7** Autologous Tissue Substitute **9** Liner **B** Resurfacing Device **J** Synthetic Substitute **K** Nonautologous Tissue Substitute	**Z** No Qualifier
9 Hip Joint, Right **B** Hip Joint, Left	**3** Percutaneous **4** Percutaneous Endoscopic	**7** Autologous Tissue Substitute **J** Synthetic Substitute **K** Nonautologous Tissue Substitute	**Z** No Qualifier
A Hip Joint, Acetabular Surface, Right CC HAC **E** Hip Joint, Acetabular Surface, Left CC HAC **R** Hip Joint, Femoral Surface, Right CC HAC **S** Hip Joint, Femoral Surface, Left CC HAC	**0** Open	**9** Liner **B** Resurfacing Device	**Z** No Qualifier
C Knee Joint, Right CC **D** Knee Joint, Left CC	**0** Open	**7** Autologous Tissue Substitute **J** Synthetic Substitute **K** Nonautologous Tissue Substitute	**Z** No Qualifier
C Knee Joint, Right CC **D** Knee Joint, Left CC	**0** Open	**9** Liner	**C** Patellar Surface **Z** No Qualifier
C Knee Joint, Right CC **D** Knee Joint, Left CC	**3** Percutaneous **4** Percutaneous Endoscopic	**7** Autologous Tissue Substitute **J** Synthetic Substitute **K** Nonautologous Tissue Substitute	**Z** No Qualifier
T Knee Joint, Femoral Surface, Right CC **U** Knee Joint, Femoral Surface, Left CC **V** Knee Joint, Tibial Surface, Right CC **W** Knee Joint, Tibial Surface, Left CC	**0** Open	**9** Liner	**Z** No Qualifier

CC 0SU909Z 0SUA09Z 0SUB09Z 0SUC09C 0SUC0JZ 0SUC4JZ 0SUD09C 0SUD0JZ 0SUD4JZ 0SUE09Z 0SUR09Z 0SUS09Z 0SUT09Z 0SUU09Z 0SUV09Z 0SUW09Z

HAC 0SU90BZ 0SUA0BZ 0SUB0BZ 0SUE0BZ 0SUR0BZ or 0SUS0BZ when reported with secondary diagnosis I26.02-I26.09, I26.92-I26.99, or I82.401-I82.4Z9

LC Limited Coverage NC Noncovered HAC HAC Associated Procedure CC Combination Cluster - See Appendix G for code lists
DRG Non-OR-Affecting MS-DRG Assignment ⊘ Non-OR-Not Affecting MS-DRG Assignment New/Revised Text in **Orange** ♂ Male ♀ Female

0 Medical and Surgical
S Lower Joints
W Revision: Correcting, to the extent possible, a portion of a malfunctioning device or the position of a displaced device

Body Part Character 4	Approach Character 5	Device Character 6	Qualifier Character 7
0 Lumbar Vertebral Joint ⦸ **3** Lumbosacral Joint ⦸	**0** Open **3** Percutaneous **4** Percutaneous Endoscopic **X** External	**0** Drainage Device **3** Infusion Device **4** Internal Fixation Device **7** Autologous Tissue Substitute **8** Spacer **A** Interbody Fusion Device **J** Synthetic Substitute **K** Nonautologous Tissue Substitute	**Z** No Qualifier
2 Lumbar Vertebral Disc ⦸ **4** Lumbosacral Disc ⦸	**0** Open **3** Percutaneous **4** Percutaneous Endoscopic **X** External	**0** Drainage Device **3** Infusion Device **7** Autologous Tissue Substitute **J** Synthetic Substitute **K** Nonautologous Tissue Substitute	**Z** No Qualifier
5 Sacrococcygeal Joint ⦸ **6** Coccygeal Joint ⦸ **7** Sacroiliac Joint, Right ⦸ **8** Sacroiliac Joint, Left ⦸	**0** Open **3** Percutaneous **4** Percutaneous Endoscopic **X** External	**0** Drainage Device **3** Infusion Device **4** Internal Fixation Device **7** Autologous Tissue Substitute **8** Spacer **J** Synthetic Substitute **K** Nonautologous Tissue Substitute	**Z** No Qualifier
9 Hip Joint, Right ⦸ **B** Hip Joint, Left ⦸	**0** Open	**0** Drainage Device **3** Infusion Device **4** Internal Fixation Device **5** External Fixation Device **7** Autologous Tissue Substitute **8** Spacer **9** Liner **B** Resurfacing Device **J** Synthetic Substitute **K** Nonautologous Tissue Substitute	**Z** No Qualifier
9 Hip Joint, Right ⦸ **B** Hip Joint, Left ⦸	**3** Percutaneous **4** Percutaneous Endoscopic **X** External	**0** Drainage Device **3** Infusion Device **4** Internal Fixation Device **5** External Fixation Device **7** Autologous Tissue Substitute **8** Spacer **J** Synthetic Substitute **K** Nonautologous Tissue Substitute	**Z** No Qualifier
A Hip Joint, Acetabular Surface, Right ⦸ **E** Hip Joint, Acetabular Surface, Left ⦸ **R** Hip Joint, Femoral Surface, Right ⦸ **S** Hip Joint, Femoral Surface, Left ⦸ **T** Knee Joint, Femoral Surface, Right ⦸ **U** Knee Joint, Femoral Surface, Left ⦸ **V** Knee Joint, Tibial Surface, Right ⦸ **W** Knee Joint, Tibial Surface, Left ⦸	**0** Open **3** Percutaneous **4** Percutaneous Endoscopic **X** External	**J** Synthetic Substitute	**Z** No Qualifier

0SW continued on next page

0SW continued from previous page

0 Medical and Surgical
S Lower Joints
W Revision: Correcting, to the extent possible, a portion of a malfunctioning device or the position of a displaced device

Body Part Character 4	Approach Character 5	Device Character 6	Qualifier Character 7
C Knee Joint, Right ⊘ **D** Knee Joint, Left ⊘	**0** Open	**0** Drainage Device **3** Infusion Device **4** Internal Fixation Device **5** External Fixation Device **7** Autologous Tissue Substitute **8** Spacer **9** Liner **K** Nonautologous Tissue Substitute	**Z** No Qualifier
C Knee Joint, Right ⊘ D Knee Joint, Left ⊘	0 Open	J Synthetic Substitute	C Patellar Surface Z No Qualifier
C Knee Joint, Right ⊘ **D** Knee Joint, Left ⊘	**3** Percutaneous **4** Percutaneous Endoscopic **X** External	**0** Drainage Device **3** Infusion Device **4** Internal Fixation Device **5** External Fixation Device **7** Autologous Tissue Substitute **8** Spacer **K** Nonautologous Tissue Substitute	**Z** No Qualifier
C Knee Joint, Right ⊘ D Knee Joint, Left ⊘	3 Percutaneous 4 Percutaneous Endoscopic X External	J Synthetic Substitute	C Patellar Surface Z No Qualifier
F Ankle Joint, Right ⊘ **G** Ankle Joint, Left ⊘ **H** Tarsal Joint, Right ⊘ **J** Tarsal Joint, Left ⊘ **K** Metatarsal-Tarsal Joint, Right ⊘ **L** Metatarsal-Tarsal Joint, Left ⊘ **M** Metatarsal-Phalangeal Joint, Right ⊘ **N** Metatarsal-Phalangeal Joint, Left ⊘ **P** Toe Phalangeal Joint, Right ⊘ **Q** Toe Phalangeal Joint, Left ⊘	**0** Open **3** Percutaneous **4** Percutaneous Endoscopic **X** External	**0** Drainage Device **3** Infusion Device **4** Internal Fixation Device **5** External Fixation Device **7** Autologous Tissue Substitute **8** Spacer **J** Synthetic Substitute **K** Nonautologous Tissue Substitute	**Z** No Qualifier

⊘ 0SW0X0Z 0SW0X3Z 0SW0X4Z 0SW0X7Z 0SW0X8Z 0SW0XAZ 0SW0XJZ 0SW0XKZ 0SW2X0Z 0SW2X3Z 0SW2X7Z 0SW2XJZ 0SW2XKZ
0SW3X0Z 0SW3X3Z 0SW3X4Z 0SW3X7Z 0SW3X8Z 0SW3XAZ 0SW3XJZ 0SW3XKZ 0SW4X0Z 0SW4X3Z 0SW4X7Z 0SW4XJZ 0SW4XKZ
0SW5X0Z 0SW5X3Z 0SW5X4Z 0SW5X7Z 0SW5X8Z 0SW5XJZ 0SW5XKZ 0SW6X0Z 0SW6X3Z 0SW6X4Z 0SW6X7Z 0SW6X8Z 0SW6XJZ
0SW6XKZ 0SW7X0Z 0SW7X3Z 0SW7X4Z 0SW7X7Z 0SW7X8Z 0SW7XJZ 0SW7XKZ 0SW8X0Z 0SW8X3Z 0SW8X4Z 0SW8X7Z 0SW8X8Z
0SW8XJZ 0SW8XKZ 0SW9X0Z 0SW9X3Z 0SW9X4Z 0SW9X5Z 0SW9X7Z 0SW9X8Z 0SW9XJZ 0SW9XKZ 0SWA0JZ 0SWA3JZ 0SWA4JZ
0SWAXJZ 0SWBX0Z 0SWBX3Z 0SWBX4Z 0SWBX5Z 0SWBX7Z 0SWBX8Z 0SWBXJZ 0SWBXKZ 0SWC0JC 0SWC3JC 0SWC4JC 0SWCX0Z
0SWCX3Z 0SWCX4Z 0SWCX5Z 0SWCX7Z 0SWCX8Z 0SWCXJC 0SWCXJZ 0SWCXKZ 0SWD0JC 0SWD3JC 0SWD4JC 0SWDX0Z 0SWDX3Z
0SWDX4Z 0SWDX5Z 0SWDX7Z 0SWDX8Z 0SWDXJC 0SWDXJZ 0SWDXKZ 0SWE0JZ 0SWE3JZ 0SWE4JZ 0SWEXJZ 0SWFX0Z 0SWFX3Z
0SWFX4Z 0SWFX5Z 0SWFX7Z 0SWFX8Z 0SWFXJZ 0SWFXKZ 0SWGX0Z 0SWGX3Z 0SWGX4Z 0SWGX5Z 0SWGX7Z 0SWGX8Z 0SWGXJZ
0SWGXKZ 0SWHX0Z 0SWHX3Z 0SWHX4Z 0SWHX5Z 0SWHX7Z 0SWHX8Z 0SWHXJZ 0SWHXKZ 0SWJX0Z 0SWJX3Z 0SWJX4Z 0SWJX5Z
0SWJX7Z 0SWJX8Z 0SWJXJZ 0SWJXKZ 0SWKX0Z 0SWKX3Z 0SWKX4Z 0SWKX5Z 0SWKX7Z 0SWKX8Z 0SWKXJZ 0SWKXKZ 0SWLX0Z
0SWLX3Z 0SWLX4Z 0SWLX5Z 0SWLX7Z 0SWLX8Z 0SWLXJZ 0SWLXKZ 0SWMX0Z 0SWMX3Z 0SWMX4Z 0SWMX5Z 0SWMX7Z 0SWMX8Z
0SWMXJZ 0SWMXKZ 0SWNX0Z 0SWNX3Z 0SWNX4Z 0SWNX5Z 0SWNX7Z 0SWNX8Z 0SWNXJZ 0SWNXKZ 0SWPX0Z 0SWPX3Z 0SWPX4Z
0SWPX5Z 0SWPX7Z 0SWPX8Z 0SWPXJZ 0SWPXKZ 0SWQX0Z 0SWQX3Z 0SWQX4Z 0SWQX5Z 0SWQX7Z 0SWQX8Z 0SWQXJZ 0SWQXKZ
0SWR0JZ 0SWR3JZ 0SWR4JZ 0SWRXJZ 0SWS0JZ 0SWS3JZ 0SWS4JZ 0SWSXJZ 0SWT0JZ 0SWT3JZ 0SWT4JZ 0SWTXJZ 0SWU0JZ
0SWU3JZ 0SWU4JZ 0SWUXJZ 0SWV0JZ 0SWV3JZ 0SWV4JZ 0SWVXJZ 0SWW0JZ 0SWW3JZ 0SWW4JZ 0SWWXJZ

Urinary System 0T1-0TY

0 Medical and Surgical
T Urinary System
1 Bypass: Altering the route of passage of the contents of a tubular body part

Body Part Character 4	Approach Character 5	Device Character 6	Qualifier Character 7
3 Kidney Pelvis, Right **4** Kidney Pelvis, Left	**0** Open **4** Percutaneous Endoscopic	**7** Autologous Tissue Substitute **J** Synthetic Substitute **K** Nonautologous Tissue Substitute **Z** No Device	**3** Kidney Pelvis, Right **4** Kidney Pelvis, Left **6** Ureter, Right **7** Ureter, Left **8** Colon **9** Colocutaneous **A** Ileum **B** Bladder **C** Ileocutaneous **D** Cutaneous
3 Kidney Pelvis, Right **4** Kidney Pelvis, Left	**3** Percutaneous	**J** Synthetic Substitute	**D** Cutaneous
6 Ureter, Right **7** Ureter, Left **8** Ureters, Bilateral	**0** Open **4** Percutaneous Endoscopic	**7** Autologous Tissue Substitute **J** Synthetic Substitute **K** Nonautologous Tissue Substitute **Z** No Device	**6** Ureter, Right **7** Ureter, Left **8** Colon **9** Colocutaneous **A** Ileum **B** Bladder **C** Ileocutaneous **D** Cutaneous
6 Ureter, Right **7** Ureter, Left **8** Ureters, Bilateral	**3** Percutaneous	**J** Synthetic Substitute	**D** Cutaneous
B Bladder	**0** Open **4** Percutaneous Endoscopic	**7** Autologous Tissue Substitute **J** Synthetic Substitute **K** Nonautologous Tissue Substitute **Z** No Device	**9** Colocutaneous **C** Ileocutaneous **D** Cutaneous
B Bladder	**3** Percutaneous	**J** Synthetic Substitute	**D** Cutaneous

0 Medical and Surgical
T Urinary System
2 Change: Taking out or off a device from a body part and putting back an identical or similar device in or on the same body part without cutting or puncturing the skin or a mucous membrane

Body Part Character 4	Approach Character 5	Device Character 6	Qualifier Character 7
5 Kidney ⃠ **9** Ureter ⃠ **B** Bladder ⃠ **D** Urethra ⃠	**X** External	**0** Drainage Device **Y** Other Device	**Z** No Qualifier

⃠ 0T25X0Z 0T25XYZ 0T29X0Z 0T29XYZ 0T2BX0Z 0T2BXYZ 0T2DX0Z 0T2DXYZ

0 Medical and Surgical
T Urinary System
5 Destruction: Physical eradication of all or a portion of a body part by the direct use of energy, force, or a destructive agent

Body Part Character 4	Approach Character 5	Device Character 6	Qualifier Character 7
0 Kidney, Right 1 Kidney, Left 3 Kidney Pelvis, Right 4 Kidney Pelvis, Left 6 Ureter, Right 7 Ureter, Left B Bladder C Bladder Neck	0 Open 3 Percutaneous 4 Percutaneous Endoscopic 7 Via Natural or Artificial Opening 8 Via Natural or Artificial Opening Endoscopic	Z No Device	Z No Qualifier
D Urethra ⦸	0 Open 3 Percutaneous 4 Percutaneous Endoscopic 7 Via Natural or Artificial Opening 8 Via Natural or Artificial Opening Endoscopic X External	Z No Device	Z No Qualifier

⦸ 0T5D0ZZ 0T5D3ZZ 0T5D4ZZ 0T5D7ZZ 0T5D8ZZ 0T5DXZZ

0 Medical and Surgical
T Urinary System
7 Dilation: Expanding an orifice or the lumen of a tubular body part

Body Part Character 4	Approach Character 5	Device Character 6	Qualifier Character 7
3 Kidney Pelvis, Right 4 Kidney Pelvis, Left 6 Ureter, Right ⦸ 7 Ureter, Left ⦸ 8 Ureters, Bilateral ⦸ B Bladder C Bladder Neck ⦸ D Urethra ⦸	0 Open 3 Percutaneous 4 Percutaneous Endoscopic 7 Via Natural or Artificial Opening 8 Via Natural or Artificial Opening Endoscopic	D Intraluminal Device Z No Device	Z No Qualifier

⦸ 0T760DZ 0T763DZ 0T764DZ 0T767DZ 0T768DZ 0T770DZ 0T773DZ 0T774DZ 0T777DZ 0T778DZ 0T780DZ 0T783DZ 0T784DZ 0T787DZ 0T787ZZ 0T788DZ 0T788ZZ 0T7C0DZ 0T7C0ZZ 0T7C3DZ 0T7C3ZZ 0T7C4DZ 0T7C4ZZ 0T7C7DZ 0T7C7ZZ 0T7C8DZ 0T7C8ZZ 0T7D0DZ 0T7D3DZ 0T7D4DZ 0T7D7DZ 0T7D7ZZ 0T7D8DZ 0T7D8ZZ

0 Medical and Surgical
T Urinary System
8 Division: Cutting into a body part, without draining fluids and/or gases from the body part, in order to separate or transect a body part

Body Part Character 4	Approach Character 5	Device Character 6	Qualifier Character 7
2 Kidneys, Bilateral C Bladder Neck	0 Open 3 Percutaneous 4 Percutaneous Endoscopic	Z No Device	Z No Qualifier

0 Medical and Surgical
T Urinary System
9 Drainage: Taking or letting out fluids and/or gases from a body part

Body Part Character 4	Approach Character 5	Device Character 6	Qualifier Character 7
0 Kidney, Right ⦸ **1** Kidney, Left ⦸ **3** Kidney Pelvis, Right ⦸ **4** Kidney Pelvis, Left ⦸ **6** Ureter, Right ⦸ **7** Ureter, Left ⦸ **8** Ureters, Bilateral ⦸ **B** Bladder ⦸ **C** Bladder Neck ⦸	**0** Open **3** Percutaneous **4** Percutaneous Endoscopic **7** Via Natural or Artificial Opening **8** Via Natural or Artificial Opening Endoscopic	**0** Drainage Device	**Z** No Qualifier
0 Kidney, Right ⦸ **1** Kidney, Left ⦸ **3** Kidney Pelvis, Right ⦸ **4** Kidney Pelvis, Left ⦸ **6** Ureter, Right ⦸ **7** Ureter, Left ⦸ **8** Ureters, Bilateral ⦸ **B** Bladder ⦸ **C** Bladder Neck ⦸	**0** Open **3** Percutaneous **4** Percutaneous Endoscopic **7** Via Natural or Artificial Opening **8** Via Natural or Artificial Opening Endoscopic	**Z** No Device	**X** Diagnostic **Z** No Qualifier
D Urethra ⦸	**0** Open **3** Percutaneous **4** Percutaneous Endoscopic **7** Via Natural or Artificial Opening **8** Via Natural or Artificial Opening Endoscopic **X** External	**0** Drainage Device	**Z** No Qualifier
D Urethra ⦸	**0** Open **3** Percutaneous **4** Percutaneous Endoscopic **7** Via Natural or Artificial Opening **8** Via Natural or Artificial Opening Endoscopic **X** External	**Z** No Device	**X** Diagnostic **Z** No Qualifier

⦸ 0T9030Z 0T903ZX 0T903ZZ 0T904ZX 0T904ZZ 0T907ZX 0T908ZX 0T9130Z 0T913ZX 0T913ZZ 0T914ZX 0T914ZZ 0T917ZX 0T918ZX 0T9330Z 0T933ZX 0T933ZZ 0T934ZX 0T934ZZ 0T937ZX 0T938ZX 0T9430Z 0T943ZX 0T943ZZ 0T944ZX 0T944ZZ 0T947ZX 0T948ZX 0T9600Z 0T9630Z 0T963ZX 0T963ZZ 0T9640Z 0T964ZX 0T9670Z 0T967ZX 0T9680Z 0T968ZX 0T9700Z 0T9730Z 0T973ZX 0T973ZZ 0T9740Z 0T974ZX 0T9770Z 0T977ZX 0T9780Z 0T978ZX 0T9800Z 0T9830Z 0T983ZX 0T983ZZ 0T9840Z 0T984ZX 0T9870Z 0T987ZX 0T9880Z 0T988ZX 0T9B30Z 0T9B3ZZ 0T9B40Z 0T9B4ZZ 0T9B70Z 0T9B7ZZ 0T9B80Z 0T9B8ZZ 0T9C30Z 0T9C3ZZ 0T9C40Z 0T9C4ZZ 0T9C70Z 0T9C7ZZ 0T9C80Z 0T9C8ZZ 0T9D0ZX 0T9D30Z 0T9D3ZX 0T9D3ZZ 0T9D4ZX 0T9D7ZX 0T9D8ZX 0T9DXZX

0 Medical and Surgical
T Urinary System
B Excision: Cutting out or off, without replacement, a portion of a body part

Body Part Character 4	Approach Character 5	Device Character 6	Qualifier Character 7
0 Kidney, Right ⦸ **1** Kidney, Left ⦸ **3** Kidney Pelvis, Right ⦸ **4** Kidney Pelvis, Left ⦸ **6** Ureter, Right ⦸ **7** Ureter, Left ⦸ **B** Bladder **C** Bladder Neck	**0** Open **3** Percutaneous **4** Percutaneous Endoscopic **7** Via Natural or Artificial Opening **8** Via Natural or Artificial Opening Endoscopic	**Z** No Device	**X** Diagnostic **Z** No Qualifier
D Urethra ⦸	**0** Open **3** Percutaneous **4** Percutaneous Endoscopic **7** Via Natural or Artificial Opening **8** Via Natural or Artificial Opening Endoscopic **X** External	**Z** No Device	**X** Diagnostic **Z** No Qualifier

0TB continued on next page

0TB continued from previous page

⦸ 0TB03ZX 0TB04ZX 0TB07ZX 0TB08ZX 0TB13ZX 0TB14ZX 0TB17ZX 0TB18ZX 0TB33ZX 0TB34ZX 0TB37ZX 0TB38ZX 0TB43ZX 0TB44ZX 0TB47ZX 0TB48ZX 0TB63ZX 0TB64ZX 0TB67ZX 0TB68ZX 0TB73ZX 0TB74ZX 0TB77ZX 0TB78ZX 0TBD0ZX 0TBD3ZX 0TBD4ZX 0TBD7ZX 0TBD8ZX 0TBDXZX

0 Medical and Surgical
T Urinary System
C Extirpation: Taking or cutting out solid matter from a body part

Body Part Character 4	Approach Character 5	Device Character 6	Qualifier Character 7
0 Kidney, Right **1** Kidney, Left **3** Kidney Pelvis, Right **4** Kidney Pelvis, Left **6** Ureter, Right **7** Ureter, Left **B** Bladder ⦸ **C** Bladder Neck ⦸	**0** Open **3** Percutaneous **4** Percutaneous Endoscopic **7** Via Natural or Artificial Opening **8** Via Natural or Artificial Opening Endoscopic	**Z** No Device	**Z** No Qualifier
D Urethra ⦸	**0** Open **3** Percutaneous **4** Percutaneous Endoscopic **7** Via Natural or Artificial Opening **8** Via Natural or Artificial Opening Endoscopic **X** External	**Z** No Device	**Z** No Qualifier

⦸ 0TCB7ZZ 0TCB8ZZ 0TCC7ZZ 0TCC8ZZ 0TCD7ZZ 0TCD8ZZ 0TCDXZZ

0 Medical and Surgical
T Urinary System
D Extraction: Pulling or stripping out or off all or a portion of a body part by the use of force

Body Part Character 4	Approach Character 5	Device Character 6	Qualifier Character 7
0 Kidney, Right **1** Kidney, Left	**0** Open **3** Percutaneous **4** Percutaneous Endoscopic	**Z** No Device	**Z** No Qualifier

0 Medical and Surgical
T Urinary System
F Fragmentation: Breaking solid matter in a body part into pieces

Body Part Character 4	Approach Character 5	Device Character 6	Qualifier Character 7
3 Kidney Pelvis, Right ⦸ DRG **4** Kidney Pelvis, Left ⦸ DRG **6** Ureter, Right ⦸ DRG **7** Ureter, Left ⦸ DRG **B** Bladder ⦸ DRG **C** Bladder Neck ⦸ DRG **D** Urethra NC ⦸	**0** Open **3** Percutaneous **4** Percutaneous Endoscopic **7** Via Natural or Artificial Opening **8** Via Natural or Artificial Opening Endoscopic **X** External	**Z** No Device	**Z** No Qualifier

⦸ 0TF30ZZ 0TF37ZZ 0TF38ZZ 0TF40ZZ 0TF47ZZ 0TF48ZZ 0TF60ZZ 0TF63ZZ 0TF64ZZ 0TF67ZZ 0TF68ZZ 0TF70ZZ 0TF73ZZ 0TF74ZZ 0TF77ZZ 0TF78ZZ 0TFB0ZZ 0TFB3ZZ 0TFB4ZZ 0TFB7ZZ 0TFB8ZZ 0TFC0ZZ 0TFC3ZZ 0TFC4ZZ 0TFC7ZZ 0TFC8ZZ 0TFD0ZZ 0TFD3ZZ 0TFD4ZZ 0TFD7ZZ 0TFD8ZZ 0TFDXZZ

NC 0TFDXZZ

DRG 0TF3XZZ 0TF4XZZ 0TF6XZZ 0TF7XZZ 0TFBXZZ 0TFCXZZ

0 Medical and Surgical
T Urinary System
H Insertion: Putting in a nonbiological appliance that monitors, assists, performs, or prevents a physiological function but does not physically take the place of a body part

Body Part Character 4	Approach Character 5	Device Character 6	Qualifier Character 7
5 Kidney ⦸	**0** Open **3** Percutaneous **4** Percutaneous Endoscopic **7** Via Natural or Artificial Opening **8** Via Natural or Artificial Opening Endoscopic	**2** Monitoring Device **3** Infusion Device	**Z** No Qualifier
9 Ureter ⦸ CC	**0** Open **3** Percutaneous **4** Percutaneous Endoscopic **7** Via Natural or Artificial Opening **8** Via Natural or Artificial Opening Endoscopic	**2** Monitoring Device **3** Infusion Device **M** Stimulator Lead	**Z** No Qualifier
B Bladder NC ⦸ CC	**0** Open **3** Percutaneous **4** Percutaneous Endoscopic **7** Via Natural or Artificial Opening **8** Via Natural or Artificial Opening Endoscopic	**2** Monitoring Device **3** Infusion Device **L** Artificial Sphincter **M** Stimulator Lead	**Z** No Qualifier
C Bladder Neck	**0** Open **3** Percutaneous **4** Percutaneous Endoscopic **7** Via Natural or Artificial Opening **8** Via Natural or Artificial Opening Endoscopic	**L** Artificial Sphincter	**Z** No Qualifier
D Urethra ⦸	**0** Open **3** Percutaneous **4** Percutaneous Endoscopic **7** Via Natural or Artificial Opening **8** Via Natural or Artificial Opening Endoscopic **X** External	**2** Monitoring Device **3** Infusion Device **L** Artificial Sphincter	**Z** No Qualifier

⦸ 0TH503Z 0TH533Z 0TH543Z 0TH572Z 0TH573Z 0TH582Z 0TH583Z 0TH903Z 0TH933Z 0TH943Z 0TH972Z 0TH973Z 0TH982Z 0TH983Z 0THB03Z 0THB33Z 0THB43Z 0THB72Z 0THB73Z 0THB82Z 0THB83Z 0THD03Z 0THD33Z 0THD43Z 0THD72Z 0THD73Z 0THD82Z 0THD83Z 0THDX3Z

CC 0TH90MZ 0TH93MZ 0TH94MZ 0TH97MZ 0TH98MZ 0THB0MZ 0THB3MZ 0THB4MZ 0THB7MZ 0THB8MZ

NC 0THB0MZ 0THB3MZ 0THB4MZ 0THB7MZ 0THB8MZ

0 Medical and Surgical
T Urinary System
J Inspection: Visually and/or manually exploring a body part

Body Part Character 4	Approach Character 5	Device Character 6	Qualifier Character 7
5 Kidney ⦸ **9** Ureter ⦸ **B** Bladder ⦸ **D** Urethra ⦸	**0** Open **3** Percutaneous **4** Percutaneous Endoscopic **7** Via Natural or Artificial Opening **8** Via Natural or Artificial Opening Endoscopic **X** External	**Z** No Device	**Z** No Qualifier

⦸ 0TJ53ZZ 0TJ54ZZ 0TJ57ZZ 0TJ58ZZ 0TJ5XZZ 0TJ93ZZ 0TJ94ZZ 0TJ97ZZ 0TJ98ZZ 0TJ9XZZ 0TJB3ZZ 0TJB7ZZ 0TJB8ZZ 0TJBXZZ 0TJD3ZZ 0TJD4ZZ 0TJD7ZZ 0TJD8ZZ 0TJDXZZ

0 Medical and Surgical
T Urinary System
L Occlusion: Completely closing an orifice or the lumen of a tubular body part

Body Part Character 4	Approach Character 5	Device Character 6	Qualifier Character 7
3 Kidney Pelvis, Right **4** Kidney Pelvis, Left **6** Ureter, Right **7** Ureter, Left **B** Bladder **C** Bladder Neck	**0** Open **3** Percutaneous **4** Percutaneous Endoscopic	**C** Extraluminal Device **D** Intraluminal Device **Z** No Device	**Z** No Qualifier
3 Kidney Pelvis, Right **4** Kidney Pelvis, Left **6** Ureter, Right **7** Ureter, Left **B** Bladder **C** Bladder Neck	**7** Via Natural or Artificial Opening **8** Via Natural or Artificial Opening Endoscopic	**D** Intraluminal Device **Z** No Device	**Z** No Qualifier
D Urethra	**0** Open **3** Percutaneous **4** Percutaneous Endoscopic **X** External	**C** Extraluminal Device **D** Intraluminal Device **Z** No Device	**Z** No Qualifier
D Urethra	**7** Via Natural or Artificial Opening **8** Via Natural or Artificial Opening Endoscopic	**D** Intraluminal Device **Z** No Device	**Z** No Qualifier

0 Medical and Surgical
T Urinary System
M Reattachment: Putting back in or on all or a portion of a separated body part to its normal location or other suitable location

Body Part Character 4	Approach Character 5	Device Character 6	Qualifier Character 7
0 Kidney, Right **1** Kidney, Left **2** Kidneys, Bilateral **3** Kidney Pelvis, Right **4** Kidney Pelvis, Left **6** Ureter, Right **7** Ureter, Left **8** Ureters, Bilateral **B** Bladder **C** Bladder Neck **D** Urethra	**0** Open **4** Percutaneous Endoscopic	**Z** No Device	**Z** No Qualifier

0 Medical and Surgical
T Urinary System
N Release: Freeing a body part from an abnormal physical constraint by cutting or by the use of force

Body Part Character 4	Approach Character 5	Device Character 6	Qualifier Character 7
0 Kidney, Right **1** Kidney, Left **3** Kidney Pelvis, Right **4** Kidney Pelvis, Left **6** Ureter, Right **7** Ureter, Left **B** Bladder **C** Bladder Neck	**0** Open **3** Percutaneous **4** Percutaneous Endoscopic **7** Via Natural or Artificial Opening **8** Via Natural or Artificial Opening Endoscopic	**Z** No Device	**Z** No Qualifier
D Urethra	**0** Open **3** Percutaneous **4** Percutaneous Endoscopic **7** Via Natural or Artificial Opening **8** Via Natural or Artificial Opening Endoscopic **X** External	**Z** No Device	**Z** No Qualifier

0 Medical and Surgical
T Urinary System
P Removal: Taking out or off a device from a body part

Body Part Character 4	Approach Character 5	Device Character 6	Qualifier Character 7
5 Kidney ⊘	**0** Open **3** Percutaneous **4** Percutaneous Endoscopic **7** Via Natural or Artificial Opening **8** Via Natural or Artificial Opening Endoscopic	**0** Drainage Device **2** Monitoring Device **3** Infusion Device **7** Autologous Tissue Substitute **C** Extraluminal Device **D** Intraluminal Device **J** Synthetic Substitute **K** Nonautologous Tissue Substitute	**Z** No Qualifier
5 Kidney ⊘	**X** External	**0** Drainage Device **2** Monitoring Device **3** Infusion Device **D** Intraluminal Device	**Z** No Qualifier
9 Ureter ⊘ CC	**0** Open **3** Percutaneous **4** Percutaneous Endoscopic **7** Via Natural or Artificial Opening **8** Via Natural or Artificial Opening Endoscopic	**0** Drainage Device **2** Monitoring Device **3** Infusion Device **7** Autologous Tissue Substitute **C** Extraluminal Device **D** Intraluminal Device **J** Synthetic Substitute **K** Nonautologous Tissue Substitute **M** Stimulator Lead	**Z** No Qualifier
9 Ureter ⊘	**X** External	**0** Drainage Device **2** Monitoring Device **3** Infusion Device **D** Intraluminal Device **M** Stimulator Lead	**Z** No Qualifier
B Bladder NC ⊘ CC	**0** Open **3** Percutaneous **4** Percutaneous Endoscopic **7** Via Natural or Artificial Opening **8** Via Natural or Artificial Opening Endoscopic	**0** Drainage Device **2** Monitoring Device **3** Infusion Device **7** Autologous Tissue Substitute **C** Extraluminal Device **D** Intraluminal Device **J** Synthetic Substitute **K** Nonautologous Tissue Substitute **L** Artificial Sphincter **M** Stimulator Lead	**Z** No Qualifier
B Bladder ⊘	**X** External	**0** Drainage Device **2** Monitoring Device **3** Infusion Device **D** Intraluminal Device **L** Artificial Sphincter **M** Stimulator Lead	**Z** No Qualifier
D Urethra ⊘	**0** Open **3** Percutaneous **4** Percutaneous Endoscopic **7** Via Natural or Artificial Opening **8** Via Natural or Artificial Opening Endoscopic	**0** Drainage Device **2** Monitoring Device **3** Infusion Device **7** Autologous Tissue Substitute **C** Extraluminal Device **D** Intraluminal Device **J** Synthetic Substitute **K** Nonautologous Tissue Substitute **L** Artificial Sphincter	**Z** No Qualifier

0TP continued on next page

0 Medical and Surgical
T Urinary System
P Removal: Taking out or off a device from a body part

0TP continued from previous page

Body Part Character 4	Approach Character 5	Device Character 6	Qualifier Character 7
D Urethra ⊘	**X** External	**0** Drainage Device **2** Monitoring Device **3** Infusion Device **D** Intraluminal Device **L** Artificial Sphincter	**Z** No Qualifier

⊘ 0TP570Z 0TP572Z 0TP573Z 0TP57DZ 0TP580Z 0TP582Z 0TP583Z 0TP58DZ 0TP5X0Z 0TP5X2Z 0TP5X3Z 0TP5XDZ 0TP970Z 0TP972Z 0TP973Z 0TP97DZ 0TP980Z 0TP982Z 0TP983Z 0TP98DZ 0TP9X0Z 0TP9X2Z 0TP9X3Z 0TP9XDZ 0TPB70Z 0TPB72Z 0TPB73Z 0TPB7DZ 0TPB80Z 0TPB82Z 0TPB83Z 0TPB8DZ 0TPBX0Z 0TPBX2Z 0TPBX3Z 0TPBXDZ 0TPBXLZ 0TPD70Z 0TPD72Z 0TPD73Z 0TPD7DZ 0TPD80Z 0TPD82Z 0TPD83Z 0TPD8DZ 0TPDX0Z 0TPDX2Z 0TPDX3Z 0TPDXDZ

CC 0TP90MZ 0TP93MZ 0TP94MZ 0TP97MZ 0TP98MZ 0TPB0MZ 0TPB3MZ 0TPB4MZ 0TPB7MZ 0TPB8MZ

NC 0TPB0MZ 0TPB3MZ 0TPB4MZ 0TPB7MZ 0TPB8MZ

0 Medical and Surgical
T Urinary System
Q Repair: Restoring, to the extent possible, a body part to its normal anatomic structure and function

Body Part Character 4	Approach Character 5	Device Character 6	Qualifier Character 7
0 Kidney, Right CC **1** Kidney, Left CC **3** Kidney Pelvis, Right CC **4** Kidney Pelvis, Left CC **6** Ureter, Right CC **7** Ureter, Left CC **B** Bladder CC **C** Bladder Neck ⊘	**0** Open **3** Percutaneous **4** Percutaneous Endoscopic **7** Via Natural or Artificial Opening **8** Via Natural or Artificial Opening Endoscopic	**Z** No Device	**Z** No Qualifier
D Urethra CC	**0** Open **3** Percutaneous **4** Percutaneous Endoscopic **7** Via Natural or Artificial Opening **8** Via Natural or Artificial Opening Endoscopic **X** External	**Z** No Device	**Z** No Qualifier

⊘ 0TQC0ZZ 0TQC3ZZ 0TQC4ZZ 0TQC7ZZ 0TQC8ZZ

CC 0TQ00ZZ 0TQ03ZZ 0TQ04ZZ 0TQ10ZZ 0TQ13ZZ 0TQ14ZZ 0TQ30ZZ 0TQ33ZZ 0TQ34ZZ 0TQ40ZZ 0TQ43ZZ 0TQ44ZZ 0TQ60ZZ 0TQ63ZZ 0TQ64ZZ 0TQ70ZZ 0TQ73ZZ 0TQ74ZZ 0TQB0ZZ 0TQB3ZZ 0TQB4ZZ 0TQD0ZZ 0TQD3ZZ 0TQD4ZZ

0 Medical and Surgical
T Urinary System
R Replacement: Putting in or on biological or synthetic material that physically takes the place and/or function of all or a portion of a body part

Body Part Character 4	Approach Character 5	Device Character 6	Qualifier Character 7
3 Kidney Pelvis, Right **4** Kidney Pelvis, Left **6** Ureter, Right **7** Ureter, Left **B** Bladder CC **C** Bladder Neck	**0** Open **4** Percutaneous Endoscopic **7** Via Natural or Artificial Opening **8** Via Natural or Artificial Opening Endoscopic	**7** Autologous Tissue Substitute **J** Synthetic Substitute **K** Nonautologous Tissue Substitute	**Z** No Qualifier
D Urethra	**0** Open **4** Percutaneous Endoscopic **7** Via Natural or Artificial Opening **8** Via Natural or Artificial Opening Endoscopic **X** External	**7** Autologous Tissue Substitute **J** Synthetic Substitute **K** Nonautologous Tissue Substitute	**Z** No Qualifier

CC 0TRB07Z

0 Medical and Surgical
T Urinary System
S Reposition: Moving to its normal location, or other suitable location, all or a portion of a body part

Body Part Character 4	Approach Character 5	Device Character 6	Qualifier Character 7
0 Kidney, Right **1** Kidney, Left **2** Kidneys, Bilateral **3** Kidney Pelvis, Right **4** Kidney Pelvis, Left **6** Ureter, Right **7** Ureter, Left **8** Ureters, Bilateral **B** Bladder **C** Bladder Neck **D** Urethra	**0** Open **4** Percutaneous Endoscopic	**Z** No Device	**Z** No Qualifier

0 Medical and Surgical
T Urinary System
T Resection: Cutting out or off, without replacement, all of a body part

Body Part Character 4	Approach Character 5	Device Character 6	Qualifier Character 7
0 Kidney, Right **1** Kidney, Left **2** Kidneys, Bilateral	**0** Open **4** Percutaneous Endoscopic	**Z** No Device	**Z** No Qualifier
3 Kidney Pelvis, Right **4** Kidney Pelvis, Left **6** Ureter, Right **7** Ureter, Left **B** Bladder CC **C** Bladder Neck **D** Urethra ⃠ CC DRG	**0** Open **4** Percutaneous Endoscopic **7** Via Natural or Artificial Opening **8** Via Natural or Artificial Opening Endoscopic	**Z** No Device	**Z** No Qualifier

⃠ 0TTD4ZZ 0TTD7ZZ 0TTD8ZZ
CC 0TTB0ZZ 0TTB4ZZ 0TTB7ZZ 0TTB8ZZ 0TTD0ZZ
DRG 0TTD0ZZ

0 Medical and Surgical
T Urinary System
U Supplement: Putting in or on biological or synthetic material that physically reinforces and/or augments the function of a portion of a body part

Body Part Character 4	Approach Character 5	Device Character 6	Qualifier Character 7
3 Kidney Pelvis, Right **4** Kidney Pelvis, Left **6** Ureter, Right **7** Ureter, Left **B** Bladder **C** Bladder Neck	**0** Open **4** Percutaneous Endoscopic **7** Via Natural or Artificial Opening **8** Via Natural or Artificial Opening Endoscopic	**7** Autologous Tissue Substitute **J** Synthetic Substitute **K** Nonautologous Tissue Substitute	**Z** No Qualifier
D Urethra	**0** Open **4** Percutaneous Endoscopic **7** Via Natural or Artificial Opening **8** Via Natural or Artificial Opening Endoscopic **X** External	**7** Autologous Tissue Substitute **J** Synthetic Substitute **K** Nonautologous Tissue Substitute	**Z** No Qualifier

0 Medical and Surgical
T Urinary System
V Restriction: Partially closing an orifice or the lumen of a tubular body part

Body Part Character 4	Approach Character 5	Device Character 6	Qualifier Character 7
3 Kidney Pelvis, Right **4** Kidney Pelvis, Left **6** Ureter, Right **7** Ureter, Left **B** Bladder **C** Bladder Neck	**0** Open **3** Percutaneous **4** Percutaneous Endoscopic	**C** Extraluminal Device **D** Intraluminal Device **Z** No Device	**Z** No Qualifier
3 Kidney Pelvis, Right **4** Kidney Pelvis, Left **6** Ureter, Right **7** Ureter, Left **B** Bladder **C** Bladder Neck	**7** Via Natural or Artificial Opening **8** Via Natural or Artificial Opening Endoscopic	**D** Intraluminal Device **Z** No Device	**Z** No Qualifier
D Urethra	**0** Open **3** Percutaneous **4** Percutaneous Endoscopic	**C** Extraluminal Device **D** Intraluminal Device **Z** No Device	**Z** No Qualifier
D Urethra	**7** Via Natural or Artificial Opening **8** Via Natural or Artificial Opening Endoscopic	**D** Intraluminal Device **Z** No Device	**Z** No Qualifier
D Urethra	**X** External	**Z** No Device	**Z** No Qualifier

0 Medical and Surgical
T Urinary System
W Revision: Correcting, to the extent possible, a portion of a malfunctioning device or the position of a displaced device

Body Part Character 4	Approach Character 5	Device Character 6	Qualifier Character 7
5 Kidney ⃠	**0** Open **3** Percutaneous **4** Percutaneous Endoscopic **7** Via Natural or Artificial Opening **8** Via Natural or Artificial Opening Endoscopic **X** External	**0** Drainage Device **2** Monitoring Device **3** Infusion Device **7** Autologous Tissue Substitute **C** Extraluminal Device **D** Intraluminal Device **J** Synthetic Substitute **K** Nonautologous Tissue Substitute	**Z** No Qualifier
9 Ureter ⃠	**0** Open **3** Percutaneous **4** Percutaneous Endoscopic **7** Via Natural or Artificial Opening **8** Via Natural or Artificial Opening Endoscopic **X** External	**0** Drainage Device **2** Monitoring Device **3** Infusion Device **7** Autologous Tissue Substitute **C** Extraluminal Device **D** Intraluminal Device **J** Synthetic Substitute **K** Nonautologous Tissue Substitute **M** Stimulator Lead	**Z** No Qualifier
B Bladder ⃠	**0** Open **3** Percutaneous **4** Percutaneous Endoscopic **7** Via Natural or Artificial Opening **8** Via Natural or Artificial Opening Endoscopic **X** External	**0** Drainage Device **2** Monitoring Device **3** Infusion Device **7** Autologous Tissue Substitute **C** Extraluminal Device **D** Intraluminal Device **J** Synthetic Substitute **K** Nonautologous Tissue Substitute **L** Artificial Sphincter **M** Stimulator Lead	**Z** No Qualifier
D Urethra ⃠	**0** Open **3** Percutaneous **4** Percutaneous Endoscopic **7** Via Natural or Artificial Opening **8** Via Natural or Artificial Opening Endoscopic **X** External	**0** Drainage Device **2** Monitoring Device **3** Infusion Device **7** Autologous Tissue Substitute **C** Extraluminal Device **D** Intraluminal Device **J** Synthetic Substitute **K** Nonautologous Tissue Substitute **L** Artificial Sphincter	**Z** No Qualifier

⃠ 0TW5X0Z 0TW5X2Z 0TW5X3Z 0TW5X7Z 0TW5XCZ 0TW5XDZ 0TW5XJZ 0TW5XKZ 0TW9X0Z 0TW9X2Z 0TW9X3Z 0TW9X7Z 0TW9XCZ 0TW9XDZ 0TW9XJZ 0TW9XKZ 0TW9XMZ 0TWBX0Z 0TWBX2Z 0TWBX3Z 0TWBX7Z 0TWBXCZ 0TWBXDZ 0TWBXJZ 0TWBXKZ 0TWBXLZ 0TWBXMZ 0TWDX0Z 0TWDX2Z 0TWDX3Z 0TWDX7Z 0TWDXCZ 0TWDXDZ 0TWDXJZ 0TWDXKZ 0TWDXLZ

0 Medical and Surgical
T Urinary System
Y Transplantation: Putting in or on all or a portion of a living body part taken from another individual or animal to physically take the place and/or function of all or a portion of a similar body part

Body Part Character 4	Approach Character 5	Device Character 6	Qualifier Character 7
0 Kidney, Right LC CC **1** Kidney, Left LC CC	**0** Open	**Z** No Device	**0** Allogeneic **1** Syngeneic **2** Zooplastic

LC 0TY00Z0 0TY00Z1 0TY00Z2 0TY10Z0 0TY10Z1 0TY10Z2
CC 0TY00Z0 0TY00Z1 0TY00Z2 0TY10Z0 0TY10Z1 0TY10Z2

Female Reproductive System 0U1-0UY

0 Medical and Surgical
U Female Reproductive System
1 Bypass: Altering the route of passage of the contents of a tubular body part

Body Part Character 4	Approach Character 5	Device Character 6	Qualifier Character 7
5 Fallopian Tube, Right ♀ **6** Fallopian Tube, Left ♀	**0** Open **4** Percutaneous Endoscopic	**7** Autologous Tissue Substitute **J** Synthetic Substitute **K** Nonautologous Tissue Substitute **Z** No Device	**5** Fallopian Tube, Right **6** Fallopian Tube, Left **9** Uterus

♀ 0U15075 0U15076 0U15079 0U150J5 0U150J6 0U150J9 0U150K5 0U150K6 0U150K9 0U150Z5 0U150Z6 0U150Z9 0U15475 0U15476 0U15479 0U154J5 0U154J6 0U154J9 0U154K5 0U154K6 0U154K9 0U154Z5 0U154Z6 0U154Z9 0U16075 0U16076 0U16079 0U160J5 0U160J6 0U160J9 0U160K5 0U160K6 0U160K9 0U160Z5 0U160Z6 0U160Z9 0U16475 0U16476 0U16479 0U164J5 0U164J6 0U164J9 0U164K5 0U164K6 0U164K9 0U164Z5 0U164Z6 0U164Z9

0 Medical and Surgical
U Female Reproductive System
2 Change: Taking out or off a device from a body part and putting back an identical or similar device in or on the same body part without cutting or puncturing the skin or a mucous membrane

Body Part Character 4	Approach Character 5	Device Character 6	Qualifier Character 7
3 Ovary ⦸ ♀ **8** Fallopian Tube ⦸ ♀ **M** Vulva ⦸ ♀	**X** External	**0** Drainage Device **Y** Other Device	**Z** No Qualifier
D Uterus and Cervix ⦸ ♀	**X** External	**0** Drainage Device **H** Contraceptive Device **Y** Other Device	**Z** No Qualifier
H Vagina and Cul-de-sac ⦸ ♀	**X** External	**0** Drainage Device **G** Intraluminal Device, Pessary **Y** Other Device	**Z** No Qualifier

♀ 0U23X0Z 0U23XYZ 0U28X0Z 0U28XYZ 0U2DX0Z 0U2DXHZ 0U2DXYZ 0U2HX0Z 0U2HXGZ 0U2HXYZ 0U2MX0Z 0U2MXYZ
⦸ 0U23X0Z 0U23XYZ 0U28X0Z 0U28XYZ 0U2DX0Z 0U2DXHZ 0U2DXYZ 0U2HX0Z 0U2HXGZ 0U2HXYZ 0U2MX0Z 0U2MXYZ

0 Medical and Surgical
U Female Reproductive System
5 Destruction: Physical eradication of all or a portion of a body part by the direct use of energy, force, or a destructive agent

Body Part Character 4	Approach Character 5	Device Character 6	Qualifier Character 7
0 Ovary, Right ♀ **1** Ovary, Left ♀ **2** Ovaries, Bilateral ♀ **4** Uterine Supporting Structure ♀	**0** Open **3** Percutaneous **4** Percutaneous Endoscopic	**Z** No Device	**Z** No Qualifier
5 Fallopian Tube, Right ♀ **6** Fallopian Tube, Left ♀ **7** Fallopian Tubes, Bilateral NC ♀ **9** Uterus ♀ **B** Endometrium ♀ **C** Cervix ♀ **F** Cul-de-sac ♀	**0** Open **3** Percutaneous **4** Percutaneous Endoscopic **7** Via Natural or Artificial Opening **8** Via Natural or Artificial Opening Endoscopic	**Z** No Device	**Z** No Qualifier
G Vagina ♀ **K** Hymen ♀	**0** Open **3** Percutaneous **4** Percutaneous Endoscopic **7** Via Natural or Artificial Opening **8** Via Natural or Artificial Opening Endoscopic **X** External	**Z** No Device	**Z** No Qualifier

0U5 continued on next page

LC Limited Coverage NC Noncovered HAC HAC Associated Procedure CC Combination Cluster - See Appendix G for code lists
DRG Non-OR-Affecting MS-DRG Assignment ⦸ Non-OR-Not Affecting MS-DRG Assignment New/Revised Text in **Orange** ♂ Male ♀ Female

0 Medical and Surgical 0U5 continued from previous page
U Female Reproductive System
5 Destruction: Physical eradication of all or a portion of a body part by the direct use of energy, force, or a destructive agent

Body Part Character 4	Approach Character 5	Device Character 6	Qualifier Character 7
J Clitoris ♀ **L** Vestibular Gland ♀ **M** Vulva ♀	**0** Open **X** External	**Z** No Device	**Z** No Qualifier

♀ 0U500ZZ 0U503ZZ 0U504ZZ 0U510ZZ 0U513ZZ 0U514ZZ 0U520ZZ 0U523ZZ 0U524ZZ 0U540ZZ 0U543ZZ 0U544ZZ 0U550ZZ 0U553ZZ 0U554ZZ 0U557ZZ 0U558ZZ 0U560ZZ 0U563ZZ 0U564ZZ 0U567ZZ 0U568ZZ 0U570ZZ 0U573ZZ 0U574ZZ 0U577ZZ 0U578ZZ 0U590ZZ 0U593ZZ 0U594ZZ 0U597ZZ 0U598ZZ 0U5B0ZZ 0U5B3ZZ 0U5B4ZZ 0U5B7ZZ 0U5B8ZZ 0U5C0ZZ 0U5C3ZZ 0U5C4ZZ 0U5C7ZZ 0U5C8ZZ 0U5F0ZZ 0U5F3ZZ 0U5F4ZZ 0U5F7ZZ 0U5F8ZZ 0U5G0ZZ 0U5G3ZZ 0U5G4ZZ 0U5G7ZZ 0U5G8ZZ 0U5GXZZ 0U5J0ZZ 0U5JXZZ 0U5K0ZZ 0U5K3ZZ 0U5K4ZZ 0U5K7ZZ 0U5K8ZZ 0U5KXZZ 0U5L0ZZ 0U5LXZZ 0U5M0ZZ 0U5MXZZ

NC 0U570ZZ 0U573ZZ 0U574ZZ 0U577ZZ or 0U578ZZ when diagnosis code Z30.2 is listed as the principal diagnosis

0 Medical and Surgical
U Female Reproductive System
7 Dilation: Expanding an orifice or the lumen of a tubular body part

Body Part Character 4	Approach Character 5	Device Character 6	Qualifier Character 7
5 Fallopian Tube, Right ♀ **6** Fallopian Tube, Left ♀ **7** Fallopian Tubes, Bilateral ♀ **9** Uterus ♀ **C** Cervix ⊘ ♀ **G** Vagina ⊘ ♀	**0** Open **3** Percutaneous **4** Percutaneous Endoscopic **7** Via Natural or Artificial Opening **8** Via Natural or Artificial Opening Endoscopic	**D** Intraluminal Device **Z** No Device	**Z** No Qualifier
K Hymen ♀	**0** Open **3** Percutaneous **4** Percutaneous Endoscopic **7** Via Natural or Artificial Opening **8** Via Natural or Artificial Opening Endoscopic **X** External	**D** Intraluminal Device **Z** No Device	**Z** No Qualifier

♀ 0U750DZ 0U750ZZ 0U753DZ 0U753ZZ 0U754DZ 0U754ZZ 0U757DZ 0U757ZZ 0U758DZ 0U758ZZ 0U760DZ 0U760ZZ 0U763DZ 0U763ZZ 0U764DZ 0U764ZZ 0U767DZ 0U767ZZ 0U768DZ 0U768ZZ 0U770DZ 0U770ZZ 0U773DZ 0U773ZZ 0U774DZ 0U774ZZ 0U777DZ 0U777ZZ 0U778DZ 0U778ZZ 0U790DZ 0U790ZZ 0U793DZ 0U793ZZ 0U794DZ 0U794ZZ 0U797DZ 0U797ZZ 0U798DZ 0U798ZZ 0U7C0DZ 0U7C0ZZ 0U7C3DZ 0U7C3ZZ 0U7C4DZ 0U7C4ZZ 0U7C7DZ 0U7C7ZZ 0U7C8DZ 0U7C8ZZ 0U7G0DZ 0U7G0ZZ 0U7G3DZ 0U7G3ZZ 0U7G4DZ 0U7G4ZZ 0U7G7DZ 0U7G7ZZ 0U7G8DZ 0U7G8ZZ 0U7K0DZ 0U7K0ZZ 0U7K3DZ 0U7K3ZZ 0U7K4DZ 0U7K4ZZ 0U7K7DZ 0U7K7ZZ 0U7K8DZ 0U7K8ZZ 0U7KXDZ 0U7KXZZ

⊘ 0U7C0DZ 0U7C0ZZ 0U7C3DZ 0U7C3ZZ 0U7C4DZ 0U7C4ZZ 0U7C7DZ 0U7C7ZZ 0U7C8DZ 0U7C8ZZ 0U7G7DZ 0U7G7ZZ 0U7G8DZ 0U7G8ZZ

0 Medical and Surgical
U Female Reproductive System
8 Division: Cutting into a body part, without draining fluids and/or gases from the body part, in order to separate or transect a body part

Body Part Character 4	Approach Character 5	Device Character 6	Qualifier Character 7
0 Ovary, Right ♀ **1** Ovary, Left ♀ **2** Ovaries, Bilateral ♀ **4** Uterine Supporting Structure ♀	**0** Open **3** Percutaneous **4** Percutaneous Endoscopic	**Z** No Device	**Z** No Qualifier
K Hymen ⊘ ♀	**7** Via Natural or Artificial Opening **8** Via Natural or Artificial Opening Endoscopic **X** External	**Z** No Device	**Z** No Qualifier

♀ 0U800ZZ 0U803ZZ 0U804ZZ 0U810ZZ 0U813ZZ 0U814ZZ 0U820ZZ 0U823ZZ 0U824ZZ 0U840ZZ 0U843ZZ 0U844ZZ 0U8K7ZZ 0U8K8ZZ 0U8KXZZ

⊘ 0U8K7ZZ 0U8K8ZZ 0U8KXZZ

LC Limited Coverage NC Noncovered HAC HAC Associated Procedure CC Combination Cluster - See Appendix G for code lists
DRG Non-OR-Affecting MS-DRG Assignment ⊘ Non-OR-Not Affecting MS-DRG Assignment New/Revised Text in **Orange** ♂ Male ♀ Female

0 Medical and Surgical
U Female Reproductive System
9 Drainage: Taking or letting out fluids and/or gases from a body part

Body Part Character 4	Approach Character 5	Device Character 6	Qualifier Character 7
0 Ovary, Right ⃠ ♀ **1** Ovary, Left ⃠ ♀ **2** Ovaries, Bilateral ♀ ⃠	**0** Open **3** Percutaneous **4** Percutaneous Endoscopic	**0** Drainage Device	**Z** No Qualifier
0 Ovary, Right ⃠ ♀ **1** Ovary, Left ♀ ⃠ **2** Ovaries, Bilateral ♀ ⃠	**0** Open **3** Percutaneous **4** Percutaneous Endoscopic	**Z** No Device	**X** Diagnostic **Z** No Qualifier
0 Ovary, Right ♀ **1** Ovary, Left ♀ **2** Ovaries, Bilateral ♀	**X** External	**Z** No Device	**Z** No Qualifier
4 Uterine Supporting Structure ⃠ ♀	**0** Open **3** Percutaneous **4** Percutaneous Endoscopic	**0** Drainage Device	**Z** No Qualifier
4 Uterine Supporting Structure ⃠ ♀	**0** Open **3** Percutaneous **4** Percutaneous Endoscopic	**Z** No Device	**X** Diagnostic **Z** No Qualifier
5 Fallopian Tube, Right ⃠ ♀ **6** Fallopian Tube, Left ⃠ ♀ **7** Fallopian Tubes, Bilateral ⃠ ♀ **9** Uterus ⃠ ♀ **C** Cervix ⃠ ♀ **F** Cul-de-sac ⃠ ♀	**0** Open **3** Percutaneous **4** Percutaneous Endoscopic **7** Via Natural or Artificial Opening **8** Via Natural or Artificial Opening Endoscopic	**0** Drainage Device	**Z** No Qualifier
5 Fallopian Tube, Right ⃠ ♀ **6** Fallopian Tube, Left ⃠ ♀ **7** Fallopian Tubes, Bilateral ⃠ ♀ **9** Uterus ⃠ ♀ **C** Cervix ⃠ ♀ **F** Cul-de-sac ⃠ ♀	**0** Open **3** Percutaneous **4** Percutaneous Endoscopic **7** Via Natural or Artificial Opening **8** Via Natural or Artificial Opening Endoscopic	**Z** No Device	**X** Diagnostic **Z** No Qualifier
G Vagina ⃠ ♀ **K** Hymen ⃠ ♀	**0** Open **3** Percutaneous **4** Percutaneous Endoscopic **7** Via Natural or Artificial Opening **8** Via Natural or Artificial Opening Endoscopic **X** External	**0** Drainage Device	**Z** No Qualifier
G Vagina ⃠ ♀ **K** Hymen ⃠ ♀	**0** Open **3** Percutaneous **4** Percutaneous Endoscopic **7** Via Natural or Artificial Opening **8** Via Natural or Artificial Opening Endoscopic **X** External	**Z** No Device	**X** Diagnostic **Z** No Qualifier
J Clitoris ♀ **L** Vestibular Gland ⃠ ♀ **M** Vulva ♀	**0** Open **X** External	**0** Drainage Device	**Z** No Qualifier
J Clitoris ♀ **L** Vestibular Gland ⃠ ♀ **M** Vulva ♀	**0** Open **X** External	**Z** No Device	**X** Diagnostic **Z** No Qualifier

♀ 0U9000Z 0U900ZX 0U900ZZ 0U9030Z 0U903ZX 0U903ZZ 0U9040Z 0U904ZX 0U904ZZ 0U90XZZ 0U9100Z 0U910ZX 0U910ZZ 0U9130Z 0U913ZX 0U913ZZ 0U9140Z 0U914ZX 0U914ZZ 0U91XZZ 0U9200Z 0U920ZX 0U920ZZ 0U9230Z 0U923ZX 0U923ZZ 0U9240Z 0U924ZX 0U924ZZ 0U92XZZ 0U9400Z 0U940ZX 0U940ZZ 0U9430Z 0U943ZX 0U943ZZ 0U9440Z 0U944ZX 0U944ZZ 0U9500Z 0U950ZX 0U950ZZ 0U9530Z 0U953ZX 0U953ZZ 0U9540Z 0U954ZX 0U954ZZ 0U9570Z 0U957ZX 0U957ZZ 0U9580Z 0U958ZX 0U958ZZ 0U9600Z 0U960ZX 0U960ZZ 0U9630Z 0U963ZX 0U963ZZ 0U9640Z 0U964ZX 0U964ZZ 0U9670Z 0U967ZX 0U967ZZ 0U9680Z 0U968ZX 0U968ZZ 0U9700Z 0U970ZX 0U970ZZ 0U9730Z 0U973ZX 0U973ZZ 0U9740Z 0U974ZX 0U974ZZ 0U9770Z 0U977ZX 0U977ZZ 0U9780Z 0U978ZX 0U978ZZ 0U9900Z 0U990ZX 0U990ZZ 0U9930Z 0U993ZX 0U993ZZ 0U9940Z 0U994ZX 0U994ZZ 0U9970Z 0U997ZX 0U997ZZ 0U9980Z 0U998ZX 0U998ZZ 0U9C00Z 0U9C0ZX 0U9C0ZZ 0U9C30Z 0U9C3ZX 0U9C3ZZ 0U9C40Z 0U9C4ZX 0U9C4ZZ 0U9C70Z 0U9C7ZX 0U9C7ZZ 0U9C80Z 0U9C8ZX 0U9C8ZZ 0U9F00Z 0U9F0ZX 0U9F0ZZ 0U9F30Z 0U9F3ZX 0U9F3ZZ 0U9F40Z 0U9F4ZX 0U9F4ZZ 0U9F70Z 0U9F7ZX 0U9F7ZZ 0U9F80Z 0U9F8ZX 0U9F8ZZ 0U9G00Z

0U9 continued on next page

0U9 continued from previous page

0U9G0ZX 0U9G0ZZ 0U9G30Z 0U9G3ZX 0U9G3ZZ 0U9G40Z 0U9G4ZX 0U9G4ZZ 0U9G70Z 0U9G7ZX 0U9G7ZZ 0U9G80Z 0U9G8ZX
0U9G8ZZ 0U9GX0Z 0U9GXZX 0U9GXZZ 0U9J00Z 0U9J0ZX 0U9J0ZZ 0U9JX0Z 0U9JXZX 0U9JXZZ 0U9K00Z 0U9K0ZX 0U9K0ZZ
0U9K30Z 0U9K3ZX 0U9K3ZZ 0U9K40Z 0U9K4ZX 0U9K4ZZ 0U9K70Z 0U9K7ZX 0U9K7ZZ 0U9K80Z 0U9K8ZX 0U9K8ZZ 0U9KX0Z
0U9KXZX 0U9KXZZ 0U9L00Z 0U9L0ZX 0U9L0ZZ 0U9LX0Z 0U9LXZX 0U9LXZZ 0U9M00Z 0U9M0ZX 0U9M0ZZ 0U9MX0Z 0U9MXZX
0U9MXZZ

⃠ 0U9030Z 0U903ZZ 0U9130Z 0U913ZZ 0U9230Z 0U923ZZ 0U9430Z 0U943ZZ 0U9530Z 0U953ZZ 0U954ZZ 0U957ZZ 0U958ZZ
0U9630Z 0U963ZZ 0U964ZZ 0U967ZZ 0U968ZZ 0U9730Z 0U973ZZ 0U974ZZ 0U977ZZ 0U978ZZ 0U9930Z 0U993ZZ 0U9C30Z
0U9C3ZZ 0U9F30Z 0U9F3ZZ 0U9F40Z 0U9F4ZZ 0U9G30Z 0U9G3ZZ 0U9K00Z 0U9K0ZZ 0U9K30Z 0U9K3ZZ 0U9K40Z 0U9K4ZZ
0U9K70Z 0U9K7ZZ 0U9K80Z 0U9K8ZZ 0U9KX0Z 0U9KXZZ 0U9L00Z 0U9L0ZZ 0U9LX0Z 0U9LXZZ

0 Medical and Surgical
U Female Reproductive System
B Excision: Cutting out or off, without replacement, a portion of a body part

Body Part Character 4	Approach Character 5	Device Character 6	Qualifier Character 7
0 Ovary, Right ♀ **1** Ovary, Left ♀ **2** Ovaries, Bilateral ♀ **4** Uterine Supporting Structure ♀ **5** Fallopian Tube, Right ♀ **6** Fallopian Tube, Left ♀ **7** Fallopian Tubes, Bilateral ♀ **9** Uterus ♀ **C** Cervix ♀ **F** Cul-de-sac ♀	**0** Open **3** Percutaneous **4** Percutaneous Endoscopic **7** Via Natural or Artificial Opening **8** Via Natural or Artificial Opening Endoscopic	**Z** No Device	**X** Diagnostic **Z** No Qualifier
G Vagina ♀ **K** Hymen ♀	**0** Open **3** Percutaneous **4** Percutaneous Endoscopic **7** Via Natural or Artificial Opening **8** Via Natural or Artificial Opening Endoscopic **X** External	**Z** No Device	**X** Diagnostic **Z** No Qualifier
J Clitoris ♀ **L** Vestibular Gland ♀ **M** Vulva ♀	**0** Open **X** External	**Z** No Device	**X** Diagnostic **Z** No Qualifier

♀ 0UB00ZX 0UB00ZZ 0UB03ZX 0UB03ZZ 0UB04ZX 0UB04ZZ 0UB07ZX 0UB07ZZ 0UB08ZX 0UB08ZZ 0UB10ZX 0UB10ZZ 0UB13ZX
0UB13ZZ 0UB14ZX 0UB14ZZ 0UB17ZX 0UB17ZZ 0UB18ZX 0UB18ZZ 0UB20ZX 0UB20ZZ 0UB23ZX 0UB23ZZ 0UB24ZX 0UB24ZZ
0UB27ZX 0UB27ZZ 0UB28ZX 0UB28ZZ 0UB40ZX 0UB40ZZ 0UB43ZX 0UB43ZZ 0UB44ZX 0UB44ZZ 0UB47ZX 0UB47ZZ 0UB48ZX
0UB48ZZ 0UB50ZX 0UB50ZZ 0UB53ZX 0UB53ZZ 0UB54ZX 0UB54ZZ 0UB57ZX 0UB57ZZ 0UB58ZX 0UB58ZZ 0UB60ZX 0UB60ZZ
0UB63ZX 0UB63ZZ 0UB64ZX 0UB64ZZ 0UB67ZX 0UB67ZZ 0UB68ZX 0UB68ZZ 0UB70ZX 0UB70ZZ 0UB73ZX 0UB73ZZ 0UB74ZX
0UB74ZZ 0UB77ZX 0UB77ZZ 0UB78ZX 0UB78ZZ 0UB90ZX 0UB90ZZ 0UB93ZX 0UB93ZZ 0UB94ZX 0UB94ZZ 0UB97ZX 0UB97ZZ
0UB98ZX 0UB98ZZ 0UBC0ZX 0UBC0ZZ 0UBC3ZX 0UBC3ZZ 0UBC4ZX 0UBC4ZZ 0UBC7ZX 0UBC7ZZ 0UBC8ZX 0UBC8ZZ 0UBF0ZX
0UBF0ZZ 0UBF3ZX 0UBF3ZZ 0UBF4ZX 0UBF4ZZ 0UBF7ZX 0UBF7ZZ 0UBF8ZX 0UBF8ZZ 0UBG0ZX 0UBG0ZZ 0UBG3ZX 0UBG3ZZ
0UBG4ZX 0UBG4ZZ 0UBG7ZX 0UBG7ZZ 0UBG8ZX 0UBG8ZZ 0UBGXZX 0UBGXZZ 0UBJ0ZX 0UBJ0ZZ 0UBJXZX 0UBJXZZ 0UBK0ZX
0UBK0ZZ 0UBK3ZX 0UBK3ZZ 0UBK4ZX 0UBK4ZZ 0UBK7ZX 0UBK7ZZ 0UBK8ZX 0UBK8ZZ 0UBKXZX 0UBKXZZ 0UBL0ZX 0UBL0ZZ
0UBLXZX 0UBLXZZ 0UBM0ZX 0UBM0ZZ 0UBMXZX 0UBMXZZ

0 Medical and Surgical
U Female Reproductive System
C Extirpation: Taking or cutting out solid matter from a body part

Body Part Character 4	Approach Character 5	Device Character 6	Qualifier Character 7
0 Ovary, Right ♀ 1 Ovary, Left ♀ 2 Ovaries, Bilateral ♀ 4 Uterine Supporting Structure ♀	0 Open 3 Percutaneous 4 Percutaneous Endoscopic	Z No Device	Z No Qualifier
5 Fallopian Tube, Right ♀ 6 Fallopian Tube, Left ♀ 7 Fallopian Tubes, Bilateral ♀ 9 Uterus ⦸ ♀ B Endometrium ♀ C Cervix ♀ F Cul-de-sac ♀	0 Open 3 Percutaneous 4 Percutaneous Endoscopic 7 Via Natural or Artificial Opening 8 Via Natural or Artificial Opening Endoscopic	Z No Device	Z No Qualifier
G Vagina ⦸ ♀ K Hymen ⦸ ♀	0 Open 3 Percutaneous 4 Percutaneous Endoscopic 7 Via Natural or Artificial Opening 8 Via Natural or Artificial Opening Endoscopic X External	Z No Device	Z No Qualifier
J Clitoris ♀ L Vestibular Gland ♀ M Vulva ⦸ ♀	0 Open X External	Z No Device	Z No Qualifier

♀ 0UC00ZZ 0UC03ZZ 0UC04ZZ 0UC10ZZ 0UC13ZZ 0UC14ZZ 0UC20ZZ 0UC23ZZ 0UC24ZZ 0UC40ZZ 0UC43ZZ 0UC44ZZ 0UC50ZZ 0UC53ZZ 0UC54ZZ 0UC57ZZ 0UC58ZZ 0UC60ZZ 0UC63ZZ 0UC64ZZ 0UC67ZZ 0UC68ZZ 0UC70ZZ 0UC73ZZ 0UC74ZZ 0UC77ZZ 0UC78ZZ 0UC90ZZ 0UC93ZZ 0UC94ZZ 0UC97ZZ 0UC98ZZ 0UCB0ZZ 0UCB3ZZ 0UCB4ZZ 0UCB7ZZ 0UCB8ZZ 0UCC0ZZ 0UCC3ZZ 0UCC4ZZ 0UCC7ZZ 0UCC8ZZ 0UCF0ZZ 0UCF3ZZ 0UCF4ZZ 0UCF7ZZ 0UCF8ZZ 0UCG0ZZ 0UCG3ZZ 0UCG4ZZ 0UCG7ZZ 0UCG8ZZ 0UCGXZZ 0UCJ0ZZ 0UCJXZZ 0UCK0ZZ 0UCK3ZZ 0UCK4ZZ 0UCK7ZZ 0UCK8ZZ 0UCKXZZ 0UCL0ZZ 0UCLXZZ 0UCM0ZZ 0UCMXZZ

⦸ 0UC97ZZ 0UC98ZZ 0UCG7ZZ 0UCG8ZZ 0UCGXZZ 0UCK0ZZ 0UCK3ZZ 0UCK4ZZ 0UCK7ZZ 0UCK8ZZ 0UCKXZZ 0UCMXZZ

0 Medical and Surgical
U Female Reproductive System
D Extraction: Pulling or stripping out or off all or a portion of a body part by the use of force

Body Part Character 4	Approach Character 5	Device Character 6	Qualifier Character 7
B Endometrium ♀	7 Via Natural or Artificial Opening 8 Via Natural or Artificial Opening Endoscopic	Z No Device	X Diagnostic Z No Qualifier
N Ova ♀	0 Open 3 Percutaneous 4 Percutaneous Endoscopic	Z No Device	Z No Qualifier

♀ 0UDB7ZX 0UDB7ZZ 0UDB8ZX 0UDB8ZZ 0UDN0ZZ 0UDN3ZZ 0UDN4ZZ

0 Medical and Surgical
U Female Reproductive System
F Fragmentation: Breaking solid matter in a body part into pieces

Body Part Character 4	Approach Character 5	Device Character 6	Qualifier Character 7
5 Fallopian Tube, Right NC ⦸ ♀ 6 Fallopian Tube, Left NC ⦸ ♀ 7 Fallopian Tubes, Bilateral NC ⦸ ♀ 9 Uterus NC ⦸ ♀	0 Open 3 Percutaneous 4 Percutaneous Endoscopic 7 Via Natural or Artificial Opening 8 Via Natural or Artificial Opening Endoscopic X External	Z No Device	Z No Qualifier

♀ 0UF50ZZ 0UF53ZZ 0UF54ZZ 0UF57ZZ 0UF58ZZ 0UF5XZZ 0UF60ZZ 0UF63ZZ 0UF64ZZ 0UF67ZZ 0UF68ZZ 0UF6XZZ 0UF70ZZ 0UF73ZZ 0UF74ZZ 0UF77ZZ 0UF78ZZ 0UF7XZZ 0UF90ZZ 0UF93ZZ 0UF94ZZ 0UF97ZZ 0UF98ZZ 0UF9XZZ

⦸ 0UF5XZZ 0UF6XZZ 0UF7XZZ 0UF9XZZ

NC 0UF5XZZ 0UF6XZZ 0UF7XZZ 0UF9XZZ

LC Limited Coverage NC Noncovered HAC HAC Associated Procedure CC Combination Cluster - See Appendix G for code lists
DRG Non-OR-Affecting MS-DRG Assignment ⦸ Non-OR-Not Affecting MS-DRG Assignment New/Revised Text in **Orange** ♂ Male ♀ Female

0 Medical and Surgical
U Female Reproductive System
H Insertion: Putting in a nonbiological appliance that monitors, assists, performs, or prevents a physiological function but does not physically take the place of a body part

Body Part Character 4	Approach Character 5	Device Character 6	Qualifier Character 7
3 Ovary ⊘ ♀	**0** Open **3** Percutaneous **4** Percutaneous Endoscopic	**3** Infusion Device	**Z** No Qualifier
8 Fallopian Tube ⊘ ♀ **D** Uterus and Cervix ⊘ ♀ **H** Vagina and Cul-de-sac ⊘ ♀	**0** Open **3** Percutaneous **4** Percutaneous Endoscopic **7** Via Natural or Artificial Opening **8** Via Natural or Artificial Opening Endoscopic	**3** Infusion Device	**Z** No Qualifier
9 Uterus ⊘ ♀	**7** Via Natural or Artificial Opening **8** Via Natural or Artificial Opening Endoscopic	**H** Contraceptive Device	**Z** No Qualifier
C Cervix ♀	**0** Open **3** Percutaneous **4** Percutaneous Endoscopic	**1** Radioactive Element	**Z** No Qualifier
C Cervix ⊘ ♀	**7** Via Natural or Artificial Opening **8** Via Natural or Artificial Opening Endoscopic	**1** Radioactive Element **H** Contraceptive Device	**Z** No Qualifier
F Cul-de-sac ⊘ ♀	**7** Via Natural or Artificial Opening **8** Via Natural or Artificial Opening Endoscopic	**G** Intraluminal Device, Pessary	**Z** No Qualifier
G Vagina ♀	**0** Open **3** Percutaneous **4** Percutaneous Endoscopic **X** External	**1** Radioactive Element	**Z** No Qualifier
G Vagina ⊘ ♀	**7** Via Natural or Artificial Opening **8** Via Natural or Artificial Opening Endoscopic	**1** Radioactive Element **G** Intraluminal Device, Pessary	**Z** No Qualifier

♀ 0UH303Z 0UH333Z 0UH343Z 0UH803Z 0UH833Z 0UH843Z 0UH873Z 0UH883Z 0UH97HZ 0UH98HZ 0UHC01Z 0UHC31Z 0UHC41Z 0UHC71Z 0UHC7HZ 0UHC81Z 0UHC8HZ 0UHD03Z 0UHD33Z 0UHD43Z 0UHD73Z 0UHD83Z 0UHF7GZ 0UHF8GZ 0UHG01Z 0UHG31Z 0UHG41Z 0UHG71Z 0UHG7GZ 0UHG81Z 0UHG8GZ 0UHGX1Z 0UHH03Z 0UHH33Z 0UHH43Z 0UHH73Z 0UHH83Z

⊘ 0UH303Z 0UH333Z 0UH343Z 0UH803Z 0UH833Z 0UH843Z 0UH873Z 0UH883Z 0UH97HZ 0UH98HZ 0UHC7HZ 0UHC8HZ 0UHD03Z 0UHD33Z 0UHD43Z 0UHD73Z 0UHD83Z 0UHF7GZ 0UHF8GZ 0UHG7GZ 0UHG8GZ 0UHH73Z 0UHH83Z

0 Medical and Surgical
U Female Reproductive System
J Inspection: Visually and/or manually exploring a body part

Body Part Character 4	Approach Character 5	Device Character 6	Qualifier Character 7
3 Ovary ⊘ ♀	**0** Open **3** Percutaneous **4** Percutaneous Endoscopic **X** External	**Z** No Device	**Z** No Qualifier
8 Fallopian Tube ⊘ ♀ **D** Uterus and Cervix ⊘ ♀ **H** Vagina and Cul-de-sac ⊘ ♀	**0** Open **3** Percutaneous **4** Percutaneous Endoscopic **7** Via Natural or Artificial Opening **8** Via Natural or Artificial Opening Endoscopic **X** External	**Z** No Device	**Z** No Qualifier
M Vulva ⊘ ♀	**0** Open **X** External	**Z** No Device	**Z** No Qualifier

♀ 0UJ30ZZ 0UJ33ZZ 0UJ34ZZ 0UJ3XZZ 0UJ80ZZ 0UJ83ZZ 0UJ84ZZ 0UJ87ZZ 0UJ88ZZ 0UJ8XZZ 0UJD0ZZ 0UJD3ZZ 0UJD4ZZ 0UJD7ZZ 0UJD8ZZ 0UJDXZZ 0UJH0ZZ 0UJH3ZZ 0UJH4ZZ 0UJH7ZZ 0UJH8ZZ 0UJHXZZ 0UJM0ZZ 0UJMXZZ

⊘ 0UJ33ZZ 0UJ3XZZ 0UJ83ZZ 0UJ87ZZ 0UJ88ZZ 0UJ8XZZ 0UJD3ZZ 0UJD7ZZ 0UJD8ZZ 0UJDXZZ 0UJH3ZZ 0UJH7ZZ 0UJH8ZZ 0UJHXZZ 0UJMXZZ

LC Limited Coverage NC Noncovered HAC HAC Associated Procedure CC Combination Cluster - See Appendix G for code lists
DRG Non-OR-Affecting MS-DRG Assignment ⊘ Non-OR-Not Affecting MS-DRG Assignment New/Revised Text in **Orange** ♂ Male ♀ Female

0 Medical and Surgical
U Female Reproductive System
L Occlusion: Completely closing an orifice or the lumen of a tubular body part

Body Part Character 4	Approach Character 5	Device Character 6	Qualifier Character 7
5 Fallopian Tube, Right ♀ **6** Fallopian Tube, Left ♀ **7** Fallopian Tubes, Bilateral NC ♀	**0** Open **3** Percutaneous **4** Percutaneous Endoscopic	**C** Extraluminal Device **D** Intraluminal Device **Z** No Device	**Z** No Qualifier
5 Fallopian Tube, Right ♀ **6** Fallopian Tube, Left ♀ **7** Fallopian Tubes, Bilateral NC ♀	**7** Via Natural or Artificial Opening **8** Via Natural or Artificial Opening Endoscopic	**D** Intraluminal Device **Z** No Device	**Z** No Qualifier
F Cul-de-sac ♀ **G** Vagina ♀	**7** Via Natural or Artificial Opening **8** Via Natural or Artificial Opening Endoscopic	**D** Intraluminal Device **Z** No Device	**Z** No Qualifier

♀ 0UL50CZ 0UL50DZ 0UL50ZZ 0UL53CZ 0UL53DZ 0UL53ZZ 0UL54CZ 0UL54DZ 0UL54ZZ 0UL57DZ 0UL57ZZ 0UL58DZ 0UL58ZZ 0UL60CZ 0UL60DZ 0UL60ZZ 0UL63CZ 0UL63DZ 0UL63ZZ 0UL64CZ 0UL64DZ 0UL64ZZ 0UL67DZ 0UL67ZZ 0UL68DZ 0UL68ZZ 0UL70CZ 0UL70DZ 0UL70ZZ 0UL73CZ 0UL73DZ 0UL73ZZ 0UL74CZ 0UL74DZ 0UL74ZZ 0UL77DZ 0UL77ZZ 0UL78DZ 0UL78ZZ 0ULF7DZ 0ULF7ZZ 0ULF8DZ 0ULF8ZZ 0ULG7DZ 0ULG7ZZ 0ULG8DZ 0ULG8ZZ

NC 0UL70CZ 0UL70DZ 0UL70ZZ 0UL73CZ 0UL73DZ 0UL73ZZ 0UL74CZ 0UL74DZ 0UL74ZZ 0UL77DZ 0UL77ZZ 0UL78DZ 0UL78ZZ
Codes with the NC symbol are identified as noncovered procedures only when diagnosis code Z30.2 is listed as the principal diagnosis.

0 Medical and Surgical
U Female Reproductive System
M Reattachment: Putting back in or on all or a portion of a separated body part to its normal location or other suitable location

Body Part Character 4	Approach Character 5	Device Character 6	Qualifier Character 7
0 Ovary, Right ♀ **1** Ovary, Left ♀ **2** Ovaries, Bilateral ♀ **4** Uterine Supporting Structure ♀ **5** Fallopian Tube, Right ♀ **6** Fallopian Tube, Left ♀ **7** Fallopian Tubes, Bilateral ♀ **9** Uterus ♀ **C** Cervix ♀ **F** Cul-de-sac ♀ **G** Vagina ♀	**0** Open **4** Percutaneous Endoscopic	**Z** No Device	**Z** No Qualifier
J Clitoris ♀ **M** Vulva ♀	**X** External	**Z** No Device	**Z** No Qualifier
K Hymen ♀	**0** Open **4** Percutaneous Endoscopic **X** External	**Z** No Device	**Z** No Qualifier

♀ 0UM00ZZ 0UM04ZZ 0UM10ZZ 0UM14ZZ 0UM20ZZ 0UM24ZZ 0UM40ZZ 0UM44ZZ 0UM50ZZ 0UM54ZZ 0UM60ZZ 0UM64ZZ 0UM70ZZ 0UM74ZZ 0UM90ZZ 0UM94ZZ 0UMC0ZZ 0UMC4ZZ 0UMF0ZZ 0UMF4ZZ 0UMG0ZZ 0UMG4ZZ 0UMJXZZ 0UMK0ZZ 0UMK4ZZ 0UMKXZZ 0UMMXZZ

0 Medical and Surgical
U Female Reproductive System
N Release: Freeing a body part from an abnormal physical constraint by cutting or by the use of force

Body Part Character 4	Approach Character 5	Device Character 6	Qualifier Character 7
0 Ovary, Right ♀ **1** Ovary, Left ♀ **2** Ovaries, Bilateral ♀ **4** Uterine Supporting Structure ♀	**0** Open **3** Percutaneous **4** Percutaneous Endoscopic	**Z** No Device	**Z** No Qualifier
5 Fallopian Tube, Right ♀ **6** Fallopian Tube, Left ♀ **7** Fallopian Tubes, Bilateral ♀ **9** Uterus ♀ **C** Cervix ♀ **F** Cul-de-sac ♀	**0** Open **3** Percutaneous **4** Percutaneous Endoscopic **7** Via Natural or Artificial Opening **8** Via Natural or Artificial Opening Endoscopic	**Z** No Device	**Z** No Qualifier
G Vagina ♀ **K** Hymen ♀	**0** Open **3** Percutaneous **4** Percutaneous Endoscopic **7** Via Natural or Artificial Opening **8** Via Natural or Artificial Opening Endoscopic **X** External	**Z** No Device	**Z** No Qualifier
J Clitoris ♀ **L** Vestibular Gland ♀ **M** Vulva ♀	**0** Open **X** External	**Z** No Device	**Z** No Qualifier

♀ 0UN00ZZ 0UN03ZZ 0UN04ZZ 0UN10ZZ 0UN13ZZ 0UN14ZZ 0UN20ZZ 0UN23ZZ 0UN24ZZ 0UN40ZZ 0UN43ZZ 0UN44ZZ 0UN50ZZ 0UN53ZZ 0UN54ZZ 0UN57ZZ 0UN58ZZ 0UN60ZZ 0UN63ZZ 0UN64ZZ 0UN67ZZ 0UN68ZZ 0UN70ZZ 0UN73ZZ 0UN74ZZ 0UN77ZZ 0UN78ZZ 0UN90ZZ 0UN93ZZ 0UN94ZZ 0UN97ZZ 0UN98ZZ 0UNC0ZZ 0UNC3ZZ 0UNC4ZZ 0UNC7ZZ 0UNC8ZZ 0UNF0ZZ 0UNF3ZZ 0UNF4ZZ 0UNF7ZZ 0UNF8ZZ 0UNG0ZZ 0UNG3ZZ 0UNG4ZZ 0UNG7ZZ 0UNG8ZZ 0UNGXZZ 0UNJ0ZZ 0UNJXZZ 0UNK0ZZ 0UNK3ZZ 0UNK4ZZ 0UNK7ZZ 0UNK8ZZ 0UNKXZZ 0UNL0ZZ 0UNLXZZ 0UNM0ZZ 0UNMXZZ

0 Medical and Surgical
U Female Reproductive System
P Removal: Taking out or off a device from a body part

Body Part Character 4	Approach Character 5	Device Character 6	Qualifier Character 7
3 Ovary ⊘ ♀	**0** Open **3** Percutaneous **4** Percutaneous Endoscopic **X** External	**0** Drainage Device **3** Infusion Device	**Z** No Qualifier
8 Fallopian Tube ♀ ⊘	**0** Open **3** Percutaneous **4** Percutaneous Endoscopic **7** Via Natural or Artificial Opening **8** Via Natural or Artificial Opening Endoscopic	**0** Drainage Device **3** Infusion Device **7** Autologous Tissue Substitute **C** Extraluminal Device **D** Intraluminal Device **J** Synthetic Substitute **K** Nonautologous Tissue Substitute	**Z** No Qualifier
8 Fallopian Tube ⊘ ♀	**X** External	**0** Drainage Device **3** Infusion Device **D** Intraluminal Device	**Z** No Qualifier
D Uterus and Cervix ⊘ ♀	**0** Open **3** Percutaneous **4** Percutaneous Endoscopic **7** Via Natural or Artificial Opening **8** Via Natural or Artificial Opening Endoscopic	**0** Drainage Device **1** Radioactive Element **3** Infusion Device **7** Autologous Tissue Substitute **C** Extraluminal Device **D** Intraluminal Device **H** Contraceptive Device **J** Synthetic Substitute **K** Nonautologous Tissue Substitute	**Z** No Qualifier

0UP continued on next page

0UP continued from previous page

0 Medical and Surgical
U Female Reproductive System
P Removal: Taking out or off a device from a body part

Body Part Character 4	Approach Character 5	Device Character 6	Qualifier Character 7
D Uterus and Cervix ⃠ ♀	**X** External	**0** Drainage Device **3** Infusion Device **D** Intraluminal Device **H** Contraceptive Device	**Z** No Qualifier
H Vagina and Cul-de-sac ⃠ ♀	**0** Open **3** Percutaneous **4** Percutaneous Endoscopic **7** Via Natural or Artificial Opening **8** Via Natural or Artificial Opening Endoscopic	**0** Drainage Device **1** Radioactive Element **3** Infusion Device **7** Autologous Tissue Substitute **D** Intraluminal Device **J** Synthetic Substitute **K** Nonautologous Tissue Substitute	**Z** No Qualifier
H Vagina and Cul-de-sac ⃠ ♀	**X** External	**0** Drainage Device **1** Radioactive Element **3** Infusion Device **D** Intraluminal Device	**Z** No Qualifier
M Vulva ♀	**0** Open	**0** Drainage Device **7** Autologous Tissue Substitute **J** Synthetic Substitute **K** Nonautologous Tissue Substitute	**Z** No Qualifier
M Vulva ⃠ ♀	**X** External	**0** Drainage Device	**Z** No Qualifier

♀ 0UP300Z 0UP303Z 0UP330Z 0UP333Z 0UP340Z 0UP343Z 0UP3X0Z 0UP3X3Z 0UP800Z 0UP803Z 0UP807Z 0UP80CZ 0UP80DZ 0UP80JZ 0UP80KZ 0UP830Z 0UP833Z 0UP837Z 0UP83CZ 0UP83DZ 0UP83JZ 0UP83KZ 0UP840Z 0UP843Z 0UP847Z 0UP84CZ 0UP84DZ 0UP84JZ 0UP84KZ 0UP870Z 0UP873Z 0UP877Z 0UP87CZ 0UP87DZ 0UP87JZ 0UP87KZ 0UP880Z 0UP883Z 0UP887Z 0UP88CZ 0UP88DZ 0UP88JZ 0UP88KZ 0UP8X0Z 0UP8X3Z 0UP8XDZ 0UPD00Z 0UPD01Z 0UPD03Z 0UPD07Z 0UPD0CZ 0UPD0DZ 0UPD0HZ 0UPD0JZ 0UPD0KZ 0UPD30Z 0UPD31Z 0UPD33Z 0UPD37Z 0UPD3CZ 0UPD3DZ 0UPD3HZ 0UPD3JZ 0UPD3KZ 0UPD40Z 0UPD41Z 0UPD43Z 0UPD47Z 0UPD4CZ 0UPD4DZ 0UPD4HZ 0UPD4JZ 0UPD4KZ 0UPD70Z 0UPD71Z 0UPD73Z 0UPD77Z 0UPD7CZ 0UPD7DZ 0UPD7HZ 0UPD7JZ 0UPD7KZ 0UPD80Z 0UPD81Z 0UPD83Z 0UPD87Z 0UPD8CZ 0UPD8DZ 0UPD8HZ 0UPD8JZ 0UPD8KZ 0UPDX0Z 0UPDX3Z 0UPDXDZ 0UPDXHZ 0UPH00Z 0UPH01Z 0UPH03Z 0UPH07Z 0UPH0DZ 0UPH0JZ 0UPH0KZ 0UPH30Z 0UPH31Z 0UPH33Z 0UPH37Z 0UPH3DZ 0UPH3JZ 0UPH3KZ 0UPH40Z 0UPH41Z 0UPH43Z 0UPH47Z 0UPH4DZ 0UPH4JZ 0UPH4KZ 0UPH70Z 0UPH71Z 0UPH73Z 0UPH77Z 0UPH7DZ 0UPH7JZ 0UPH7KZ 0UPH80Z 0UPH81Z 0UPH83Z 0UPH87Z 0UPH8DZ 0UPH8JZ 0UPH8KZ 0UPHX0Z 0UPHX1Z 0UPHX3Z 0UPHXDZ 0UPM00Z 0UPM07Z 0UPM0JZ 0UPM0KZ 0UPMX0Z

⃠ 0UP3X0Z 0UP3X3Z 0UP870Z 0UP873Z 0UP87DZ 0UP880Z 0UP883Z 0UP88DZ 0UP8X0Z 0UP8X3Z 0UP8XDZ 0UPD3CZ 0UPD4CZ 0UPD70Z 0UPD73Z 0UPD7CZ 0UPD7DZ 0UPD7HZ 0UPD80Z 0UPD83Z 0UPD8CZ 0UPD8DZ 0UPD8HZ 0UPDX0Z 0UPDX3Z 0UPDXDZ 0UPDXHZ 0UPH70Z 0UPH73Z 0UPH7DZ 0UPH80Z 0UPH83Z 0UPH8DZ 0UPHX0Z 0UPHX1Z 0UPHX3Z 0UPHXDZ 0UPMX0Z

0 Medical and Surgical
U Female Reproductive System
Q Repair: Restoring, to the extent possible, a body part to its normal anatomic structure and function

Body Part Character 4	Approach Character 5	Device Character 6	Qualifier Character 7
0 Ovary, Right CC ♀ **1** Ovary, Left CC ♀ **2** Ovaries, Bilateral CC ♀ **4** Uterine Supporting Structure ♀	**0** Open **3** Percutaneous **4** Percutaneous Endoscopic	**Z** No Device	**Z** No Qualifier
5 Fallopian Tube, Right CC ♀ **6** Fallopian Tube, Left CC ♀ **7** Fallopian Tubes, Bilateral CC ♀ **9** Uterus ♀ **C** Cervix ♀ **F** Cul-de-sac ♀	**0** Open **3** Percutaneous **4** Percutaneous Endoscopic **7** Via Natural or Artificial Opening **8** Via Natural or Artificial Opening Endoscopic	**Z** No Device	**Z** No Qualifier
G Vagina ♀ **K** Hymen ♀	**0** Open **3** Percutaneous **4** Percutaneous Endoscopic **7** Via Natural or Artificial Opening **8** Via Natural or Artificial Opening Endoscopic **X** External	**Z** No Device	**Z** No Qualifier
J Clitoris ♀ **L** Vestibular Gland ♀ **M** Vulva CC ♀	**0** Open **X** External	**Z** No Device	**Z** No Qualifier

♀ 0UQ00ZZ 0UQ03ZZ 0UQ04ZZ 0UQ10ZZ 0UQ13ZZ 0UQ14ZZ 0UQ20ZZ 0UQ23ZZ 0UQ24ZZ 0UQ40ZZ 0UQ43ZZ 0UQ44ZZ 0UQ50ZZ 0UQ53ZZ 0UQ54ZZ 0UQ57ZZ 0UQ58ZZ 0UQ60ZZ 0UQ63ZZ 0UQ64ZZ 0UQ67ZZ 0UQ68ZZ 0UQ70ZZ 0UQ73ZZ 0UQ74ZZ 0UQ77ZZ 0UQ78ZZ 0UQ90ZZ 0UQ93ZZ 0UQ94ZZ 0UQ97ZZ 0UQ98ZZ 0UQC0ZZ 0UQC3ZZ 0UQC4ZZ 0UQC7ZZ 0UQC8ZZ 0UQF0ZZ 0UQF3ZZ 0UQF4ZZ 0UQF7ZZ 0UQF8ZZ 0UQG0ZZ 0UQG3ZZ 0UQG4ZZ 0UQG7ZZ 0UQG8ZZ 0UQGXZZ 0UQJ0ZZ 0UQJXZZ 0UQK0ZZ 0UQK3ZZ 0UQK4ZZ 0UQK7ZZ 0UQK8ZZ 0UQKXZZ 0UQL0ZZ 0UQLXZZ 0UQM0ZZ 0UQMXZZ

CC 0UQ00ZZ 0UQ03ZZ 0UQ04ZZ 0UQ10ZZ 0UQ13ZZ 0UQ14ZZ 0UQ20ZZ 0UQ23ZZ 0UQ24ZZ 0UQ50ZZ 0UQ53ZZ 0UQ54ZZ 0UQ60ZZ 0UQ63ZZ 0UQ64ZZ 0UQ70ZZ 0UQ73ZZ 0UQ74ZZ 0UQM0ZZ 0UQMXZZ

0 Medical and Surgical
U Female Reproductive System
S Reposition: Moving to its normal location, or other suitable location, all or a portion of a body part

Body Part Character 4	Approach Character 5	Device Character 6	Qualifier Character 7
0 Ovary, Right ♀ **1** Ovary, Left ♀ **2** Ovaries, Bilateral ♀ **4** Uterine Supporting Structure ♀ **5** Fallopian Tube, Right ♀ **6** Fallopian Tube, Left ♀ **7** Fallopian Tubes, Bilateral ♀ **C** Cervix ♀ **F** Cul-de-sac ♀	**0** Open **4** Percutaneous Endoscopic	**Z** No Device	**Z** No Qualifier
9 Uterus ⊘ ♀ **G** Vagina ♀	**0** Open **4** Percutaneous Endoscopic **X** External	**Z** No Device	**Z** No Qualifier

♀ 0US00ZZ 0US04ZZ 0US10ZZ 0US14ZZ 0US20ZZ 0US24ZZ 0US40ZZ 0US44ZZ 0US50ZZ 0US54ZZ 0US60ZZ 0US64ZZ 0US70ZZ 0US74ZZ 0US90ZZ 0US94ZZ 0US9XZZ 0USC0ZZ 0USC4ZZ 0USF0ZZ 0USF4ZZ 0USG0ZZ 0USG4ZZ 0USGXZZ

⊘ 0US9XZZ

0 Medical and Surgical
U Female Reproductive System
T Resection: Cutting out or off, without replacement, all of a body part

Body Part Character 4	Approach Character 5	Device Character 6	Qualifier Character 7
0 Ovary, Right CC ♀ **1** Ovary, Left CC ♀ **2** Ovaries, Bilateral CC ♀ **5** Fallopian Tube, Right CC ♀ **6** Fallopian Tube, Left CC ♀ **7** Fallopian Tubes, Bilateral CC ♀ **9** Uterus CC ♀	**0** Open **4** Percutaneous Endoscopic **7** Via Natural or Artificial Opening **8** Via Natural or Artificial Opening Endoscopic **F** Via Natural or Artificial Opening With Percutaneous Endoscopic Assistance	**Z** No Device	**Z** No Qualifier
4 Uterine Supporting Structure CC ♀ **C** Cervix CC ♀ **F** Cul-de-sac ♀ **G** Vagina CC ♀	**0** Open **4** Percutaneous Endoscopic **7** Via Natural or Artificial Opening **8** Via Natural or Artificial Opening Endoscopic	**Z** No Device	**Z** No Qualifier
J Clitoris ♀ **L** Vestibular Gland ♀ **M** Vulva CC ♀	**0** Open **X** External	**Z** No Device	**Z** No Qualifier
K Hymen ♀	**0** Open **4** Percutaneous Endoscopic **7** Via Natural or Artificial Opening **8** Via Natural or Artificial Opening Endoscopic **X** External	**Z** No Device	**Z** No Qualifier

♀ 0UT00ZZ 0UT04ZZ 0UT07ZZ 0UT08ZZ 0UT0FZZ 0UT10ZZ 0UT14ZZ 0UT17ZZ 0UT18ZZ 0UT1FZZ 0UT20ZZ 0UT24ZZ 0UT27ZZ 0UT28ZZ 0UT2FZZ 0UT40ZZ 0UT44ZZ 0UT47ZZ 0UT48ZZ 0UT50ZZ 0UT54ZZ 0UT57ZZ 0UT58ZZ 0UT5FZZ 0UT60ZZ 0UT64ZZ 0UT67ZZ 0UT68ZZ 0UT6FZZ 0UT70ZZ 0UT74ZZ 0UT77ZZ 0UT78ZZ 0UT7FZZ 0UT90ZZ 0UT94ZZ 0UT97ZZ 0UT98ZZ 0UT9FZZ 0UTC0ZZ 0UTC4ZZ 0UTC7ZZ 0UTC8ZZ 0UTF0ZZ 0UTF4ZZ 0UTF7ZZ 0UTF8ZZ 0UTG0ZZ 0UTG4ZZ 0UTG7ZZ 0UTG8ZZ 0UTJ0ZZ 0UTJXZZ 0UTK0ZZ 0UTK4ZZ 0UTK7ZZ 0UTK8ZZ 0UTKXZZ 0UTL0ZZ 0UTLXZZ 0UTM0ZZ 0UTMXZZ

CC 0UT00ZZ 0UT04ZZ 0UT10ZZ 0UT14ZZ 0UT20ZZ 0UT24ZZ 0UT40ZZ 0UT44ZZ 0UT47ZZ 0UT48ZZ 0UT50ZZ 0UT54ZZ 0UT60ZZ 0UT64ZZ 0UT70ZZ 0UT74ZZ 0UT90ZZ 0UT94ZZ 0UT97ZZ 0UT98ZZ 0UT9FZZ 0UTC0ZZ 0UTC4ZZ 0UTC7ZZ 0UTC8ZZ 0UTG0ZZ 0UTM0ZZ 0UTMXZZ

0 Medical and Surgical
U Female Reproductive System
U Supplement: Putting in or on biological or synthetic material that physically reinforces and/or augments the function of a portion of a body part

Body Part Character 4	Approach Character 5	Device Character 6	Qualifier Character 7
4 Uterine Supporting Structure ♀	**0** Open **4** Percutaneous Endoscopic	**7** Autologous Tissue Substitute **J** Synthetic Substitute **K** Nonautologous Tissue Substitute	**Z** No Qualifier
5 Fallopian Tube, Right ♀ **6** Fallopian Tube, Left ♀ **7** Fallopian Tubes, Bilateral ♀ **F** Cul-de-sac ♀	**0** Open **4** Percutaneous Endoscopic **7** Via Natural or Artificial Opening **8** Via Natural or Artificial Opening Endoscopic	**7** Autologous Tissue Substitute **J** Synthetic Substitute **K** Nonautologous Tissue Substitute	**Z** No Qualifier
G Vagina ♀ **K** Hymen ♀	**0** Open **4** Percutaneous Endoscopic **7** Via Natural or Artificial Opening **8** Via Natural or Artificial Opening Endoscopic **X** External	**7** Autologous Tissue Substitute **J** Synthetic Substitute **K** Nonautologous Tissue Substitute	**Z** No Qualifier
J Clitoris ♀ **M** Vulva ♀	**0** Open **X** External	**7** Autologous Tissue Substitute **J** Synthetic Substitute **K** Nonautologous Tissue Substitute	**Z** No Qualifier

♀ 0UU407Z 0UU40JZ 0UU40KZ 0UU447Z 0UU44JZ 0UU44KZ 0UU507Z 0UU50JZ 0UU50KZ 0UU547Z 0UU54JZ 0UU54KZ 0UU577Z 0UU57JZ 0UU57KZ 0UU587Z 0UU58JZ 0UU58KZ 0UU607Z 0UU60JZ 0UU60KZ 0UU647Z 0UU64JZ 0UU64KZ 0UU677Z 0UU67JZ

0UU continued on next page

0UU continued from previous page

0UU67KZ 0UU687Z 0UU68JZ 0UU68KZ 0UU707Z 0UU70JZ 0UU70KZ 0UU747Z 0UU74JZ 0UU74KZ 0UU777Z 0UU77JZ 0UU77KZ
0UU787Z 0UU78JZ 0UU78KZ 0UUF07Z 0UUF0JZ 0UUF0KZ 0UUF47Z 0UUF4JZ 0UUF4KZ 0UUF77Z 0UUF7JZ 0UUF7KZ 0UUF87Z
0UUF8JZ 0UUF8KZ 0UUG07Z 0UUG0JZ 0UUG0KZ 0UUG47Z 0UUG4JZ 0UUG4KZ 0UUG77Z 0UUG7JZ 0UUG7KZ 0UUG87Z 0UUG8JZ
0UUG8KZ 0UUGX7Z 0UUGXJZ 0UUGXKZ 0UUJ07Z 0UUJ0JZ 0UUJ0KZ 0UUJX7Z 0UUJXJZ 0UUJXKZ 0UUK07Z 0UUK0JZ 0UUK0KZ
0UUK47Z 0UUK4JZ 0UUK4KZ 0UUK77Z 0UUK7JZ 0UUK7KZ 0UUK87Z 0UUK8JZ 0UUK8KZ 0UUKX7Z 0UUKXJZ 0UUKXKZ 0UUM07Z
0UUM0JZ 0UUM0KZ 0UUMX7Z 0UUMXJZ 0UUMXKZ

0 Medical and Surgical
U Female Reproductive System
V Restriction: Partially closing an orifice or the lumen of a tubular body part

Body Part Character 4	Approach Character 5	Device Character 6	Qualifier Character 7
C Cervix ♀	**0** Open **3** Percutaneous **4** Percutaneous Endoscopic	**C** Extraluminal Device **D** Intraluminal Device **Z** No Device	**Z** No Qualifier
C Cervix ♀	**7** Via Natural or Artificial Opening **8** Via Natural or Artificial Opening Endoscopic	**D** Intraluminal Device **Z** No Device	**Z** No Qualifier

♀ 0UVC0CZ 0UVC0DZ 0UVC0ZZ 0UVC3CZ 0UVC3DZ 0UVC3ZZ 0UVC4CZ 0UVC4DZ 0UVC4ZZ 0UVC7DZ 0UVC7ZZ 0UVC8DZ 0UVC8ZZ

0 Medical and Surgical
U Female Reproductive System
W Revision: Correcting, to the extent possible, a portion of a malfunctioning device or the position of a displaced device

Body Part Character 4	Approach Character 5	Device Character 6	Qualifier Character 7
3 Ovary ⊘ ♀	**0** Open **3** Percutaneous **4** Percutaneous Endoscopic **X** External	**0** Drainage Device **3** Infusion Device	**Z** No Qualifier
8 Fallopian Tube ⊘ ♀	**0** Open **3** Percutaneous **4** Percutaneous Endoscopic **7** Via Natural or Artificial Opening **8** Via Natural or Artificial Opening Endoscopic **X** External	**0** Drainage Device **3** Infusion Device **7** Autologous Tissue Substitute **C** Extraluminal Device **D** Intraluminal Device **J** Synthetic Substitute **K** Nonautologous Tissue Substitute	**Z** No Qualifier
D Uterus and Cervix ♀	**0** Open **3** Percutaneous **4** Percutaneous Endoscopic **7** Via Natural or Artificial Opening **8** Via Natural or Artificial Opening Endoscopic	**0** Drainage Device **1** Radioactive Element **3** Infusion Device **7** Autologous Tissue Substitute **C** Extraluminal Device **D** Intraluminal Device **H** Contraceptive Device **J** Synthetic Substitute **K** Nonautologous Tissue Substitute	**Z** No Qualifier
D Uterus and Cervix ⊘ ♀	**X** External	**0** Drainage Device **3** Infusion Device **7** Autologous Tissue Substitute **C** Extraluminal Device **D** Intraluminal Device **H** Contraceptive Device **J** Synthetic Substitute **K** Nonautologous Tissue Substitute	**Z** No Qualifier

0UW continued on next page

0UW continued from previous page

0 Medical and Surgical
U Female Reproductive System
W Revision: Correcting, to the extent possible, a portion of a malfunctioning device or the position of a displaced device

Body Part Character 4	Approach Character 5	Device Character 6	Qualifier Character 7
H Vagina and Cul-de-sac ♀	**0** Open **3** Percutaneous **4** Percutaneous Endoscopic **7** Via Natural or Artificial Opening **8** Via Natural or Artificial Opening Endoscopic	**0** Drainage Device **1** Radioactive Element **3** Infusion Device **7** Autologous Tissue Substitute **D** Intraluminal Device **J** Synthetic Substitute **K** Nonautologous Tissue Substitute	**Z** No Qualifier
H Vagina and Cul-de-sac ⃠ ♀	**X** External	**0** Drainage Device **3** Infusion Device **7** Autologous Tissue Substitute **D** Intraluminal Device **J** Synthetic Substitute **K** Nonautologous Tissue Substitute	**Z** No Qualifier
M Vulva ⃠ ♀	**0** Open **X** External	**0** Drainage Device **7** Autologous Tissue Substitute **J** Synthetic Substitute **K** Nonautologous Tissue Substitute	**Z** No Qualifier

♀ 0UW300Z 0UW303Z 0UW330Z 0UW333Z 0UW340Z 0UW343Z 0UW3X0Z 0UW3X3Z 0UW800Z 0UW803Z 0UW807Z 0UW80CZ 0UW80DZ 0UW80JZ 0UW80KZ 0UW830Z 0UW833Z 0UW837Z 0UW83CZ 0UW83DZ 0UW83JZ 0UW83KZ 0UW840Z 0UW843Z 0UW847Z 0UW84CZ 0UW84DZ 0UW84JZ 0UW84KZ 0UW870Z 0UW873Z 0UW877Z 0UW87CZ 0UW87DZ 0UW87JZ 0UW87KZ 0UW880Z 0UW883Z 0UW887Z 0UW88CZ 0UW88DZ 0UW88JZ 0UW88KZ 0UW8X0Z 0UW8X3Z 0UW8X7Z 0UW8XCZ 0UW8XDZ 0UW8XJZ 0UW8XKZ 0UWD00Z 0UWD01Z 0UWD03Z 0UWD07Z 0UWD0CZ 0UWD0DZ 0UWD0HZ 0UWD0JZ 0UWD0KZ 0UWD30Z 0UWD31Z 0UWD33Z 0UWD37Z 0UWD3CZ 0UWD3DZ 0UWD3HZ 0UWD3JZ 0UWD3KZ 0UWD40Z 0UWD41Z 0UWD43Z 0UWD47Z 0UWD4CZ 0UWD4DZ 0UWD4HZ 0UWD4JZ 0UWD4KZ 0UWD70Z 0UWD71Z 0UWD73Z 0UWD77Z 0UWD7CZ 0UWD7DZ 0UWD7HZ 0UWD7JZ 0UWD7KZ 0UWD80Z 0UWD81Z 0UWD83Z 0UWD87Z 0UWD8CZ 0UWD8DZ 0UWD8HZ 0UWD8JZ 0UWD8KZ 0UWDX0Z 0UWDX3Z 0UWDX7Z 0UWDXCZ 0UWDXDZ 0UWDXHZ 0UWDXJZ 0UWDXKZ 0UWH00Z 0UWH01Z 0UWH03Z 0UWH07Z 0UWH0DZ 0UWH0JZ 0UWH0KZ 0UWH30Z 0UWH31Z 0UWH33Z 0UWH37Z 0UWH3DZ 0UWH3JZ 0UWH3KZ 0UWH40Z 0UWH41Z 0UWH43Z 0UWH47Z 0UWH4DZ 0UWH4JZ 0UWH4KZ 0UWH70Z 0UWH71Z 0UWH73Z 0UWH77Z 0UWH7DZ 0UWH7JZ 0UWH7KZ 0UWH80Z 0UWH81Z 0UWH83Z 0UWH87Z 0UWH8DZ 0UWH8JZ 0UWH8KZ 0UWHX0Z 0UWHX3Z 0UWHX7Z 0UWHXDZ 0UWHXJZ 0UWHXKZ 0UWM00Z 0UWM07Z 0UWM0JZ 0UWM0KZ 0UWMX0Z 0UWMX7Z 0UWMXJZ 0UWMXKZ

⃠ 0UW3X0Z 0UW3X3Z 0UW8X0Z 0UW8X3Z 0UW8X7Z 0UW8XCZ 0UW8XDZ 0UW8XJZ 0UW8XKZ 0UWDX0Z 0UWDX3Z 0UWDX7Z 0UWDXCZ 0UWDXDZ 0UWDXHZ 0UWDXJZ 0UWDXKZ 0UWHX0Z 0UWHX3Z 0UWHX7Z 0UWHXDZ 0UWHXJZ 0UWHXKZ 0UWMX0Z 0UWMX7Z 0UWMXJZ 0UWMXKZ

0 Medical and Surgical
U Female Reproductive System
Y Transplantation: Putting in or on all or a portion of a living body part taken from another individual or animal to physically take the place and/or function of all or a portion of a similar body part

Body Part Character 4	Approach Character 5	Device Character 6	Qualifier Character 7
0 Ovary, Right ♀ **1** Ovary, Left ♀	**0** Open	**Z** No Device	**0** Allogeneic **1** Syngeneic **2** Zooplastic

♀ 0UY00Z0 0UY00Z1 0UY00Z2 0UY10Z0 0UY10Z1 0UY10Z2

Male Reproductive System 0V1-0VW

0 Medical and Surgical
V Male Reproductive System
1 Bypass: Altering the route of passage of the contents of a tubular body part

Body Part Character 4	Approach Character 5	Device Character 6	Qualifier Character 7
N Vas Deferens, Right ♂ **P** Vas Deferens, Left ♂ **Q** Vas Deferens, Bilateral ♂	**0** Open **4** Percutaneous Endoscopic	**7** Autologous Tissue Substitute **J** Synthetic Substitute **K** Nonautologous Tissue Substitute **Z** No Device	**J** Epididymis, Right **K** Epididymis, Left **N** Vas Deferens, Right **P** Vas Deferens, Left

♂ 0V1N07J 0V1N07K 0V1N07N 0V1N07P 0V1N0JJ 0V1N0JK 0V1N0JN 0V1N0JP 0V1N0KJ 0V1N0KK 0V1N0KN 0V1N0KP 0V1N0ZJ 0V1N0ZK 0V1N0ZN 0V1N0ZP 0V1N47J 0V1N47K 0V1N47N 0V1N47P 0V1N4JJ 0V1N4JK 0V1N4JN 0V1N4JP 0V1N4KJ 0V1N4KK 0V1N4KN 0V1N4KP 0V1N4ZJ 0V1N4ZK 0V1N4ZN 0V1N4ZP 0V1P07J 0V1P07K 0V1P07N 0V1P07P 0V1P0JJ 0V1P0JK 0V1P0JN 0V1P0JP 0V1P0KJ 0V1P0KK 0V1P0KN 0V1P0KP 0V1P0ZJ 0V1P0ZK 0V1P0ZN 0V1P0ZP 0V1P47J 0V1P47K 0V1P47N 0V1P47P 0V1P4JJ 0V1P4JK 0V1P4JN 0V1P4JP 0V1P4KJ 0V1P4KK 0V1P4KN 0V1P4KP 0V1P4ZJ 0V1P4ZK 0V1P4ZN 0V1P4ZP 0V1Q07J 0V1Q07K 0V1Q07N 0V1Q07P 0V1Q0JJ 0V1Q0JK 0V1Q0JN 0V1Q0JP 0V1Q0KJ 0V1Q0KK 0V1Q0KN 0V1Q0KP 0V1Q0ZJ 0V1Q0ZK 0V1Q0ZN 0V1Q0ZP 0V1Q47J 0V1Q47K 0V1Q47N 0V1Q47P 0V1Q4JJ 0V1Q4JK 0V1Q4JN 0V1Q4JP 0V1Q4KJ 0V1Q4KK 0V1Q4KN 0V1Q4KP 0V1Q4ZJ 0V1Q4ZK 0V1Q4ZN 0V1Q4ZP

0 Medical and Surgical
V Male Reproductive System
2 Change: Taking out or off a device from a body part and putting back an identical or similar device in or on the same body part without cutting or puncturing the skin or a mucous membrane

Body Part Character 4	Approach Character 5	Device Character 6	Qualifier Character 7
4 Prostate and Seminal Vesicles ⊘ ♂ **8** Scrotum and Tunica Vaginalis ⊘ ♂ **D** Testis ⊘ ♂ **M** Epididymis and Spermatic Cord ⊘ ♂ **R** Vas Deferens ⊘ ♂ **S** Penis ⊘ ♂	**X** External	**0** Drainage Device **Y** Other Device	**Z** No Qualifier

♂ 0V24X0Z 0V24XYZ 0V28X0Z 0V28XYZ 0V2DX0Z 0V2DXYZ 0V2MX0Z 0V2MXYZ 0V2RX0Z 0V2RXYZ 0V2SX0Z 0V2SXYZ
⊘ 0V24X0Z 0V24XYZ 0V28X0Z 0V28XYZ 0V2DX0Z 0V2DXYZ 0V2MX0Z 0V2MXYZ 0V2RX0Z 0V2RXYZ 0V2SX0Z 0V2SXYZ

0 Medical and Surgical
V Male Reproductive System
5 Destruction: Physical eradication of all or a portion of a body part by the direct use of energy, force, or a destructive agent

Body Part Character 4	Approach Character 5	Device Character 6	Qualifier Character 7
0 Prostate ♂	**0** Open **3** Percutaneous **4** Percutaneous Endoscopic **7** Via Natural or Artificial Opening **8** Via Natural or Artificial Opening Endoscopic	**Z** No Device	**Z** No Qualifier
1 Seminal Vesicle, Right ♂ **2** Seminal Vesicle, Left ♂ **3** Seminal Vesicles, Bilateral ♂ **6** Tunica Vaginalis, Right ♂ **7** Tunica Vaginalis, Left ♂ **9** Testis, Right ♂ **B** Testis, Left ♂ **C** Testes, Bilateral ♂ **F** Spermatic Cord, Right ♂ **G** Spermatic Cord, Left ♂ **H** Spermatic Cords, Bilateral ♂ **J** Epididymis, Right ♂ **K** Epididymis, Left ♂ **L** Epididymis, Bilateral ♂ **N** Vas Deferens, Right NC ⃠ ♂ **P** Vas Deferens, Left NC ⃠ ♂ **Q** Vas Deferens, Bilateral NC ⃠ ♂	**0** Open **3** Percutaneous **4** Percutaneous Endoscopic	**Z** No Device	**Z** No Qualifier
5 Scrotum ⃠ ♂ **S** Penis ♂ **T** Prepuce ♂	**0** Open **3** Percutaneous **4** Percutaneous Endoscopic **X** External	**Z** No Device	**Z** No Qualifier

♂ 0V500ZZ 0V503ZZ 0V504ZZ 0V507ZZ 0V508ZZ 0V510ZZ 0V513ZZ 0V514ZZ 0V520ZZ 0V523ZZ 0V524ZZ 0V530ZZ 0V533ZZ 0V534ZZ 0V550ZZ 0V553ZZ 0V554ZZ 0V55XZZ 0V560ZZ 0V563ZZ 0V564ZZ 0V570ZZ 0V573ZZ 0V574ZZ 0V590ZZ 0V593ZZ 0V594ZZ 0V5B0ZZ 0V5B3ZZ 0V5B4ZZ 0V5C0ZZ 0V5C3ZZ 0V5C4ZZ 0V5F0ZZ 0V5F3ZZ 0V5F4ZZ 0V5G0ZZ 0V5G3ZZ 0V5G4ZZ 0V5H0ZZ 0V5H3ZZ 0V5H4ZZ 0V5J0ZZ 0V5J3ZZ 0V5J4ZZ 0V5K0ZZ 0V5K3ZZ 0V5K4ZZ 0V5L0ZZ 0V5L3ZZ 0V5L4ZZ 0V5N0ZZ 0V5N3ZZ 0V5N4ZZ 0V5P0ZZ 0V5P3ZZ 0V5P4ZZ 0V5Q0ZZ 0V5Q3ZZ 0V5Q4ZZ 0V5S0ZZ 0V5S3ZZ 0V5S4ZZ 0V5SXZZ 0V5T0ZZ 0V5T3ZZ 0V5T4ZZ 0V5TXZZ

⃠ 0V550ZZ 0V553ZZ 0V554ZZ 0V55XZZ 0V5N0ZZ 0V5N3ZZ 0V5N4ZZ 0V5P0ZZ 0V5P3ZZ 0V5P4ZZ 0V5Q0ZZ 0V5Q3ZZ 0V5Q4ZZ

NC 0V5N0ZZ 0V5N3ZZ 0V5N4ZZ 0V5P0ZZ 0V5P3ZZ 0V5P4ZZ 0V5Q0ZZ 0V5Q3ZZ or 0V5Q4ZZ when diagnosis code Z30.2 is listed as the principal diagnosis

0 Medical and Surgical
V Male Reproductive System
7 Dilation: Expanding an orifice or the lumen of a tubular body part

Body Part Character 4	Approach Character 5	Device Character 6	Qualifier Character 7
N Vas Deferens, Right ♂ **P** Vas Deferens, Left ♂ **Q** Vas Deferens, Bilateral ♂	**0** Open **3** Percutaneous **4** Percutaneous Endoscopic	**D** Intraluminal Device **Z** No Device	**Z** No Qualifier

♂ 0V7N0DZ 0V7N0ZZ 0V7N3DZ 0V7N3ZZ 0V7N4DZ 0V7N4ZZ 0V7P0DZ 0V7P0ZZ 0V7P3DZ 0V7P3ZZ 0V7P4DZ 0V7P4ZZ 0V7Q0DZ 0V7Q0ZZ 0V7Q3DZ 0V7Q3ZZ 0V7Q4DZ 0V7Q4ZZ

0 Medical and Surgical
V Male Reproductive System
9 Drainage: Taking or letting out fluids and/or gases from a body part

Body Part Character 4	Approach Character 5	Device Character 6	Qualifier Character 7
0 Prostate ⊘ ♂	**0** Open **3** Percutaneous **4** Percutaneous Endoscopic **7** Via Natural or Artificial Opening **8** Via Natural or Artificial Opening Endoscopic	**0** Drainage Device	**Z** No Qualifier
0 Prostate ⊘ ♂	**0** Open **3** Percutaneous **4** Percutaneous Endoscopic **7** Via Natural or Artificial Opening **8** Via Natural or Artificial Opening Endoscopic	**Z** No Device	**X** Diagnostic **Z** No Qualifier
1 Seminal Vesicle, Right ⊘ ♂ **2** Seminal Vesicle, Left ⊘ ♂ **3** Seminal Vesicles, Bilateral ⊘ ♂ **6** Tunica Vaginalis, Right ⊘ ♂ **7** Tunica Vaginalis, Left ⊘ ♂ **9** Testis, Right ⊘ ♂ **B** Testis, Left ⊘ ♂ **C** Testes, Bilateral ⊘ ♂ **F** Spermatic Cord, Right ⊘ ♂ **G** Spermatic Cord, Left ⊘ ♂ **H** Spermatic Cords, Bilateral ⊘ ♂ **J** Epididymis, Right ⊘ ♂ **K** Epididymis, Left ⊘ ♂ **L** Epididymis, Bilateral ⊘ ♂ **N** Vas Deferens, Right ⊘ ♂ **P** Vas Deferens, Left ⊘ ♂ **Q** Vas Deferens, Bilateral ⊘ ♂	**0** Open **3** Percutaneous **4** Percutaneous Endoscopic	**0** Drainage Device	**Z** No Qualifier
1 Seminal Vesicle, Right ⊘ ♂ **2** Seminal Vesicle, Left ⊘ ♂ **3** Seminal Vesicles, Bilateral ⊘ ♂ **6** Tunica Vaginalis, Right ⊘ ♂ **7** Tunica Vaginalis, Left ⊘ ♂ **9** Testis, Right ⊘ ♂ **B** Testis, Left ⊘ ♂ **C** Testes, Bilateral ⊘ ♂ **F** Spermatic Cord, Right ⊘ ♂ **G** Spermatic Cord, Left ⊘ ♂ **H** Spermatic Cords, Bilateral ⊘ ♂ **J** Epididymis, Right ⊘ ♂ **K** Epididymis, Left ⊘ ♂ **L** Epididymis, Bilateral ⊘ ♂ **N** Vas Deferens, Right ⊘ ♂ **P** Vas Deferens, Left ⊘ ♂ **Q** Vas Deferens, Bilateral ⊘ ♂	**0** Open **3** Percutaneous **4** Percutaneous Endoscopic	**Z** No Device	**X** Diagnostic **Z** No Qualifier
5 Scrotum ⊘ ♂ **S** Penis ⊘ ♂ **T** Prepuce ⊘ ♂	**0** Open **3** Percutaneous **4** Percutaneous Endoscopic **X** External	**0** Drainage Device	**Z** No Qualifier
5 Scrotum ⊘ ♂ **S** Penis ⊘ ♂ **T** Prepuce ⊘ ♂	**0** Open **3** Percutaneous **4** Percutaneous Endoscopic **X** External	**Z** No Device	**X** Diagnostic **Z** No Qualifier

♂ 0V9000Z 0V900ZX 0V900ZZ 0V9030Z 0V903ZX 0V903ZZ 0V9040Z 0V904ZX 0V904ZZ 0V9070Z 0V907ZX 0V907ZZ 0V9080Z 0V908ZX 0V908ZZ 0V9100Z 0V910ZX 0V910ZZ 0V9130Z 0V913ZX 0V913ZZ 0V9140Z 0V914ZX 0V914ZZ 0V9200Z 0V920ZX 0V920ZZ 0V9230Z 0V923ZX 0V923ZZ 0V9240Z 0V924ZX 0V924ZZ 0V9300Z 0V930ZX 0V930ZZ 0V9330Z 0V933ZX 0V933ZZ 0V9340Z 0V934ZX 0V934ZZ 0V9500Z 0V950ZX 0V950ZZ 0V9530Z 0V953ZX 0V953ZZ 0V9540Z 0V954ZX 0V954ZZ 0V95X0Z

0V9 continued on next page

0V9 continued from previous page

0V95XZX 0V95XZZ 0V9600Z 0V960ZX 0V960ZZ 0V9630Z 0V963ZX 0V963ZZ 0V9640Z 0V964ZX 0V964ZZ 0V9700Z 0V970ZX
0V970ZZ 0V9730Z 0V973ZX 0V973ZZ 0V9740Z 0V974ZX 0V974ZZ 0V9900Z 0V990ZX 0V990ZZ 0V9930Z 0V993ZX 0V993ZZ
0V9940Z 0V994ZX 0V994ZZ 0V9B00Z 0V9B0ZX 0V9B0ZZ 0V9B30Z 0V9B3ZX 0V9B3ZZ 0V9B40Z 0V9B4ZX 0V9B4ZZ 0V9C00Z
0V9C0ZX 0V9C0ZZ 0V9C30Z 0V9C3ZX 0V9C3ZZ 0V9C40Z 0V9C4ZX 0V9C4ZZ 0V9F00Z 0V9F0ZX 0V9F0ZZ 0V9F30Z 0V9F3ZX
0V9F3ZZ 0V9F40Z 0V9F4ZX 0V9F4ZZ 0V9G00Z 0V9G0ZX 0V9G0ZZ 0V9G30Z 0V9G3ZX 0V9G3ZZ 0V9G40Z 0V9G4ZX 0V9G4ZZ
0V9H00Z 0V9H0ZX 0V9H0ZZ 0V9H30Z 0V9H3ZX 0V9H3ZZ 0V9H40Z 0V9H4ZX 0V9H4ZZ 0V9J00Z 0V9J0ZX 0V9J0ZZ 0V9J30Z
0V9J3ZX 0V9J3ZZ 0V9J40Z 0V9J4ZX 0V9J4ZZ 0V9K00Z 0V9K0ZX 0V9K0ZZ 0V9K30Z 0V9K3ZX 0V9K3ZZ 0V9K40Z 0V9K4ZX
0V9K4ZZ 0V9L00Z 0V9L0ZX 0V9L0ZZ 0V9L30Z 0V9L3ZX 0V9L3ZZ 0V9L40Z 0V9L4ZX 0V9L4ZZ 0V9N00Z 0V9N0ZX 0V9N0ZZ
0V9N30Z 0V9N3ZX 0V9N3ZZ 0V9N40Z 0V9N4ZX 0V9N4ZZ 0V9P00Z 0V9P0ZX 0V9P0ZZ 0V9P30Z 0V9P3ZX 0V9P3ZZ 0V9P40Z
0V9P4ZX 0V9P4ZZ 0V9Q00Z 0V9Q0ZX 0V9Q0ZZ 0V9Q30Z 0V9Q3ZX 0V9Q3ZZ 0V9Q40Z 0V9Q4ZX 0V9Q4ZZ 0V9S00Z 0V9S0ZX
0V9S0ZZ 0V9S30Z 0V9S3ZX 0V9S3ZZ 0V9S40Z 0V9S4ZX 0V9S4ZZ 0V9SX0Z 0V9SXZX 0V9SXZZ 0V9T00Z 0V9T0ZX 0V9T0ZZ
0V9T30Z 0V9T3ZX 0V9T3ZZ 0V9T40Z 0V9T4ZX 0V9T4ZZ 0V9TX0Z 0V9TXZX 0V9TXZZ

⦸ 0V9030Z 0V903ZX 0V903ZZ 0V9040Z 0V904ZX 0V904ZZ 0V907ZX 0V908ZX 0V9130Z 0V913ZX 0V913ZZ 0V9140Z 0V914ZX
0V914ZZ 0V9230Z 0V923ZX 0V923ZZ 0V9240Z 0V924ZX 0V924ZZ 0V9330Z 0V933ZX 0V933ZZ 0V9340Z 0V934ZX 0V934ZZ
0V9500Z 0V950ZX 0V950ZZ 0V9530Z 0V953ZX 0V953ZZ 0V9540Z 0V954ZX 0V954ZZ 0V95X0Z 0V95XZX 0V95XZZ 0V9600Z
0V960ZX 0V960ZZ 0V9630Z 0V963ZX 0V963ZZ 0V9640Z 0V964ZX 0V964ZZ 0V9700Z 0V970ZX 0V970ZZ 0V9730Z 0V973ZX
0V973ZZ 0V9740Z 0V974ZX 0V974ZZ 0V9930Z 0V993ZX 0V993ZZ 0V9940Z 0V994ZX 0V994ZZ 0V9B30Z 0V9B3ZX 0V9B3ZZ
0V9B40Z 0V9B4ZX 0V9B4ZZ 0V9C30Z 0V9C3ZX 0V9C3ZZ 0V9C40Z 0V9C4ZX 0V9C4ZZ 0V9F00Z 0V9F0ZX 0V9F0ZZ 0V9F30Z
0V9F3ZX 0V9F3ZZ 0V9F40Z 0V9F4ZX 0V9F4ZZ 0V9G00Z 0V9G0ZX 0V9G0ZZ 0V9G30Z 0V9G3ZX 0V9G3ZZ 0V9G40Z 0V9G4ZX
0V9G4ZZ 0V9H00Z 0V9H0ZX 0V9H0ZZ 0V9H30Z 0V9H3ZX 0V9H3ZZ 0V9H40Z 0V9H4ZX 0V9H4ZZ 0V9J0ZX 0V9J30Z 0V9J3ZX
0V9J3ZZ 0V9J4ZX 0V9K0ZX 0V9K30Z 0V9K3ZX 0V9K3ZZ 0V9K4ZX 0V9L0ZX 0V9L30Z 0V9L3ZX 0V9L3ZZ 0V9L4ZX 0V9N00Z
0V9N0ZX 0V9N0ZZ 0V9N30Z 0V9N3ZX 0V9N3ZZ 0V9N40Z 0V9N4ZX 0V9N4ZZ 0V9P00Z 0V9P0ZX 0V9P0ZZ 0V9P30Z 0V9P3ZX
0V9P3ZZ 0V9P40Z 0V9P4ZX 0V9P4ZZ 0V9Q00Z 0V9Q0ZX 0V9Q0ZZ 0V9Q30Z 0V9Q3ZX 0V9Q3ZZ 0V9Q40Z 0V9Q4ZX 0V9Q4ZZ
0V9S30Z 0V9S3ZZ 0V9T30Z 0V9T3ZZ

0 Medical and Surgical
V Male Reproductive System
B Excision: Cutting out or off, without replacement, a portion of a body part

Body Part Character 4	Approach Character 5	Device Character 6	Qualifier Character 7
0 Prostate ⦸ ♂	**0** Open **3** Percutaneous **4** Percutaneous Endoscopic **7** Via Natural or Artificial Opening **8** Via Natural or Artificial Opening Endoscopic	**Z** No Device	**X** Diagnostic **Z** No Qualifier
1 Seminal Vesicle, Right ⦸ ♂ **2** Seminal Vesicle, Left ⦸ ♂ **3** Seminal Vesicles, Bilateral ⦸ ♂ **6** Tunica Vaginalis, Right ⦸ ♂ **7** Tunica Vaginalis, Left ⦸ ♂ **9** Testis, Right ⦸ ♂ **B** Testis, Left ⦸ ♂ **C** Testes, Bilateral ⦸ ♂ **F** Spermatic Cord, Right ⦸ ♂ **G** Spermatic Cord, Left ⦸ ♂ **H** Spermatic Cords, Bilateral ⦸ ♂ **J** Epididymis, Right ⦸ ♂ **K** Epididymis, Left ⦸ ♂ **L** Epididymis, Bilateral ⦸ ♂ **N** Vas Deferens, Right NC ⦸ ♂ **P** Vas Deferens, Left NC ⦸ ♂ **Q** Vas Deferens, Bilateral NC ⦸ ♂	**0** Open **3** Percutaneous **4** Percutaneous Endoscopic	**Z** No Device	**X** Diagnostic **Z** No Qualifier
5 Scrotum ⦸ ♂ **S** Penis ♂ **T** Prepuce ♂	**0** Open **3** Percutaneous **4** Percutaneous Endoscopic **X** External	**Z** No Device	**X** Diagnostic **Z** No Qualifier

♂ 0VB00ZX 0VB00ZZ 0VB03ZX 0VB03ZZ 0VB04ZX 0VB04ZZ 0VB07ZX 0VB07ZZ 0VB08ZX 0VB08ZZ 0VB10ZX 0VB10ZZ 0VB13ZX
0VB13ZZ 0VB14ZX 0VB14ZZ 0VB20ZX 0VB20ZZ 0VB23ZX 0VB23ZZ 0VB24ZX 0VB24ZZ 0VB30ZX 0VB30ZZ 0VB33ZX 0VB33ZZ
0VB34ZX 0VB34ZZ 0VB50ZX 0VB50ZZ 0VB53ZX 0VB53ZZ 0VB54ZX 0VB54ZZ 0VB5XZX 0VB5XZZ 0VB60ZX 0VB60ZZ 0VB63ZX
0VB63ZZ 0VB64ZX 0VB64ZZ 0VB70ZX 0VB70ZZ 0VB73ZX 0VB73ZZ 0VB74ZX 0VB74ZZ 0VB90ZX 0VB90ZZ 0VB93ZX 0VB93ZZ
0VB94ZX 0VB94ZZ 0VBB0ZX 0VBB0ZZ 0VBB3ZX 0VBB3ZZ 0VBB4ZX 0VBB4ZZ 0VBC0ZX 0VBC0ZZ 0VBC3ZX 0VBC3ZZ 0VBC4ZX
0VBC4ZZ 0VBF0ZX 0VBF0ZZ 0VBF3ZX 0VBF3ZZ 0VBF4ZX 0VBF4ZZ 0VBG0ZX 0VBG0ZZ 0VBG3ZX 0VBG3ZZ 0VBG4ZX 0VBG4ZZ
0VBH0ZX 0VBH0ZZ 0VBH3ZX 0VBH3ZZ 0VBH4ZX 0VBH4ZZ 0VBJ0ZX 0VBJ0ZZ 0VBJ3ZX 0VBJ3ZZ 0VBJ4ZX 0VBJ4ZZ 0VBK0ZX
0VBK0ZZ 0VBK3ZX 0VBK3ZZ 0VBK4ZX 0VBK4ZZ 0VBL0ZX 0VBL0ZZ 0VBL3ZX 0VBL3ZZ 0VBL4ZX 0VBL4ZZ 0VBN0ZX 0VBN0ZZ

0VB continued on next page

0VB continued from previous page

0VBN3ZX 0VBN3ZZ 0VBN4ZX 0VBN4ZZ 0VBP0ZX 0VBP0ZZ 0VBP3ZX 0VBP3ZZ 0VBP4ZX 0VBP4ZZ 0VBQ0ZX 0VBQ0ZZ 0VBQ3ZX 0VBQ3ZZ 0VBQ4ZX 0VBQ4ZZ 0VBS0ZX 0VBS0ZZ 0VBS3ZX 0VBS3ZZ 0VBS4ZX 0VBS4ZZ 0VBSXZX 0VBSXZZ 0VBT0ZX 0VBT0ZZ 0VBT3ZX 0VBT3ZZ 0VBT4ZX 0VBT4ZZ 0VBTXZX 0VBTXZZ

⦸ 0VB03ZX 0VB04ZX 0VB07ZX 0VB08ZX 0VB13ZX 0VB14ZX 0VB23ZX 0VB24ZX 0VB33ZX 0VB34ZX 0VB50ZX 0VB50ZZ 0VB53ZX 0VB53ZZ 0VB54ZX 0VB54ZZ 0VB5XZX 0VB5XZZ 0VB60ZX 0VB63ZX 0VB64ZX 0VB70ZX 0VB73ZX 0VB74ZX 0VB93ZX 0VB94ZX 0VBB3ZX 0VBB4ZX 0VBC3ZX 0VBC4ZX 0VBF0ZX 0VBF3ZX 0VBF4ZX 0VBG0ZX 0VBG3ZX 0VBG4ZX 0VBH0ZX 0VBH3ZX 0VBH4ZX 0VBJ0ZX 0VBJ3ZX 0VBJ4ZX 0VBK0ZX 0VBK3ZX 0VBK4ZX 0VBL0ZX 0VBL3ZX 0VBL4ZX 0VBN0ZX 0VBN0ZZ 0VBN3ZX 0VBN3ZZ 0VBN4ZX 0VBN4ZZ 0VBP0ZX 0VBP0ZZ 0VBP3ZX 0VBP3ZZ 0VBP4ZX 0VBP4ZZ 0VBQ0ZX 0VBQ0ZZ 0VBQ3ZX 0VBQ3ZZ 0VBQ4ZX 0VBQ4ZZ

NC 0VBN0ZZ 0VBN3ZZ 0VBN4ZZ 0VBP0ZZ 0VBP3ZZ 0VBP4ZZ 0VBQ0ZZ 0VBQ3ZZ or 0VBQ4ZZ when diagnosis code Z30.2 is listed as the principal diagnosis

0 Medical and Surgical
V Male Reproductive System
C Extirpation: Taking or cutting out solid matter from a body part

Body Part Character 4	Approach Character 5	Device Character 6	Qualifier Character 7
0 Prostate ♂	**0** Open **3** Percutaneous **4** Percutaneous Endoscopic **7** Via Natural or Artificial Opening **8** Via Natural or Artificial Opening Endoscopic	**Z** No Device	**Z** No Qualifier
1 Seminal Vesicle, Right ♂ **2** Seminal Vesicle, Left ♂ **3** Seminal Vesicles, Bilateral ♂ **6** Tunica Vaginalis, Right ⦸ ♂ **7** Tunica Vaginalis, Left ⦸ ♂ **9** Testis, Right ♂ **B** Testis, Left ♂ **C** Testes, Bilateral ♂ **F** Spermatic Cord, Right ♂ **G** Spermatic Cord, Left ♂ **H** Spermatic Cords, Bilateral ♂ **J** Epididymis, Right ♂ **K** Epididymis, Left ♂ **L** Epididymis, Bilateral ♂ **N** Vas Deferens, Right ⦸ ♂ **P** Vas Deferens, Left ⦸ ♂ **Q** Vas Deferens, Bilateral ⦸ ♂	**0** Open **3** Percutaneous **4** Percutaneous Endoscopic	**Z** No Device	**Z** No Qualifier
5 Scrotum ⦸ ♂ **S** Penis ⦸ ♂ **T** Prepuce ♂	**0** Open **3** Percutaneous **4** Percutaneous Endoscopic **X** External	**Z** No Device	**Z** No Qualifier

♂ 0VC00ZZ 0VC03ZZ 0VC04ZZ 0VC07ZZ 0VC08ZZ 0VC10ZZ 0VC13ZZ 0VC14ZZ 0VC20ZZ 0VC23ZZ 0VC24ZZ 0VC30ZZ 0VC33ZZ 0VC34ZZ 0VC50ZZ 0VC53ZZ 0VC54ZZ 0VC5XZZ 0VC60ZZ 0VC63ZZ 0VC64ZZ 0VC70ZZ 0VC73ZZ 0VC74ZZ 0VC90ZZ 0VC93ZZ 0VC94ZZ 0VCB0ZZ 0VCB3ZZ 0VCB4ZZ 0VCC0ZZ 0VCC3ZZ 0VCC4ZZ 0VCF0ZZ 0VCF3ZZ 0VCF4ZZ 0VCG0ZZ 0VCG3ZZ 0VCG4ZZ 0VCH0ZZ 0VCH3ZZ 0VCH4ZZ 0VCJ0ZZ 0VCJ3ZZ 0VCJ4ZZ 0VCK0ZZ 0VCK3ZZ 0VCK4ZZ 0VCL0ZZ 0VCL3ZZ 0VCL4ZZ 0VCN0ZZ 0VCN3ZZ 0VCN4ZZ 0VCP0ZZ 0VCP3ZZ 0VCP4ZZ 0VCQ0ZZ 0VCQ3ZZ 0VCQ4ZZ 0VCS0ZZ 0VCS3ZZ 0VCS4ZZ 0VCSXZZ 0VCT0ZZ 0VCT3ZZ 0VCT4ZZ 0VCTXZZ

⦸ 0VC50ZZ 0VC53ZZ 0VC54ZZ 0VC5XZZ 0VC60ZZ 0VC63ZZ 0VC64ZZ 0VC70ZZ 0VC73ZZ 0VC74ZZ 0VCN0ZZ 0VCN3ZZ 0VCN4ZZ 0VCP0ZZ 0VCP3ZZ 0VCP4ZZ 0VCQ0ZZ 0VCQ3ZZ 0VCQ4ZZ 0VCSXZZ

0 Medical and Surgical
V Male Reproductive System
H Insertion: Putting in a nonbiological appliance that monitors, assists, performs, or prevents a physiological function but does not physically take the place of a body part

Body Part Character 4	Approach Character 5	Device Character 6	Qualifier Character 7
0 Prostate ♂	**0** Open **3** Percutaneous **4** Percutaneous Endoscopic **7** Via Natural or Artificial Opening **8** Via Natural or Artificial Opening Endoscopic	**1** Radioactive Element	**Z** No Qualifier
4 Prostate and Seminal Vesicles ⊘ ♂ **8** Scrotum and Tunica Vaginalis ⊘ ♂ **D** Testis ⊘ ♂ **M** Epididymis and Spermatic Cord ⊘ ♂ **R** Vas Deferens ⊘ ♂	**0** Open **3** Percutaneous **4** Percutaneous Endoscopic **7** Via Natural or Artificial Opening **8** Via Natural or Artificial Opening Endoscopic	**3** Infusion Device	**Z** No Qualifier
S Penis ⊘ ♂	**0** Open **3** Percutaneous **4** Percutaneous Endoscopic **X** External	**3** Infusion Device	**Z** No Qualifier

♂ 0VH001Z 0VH031Z 0VH041Z 0VH071Z 0VH081Z 0VH403Z 0VH433Z 0VH443Z 0VH473Z 0VH483Z 0VH803Z 0VH833Z 0VH843Z 0VH873Z 0VH883Z 0VHD03Z 0VHD33Z 0VHD43Z 0VHD73Z 0VHD83Z 0VHM03Z 0VHM33Z 0VHM43Z 0VHM73Z 0VHM83Z 0VHR03Z 0VHR33Z 0VHR43Z 0VHR73Z 0VHR83Z 0VHS03Z 0VHS33Z 0VHS43Z 0VHSX3Z

⊘ 0VH403Z 0VH433Z 0VH443Z 0VH473Z 0VH483Z 0VH803Z 0VH833Z 0VH843Z 0VH873Z 0VH883Z 0VHD03Z 0VHD33Z 0VHD43Z 0VHD73Z 0VHD83Z 0VHM03Z 0VHM33Z 0VHM43Z 0VHM73Z 0VHM83Z 0VHR03Z 0VHR33Z 0VHR43Z 0VHR73Z 0VHR83Z 0VHS03Z 0VHS33Z 0VHS43Z 0VHSX3Z

0 Medical and Surgical
V Male Reproductive System
J Inspection: Visually and/or manually exploring a body part

Body Part Character 4	Approach Character 5	Device Character 6	Qualifier Character 7
4 Prostate and Seminal Vesicles ⊘ ♂ **8** Scrotum and Tunica Vaginalis ⊘ ♂ **D** Testis ⊘ ♂ **M** Epididymis and Spermatic Cord ⊘ ♂ **R** Vas Deferens ⊘ ♂ **S** Penis ⊘ ♂	**0** Open **3** Percutaneous **4** Percutaneous Endoscopic **X** External	**Z** No Device	**Z** No Qualifier

♂ 0VJ40ZZ 0VJ43ZZ 0VJ44ZZ 0VJ4XZZ 0VJ80ZZ 0VJ83ZZ 0VJ84ZZ 0VJ8XZZ 0VJD0ZZ 0VJD3ZZ 0VJD4ZZ 0VJDXZZ 0VJM0ZZ 0VJM3ZZ 0VJM4ZZ 0VJMXZZ 0VJR0ZZ 0VJR3ZZ 0VJR4ZZ 0VJRXZZ 0VJS0ZZ 0VJS3ZZ 0VJS4ZZ 0VJSXZZ

⊘ 0VJ43ZZ 0VJ4XZZ 0VJ80ZZ 0VJ83ZZ 0VJ84ZZ 0VJ8XZZ 0VJD3ZZ 0VJDXZZ 0VJM3ZZ 0VJMXZZ 0VJR3ZZ 0VJRXZZ 0VJS0ZZ 0VJS3ZZ 0VJS4ZZ 0VJSXZZ

0 Medical and Surgical
V Male Reproductive System
L Occlusion: Completely closing an orifice or the lumen of a tubular body part

Body Part Character 4	Approach Character 5	Device Character 6	Qualifier Character 7
F Spermatic Cord, Right NC ⊘ ♂ **G** Spermatic Cord, Left NC ⊘ ♂ **H** Spermatic Cords, Bilateral NC ⊘ ♂ **N** Vas Deferens, Right NC ⊘ ♂ **P** Vas Deferens, Left NC ⊘ ♂ **Q** Vas Deferens, Bilateral NC ⊘ ♂	**0** Open **3** Percutaneous **4** Percutaneous Endoscopic	**C** Extraluminal Device **D** Intraluminal Device **Z** No Device	**Z** No Qualifier

♂ 0VLF0CZ 0VLF0DZ 0VLF0ZZ 0VLF3CZ 0VLF3DZ 0VLF3ZZ 0VLF4CZ 0VLF4DZ 0VLF4ZZ 0VLG0CZ 0VLG0DZ 0VLG0ZZ 0VLG3CZ 0VLG3DZ 0VLG3ZZ 0VLG4CZ 0VLG4DZ 0VLG4ZZ 0VLH0CZ 0VLH0DZ 0VLH0ZZ 0VLH3CZ 0VLH3DZ 0VLH3ZZ 0VLH4CZ 0VLH4DZ 0VLH4ZZ 0VLN0CZ 0VLN0DZ 0VLN0ZZ 0VLN3CZ 0VLN3DZ 0VLN3ZZ 0VLN4CZ 0VLN4DZ 0VLN4ZZ 0VLP0CZ 0VLP0DZ 0VLP0ZZ 0VLP3CZ 0VLP3DZ 0VLP3ZZ 0VLP4CZ 0VLP4DZ 0VLP4ZZ 0VLQ0CZ 0VLQ0DZ 0VLQ0ZZ 0VLQ3CZ 0VLQ3DZ 0VLQ3ZZ 0VLQ4CZ 0VLQ4DZ 0VLQ4ZZ

⊘ 0VLF0CZ 0VLF0DZ 0VLF0ZZ 0VLF3CZ 0VLF3DZ 0VLF3ZZ 0VLF4CZ 0VLF4DZ 0VLF4ZZ 0VLG0CZ 0VLG0DZ 0VLG0ZZ 0VLG3CZ 0VLG3DZ 0VLG3ZZ 0VLG4CZ 0VLG4DZ 0VLG4ZZ 0VLH0CZ 0VLH0DZ 0VLH0ZZ 0VLH3CZ 0VLH3DZ 0VLH3ZZ 0VLH4CZ 0VLH4DZ 0VLH4ZZ 0VLN0CZ 0VLN0ZZ 0VLN3CZ 0VLN3ZZ 0VLN4CZ 0VLN4ZZ 0VLP0CZ 0VLP0ZZ 0VLP3CZ 0VLP3ZZ 0VLP4CZ 0VLP4ZZ 0VLQ0CZ 0VLQ0ZZ 0VLQ3CZ 0VLQ3ZZ 0VLQ4CZ 0VLQ4ZZ

NC 0VLF0CZ 0VLF0DZ 0VLF0ZZ 0VLF3CZ 0VLF3DZ 0VLF3ZZ 0VLF4CZ 0VLF4DZ 0VLF4ZZ 0VLG0CZ 0VLG0DZ 0VLG0ZZ 0VLG3CZ 0VLG3DZ 0VLG3ZZ 0VLG4CZ 0VLG4DZ 0VLG4ZZ 0VLH0CZ 0VLH0DZ 0VLH0ZZ 0VLH3CZ 0VLH3DZ 0VLH3ZZ 0VLH4CZ 0VLH4DZ 0VLH4ZZ 0VLN0CZ 0VLN0ZZ 0VLN3CZ 0VLN3ZZ 0VLN4CZ 0VLN4ZZ 0VLP0CZ 0VLP0ZZ 0VLP3CZ 0VLP3ZZ 0VLP4CZ 0VLP4ZZ 0VLQ0CZ 0VLQ0ZZ 0VLQ3CZ 0VLQ3ZZ 0VLQ4CZ or 0VLQ4ZZ Codes with the NC symbol are identified as noncovered procedures only when diagnosis code Z30.2 is listed as the principal diagnosis.

0 Medical and Surgical
V Male Reproductive System
M Reattachment: Putting back in or on all or a portion of a separated body part to its normal location or other suitable location

Body Part Character 4	Approach Character 5	Device Character 6	Qualifier Character 7
5 Scrotum ♂ **S** Penis ♂	**X** External	**Z** No Device	**Z** No Qualifier
6 Tunica Vaginalis, Right ♂ **7** Tunica Vaginalis, Left ♂ **9** Testis, Right ♂ **B** Testis, Left ♂ **C** Testes, Bilateral ♂ **F** Spermatic Cord, Right ♂ **G** Spermatic Cord, Left ♂ **H** Spermatic Cords, Bilateral ♂	**0** Open **4** Percutaneous Endoscopic	**Z** No Device	**Z** No Qualifier

♂ 0VM5XZZ 0VM60ZZ 0VM64ZZ 0VM70ZZ 0VM74ZZ 0VM90ZZ 0VM94ZZ 0VMB0ZZ 0VMB4ZZ 0VMC0ZZ 0VMC4ZZ 0VMF0ZZ 0VMF4ZZ 0VMG0ZZ 0VMG4ZZ 0VMH0ZZ 0VMH4ZZ 0VMSXZZ

LC Limited Coverage NC Noncovered HAC HAC Associated Procedure CC Combination Cluster - See Appendix G for code lists
DRG Non-OR-Affecting MS-DRG Assignment ⊘ Non-OR-Not Affecting MS-DRG Assignment New/Revised Text in **Orange** ♂ Male ♀ Female

0 Medical and Surgical
V Male Reproductive System
N Release: Freeing a body part from an abnormal physical constraint by cutting or by the use of force

Body Part Character 4	Approach Character 5	Device Character 6	Qualifier Character 7
0 Prostate ♂	**0** Open **3** Percutaneous **4** Percutaneous Endoscopic **7** Via Natural or Artificial Opening **8** Via Natural or Artificial Opening Endoscopic	**Z** No Device	**Z** No Qualifier
1 Seminal Vesicle, Right ♂ **2** Seminal Vesicle, Left ♂ **3** Seminal Vesicles, Bilateral ♂ **6** Tunica Vaginalis, Right ♂ **7** Tunica Vaginalis, Left ♂ **9** Testis, Right ⃠ ♂ **B** Testis, Left ⃠ ♂ **C** Testes, Bilateral ⃠ ♂ **F** Spermatic Cord, Right ♂ **G** Spermatic Cord, Left ♂ **H** Spermatic Cords, Bilateral ♂ **J** Epididymis, Right ♂ **K** Epididymis, Left ♂ **L** Epididymis, Bilateral ♂ **N** Vas Deferens, Right ♂ **P** Vas Deferens, Left ♂ **Q** Vas Deferens, Bilateral ♂	**0** Open **3** Percutaneous **4** Percutaneous Endoscopic	**Z** No Device	**Z** No Qualifier
5 Scrotum ♂ **S** Penis ♂ **T** Prepuce ⃠ ♂	**0** Open **3** Percutaneous **4** Percutaneous Endoscopic **X** External	**Z** No Device	**Z** No Qualifier

♂ 0VN00ZZ 0VN03ZZ 0VN04ZZ 0VN07ZZ 0VN08ZZ 0VN10ZZ 0VN13ZZ 0VN14ZZ 0VN20ZZ 0VN23ZZ 0VN24ZZ 0VN30ZZ 0VN33ZZ 0VN34ZZ 0VN50ZZ 0VN53ZZ 0VN54ZZ 0VN5XZZ 0VN60ZZ 0VN63ZZ 0VN64ZZ 0VN70ZZ 0VN73ZZ 0VN74ZZ 0VN90ZZ 0VN93ZZ 0VN94ZZ 0VNB0ZZ 0VNB3ZZ 0VNB4ZZ 0VNC0ZZ 0VNC3ZZ 0VNC4ZZ 0VNF0ZZ 0VNF3ZZ 0VNF4ZZ 0VNG0ZZ 0VNG3ZZ 0VNG4ZZ 0VNH0ZZ 0VNH3ZZ 0VNH4ZZ 0VNJ0ZZ 0VNJ3ZZ 0VNJ4ZZ 0VNK0ZZ 0VNK3ZZ 0VNK4ZZ 0VNL0ZZ 0VNL3ZZ 0VNL4ZZ 0VNN0ZZ 0VNN3ZZ 0VNN4ZZ 0VNP0ZZ 0VNP3ZZ 0VNP4ZZ 0VNQ0ZZ 0VNQ3ZZ 0VNQ4ZZ 0VNS0ZZ 0VNS3ZZ 0VNS4ZZ 0VNSXZZ 0VNT0ZZ 0VNT3ZZ 0VNT4ZZ 0VNTXZZ

⃠ 0VN90ZZ 0VN93ZZ 0VN94ZZ 0VNB0ZZ 0VNB3ZZ 0VNB4ZZ 0VNC0ZZ 0VNC3ZZ 0VNC4ZZ 0VNT0ZZ 0VNT3ZZ 0VNT4ZZ 0VNTXZZ

0 Medical and Surgical
V Male Reproductive System
P Removal: Taking out or off a device from a body part

Body Part Character 4	Approach Character 5	Device Character 6	Qualifier Character 7
4 Prostate and Seminal Vesicles ⃠ ♂	**0** Open **3** Percutaneous **4** Percutaneous Endoscopic **7** Via Natural or Artificial Opening **8** Via Natural or Artificial Opening Endoscopic	**0** Drainage Device **1** Radioactive Element **3** Infusion Device **7** Autologous Tissue Substitute **J** Synthetic Substitute **K** Nonautologous Tissue Substitute	**Z** No Qualifier
4 Prostate and Seminal Vesicles ⃠ ♂	**X** External	**0** Drainage Device **1** Radioactive Element **3** Infusion Device	**Z** No Qualifier
8 Scrotum and Tunica Vaginalis ⃠ ♂ **D** Testis ⃠ ♂ **S** Penis ⃠ ♂	**0** Open **3** Percutaneous **4** Percutaneous Endoscopic **7** Via Natural or Artificial Opening **8** Via Natural or Artificial Opening Endoscopic	**0** Drainage Device **3** Infusion Device **7** Autologous Tissue Substitute **J** Synthetic Substitute **K** Nonautologous Tissue Substitute	**Z** No Qualifier
8 Scrotum and Tunica Vaginalis ⃠ ♂ **D** Testis ⃠ ♂ **S** Penis ⃠ ♂	**X** External	**0** Drainage Device **3** Infusion Device	**Z** No Qualifier
M Epididymis and Spermatic Cord ⃠ ♂	**0** Open **3** Percutaneous **4** Percutaneous Endoscopic **7** Via Natural or Artificial Opening **8** Via Natural or Artificial Opening Endoscopic	**0** Drainage Device **3** Infusion Device **7** Autologous Tissue Substitute **C** Extraluminal Device **J** Synthetic Substitute **K** Nonautologous Tissue Substitute	**Z** No Qualifier
M Epididymis and Spermatic Cord ⃠ ♂	**X** External	**0** Drainage Device **3** Infusion Device	**Z** No Qualifier
R Vas Deferens ⃠ ♂	**0** Open **3** Percutaneous **4** Percutaneous Endoscopic **7** Via Natural or Artificial Opening **8** Via Natural or Artificial Opening Endoscopic	**0** Drainage Device **3** Infusion Device **7** Autologous Tissue Substitute **C** Extraluminal Device **D** Intraluminal Device **J** Synthetic Substitute **K** Nonautologous Tissue Substitute	**Z** No Qualifier
R Vas Deferens ⃠ ♂	**X** External	**0** Drainage Device **3** Infusion Device **D** Intraluminal Device	**Z** No Qualifier

♂ 0VP400Z 0VP401Z 0VP403Z 0VP407Z 0VP40JZ 0VP40KZ 0VP430Z 0VP431Z 0VP433Z 0VP437Z 0VP43JZ 0VP43KZ 0VP440Z 0VP441Z 0VP443Z 0VP447Z 0VP44JZ 0VP44KZ 0VP470Z 0VP471Z 0VP473Z 0VP477Z 0VP47JZ 0VP47KZ 0VP480Z 0VP481Z 0VP483Z 0VP487Z 0VP48JZ 0VP48KZ 0VP4X0Z 0VP4X1Z 0VP4X3Z 0VP800Z 0VP803Z 0VP807Z 0VP80JZ 0VP80KZ 0VP830Z 0VP833Z 0VP837Z 0VP83JZ 0VP83KZ 0VP840Z 0VP843Z 0VP847Z 0VP84JZ 0VP84KZ 0VP870Z 0VP873Z 0VP877Z 0VP87JZ 0VP87KZ 0VP880Z 0VP883Z 0VP887Z 0VP88JZ 0VP88KZ 0VP8X0Z 0VP8X3Z 0VPD00Z 0VPD03Z 0VPD07Z 0VPD0JZ 0VPD0KZ 0VPD30Z 0VPD33Z 0VPD37Z 0VPD3JZ 0VPD3KZ 0VPD40Z 0VPD43Z 0VPD47Z 0VPD4JZ 0VPD4KZ 0VPD70Z 0VPD73Z 0VPD77Z 0VPD7JZ 0VPD7KZ 0VPD80Z 0VPD83Z 0VPD87Z 0VPD8JZ 0VPD8KZ 0VPDX0Z 0VPDX3Z 0VPM00Z 0VPM03Z 0VPM07Z 0VPM0CZ 0VPM0JZ 0VPM0KZ 0VPM30Z 0VPM33Z 0VPM37Z 0VPM3CZ 0VPM3JZ 0VPM3KZ 0VPM40Z 0VPM43Z 0VPM47Z 0VPM4CZ 0VPM4JZ 0VPM4KZ 0VPM70Z 0VPM73Z 0VPM77Z 0VPM7CZ 0VPM7JZ 0VPM7KZ 0VPM80Z 0VPM83Z 0VPM87Z 0VPM8CZ 0VPM8JZ 0VPM8KZ 0VPMX0Z 0VPMX3Z 0VPR00Z 0VPR03Z 0VPR07Z 0VPR0CZ 0VPR0DZ 0VPR0JZ 0VPR0KZ 0VPR30Z 0VPR33Z 0VPR37Z 0VPR3CZ 0VPR3DZ 0VPR3JZ 0VPR3KZ 0VPR40Z 0VPR43Z 0VPR47Z 0VPR4CZ 0VPR4DZ 0VPR4JZ 0VPR4KZ 0VPR70Z 0VPR73Z 0VPR77Z 0VPR7CZ 0VPR7DZ 0VPR7JZ 0VPR7KZ 0VPR80Z 0VPR83Z 0VPR87Z 0VPR8CZ 0VPR8DZ 0VPR8JZ 0VPR8KZ 0VPRX0Z 0VPRX3Z 0VPRXDZ 0VPS00Z 0VPS03Z 0VPS07Z 0VPS0JZ 0VPS0KZ 0VPS30Z 0VPS33Z 0VPS37Z 0VPS3JZ 0VPS3KZ 0VPS40Z 0VPS43Z 0VPS47Z 0VPS4JZ 0VPS4KZ 0VPS70Z 0VPS73Z 0VPS77Z 0VPS7JZ 0VPS7KZ 0VPS80Z 0VPS83Z 0VPS87Z 0VPS8JZ 0VPS8KZ 0VPSX0Z 0VPSX3Z

⃠ 0VP470Z 0VP473Z 0VP480Z 0VP483Z 0VP4X0Z 0VP4X1Z 0VP4X3Z 0VP800Z 0VP803Z 0VP807Z 0VP80JZ 0VP80KZ 0VP830Z 0VP833Z 0VP837Z 0VP83JZ 0VP83KZ 0VP840Z 0VP843Z 0VP847Z 0VP84JZ 0VP84KZ 0VP870Z 0VP873Z 0VP877Z 0VP87JZ 0VP87KZ 0VP880Z 0VP883Z 0VP887Z 0VP88JZ 0VP88KZ 0VP8X0Z 0VP8X3Z 0VPD70Z 0VPD73Z 0VPD80Z 0VPD83Z 0VPDX0Z 0VPDX3Z 0VPM70Z 0VPM73Z 0VPM80Z 0VPM83Z 0VPMX0Z 0VPMX3Z 0VPR00Z 0VPR03Z 0VPR07Z 0VPR0CZ 0VPR0JZ 0VPR0KZ 0VPR30Z 0VPR33Z 0VPR37Z 0VPR3CZ 0VPR3JZ 0VPR3KZ 0VPR40Z 0VPR43Z 0VPR47Z 0VPR4CZ 0VPR4JZ 0VPR4KZ 0VPR70Z 0VPR73Z 0VPR77Z 0VPR7CZ 0VPR7DZ 0VPR7JZ 0VPR7KZ 0VPR80Z 0VPR83Z 0VPR87Z 0VPR8CZ 0VPR8DZ 0VPR8JZ 0VPR8KZ 0VPRX0Z 0VPRX3Z 0VPRXDZ 0VPS70Z 0VPS73Z 0VPS80Z 0VPS83Z 0VPSX0Z 0VPSX3Z

0 Medical and Surgical
V Male Reproductive System
Q Repair: Restoring, to the extent possible, a body part to its normal anatomic structure and function

Body Part Character 4	Approach Character 5	Device Character 6	Qualifier Character 7
0 Prostate ♂	0 Open 3 Percutaneous 4 Percutaneous Endoscopic 7 Via Natural or Artificial Opening 8 Via Natural or Artificial Opening Endoscopic	Z No Device	Z No Qualifier
1 Seminal Vesicle, Right ♂ 2 Seminal Vesicle, Left ♂ 3 Seminal Vesicles, Bilateral ♂ 6 Tunica Vaginalis, Right ⃠ ♂ 7 Tunica Vaginalis, Left ⃠ ♂ 9 Testis, Right ♂ B Testis, Left ♂ C Testes, Bilateral ♂ F Spermatic Cord, Right ♂ G Spermatic Cord, Left ♂ H Spermatic Cords, Bilateral ♂ J Epididymis, Right ♂ K Epididymis, Left ♂ L Epididymis, Bilateral ♂ N Vas Deferens, Right ♂ P Vas Deferens, Left ♂ Q Vas Deferens, Bilateral ♂	0 Open 3 Percutaneous 4 Percutaneous Endoscopic	Z No Device	Z No Qualifier
5 Scrotum ⃠ ♂ S Penis ♂ T Prepuce ♂	0 Open 3 Percutaneous 4 Percutaneous Endoscopic X External	Z No Device	Z No Qualifier

♂ 0VQ00ZZ 0VQ03ZZ 0VQ04ZZ 0VQ07ZZ 0VQ08ZZ 0VQ10ZZ 0VQ13ZZ 0VQ14ZZ 0VQ20ZZ 0VQ23ZZ 0VQ24ZZ 0VQ30ZZ 0VQ33ZZ 0VQ34ZZ 0VQ50ZZ 0VQ53ZZ 0VQ54ZZ 0VQ5XZZ 0VQ60ZZ 0VQ63ZZ 0VQ64ZZ 0VQ70ZZ 0VQ73ZZ 0VQ74ZZ 0VQ90ZZ 0VQ93ZZ 0VQ94ZZ 0VQB0ZZ 0VQB3ZZ 0VQB4ZZ 0VQC0ZZ 0VQC3ZZ 0VQC4ZZ 0VQF0ZZ 0VQF3ZZ 0VQF4ZZ 0VQG0ZZ 0VQG3ZZ 0VQG4ZZ 0VQH0ZZ 0VQH3ZZ 0VQH4ZZ 0VQJ0ZZ 0VQJ3ZZ 0VQJ4ZZ 0VQK0ZZ 0VQK3ZZ 0VQK4ZZ 0VQL0ZZ 0VQL3ZZ 0VQL4ZZ 0VQN0ZZ 0VQN3ZZ 0VQN4ZZ 0VQP0ZZ 0VQP3ZZ 0VQP4ZZ 0VQQ0ZZ 0VQQ3ZZ 0VQQ4ZZ 0VQS0ZZ 0VQS3ZZ 0VQS4ZZ 0VQSXZZ 0VQT0ZZ 0VQT3ZZ 0VQT4ZZ 0VQTXZZ

⃠ 0VQ50ZZ 0VQ53ZZ 0VQ54ZZ 0VQ5XZZ 0VQ60ZZ 0VQ63ZZ 0VQ64ZZ 0VQ70ZZ 0VQ73ZZ 0VQ74ZZ

0 Medical and Surgical
V Male Reproductive System
R Replacement: Putting in or on biological or synthetic material that physically takes the place and/or function of all or a portion of a body part

Body Part Character 4	Approach Character 5	Device Character 6	Qualifier Character 7
9 Testis, Right ♂ B Testis, Left ♂ C Testes, Bilateral ♂	0 Open	J Synthetic Substitute	Z No Qualifier

♂ 0VR90JZ 0VRB0JZ 0VRC0JZ

0 Medical and Surgical
V Male Reproductive System
S Reposition: Moving to its normal location, or other suitable location, all or a portion of a body part

Body Part Character 4	Approach Character 5	Device Character 6	Qualifier Character 7
9 Testis, Right ♂ B Testis, Left ♂ C Testes, Bilateral ♂ F Spermatic Cord, Right ♂ G Spermatic Cord, Left ♂ H Spermatic Cords, Bilateral ♂	0 Open 3 Percutaneous 4 Percutaneous Endoscopic	Z No Device	Z No Qualifier

♂ 0VS90ZZ 0VS93ZZ 0VS94ZZ 0VSB0ZZ 0VSB3ZZ 0VSB4ZZ 0VSC0ZZ 0VSC3ZZ 0VSC4ZZ 0VSF0ZZ 0VSF3ZZ 0VSF4ZZ 0VSG0ZZ 0VSG3ZZ 0VSG4ZZ 0VSH0ZZ 0VSH3ZZ 0VSH4ZZ

LC Limited Coverage NC Noncovered HAC HAC Associated Procedure CC Combination Cluster - See Appendix G for code lists
DRG Non-OR-Affecting MS-DRG Assignment ⃠ Non-OR-Not Affecting MS-DRG Assignment New/Revised Text in **Orange** ♂ Male ♀ Female

0 Medical and Surgical
V Male Reproductive System
T Resection: Cutting out or off, without replacement, all of a body part

Body Part Character 4	Approach Character 5	Device Character 6	Qualifier Character 7
0 Prostate CC ♂	**0** Open **4** Percutaneous Endoscopic **7** Via Natural or Artificial Opening **8** Via Natural or Artificial Opening Endoscopic	**Z** No Device	**Z** No Qualifier
1 Seminal Vesicle, Right ♂ **2** Seminal Vesicle, Left ♂ **3** Seminal Vesicles, Bilateral CC ♂ **6** Tunica Vaginalis, Right ♂ **7** Tunica Vaginalis, Left ♂ **9** Testis, Right ♂ **B** Testis, Left ♂ **C** Testes, Bilateral ♂ **F** Spermatic Cord, Right ♂ **G** Spermatic Cord, Left ♂ **H** Spermatic Cords, Bilateral ♂ **J** Epididymis, Right ♂ **K** Epididymis, Left ♂ **L** Epididymis, Bilateral ♂ **N** Vas Deferens, Right NC ⊘ ♂ **P** Vas Deferens, Left NC ⊘ ♂ **Q** Vas Deferens, Bilateral NC ⊘ ♂	**0** Open **4** Percutaneous Endoscopic	**Z** No Device	**Z** No Qualifier
5 Scrotum ⊘ ♂ **S** Penis ♂ **T** Prepuce ⊘ ♂	**0** Open **4** Percutaneous Endoscopic **X** External	**Z** No Device	**Z** No Qualifier

♂ 0VT00ZZ 0VT04ZZ 0VT07ZZ 0VT08ZZ 0VT10ZZ 0VT14ZZ 0VT20ZZ 0VT24ZZ 0VT30ZZ 0VT34ZZ 0VT50ZZ 0VT54ZZ 0VT5XZZ 0VT60ZZ 0VT64ZZ 0VT70ZZ 0VT74ZZ 0VT90ZZ 0VT94ZZ 0VTB0ZZ 0VTB4ZZ 0VTC0ZZ 0VTC4ZZ 0VTF0ZZ 0VTF4ZZ 0VTG0ZZ 0VTG4ZZ 0VTH0ZZ 0VTH4ZZ 0VTJ0ZZ 0VTJ4ZZ 0VTK0ZZ 0VTK4ZZ 0VTL0ZZ 0VTL4ZZ 0VTN0ZZ 0VTN4ZZ 0VTP0ZZ 0VTP4ZZ 0VTQ0ZZ 0VTQ4ZZ 0VTS0ZZ 0VTS4ZZ 0VTSXZZ 0VTT0ZZ 0VTT4ZZ 0VTTXZZ

⊘ 0VT50ZZ 0VT54ZZ 0VT5XZZ 0VTN0ZZ 0VTN4ZZ 0VTP0ZZ 0VTP4ZZ 0VTQ0ZZ 0VTQ4ZZ 0VTT0ZZ 0VTT4ZZ 0VTTXZZ

CC 0VT00ZZ 0VT04ZZ 0VT07ZZ 0VT08ZZ 0VT30ZZ 0VT34ZZ

NC 0VTN0ZZ 0VTN4ZZ 0VTP0ZZ 0VTP4ZZ 0VTQ0ZZ or 0VTQ4ZZ when diagnosis code Z30.2 is listed as the principal diagnosis

0 Medical and Surgical
V Male Reproductive System
U Supplement: Putting in or on biological or synthetic material that physically reinforces and/or augments the function of a portion of a body part

Body Part Character 4	Approach Character 5	Device Character 6	Qualifier Character 7
1 Seminal Vesicle, Right ♂ **2** Seminal Vesicle, Left ♂ **3** Seminal Vesicles, Bilateral ♂ **6** Tunica Vaginalis, Right ♂ **7** Tunica Vaginalis, Left ♂ **F** Spermatic Cord, Right ♂ **G** Spermatic Cord, Left ♂ **H** Spermatic Cords, Bilateral ♂ **J** Epididymis, Right ♂ **K** Epididymis, Left ♂ **L** Epididymis, Bilateral ♂ **N** Vas Deferens, Right ♂ **P** Vas Deferens, Left ♂ **Q** Vas Deferens, Bilateral ♂	**0** Open **4** Percutaneous Endoscopic	**7** Autologous Tissue Substitute **J** Synthetic Substitute **K** Nonautologous Tissue Substitute	**Z** No Qualifier
5 Scrotum ♂ **S** Penis ⃠ ♂ **T** Prepuce ♂	**0** Open **4** Percutaneous Endoscopic **X** External	**7** Autologous Tissue Substitute **J** Synthetic Substitute **K** Nonautologous Tissue Substitute	**Z** No Qualifier
9 Testis, Right ♂ **B** Testis, Left ♂ **C** Testes, Bilateral ♂	**0** Open	**7** Autologous Tissue Substitute **J** Synthetic Substitute **K** Nonautologous Tissue Substitute	**Z** No Qualifier

♂ 0VU107Z 0VU10JZ 0VU10KZ 0VU147Z 0VU14JZ 0VU14KZ 0VU207Z 0VU20JZ 0VU20KZ 0VU247Z 0VU24JZ 0VU24KZ 0VU307Z 0VU30JZ 0VU30KZ 0VU347Z 0VU34JZ 0VU34KZ 0VU507Z 0VU50JZ 0VU50KZ 0VU547Z 0VU54JZ 0VU54KZ 0VU5X7Z 0VU5XJZ 0VU5XKZ 0VU607Z 0VU60JZ 0VU60KZ 0VU647Z 0VU64JZ 0VU64KZ 0VU707Z 0VU70JZ 0VU70KZ 0VU747Z 0VU74JZ 0VU74KZ 0VU907Z 0VU90JZ 0VU90KZ 0VUB07Z 0VUB0JZ 0VUB0KZ 0VUC07Z 0VUC0JZ 0VUC0KZ 0VUF07Z 0VUF0JZ 0VUF0KZ 0VUF47Z 0VUF4JZ 0VUF4KZ 0VUG07Z 0VUG0JZ 0VUG0KZ 0VUG47Z 0VUG4JZ 0VUG4KZ 0VUH07Z 0VUH0JZ 0VUH0KZ 0VUH47Z 0VUH4JZ 0VUH4KZ 0VUJ07Z 0VUJ0JZ 0VUJ0KZ 0VUJ47Z 0VUJ4JZ 0VUJ4KZ 0VUK07Z 0VUK0JZ 0VUK0KZ 0VUK47Z 0VUK4JZ 0VUK4KZ 0VUL07Z 0VUL0JZ 0VUL0KZ 0VUL47Z 0VUL4JZ 0VUL4KZ 0VUN07Z 0VUN0JZ 0VUN0KZ 0VUN47Z 0VUN4JZ 0VUN4KZ 0VUP07Z 0VUP0JZ 0VUP0KZ 0VUP47Z 0VUP4JZ 0VUP4KZ 0VUQ07Z 0VUQ0JZ 0VUQ0KZ 0VUQ47Z 0VUQ4JZ 0VUQ4KZ 0VUS07Z 0VUS0JZ 0VUS0KZ 0VUS47Z 0VUS4JZ 0VUS4KZ 0VUSX7Z 0VUSXJZ 0VUSXKZ 0VUT07Z 0VUT0JZ 0VUT0KZ 0VUT47Z 0VUT4JZ 0VUT4KZ 0VUTX7Z 0VUTXJZ 0VUTXKZ

⃠ 0VUSX7Z 0VUSXJZ 0VUSXKZ

0 Medical and Surgical
V Male Reproductive System
W Revision: Correcting, to the extent possible, a portion of a malfunctioning device or the position of a displaced device

Body Part Character 4	Approach Character 5	Device Character 6	Qualifier Character 7
4 Prostate and Seminal Vesicles ⦸ ♂ **8** Scrotum and Tunica Vaginalis ⦸ ♂ **D** Testis ⦸ ♂ **S** Penis ⦸ ♂	**0** Open **3** Percutaneous **4** Percutaneous Endoscopic **7** Via Natural or Artificial Opening **8** Via Natural or Artificial Opening Endoscopic **X** External	**0** Drainage Device **3** Infusion Device **7** Autologous Tissue Substitute **J** Synthetic Substitute **K** Nonautologous Tissue Substitute	**Z** No Qualifier
M Epididymis and Spermatic Cord ⦸ ♂	**0** Open **3** Percutaneous **4** Percutaneous Endoscopic **7** Via Natural or Artificial Opening **8** Via Natural or Artificial Opening Endoscopic **X** External	**0** Drainage Device **3** Infusion Device **7** Autologous Tissue Substitute **C** Extraluminal Device **J** Synthetic Substitute **K** Nonautologous Tissue Substitute	**Z** No Qualifier
R Vas Deferens ⦸ ♂	**0** Open **3** Percutaneous **4** Percutaneous Endoscopic **7** Via Natural or Artificial Opening **8** Via Natural or Artificial Opening Endoscopic **X** External	**0** Drainage Device **3** Infusion Device **7** Autologous Tissue Substitute **C** Extraluminal Device **D** Intraluminal Device **J** Synthetic Substitute **K** Nonautologous Tissue Substitute	**Z** No Qualifier

♂ 0VW400Z 0VW403Z 0VW407Z 0VW40JZ 0VW40KZ 0VW430Z 0VW433Z 0VW437Z 0VW43JZ 0VW43KZ 0VW440Z 0VW443Z 0VW447Z 0VW44JZ 0VW44KZ 0VW470Z 0VW473Z 0VW477Z 0VW47JZ 0VW47KZ 0VW480Z 0VW483Z 0VW487Z 0VW48JZ 0VW48KZ 0VW4X0Z 0VW4X3Z 0VW4X7Z 0VW4XJZ 0VW4XKZ 0VW800Z 0VW803Z 0VW807Z 0VW80JZ 0VW80KZ 0VW830Z 0VW833Z 0VW837Z 0VW83JZ 0VW83KZ 0VW840Z 0VW843Z 0VW847Z 0VW84JZ 0VW84KZ 0VW870Z 0VW873Z 0VW877Z 0VW87JZ 0VW87KZ 0VW880Z 0VW883Z 0VW887Z 0VW88JZ 0VW88KZ 0VW8X0Z 0VW8X3Z 0VW8X7Z 0VW8XJZ 0VW8XKZ 0VWD00Z 0VWD03Z 0VWD07Z 0VWD0JZ 0VWD0KZ 0VWD30Z 0VWD33Z 0VWD37Z 0VWD3JZ 0VWD3KZ 0VWD40Z 0VWD43Z 0VWD47Z 0VWD4JZ 0VWD4KZ 0VWD70Z 0VWD73Z 0VWD77Z 0VWD7JZ 0VWD7KZ 0VWD80Z 0VWD83Z 0VWD87Z 0VWD8JZ 0VWD8KZ 0VWDX0Z 0VWDX3Z 0VWDX7Z 0VWDXJZ 0VWDXKZ 0VWM00Z 0VWM03Z 0VWM07Z 0VWM0CZ 0VWM0JZ 0VWM0KZ 0VWM30Z 0VWM33Z 0VWM37Z 0VWM3CZ 0VWM3JZ 0VWM3KZ 0VWM40Z 0VWM43Z 0VWM47Z 0VWM4CZ 0VWM4JZ 0VWM4KZ 0VWM70Z 0VWM73Z 0VWM77Z 0VWM7CZ 0VWM7JZ 0VWM7KZ 0VWM80Z 0VWM83Z 0VWM87Z 0VWM8CZ 0VWM8JZ 0VWM8KZ 0VWMX0Z 0VWMX3Z 0VWMX7Z 0VWMXCZ 0VWMXJZ 0VWMXKZ 0VWR00Z 0VWR03Z 0VWR07Z 0VWR0CZ 0VWR0DZ 0VWR0JZ 0VWR0KZ 0VWR30Z 0VWR33Z 0VWR37Z 0VWR3CZ 0VWR3DZ 0VWR3JZ 0VWR3KZ 0VWR40Z 0VWR43Z 0VWR47Z 0VWR4CZ 0VWR4DZ 0VWR4JZ 0VWR4KZ 0VWR70Z 0VWR73Z 0VWR77Z 0VWR7CZ 0VWR7DZ 0VWR7JZ 0VWR7KZ 0VWR80Z 0VWR83Z 0VWR87Z 0VWR8CZ 0VWR8DZ 0VWR8JZ 0VWR8KZ 0VWRX0Z 0VWRX3Z 0VWRX7Z 0VWRXCZ 0VWRXDZ 0VWRXJZ 0VWRXKZ 0VWS00Z 0VWS03Z 0VWS07Z 0VWS0JZ 0VWS0KZ 0VWS30Z 0VWS33Z 0VWS37Z 0VWS3JZ 0VWS3KZ 0VWS40Z 0VWS43Z 0VWS47Z 0VWS4JZ 0VWS4KZ 0VWS70Z 0VWS73Z 0VWS77Z 0VWS7JZ 0VWS7KZ 0VWS80Z 0VWS83Z 0VWS87Z 0VWS8JZ 0VWS8KZ 0VWSX0Z 0VWSX3Z 0VWSX7Z 0VWSXJZ 0VWSXKZ

⦸ 0VW4X0Z 0VW4X3Z 0VW4X7Z 0VW4XJZ 0VW4XKZ 0VW800Z 0VW803Z 0VW807Z 0VW80JZ 0VW80KZ 0VW830Z 0VW833Z 0VW837Z 0VW83JZ 0VW83KZ 0VW840Z 0VW843Z 0VW847Z 0VW84JZ 0VW84KZ 0VW870Z 0VW873Z 0VW877Z 0VW87JZ 0VW87KZ 0VW880Z 0VW883Z 0VW887Z 0VW88JZ 0VW88KZ 0VW8X0Z 0VW8X3Z 0VW8X7Z 0VW8XJZ 0VW8XKZ 0VWDX0Z 0VWDX3Z 0VWDX7Z 0VWDXJZ 0VWDXKZ 0VWMX0Z 0VWMX3Z 0VWMX7Z 0VWMXCZ 0VWMXJZ 0VWMXKZ 0VWR00Z 0VWR03Z 0VWR07Z 0VWR0CZ 0VWR0DZ 0VWR0JZ 0VWR0KZ 0VWR30Z 0VWR33Z 0VWR37Z 0VWR3CZ 0VWR3DZ 0VWR3JZ 0VWR3KZ 0VWR40Z 0VWR43Z 0VWR47Z 0VWR4CZ 0VWR4DZ 0VWR4JZ 0VWR4KZ 0VWR70Z 0VWR73Z 0VWR77Z 0VWR7CZ 0VWR7DZ 0VWR7JZ 0VWR7KZ 0VWR80Z 0VWR83Z 0VWR87Z 0VWR8CZ 0VWR8DZ 0VWR8JZ 0VWR8KZ 0VWRX0Z 0VWRX3Z 0VWRX7Z 0VWRXCZ 0VWRXDZ 0VWRXJZ 0VWRXKZ 0VWSX0Z 0VWSX3Z 0VWSX7Z 0VWSXJZ 0VWSXKZ

Anatomical Regions, General 0W0-0WY

0 Medical and Surgical
W Anatomical Regions, General
0 Alteration: Modifying the anatomic structure of a body part without affecting the function of the body part

Body Part Character 4	Approach Character 5	Device Character 6	Qualifier Character 7
0 Head **2** Face **4** Upper Jaw **5** Lower Jaw **6** Neck **8** Chest Wall **F** Abdominal Wall **K** Upper Back **L** Lower Back **M** Perineum, Male ♂ **N** Perineum, Female ♀	**0** Open **3** Percutaneous **4** Percutaneous Endoscopic	**7** Autologous Tissue Substitute **J** Synthetic Substitute **K** Nonautologous Tissue Substitute **Z** No Device	**Z** No Qualifier

♂ 0W0M07Z 0W0M0JZ 0W0M0KZ 0W0M0ZZ 0W0M37Z 0W0M3JZ 0W0M3KZ 0W0M3ZZ 0W0M47Z 0W0M4JZ 0W0M4KZ 0W0M4ZZ
♀ 0W0N07Z 0W0N0JZ 0W0N0KZ 0W0N0ZZ 0W0N37Z 0W0N3JZ 0W0N3KZ 0W0N3ZZ 0W0N47Z 0W0N4JZ 0W0N4KZ 0W0N4ZZ

0 Medical and Surgical
W Anatomical Regions, General
1 Bypass: Altering the route of passage of the contents of a tubular body part

Body Part Character 4	Approach Character 5	Device Character 6	Qualifier Character 7
1 Cranial Cavity	**0** Open	**J** Synthetic Substitute	**9** Pleural Cavity, Right **B** Pleural Cavity, Left **G** Peritoneal Cavity **J** Pelvic Cavity
9 Pleural Cavity, Right ⦸ **B** Pleural Cavity, Left ⦸ **G** Peritoneal Cavity ⦸ **J** Pelvic Cavity ⦸	**0** Open **4** Percutaneous Endoscopic	**J** Synthetic Substitute	**4** Cutaneous **9** Pleural Cavity, Right **B** Pleural Cavity, Left **G** Peritoneal Cavity **J** Pelvic Cavity **Y** Lower Vein
9 Pleural Cavity, Right ⦸ **B** Pleural Cavity, Left ⦸ **G** Peritoneal Cavity **J** Pelvic Cavity ⦸	**3** Percutaneous	**J** Synthetic Substitute	**4** Cutaneous

⦸ 0W190J4 0W190JG 0W190JY 0W193J4 0W194J4 0W194JG 0W194JY 0W1B0J4 0W1B0JG 0W1B0JY 0W1B3J4 0W1B4J4 0W1B4JG 0W1B4JY 0W1G0J9 0W1G0JB 0W1G0JG 0W1G0JJ 0W1G4J9 0W1G4JB 0W1G4JG 0W1G4JJ 0W1J0J4 0W1J0JY 0W1J3J4 0W1J4J4 0W1J4JY

0 Medical and Surgical
W Anatomical Regions, General
2 Change: Taking out or off a device from a body part and putting back an identical or similar device in or on the same body part without cutting or puncturing the skin or a mucous membrane

Body Part Character 4	Approach Character 5	Device Character 6	Qualifier Character 7
0 Head ⊘ **1** Cranial Cavity ⊘ **2** Face ⊘ **4** Upper Jaw ⊘ **5** Lower Jaw ⊘ **6** Neck ⊘ **8** Chest Wall ⊘ **9** Pleural Cavity, Right ⊘ **B** Pleural Cavity, Left ⊘ **C** Mediastinum ⊘ **D** Pericardial Cavity ⊘ **F** Abdominal Wall ⊘ **G** Peritoneal Cavity ⊘ **H** Retroperitoneum ⊘ **J** Pelvic Cavity ⊘ **K** Upper Back ⊘ **L** Lower Back ⊘ **M** Perineum, Male ♂ ⊘ **N** Perineum, Female ♀ ⊘	**X** External	**0** Drainage Device **Y** Other Device	**Z** No Qualifier

♂ 0W2MX0Z 0W2MXYZ
♀ 0W2NX0Z 0W2NXYZ
⊘ 0W20X0Z 0W20XYZ 0W21X0Z 0W21XYZ 0W22X0Z 0W22XYZ 0W24X0Z 0W24XYZ 0W25X0Z 0W25XYZ 0W26X0Z 0W26XYZ 0W28X0Z 0W28XYZ 0W29X0Z 0W29XYZ 0W2BX0Z 0W2BXYZ 0W2CX0Z 0W2CXYZ 0W2DX0Z 0W2DXYZ 0W2FX0Z 0W2FXYZ 0W2GX0Z 0W2GXYZ 0W2HX0Z 0W2HXYZ 0W2JX0Z 0W2JXYZ 0W2KX0Z 0W2KXYZ 0W2LX0Z 0W2LXYZ 0W2MX0Z 0W2MXYZ 0W2NX0Z 0W2NXYZ

0 Medical and Surgical
W Anatomical Regions, General
3 Control: Stopping, or attempting to stop, postprocedural or other acute bleeding

Body Part Character 4	Approach Character 5	Device Character 6	Qualifier Character 7
0 Head **1** Cranial Cavity **2** Face **4** Upper Jaw **5** Lower Jaw **6** Neck **8** Chest Wall **9** Pleural Cavity, Right **B** Pleural Cavity, Left **C** Mediastinum **D** Pericardial Cavity **F** Abdominal Wall **G** Peritoneal Cavity ⊘ **H** Retroperitoneum **J** Pelvic Cavity **K** Upper Back **L** Lower Back **M** Perineum, Male ♂ **N** Perineum, Female ♀	**0** Open **3** Percutaneous **4** Percutaneous Endoscopic	**Z** No Device	**Z** No Qualifier
3 Oral Cavity and Throat	**0** Open **3** Percutaneous **4** Percutaneous Endoscopic **7** Via Natural or Artificial Opening **8** Via Natural or Artificial Opening Endoscopic **X** External	**Z** No Device	**Z** No Qualifier
P Gastrointestinal Tract ⊘ **Q** Respiratory Tract **R** Genitourinary Tract	**0** Open **3** Percutaneous **4** Percutaneous Endoscopic **7** Via Natural or Artificial Opening **8** Via Natural or Artificial Opening Endoscopic	**Z** No Device	**Z** No Qualifier

♂ 0W3M0ZZ 0W3M3ZZ 0W3M4ZZ
♀ 0W3N0ZZ 0W3N3ZZ 0W3N4ZZ
⊘ 0W3G0ZZ 0W3P8ZZ

0 Medical and Surgical
W Anatomical Regions, General
4 Creation: Putting in or on biological or synthetic material to form a new body part that to the extent possible replicates the anatomic structure or function of an absent body part

Body Part Character 4	Approach Character 5	Device Character 6	Qualifier Character 7
M Perineum, Male ♂ NC	**0** Open	**7** Autologous Tissue Substitute **J** Synthetic Substitute **K** Nonautologous Tissue Substitute **Z** No Device	**0** Vagina
N Perineum, Female ♀ NC	**0** Open	**7** Autologous Tissue Substitute **J** Synthetic Substitute **K** Nonautologous Tissue Substitute **Z** No Device	**1** Penis

♂ 0W4M070 0W4M0J0 0W4M0K0 0W4M0Z0
♀ 0W4N071 0W4N0J1 0W4N0K1 0W4N0Z1
NC 0W4M070 0W4M0J0 0W4M0K0 0W4M0Z0 0W4N071 0W4N0J1 0W4N0K1 0W4N0Z1

0 Medical and Surgical
W Anatomical Regions, General
8 Division: Cutting into a body part, without draining fluids and/or gases from the body part, in order to separate or transect a body part

Body Part Character 4	Approach Character 5	Device Character 6	Qualifier Character 7
N Perineum, Female ♀ ⦸	**X** External	**Z** No Device	**Z** No Qualifier

♀ 0W8NXZZ
⦸ 0W8NXZZ

0 Medical and Surgical
W Anatomical Regions, General
9 Drainage: Taking or letting out fluids and/or gases from a body part

Body Part Character 4	Approach Character 5	Device Character 6	Qualifier Character 7
0 Head ⦸ **1** Cranial Cavity ⦸ **2** Face ⦸ **3** Oral Cavity and Throat ⦸ **4** Upper Jaw ⦸ **5** Lower Jaw ⦸ **6** Neck ⦸ **8** Chest Wall ⦸ **9** Pleural Cavity, Right ⦸ **B** Pleural Cavity, Left ⦸ **C** Mediastinum **D** Pericardial Cavity ⦸ **F** Abdominal Wall ⦸ **G** Peritoneal Cavity ⦸ **H** Retroperitoneum **J** Pelvic Cavity ⦸ **K** Upper Back ⦸ **L** Lower Back ⦸ **M** Perineum, Male ♂ ⦸ **N** Perineum, Female ♀	**0** Open **3** Percutaneous **4** Percutaneous Endoscopic	**0** Drainage Device	**Z** No Qualifier

0W9 continued on next page

0W9 continued from previous page

0 Medical and Surgical
W Anatomical Regions, General
9 Drainage: Taking or letting out fluids and/or gases from a body part

Body Part Character 4	Approach Character 5	Device Character 6	Qualifier Character 7
0 Head ⊘ **1** Cranial Cavity ⊘ **2** Face ⊘ **3** Oral Cavity and Throat ⊘ **4** Upper Jaw ⊘ **5** Lower Jaw ⊘ **6** Neck ⊘ **8** Chest Wall ⊘ **9** Pleural Cavity, Right ⊘ **B** Pleural Cavity, Left ⊘ **C** Mediastinum ⊘ **D** Pericardial Cavity ⊘ **F** Abdominal Wall ⊘ **G** Peritoneal Cavity ⊘ **H** Retroperitoneum ⊘ **J** Pelvic Cavity ⊘ **K** Upper Back ⊘ **L** Lower Back ⊘ **M** Perineum, Male ♂ ⊘ **N** Perineum, Female ♀ ⊘	**0** Open **3** Percutaneous **4** Percutaneous Endoscopic	**Z** No Device	**X** Diagnostic **Z** No Qualifier

♂ 0W9M00Z 0W9M0ZX 0W9M0ZZ 0W9M30Z 0W9M3ZX 0W9M3ZZ 0W9M40Z 0W9M4ZX 0W9M4ZZ

♀ 0W9N00Z 0W9N0ZX 0W9N0ZZ 0W9N30Z 0W9N3ZX 0W9N3ZZ 0W9N40Z 0W9N4ZZ

⊘ 0W9000Z 0W900ZX 0W900ZZ 0W9030Z 0W903ZX 0W903ZZ 0W9040Z 0W904ZX 0W904ZZ 0W9130Z 0W913ZX 0W913ZZ 0W9140Z 0W914ZX 0W914ZZ 0W920ZX 0W9230Z 0W923ZX 0W923ZZ 0W924ZX 0W930ZX 0W9330Z 0W933ZX 0W933ZZ 0W934ZX 0W940ZX 0W9430Z 0W943ZX 0W943ZZ 0W944ZX 0W950ZX 0W9530Z 0W953ZX 0W953ZZ 0W954ZX 0W960ZX 0W9630Z 0W963ZX 0W963ZZ 0W964ZX 0W9800Z 0W980ZX 0W980ZZ 0W9830Z 0W983ZX 0W983ZZ 0W9840Z 0W984ZX 0W984ZZ 0W9900Z 0W990ZX 0W990ZZ 0W9930Z 0W993ZX 0W993ZZ 0W9940Z 0W994ZX 0W994ZZ 0W9B00Z 0W9B0ZX 0W9B0ZZ 0W9B30Z 0W9B3ZX 0W9B3ZZ 0W9B40Z 0W9B4ZX 0W9B4ZZ 0W9C30Z 0W9C3ZX 0W9C3ZZ 0W9C4ZX 0W9D30Z 0W9D3ZX 0W9D3ZZ 0W9D40Z 0W9D4ZX 0W9D4ZZ 0W9F30Z 0W9F3ZZ 0W9F40Z 0W9F4ZZ 0W9G30Z 0W9G3ZZ 0W9G40Z 0W9G4ZZ 0W9H30Z 0W9H3ZZ 0W9J30Z 0W9J3ZZ 0W9K00Z 0W9K0ZX 0W9K0ZZ 0W9K30Z 0W9K3ZX 0W9K3ZZ 0W9K40Z 0W9K4ZX 0W9K4ZZ 0W9L00Z 0W9L0ZX 0W9L0ZZ 0W9L30Z 0W9L3ZX 0W9L3ZZ 0W9L40Z 0W9L4ZX 0W9L4ZZ 0W9M00Z 0W9M0ZX 0W9M0ZZ 0W9M30Z 0W9M3ZX 0W9M3ZZ 0W9M40Z 0W9M4ZX 0W9M4ZZ 0W9N0ZX 0W9N30Z 0W9N3ZX 0W9N3ZZ 0W9N4ZX

0 Medical and Surgical
W Anatomical Regions, General
B Excision: Cutting out or off, without replacement, a portion of a body part

Body Part Character 4	Approach Character 5	Device Character 6	Qualifier Character 7
0 Head ⊘ **2** Face ⊘ **4** Upper Jaw ⊘ **5** Lower Jaw ⊘ **8** Chest Wall ⊘ **K** Upper Back ⊘ **L** Lower Back ⊘ **M** Perineum, Male ♂ ⊘ **N** Perineum, Female ♀	**0** Open **3** Percutaneous **4** Percutaneous Endoscopic **X** External	**Z** No Device	**X** Diagnostic **Z** No Qualifier
6 Neck ⊘ **F** Abdominal Wall	**0** Open **3** Percutaneous **4** Percutaneous Endoscopic	**Z** No Device	**X** Diagnostic **Z** No Qualifier
6 Neck ⊘ **F** Abdominal Wall	**X** External	**Z** No Device	**2** Stoma **X** Diagnostic **Z** No Qualifier
C Mediastinum ⊘ **H** Retroperitoneum ⊘	**0** Open **3** Percutaneous **4** Percutaneous Endoscopic	**Z** No Device	**X** Diagnostic **Z** No Qualifier

♂ 0WBM0ZX 0WBM0ZZ 0WBM3ZX 0WBM3ZZ 0WBM4ZX 0WBM4ZZ 0WBMXZX 0WBMXZZ

♀ 0WBN0ZX 0WBN0ZZ 0WBN3ZX 0WBN3ZZ 0WBN4ZX 0WBN4ZZ 0WBNXZX 0WBNXZZ

0WB continued on next page

0WB continued from previous page

⊘ 0WB00ZX 0WB03ZX 0WB04ZX 0WB0XZX 0WB20ZX 0WB23ZX 0WB24ZX 0WB2XZX 0WB40ZX 0WB43ZX 0WB44ZX 0WB4XZX 0WB50ZX 0WB53ZX 0WB54ZX 0WB5XZX 0WB60ZX 0WB63ZX 0WB64ZX 0WB6XZX 0WB80ZX 0WB83ZX 0WB84ZX 0WB8XZX 0WBC3ZX 0WBC4ZX 0WBH3ZX 0WBH4ZX 0WBK0ZX 0WBK3ZX 0WBK4ZX 0WBKXZX 0WBL0ZX 0WBL3ZX 0WBL4ZX 0WBLXZX 0WBM0ZX 0WBM3ZX 0WBM4ZX 0WBMXZX

0 Medical and Surgical
W Anatomical Regions, General
C Extirpation: Taking or cutting out solid matter from a body part

Body Part Character 4	Approach Character 5	Device Character 6	Qualifier Character 7
1 Cranial Cavity ⊘ **3** Oral Cavity and Throat ⊘ **9** Pleural Cavity, Right ⊘ **B** Pleural Cavity, Left ⊘ **C** Mediastinum ⊘ **D** Pericardial Cavity ⊘ **G** Peritoneal Cavity ⊘ **J** Pelvic Cavity ⊘	**0** Open **3** Percutaneous **4** Percutaneous Endoscopic **X** External	**Z** No Device	**Z** No Qualifier
P Gastrointestinal Tract ⊘ **Q** Respiratory Tract ⊘ **R** Genitourinary Tract ⊘	**0** Open **3** Percutaneous **4** Percutaneous Endoscopic **7** Via Natural or Artificial Opening **8** Via Natural or Artificial Opening Endoscopic **X** External	**Z** No Device	**Z** No Qualifier

⊘ 0WC1XZZ 0WC3XZZ 0WC90ZZ 0WC93ZZ 0WC94ZZ 0WC9XZZ 0WCB0ZZ 0WCB3ZZ 0WCB4ZZ 0WCBXZZ 0WCCXZZ 0WCDXZZ 0WCGXZZ 0WCJXZZ 0WCP7ZZ 0WCP8ZZ 0WCPXZZ 0WCQ0ZZ 0WCQ3ZZ 0WCQ4ZZ 0WCQXZZ 0WCR7ZZ 0WCR8ZZ 0WCRXZZ

0 Medical and Surgical
W Anatomical Regions, General
F Fragmentation: Breaking solid matter in a body part into pieces

Body Part Character 4	Approach Character 5	Device Character 6	Qualifier Character 7
1 Cranial Cavity NC ⊘ **3** Oral Cavity and Throat NC ⊘ **9** Pleural Cavity, Right NC ⊘ **B** Pleural Cavity, Left NC ⊘ **C** Mediastinum NC ⊘ **D** Pericardial Cavity **G** Peritoneal Cavity NC ⊘ **J** Pelvic Cavity NC ⊘	**0** Open **3** Percutaneous **4** Percutaneous Endoscopic **X** External	**Z** No Device	**Z** No Qualifier
P Gastrointestinal Tract NC ⊘ **Q** Respiratory Tract NC ⊘ **R** Genitourinary Tract ⊘ DRG	**0** Open **3** Percutaneous **4** Percutaneous Endoscopic **7** Via Natural or Artificial Opening **8** Via Natural or Artificial Opening Endoscopic **X** External	**Z** No Device	**Z** No Qualifier

⊘ 0WF1XZZ 0WF3XZZ 0WF9XZZ 0WFBXZZ 0WFCXZZ 0WFGXZZ 0WFJ0ZZ 0WFJ3ZZ 0WFJ4ZZ 0WFJXZZ 0WFP0ZZ 0WFP3ZZ 0WFP4ZZ 0WFP7ZZ 0WFP8ZZ 0WFPXZZ 0WFQXZZ 0WFR0ZZ 0WFR3ZZ 0WFR4ZZ 0WFR7ZZ 0WFR8ZZ

NC 0WF1XZZ 0WF3XZZ 0WF9XZZ 0WFBXZZ 0WFCXZZ 0WFGXZZ 0WFJXZZ 0WFPXZZ 0WFQXZZ

DRG 0WFRXZZ

0 Medical and Surgical
W Anatomical Regions, General
H Insertion: Putting in a nonbiological appliance that monitors, assists, performs, or prevents a physiological function but does not physically take the place of a body part

Body Part Character 4	Approach Character 5	Device Character 6	Qualifier Character 7
0 Head DRG **1** Cranial Cavity ⊘ **2** Face DRG **3** Oral Cavity and Throat **4** Upper Jaw DRG **5** Lower Jaw DRG **6** Neck DRG **8** Chest Wall ⊘ **9** Pleural Cavity, Right ⊘ **B** Pleural Cavity, Left ⊘ **C** Mediastinum **D** Pericardial Cavity **F** Abdominal Wall **G** Peritoneal Cavity **H** Retroperitoneum **J** Pelvic Cavity **K** Upper Back DRG **L** Lower Back DRG **M** Perineum, Male ♂ DRG **N** Perineum, Female ♀	**0** Open **3** Percutaneous **4** Percutaneous Endoscopic	**1** Radioactive Element **3** Infusion Device **Y** Other Device	**Z** No Qualifier
P Gastrointestinal Tract ⊘ **Q** Respiratory Tract ⊘ **R** Genitourinary Tract ⊘	**0** Open **3** Percutaneous **4** Percutaneous Endoscopic **7** Via Natural or Artificial Opening **8** Via Natural or Artificial Opening Endoscopic	**1** Radioactive Element **3** Infusion Device **Y** Other Device	**Z** No Qualifier

♀ 0WHN03Z 0WHN0YZ 0WHN33Z 0WHN3YZ 0WHN43Z 0WHN4YZ

⊘ 0WH103Z 0WH133Z 0WH143Z 0WH803Z 0WH80YZ 0WH833Z 0WH83YZ 0WH843Z 0WH84YZ 0WH903Z 0WH90YZ 0WH933Z 0WH93YZ 0WH943Z 0WH94YZ 0WHB03Z 0WHB0YZ 0WHB33Z 0WHB3YZ 0WHB43Z 0WHB4YZ 0WHP0YZ 0WHP33Z 0WHP3YZ 0WHP43Z 0WHP4YZ 0WHP73Z 0WHP7YZ 0WHP83Z 0WHP8YZ 0WHQ03Z 0WHQ0YZ 0WHQ73Z 0WHQ7YZ 0WHQ83Z 0WHQ8YZ 0WHR03Z 0WHR0YZ 0WHR33Z 0WHR3YZ 0WHR43Z 0WHR4YZ 0WHR73Z 0WHR7YZ 0WHR83Z 0WHR8YZ

DRG 0WH003Z 0WH00YZ 0WH033Z 0WH03YZ 0WH043Z 0WH04YZ 0WH203Z 0WH20YZ 0WH233Z 0WH23YZ 0WH243Z 0WH24YZ 0WH403Z 0WH40YZ 0WH433Z 0WH43YZ 0WH443Z 0WH44YZ 0WH503Z 0WH50YZ 0WH533Z 0WH53YZ 0WH543Z 0WH54YZ 0WH603Z 0WH60YZ 0WH633Z 0WH63YZ 0WH643Z 0WH64YZ 0WHK03Z 0WHK0YZ 0WHK33Z 0WHK3YZ 0WHK43Z 0WHK4YZ 0WHL03Z 0WHL0YZ 0WHL33Z 0WHL3YZ 0WHL43Z 0WHL4YZ 0WHM03Z 0WHM0YZ 0WHM33Z 0WHM3YZ 0WHM43Z 0WHM4YZ

0 Medical and Surgical
W Anatomical Regions, General
J Inspection: Visually and/or manually exploring a body part

Body Part Character 4	Approach Character 5	Device Character 6	Qualifier Character 7
0 Head ⦸ DRG **2** Face ⦸ DRG **3** Oral Cavity and Throat ⦸ **4** Upper Jaw ⦸ DRG **5** Lower Jaw ⦸ DRG **6** Neck ⦸ **8** Chest Wall ⦸ **F** Abdominal Wall ⦸ **K** Upper Back ⦸ DRG **L** Lower Back ⦸ DRG **M** Perineum, Male ♂ ⦸ DRG **N** Perineum, Female ♀ ⦸	**0** Open **3** Percutaneous **4** Percutaneous Endoscopic **X** External	**Z** No Device	**Z** No Qualifier
1 Cranial Cavity ⦸ **9** Pleural Cavity, Right ⦸ **B** Pleural Cavity, Left ⦸ **C** Mediastinum ⦸ **D** Pericardial Cavity ⦸ **G** Peritoneal Cavity ⦸ **H** Retroperitoneum ⦸ **J** Pelvic Cavity ⦸	**0** Open **3** Percutaneous **4** Percutaneous Endoscopic	**Z** No Device	**Z** No Qualifier
P Gastrointestinal Tract ⦸ **Q** Respiratory Tract ⦸ **R** Genitourinary Tract ⦸	**0** Open **3** Percutaneous **4** Percutaneous Endoscopic **7** Via Natural or Artificial Opening **8** Via Natural or Artificial Opening Endoscopic	**Z** No Device	**Z** No Qualifier

♂ 0WJM0ZZ 0WJM3ZZ 0WJM4ZZ 0WJMXZZ

♀ 0WJN0ZZ 0WJN3ZZ 0WJN4ZZ 0WJNXZZ

⦸ 0WJ03ZZ 0WJ04ZZ 0WJ0XZZ 0WJ13ZZ 0WJ23ZZ 0WJ24ZZ 0WJ2XZZ 0WJ30ZZ 0WJ33ZZ 0WJ34ZZ 0WJ3XZZ 0WJ43ZZ 0WJ44ZZ 0WJ4XZZ 0WJ53ZZ 0WJ54ZZ 0WJ5XZZ 0WJ63ZZ 0WJ6XZZ 0WJ83ZZ 0WJ8XZZ 0WJ93ZZ 0WJB3ZZ 0WJC3ZZ 0WJD0ZZ 0WJD3ZZ 0WJF3ZZ 0WJFXZZ 0WJG3ZZ 0WJH3ZZ 0WJJ3ZZ 0WJK3ZZ 0WJK4ZZ 0WJKXZZ 0WJL3ZZ 0WJL4ZZ 0WJLXZZ 0WJM3ZZ 0WJMXZZ 0WJN3ZZ 0WJNXZZ 0WJP3ZZ 0WJP7ZZ 0WJP8ZZ 0WJQ3ZZ 0WJQ7ZZ 0WJQ8ZZ 0WJR3ZZ 0WJR7ZZ 0WJR8ZZ

DRG 0WJ00ZZ 0WJ20ZZ 0WJ40ZZ 0WJ50ZZ 0WJK0ZZ 0WJL0ZZ 0WJM0ZZ 0WJM4ZZ

0 Medical and Surgical
W Anatomical Regions, General
M Reattachment: Putting back in or on all or a portion of a separated body part to its normal location or other suitable location

Body Part Character 4	Approach Character 5	Device Character 6	Qualifier Character 7
2 Face **4** Upper Jaw **5** Lower Jaw **6** Neck **8** Chest Wall **F** Abdominal Wall **K** Upper Back **L** Lower Back **M** Perineum, Male ♂ **N** Perineum, Female ♀	**0** Open	**Z** No Device	**Z** No Qualifier

♂ 0WMM0ZZ

♀ 0WMN0ZZ

LC Limited Coverage NC Noncovered HAC HAC Associated Procedure CC Combination Cluster - See Appendix G for code lists
DRG Non-OR-Affecting MS-DRG Assignment ⦸ Non-OR-Not Affecting MS-DRG Assignment New/Revised Text in **Orange** ♂ Male ♀ Female

0 Medical and Surgical
W Anatomical Regions, General
P Removal: Taking out or off a device from a body part

Body Part Character 4	Approach Character 5	Device Character 6	Qualifier Character 7
0 Head ⊘ **2** Face ⊘ **4** Upper Jaw ⊘ **5** Lower Jaw ⊘ **6** Neck ⊘ **8** Chest Wall ⊘ **C** Mediastinum ⊘ **F** Abdominal Wall ⊘ **K** Upper Back ⊘ **L** Lower Back ⊘ **M** Perineum, Male ♂ ⊘ **N** Perineum, Female ♀ ⊘	**0** Open **3** Percutaneous **4** Percutaneous Endoscopic **X** External	**0** Drainage Device **1** Radioactive Element **3** Infusion Device **7** Autologous Tissue Substitute **J** Synthetic Substitute **K** Nonautologous Tissue Substitute **Y** Other Device	**Z** No Qualifier
1 Cranial Cavity ⊘ **9** Pleural Cavity, Right ⊘ **B** Pleural Cavity, Left ⊘ **G** Peritoneal Cavity ⊘ **J** Pelvic Cavity ⊘	**0** Open **3** Percutaneous **4** Percutaneous Endoscopic	**0** Drainage Device **1** Radioactive Element **3** Infusion Device **J** Synthetic Substitute **Y** Other Device	**Z** No Qualifier
1 Cranial Cavity ⊘ **9** Pleural Cavity, Right ⊘ **B** Pleural Cavity, Left ⊘ **G** Peritoneal Cavity ⊘ **J** Pelvic Cavity ⊘	**X** External	**0** Drainage Device **1** Radioactive Element **3** Infusion Device	**Z** No Qualifier
D Pericardial Cavity ⊘ **H** Retroperitoneum ⊘	**0** Open **3** Percutaneous **4** Percutaneous Endoscopic	**0** Drainage Device **1** Radioactive Element **3** Infusion Device **Y** Other Device	**Z** No Qualifier
D Pericardial Cavity ⊘ **H** Retroperitoneum ⊘	**X** External	**0** Drainage Device **1** Radioactive Element **3** Infusion Device	**Z** No Qualifier
P Gastrointestinal Tract ⊘ **Q** Respiratory Tract ⊘ **R** Genitourinary Tract ⊘	**0** Open **3** Percutaneous **4** Percutaneous Endoscopic **7** Via Natural or Artificial Opening **8** Via Natural or Artificial Opening Endoscopic **X** External	**1** Radioactive Element **3** Infusion Device **Y** Other Device	**Z** No Qualifier

♂ 0WPM00Z 0WPM01Z 0WPM03Z 0WPM07Z 0WPM0JZ 0WPM0KZ 0WPM0YZ 0WPM30Z 0WPM31Z 0WPM33Z 0WPM37Z 0WPM3JZ 0WPM3KZ 0WPM3YZ 0WPM40Z 0WPM41Z 0WPM43Z 0WPM47Z 0WPM4JZ 0WPM4KZ 0WPM4YZ 0WPMX0Z 0WPMX1Z 0WPMX3Z 0WPMX7Z 0WPMXJZ 0WPMXKZ 0WPMXYZ

♀ 0WPN00Z 0WPN01Z 0WPN03Z 0WPN07Z 0WPN0JZ 0WPN0KZ 0WPN0YZ 0WPN30Z 0WPN31Z 0WPN33Z 0WPN37Z 0WPN3JZ 0WPN3KZ 0WPN3YZ 0WPN40Z 0WPN41Z 0WPN43Z 0WPN47Z 0WPN4JZ 0WPN4KZ 0WPN4YZ 0WPNX0Z 0WPNX1Z 0WPNX3Z 0WPNX7Z 0WPNXJZ 0WPNXKZ 0WPNXYZ

⊘ 0WP000Z 0WP001Z 0WP003Z 0WP007Z 0WP00JZ 0WP00KZ 0WP00YZ 0WP030Z 0WP031Z 0WP033Z 0WP037Z 0WP03JZ 0WP03KZ 0WP03YZ 0WP040Z 0WP041Z 0WP043Z 0WP047Z 0WP04JZ 0WP04KZ 0WP04YZ 0WP0X0Z 0WP0X1Z 0WP0X3Z 0WP0X7Z 0WP0XJZ 0WP0XKZ 0WP0XYZ 0WP103Z 0WP133Z 0WP143Z 0WP1X0Z 0WP1X1Z 0WP1X3Z 0WP200Z 0WP201Z 0WP203Z 0WP207Z 0WP20JZ 0WP20KZ 0WP20YZ 0WP230Z 0WP231Z 0WP233Z 0WP237Z 0WP23JZ 0WP23KZ 0WP23YZ 0WP240Z 0WP241Z 0WP243Z 0WP247Z 0WP24JZ 0WP24KZ 0WP24YZ 0WP2X0Z 0WP2X1Z 0WP2X3Z 0WP2X7Z 0WP2XJZ 0WP2XKZ 0WP2XYZ 0WP400Z 0WP401Z 0WP403Z 0WP407Z 0WP40JZ 0WP40KZ 0WP40YZ 0WP430Z 0WP431Z 0WP433Z 0WP437Z 0WP43JZ 0WP43KZ 0WP43YZ 0WP440Z 0WP441Z 0WP443Z 0WP447Z 0WP44JZ 0WP44KZ 0WP44YZ 0WP4X0Z 0WP4X1Z 0WP4X3Z 0WP4X7Z 0WP4XJZ 0WP4XKZ 0WP4XYZ 0WP500Z 0WP501Z 0WP503Z 0WP507Z 0WP50JZ 0WP50KZ 0WP50YZ 0WP530Z 0WP531Z 0WP533Z 0WP537Z 0WP53JZ 0WP53KZ 0WP53YZ 0WP540Z 0WP541Z 0WP543Z 0WP547Z 0WP54JZ 0WP54KZ 0WP54YZ 0WP5X0Z 0WP5X1Z 0WP5X3Z 0WP5X7Z 0WP5XJZ 0WP5XKZ 0WP5XYZ 0WP600Z 0WP601Z 0WP603Z 0WP607Z 0WP60JZ 0WP60KZ 0WP60YZ 0WP630Z 0WP631Z 0WP633Z 0WP637Z 0WP63JZ 0WP63KZ 0WP63YZ 0WP640Z 0WP641Z 0WP643Z 0WP647Z 0WP64JZ 0WP64KZ 0WP64YZ 0WP6X0Z 0WP6X1Z 0WP6X3Z 0WP6X7Z 0WP6XJZ 0WP6XKZ 0WP6XYZ 0WP800Z 0WP801Z 0WP803Z 0WP807Z 0WP80JZ 0WP80KZ 0WP80YZ 0WP830Z 0WP831Z 0WP833Z 0WP837Z 0WP83JZ 0WP83KZ 0WP83YZ 0WP840Z 0WP841Z 0WP843Z 0WP847Z 0WP84JZ 0WP84KZ 0WP84YZ 0WP8X0Z 0WP8X1Z 0WP8X3Z 0WP8X7Z 0WP8XJZ 0WP8XKZ 0WP8XYZ 0WP900Z 0WP901Z 0WP903Z 0WP90JZ 0WP90YZ 0WP930Z 0WP931Z 0WP933Z 0WP93JZ 0WP93YZ 0WP940Z 0WP941Z 0WP943Z 0WP94JZ 0WP94YZ 0WP9X0Z 0WP9X1Z 0WP9X3Z 0WPB00Z 0WPB01Z 0WPB03Z 0WPB0JZ 0WPB0YZ 0WPB30Z 0WPB31Z 0WPB33Z 0WPB3JZ 0WPB3YZ 0WPB40Z 0WPB41Z 0WPB43Z 0WPB4JZ 0WPB4YZ 0WPBX0Z 0WPBX1Z 0WPBX3Z 0WPCX0Z 0WPCX1Z 0WPCX3Z 0WPCX7Z 0WPCXJZ 0WPCXKZ 0WPCXYZ 0WPDX0Z 0WPDX1Z 0WPDX3Z 0WPFX0Z 0WPFX1Z 0WPFX3Z 0WPFX7Z 0WPFXJZ 0WPFXKZ 0WPFXYZ 0WPGX0Z 0WPGX1Z 0WPGX3Z 0WPHX0Z 0WPHX1Z 0WPHX3Z 0WPJ00Z 0WPJ01Z 0WPJ03Z 0WPJ0JZ 0WPJ0YZ 0WPJ30Z 0WPJ31Z 0WPJ33Z 0WPJ3JZ 0WPJ3YZ 0WPJ40Z 0WPJ41Z 0WPJ43Z 0WPJ4JZ

0WP continued on next page

0WP continued from previous page

0WPJ4YZ 0WPJX0Z 0WPJX1Z 0WPJX3Z 0WPK00Z 0WPK01Z 0WPK03Z 0WPK07Z 0WPK0JZ 0WPK0KZ 0WPK0YZ 0WPK30Z 0WPK31Z
0WPK33Z 0WPK37Z 0WPK3JZ 0WPK3KZ 0WPK3YZ 0WPK40Z 0WPK41Z 0WPK43Z 0WPK47Z 0WPK4JZ 0WPK4KZ 0WPK4YZ 0WPKX0Z
0WPKX1Z 0WPKX3Z 0WPKX7Z 0WPKXJZ 0WPKXKZ 0WPKXYZ 0WPL00Z 0WPL01Z 0WPL03Z 0WPL07Z 0WPL0JZ 0WPL0KZ 0WPL0YZ
0WPL30Z 0WPL31Z 0WPL33Z 0WPL37Z 0WPL3JZ 0WPL3KZ 0WPL3YZ 0WPL40Z 0WPL41Z 0WPL43Z 0WPL47Z 0WPL4JZ 0WPL4KZ
0WPL4YZ 0WPLX0Z 0WPLX1Z 0WPLX3Z 0WPLX7Z 0WPLXJZ 0WPLXKZ 0WPLXYZ 0WPM00Z 0WPM01Z 0WPM03Z 0WPM0JZ 0WPM0YZ
0WPM30Z 0WPM31Z 0WPM33Z 0WPM3JZ 0WPM3YZ 0WPM40Z 0WPM41Z 0WPM43Z 0WPM4JZ 0WPM4YZ 0WPMX0Z 0WPMX1Z 0WPMX3Z
0WPMXYZ 0WPNX0Z 0WPNX1Z 0WPNX3Z 0WPNX7Z 0WPNXJZ 0WPNXKZ 0WPNXYZ 0WPP31Z 0WPP33Z 0WPP3YZ 0WPP41Z 0WPP43Z
0WPP4YZ 0WPP71Z 0WPP73Z 0WPP7YZ 0WPP81Z 0WPP83Z 0WPP8YZ 0WPPX1Z 0WPPX3Z 0WPPXYZ 0WPQ01Z 0WPQ03Z 0WPQ0YZ
0WPQ73Z 0WPQ83Z 0WPQ8YZ 0WPQX1Z 0WPQX3Z 0WPQXYZ 0WPR01Z 0WPR03Z 0WPR0YZ 0WPR31Z 0WPR33Z 0WPR3YZ 0WPR41Z
0WPR43Z 0WPR4YZ 0WPR71Z 0WPR73Z 0WPR7YZ 0WPR81Z 0WPR83Z 0WPR8YZ 0WPRX1Z 0WPRX3Z 0WPRXYZ

0 Medical and Surgical
W Anatomical Regions, General
Q Repair: Restoring, to the extent possible, a body part to its normal anatomic structure and function

Body Part Character 4	Approach Character 5	Device Character 6	Qualifier Character 7
0 Head **2** Face **4** Upper Jaw **5** Lower Jaw **8** Chest Wall CC **K** Upper Back **L** Lower Back **M** Perineum, Male ♂ **N** Perineum, Female ♀ ⊘ CC	**0** Open **3** Percutaneous **4** Percutaneous Endoscopic **X** External	**Z** No Device	**Z** No Qualifier
6 Neck **F** Abdominal Wall	**0** Open **3** Percutaneous **4** Percutaneous Endoscopic	**Z** No Device	**Z** No Qualifier
6 Neck **F** Abdominal Wall CC	**X** External	**Z** No Device	**2** Stoma **Z** No Qualifier
C Mediastinum CC	**0** Open **3** Percutaneous **4** Percutaneous Endoscopic	**Z** No Device	**Z** No Qualifier

♂ 0WQM0ZZ 0WQM3ZZ 0WQM4ZZ 0WQMXZZ
♀ 0WQN0ZZ 0WQN3ZZ 0WQN4ZZ 0WQNXZZ
⊘ 0WQNXZZ
CC 0WQ80ZZ 0WQ83ZZ 0WQ84ZZ 0WQC0ZZ 0WQC3ZZ 0WQC4ZZ 0WQFXZ2 0WQFXZZ 0WQN0ZZ 0WQN3ZZ 0WQN4ZZ

0 Medical and Surgical
W Anatomical Regions, General
U Supplement: Putting in or on biological or synthetic material that physically reinforces and/or augments the function of a portion of a body part

Body Part Character 4	Approach Character 5	Device Character 6	Qualifier Character 7
0 Head **2** Face **4** Upper Jaw **5** Lower Jaw **6** Neck **8** Chest Wall **C** Mediastinum **F** Abdominal Wall **K** Upper Back **L** Lower Back **M** Perineum, Male ♂ **N** Perineum, Female ♀	**0** Open **4** Percutaneous Endoscopic	**7** Autologous Tissue Substitute **J** Synthetic Substitute **K** Nonautologous Tissue Substitute	**Z** No Qualifier

♂ 0WUM07Z 0WUM0JZ 0WUM0KZ 0WUM47Z 0WUM4JZ 0WUM4KZ
♀ 0WUN07Z 0WUN0JZ 0WUN0KZ 0WUN47Z 0WUN4JZ 0WUN4KZ

0 Medical and Surgical
W Anatomical Regions, General
W Revision: Correcting, to the extent possible, a portion of a malfunctioning device or the position of a displaced device

Body Part Character 4	Approach Character 5	Device Character 6	Qualifier Character 7
0 Head ⦸ DRG **2** Face ⦸ DRG **4** Upper Jaw ⦸ DRG **5** Lower Jaw ⦸ DRG **6** Neck ⦸ DRG **8** Chest Wall ⦸ **C** Mediastinum ⦸ **F** Abdominal Wall ⦸ **K** Upper Back ⦸ DRG **L** Lower Back ⦸ DRG **M** Perineum, Male ♂ ⦸ DRG **N** Perineum, Female ♀ ⦸	**0** Open **3** Percutaneous **4** Percutaneous Endoscopic **X** External	**0** Drainage Device **1** Radioactive Element **3** Infusion Device **7** Autologous Tissue Substitute **J** Synthetic Substitute **K** Nonautologous Tissue Substitute **Y** Other Device	**Z** No Qualifier
1 Cranial Cavity ⦸ **9** Pleural Cavity, Right ⦸ **B** Pleural Cavity, Left ⦸ **G** Peritoneal Cavity ⦸ **J** Pelvic Cavity ⦸	**0** Open **3** Percutaneous **4** Percutaneous Endoscopic **X** External	**0** Drainage Device **1** Radioactive Element **3** Infusion Device **J** Synthetic Substitute **Y** Other Device	**Z** No Qualifier
D Pericardial Cavity ⦸ **H** Retroperitoneum ⦸	**0** Open **3** Percutaneous **4** Percutaneous Endoscopic **X** External	**0** Drainage Device **1** Radioactive Element **3** Infusion Device **Y** Other Device	**Z** No Qualifier
P Gastrointestinal Tract ⦸ **Q** Respiratory Tract ⦸ **R** Genitourinary Tract ⦸	**0** Open **3** Percutaneous **4** Percutaneous Endoscopic **7** Via Natural or Artificial Opening **8** Via Natural or Artificial Opening Endoscopic **X** External	**1** Radioactive Element **3** Infusion Device **Y** Other Device	**Z** No Qualifier

♂ 0WWM00Z 0WWM01Z 0WWM03Z 0WWM07Z 0WWM0JZ 0WWM0KZ 0WWM0YZ 0WWM30Z 0WWM31Z 0WWM33Z 0WWM37Z 0WWM3JZ 0WWM3KZ 0WWM3YZ 0WWM40Z 0WWM41Z 0WWM43Z 0WWM47Z 0WWM4JZ 0WWM4KZ 0WWM4YZ 0WWMX0Z 0WWMX1Z 0WWMX3Z 0WWMX7Z 0WWMXJZ 0WWMXKZ 0WWMXYZ

♀ 0WWN00Z 0WWN01Z 0WWN03Z 0WWN07Z 0WWN0JZ 0WWN0KZ 0WWN0YZ 0WWN30Z 0WWN31Z 0WWN33Z 0WWN37Z 0WWN3JZ 0WWN3KZ 0WWN3YZ 0WWN40Z 0WWN41Z 0WWN43Z 0WWN47Z 0WWN4JZ 0WWN4KZ 0WWN4YZ 0WWNX0Z 0WWNX1Z 0WWNX3Z 0WWNX7Z 0WWNXJZ 0WWNXKZ 0WWNXYZ

⦸ 0WW0X0Z 0WW0X1Z 0WW0X3Z 0WW0X7Z 0WW0XJZ 0WW0XKZ 0WW0XYZ 0WW1X0Z 0WW1X1Z 0WW1X3Z 0WW1XJZ 0WW1XYZ 0WW2X0Z 0WW2X1Z 0WW2X3Z 0WW2X7Z 0WW2XJZ 0WW2XKZ 0WW2XYZ 0WW4X0Z 0WW4X1Z 0WW4X3Z 0WW4X7Z 0WW4XJZ 0WW4XKZ 0WW4XYZ 0WW5X0Z 0WW5X1Z 0WW5X3Z 0WW5X7Z 0WW5XJZ 0WW5XKZ 0WW5XYZ 0WW6X0Z 0WW6X1Z 0WW6X3Z 0WW6X7Z 0WW6XJZ 0WW6XKZ 0WW6XYZ 0WW800Z 0WW801Z 0WW803Z 0WW807Z 0WW80JZ 0WW80KZ 0WW80YZ 0WW830Z 0WW831Z 0WW833Z 0WW837Z 0WW83JZ 0WW83KZ 0WW83YZ 0WW840Z 0WW841Z 0WW843Z 0WW847Z 0WW84JZ 0WW84KZ 0WW84YZ 0WW8X0Z 0WW8X1Z 0WW8X3Z 0WW8X7Z 0WW8XJZ 0WW8XKZ 0WW8XYZ 0WW900Z 0WW901Z 0WW903Z 0WW90JZ 0WW90YZ 0WW930Z 0WW931Z 0WW933Z 0WW93JZ 0WW93YZ 0WW940Z 0WW941Z 0WW943Z 0WW94JZ 0WW94YZ 0WW9X0Z 0WW9X1Z 0WW9X3Z 0WW9XJZ 0WW9XYZ 0WWB00Z 0WWB01Z 0WWB03Z 0WWB0JZ 0WWB0YZ 0WWB30Z 0WWB31Z 0WWB33Z 0WWB3JZ 0WWB3YZ 0WWB40Z 0WWB41Z 0WWB43Z 0WWB4JZ 0WWB4YZ 0WWBX0Z 0WWBX1Z 0WWBX3Z 0WWBXJZ 0WWBXYZ 0WWCX0Z 0WWCX1Z 0WWCX3Z 0WWCX7Z 0WWCXJZ 0WWCXKZ 0WWCXYZ 0WWDX0Z 0WWDX1Z 0WWDX3Z 0WWDXYZ 0WWFX0Z 0WWFX1Z 0WWFX3Z 0WWFX7Z 0WWFXJZ 0WWFXKZ 0WWFXYZ 0WWGX0Z 0WWGX1Z 0WWGX3Z 0WWGXJZ 0WWGXYZ 0WWHX0Z 0WWHX1Z 0WWHX3Z 0WWHXYZ 0WWJX0Z 0WWJX1Z 0WWJX3Z 0WWJXJZ 0WWJXYZ 0WWKX0Z 0WWKX1Z 0WWKX3Z 0WWKX7Z 0WWKXJZ 0WWKXKZ 0WWKXYZ 0WWLX0Z 0WWLX1Z 0WWLX3Z 0WWLX7Z 0WWLXJZ 0WWLXKZ 0WWLXYZ 0WWMX0Z 0WWMX1Z 0WWMX3Z 0WWMX7Z 0WWMXJZ 0WWMXKZ 0WWMXYZ 0WWNX0Z 0WWNX1Z 0WWNX3Z 0WWNX7Z 0WWNXJZ 0WWNXKZ 0WWNXYZ 0WWP31Z 0WWP33Z 0WWP3YZ 0WWP41Z 0WWP43Z 0WWP4YZ 0WWP71Z 0WWP73Z 0WWP7YZ 0WWP81Z 0WWP83Z 0WWP8YZ 0WWPX1Z 0WWPX3Z 0WWPXYZ 0WWQ01Z 0WWQ03Z 0WWQ0YZ 0WWQX1Z 0WWQX3Z 0WWQXYZ 0WWR01Z 0WWR03Z 0WWR0YZ 0WWR31Z 0WWR33Z 0WWR3YZ 0WWR41Z 0WWR43Z 0WWR4YZ 0WWR71Z 0WWR73Z 0WWR7YZ 0WWR81Z 0WWR83Z 0WWR8YZ 0WWRX1Z 0WWRX3Z 0WWRXYZ

DRG 0WW000Z 0WW001Z 0WW003Z 0WW007Z 0WW00JZ 0WW00KZ 0WW00YZ 0WW030Z 0WW031Z 0WW033Z 0WW037Z 0WW03JZ 0WW03KZ 0WW03YZ 0WW040Z 0WW041Z 0WW043Z 0WW047Z 0WW04JZ 0WW04KZ 0WW04YZ 0WW200Z 0WW201Z 0WW203Z 0WW207Z 0WW20JZ 0WW20KZ 0WW20YZ 0WW230Z 0WW231Z 0WW233Z 0WW237Z 0WW23JZ 0WW23KZ 0WW23YZ 0WW240Z 0WW241Z 0WW243Z 0WW247Z 0WW24JZ 0WW24KZ 0WW24YZ 0WW400Z 0WW401Z 0WW403Z 0WW407Z 0WW40JZ 0WW40KZ 0WW40YZ 0WW430Z 0WW431Z 0WW433Z 0WW437Z 0WW43JZ 0WW43KZ 0WW43YZ 0WW440Z 0WW441Z 0WW443Z 0WW447Z 0WW44JZ 0WW44KZ 0WW44YZ 0WW500Z 0WW501Z 0WW503Z 0WW507Z 0WW50JZ 0WW50KZ 0WW50YZ 0WW530Z 0WW531Z 0WW533Z 0WW537Z 0WW53JZ 0WW53KZ 0WW53YZ 0WW540Z 0WW541Z 0WW543Z 0WW547Z 0WW54JZ 0WW54KZ 0WW54YZ 0WW600Z 0WW601Z 0WW603Z 0WW607Z 0WW60JZ 0WW60KZ 0WW60YZ 0WW630Z 0WW631Z 0WW633Z 0WW637Z 0WW63JZ 0WW63KZ 0WW63YZ 0WW640Z 0WW641Z 0WW643Z 0WW647Z 0WW64JZ 0WW64KZ 0WW64YZ 0WWK00Z 0WWK01Z 0WWK03Z 0WWK07Z 0WWK0JZ 0WWK0KZ 0WWK0YZ 0WWK30Z 0WWK31Z 0WWK33Z 0WWK37Z 0WWK3JZ 0WWK3KZ 0WWK3YZ 0WWK40Z 0WWK41Z 0WWK43Z 0WWK47Z 0WWK4JZ 0WWK4KZ 0WWK4YZ 0WWL00Z 0WWL01Z 0WWL03Z 0WWL07Z 0WWL0JZ 0WWL0KZ 0WWL0YZ 0WWL30Z 0WWL31Z 0WWL33Z 0WWL37Z 0WWL3JZ 0WWL3KZ 0WWL3YZ 0WWL40Z 0WWL41Z 0WWL43Z 0WWL47Z 0WWL4JZ 0WWL4KZ 0WWL4YZ 0WWM00Z 0WWM01Z 0WWM03Z 0WWM0JZ 0WWM0YZ 0WWM30Z 0WWM31Z 0WWM33Z 0WWM3JZ 0WWM3YZ 0WWM40Z 0WWM41Z 0WWM43Z 0WWM4JZ 0WWM4YZ

0 Medical and Surgical
W Anatomical Regions, General
Y Transplantation: Putting in or on all or a portion of a living body part taken from another individual or animal to physically take the place and/or function of all or a portion of a similar body part

Body Part Character 4	Approach Character 5	Device Character 6	Qualifier Character 7
2 Face ⃠	0 Open	Z No Device	0 Allogeneic 1 Syngeneic

⃠ 0WY20Z0 0WY20Z1

Anatomical Regions, Upper Extremities 0X0-0XY

0 Medical and Surgical
X Anatomical Regions, Upper Extremities
0 Alteration: Modifying the anatomic structure of a body part without affecting the function of the body part

Body Part Character 4	Approach Character 5	Device Character 6	Qualifier Character 7
2 Shoulder Region, Right 3 Shoulder Region, Left 4 Axilla, Right 5 Axilla, Left 6 Upper Extremity, Right 7 Upper Extremity, Left 8 Upper Arm, Right 9 Upper Arm, Left B Elbow Region, Right C Elbow Region, Left D Lower Arm, Right F Lower Arm, Left G Wrist Region, Right H Wrist Region, Left	0 Open 3 Percutaneous 4 Percutaneous Endoscopic	7 Autologous Tissue Substitute J Synthetic Substitute K Nonautologous Tissue Substitute Z No Device	Z No Qualifier

0 Medical and Surgical
X Anatomical Regions, Upper Extremities
2 Change: Taking out or off a device from a body part and putting back an identical or similar device in or on the same body part without cutting or puncturing the skin or a mucous membrane

Body Part Character 4	Approach Character 5	Device Character 6	Qualifier Character 7
6 Upper Extremity, Right ⦸ 7 Upper Extremity, Left ⦸	X External	0 Drainage Device Y Other Device	Z No Qualifier

⦸ 0X26X0Z 0X26XYZ 0X27X0Z 0X27XYZ

0 Medical and Surgical
X Anatomical Regions, Upper Extremities
3 Control: Stopping, or attempting to stop, postprocedural or other acute bleeding

Body Part Character 4	Approach Character 5	Device Character 6	Qualifier Character 7
2 Shoulder Region, Right 3 Shoulder Region, Left 4 Axilla, Right 5 Axilla, Left 6 Upper Extremity, Right 7 Upper Extremity, Left 8 Upper Arm, Right 9 Upper Arm, Left B Elbow Region, Right C Elbow Region, Left D Lower Arm, Right F Lower Arm, Left G Wrist Region, Right H Wrist Region, Left J Hand, Right K Hand, Left	0 Open 3 Percutaneous 4 Percutaneous Endoscopic	Z No Device	Z No Qualifier

0 Medical and Surgical
X Anatomical Regions, Upper Extremities
6 Detachment: Cutting off all or a portion of the upper or lower extremities

Body Part Character 4	Approach Character 5	Device Character 6	Qualifier Character 7
0 Forequarter, Right **1** Forequarter, Left **2** Shoulder Region, Right **3** Shoulder Region, Left **B** Elbow Region, Right **C** Elbow Region, Left	**0** Open	**Z** No Device	**Z** No Qualifier
8 Upper Arm, Right **9** Upper Arm, Left **D** Lower Arm, Right **F** Lower Arm, Left	**0** Open	**Z** No Device	**1** High **2** Mid **3** Low
J Hand, Right **K** Hand, Left	**0** Open	**Z** No Device	**0** Complete **4** Complete 1st Ray **5** Complete 2nd Ray **6** Complete 3rd Ray **7** Complete 4th Ray **8** Complete 5th Ray **9** Partial 1st Ray **B** Partial 2nd Ray **C** Partial 3rd Ray **D** Partial 4th Ray **F** Partial 5th Ray
L Thumb, Right **M** Thumb, Left **N** Index Finger, Right **P** Index Finger, Left **Q** Middle Finger, Right **R** Middle Finger, Left **S** Ring Finger, Right **T** Ring Finger, Left **V** Little Finger, Right **W** Little Finger, Left	**0** Open	**Z** No Device	**0** Complete **1** High **2** Mid **3** Low

0 Medical and Surgical
X Anatomical Regions, Upper Extremities
9 Drainage: Taking or letting out fluids and/or gases from a body part

Body Part Character 4	Approach Character 5	Device Character 6	Qualifier Character 7
2 Shoulder Region, Right ⊘ **3** Shoulder Region, Left ⊘ **4** Axilla, Right ⊘ **5** Axilla, Left ⊘ **6** Upper Extremity, Right ⊘ **7** Upper Extremity, Left ⊘ **8** Upper Arm, Right ⊘ **9** Upper Arm, Left ⊘ **B** Elbow Region, Right ⊘ **C** Elbow Region, Left ⊘ **D** Lower Arm, Right ⊘ **F** Lower Arm, Left ⊘ **G** Wrist Region, Right ⊘ **H** Wrist Region, Left ⊘ **J** Hand, Right ⊘ **K** Hand, Left ⊘	**0** Open **3** Percutaneous **4** Percutaneous Endoscopic	**0** Drainage Device	**Z** No Qualifier
2 Shoulder Region, Right ⊘ **3** Shoulder Region, Left ⊘ **4** Axilla, Right ⊘ **5** Axilla, Left ⊘ **6** Upper Extremity, Right ⊘ **7** Upper Extremity, Left ⊘ **8** Upper Arm, Right ⊘ **9** Upper Arm, Left ⊘ **B** Elbow Region, Right ⊘ **C** Elbow Region, Left ⊘ **D** Lower Arm, Right ⊘ **F** Lower Arm, Left ⊘ **G** Wrist Region, Right ⊘ **H** Wrist Region, Left ⊘ **J** Hand, Right ⊘ **K** Hand, Left ⊘	**0** Open **3** Percutaneous **4** Percutaneous Endoscopic	**Z** No Device	**X** Diagnostic **Z** No Qualifier

⊘ 0X9200Z 0X920ZX 0X920ZZ 0X9230Z 0X923ZX 0X923ZZ 0X9240Z 0X924ZX 0X924ZZ 0X9300Z 0X930ZX 0X930ZZ 0X9330Z 0X933ZX 0X933ZZ 0X9340Z 0X934ZX 0X934ZZ 0X9400Z 0X940ZX 0X940ZZ 0X9430Z 0X943ZX 0X943ZZ 0X9440Z 0X944ZX 0X944ZZ 0X9500Z 0X950ZX 0X950ZZ 0X9530Z 0X953ZX 0X953ZZ 0X9540Z 0X954ZX 0X954ZZ 0X9600Z 0X960ZX 0X960ZZ 0X9630Z 0X963ZX 0X963ZZ 0X9640Z 0X964ZX 0X964ZZ 0X9700Z 0X970ZX 0X970ZZ 0X9730Z 0X973ZX 0X973ZZ 0X9740Z 0X974ZX 0X974ZZ 0X9800Z 0X980ZX 0X980ZZ 0X9830Z 0X983ZX 0X983ZZ 0X9840Z 0X984ZX 0X984ZZ 0X9900Z 0X990ZX 0X990ZZ 0X9930Z 0X993ZX 0X993ZZ 0X9940Z 0X994ZX 0X994ZZ 0X9B00Z 0X9B0ZX 0X9B0ZZ 0X9B30Z 0X9B3ZX 0X9B3ZZ 0X9B40Z 0X9B4ZX 0X9B4ZZ 0X9C00Z 0X9C0ZX 0X9C0ZZ 0X9C30Z 0X9C3ZX 0X9C3ZZ 0X9C40Z 0X9C4ZX 0X9C4ZZ 0X9D00Z 0X9D0ZX 0X9D0ZZ 0X9D30Z 0X9D3ZX 0X9D3ZZ 0X9D40Z 0X9D4ZX 0X9D4ZZ 0X9F00Z 0X9F0ZX 0X9F0ZZ 0X9F30Z 0X9F3ZX 0X9F3ZZ 0X9F40Z 0X9F4ZX 0X9F4ZZ 0X9G00Z 0X9G0ZX 0X9G0ZZ 0X9G30Z 0X9G3ZX 0X9G3ZZ 0X9G40Z 0X9G4ZX 0X9G4ZZ 0X9H00Z 0X9H0ZX 0X9H0ZZ 0X9H30Z 0X9H3ZX 0X9H3ZZ 0X9H40Z 0X9H4ZX 0X9H4ZZ 0X9J00Z 0X9J0ZX 0X9J0ZZ 0X9J30Z 0X9J3ZX 0X9J3ZZ 0X9J40Z 0X9J4ZX 0X9J4ZZ 0X9K00Z 0X9K0ZX 0X9K0ZZ 0X9K30Z 0X9K3ZX 0X9K3ZZ 0X9K40Z 0X9K4ZX 0X9K4ZZ

0 Medical and Surgical
X Anatomical Regions, Upper Extremities
B Excision: Cutting out or off, without replacement, a portion of a body part

Body Part Character 4	Approach Character 5	Device Character 6	Qualifier Character 7
2 Shoulder Region, Right ⊘	**0** Open	**Z** No Device	**X** Diagnostic
3 Shoulder Region, Left ⊘	**3** Percutaneous		**Z** No Qualifier
4 Axilla, Right ⊘	**4** Percutaneous Endoscopic		
5 Axilla, Left ⊘			
6 Upper Extremity, Right ⊘			
7 Upper Extremity, Left ⊘			
8 Upper Arm, Right ⊘			
9 Upper Arm, Left ⊘			
B Elbow Region, Right ⊘			
C Elbow Region, Left ⊘			
D Lower Arm, Right ⊘			
F Lower Arm, Left ⊘			
G Wrist Region, Right ⊘			
H Wrist Region, Left ⊘			
J Hand, Right ⊘			
K Hand, Left ⊘			

⊘ 0XB20ZX 0XB23ZX 0XB24ZX 0XB30ZX 0XB33ZX 0XB34ZX 0XB40ZX 0XB43ZX 0XB44ZX 0XB50ZX 0XB53ZX 0XB54ZX 0XB60ZX 0XB63ZX 0XB64ZX 0XB70ZX 0XB73ZX 0XB74ZX 0XB80ZX 0XB83ZX 0XB84ZX 0XB90ZX 0XB93ZX 0XB94ZX 0XBB0ZX 0XBB3ZX 0XBB4ZX 0XBC0ZX 0XBC3ZX 0XBC4ZX 0XBD0ZX 0XBD3ZX 0XBD4ZX 0XBF0ZX 0XBF3ZX 0XBF4ZX 0XBG0ZX 0XBG3ZX 0XBG4ZX 0XBH0ZX 0XBH3ZX 0XBH4ZX 0XBJ0ZX 0XBJ3ZX 0XBJ4ZX 0XBK0ZX 0XBK3ZX 0XBK4ZX

0 Medical and Surgical
X Anatomical Regions, Upper Extremities
H Insertion: Putting in a nonbiological appliance that monitors, assists, performs, or prevents a physiological function but does not physically take the place of a body part

Body Part Character 4	Approach Character 5	Device Character 6	Qualifier Character 7
2 Shoulder Region, Right DRG	**0** Open	**1** Radioactive Element	**Z** No Qualifier
3 Shoulder Region, Left DRG	**3** Percutaneous	**3** Infusion Device	
4 Axilla, Right DRG	**4** Percutaneous Endoscopic	**Y** Other Device	
5 Axilla, Left DRG			
6 Upper Extremity, Right DRG			
7 Upper Extremity, Left DRG			
8 Upper Arm, Right DRG			
9 Upper Arm, Left DRG			
B Elbow Region, Right DRG			
C Elbow Region, Left DRG			
D Lower Arm, Right DRG			
F Lower Arm, Left DRG			
G Wrist Region, Right DRG			
H Wrist Region, Left DRG			
J Hand, Right DRG			
K Hand, Left DRG			

DRG 0XH203Z 0XH20YZ 0XH233Z 0XH23YZ 0XH243Z 0XH24YZ 0XH303Z 0XH30YZ 0XH333Z 0XH33YZ 0XH343Z 0XH34YZ 0XH403Z 0XH40YZ 0XH433Z 0XH43YZ 0XH443Z 0XH44YZ 0XH503Z 0XH50YZ 0XH533Z 0XH53YZ 0XH543Z 0XH54YZ 0XH603Z 0XH60YZ 0XH633Z 0XH63YZ 0XH643Z 0XH64YZ 0XH703Z 0XH70YZ 0XH733Z 0XH73YZ 0XH743Z 0XH74YZ 0XH803Z 0XH80YZ 0XH833Z 0XH83YZ 0XH843Z 0XH84YZ 0XH903Z 0XH90YZ 0XH933Z 0XH93YZ 0XH943Z 0XH94YZ 0XHB03Z 0XHB0YZ 0XHB33Z 0XHB3YZ 0XHB43Z 0XHB4YZ 0XHC03Z 0XHC0YZ 0XHC33Z 0XHC3YZ 0XHC43Z 0XHC4YZ 0XHD03Z 0XHD0YZ 0XHD33Z 0XHD3YZ 0XHD43Z 0XHD4YZ 0XHF03Z 0XHF0YZ 0XHF33Z 0XHF3YZ 0XHF43Z 0XHF4YZ 0XHG03Z 0XHG0YZ 0XHG33Z 0XHG3YZ 0XHG43Z 0XHG4YZ 0XHH03Z 0XHH0YZ 0XHH33Z 0XHH3YZ 0XHH43Z 0XHH4YZ 0XHJ03Z 0XHJ0YZ 0XHJ33Z 0XHJ3YZ 0XHJ43Z 0XHJ4YZ 0XHK03Z 0XHK0YZ 0XHK33Z 0XHK3YZ 0XHK43Z 0XHK4YZ

0 Medical and Surgical
X Anatomical Regions, Upper Extremities
J Inspection: Visually and/or manually exploring a body part

Body Part Character 4	Approach Character 5	Device Character 6	Qualifier Character 7
2 Shoulder Region, Right ⊘ DRG **3** Shoulder Region, Left ⊘ DRG **4** Axilla, Right ⊘ DRG **5** Axilla, Left ⊘ DRG **6** Upper Extremity, Right ⊘ DRG **7** Upper Extremity, Left ⊘ DRG **8** Upper Arm, Right ⊘ DRG **9** Upper Arm, Left ⊘ DRG **B** Elbow Region, Right ⊘ DRG **C** Elbow Region, Left ⊘ DRG **D** Lower Arm, Right ⊘ DRG **F** Lower Arm, Left ⊘ DRG **G** Wrist Region, Right ⊘ DRG **H** Wrist Region, Left ⊘ DRG **J** Hand, Right ⊘ DRG **K** Hand, Left ⊘ DRG	**0** Open **3** Percutaneous **4** Percutaneous Endoscopic **X** External	**Z** No Device	**Z** No Qualifier

⊘ 0XJ23ZZ 0XJ24ZZ 0XJ2XZZ 0XJ33ZZ 0XJ34ZZ 0XJ3XZZ 0XJ43ZZ 0XJ44ZZ 0XJ4XZZ 0XJ53ZZ 0XJ54ZZ 0XJ5XZZ 0XJ63ZZ 0XJ64ZZ 0XJ6XZZ 0XJ73ZZ 0XJ74ZZ 0XJ7XZZ 0XJ83ZZ 0XJ84ZZ 0XJ8XZZ 0XJ93ZZ 0XJ94ZZ 0XJ9XZZ 0XJB3ZZ 0XJB4ZZ 0XJBXZZ 0XJC3ZZ 0XJC4ZZ 0XJCXZZ 0XJD3ZZ 0XJD4ZZ 0XJDXZZ 0XJF3ZZ 0XJF4ZZ 0XJFXZZ 0XJG3ZZ 0XJG4ZZ 0XJGXZZ 0XJH3ZZ 0XJH4ZZ 0XJHXZZ 0XJJ3ZZ 0XJJXZZ 0XJK3ZZ 0XJKXZZ

DRG 0XJ20ZZ 0XJ30ZZ 0XJ40ZZ 0XJ50ZZ 0XJ60ZZ 0XJ70ZZ 0XJ80ZZ 0XJ90ZZ 0XJB0ZZ 0XJC0ZZ 0XJD0ZZ 0XJF0ZZ 0XJG0ZZ 0XJH0ZZ 0XJJ0ZZ 0XJK0ZZ

0 Medical and Surgical
X Anatomical Regions, Upper Extremities
M Reattachment: Putting back in or on all or a portion of a separated body part to its normal location or other suitable location

Body Part Character 4	Approach Character 5	Device Character 6	Qualifier Character 7
0 Forequarter, Right **1** Forequarter, Left **2** Shoulder Region, Right **3** Shoulder Region, Left **4** Axilla, Right **5** Axilla, Left **6** Upper Extremity, Right **7** Upper Extremity, Left **8** Upper Arm, Right **9** Upper Arm, Left **B** Elbow Region, Right **C** Elbow Region, Left **D** Lower Arm, Right **F** Lower Arm, Left **G** Wrist Region, Right **H** Wrist Region, Left **J** Hand, Right **K** Hand, Left **L** Thumb, Right **M** Thumb, Left **N** Index Finger, Right **P** Index Finger, Left **Q** Middle Finger, Right **R** Middle Finger, Left **S** Ring Finger, Right **T** Ring Finger, Left **V** Little Finger, Right **W** Little Finger, Left	**0** Open	**Z** No Device	**Z** No Qualifier

LC Limited Coverage NC Noncovered HAC HAC Associated Procedure CC Combination Cluster - See Appendix G for code lists
DRG Non-OR-Affecting MS-DRG Assignment ⊘ Non-OR-Not Affecting MS-DRG Assignment New/Revised Text in **Orange** ♂ Male ♀ Female

0 Medical and Surgical
X Anatomical Regions, Upper Extremities
P Removal: Taking out or off a device from a body part

Body Part Character 4	Approach Character 5	Device Character 6	Qualifier Character 7
6 Upper Extremity, Right ⊘ 7 Upper Extremity, Left ⊘	0 Open 3 Percutaneous 4 Percutaneous Endoscopic X External	0 Drainage Device 1 Radioactive Element 3 Infusion Device 7 Autologous Tissue Substitute J Synthetic Substitute K Nonautologous Tissue Substitute Y Other Device	Z No Qualifier

⊘ 0XP600Z 0XP601Z 0XP603Z 0XP607Z 0XP60JZ 0XP60KZ 0XP60YZ 0XP630Z 0XP631Z 0XP633Z 0XP637Z 0XP63JZ 0XP63KZ 0XP63YZ 0XP640Z 0XP641Z 0XP643Z 0XP647Z 0XP64JZ 0XP64KZ 0XP64YZ 0XP6X0Z 0XP6X1Z 0XP6X3Z 0XP6X7Z 0XP6XJZ 0XP6XKZ 0XP6XYZ 0XP700Z 0XP701Z 0XP703Z 0XP707Z 0XP70JZ 0XP70KZ 0XP70YZ 0XP730Z 0XP731Z 0XP733Z 0XP737Z 0XP73JZ 0XP73KZ 0XP73YZ 0XP740Z 0XP741Z 0XP743Z 0XP747Z 0XP74JZ 0XP74KZ 0XP74YZ 0XP7X0Z 0XP7X1Z 0XP7X3Z 0XP7X7Z 0XP7XJZ 0XP7XKZ 0XP7XYZ

0 Medical and Surgical
X Anatomical Regions, Upper Extremities
Q Repair: Restoring, to the extent possible, a body part to its normal anatomic structure and function

Body Part Character 4	Approach Character 5	Device Character 6	Qualifier Character 7
2 Shoulder Region, Right 3 Shoulder Region, Left 4 Axilla, Right 5 Axilla, Left 6 Upper Extremity, Right 7 Upper Extremity, Left 8 Upper Arm, Right 9 Upper Arm, Left B Elbow Region, Right C Elbow Region, Left D Lower Arm, Right F Lower Arm, Left G Wrist Region, Right H Wrist Region, Left J Hand, Right K Hand, Left L Thumb, Right M Thumb, Left N Index Finger, Right P Index Finger, Left Q Middle Finger, Right R Middle Finger, Left S Ring Finger, Right T Ring Finger, Left V Little Finger, Right W Little Finger, Left	0 Open 3 Percutaneous 4 Percutaneous Endoscopic X External	Z No Device	Z No Qualifier

0 Medical and Surgical
X Anatomical Regions, Upper Extremities
R Replacement: Putting in or on biological or synthetic material that physically takes the place and/or function of all or a portion of a body part

Body Part Character 4	Approach Character 5	Device Character 6	Qualifier Character 7
L Thumb, Right M Thumb, Left	0 Open 4 Percutaneous Endoscopic	7 Autologous Tissue Substitute	N Toe, Right P Toe, Left

0 Medical and Surgical
X Anatomical Regions, Upper Extremities
U Supplement: Putting in or on biological or synthetic material that physically reinforces and/or augments the function of a portion of a body part

Body Part Character 4	Approach Character 5	Device Character 6	Qualifier Character 7
2 Shoulder Region, Right **3** Shoulder Region, Left **4** Axilla, Right **5** Axilla, Left **6** Upper Extremity, Right **7** Upper Extremity, Left **8** Upper Arm, Right **9** Upper Arm, Left **B** Elbow Region, Right **C** Elbow Region, Left **D** Lower Arm, Right **F** Lower Arm, Left **G** Wrist Region, Right **H** Wrist Region, Left **J** Hand, Right **K** Hand, Left **L** Thumb, Right **M** Thumb, Left **N** Index Finger, Right **P** Index Finger, Left **Q** Middle Finger, Right **R** Middle Finger, Left **S** Ring Finger, Right **T** Ring Finger, Left **V** Little Finger, Right **W** Little Finger, Left	**0** Open **4** Percutaneous Endoscopic	**7** Autologous Tissue Substitute **J** Synthetic Substitute **K** Nonautologous Tissue Substitute	**Z** No Qualifier

0 Medical and Surgical
X Anatomical Regions, Upper Extremities
W Revision: Correcting, to the extent possible, a portion of a malfunctioning device or the position of a displaced device

Body Part Character 4	Approach Character 5	Device Character 6	Qualifier Character 7
6 Upper Extremity, Right ⊘ DRG **7** Upper Extremity, Left ⊘ DRG	**0** Open **3** Percutaneous **4** Percutaneous Endoscopic **X** External	**0** Drainage Device **3** Infusion Device **7** Autologous Tissue Substitute **J** Synthetic Substitute **K** Nonautologous Tissue Substitute **Y** Other Device	**Z** No Qualifier

⊘ 0XW6X0Z 0XW6X3Z 0XW6X7Z 0XW6XJZ 0XW6XKZ 0XW6XYZ 0XW7X0Z 0XW7X3Z 0XW7X7Z 0XW7XJZ 0XW7XKZ 0XW7XYZ

DRG 0XW600Z 0XW603Z 0XW607Z 0XW60JZ 0XW60KZ 0XW60YZ 0XW630Z 0XW633Z 0XW637Z 0XW63JZ 0XW63KZ 0XW63YZ 0XW640Z 0XW643Z 0XW647Z 0XW64JZ 0XW64KZ 0XW64YZ 0XW700Z 0XW703Z 0XW707Z 0XW70JZ 0XW70KZ 0XW70YZ 0XW730Z 0XW733Z 0XW737Z 0XW73JZ 0XW73KZ 0XW73YZ 0XW740Z 0XW743Z 0XW747Z 0XW74JZ 0XW74KZ 0XW74YZ

0 Medical and Surgical
X Anatomical Regions, Upper Extremities
X Transfer: Moving, without taking out, all or a portion of a body part to another location to take over the function of all or a portion of a body part

Body Part Character 4	Approach Character 5	Device Character 6	Qualifier Character 7
N Index Finger, Right	**0** Open	**Z** No Device	**L** Thumb, Right
P Index Finger, Left	**0** Open	**Z** No Device	**M** Thumb, Left

LC Limited Coverage NC Noncovered HAC HAC Associated Procedure CC Combination Cluster - See Appendix G for code lists
DRG Non-OR-Affecting MS-DRG Assignment ⊘ Non-OR-Not Affecting MS-DRG Assignment New/Revised Text in **Orange** ♂ Male ♀ Female

0 Medical and Surgical
X Anatomical Regions, Upper Extremities
Y Transplantation: Putting in or on all or a portion of a living body part taken from another individual or animal to physically take the place and/or function of all or a portion of a similar body part

Body Part Character 4	Approach Character 5	Device Character 6	Qualifier Character 7
J Hand, Right ⃠ K Hand, Left ⃠	0 Open	Z No Device	0 Allogeneic 1 Syngeneic

⃠ 0XYJ0Z0 0XYJ0Z1 0XYK0Z0 0XYK0Z1

Anatomical Regions, Lower Extremities 0Y0-0YW

0 Medical and Surgical
Y Anatomical Regions, Lower Extremities
0 Alteration: Modifying the anatomic structure of a body part without affecting the function of the body part

Body Part Character 4	Approach Character 5	Device Character 6	Qualifier Character 7
0 Buttock, Right **1** Buttock, Left **9** Lower Extremity, Right **B** Lower Extremity, Left **C** Upper Leg, Right **D** Upper Leg, Left **F** Knee Region, Right **G** Knee Region, Left **H** Lower Leg, Right **J** Lower Leg, Left **K** Ankle Region, Right **L** Ankle Region, Left	**0** Open **3** Percutaneous **4** Percutaneous Endoscopic	**7** Autologous Tissue Substitute **J** Synthetic Substitute **K** Nonautologous Tissue Substitute **Z** No Device	**Z** No Qualifier

0 Medical and Surgical
Y Anatomical Regions, Lower Extremities
2 Change: Taking out or off a device from a body part and putting back an identical or similar device in or on the same body part without cutting or puncturing the skin or a mucous membrane

Body Part Character 4	Approach Character 5	Device Character 6	Qualifier Character 7
9 Lower Extremity, Right ⦸ **B** Lower Extremity, Left ⦸	**X** External	**0** Drainage Device **Y** Other Device	**Z** No Qualifier

⦸ 0Y29X0Z 0Y29XYZ 0Y2BX0Z 0Y2BXYZ

0 Medical and Surgical
Y Anatomical Regions, Lower Extremities
3 Control: Stopping, or attempting to stop, postprocedural or other acute bleeding

Body Part Character 4	Approach Character 5	Device Character 6	Qualifier Character 7
0 Buttock, Right **1** Buttock, Left **5** Inguinal Region, Right **6** Inguinal Region, Left **7** Femoral Region, Right **8** Femoral Region, Left **9** Lower Extremity, Right **B** Lower Extremity, Left **C** Upper Leg, Right **D** Upper Leg, Left **F** Knee Region, Right **G** Knee Region, Left **H** Lower Leg, Right **J** Lower Leg, Left **K** Ankle Region, Right **L** Ankle Region, Left **M** Foot, Right **N** Foot, Left	**0** Open **3** Percutaneous **4** Percutaneous Endoscopic	**Z** No Device	**Z** No Qualifier

0 Medical and Surgical
Y Anatomical Regions, Lower Extremities
6 Detachment: Cutting off all or a portion of the upper or lower extremities

Body Part Character 4	Approach Character 5	Device Character 6	Qualifier Character 7
2 Hindquarter, Right **3** Hindquarter, Left **4** Hindquarter, Bilateral **7** Femoral Region, Right **8** Femoral Region, Left **F** Knee Region, Right **G** Knee Region, Left	**0** Open	**Z** No Device	**Z** No Qualifier
C Upper Leg, Right **D** Upper Leg, Left **H** Lower Leg, Right **J** Lower Leg, Left	**0** Open	**Z** No Device	**1** High **2** Mid **3** Low
M Foot, Right **N** Foot, Left	**0** Open	**Z** No Device	**0** Complete **4** Complete 1st Ray **5** Complete 2nd Ray **6** Complete 3rd Ray **7** Complete 4th Ray **8** Complete 5th Ray **9** Partial 1st Ray **B** Partial 2nd Ray **C** Partial 3rd Ray **D** Partial 4th Ray **F** Partial 5th Ray
P 1st Toe, Right **Q** 1st Toe, Left **R** 2nd Toe, Right **S** 2nd Toe, Left **T** 3rd Toe, Right **U** 3rd Toe, Left **V** 4th Toe, Right **W** 4th Toe, Left **X** 5th Toe, Right **Y** 5th Toe, Left	**0** Open	**Z** No Device	**0** Complete **1** High **2** Mid **3** Low

0 Medical and Surgical
Y Anatomical Regions, Lower Extremities
9 Drainage: Taking or letting out fluids and/or gases from a body part

Body Part Character 4	Approach Character 5	Device Character 6	Qualifier Character 7
0 Buttock, Right ⦸ **1** Buttock, Left ⦸ **5** Inguinal Region, Right ⦸ **6** Inguinal Region, Left ⦸ **7** Femoral Region, Right ⦸ **8** Femoral Region, Left ⦸ **9** Lower Extremity, Right ⦸ **B** Lower Extremity, Left ⦸ **C** Upper Leg, Right ⦸ **D** Upper Leg, Left ⦸ **F** Knee Region, Right ⦸ **G** Knee Region, Left ⦸ **H** Lower Leg, Right ⦸ **J** Lower Leg, Left ⦸ **K** Ankle Region, Right ⦸ **L** Ankle Region, Left ⦸ **M** Foot, Right ⦸ **N** Foot, Left ⦸	**0** Open **3** Percutaneous **4** Percutaneous Endoscopic	**0** Drainage Device	**Z** No Qualifier
0 Buttock, Right ⦸ **1** Buttock, Left ⦸ **5** Inguinal Region, Right ⦸ **6** Inguinal Region, Left ⦸ **7** Femoral Region, Right ⦸ **8** Femoral Region, Left ⦸ **9** Lower Extremity, Right ⦸ **B** Lower Extremity, Left ⦸ **C** Upper Leg, Right ⦸ **D** Upper Leg, Left ⦸ **F** Knee Region, Right ⦸ **G** Knee Region, Left ⦸ **H** Lower Leg, Right ⦸ **J** Lower Leg, Left ⦸ **K** Ankle Region, Right ⦸ **L** Ankle Region, Left ⦸ **M** Foot, Right ⦸ **N** Foot, Left ⦸	**0** Open **3** Percutaneous **4** Percutaneous Endoscopic	**Z** No Device	**X** Diagnostic **Z** No Qualifier

⦸ 0Y9000Z 0Y900ZX 0Y900ZZ 0Y9030Z 0Y903ZX 0Y903ZZ 0Y9040Z 0Y904ZX 0Y904ZZ 0Y9100Z 0Y910ZX 0Y910ZZ 0Y9130Z
0Y913ZX 0Y913ZZ 0Y9140Z 0Y914ZX 0Y914ZZ 0Y9530Z 0Y953ZZ 0Y9630Z 0Y963ZZ 0Y9700Z 0Y970ZX 0Y970ZZ 0Y9730Z
0Y973ZX 0Y973ZZ 0Y9740Z 0Y974ZX 0Y974ZZ 0Y9800Z 0Y980ZX 0Y980ZZ 0Y9830Z 0Y983ZX 0Y983ZZ 0Y9840Z 0Y984ZX
0Y984ZZ 0Y9900Z 0Y990ZX 0Y990ZZ 0Y9930Z 0Y993ZX 0Y993ZZ 0Y9940Z 0Y994ZX 0Y994ZZ 0Y9B00Z 0Y9B0ZX 0Y9B0ZZ
0Y9B30Z 0Y9B3ZX 0Y9B3ZZ 0Y9B40Z 0Y9B4ZX 0Y9B4ZZ 0Y9C00Z 0Y9C0ZX 0Y9C0ZZ 0Y9C30Z 0Y9C3ZX 0Y9C3ZZ 0Y9C40Z
0Y9C4ZX 0Y9C4ZZ 0Y9D00Z 0Y9D0ZX 0Y9D0ZZ 0Y9D30Z 0Y9D3ZX 0Y9D3ZZ 0Y9D40Z 0Y9D4ZX 0Y9D4ZZ 0Y9F00Z 0Y9F0ZX
0Y9F0ZZ 0Y9F30Z 0Y9F3ZX 0Y9F3ZZ 0Y9F40Z 0Y9F4ZX 0Y9F4ZZ 0Y9G00Z 0Y9G0ZX 0Y9G0ZZ 0Y9G30Z 0Y9G3ZX 0Y9G3ZZ
0Y9G40Z 0Y9G4ZX 0Y9G4ZZ 0Y9H00Z 0Y9H0ZX 0Y9H0ZZ 0Y9H30Z 0Y9H3ZX 0Y9H3ZZ 0Y9H40Z 0Y9H4ZX 0Y9H4ZZ 0Y9J00Z
0Y9J0ZX 0Y9J0ZZ 0Y9J30Z 0Y9J3ZX 0Y9J3ZZ 0Y9J40Z 0Y9J4ZX 0Y9J4ZZ 0Y9K00Z 0Y9K0ZX 0Y9K0ZZ 0Y9K30Z 0Y9K3ZX
0Y9K3ZZ 0Y9K40Z 0Y9K4ZX 0Y9K4ZZ 0Y9L00Z 0Y9L0ZX 0Y9L0ZZ 0Y9L30Z 0Y9L3ZX 0Y9L3ZZ 0Y9L40Z 0Y9L4ZX 0Y9L4ZZ
0Y9M00Z 0Y9M0ZX 0Y9M0ZZ 0Y9M30Z 0Y9M3ZX 0Y9M3ZZ 0Y9M40Z 0Y9M4ZX 0Y9M4ZZ 0Y9N00Z 0Y9N0ZX 0Y9N0ZZ 0Y9N30Z
0Y9N3ZX 0Y9N3ZZ 0Y9N40Z 0Y9N4ZX 0Y9N4ZZ

0 Medical and Surgical
Y Anatomical Regions, Lower Extremities
B Excision: Cutting out or off, without replacement, a portion of a body part

Body Part Character 4	Approach Character 5	Device Character 6	Qualifier Character 7
0 Buttock, Right ⊘	**0** Open	**Z** No Device	**X** Diagnostic
1 Buttock, Left ⊘	**3** Percutaneous		**Z** No Qualifier
5 Inguinal Region, Right	**4** Percutaneous Endoscopic		
6 Inguinal Region, Left			
7 Femoral Region, Right			
8 Femoral Region, Left			
9 Lower Extremity, Right ⊘			
B Lower Extremity, Left ⊘			
C Upper Leg, Right ⊘			
D Upper Leg, Left ⊘			
F Knee Region, Right ⊘			
G Knee Region, Left ⊘			
H Lower Leg, Right ⊘			
J Lower Leg, Left ⊘			
K Ankle Region, Right ⊘			
L Ankle Region, Left ⊘			
M Foot, Right ⊘			
N Foot, Left ⊘			

⊘ 0YB00ZX 0YB03ZX 0YB04ZX 0YB10ZX 0YB13ZX 0YB14ZX 0YB90ZX 0YB93ZX 0YB94ZX 0YBB0ZX 0YBB3ZX 0YBB4ZX 0YBC0ZX 0YBC3ZX 0YBC4ZX 0YBD0ZX 0YBD3ZX 0YBD4ZX 0YBF0ZX 0YBF3ZX 0YBF4ZX 0YBG0ZX 0YBG3ZX 0YBG4ZX 0YBH0ZX 0YBH3ZX 0YBH4ZX 0YBJ0ZX 0YBJ3ZX 0YBJ4ZX 0YBK0ZX 0YBK3ZX 0YBK4ZX 0YBL0ZX 0YBL3ZX 0YBL4ZX 0YBM0ZX 0YBM3ZX 0YBM4ZX 0YBN0ZX 0YBN3ZX 0YBN4ZX

0 Medical and Surgical
Y Anatomical Regions, Lower Extremities
H Insertion: Putting in a nonbiological appliance that monitors, assists, performs, or prevents a physiological function but does not physically take the place of a body part

Body Part Character 4	Approach Character 5	Device Character 6	Qualifier Character 7
0 Buttock, Right DRG	**0** Open	**1** Radioactive Element	**Z** No Qualifier
1 Buttock, Left DRG	**3** Percutaneous	**3** Infusion Device	
5 Inguinal Region, Right DRG	**4** Percutaneous Endoscopic	**Y** Other Device	
6 Inguinal Region, Left DRG			
7 Femoral Region, Right DRG			
8 Femoral Region, Left DRG			
9 Lower Extremity, Right DRG			
B Lower Extremity, Left DRG			
C Upper Leg, Right DRG			
D Upper Leg, Left DRG			
F Knee Region, Right DRG			
G Knee Region, Left DRG			
H Lower Leg, Right DRG			
J Lower Leg, Left DRG			
K Ankle Region, Right DRG			
L Ankle Region, Left DRG			
M Foot, Right DRG			
N Foot, Left DRG			

DRG 0YH003Z 0YH00YZ 0YH033Z 0YH03YZ 0YH043Z 0YH04YZ 0YH103Z 0YH10YZ 0YH133Z 0YH13YZ 0YH143Z 0YH14YZ 0YH503Z 0YH50YZ 0YH533Z 0YH53YZ 0YH543Z 0YH54YZ 0YH603Z 0YH60YZ 0YH633Z 0YH63YZ 0YH643Z 0YH64YZ 0YH703Z 0YH70YZ 0YH733Z 0YH73YZ 0YH743Z 0YH74YZ 0YH803Z 0YH80YZ 0YH833Z 0YH83YZ 0YH843Z 0YH84YZ 0YH903Z 0YH90YZ 0YH933Z 0YH93YZ 0YH943Z 0YH94YZ 0YHB03Z 0YHB0YZ 0YHB33Z 0YHB3YZ 0YHB43Z 0YHB4YZ 0YHC03Z 0YHC0YZ 0YHC33Z 0YHC3YZ 0YHC43Z 0YHC4YZ 0YHD03Z 0YHD0YZ 0YHD33Z 0YHD3YZ 0YHD43Z 0YHD4YZ 0YHF03Z 0YHF0YZ 0YHF33Z 0YHF3YZ 0YHF43Z 0YHF4YZ 0YHG03Z 0YHG0YZ 0YHG33Z 0YHG3YZ 0YHG43Z 0YHG4YZ 0YHH03Z 0YHH0YZ 0YHH33Z 0YHH3YZ 0YHH43Z 0YHH4YZ 0YHJ03Z 0YHJ0YZ 0YHJ33Z 0YHJ3YZ 0YHJ43Z 0YHJ4YZ 0YHK03Z 0YHK0YZ 0YHK33Z 0YHK3YZ 0YHK43Z 0YHK4YZ 0YHL03Z 0YHL0YZ 0YHL33Z 0YHL3YZ 0YHL43Z 0YHL4YZ 0YHM03Z 0YHM0YZ 0YHM33Z 0YHM3YZ 0YHM43Z 0YHM4YZ 0YHN03Z 0YHN0YZ 0YHN33Z 0YHN3YZ 0YHN43Z 0YHN4YZ

0 Medical and Surgical
Y Anatomical Regions, Lower Extremities
J Inspection: Visually and/or manually exploring a body part

Body Part Character 4	Approach Character 5	Device Character 6	Qualifier Character 7
0 Buttock, Right ⦸ DRG	**0** Open	**Z** No Device	**Z** No Qualifier
1 Buttock, Left ⦸ DRG	**3** Percutaneous		
5 Inguinal Region, Right ⦸	**4** Percutaneous Endoscopic		
6 Inguinal Region, Left ⦸	**X** External		
7 Femoral Region, Right ⦸			
8 Femoral Region, Left ⦸ DRG			
9 Lower Extremity, Right ⦸ DRG			
A Inguinal Region, Bilateral ⦸			
B Lower Extremity, Left ⦸ DRG			
C Upper Leg, Right ⦸ DRG			
D Upper Leg, Left ⦸ DRG			
E Femoral Region, Bilateral ⦸ DRG			
F Knee Region, Right ⦸ DRG			
G Knee Region, Left ⦸ DRG			
H Lower Leg, Right ⦸ DRG			
J Lower Leg, Left ⦸ DRG			
K Ankle Region, Right ⦸ DRG			
L Ankle Region, Left ⦸ DRG			
M Foot, Right ⦸ DRG			
N Foot, Left ⦸ DRG			

⦸ 0YJ03ZZ 0YJ04ZZ 0YJ0XZZ 0YJ13ZZ 0YJ14ZZ 0YJ1XZZ 0YJ53ZZ 0YJ5XZZ 0YJ63ZZ 0YJ6XZZ 0YJ73ZZ 0YJ7XZZ 0YJ83ZZ 0YJ8XZZ 0YJ93ZZ 0YJ94ZZ 0YJ9XZZ 0YJA3ZZ 0YJAXZZ 0YJB3ZZ 0YJB4ZZ 0YJBXZZ 0YJC3ZZ 0YJC4ZZ 0YJCXZZ 0YJD3ZZ 0YJD4ZZ 0YJDXZZ 0YJE3ZZ 0YJEXZZ 0YJF3ZZ 0YJF4ZZ 0YJFXZZ 0YJG3ZZ 0YJG4ZZ 0YJGXZZ 0YJH3ZZ 0YJH4ZZ 0YJHXZZ 0YJJ3ZZ 0YJJ4ZZ 0YJJXZZ 0YJK3ZZ 0YJK4ZZ 0YJKXZZ 0YJL3ZZ 0YJL4ZZ 0YJLXZZ 0YJM3ZZ 0YJM4ZZ 0YJMXZZ 0YJN3ZZ 0YJN4ZZ 0YJNXZZ

DRG 0YJ00ZZ 0YJ10ZZ 0YJ80ZZ 0YJ90ZZ 0YJB0ZZ 0YJC0ZZ 0YJD0ZZ 0YJE0ZZ 0YJF0ZZ 0YJG0ZZ 0YJH0ZZ 0YJJ0ZZ 0YJK0ZZ 0YJL0ZZ 0YJM0ZZ 0YJN0ZZ

0 Medical and Surgical
Y Anatomical Regions, Lower Extremities
M Reattachment: Putting back in or on all or a portion of a separated body part to its normal location or other suitable location

Body Part Character 4	Approach Character 5	Device Character 6	Qualifier Character 7
0 Buttock, Right **1** Buttock, Left **2** Hindquarter, Right **3** Hindquarter, Left **4** Hindquarter, Bilateral **5** Inguinal Region, Right **6** Inguinal Region, Left **7** Femoral Region, Right **8** Femoral Region, Left **9** Lower Extremity, Right **B** Lower Extremity, Left **C** Upper Leg, Right **D** Upper Leg, Left **F** Knee Region, Right **G** Knee Region, Left **H** Lower Leg, Right **J** Lower Leg, Left **K** Ankle Region, Right **L** Ankle Region, Left **M** Foot, Right **N** Foot, Left **P** 1st Toe, Right **Q** 1st Toe, Left **R** 2nd Toe, Right **S** 2nd Toe, Left **T** 3rd Toe, Right **U** 3rd Toe, Left **V** 4th Toe, Right **W** 4th Toe, Left **X** 5th Toe, Right **Y** 5th Toe, Left	**0** Open	**Z** No Device	**Z** No Qualifier

0 Medical and Surgical
Y Anatomical Regions, Lower Extremities
P Removal: Taking out or off a device from a body part

Body Part Character 4	Approach Character 5	Device Character 6	Qualifier Character 7
9 Lower Extremity, Right ⃠ **B** Lower Extremity, Left ⃠	**0** Open **3** Percutaneous **4** Percutaneous Endoscopic **X** External	**0** Drainage Device **1** Radioactive Element **3** Infusion Device **7** Autologous Tissue Substitute **J** Synthetic Substitute **K** Nonautologous Tissue Substitute **Y** Other Device	**Z** No Qualifier

⃠ 0YP900Z 0YP901Z 0YP903Z 0YP907Z 0YP90JZ 0YP90KZ 0YP90YZ 0YP930Z 0YP931Z 0YP933Z 0YP937Z 0YP93JZ 0YP93KZ 0YP93YZ 0YP940Z 0YP941Z 0YP943Z 0YP947Z 0YP94JZ 0YP94KZ 0YP94YZ 0YP9X0Z 0YP9X1Z 0YP9X3Z 0YP9X7Z 0YP9XJZ 0YP9XKZ 0YP9XYZ 0YPB00Z 0YPB01Z 0YPB03Z 0YPB07Z 0YPB0JZ 0YPB0KZ 0YPB0YZ 0YPB30Z 0YPB31Z 0YPB33Z 0YPB37Z 0YPB3JZ 0YPB3KZ 0YPB3YZ 0YPB40Z 0YPB41Z 0YPB43Z 0YPB47Z 0YPB4JZ 0YPB4KZ 0YPB4YZ 0YPBX0Z 0YPBX1Z 0YPBX3Z 0YPBX7Z 0YPBXJZ 0YPBXKZ 0YPBXYZ

0 Medical and Surgical
Y Anatomical Regions, Lower Extremities
Q Repair: Restoring, to the extent possible, a body part to its normal anatomic structure and function

Body Part Character 4	Approach Character 5	Device Character 6	Qualifier Character 7
0 Buttock, Right	**0** Open	**Z** No Device	**Z** No Qualifier
1 Buttock, Left	**3** Percutaneous		
5 Inguinal Region, Right ⊘	**4** Percutaneous Endoscopic		
6 Inguinal Region, Left ⊘	**X** External		
7 Femoral Region, Right ⊘			
8 Femoral Region, Left ⊘			
9 Lower Extremity, Right			
A Inguinal Region, Bilateral ⊘			
B Lower Extremity, Left			
C Upper Leg, Right			
D Upper Leg, Left			
E Femoral Region, Bilateral ⊘			
F Knee Region, Right			
G Knee Region, Left			
H Lower Leg, Right			
J Lower Leg, Left			
K Ankle Region, Right			
L Ankle Region, Left			
M Foot, Right			
N Foot, Left			
P 1st Toe, Right			
Q 1st Toe, Left			
R 2nd Toe, Right			
S 2nd Toe, Left			
T 3rd Toe, Right			
U 3rd Toe, Left			
V 4th Toe, Right			
W 4th Toe, Left			
X 5th Toe, Right			
Y 5th Toe, Left			

⊘ 0YQ5XZZ 0YQ6XZZ 0YQ7XZZ 0YQ8XZZ 0YQAXZZ 0YQEXZZ

0 Medical and Surgical
Y Anatomical Regions, Lower Extremities
U Supplement: Putting in or on biological or synthetic material that physically reinforces and/or augments the function of a portion of a body part

Body Part Character 4	Approach Character 5	Device Character 6	Qualifier Character 7
0 Buttock, Right **1** Buttock, Left **5** Inguinal Region, Right **6** Inguinal Region, Left **7** Femoral Region, Right **8** Femoral Region, Left **9** Lower Extremity, Right **A** Inguinal Region, Bilateral **B** Lower Extremity, Left **C** Upper Leg, Right **D** Upper Leg, Left **E** Femoral Region, Bilateral **F** Knee Region, Right **G** Knee Region, Left **H** Lower Leg, Right **J** Lower Leg, Left **K** Ankle Region, Right **L** Ankle Region, Left **M** Foot, Right **N** Foot, Left **P** 1st Toe, Right **Q** 1st Toe, Left **R** 2nd Toe, Right **S** 2nd Toe, Left **T** 3rd Toe, Right **U** 3rd Toe, Left **V** 4th Toe, Right **W** 4th Toe, Left **X** 5th Toe, Right **Y** 5th Toe, Left	**0** Open **4** Percutaneous Endoscopic	**7** Autologous Tissue Substitute **J** Synthetic Substitute **K** Nonautologous Tissue Substitute	**Z** No Qualifier

0 Medical and Surgical
Y Anatomical Regions, Lower Extremities
W Revision: Correcting, to the extent possible, a portion of a malfunctioning device or the position of a displaced device

Body Part Character 4	Approach Character 5	Device Character 6	Qualifier Character 7
9 Lower Extremity, Right ⊘ DRG **B** Lower Extremity, Left ⊘ DRG	**0** Open **3** Percutaneous **4** Percutaneous Endoscopic **X** External	**0** Drainage Device **3** Infusion Device **7** Autologous Tissue Substitute **J** Synthetic Substitute **K** Nonautologous Tissue Substitute **Y** Other Device	**Z** No Qualifier

⊘ 0YW9X0Z 0YW9X3Z 0YW9X7Z 0YW9XJZ 0YW9XKZ 0YW9XYZ 0YWBX0Z 0YWBX3Z 0YWBX7Z 0YWBXJZ 0YWBXKZ 0YWBXYZ

DRG 0YW900Z 0YW903Z 0YW907Z 0YW90JZ 0YW90KZ 0YW90YZ 0YW930Z 0YW933Z 0YW937Z 0YW93JZ 0YW93KZ 0YW93YZ 0YW940Z 0YW943Z 0YW947Z 0YW94JZ 0YW94KZ 0YW94YZ 0YWB00Z 0YWB03Z 0YWB07Z 0YWB0JZ 0YWB0KZ 0YWB0YZ 0YWB30Z 0YWB33Z 0YWB37Z 0YWB3JZ 0YWB3KZ 0YWB3YZ 0YWB40Z 0YWB43Z 0YWB47Z 0YWB4JZ 0YWB4KZ 0YWB4YZ

Obstetrics 102-10Y

1 Obstetrics
0 Pregnancy
2 Change: Taking out or off a device from a body part and putting back an identical or similar device in or on the same body part without cutting or puncturing the skin or a mucous membrane

Body Part Character 4	Approach Character 5	Device Character 6	Qualifier Character 7
0 Products of Conception ⦸ ♀	7 Via Natural or Artificial Opening	3 Monitoring Electrode Y Other Device	Z No Qualifier

♀ 102073Z 10207YZ
⦸ 102073Z 10207YZ

1 Obstetrics
0 Pregnancy
9 Drainage: Taking or letting out fluids and/or gases from a body part

Body Part Character 4	Approach Character 5	Device Character 6	Qualifier Character 7
0 Products of Conception ⦸ ♀	0 Open 3 Percutaneous 4 Percutaneous Endoscopic 7 Via Natural or Artificial Opening 8 Via Natural or Artificial Opening Endoscopic	Z No Device	9 Fetal Blood A Fetal Cerebrospinal Fluid B Fetal Fluid, Other C Amniotic Fluid, Therapeutic D Fluid, Other U Amniotic Fluid, Diagnostic

♀ 10900Z9 10900ZA 10900ZB 10900ZC 10900ZD 10900ZU 10903Z9 10903ZA 10903ZB 10903ZC 10903ZD 10903ZU 10904Z9 10904ZA 10904ZB 10904ZC 10904ZD 10904ZU 10907Z9 10907ZA 10907ZB 10907ZC 10907ZD 10907ZU 10908Z9 10908ZA 10908ZB 10908ZC 10908ZD 10908ZU
⦸ 10900Z9 10900ZA 10900ZB 10900ZC 10900ZD 10900ZU 10903Z9 10903ZA 10903ZB 10903ZC 10903ZD 10903ZU 10904Z9 10904ZA 10904ZB 10904ZC 10904ZD 10904ZU 10907Z9 10907ZA 10907ZB 10907ZC 10907ZD 10907ZU 10908Z9 10908ZA 10908ZB 10908ZC 10908ZD 10908ZU

1 Obstetrics
0 Pregnancy
A Abortion: Artificially terminating a pregnancy

Body Part Character 4	Approach Character 5	Device Character 6	Qualifier Character 7
0 Products of Conception ♀	0 Open 3 Percutaneous 4 Percutaneous Endoscopic 8 Via Natural or Artificial Opening Endoscopic	Z No Device	Z No Qualifier
0 Products of Conception ⦸ DRG ♀	7 Via Natural or Artificial Opening	Z No Device	6 Vacuum W Laminaria X Abortifacient Z No Qualifier

♀ 10A00ZZ 10A03ZZ 10A04ZZ 10A07Z6 10A07ZW 10A07ZX 10A07ZZ 10A08ZZ
⦸ 10A07ZW 10A07ZX
DRG 10A07Z6

1 Obstetrics
0 Pregnancy
D Extraction: Pulling or stripping out or off all or a portion of a body part by the use of force

Body Part Character 4	Approach Character 5	Device Character 6	Qualifier Character 7
0 Products of Conception ♀	**0** Open	**Z** No Device	**0** Classical **1** Low Cervical **2** Extraperitoneal
0 Products of Conception CC DRG ♀	**7** Via Natural or Artificial Opening	**Z** No Device	**3** Low Forceps **4** Mid Forceps **5** High Forceps **6** Vacuum **7** Internal Version **8** Other
1 Products of Conception, Retained ♀ **2** Products of Conception, Ectopic ♀	**7** Via Natural or Artificial Opening **8** Via Natural or Artificial Opening Endoscopic	**Z** No Device	**Z** No Qualifier

♀ 10D00Z0 10D00Z1 10D00Z2 10D07Z3 10D07Z4 10D07Z5 10D07Z6 10D07Z7 10D07Z8 10D17ZZ 10D18ZZ 10D27ZZ 10D28ZZ
DRG 10D07Z3 10D07Z4 10D07Z5 10D07Z6 10D07Z7 10D07Z8
CC 10D07Z3 10D07Z4 10D07Z5 10D07Z6

1 Obstetrics
0 Pregnancy
E Delivery: Assisting the passage of the products of conception from the genital canal

Body Part Character 4	Approach Character 5	Device Character 6	Qualifier Character 7
0 Products of Conception CC DRG ♀	**X** External	**Z** No Device	**Z** No Qualifier

♀ 10E0XZZ
DRG 10E0XZZ
CC 10E0XZZ

1 Obstetrics
0 Pregnancy
H Insertion: Putting in a nonbiological appliance that monitors, assists, performs, or prevents a physiological function but does not physically take the place of a body part

Body Part Character 4	Approach Character 5	Device Character 6	Qualifier Character 7
0 Products of Conception ⊘ ♀	**0** Open **7** Via Natural or Artificial Opening	**3** Monitoring Electrode **Y** Other Device	**Z** No Qualifier

♀ 10H003Z 10H00YZ 10H073Z 10H07YZ
⊘ 10H073Z 10H07YZ

1 Obstetrics
0 Pregnancy
J Inspection: Visually and/or manually exploring a body part

Body Part Character 4	Approach Character 5	Device Character 6	Qualifier Character 7
0 Products of Conception ⊘ ♀ **1** Products of Conception, Retained ⊘ ♀ **2** Products of Conception, Ectopic ⊘ ♀	**0** Open **3** Percutaneous **4** Percutaneous Endoscopic **7** Via Natural or Artificial Opening **8** Via Natural or Artificial Opening Endoscopic **X** External	**Z** No Device	**Z** No Qualifier

♀ 10J00ZZ 10J03ZZ 10J04ZZ 10J07ZZ 10J08ZZ 10J0XZZ 10J10ZZ 10J13ZZ 10J14ZZ 10J17ZZ 10J18ZZ 10J1XZZ 10J20ZZ 10J23ZZ 10J24ZZ 10J27ZZ 10J28ZZ 10J2XZZ
⊘ 10J00ZZ 10J03ZZ 10J04ZZ 10J07ZZ 10J08ZZ 10J0XZZ 10J10ZZ 10J13ZZ 10J14ZZ 10J17ZZ 10J18ZZ 10J1XZZ 10J20ZZ 10J23ZZ 10J24ZZ 10J27ZZ 10J28ZZ 10J2XZZ

LC Limited Coverage NC Noncovered HAC HAC Associated Procedure CC Combination Cluster - See Appendix G for code lists
DRG Non-OR-Affecting MS-DRG Assignment ⊘ Non-OR-Not Affecting MS-DRG Assignment New/Revised Text in **Orange** ♂ Male ♀ Female

1 Obstetrics
0 Pregnancy
P Removal: Taking out or off a device from a body part, region or orifice

Body Part Character 4	Approach Character 5	Device Character 6	Qualifier Character 7
0 Products of Conception ♀	**0** Open **7** Via Natural or Artificial Opening	**3** Monitoring Electrode **Y** Other Device	**Z** No Qualifier

♀ 10P003Z 10P00YZ 10P073Z 10P07YZ

1 Obstetrics
0 Pregnancy
Q Repair: Restoring, to the extent possible, a body part to its normal anatomic structure and function

Body Part Character 4	Approach Character 5	Device Character 6	Qualifier Character 7
0 Products of Conception ⦸ ♀	**0** Open **3** Percutaneous **4** Percutaneous Endoscopic **7** Via Natural or Artificial Opening **8** Via Natural or Artificial Opening Endoscopic	**Y** Other Device **Z** No Device	**E** Nervous System **F** Cardiovascular System **G** Lymphatics and Hemic **H** Eye **J** Ear, Nose and Sinus **K** Respiratory System **L** Mouth and Throat **M** Gastrointestinal System **N** Hepatobiliary and Pancreas **P** Endocrine System **Q** Skin **R** Musculoskeletal System **S** Urinary System **T** Female Reproductive System **V** Male Reproductive System **Y** Other Body System

♀ 10Q00YE 10Q00YF 10Q00YG 10Q00YH 10Q00YJ 10Q00YK 10Q00YL 10Q00YM 10Q00YN 10Q00YP 10Q00YQ 10Q00YR 10Q00YS
10Q00YT 10Q00YV 10Q00YY 10Q00ZE 10Q00ZF 10Q00ZG 10Q00ZH 10Q00ZJ 10Q00ZK 10Q00ZL 10Q00ZM 10Q00ZN 10Q00ZP
10Q00ZQ 10Q00ZR 10Q00ZS 10Q00ZT 10Q00ZV 10Q00ZY 10Q03YE 10Q03YF 10Q03YG 10Q03YH 10Q03YJ 10Q03YK 10Q03YL
10Q03YM 10Q03YN 10Q03YP 10Q03YQ 10Q03YR 10Q03YS 10Q03YT 10Q03YV 10Q03YY 10Q03ZE 10Q03ZF 10Q03ZG 10Q03ZH
10Q03ZJ 10Q03ZK 10Q03ZL 10Q03ZM 10Q03ZN 10Q03ZP 10Q03ZQ 10Q03ZR 10Q03ZS 10Q03ZT 10Q03ZV 10Q03ZY 10Q04YE
10Q04YF 10Q04YG 10Q04YH 10Q04YJ 10Q04YK 10Q04YL 10Q04YM 10Q04YN 10Q04YP 10Q04YQ 10Q04YR 10Q04YS 10Q04YT
10Q04YV 10Q04YY 10Q04ZE 10Q04ZF 10Q04ZG 10Q04ZH 10Q04ZJ 10Q04ZK 10Q04ZL 10Q04ZM 10Q04ZN 10Q04ZP 10Q04ZQ
10Q04ZR 10Q04ZS 10Q04ZT 10Q04ZV 10Q04ZY 10Q07YE 10Q07YF 10Q07YG 10Q07YH 10Q07YJ 10Q07YK 10Q07YL 10Q07YM
10Q07YN 10Q07YP 10Q07YQ 10Q07YR 10Q07YS 10Q07YT 10Q07YV 10Q07YY 10Q07ZE 10Q07ZF 10Q07ZG 10Q07ZH 10Q07ZJ
10Q07ZK 10Q07ZL 10Q07ZM 10Q07ZN 10Q07ZP 10Q07ZQ 10Q07ZR 10Q07ZS 10Q07ZT 10Q07ZV 10Q07ZY 10Q08YE 10Q08YF
10Q08YG 10Q08YH 10Q08YJ 10Q08YK 10Q08YL 10Q08YM 10Q08YN 10Q08YP 10Q08YQ 10Q08YR 10Q08YS 10Q08YT 10Q08YV
10Q08YY 10Q08ZE 10Q08ZF 10Q08ZG 10Q08ZH 10Q08ZJ 10Q08ZK 10Q08ZL 10Q08ZM 10Q08ZN 10Q08ZP 10Q08ZQ 10Q08ZR
10Q08ZS 10Q08ZT 10Q08ZV 10Q08ZY

⦸ 10Q00YE 10Q00YF 10Q00YG 10Q00YH 10Q00YJ 10Q00YK 10Q00YL 10Q00YM 10Q00YN 10Q00YP 10Q00YQ 10Q00YR 10Q00YS
10Q00YT 10Q00YV 10Q00YY 10Q00ZE 10Q00ZF 10Q00ZG 10Q00ZH 10Q00ZJ 10Q00ZK 10Q00ZL 10Q00ZM 10Q00ZN 10Q00ZP
10Q00ZQ 10Q00ZR 10Q00ZS 10Q00ZT 10Q00ZV 10Q00ZY 10Q03YE 10Q03YF 10Q03YG 10Q03YH 10Q03YJ 10Q03YK 10Q03YL
10Q03YM 10Q03YN 10Q03YP 10Q03YQ 10Q03YR 10Q03YS 10Q03YT 10Q03YV 10Q03YY 10Q03ZE 10Q03ZF 10Q03ZG 10Q03ZH
10Q03ZJ 10Q03ZK 10Q03ZL 10Q03ZM 10Q03ZN 10Q03ZP 10Q03ZQ 10Q03ZR 10Q03ZS 10Q03ZT 10Q03ZV 10Q03ZY 10Q04YE
10Q04YF 10Q04YG 10Q04YH 10Q04YJ 10Q04YK 10Q04YL 10Q04YM 10Q04YN 10Q04YP 10Q04YQ 10Q04YR 10Q04YS 10Q04YT
10Q04YV 10Q04YY 10Q04ZE 10Q04ZF 10Q04ZG 10Q04ZH 10Q04ZJ 10Q04ZK 10Q04ZL 10Q04ZM 10Q04ZN 10Q04ZP 10Q04ZQ
10Q04ZR 10Q04ZS 10Q04ZT 10Q04ZV 10Q04ZY 10Q07YE 10Q07YF 10Q07YG 10Q07YH 10Q07YJ 10Q07YK 10Q07YL 10Q07YM
10Q07YN 10Q07YP 10Q07YQ 10Q07YR 10Q07YS 10Q07YT 10Q07YV 10Q07YY 10Q07ZE 10Q07ZF 10Q07ZG 10Q07ZH 10Q07ZJ
10Q07ZK 10Q07ZL 10Q07ZM 10Q07ZN 10Q07ZP 10Q07ZQ 10Q07ZR 10Q07ZS 10Q07ZT 10Q07ZV 10Q07ZY 10Q08YE 10Q08YF
10Q08YG 10Q08YH 10Q08YJ 10Q08YK 10Q08YL 10Q08YM 10Q08YN 10Q08YP 10Q08YQ 10Q08YR 10Q08YS 10Q08YT 10Q08YV
10Q08YY 10Q08ZE 10Q08ZF 10Q08ZG 10Q08ZH 10Q08ZJ 10Q08ZK 10Q08ZL 10Q08ZM 10Q08ZN 10Q08ZP 10Q08ZQ 10Q08ZR
10Q08ZS 10Q08ZT 10Q08ZV 10Q08ZY

1 Obstetrics
0 Pregnancy
S Reposition: Moving to its normal location, or other suitable location, all or a portion of a body part

Body Part Character 4	Approach Character 5	Device Character 6	Qualifier Character 7
0 Products of Conception ⦸ DRG ♀	**7** Via Natural or Artificial Opening **X** External	**Z** No Device	**Z** No Qualifier
2 Products of Conception, Ectopic ♀	**0** Open **3** Percutaneous **4** Percutaneous Endoscopic **7** Via Natural or Artificial Opening **8** Via Natural or Artificial Opening Endoscopic	**Z** No Device	**Z** No Qualifier

♀ 10S07ZZ 10S0XZZ 10S20ZZ 10S23ZZ 10S24ZZ 10S27ZZ 10S28ZZ
⦸ 10S0XZZ
DRG 10S07ZZ

1 Obstetrics
0 Pregnancy
T Resection: Cutting out or off, without replacement, all of a body part

Body Part Character 4	Approach Character 5	Device Character 6	Qualifier Character 7
2 Products of Conception, Ectopic ♀	**0** Open **3** Percutaneous **4** Percutaneous Endoscopic **7** Via Natural or Artificial Opening **8** Via Natural or Artificial Opening Endoscopic	**Z** No Device	**Z** No Qualifier

♀ 10T20ZZ 10T23ZZ 10T24ZZ 10T27ZZ 10T28ZZ

1 Obstetrics
0 Pregnancy
Y Transplantation: Putting in or on all or a portion of a living body part taken from another individual or animal to physically take the place and/or function of all or a portion of a similar body part

Body Part Character 4	Approach Character 5	Device Character 6	Qualifier Character 7
0 Products of Conception ⦸ ♀	**3** Percutaneous **4** Percutaneous Endoscopic **7** Via Natural or Artificial Opening	**Z** No Device	**E** Nervous System **F** Cardiovascular System **G** Lymphatics and Hemic **H** Eye **J** Ear, Nose and Sinus **K** Respiratory System **L** Mouth and Throat **M** Gastrointestinal System **N** Hepatobiliary and Pancreas **P** Endocrine System **Q** Skin **R** Musculoskeletal System **S** Urinary System **T** Female Reproductive System **V** Male Reproductive System **Y** Other Body System

♀ 10Y03ZE 10Y03ZF 10Y03ZG 10Y03ZH 10Y03ZJ 10Y03ZK 10Y03ZL 10Y03ZM 10Y03ZN 10Y03ZP 10Y03ZQ 10Y03ZR 10Y03ZS
10Y03ZT 10Y03ZV 10Y03ZY 10Y04ZE 10Y04ZF 10Y04ZG 10Y04ZH 10Y04ZJ 10Y04ZK 10Y04ZL 10Y04ZM 10Y04ZN 10Y04ZP
10Y04ZQ 10Y04ZR 10Y04ZS 10Y04ZT 10Y04ZV 10Y04ZY 10Y07ZE 10Y07ZF 10Y07ZG 10Y07ZH 10Y07ZJ 10Y07ZK 10Y07ZL
10Y07ZM 10Y07ZN 10Y07ZP 10Y07ZQ 10Y07ZR 10Y07ZS 10Y07ZT 10Y07ZV 10Y07ZY
⦸ 10Y03ZE 10Y03ZF 10Y03ZG 10Y03ZH 10Y03ZJ 10Y03ZK 10Y03ZL 10Y03ZM 10Y03ZN 10Y03ZP 10Y03ZQ 10Y03ZR 10Y03ZS
10Y03ZT 10Y03ZV 10Y03ZY 10Y04ZE 10Y04ZF 10Y04ZG 10Y04ZH 10Y04ZJ 10Y04ZK 10Y04ZL 10Y04ZM 10Y04ZN 10Y04ZP
10Y04ZQ 10Y04ZR 10Y04ZS 10Y04ZT 10Y04ZV 10Y04ZY 10Y07ZE 10Y07ZF 10Y07ZG 10Y07ZH 10Y07ZJ 10Y07ZK 10Y07ZL
10Y07ZM 10Y07ZN 10Y07ZP 10Y07ZQ 10Y07ZR 10Y07ZS 10Y07ZT 10Y07ZV 10Y07ZY

Placement-Anatomical Regions 2W0-2W6

2 Placement
W Anatomical Regions
0 Change: Taking out or off a device from a body part and putting back an identical or similar device in or on the same body part without cutting or puncturing the skin or a mucous membrane

Body Region Character 4	Approach Character 5	Device Character 6	Qualifier Character 7
0 Head ⊘ **2** Neck ⊘ **3** Abdominal Wall ⊘ **4** Chest Wall ⊘ **5** Back ⊘ **6** Inguinal Region, Right ⊘ **7** Inguinal Region, Left ⊘ **8** Upper Extremity, Right ⊘ **9** Upper Extremity, Left ⊘ **A** Upper Arm, Right ⊘ **B** Upper Arm, Left ⊘ **C** Lower Arm, Right ⊘ **D** Lower Arm, Left ⊘ **E** Hand, Right ⊘ **F** Hand, Left ⊘ **G** Thumb, Right ⊘ **H** Thumb, Left ⊘ **J** Finger, Right ⊘ **K** Finger, Left ⊘ **L** Lower Extremity, Right ⊘ **M** Lower Extremity, Left ⊘ **N** Upper Leg, Right ⊘ **P** Upper Leg, Left ⊘ **Q** Lower Leg, Right ⊘ **R** Lower Leg, Left ⊘ **S** Foot, Right ⊘ **T** Foot, Left ⊘ **U** Toe, Right ⊘ **V** Toe, Left ⊘	**X** External	**0** Traction Apparatus **1** Splint **2** Cast **3** Brace **4** Bandage **5** Packing Material **6** Pressure Dressing **7** Intermittent Pressure Device **Y** Other Device	**Z** No Qualifier
1 Face ⊘	**X** External	**0** Traction Apparatus **1** Splint **2** Cast **3** Brace **4** Bandage **5** Packing Material **6** Pressure Dressing **7** Intermittent Pressure Device **9** Wire **Y** Other Device	**Z** No Qualifier

⊘ 2W00X0Z 2W00X1Z 2W00X2Z 2W00X3Z 2W00X4Z 2W00X5Z 2W00X6Z 2W00X7Z 2W00XYZ 2W01X0Z 2W01X1Z 2W01X2Z 2W01X3Z
2W01X4Z 2W01X5Z 2W01X6Z 2W01X7Z 2W01X9Z 2W01XYZ 2W02X0Z 2W02X1Z 2W02X2Z 2W02X3Z 2W02X4Z 2W02X5Z 2W02X6Z
2W02X7Z 2W02XYZ 2W03X0Z 2W03X1Z 2W03X2Z 2W03X3Z 2W03X4Z 2W03X5Z 2W03X6Z 2W03X7Z 2W03XYZ 2W04X0Z 2W04X1Z
2W04X2Z 2W04X3Z 2W04X4Z 2W04X5Z 2W04X6Z 2W04X7Z 2W04XYZ 2W05X0Z 2W05X1Z 2W05X2Z 2W05X3Z 2W05X4Z 2W05X5Z
2W05X6Z 2W05X7Z 2W05XYZ 2W06X0Z 2W06X1Z 2W06X2Z 2W06X3Z 2W06X4Z 2W06X5Z 2W06X6Z 2W06X7Z 2W06XYZ 2W07X0Z
2W07X1Z 2W07X2Z 2W07X3Z 2W07X4Z 2W07X5Z 2W07X6Z 2W07X7Z 2W07XYZ 2W08X0Z 2W08X1Z 2W08X2Z 2W08X3Z 2W08X4Z
2W08X5Z 2W08X6Z 2W08X7Z 2W08XYZ 2W09X0Z 2W09X1Z 2W09X2Z 2W09X3Z 2W09X4Z 2W09X5Z 2W09X6Z 2W09X7Z 2W09XYZ
2W0AX0Z 2W0AX1Z 2W0AX2Z 2W0AX3Z 2W0AX4Z 2W0AX5Z 2W0AX6Z 2W0AX7Z 2W0AXYZ 2W0BX0Z 2W0BX1Z 2W0BX2Z 2W0BX3Z
2W0BX4Z 2W0BX5Z 2W0BX6Z 2W0BX7Z 2W0BXYZ 2W0CX0Z 2W0CX1Z 2W0CX2Z 2W0CX3Z 2W0CX4Z 2W0CX5Z 2W0CX6Z 2W0CX7Z
2W0CXYZ 2W0DX0Z 2W0DX1Z 2W0DX2Z 2W0DX3Z 2W0DX4Z 2W0DX5Z 2W0DX6Z 2W0DX7Z 2W0DXYZ 2W0EX0Z 2W0EX1Z 2W0EX2Z
2W0EX3Z 2W0EX4Z 2W0EX5Z 2W0EX6Z 2W0EX7Z 2W0EXYZ 2W0FX0Z 2W0FX1Z 2W0FX2Z 2W0FX3Z 2W0FX4Z 2W0FX5Z 2W0FX6Z
2W0FX7Z 2W0FXYZ 2W0GX0Z 2W0GX1Z 2W0GX2Z 2W0GX3Z 2W0GX4Z 2W0GX5Z 2W0GX6Z 2W0GX7Z 2W0GXYZ 2W0HX0Z 2W0HX1Z
2W0HX2Z 2W0HX3Z 2W0HX4Z 2W0HX5Z 2W0HX6Z 2W0HX7Z 2W0HXYZ 2W0JX0Z 2W0JX1Z 2W0JX2Z 2W0JX3Z 2W0JX4Z 2W0JX5Z
2W0JX6Z 2W0JX7Z 2W0JXYZ 2W0KX0Z 2W0KX1Z 2W0KX2Z 2W0KX3Z 2W0KX4Z 2W0KX5Z 2W0KX6Z 2W0KX7Z 2W0KXYZ 2W0LX0Z
2W0LX1Z 2W0LX2Z 2W0LX3Z 2W0LX4Z 2W0LX5Z 2W0LX6Z 2W0LX7Z 2W0LXYZ 2W0MX0Z 2W0MX1Z 2W0MX2Z 2W0MX3Z 2W0MX4Z
2W0MX5Z 2W0MX6Z 2W0MX7Z 2W0MXYZ 2W0NX0Z 2W0NX1Z 2W0NX2Z 2W0NX3Z 2W0NX4Z 2W0NX5Z 2W0NX6Z 2W0NX7Z 2W0NXYZ
2W0PX0Z 2W0PX1Z 2W0PX2Z 2W0PX3Z 2W0PX4Z 2W0PX5Z 2W0PX6Z 2W0PX7Z 2W0PXYZ 2W0QX0Z 2W0QX1Z 2W0QX2Z 2W0QX3Z
2W0QX4Z 2W0QX5Z 2W0QX6Z 2W0QX7Z 2W0QXYZ 2W0RX0Z 2W0RX1Z 2W0RX2Z 2W0RX3Z 2W0RX4Z 2W0RX5Z 2W0RX6Z 2W0RX7Z
2W0RXYZ 2W0SX0Z 2W0SX1Z 2W0SX2Z 2W0SX3Z 2W0SX4Z 2W0SX5Z 2W0SX6Z 2W0SX7Z 2W0SXYZ 2W0TX0Z 2W0TX1Z 2W0TX2Z
2W0TX3Z 2W0TX4Z 2W0TX5Z 2W0TX6Z 2W0TX7Z 2W0TXYZ 2W0UX0Z 2W0UX1Z 2W0UX2Z 2W0UX3Z 2W0UX4Z 2W0UX5Z 2W0UX6Z
2W0UX7Z 2W0UXYZ 2W0VX0Z 2W0VX1Z 2W0VX2Z 2W0VX3Z 2W0VX4Z 2W0VX5Z 2W0VX6Z 2W0VX7Z 2W0VXYZ

LC Limited Coverage NC Noncovered HAC HAC Associated Procedure CC Combination Cluster - See Appendix G for code lists
DRG Non-OR-Affecting MS-DRG Assignment ⊘ Non-OR-Not Affecting MS-DRG Assignment New/Revised Text in **Orange** ♂ Male ♀ Female

2 Placement
W Anatomical Regions
1 Compression: Putting pressure on a body region

Body Region Character 4	Approach Character 5	Device Character 6	Qualifier Character 7
0 Head ⃠ **1** Face ⃠ **2** Neck ⃠ **3** Abdominal Wall ⃠ **4** Chest Wall ⃠ **5** Back ⃠ **6** Inguinal Region, Right ⃠ **7** Inguinal Region, Left ⃠ **8** Upper Extremity, Right ⃠ **9** Upper Extremity, Left ⃠ **A** Upper Arm, Right ⃠ **B** Upper Arm, Left ⃠ **C** Lower Arm, Right ⃠ **D** Lower Arm, Left ⃠ **E** Hand, Right ⃠ **F** Hand, Left ⃠ **G** Thumb, Right ⃠ **H** Thumb, Left ⃠ **J** Finger, Right ⃠ **K** Finger, Left ⃠ **L** Lower Extremity, Right ⃠ **M** Lower Extremity, Left ⃠ **N** Upper Leg, Right ⃠ **P** Upper Leg, Left ⃠ **Q** Lower Leg, Right ⃠ **R** Lower Leg, Left ⃠ **S** Foot, Right ⃠ **T** Foot, Left ⃠ **U** Toe, Right ⃠ **V** Toe, Left ⃠	**X** External	**6** Pressure Dressing **7** Intermittent Pressure Device	**Z** No Qualifier

⃠ 2W10X6Z 2W10X7Z 2W11X6Z 2W11X7Z 2W12X6Z 2W12X7Z 2W13X6Z 2W13X7Z 2W14X6Z 2W14X7Z 2W15X6Z 2W15X7Z 2W16X6Z 2W16X7Z 2W17X6Z 2W17X7Z 2W18X6Z 2W18X7Z 2W19X6Z 2W19X7Z 2W1AX6Z 2W1AX7Z 2W1BX6Z 2W1BX7Z 2W1CX6Z 2W1CX7Z 2W1DX6Z 2W1DX7Z 2W1EX6Z 2W1EX7Z 2W1FX6Z 2W1FX7Z 2W1GX6Z 2W1GX7Z 2W1HX6Z 2W1HX7Z 2W1JX6Z 2W1JX7Z 2W1KX6Z 2W1KX7Z 2W1LX6Z 2W1LX7Z 2W1MX6Z 2W1MX7Z 2W1NX6Z 2W1NX7Z 2W1PX6Z 2W1PX7Z 2W1QX6Z 2W1QX7Z 2W1RX6Z 2W1RX7Z 2W1SX6Z 2W1SX7Z 2W1TX6Z 2W1TX7Z 2W1UX6Z 2W1UX7Z 2W1VX6Z 2W1VX7Z

2 Placement
W Anatomical Regions
2 Dressing: Putting material on a body region for protection

Body Region Character 4	Approach Character 5	Device Character 6	Qualifier Character 7
0 Head ⃠ **1** Face ⃠ **2** Neck ⃠ **3** Abdominal Wall ⃠ **4** Chest Wall ⃠ **5** Back ⃠ **6** Inguinal Region, Right ⃠ **7** Inguinal Region, Left ⃠ **8** Upper Extremity, Right ⃠ **9** Upper Extremity, Left ⃠ **A** Upper Arm, Right ⃠ **B** Upper Arm, Left ⃠ **C** Lower Arm, Right ⃠ **D** Lower Arm, Left ⃠ **E** Hand, Right ⃠ **F** Hand, Left ⃠ **G** Thumb, Right ⃠ **H** Thumb, Left ⃠ **J** Finger, Right ⃠ **K** Finger, Left ⃠ **L** Lower Extremity, Right ⃠ **M** Lower Extremity, Left ⃠ **N** Upper Leg, Right ⃠ **P** Upper Leg, Left ⃠ **Q** Lower Leg, Right ⃠ **R** Lower Leg, Left ⃠ **S** Foot, Right ⃠ **T** Foot, Left ⃠ **U** Toe, Right ⃠ **V** Toe, Left ⃠	**X** External	**4** Bandage	**Z** No Qualifier

⃠ 2W20X4Z 2W21X4Z 2W22X4Z 2W23X4Z 2W24X4Z 2W25X4Z 2W26X4Z 2W27X4Z 2W28X4Z 2W29X4Z 2W2AX4Z 2W2BX4Z 2W2CX4Z 2W2DX4Z 2W2EX4Z 2W2FX4Z 2W2GX4Z 2W2HX4Z 2W2JX4Z 2W2KX4Z 2W2LX4Z 2W2MX4Z 2W2NX4Z 2W2PX4Z 2W2QX4Z 2W2RX4Z 2W2SX4Z 2W2TX4Z 2W2UX4Z 2W2VX4Z

2 Placement
W Anatomical Regions
3 Immobilization: Limiting or preventing motion of a body region

Body Region Character 4	Approach Character 5	Device Character 6	Qualifier Character 7
0 Head ⦸ **2** Neck ⦸ **3** Abdominal Wall ⦸ **4** Chest Wall ⦸ **5** Back ⦸ **6** Inguinal Region, Right ⦸ **7** Inguinal Region, Left ⦸ **8** Upper Extremity, Right ⦸ **9** Upper Extremity, Left ⦸ **A** Upper Arm, Right ⦸ **B** Upper Arm, Left ⦸ **C** Lower Arm, Right ⦸ **D** Lower Arm, Left ⦸ **E** Hand, Right ⦸ **F** Hand, Left ⦸ **G** Thumb, Right ⦸ **H** Thumb, Left ⦸ **J** Finger, Right ⦸ **K** Finger, Left ⦸ **L** Lower Extremity, Right ⦸ **M** Lower Extremity, Left ⦸ **N** Upper Leg, Right ⦸ **P** Upper Leg, Left ⦸ **Q** Lower Leg, Right ⦸ **R** Lower Leg, Left ⦸ **S** Foot, Right ⦸ **T** Foot, Left ⦸ **U** Toe, Right ⦸ **V** Toe, Left ⦸	**X** External	**1** Splint **2** Cast **3** Brace **Y** Other Device	**Z** No Qualifier
1 Face ⦸	**X** External	**1** Splint **2** Cast **3** Brace **9** Wire **Y** Other Device	**Z** No Qualifier

⦸ 2W30X1Z 2W30X2Z 2W30X3Z 2W30XYZ 2W31X1Z 2W31X2Z 2W31X3Z 2W31X9Z 2W31XYZ 2W32X1Z 2W32X2Z 2W32X3Z 2W32XYZ
2W33X1Z 2W33X2Z 2W33X3Z 2W33XYZ 2W34X1Z 2W34X2Z 2W34X3Z 2W34XYZ 2W35X1Z 2W35X2Z 2W35X3Z 2W35XYZ 2W36X1Z
2W36X2Z 2W36X3Z 2W36XYZ 2W37X1Z 2W37X2Z 2W37X3Z 2W37XYZ 2W38X1Z 2W38X2Z 2W38X3Z 2W38XYZ 2W39X1Z 2W39X2Z
2W39X3Z 2W39XYZ 2W3AX1Z 2W3AX2Z 2W3AX3Z 2W3AXYZ 2W3BX1Z 2W3BX2Z 2W3BX3Z 2W3BXYZ 2W3CX1Z 2W3CX2Z 2W3CX3Z
2W3CXYZ 2W3DX1Z 2W3DX2Z 2W3DX3Z 2W3DXYZ 2W3EX1Z 2W3EX2Z 2W3EX3Z 2W3EXYZ 2W3FX1Z 2W3FX2Z 2W3FX3Z 2W3FXYZ
2W3GX1Z 2W3GX2Z 2W3GX3Z 2W3GXYZ 2W3HX1Z 2W3HX2Z 2W3HX3Z 2W3HXYZ 2W3JX1Z 2W3JX2Z 2W3JX3Z 2W3JXYZ 2W3KX1Z
2W3KX2Z 2W3KX3Z 2W3KXYZ 2W3LX1Z 2W3LX2Z 2W3LX3Z 2W3LXYZ 2W3MX1Z 2W3MX2Z 2W3MX3Z 2W3MXYZ 2W3NX1Z 2W3NX2Z
2W3NX3Z 2W3NXYZ 2W3PX1Z 2W3PX2Z 2W3PX3Z 2W3PXYZ 2W3QX1Z 2W3QX2Z 2W3QX3Z 2W3QXYZ 2W3RX1Z 2W3RX2Z 2W3RX3Z
2W3RXYZ 2W3SX1Z 2W3SX2Z 2W3SX3Z 2W3SXYZ 2W3TX1Z 2W3TX2Z 2W3TX3Z 2W3TXYZ 2W3UX1Z 2W3UX2Z 2W3UX3Z 2W3UXYZ
2W3VX1Z 2W3VX2Z 2W3VX3Z 2W3VXYZ

2 Placement
W Anatomical Regions
4 Packing: Putting material in a body region or orifice

Body Region Character 4	Approach Character 5	Device Character 6	Qualifier Character 7
0 Head ⃠ **1** Face ⃠ **2** Neck ⃠ **3** Abdominal Wall ⃠ **4** Chest Wall ⃠ **5** Back ⃠ **6** Inguinal Region, Right ⃠ **7** Inguinal Region, Left ⃠ **8** Upper Extremity, Right ⃠ **9** Upper Extremity, Left ⃠ **A** Upper Arm, Right ⃠ **B** Upper Arm, Left ⃠ **C** Lower Arm, Right ⃠ **D** Lower Arm, Left ⃠ **E** Hand, Right ⃠ **F** Hand, Left ⃠ **G** Thumb, Right ⃠ **H** Thumb, Left ⃠ **J** Finger, Right ⃠ **K** Finger, Left ⃠ **L** Lower Extremity, Right ⃠ **M** Lower Extremity, Left ⃠ **N** Upper Leg, Right ⃠ **P** Upper Leg, Left ⃠ **Q** Lower Leg, Right ⃠ **R** Lower Leg, Left ⃠ **S** Foot, Right ⃠ **T** Foot, Left ⃠ **U** Toe, Right ⃠ **V** Toe, Left ⃠	**X** External	**5** Packing Material	**Z** No Qualifier

⃠ 2W40X5Z 2W41X5Z 2W42X5Z 2W43X5Z 2W44X5Z 2W45X5Z 2W46X5Z 2W47X5Z 2W48X5Z 2W49X5Z 2W4AX5Z 2W4BX5Z 2W4CX5Z 2W4DX5Z 2W4EX5Z 2W4FX5Z 2W4GX5Z 2W4HX5Z 2W4JX5Z 2W4KX5Z 2W4LX5Z 2W4MX5Z 2W4NX5Z 2W4PX5Z 2W4QX5Z 2W4RX5Z 2W4SX5Z 2W4TX5Z 2W4UX5Z 2W4VX5Z

2 Placement
W Anatomical Regions
5 Removal: Taking out or off a device from a body part

Body Region Character 4	Approach Character 5	Device Character 6	Qualifier Character 7
0 Head ⦸ **2** Neck ⦸ **3** Abdominal Wall ⦸ **4** Chest Wall ⦸ **5** Back ⦸ **6** Inguinal Region, Right ⦸ **7** Inguinal Region, Left ⦸ **8** Upper Extremity, Right ⦸ **9** Upper Extremity, Left ⦸ **A** Upper Arm, Right ⦸ **B** Upper Arm, Left ⦸ **C** Lower Arm, Right ⦸ **D** Lower Arm, Left ⦸ **E** Hand, Right ⦸ **F** Hand, Left ⦸ **G** Thumb, Right ⦸ **H** Thumb, Left ⦸ **J** Finger, Right ⦸ **K** Finger, Left ⦸ **L** Lower Extremity, Right ⦸ **M** Lower Extremity, Left ⦸ **N** Upper Leg, Right ⦸ **P** Upper Leg, Left ⦸ **Q** Lower Leg, Right ⦸ **R** Lower Leg, Left ⦸ **S** Foot, Right ⦸ **T** Foot, Left ⦸ **U** Toe, Right ⦸ **V** Toe, Left ⦸	**X** External	**0** Traction Apparatus **1** Splint **2** Cast **3** Brace **4** Bandage **5** Packing Material **6** Pressure Dressing **7** Intermittent Pressure Device **Y** Other Device	**Z** No Qualifier
1 Face ⦸	**X** External	**0** Traction Apparatus **1** Splint **2** Cast **3** Brace **4** Bandage **5** Packing Material **6** Pressure Dressing **7** Intermittent Pressure Device **9** Wire **Y** Other Device	**Z** No Qualifier

⦸

2W50X0Z	2W50X1Z	2W50X2Z	2W50X3Z	2W50X4Z	2W50X5Z	2W50X6Z	2W50X7Z	2W50XYZ	2W51X0Z	2W51X1Z	2W51X2Z	2W51X3Z
2W51X4Z	2W51X5Z	2W51X6Z	2W51X7Z	2W51X9Z	2W51XYZ	2W52X0Z	2W52X1Z	2W52X2Z	2W52X3Z	2W52X4Z	2W52X5Z	2W52X6Z
2W52X7Z	2W52XYZ	2W53X0Z	2W53X1Z	2W53X2Z	2W53X3Z	2W53X4Z	2W53X5Z	2W53X6Z	2W53X7Z	2W53XYZ	2W54X0Z	2W54X1Z
2W54X2Z	2W54X3Z	2W54X4Z	2W54X5Z	2W54X6Z	2W54X7Z	2W54XYZ	2W55X0Z	2W55X1Z	2W55X2Z	2W55X3Z	2W55X4Z	2W55X5Z
2W55X6Z	2W55X7Z	2W55XYZ	2W56X0Z	2W56X1Z	2W56X2Z	2W56X3Z	2W56X4Z	2W56X5Z	2W56X6Z	2W56X7Z	2W56XYZ	2W57X0Z
2W57X1Z	2W57X2Z	2W57X3Z	2W57X4Z	2W57X5Z	2W57X6Z	2W57X7Z	2W57XYZ	2W58X0Z	2W58X1Z	2W58X2Z	2W58X3Z	2W58X4Z
2W58X5Z	2W58X6Z	2W58X7Z	2W58XYZ	2W59X0Z	2W59X1Z	2W59X2Z	2W59X3Z	2W59X4Z	2W59X5Z	2W59X6Z	2W59X7Z	2W59XYZ
2W5AX0Z	2W5AX1Z	2W5AX2Z	2W5AX3Z	2W5AX4Z	2W5AX5Z	2W5AX6Z	2W5AX7Z	2W5AXYZ	2W5BX0Z	2W5BX1Z	2W5BX2Z	2W5BX3Z
2W5BX4Z	2W5BX5Z	2W5BX6Z	2W5BX7Z	2W5BXYZ	2W5CX0Z	2W5CX1Z	2W5CX2Z	2W5CX3Z	2W5CX4Z	2W5CX5Z	2W5CX6Z	2W5CX7Z
2W5CXYZ	2W5DX0Z	2W5DX1Z	2W5DX2Z	2W5DX3Z	2W5DX4Z	2W5DX5Z	2W5DX6Z	2W5DX7Z	2W5DXYZ	2W5EX0Z	2W5EX1Z	2W5EX2Z
2W5EX3Z	2W5EX4Z	2W5EX5Z	2W5EX6Z	2W5EX7Z	2W5EXYZ	2W5FX0Z	2W5FX1Z	2W5FX2Z	2W5FX3Z	2W5FX4Z	2W5FX5Z	2W5FX6Z
2W5FX7Z	2W5FXYZ	2W5GX0Z	2W5GX1Z	2W5GX2Z	2W5GX3Z	2W5GX4Z	2W5GX5Z	2W5GX6Z	2W5GX7Z	2W5GXYZ	2W5HX0Z	2W5HX1Z
2W5HX2Z	2W5HX3Z	2W5HX4Z	2W5HX5Z	2W5HX6Z	2W5HX7Z	2W5HXYZ	2W5JX0Z	2W5JX1Z	2W5JX2Z	2W5JX3Z	2W5JX4Z	2W5JX5Z
2W5JX6Z	2W5JX7Z	2W5JXYZ	2W5KX0Z	2W5KX1Z	2W5KX2Z	2W5KX3Z	2W5KX4Z	2W5KX5Z	2W5KX6Z	2W5KX7Z	2W5KXYZ	2W5LX0Z
2W5LX1Z	2W5LX2Z	2W5LX3Z	2W5LX4Z	2W5LX5Z	2W5LX6Z	2W5LX7Z	2W5LXYZ	2W5MX0Z	2W5MX1Z	2W5MX2Z	2W5MX3Z	2W5MX4Z
2W5MX5Z	2W5MX6Z	2W5MX7Z	2W5MXYZ	2W5NX0Z	2W5NX1Z	2W5NX2Z	2W5NX3Z	2W5NX4Z	2W5NX5Z	2W5NX6Z	2W5NX7Z	2W5NXYZ
2W5PX0Z	2W5PX1Z	2W5PX2Z	2W5PX3Z	2W5PX4Z	2W5PX5Z	2W5PX6Z	2W5PX7Z	2W5PXYZ	2W5QX0Z	2W5QX1Z	2W5QX2Z	2W5QX3Z
2W5QX4Z	2W5QX5Z	2W5QX6Z	2W5QX7Z	2W5QXYZ	2W5RX0Z	2W5RX1Z	2W5RX2Z	2W5RX3Z	2W5RX4Z	2W5RX5Z	2W5RX6Z	2W5RX7Z
2W5RXYZ	2W5SX0Z	2W5SX1Z	2W5SX2Z	2W5SX3Z	2W5SX4Z	2W5SX5Z	2W5SX6Z	2W5SX7Z	2W5SXYZ	2W5TX0Z	2W5TX1Z	2W5TX2Z
2W5TX3Z	2W5TX4Z	2W5TX5Z	2W5TX6Z	2W5TX7Z	2W5TXYZ	2W5UX0Z	2W5UX1Z	2W5UX2Z	2W5UX3Z	2W5UX4Z	2W5UX5Z	2W5UX6Z
2W5UX7Z	2W5UXYZ	2W5VX0Z	2W5VX1Z	2W5VX2Z	2W5VX3Z	2W5VX4Z	2W5VX5Z	2W5VX6Z	2W5VX7Z	2W5VXYZ		

LC Limited Coverage NC Noncovered HAC HAC Associated Procedure CC Combination Cluster - See Appendix G for code lists
DRG Non-OR-Affecting MS-DRG Assignment ⦸ Non-OR-Not Affecting MS-DRG Assignment New/Revised Text in **Orange** ♂ Male ♀ Female

2 Placement
W Anatomical Regions
6 Traction: Exerting a pulling force on a body region in a distal direction

Body Region Character 4	Approach Character 5	Device Character 6	Qualifier Character 7
0 Head ⦸ **1** Face ⦸ **2** Neck ⦸ **3** Abdominal Wall ⦸ **4** Chest Wall ⦸ **5** Back ⦸ **6** Inguinal Region, Right ⦸ **7** Inguinal Region, Left ⦸ **8** Upper Extremity, Right ⦸ **9** Upper Extremity, Left ⦸ **A** Upper Arm, Right ⦸ **B** Upper Arm, Left ⦸ **C** Lower Arm, Right ⦸ **D** Lower Arm, Left ⦸ **E** Hand, Right ⦸ **F** Hand, Left ⦸ **G** Thumb, Right ⦸ **H** Thumb, Left ⦸ **J** Finger, Right ⦸ **K** Finger, Left ⦸ **L** Lower Extremity, Right ⦸ **M** Lower Extremity, Left ⦸ **N** Upper Leg, Right ⦸ **P** Upper Leg, Left ⦸ **Q** Lower Leg, Right ⦸ **R** Lower Leg, Left ⦸ **S** Foot, Right ⦸ **T** Foot, Left ⦸ **U** Toe, Right ⦸ **V** Toe, Left ⦸	**X** External	**0** Traction Apparatus **Z** No Device	**Z** No Qualifier

⦸ 2W60X0Z 2W60XZZ 2W61X0Z 2W61XZZ 2W62X0Z 2W62XZZ 2W63X0Z 2W63XZZ 2W64X0Z 2W64XZZ 2W65X0Z 2W65XZZ 2W66X0Z 2W66XZZ 2W67X0Z 2W67XZZ 2W68X0Z 2W68XZZ 2W69X0Z 2W69XZZ 2W6AX0Z 2W6AXZZ 2W6BX0Z 2W6BXZZ 2W6CX0Z 2W6CXZZ 2W6DX0Z 2W6DXZZ 2W6EX0Z 2W6EXZZ 2W6FX0Z 2W6FXZZ 2W6GX0Z 2W6GXZZ 2W6HX0Z 2W6HXZZ 2W6JX0Z 2W6JXZZ 2W6KX0Z 2W6KXZZ 2W6LX0Z 2W6LXZZ 2W6MX0Z 2W6MXZZ 2W6NX0Z 2W6NXZZ 2W6PX0Z 2W6PXZZ 2W6QX0Z 2W6QXZZ 2W6RX0Z 2W6RXZZ 2W6SX0Z 2W6SXZZ 2W6TX0Z 2W6TXZZ 2W6UX0Z 2W6UXZZ 2W6VX0Z 2W6VXZZ

Placement-Anatomical Orifices 2Y0-2Y5

2 Placement
Y Anatomical Orifices
0 Change: Taking out or off a device from a body part and putting back an identical or similar device in or on the same body part without cutting or puncturing the skin or a mucous membrane

Body Region Character 4	Approach Character 5	Device Character 6	Qualifier Character 7
0 Mouth and Pharynx ⦸ **1** Nasal ⦸ **2** Ear ⦸ **3** Anorectal ⦸ **4** Female Genital Tract ⦸ ♀ **5** Urethra ⦸	**X** External	**5** Packing Material	**Z** No Qualifier

♀ 2Y04X5Z
⦸ 2Y00X5Z 2Y01X5Z 2Y02X5Z 2Y03X5Z 2Y04X5Z 2Y05X5Z

2 Placement
Y Anatomical Orifices
4 Packing: Putting material in a body region or orifice

Body Region Character 4	Approach Character 5	Device Character 6	Qualifier Character 7
0 Mouth and Pharynx ⦸ **1** Nasal ⦸ **2** Ear ⦸ **3** Anorectal ⦸ **4** Female Genital Tract ⦸ ♀ **5** Urethra ⦸	**X** External	**5** Packing Material	**Z** No Qualifier

♀ 2Y44X5Z
⦸ 2Y40X5Z 2Y41X5Z 2Y42X5Z 2Y43X5Z 2Y44X5Z 2Y45X5Z

2 Placement
Y Anatomical Orifices
5 Removal: Taking out or off a device from a body part

Body Region Character 4	Approach Character 5	Device Character 6	Qualifier Character 7
0 Mouth and Pharynx ⦸ **1** Nasal ⦸ **2** Ear ⦸ **3** Anorectal ⦸ **4** Female Genital Tract ⦸ ♀ **5** Urethra ⦸	**X** External	**5** Packing Material	**Z** No Qualifier

♀ 2Y54X5Z
⦸ 2Y50X5Z 2Y51X5Z 2Y52X5Z 2Y53X5Z 2Y54X5Z 2Y55X5Z

Administration 302-3E1

3 Administration
0 Circulatory
2 Transfusion: Putting in blood or blood products

Body System / Region Character 4	Approach Character 5	Substance Character 6	Qualifier Character 7
3 Peripheral Vein NC **4** Central Vein NC	**0** Open **3** Percutaneous	**A** Stem Cells, Embryonic	**Z** No Qualifier
3 Peripheral Vein ⃠ NC **4** Central Vein ⃠ NC	**0** Open **3** Percutaneous	**G** Bone Marrow **X** Stem Cells, Cord Blood **Y** Stem Cells, Hematopoietic	**0** Autologous **2** Allogeneic, Related **3** Allogeneic, Unrelated **4** Allogeneic, Unspecified
3 Peripheral Vein ⃠ **4** Central Vein ⃠	**0** Open **3** Percutaneous	**H** Whole Blood **J** Serum Albumin **K** Frozen Plasma **L** Fresh Plasma **M** Plasma Cryoprecipitate **N** Red Blood Cells **P** Frozen Red Cells **Q** White Cells **R** Platelets **S** Globulin **T** Fibrinogen **V** Antihemophilic Factors **W** Factor IX	**0** Autologous **1** Nonautologous
5 Peripheral Artery ⃠ NC **6** Central Artery ⃠ NC	**0** Open **3** Percutaneous	**G** Bone Marrow **H** Whole Blood **J** Serum Albumin **K** Frozen Plasma **L** Fresh Plasma **M** Plasma Cryoprecipitate **N** Red Blood Cells **P** Frozen Red Cells **Q** White Cells **R** Platelets **S** Globulin **T** Fibrinogen **V** Antihemophilic Factors **W** Factor IX **X** Stem Cells, Cord Blood **Y** Stem Cells, Hematopoietic	**0** Autologous **1** Nonautologous
7 Products of Conception, Circulatory ⃠ ♀	**3** Percutaneous **7** Via Natural or Artificial Opening	**H** Whole Blood **J** Serum Albumin **K** Frozen Plasma **L** Fresh Plasma **M** Plasma Cryoprecipitate **N** Red Blood Cells **P** Frozen Red Cells **Q** White Cells **R** Platelets **S** Globulin **T** Fibrinogen **V** Antihemophilic Factors **W** Factor IX	**1** Nonautologous
8 Vein ⃠	**0** Open **3** Percutaneous	**B** 4-Factor Prothrombin Complex Concentrate	**1** Nonautologous

♀ 30273H1 30273J1 30273K1 30273L1 30273M1 30273N1 30273P1 30273Q1 30273R1 30273S1 30273T1 30273V1 30273W1 30277H1 30277J1 30277K1 30277L1 30277M1 30277N1 30277P1 30277Q1 30277R1 30277S1 30277T1 30277V1 30277W1

⃠ 30230G2 30230G3 30230G4 30230H0 30230H1 30230J0 30230J1 30230K0 30230K1 30230L0 30230L1 30230M0 30230M1 30230N0 30230N1 30230P0 30230P1 30230Q0 30230Q1 30230R0 30230R1 30230S0 30230S1 30230T0 30230T1 30230V0 30230V1 30230W0 30230W1 30230X2 30230X3 30230X4 30230Y2 30230Y3 30230Y4 30233G2 30233G3 30233G4 30233H0 30233H1 30233J0 30233J1 30233K0 30233K1 30233L0 30233L1 30233M0 30233M1 30233N0 30233N1 30233P0 30233P1 30233Q0 30233Q1 30233R0 30233R1 30233S0 30233S1 30233T0 30233T1 30233V0 30233V1 30233W0 30233W1 30233X2 30233X3 30233X4 30233Y2 30233Y3 30233Y4 30240G2 30240G3 30240G4 30240H0 30240H1 30240J0 30240J1 30240K0

302 continued on next page

LC Limited Coverage NC Noncovered HAC HAC Associated Procedure CC Combination Cluster - See Appendix G for code lists
DRG Non-OR-Affecting MS-DRG Assignment ⃠ Non-OR-Not Affecting MS-DRG Assignment New/Revised Text in **Orange** ♂ Male ♀ Female

302 continued from previous page

30240K1 30240L0 30240L1 30240M0 30240M1 30240N0 30240N1 30240P0 30240P1 30240Q0 30240Q1 30240R0 30240R1 30240S0 30240S1 30240T0 30240T1 30240V0 30240V1 30240W0 30240W1 30240X2 30240X3 30240X4 30240Y2 30240Y3 30240Y4 30243G2 30243G3 30243G4 30243H0 30243H1 30243J0 30243J1 30243K0 30243K1 30243L0 30243L1 30243M0 30243M1 30243N0 30243N1 30243P0 30243P1 30243Q0 30243Q1 30243R0 30243R1 30243S0 30243S1 30243T0 30243T1 30243V0 30243V1 30243W0 30243W1 30243X2 30243X3 30243X4 30243Y2 30243Y3 30243Y4 30250H0 30250H1 30250J0 30250J1 30250K0 30250K1 30250L0 30250L1 30250M0 30250M1 30250N0 30250N1 30250P0 30250P1 30250Q0 30250Q1 30250R0 30250R1 30250S0 30250S1 30250T0 30250T1 30250V0 30250V1 30250W0 30250W1 30253H0 30253H1 30253J0 30253J1 30253K0 30253K1 30253L0 30253L1 30253M0 30253M1 30253N0 30253N1 30253P0 30253P1 30253Q0 30253Q1 30253R0 30253R1 30253S0 30253S1 30253T0 30253T1 30253V0 30253V1 30253W0 30253W1 30260H0 30260H1 30260J0 30260J1 30260K0 30260K1 30260L0 30260L1 30260M0 30260M1 30260N0 30260N1 30260P0 30260P1 30260Q0 30260Q1 30260R0 30260R1 30260S0 30260S1 30260T0 30260T1 30260V0 30260V1 30260W0 30260W1 30263H0 30263H1 30263J0 30263J1 30263K0 30263K1 30263L0 30263L1 30263M0 30263M1 30263N0 30263N1 30263P0 30263P1 30263Q0 30263Q1 30263R0 30263R1 30263S0 30263S1 30263T0 30263T1 30263V0 30263V1 30263W0 30263W1 30273H1 30273J1 30273K1 30273L1 30273M1 30273N1 30273P1 30273Q1 30273R1 30273S1 30273T1 30273V1 30273W1 30277H1 30277J1 30277K1 30277L1 30277M1 30277N1 30277P1 30277Q1 30277R1 30277S1 30277T1 30277V1 30277W1 30280B1 30283B1

NC 30250G1 30250Y1 30253G1 30253Y1 30260G1 30260Y1 30263G1 or 30263Y1 Codes in this list are noncovered procedures only when reported with C90.00 or C90.01 as either a principal or secondary diagnosis.

NC 30230AZ 30230G0 30230Y0 30233AZ 30233G0 30233Y0 30240AZ 30240G0 30240Y0 30243AZ 30243G0 30243Y0 30250G0 30250Y0 30253G0 30253Y0 30260G0 30260Y0 30263G0 or 30263Y0 Codes in this list are noncovered procedures only when reported with C91.00, C92.00, C92.10, C92.11, C92.40, C92.50, C92.60, C92.A0, C93.00, C94.00, or C95.00 as either a principal or secondary diagnosis.

3 Administration
C Indwelling Device
1 Irrigation: Putting in or on a cleansing substance

Body System / Region Character 4	Approach Character 5	Substance Character 6	Qualifier Character 7
Z None ⃠	**X** External	**8** Irrigating Substance	**Z** No Qualifier

⃠ 3C1ZX8Z

3 Administration
E Physiological Systems and Anatomical Regions
0 Introduction: Putting in or on a therapeutic, diagnostic, nutritional, physiological, or prophylactic substance except blood or blood products

Body System / Region Character 4	Approach Character 5	Substance Character 6	Qualifier Character 7
0 Skin and Mucous Membranes ⃠	**X** External	**0** Antineoplastic	**5** Other Antineoplastic **M** Monoclonal Antibody
0 Skin and Mucous Membranes ⃠	**X** External	**2** Anti-infective	**8** Oxazolidinones **9** Other Anti-infective
0 Skin and Mucous Membranes ⃠	**X** External	**3** Anti-inflammatory **4** Serum, Toxoid and Vaccine **B** Local Anesthetic **K** Other Diagnostic Substance **M** Pigment **N** Analgesics, Hypnotics, Sedatives **T** Destructive Agent	**Z** No Qualifier
0 Skin and Mucous Membranes ⃠	**X** External	**G** Other Therapeutic Substance	**C** Other Substance
1 Subcutaneous Tissue ⃠	**0** Open	**2** Anti-infective	**A** Anti-Infective Envelope
1 Subcutaneous Tissue ⃠	**3** Percutaneous	**0** Antineoplastic	**5** Other Antineoplastic **M** Monoclonal Antibody
1 Subcutaneous Tissue ⃠	**3** Percutaneous	**2** Anti-infective	**8** Oxazolidinones **9** Other Anti-infective **A** Anti-Infective Envelope
1 Subcutaneous Tissue ⃠	**3** Percutaneous	**3** Anti-inflammatory **4** Serum, Toxoid and Vaccine **6** Nutritional Substance **7** Electrolytic and Water Balance Substance **B** Local Anesthetic **H** Radioactive Substance **K** Other Diagnostic Substance **N** Analgesics, Hypnotics, Sedatives **T** Destructive Agent	**Z** No Qualifier
1 Subcutaneous Tissue ⃠	**3** Percutaneous	**G** Other Therapeutic Substance	**C** Other Substance

3E0 continued on next page

3 Administration
E Physiological Systems and Anatomical Regions
0 Introduction: Putting in or on a therapeutic, diagnostic, nutritional, physiological, or prophylactic substance except blood or blood products

3E0 continued from previous page

Body System / Region Character 4	Approach Character 5	Substance Character 6	Qualifier Character 7
1 Subcutaneous Tissue ⃠	3 Percutaneous	V Hormone	G Insulin J Other Hormone
2 Muscle ⃠	3 Percutaneous	0 Antineoplastic	5 Other Antineoplastic M Monoclonal Antibody
2 Muscle ⃠	3 Percutaneous	2 Anti-infective	8 Oxazolidinones 9 Other Anti-infective
2 Muscle ⃠	3 Percutaneous	3 Anti-inflammatory 4 Serum, Toxoid and Vaccine 6 Nutritional Substance 7 Electrolytic and Water Balance Substance B Local Anesthetic H Radioactive Substance K Other Diagnostic Substance N Analgesics, Hypnotics, Sedatives T Destructive Agent	Z No Qualifier
2 Muscle ⃠	3 Percutaneous	G Other Therapeutic Substance	C Other Substance
3 Peripheral Vein ⃠ DRG	0 Open	0 Antineoplastic	2 High-dose Interleukin-2 3 Low-dose Interleukin-2 5 Other Antineoplastic M Monoclonal Antibody P Clofarabine
3 Peripheral Vein ⃠ DRG	0 Open	1 Thrombolytic	6 Recombinant Human-activated Protein C 7 Other Thrombolytic
3 Peripheral Vein ⃠	0 Open	2 Anti-infective	8 Oxazolidinones 9 Other Anti-infective
3 Peripheral Vein ⃠	0 Open	3 Anti-inflammatory 4 Serum, Toxoid and Vaccine 6 Nutritional Substance 7 Electrolytic and Water Balance Substance F Intracirculatory Anesthetic H Radioactive Substance K Other Diagnostic Substance N Analgesics, Hypnotics, Sedatives P Platelet Inhibitor R Antiarrhythmic T Destructive Agent X Vasopressor	Z No Qualifier
3 Peripheral Vein ⃠	0 Open	G Other Therapeutic Substance	C Other Substance N Blood Brain Barrier Disruption
3 Peripheral Vein DRG	0 Open	U Pancreatic Islet Cells	0 Autologous 1 Nonautologous
3 Peripheral Vein ⃠	0 Open	V Hormone	G Insulin H Human B -type Natriuretic Peptide J Other Hormone
3 Peripheral Vein ⃠	0 Open	W Immunotherapeutic	K Immunostimulator L Immunosuppressive

3E0 continued on next page

3 **Administration**
E **Physiological Systems and Anatomical Regions**
0 **Introduction:** Putting in or on a therapeutic, diagnostic, nutritional, physiological, or prophylactic substance except blood or blood products

3E0 continued from previous page

Body System / Region Character 4	Approach Character 5	Substance Character 6	Qualifier Character 7
3 Peripheral Vein ⦸ DRG	3 Percutaneous	0 Antineoplastic	2 High-dose Interleukin-2 3 Low-dose Interleukin-2 5 Other Antineoplastic M Monoclonal Antibody P Clofarabine
3 Peripheral Vein ⦸ DRG	3 Percutaneous	1 Thrombolytic	6 Recombinant Human-activated Protein C 7 Other Thrombolytic
3 Peripheral Vein ⦸	3 Percutaneous	2 Anti-infective	8 Oxazolidinones 9 Other Anti-infective
3 Peripheral Vein ⦸	3 Percutaneous	3 Anti-inflammatory 4 Serum, Toxoid and Vaccine 6 Nutritional Substance 7 Electrolytic and Water Balance Substance F Intracirculatory Anesthetic H Radioactive Substance K Other Diagnostic Substance N Analgesics, Hypnotics, Sedatives P Platelet Inhibitor R Antiarrhythmic T Destructive Agent X Vasopressor	Z No Qualifier
3 Peripheral Vein ⦸	3 Percutaneous	G Other Therapeutic Substance	C Other Substance N Blood Brain Barrier Disruption Q Glucarpidase
3 Peripheral Vein DRG	3 Percutaneous	U Pancreatic Islet Cells	0 Autologous 1 Nonautologous
3 Peripheral Vein ⦸	3 Percutaneous	V Hormone	G Insulin H Human B-type Natriuretic Peptide J Other Hormone
3 Peripheral Vein ⦸	3 Percutaneous	W Immunotherapeutic	K Immunostimulator L Immunosuppressive
4 Central Vein ⦸ DRG	0 Open	0 Antineoplastic	2 High-dose Interleukin-2 3 Low-dose Interleukin-2 5 Other Antineoplastic M Monoclonal Antibody P Clofarabine
4 Central Vein ⦸ DRG	0 Open	1 Thrombolytic	6 Recombinant Human-activated Protein C 7 Other Thrombolytic
4 Central Vein ⦸	0 Open	2 Anti-infective	8 Oxazolidinones 9 Other Anti-infective

3E0 continued on next page

3E0 continued from previous page

3 Administration
E Physiological Systems and Anatomical Regions
0 Introduction: Putting in or on a therapeutic, diagnostic, nutritional, physiological, or prophylactic substance except blood or blood products

Body System / Region Character 4	Approach Character 5	Substance Character 6	Qualifier Character 7
4 Central Vein ⦸ DRG	**0** Open	**3** Anti-inflammatory **4** Serum, Toxoid and Vaccine **6** Nutritional Substance **7** Electrolytic and Water Balance Substance **F** Intracirculatory Anesthetic **H** Radioactive Substance **K** Other Diagnostic Substance **N** Analgesics, Hypnotics, Sedatives **P** Platelet Inhibitor **R** Antiarrhythmic **T** Destructive Agent **X** Vasopressor	**Z** No Qualifier
4 Central Vein ⦸	**0** Open	**G** Other Therapeutic Substance	**C** Other Substance **N** Blood Brain Barrier Disruption
4 Central Vein ⦸	**0** Open	**V** Hormone	**G** Insulin **H** Human B-type Natriuretic Peptide **J** Other Hormone
4 Central Vein ⦸	**0** Open	**W** Immunotherapeutic	**K** Immunostimulator **L** Immunosuppressive
4 Central Vein ⦸ DRG	**3** Percutaneous	**0** Antineoplastic	**2** High-dose Interleukin-2 **3** Low-dose Interleukin-2 **5** Other Antineoplastic **M** Monoclonal Antibody **P** Clofarabine
4 Central Vein ⦸ DRG	**3** Percutaneous	**1** Thrombolytic	**6** Recombinant Human-activated Protein C **7** Other Thrombolytic
4 Central Vein ⦸	**3** Percutaneous	**2** Anti-infective	**8** Oxazolidinones **9** Other Anti-infective
4 Central Vein ⦸	**3** Percutaneous	**3** Anti-inflammatory **4** Serum, Toxoid and Vaccine **6** Nutritional Substance **7** Electrolytic and Water Balance Substance **F** Intracirculatory Anesthetic **H** Radioactive Substance **K** Other Diagnostic Substance **N** Analgesics, Hypnotics, Sedatives **P** Platelet Inhibitor **R** Antiarrhythmic **T** Destructive Agent **X** Vasopressor	**Z** No Qualifier
4 Central Vein ⦸	**3** Percutaneous	**G** Other Therapeutic Substance	**C** Other Substance **N** Blood Brain Barrier Disruption **Q** Glucarpidase
4 Central Vein ⦸	**3** Percutaneous	**V** Hormone	**G** Insulin **H** Human B-type Natriuretic Peptide **J** Other Hormone
4 Central Vein ⦸	**3** Percutaneous	**W** Immunotherapeutic	**K** Immunostimulator **L** Immunosuppressive

3E0 continued on next page

3E0 continued from previous page

3 Administration
E Physiological Systems and Anatomical Regions
0 Introduction: Putting in or on a therapeutic, diagnostic, nutritional, physiological, or prophylactic substance except blood or blood products

Body System / Region Character 4	Approach Character 5	Substance Character 6	Qualifier Character 7
5 Peripheral Artery ⊘ DRG **6** Central Artery ⊘ DRG	**0** Open **3** Percutaneous	**0** Antineoplastic	**2** High-dose Interleukin-2 **3** Low-dose Interleukin-2 **5** Other Antineoplastic **M** Monoclonal Antibody **P** Clofarabine
5 Peripheral Artery ⊘ DRG **6** Central Artery ⊘ DRG	**0** Open **3** Percutaneous	**1** Thrombolytic	**6** Recombinant Human-activated Protein C **7** Other Thrombolytic
5 Peripheral Artery ⊘ **6** Central Artery ⊘	**0** Open **3** Percutaneous	**2** Anti-infective	**8** Oxazolidinones **9** Other Anti-infective
5 Peripheral Artery ⊘ **6** Central Artery ⊘	**0** Open **3** Percutaneous	**3** Anti-inflammatory **4** Serum, Toxoid and Vaccine **6** Nutritional Substance **7** Electrolytic and Water Balance Substance **F** Intracirculatory Anesthetic **H** Radioactive Substance **K** Other Diagnostic Substance **N** Analgesics, Hypnotics, Sedatives **P** Platelet Inhibitor **R** Antiarrhythmic **T** Destructive Agent **X** Vasopressor	**Z** No Qualifier
5 Peripheral Artery ⊘ **6** Central Artery ⊘	**0** Open **3** Percutaneous	**G** Other Therapeutic Substance	**C** Other Substance **N** Blood Brain Barrier Disruption
5 Peripheral Artery ⊘ **6** Central Artery ⊘	**0** Open **3** Percutaneous	**V** Hormone	**G** Insulin **H** Human B-type Natriuretic Peptide **J** Other Hormone
5 Peripheral Artery ⊘ **6** Central Artery ⊘	**0** Open **3** Percutaneous	**W** Immunotherapeutic	**K** Immunostimulator **L** Immunosuppressive
7 Coronary Artery ⊘ **8** Heart ⊘ DRG	**0** Open **3** Percutaneous	**1** Thrombolytic	**6** Recombinant Human-activated Protein C **7** Other Thrombolytic
7 Coronary Artery ⊘ **8** Heart ⊘	**0** Open **3** Percutaneous	**G** Other Therapeutic Substance	**C** Other Substance
7 Coronary Artery ⊘ **8** Heart ⊘	**0** Open **3** Percutaneous	**K** Other Diagnostic Substance **P** Platelet Inhibitor	**Z** No Qualifier
9 Nose ⊘	**3** Percutaneous **7** Via Natural or Artificial Opening **X** External	**0** Antineoplastic	**5** Other Antineoplastic **M** Monoclonal Antibody
9 Nose ⊘	**3** Percutaneous **7** Via Natural or Artificial Opening **X** External	**2** Anti-infective	**8** Oxazolidinones **9** Other Anti-infective
9 Nose ⊘	**3** Percutaneous **7** Via Natural or Artificial Opening **X** External	**3** Anti-inflammatory **4** Serum, Toxoid and Vaccine **B** Local Anesthetic **H** Radioactive Substance **K** Other Diagnostic Substance **N** Analgesics, Hypnotics, Sedatives **T** Destructive Agent	**Z** No Qualifier
9 Nose ⊘	**3** Percutaneous **7** Via Natural or Artificial Opening **X** External	**G** Other Therapeutic Substance	**C** Other Substance

3E0 continued on next page

3E0 continued from previous page

3 Administration
E Physiological Systems and Anatomical Regions
0 Introduction: Putting in or on a therapeutic, diagnostic, nutritional, physiological, or prophylactic substance except blood or blood products

Body System / Region Character 4	Approach Character 5	Substance Character 6	Qualifier Character 7
A Bone Marrow ⦸	3 Percutaneous	0 Antineoplastic	5 Other Antineoplastic M Monoclonal Antibody
A Bone Marrow ⦸	3 Percutaneous	G Other Therapeutic Substance	C Other Substance
B Ear ⦸	3 Percutaneous 7 Via Natural or Artificial Opening X External	0 Antineoplastic	4 Liquid Brachytherapy Radioisotope 5 Other Antineoplastic M Monoclonal Antibody
B Ear ⦸	3 Percutaneous 7 Via Natural or Artificial Opening X External	2 Anti-infective	8 Oxazolidinones 9 Other Anti-infective
B Ear ⦸	3 Percutaneous 7 Via Natural or Artificial Opening X External	3 Anti-inflammatory B Local Anesthetic H Radioactive Substance K Other Diagnostic Substance N Analgesics, Hypnotics, Sedatives T Destructive Agent	Z No Qualifier
B Ear	3 Percutaneous 7 Via Natural or Artificial Opening X External	G Other Therapeutic Substance	C Other Substance
C Eye ⦸	3 Percutaneous 7 Via Natural or Artificial Opening X External	0 Antineoplastic	4 Liquid Brachytherapy Radioisotope 5 Other Antineoplastic M Monoclonal Antibody
C Eye ⦸	3 Percutaneous 7 Via Natural or Artificial Opening X External	2 Anti-infective	8 Oxazolidinones 9 Other Anti-infective
C Eye ⦸	3 Percutaneous 7 Via Natural or Artificial Opening X External	3 Anti-inflammatory B Local Anesthetic H Radioactive Substance K Other Diagnostic Substance M Pigment N Analgesics, Hypnotics, Sedatives T Destructive Agent	Z No Qualifier
C Eye	3 Percutaneous 7 Via Natural or Artificial Opening X External	G Other Therapeutic Substance	C Other Substance
C Eye	3 Percutaneous 7 Via Natural or Artificial Opening X External	S Gas	F Other Gas
D Mouth and Pharynx ⦸	3 Percutaneous 7 Via Natural or Artificial Opening X External	0 Antineoplastic	4 Liquid Brachytherapy Radioisotope 5 Other Antineoplastic M Monoclonal Antibody
D Mouth and Pharynx ⦸	3 Percutaneous 7 Via Natural or Artificial Opening X External	2 Anti-infective	8 Oxazolidinones 9 Other Anti-infective

3E0 continued on next page

3E0 continued from previous page

3 Administration
E Physiological Systems and Anatomical Regions
0 Introduction: Putting in or on a therapeutic, diagnostic, nutritional, physiological, or prophylactic substance except blood or blood products

Body System / Region Character 4	Approach Character 5	Substance Character 6	Qualifier Character 7
D Mouth and Pharynx ⃠	**3** Percutaneous **7** Via Natural or Artificial Opening **X** External	**3** Anti-inflammatory **4** Serum, Toxoid and Vaccine **6** Nutritional Substance **7** Electrolytic and Water Balance Substance **B** Local Anesthetic **H** Radioactive Substance **K** Other Diagnostic Substance **N** Analgesics, Hypnotics, Sedatives **R** Antiarrhythmic **T** Destructive Agent	**Z** No Qualifier
D Mouth and Pharynx ⃠	**3** Percutaneous **7** Via Natural or Artificial Opening **X** External	**G** Other Therapeutic Substance	**C** Other Substance
E Products of Conception ⃠ ♀ **G** Upper GI ⃠ **H** Lower GI ⃠ **K** Genitourinary Tract ⃠ **N** Male Reproductive ⃠ ♂	**3** Percutaneous **7** Via Natural or Artificial Opening **8** Via Natural or Artificial Opening Endoscopic	**0** Antineoplastic	**4** Liquid Brachytherapy Radioisotope **5** Other Antineoplastic **M** Monoclonal Antibody
E Products of Conception ⃠ ♀ **G** Upper GI ⃠ **H** Lower GI ⃠ **K** Genitourinary Tract ⃠ **N** Male Reproductive ⃠ ♂	**3** Percutaneous **7** Via Natural or Artificial Opening **8** Via Natural or Artificial Opening Endoscopic	**2** Anti-infective	**8** Oxazolidinones **9** Other Anti-infective
E Products of Conception ⃠ ♀ **G** Upper GI ⃠ **H** Lower GI ⃠ **K** Genitourinary Tract ⃠ **N** Male Reproductive ⃠ ♂	**3** Percutaneous **7** Via Natural or Artificial Opening **8** Via Natural or Artificial Opening Endoscopic	**3** Anti-inflammatory **6** Nutritional Substance **7** Electrolytic and Water Balance Substance **B** Local Anesthetic **H** Radioactive Substance **K** Other Diagnostic Substance **N** Analgesics, Hypnotics, Sedatives **T** Destructive Agent	**Z** No Qualifier
E Products of Conception ⃠ ♀ **G** Upper GI ⃠ **H** Lower GI ⃠ **K** Genitourinary Tract ⃠ **N** Male Reproductive ⃠ ♂	**3** Percutaneous **7** Via Natural or Artificial Opening **8** Via Natural or Artificial Opening Endoscopic	**G** Other Therapeutic Substance	**C** Other Substance
E Products of Conception ⃠ ♀ **G** Upper GI ⃠ **H** Lower GI ⃠ **K** Genitourinary Tract ⃠ **N** Male Reproductive ⃠ ♂	**3** Percutaneous **7** Via Natural or Artificial Opening **8** Via Natural or Artificial Opening Endoscopic	**S** Gas	**F** Other Gas
F Respiratory Tract ⃠	**3** Percutaneous	**0** Antineoplastic	**4** Liquid Brachytherapy Radioisotope **5** Other Antineoplastic **M** Monoclonal Antibody
F Respiratory Tract ⃠	**3** Percutaneous	**2** Anti-infective	**8** Oxazolidinones **9** Other Anti-infective

3E0 continued on next page

3 **Administration**
E **Physiological Systems and Anatomical Regions**
0 **Introduction:** Putting in or on a therapeutic, diagnostic, nutritional, physiological, or prophylactic substance except blood or blood products

3E0 continued from previous page

Body System / Region Character 4	Approach Character 5	Substance Character 6	Qualifier Character 7
F Respiratory Tract ⃠	**3** Percutaneous	**3** Anti-inflammatory **6** Nutritional Substance **7** Electrolytic and Water Balance Substance **B** Local Anesthetic **H** Radioactive Substance **K** Other Diagnostic Substance **N** Analgesics, Hypnotics, Sedatives **T** Destructive Agent	**Z** No Qualifier
F Respiratory Tract ⃠	**3** Percutaneous	**G** Other Therapeutic Substance	**C** Other Substance
F Respiratory Tract ⃠	**3** Percutaneous	**S** Gas	**D** Nitric Oxide **F** Other Gas
F Respiratory Tract ⃠	**7** Via Natural or Artificial Opening **8** Via Natural or Artificial Opening Endoscopic	**0** Antineoplastic	**4** Liquid Brachytherapy Radioisotope **5** Other Antineoplastic **M** Monoclonal Antibody
F Respiratory Tract ⃠	**7** Via Natural or Artificial Opening **8** Via Natural or Artificial Opening Endoscopic	**2** Anti-infective	**8** Oxazolidinones **9** Other Anti-infective
F Respiratory Tract ⃠	**7** Via Natural or Artificial Opening **8** Via Natural or Artificial Opening Endoscopic	**3** Anti-inflammatory **6** Nutritional Substance **7** Electrolytic and Water Balance Substance **B** Local Anesthetic **D** Inhalation Anesthetic **H** Radioactive Substance **K** Other Diagnostic Substance **N** Analgesics, Hypnotics, Sedatives **T** Destructive Agent	**Z** No Qualifier
F Respiratory Tract ⃠	**7** Via Natural or Artificial Opening **8** Via Natural or Artificial Opening Endoscopic	**G** Other Therapeutic Substance	**C** Other Substance
F Respiratory Tract ⃠	**7** Via Natural or Artificial Opening **8** Via Natural or Artificial Opening Endoscopic	**S** Gas	**D** Nitric Oxide **F** Other Gas
J Biliary and Pancreatic Tract ⃠	**3** Percutaneous **7** Via Natural or Artificial Opening **8** Via Natural or Artificial Opening Endoscopic	**0** Antineoplastic	**4** Liquid Brachytherapy Radioisotope **5** Other Antineoplastic **M** Monoclonal Antibody
J Biliary and Pancreatic Tract ⃠	**3** Percutaneous **7** Via Natural or Artificial Opening **8** Via Natural or Artificial Opening Endoscopic	**2** Anti-infective	**8** Oxazolidinones **9** Other Anti-infective
J Biliary and Pancreatic Tract ⃠	**3** Percutaneous **7** Via Natural or Artificial Opening **8** Via Natural or Artificial Opening Endoscopic	**3** Anti-inflammatory **6** Nutritional Substance **7** Electrolytic and Water Balance Substance **B** Local Anesthetic **H** Radioactive Substance **K** Other Diagnostic Substance **N** Analgesics, Hypnotics, Sedatives **T** Destructive Agent	**Z** No Qualifier

3E0 continued on next page

3E0 continued from previous page

3 Administration
E Physiological Systems and Anatomical Regions
0 Introduction: Putting in or on a therapeutic, diagnostic, nutritional, physiological, or prophylactic substance except blood or blood products

Body System / Region Character 4	Approach Character 5	Substance Character 6	Qualifier Character 7
J Biliary and Pancreatic Tract ⊘	**3** Percutaneous **7** Via Natural or Artificial Opening **8** Via Natural or Artificial Opening Endoscopic	**G** Other Therapeutic Substance	**C** Other Substance
J Biliary and Pancreatic Tract ⊘	**3** Percutaneous **7** Via Natural or Artificial Opening **8** Via Natural or Artificial Opening Endoscopic	**S** Gas	**F** Other Gas
J Biliary and Pancreatic Tract DRG	**3** Percutaneous **7** Via Natural or Artificial Opening **8** Via Natural or Artificial Opening Endoscopic	**U** Pancreatic Islet Cells	**0** Autologous **1** Nonautologous
L Pleural Cavity ⊘ **M** Peritoneal Cavity ⊘	**0** Open	**5** Adhesion Barrier	**Z** No Qualifier
L Pleural Cavity ⊘ **M** Peritoneal Cavity ⊘	**3** Percutaneous	**0** Antineoplastic	**4** Liquid Brachytherapy Radioisotope **5** Other Antineoplastic **M** Monoclonal Antibody
L Pleural Cavity ⊘ **M** Peritoneal Cavity ⊘	**3** Percutaneous	**2** Anti-infective	**8** Oxazolidinones **9** Other Anti-infective
L Pleural Cavity ⊘ **M** Peritoneal Cavity ⊘	**3** Percutaneous	**3** Anti-inflammatory **6** Nutritional Substance **7** Electrolytic and Water Balance Substance **B** Local Anesthetic **H** Radioactive Substance **K** Other Diagnostic Substance **N** Analgesics, Hypnotics, Sedatives **T** Destructive Agent	**Z** No Qualifier
L Pleural Cavity ⊘ **M** Peritoneal Cavity ⊘	**3** Percutaneous	**G** Other Therapeutic Substance	**C** Other Substance
L Pleural Cavity ⊘ **M** Peritoneal Cavity ⊘	**3** Percutaneous	**S** Gas	**F** Other Gas
L Pleural Cavity ⊘ **M** Peritoneal Cavity ⊘	**7** Via Natural or Artificial Opening	**0** Antineoplastic	**4** Liquid Brachytherapy Radioisotope **5** Other Antineoplastic **M** Monoclonal Antibody
L Pleural Cavity ⊘ **M** Peritoneal Cavity ⊘	**7** Via Natural or ArtificialOpening	**S** Gas	**F** Other Gas
P Female Reproductive ⊘ ♀	**0** Open	**5** Adhesion Barrier	**Z** No Qualifier
P Female Reproductive ⊘ ♀	**3** Percutaneous **7** Via Natural or Artificial Opening	**0** Antineoplastic	**4** Liquid Brachytherapy Radioisotope **5** Other Antineoplastic **M** Monoclonal Antibody
P Female Reproductive ⊘ ♀	**3** Percutaneous **7** Via Natural or Artificial Opening	**2** Anti-infective	**8** Oxazolidinones **9** Other Anti-infective

3E0 continued on next page

3 Administration
3E0 continued from previous page

E Physiological Systems and Anatomical Regions

0 Introduction: Putting in or on a therapeutic, diagnostic, nutritional, physiological, or prophylactic substance except blood or blood products

Body System / Region Character 4	Approach Character 5	Substance Character 6	Qualifier Character 7
P Female Reproductive ⦸ ♀	**3** Percutaneous **7** Via Natural or Artificial Opening	**3** Anti-inflammatory **6** Nutritional Substance **7** Electrolytic and Water Balance Substance **B** Local Anesthetic **H** Radioactive Substance **K** Other Diagnostic Substance **L** Sperm **N** Analgesics, Hypnotics, Sedatives **T** Destructive Agent	**Z** No Qualifier
P Female Reproductive ⦸ ♀	**3** Percutaneous **7** Via Natural or Artificial Opening	**G** Other Therapeutic Substance	**C** Other Substance
P Female Reproductive ⦸ ♀	**3** Percutaneous **7** Via Natural or Artificial Opening	**Q** Fertilized Ovum	**0** Autologous **1** Nonautologous
P Female Reproductive ⦸ ♀	**3** Percutaneous **7** Via Natural or Artificial Opening	**S** Gas	**F** Other Gas
P Female Reproductive ⦸ ♀	**8** Via Natural or Artificial Opening Endoscopic	**0** Antineoplastic	**4** Liquid Brachytherapy Radioisotope **5** Other Antineoplastic **M** Monoclonal Antibody
P Female Reproductive ⦸ ♀	**8** Via Natural or Artificial Opening Endoscopic	**2** Anti-infective	**8** Oxazolidinones **9** Other Anti-infective
P Female Reproductive ⦸ ♀	**8** Via Natural or Artificial Opening Endoscopic	**3** Anti-inflammatory **6** Nutritional Substance **7** Electrolytic and Water Balance Substance **B** Local Anesthetic **H** Radioactive Substance **K** Other Diagnostic Substance **N** Analgesics, Hypnotics, Sedatives **T** Destructive Agent	**Z** No Qualifier
P Female Reproductive ⦸ ♀	**8** Via Natural or Artificial Opening Endoscopic	**G** Other Therapeutic Substance	**C** Other Substance
P Female Reproductive ⦸ ♀	**8** Via Natural or Artificial Opening Endoscopic	**S** Gas	**F** Other Gas
Q Cranial Cavity and Brain ⦸ DRG	**0** Open **3** Percutaneous	**0** Antineoplastic	**4** Liquid Brachytherapy Radioisotope **5** Other Antineoplastic **M** Monoclonal Antibody
Q Cranial Cavity and Brain ⦸	**0** Open **3** Percutaneous	**2** Anti-infective	**8** Oxazolidinones **9** Other Anti-infective
Q Cranial Cavity and Brain ⦸	**0** Open **3** Percutaneous	**3** Anti-inflammatory **6** Nutritional Substance **7** Electrolytic and Water Balance Substance **A** Stem Cells, Embryonic **B** Local Anesthetic **H** Radioactive Substance **K** Other Diagnostic Substance **N** Analgesics, Hypnotics, Sedatives **T** Destructive Agent	**Z** No Qualifier
Q Cranial Cavity and Brain ⦸	**0** Open **3** Percutaneous	**E** Stem Cells, Somatic	**0** Autologous **1** Nonautologous

3E0 continued on next page

3E0 continued from previous page

3 Administration
E Physiological Systems and Anatomical Regions
0 Introduction: Putting in or on a therapeutic, diagnostic, nutritional, physiological, or prophylactic substance except blood or blood products

Body System / Region Character 4	Approach Character 5	Substance Character 6	Qualifier Character 7
Q Cranial Cavity and Brain ⃠	0 Open 3 Percutaneous	G Other Therapeutic Substance	C Other Substance
Q Cranial Cavity and Brain ⃠	0 Open 3 Percutaneous	S Gas	F Other Gas
Q Cranial Cavity and Brain ⃠ DRG	7 Via Natural or Artificial Opening	0 Antineoplastic	4 Liquid Brachytherapy Radioisotope 5 Other Antineoplastic M Monoclonal Antibody
Q Cranial Cavity and Brain ⃠	7 Via Natural or Artificial Opening	S Gas	F Other Gas
R Spinal Canal ⃠	0 Open	A Stem Cells, Embryonic	Z No Qualifier
R Spinal Canal ⃠	0 Open	E Stem Cells, Somatic	0 Autologous 1 Nonautologous
R Spinal Canal ⃠ DRG	3 Percutaneous	0 Antineoplastic	2 High-dose Interleukin-2 3 Low-dose Interleukin-2 4 Liquid Brachytherapy Radioisotope 5 Other Antineoplastic M Monoclonal Antibody
R Spinal Canal ⃠	3 Percutaneous	2 Anti-infective	8 Oxazolidinones 9 Other Anti-infective
R Spinal Canal ⃠	3 Percutaneous	3 Anti-inflammatory 6 Nutritional Substance 7 Electrolytic and Water Balance Substance A Stem Cells, Embryonic B Local Anesthetic C Regional Anesthetic H Radioactive Substance K Other Diagnostic Substance N Analgesics, Hypnotics, Sedatives T Destructive Agent	Z No Qualifier
R Spinal Canal ⃠	3 Percutaneous	E Stem Cells, Somatic	0 Autologous 1 Nonautologous
R Spinal Canal ⃠	3 Percutaneous	G Other Therapeutic Substance	C Other Substance
R Spinal Canal ⃠	3 Percutaneous	S Gas	F Other Gas
R Spinal Canal ⃠	7 Via Natural or Artificial Opening	S Gas	F Other Gas
S Epidural Space ⃠ DRG	3 Percutaneous	0 Antineoplastic	2 High-dose Interleukin-2 3 Low-dose Interleukin-2 4 Liquid Brachytherapy Radioisotope 5 Other Antineoplastic M Monoclonal Antibody
S Epidural Space ⃠	3 Percutaneous	2 Anti-infective	8 Oxazolidinones 9 Other Anti-infective

3E0 continued on next page

3 Administration
E Physiological Systems and Anatomical Regions
0 Introduction: Putting in or on a therapeutic, diagnostic, nutritional, physiological, or prophylactic substance except blood or blood products

3E0 continued from previous page

Body System / Region Character 4	Approach Character 5	Substance Character 6	Qualifier Character 7
S Epidural Space ⦸	**3** Percutaneous	**3** Anti-inflammatory **6** Nutritional Substance **7** Electrolytic and Water Balance Substance **B** Local Anesthetic **C** Regional Anesthetic **H** Radioactive Substance **K** Other Diagnostic Substance **N** Analgesics, Hypnotics, Sedatives **T** Destructive Agent	**Z** No Qualifier
S Epidural Space ⦸	**3** Percutaneous	**G** Other Therapeutic Substance	**C** Other Substance
S Epidural Space ⦸	**3** Percutaneous	**S** Gas	**F** Other Gas
S Epidural Space ⦸	**7** Via Natural or Artificial Opening	**S** Gas	**F** Other Gas
T Peripheral Nerves and Plexi ⦸ **X** Cranial Nerves ⦸	**3** Percutaneous	**3** Anti-inflammatory **B** Local Anesthetic **C** Regional Anesthetic **T** Destructive Agent	**Z** No Qualifier
T Peripheral Nerves and Plexi ⦸ **X** Cranial Nerves ⦸	**3** Percutaneous	**G** Other Therapeutic Substance	**C** Other Substance
U Joints ⦸	**0** Open	**2** Anti-infective	**8** Oxazolidinones **9** Other Anti-infective
U Joints ⦸	**0** Open	**G** Other Therapeutic Substance	**B** Recombinant Bone Morphogenetic Protein
U Joints ⦸	**3** Percutaneous	**0** Antineoplastic	**4** Liquid Brachytherapy Radioisotope **5** Other Antineoplastic **M** Monoclonal Antibody
U Joints ⦸	**3** Percutaneous	**2** Anti-infective	**8** Oxazolidinones **9** Other Anti-infective
U Joints ⦸	**3** Percutaneous	**3** Anti-inflammatory **6** Nutritional Substance **7** Electrolytic and Water Balance Substance **B** Local Anesthetic **H** Radioactive Substance **K** Other Diagnostic Substance **N** Analgesics, Hypnotics, Sedatives **T** Destructive Agent	**Z** No Qualifier
U Joints ⦸	**3** Percutaneous	**G** Other Therapeutic Substance	**B** Recombinant Bone Morphogenetic Protein **C** Other Substance
U Joints ⦸	**3** Percutaneous	**S** Gas	**F** Other Gas
V Bones ⦸	**0** Open	**G** Other Therapeutic Substance	**B** Recombinant Bone Morphogenetic Protein
V Bones ⦸	**3** Percutaneous	**0** Antineoplastic	**5** Other Antineoplastic **M** Monoclonal Antibody
V Bones ⦸	**3** Percutaneous	**2** Anti-infective	**8** Oxazolidinones **9** Other Anti-infective

3E0 continued on next page

3E0 continued from previous page

3 Administration
E Physiological Systems and Anatomical Regions
0 Introduction: Putting in or on a therapeutic, diagnostic, nutritional, physiological, or prophylactic substance except blood or blood products

Body System / Region Character 4	Approach Character 5	Substance Character 6	Qualifier Character 7
V Bones ⃠	**3** Percutaneous	**3** Anti-inflammatory **6** Nutritional Substance **7** Electrolytic and Water Balance Substance **B** Local Anesthetic **H** Radioactive Substance **K** Other Diagnostic Substance **N** Analgesics, Hypnotics, Sedatives **T** Destructive Agent	**Z** No Qualifier
V Bones ⃠	**3** Percutaneous	**G** Other Therapeutic Substance	**B** Recombinant Bone Morphogenetic Protein **C** Other Substance
W Lymphatics ⃠	**3** Percutaneous	**0** Antineoplastic	**5** Other Antineoplastic **M** Monoclonal Antibody
W Lymphatics ⃠	**3** Percutaneous	**2** Anti-infective	**8** Oxazolidinones **9** Other Anti-infective
W Lymphatics ⃠	**3** Percutaneous	**3** Anti-inflammatory **6** Nutritional Substance **7** Electrolytic and Water Balance Substance **B** Local Anesthetic **H** Radioactive Substance **K** Other Diagnostic Substance **N** Analgesics, Hypnotics, Sedatives **T** Destructive Agent	**Z** No Qualifier
W Lymphatics ⃠	**3** Percutaneous	**G** Other Therapeutic Substance	**C** Other Substance
Y Pericardial Cavity ⃠	**3** Percutaneous	**0** Antineoplastic	**4** Liquid Brachytherapy Radioisotope **5** Other Antineoplastic **M** Monoclonal Antibody
Y Pericardial Cavity ⃠	**3** Percutaneous	**2** Anti-infective	**8** Oxazolidinones **9** Other Anti-infective
Y Pericardial Cavity ⃠	**3** Percutaneous	**3** Anti-inflammatory **6** Nutritional Substance **7** Electrolytic and Water Balance Substance **B** Local Anesthetic **H** Radioactive Substance **K** Other Diagnostic Substance **N** Analgesics, Hypnotics, Sedatives **T** Destructive Agent	**Z** No Qualifier
Y Pericardial Cavity ⃠	**3** Percutaneous	**G** Other Therapeutic Substance	**C** Other Substance
Y Pericardial Cavity ⃠	**3** Percutaneous	**S** Gas	**F** Other Gas
Y Pericardial Cavity ⃠	**7** Via Natural or Artificial Opening	**0** Antineoplastic	**4** Liquid Brachytherapy Radioisotope **5** Other Antineoplastic **M** Monoclonal Antibody
Y Pericardial Cavity ⃠	**7** Via Natural or Artificial Opening	**S** Gas	**F** Other Gas

♂ 3E0N304 3E0N305 3E0N30M 3E0N328 3E0N329 3E0N33Z 3E0N36Z 3E0N37Z 3E0N3BZ 3E0N3GC 3E0N3HZ 3E0N3KZ 3E0N3NZ 3E0N3SF 3E0N3TZ 3E0N704 3E0N705 3E0N70M 3E0N728 3E0N729 3E0N73Z 3E0N76Z 3E0N77Z 3E0N7BZ 3E0N7GC 3E0N7HZ 3E0N7KZ 3E0N7NZ 3E0N7SF 3E0N7TZ 3E0N804 3E0N805 3E0N80M 3E0N828 3E0N829 3E0N83Z 3E0N86Z 3E0N87Z 3E0N8BZ 3E0N8GC 3E0N8HZ 3E0N8KZ 3E0N8NZ 3E0N8SF 3E0N8TZ

♀ 3E0E304 3E0E305 3E0E30M 3E0E328 3E0E329 3E0E33Z 3E0E36Z 3E0E37Z 3E0E3BZ 3E0E3GC 3E0E3HZ 3E0E3KZ 3E0E3NZ 3E0E3SF 3E0E3TZ 3E0E704 3E0E705 3E0E70M 3E0E728 3E0E729 3E0E73Z 3E0E76Z 3E0E77Z 3E0E7BZ 3E0E7GC 3E0E7HZ

3E0 continued on next page

3E0 continued from previous page

3E0E7KZ 3E0E7NZ 3E0E7SF 3E0E7TZ 3E0E804 3E0E805 3E0E80M 3E0E828 3E0E829 3E0E83Z 3E0E86Z 3E0E87Z 3E0E8BZ
3E0E8GC 3E0E8HZ 3E0E8KZ 3E0E8NZ 3E0E8SF 3E0E8TZ 3E0P05Z 3E0P304 3E0P305 3E0P30M 3E0P328 3E0P329 3E0P33Z
3E0P36Z 3E0P37Z 3E0P3BZ 3E0P3GC 3E0P3HZ 3E0P3KZ 3E0P3LZ 3E0P3NZ 3E0P3Q0 3E0P3Q1 3E0P3SF 3E0P3TZ 3E0P704
3E0P705 3E0P70M 3E0P728 3E0P729 3E0P73Z 3E0P76Z 3E0P77Z 3E0P7BZ 3E0P7GC 3E0P7HZ 3E0P7KZ 3E0P7LZ 3E0P7NZ
3E0P7Q0 3E0P7Q1 3E0P7SF 3E0P7TZ 3E0P804 3E0P805 3E0P80M 3E0P828 3E0P829 3E0P83Z 3E0P86Z 3E0P87Z 3E0P8BZ
3E0P8GC 3E0P8HZ 3E0P8KZ 3E0P8NZ 3E0P8SF 3E0P8TZ

⦸ 3E00X05 3E00X0M 3E00X28 3E00X29 3E00X3Z 3E00X4Z 3E00XBZ 3E00XGC 3E00XKZ 3E00XMZ 3E00XNZ 3E00XTZ 3E0102A
3E01305 3E0130M 3E01328 3E01329 3E0132A 3E0133Z 3E0134Z 3E0136Z 3E0137Z 3E013BZ 3E013GC 3E013HZ 3E013KZ
3E013NZ 3E013TZ 3E013VG 3E013VJ 3E02305 3E0230M 3E02328 3E02329 3E0233Z 3E0234Z 3E0236Z 3E0237Z 3E023BZ
3E023GC 3E023HZ 3E023KZ 3E023NZ 3E023TZ 3E03003 3E03005 3E0300M 3E0300P 3E03016 3E03028 3E03029 3E0303Z
3E0304Z 3E0306Z 3E0307Z 3E030FZ 3E030GC 3E030GN 3E030HZ 3E030KZ 3E030NZ 3E030PZ 3E030RZ 3E030VG 3E030VH
3E030VJ 3E030WK 3E030WL 3E030XZ 3E03303 3E03305 3E0330M 3E0330P 3E03316 3E03328 3E03329 3E0333Z 3E0334Z
3E0336Z 3E0337Z 3E033FZ 3E033GC 3E033GN 3E033GQ 3E033HZ 3E033KZ 3E033NZ 3E033PZ 3E033RZ 3E033VG 3E033VH
3E033VJ 3E033WK 3E033WL 3E033XZ 3E04003 3E04005 3E0400M 3E0400P 3E04016 3E04028 3E04029 3E0403Z 3E0404Z
3E0406Z 3E0407Z 3E040FZ 3E040GC 3E040GN 3E040HZ 3E040KZ 3E040NZ 3E040PZ 3E040RZ 3E040VG 3E040VH 3E040VJ
3E040WK 3E040WL 3E040XZ 3E04303 3E04305 3E0430M 3E0430P 3E04316 3E04328 3E04329 3E0433Z 3E0434Z 3E0436Z
3E0437Z 3E043FZ 3E043GC 3E043GN 3E043GQ 3E043HZ 3E043KZ 3E043NZ 3E043PZ 3E043RZ 3E043VG 3E043VH 3E043VJ
3E043WK 3E043WL 3E043XZ 3E05003 3E05005 3E0500M 3E0500P 3E05016 3E05028 3E05029 3E0503Z 3E0504Z 3E0506Z
3E0507Z 3E050FZ 3E050GC 3E050GN 3E050HZ 3E050KZ 3E050NZ 3E050PZ 3E050RZ 3E050TZ 3E050VG 3E050VH 3E050VJ
3E050WK 3E050WL 3E050XZ 3E05303 3E05305 3E0530M 3E0530P 3E05316 3E05328 3E05329 3E0533Z 3E0534Z 3E0536Z
3E0537Z 3E053FZ 3E053GC 3E053GN 3E053HZ 3E053KZ 3E053NZ 3E053PZ 3E053RZ 3E053TZ 3E053VG 3E053VH 3E053VJ
3E053WK 3E053WL 3E053XZ 3E06003 3E06005 3E0600M 3E0600P 3E06016 3E06028 3E06029 3E0603Z 3E0604Z 3E0606Z
3E0607Z 3E060FZ 3E060GC 3E060GN 3E060HZ 3E060KZ 3E060NZ 3E060PZ 3E060RZ 3E060TZ 3E060VG 3E060VH 3E060VJ
3E060WK 3E060WL 3E060XZ 3E06303 3E06305 3E0630M 3E0630P 3E06316 3E06328 3E06329 3E0633Z 3E0634Z 3E0636Z
3E0637Z 3E063FZ 3E063GC 3E063GN 3E063HZ 3E063KZ 3E063NZ 3E063PZ 3E063RZ 3E063TZ 3E063VG 3E063VH 3E063VJ
3E063WK 3E063WL 3E063XZ 3E07016 3E07017 3E070GC 3E070KZ 3E070PZ 3E07316 3E07317 3E073GC 3E073KZ 3E073PZ
3E08016 3E080GC 3E080KZ 3E080PZ 3E08316 3E083GC 3E083KZ 3E083PZ 3E09305 3E0930M 3E09328 3E09329 3E0933Z
3E0934Z 3E093BZ 3E093GC 3E093HZ 3E093KZ 3E093NZ 3E093TZ 3E09705 3E0970M 3E09728 3E09729 3E0973Z 3E0974Z
3E097BZ 3E097GC 3E097HZ 3E097KZ 3E097NZ 3E097TZ 3E09X05 3E09X0M 3E09X28 3E09X29 3E09X3Z 3E09X4Z 3E09XBZ
3E09XGC 3E09XHZ 3E09XKZ 3E09XNZ 3E09XTZ 3E0A305 3E0A30M 3E0A3GC 3E0B304 3E0B305 3E0B30M 3E0B328 3E0B3NZ
3E0B704 3E0B705 3E0B70M 3E0B728 3E0B7NZ 3E0BX04 3E0BX05 3E0BX0M 3E0BX28 3E0BXNZ 3E0C304 3E0C305 3E0C30M
3E0C328 3E0C329 3E0C3NZ 3E0C704 3E0C705 3E0C70M 3E0C728 3E0C7NZ 3E0CX04 3E0CX05 3E0CX0M 3E0CX28 3E0CXNZ
3E0D304 3E0D305 3E0D30M 3E0D328 3E0D329 3E0D33Z 3E0D34Z 3E0D36Z 3E0D37Z 3E0D3BZ 3E0D3GC 3E0D3HZ 3E0D3KZ
3E0D3NZ 3E0D3RZ 3E0D3TZ 3E0D704 3E0D705 3E0D70M 3E0D728 3E0D729 3E0D73Z 3E0D74Z 3E0D76Z 3E0D77Z 3E0D7BZ
3E0D7GC 3E0D7HZ 3E0D7KZ 3E0D7NZ 3E0D7RZ 3E0D7TZ 3E0DX04 3E0DX05 3E0DX0M 3E0DX28 3E0DX29 3E0DX3Z 3E0DX4Z
3E0DX6Z 3E0DX7Z 3E0DXBZ 3E0DXGC 3E0DXHZ 3E0DXKZ 3E0DXNZ 3E0DXRZ 3E0DXTZ 3E0E304 3E0E305 3E0E30M 3E0E328
3E0E329 3E0E33Z 3E0E36Z 3E0E37Z 3E0E3BZ 3E0E3GC 3E0E3HZ 3E0E3KZ 3E0E3NZ 3E0E3SF 3E0E3TZ 3E0E704 3E0E705
3E0E70M 3E0E728 3E0E729 3E0E73Z 3E0E76Z 3E0E77Z 3E0E7BZ 3E0E7GC 3E0E7HZ 3E0E7KZ 3E0E7NZ 3E0E7SF 3E0E7TZ
3E0E804 3E0E805 3E0E80M 3E0E828 3E0E829 3E0E83Z 3E0E86Z 3E0E87Z 3E0E8BZ 3E0E8GC 3E0E8HZ 3E0E8KZ 3E0E8NZ
3E0E8SF 3E0E8TZ 3E0F304 3E0F305 3E0F30M 3E0F328 3E0F329 3E0F33Z 3E0F36Z 3E0F37Z 3E0F3BZ 3E0F3GC 3E0F3HZ
3E0F3KZ 3E0F3NZ 3E0F3SD 3E0F3SF 3E0F3TZ 3E0F704 3E0F705 3E0F70M 3E0F728 3E0F729 3E0F73Z 3E0F76Z 3E0F77Z
3E0F7BZ 3E0F7DZ 3E0F7GC 3E0F7HZ 3E0F7KZ 3E0F7NZ 3E0F7SD 3E0F7SF 3E0F7TZ 3E0F804 3E0F805 3E0F80M 3E0F828
3E0F829 3E0F83Z 3E0F86Z 3E0F87Z 3E0F8BZ 3E0F8DZ 3E0F8GC 3E0F8HZ 3E0F8KZ 3E0F8NZ 3E0F8SD 3E0F8SF 3E0F8TZ
3E0G304 3E0G305 3E0G30M 3E0G328 3E0G329 3E0G33Z 3E0G36Z 3E0G37Z 3E0G3BZ 3E0G3HZ 3E0G3KZ 3E0G3NZ 3E0G3SF
3E0G3TZ 3E0G704 3E0G705 3E0G70M 3E0G728 3E0G729 3E0G73Z 3E0G76Z 3E0G77Z 3E0G7BZ 3E0G7GC 3E0G7HZ 3E0G7KZ
3E0G7NZ 3E0G7SF 3E0G7TZ 3E0G804 3E0G805 3E0G80M 3E0G828 3E0G829 3E0G83Z 3E0G86Z 3E0G87Z 3E0G8BZ 3E0G8GC
3E0G8HZ 3E0G8KZ 3E0G8NZ 3E0G8SF 3E0G8TZ 3E0H304 3E0H305 3E0H30M 3E0H328 3E0H329 3E0H33Z 3E0H36Z 3E0H37Z
3E0H3BZ 3E0H3GC 3E0H3HZ 3E0H3KZ 3E0H3NZ 3E0H3SF 3E0H3TZ 3E0H704 3E0H705 3E0H70M 3E0H728 3E0H729 3E0H73Z
3E0H76Z 3E0H77Z 3E0H7BZ 3E0H7GC 3E0H7HZ 3E0H7KZ 3E0H7NZ 3E0H7SF 3E0H7TZ 3E0H804 3E0H805 3E0H80M 3E0H828
3E0H829 3E0H83Z 3E0H86Z 3E0H87Z 3E0H8BZ 3E0H8GC 3E0H8HZ 3E0H8KZ 3E0H8NZ 3E0H8SF 3E0H8TZ 3E0J304 3E0J305
3E0J30M 3E0J328 3E0J329 3E0J33Z 3E0J36Z 3E0J37Z 3E0J3BZ 3E0J3GC 3E0J3HZ 3E0J3KZ 3E0J3NZ 3E0J3SF 3E0J3TZ
3E0J704 3E0J705 3E0J70M 3E0J728 3E0J729 3E0J73Z 3E0J76Z 3E0J77Z 3E0J7BZ 3E0J7GC 3E0J7HZ 3E0J7KZ 3E0J7NZ
3E0J7SF 3E0J7TZ 3E0J804 3E0J805 3E0J80M 3E0J828 3E0J829 3E0J83Z 3E0J86Z 3E0J87Z 3E0J8BZ 3E0J8GC 3E0J8HZ
3E0J8KZ 3E0J8NZ 3E0J8SF 3E0J8TZ 3E0K304 3E0K305 3E0K30M 3E0K328 3E0K329 3E0K33Z 3E0K36Z 3E0K37Z 3E0K3BZ
3E0K3GC 3E0K3HZ 3E0K3KZ 3E0K3NZ 3E0K3SF 3E0K3TZ 3E0K704 3E0K705 3E0K70M 3E0K728 3E0K729 3E0K73Z 3E0K76Z
3E0K77Z 3E0K7BZ 3E0K7GC 3E0K7HZ 3E0K7KZ 3E0K7NZ 3E0K7SF 3E0K7TZ 3E0K804 3E0K805 3E0K80M 3E0K828 3E0K829
3E0K83Z 3E0K86Z 3E0K87Z 3E0K8BZ 3E0K8GC 3E0K8HZ 3E0K8KZ 3E0K8NZ 3E0K8SF 3E0K8TZ 3E0L05Z 3E0L304 3E0L305
3E0L30M 3E0L328 3E0L329 3E0L33Z 3E0L36Z 3E0L37Z 3E0L3BZ 3E0L3GC 3E0L3HZ 3E0L3KZ 3E0L3NZ 3E0L3SF 3E0L3TZ
3E0L704 3E0L705 3E0L70M 3E0L7SF 3E0M05Z 3E0M304 3E0M305 3E0M30M 3E0M328 3E0M329 3E0M33Z 3E0M36Z 3E0M37Z
3E0M3BZ 3E0M3GC 3E0M3HZ 3E0M3KZ 3E0M3NZ 3E0M3SF 3E0M3TZ 3E0M704 3E0M705 3E0M70M 3E0M7SF 3E0N304 3E0N305
3E0N30M 3E0N328 3E0N329 3E0N33Z 3E0N36Z 3E0N37Z 3E0N3BZ 3E0N3GC 3E0N3HZ 3E0N3KZ 3E0N3NZ 3E0N3SF 3E0N3TZ
3E0N704 3E0N705 3E0N70M 3E0N728 3E0N729 3E0N73Z 3E0N76Z 3E0N77Z 3E0N7BZ 3E0N7GC 3E0N7HZ 3E0N7KZ 3E0N7NZ
3E0N7SF 3E0N7TZ 3E0N804 3E0N805 3E0N80M 3E0N828 3E0N829 3E0N83Z 3E0N86Z 3E0N87Z 3E0N8BZ 3E0N8GC 3E0N8HZ
3E0N8KZ 3E0N8NZ 3E0N8SF 3E0N8TZ 3E0P05Z 3E0P304 3E0P305 3E0P30M 3E0P328 3E0P329 3E0P33Z 3E0P36Z 3E0P37Z
3E0P3BZ 3E0P3GC 3E0P3HZ 3E0P3KZ 3E0P3LZ 3E0P3NZ 3E0P3SF 3E0P3TZ 3E0P704 3E0P705 3E0P70M 3E0P728 3E0P729
3E0P76Z 3E0P77Z 3E0P7BZ 3E0P7GC 3E0P7HZ 3E0P7KZ 3E0P7LZ 3E0P7NZ 3E0P7SF 3E0P7TZ 3E0P804 3E0P805 3E0P80M
3E0P828 3E0P829 3E0P83Z 3E0P86Z 3E0P87Z 3E0P8BZ 3E0P8GC 3E0P8HZ 3E0P8KZ 3E0P8NZ 3E0P8SF 3E0P8TZ 3E0Q004
3E0Q005 3E0Q00M 3E0Q028 3E0Q029 3E0Q03Z 3E0Q06Z 3E0Q07Z 3E0Q0AZ 3E0Q0BZ 3E0Q0E0 3E0Q0E1 3E0Q0GC 3E0Q0HZ
3E0Q0KZ 3E0Q0NZ 3E0Q0SF 3E0Q0TZ 3E0Q304 3E0Q30M 3E0Q328 3E0Q329 3E0Q33Z 3E0Q36Z 3E0Q37Z 3E0Q3AZ 3E0Q3BZ
3E0Q3E0 3E0Q3E1 3E0Q3GC 3E0Q3HZ 3E0Q3KZ 3E0Q3NZ 3E0Q3SF 3E0Q3TZ 3E0Q704 3E0Q70M 3E0Q7SF 3E0R0AZ 3E0R0E0
3E0R0E1 3E0R303 3E0R304 3E0R305 3E0R30M 3E0R328 3E0R329 3E0R33Z 3E0R36Z 3E0R37Z 3E0R3AZ 3E0R3BZ 3E0R3CZ

3E0 continued on next page

LC Limited Coverage NC Noncovered HAC HAC Associated Procedure CC Combination Cluster - See Appendix G for code lists
DRG Non-OR-Affecting MS-DRG Assignment ⦸ Non-OR-Not Affecting MS-DRG Assignment New/Revised Text in Orange ♂ Male ♀ Female

3E0 continued from previous page

3E0R3E0 3E0R3E1 3E0R3GC 3E0R3HZ 3E0R3KZ 3E0R3NZ 3E0R3SF 3E0R3TZ 3E0R7SF 3E0S303 3E0S304 3E0S305 3E0S30M
3E0S328 3E0S329 3E0S33Z 3E0S36Z 3E0S37Z 3E0S3BZ 3E0S3CZ 3E0S3GC 3E0S3HZ 3E0S3KZ 3E0S3NZ 3E0S3SF 3E0S3TZ
3E0S7SF 3E0T33Z 3E0T3BZ 3E0T3CZ 3E0T3GC 3E0T3TZ 3E0U028 3E0U029 3E0U0GB 3E0U304 3E0U305 3E0U30M 3E0U328
3E0U329 3E0U33Z 3E0U36Z 3E0U37Z 3E0U3BZ 3E0U3GB 3E0U3GC 3E0U3HZ 3E0U3KZ 3E0U3NZ 3E0U3SF 3E0U3TZ 3E0V0GB
3E0V305 3E0V30M 3E0V328 3E0V329 3E0V33Z 3E0V36Z 3E0V37Z 3E0V3BZ 3E0V3GB 3E0V3GC 3E0V3HZ 3E0V3KZ 3E0V3NZ
3E0V3TZ 3E0W305 3E0W30M 3E0W328 3E0W329 3E0W33Z 3E0W36Z 3E0W37Z 3E0W3BZ 3E0W3GC 3E0W3HZ 3E0W3KZ 3E0W3NZ
3E0W3TZ 3E0X33Z 3E0X3BZ 3E0X3CZ 3E0X3GC 3E0X3TZ 3E0Y304 3E0Y305 3E0Y30M 3E0Y328 3E0Y329 3E0Y33Z 3E0Y36Z
3E0Y37Z 3E0Y3BZ 3E0Y3GC 3E0Y3HZ 3E0Y3KZ 3E0Y3NZ 3E0Y3SF 3E0Y3TZ 3E0Y704 3E0Y705 3E0Y70M 3E0Y7SF

DRG 3E03002 3E03017 3E030U0 3E030U1 3E03302 3E03317 3E033U0 3E033U1 3E04002 3E04017 3E04302 3E04317 3E05002
3E05017 3E05302 3E05317 3E06002 3E06017 3E06302 3E06317 3E08017 3E08317 3E0J3U0 3E0J3U1 3E0J7U0 3E0J7U1
3E0J8U0 3E0J8U1 3E0Q305 3E0Q705 3E0R302 3E0S302

3 Administration
E Physiological Systems and Anatomical Regions
1 Irrigation: Putting in or on a cleansing substance

Body System / Region Character 4	Approach Character 5	Substance Character 6	Qualifier Character 7
0 Skin and Mucous Membranes ⦸ **C** Eye ⦸	**3** Percutaneous **X** External	**8** Irrigating Substance	**X** Diagnostic **Z** No Qualifier
9 Nose ⦸ **B** Ear ⦸ **F** Respiratory Tract ⦸ **G** Upper GI ⦸ **H** Lower GI ⦸ **J** Biliary and Pancreatic Tract ⦸ **K** Genitourinary Tract ⦸ **N** Male Reproductive ♂ **P** Female Reproductive ⦸ ♀	**3** Percutaneous **7** Via Natural or Artificial Opening **8** Via Natural or Artificial Opening Endoscopic	**8** Irrigating Substance	**X** Diagnostic **Z** No Qualifier
L Pleural Cavity ⦸ **Q** Cranial Cavity and Brain ⦸ **R** Spinal Canal ⦸ **S** Epidural Space ⦸ **U** Joints ⦸ **Y** Pericardial Cavity ⦸	**3** Percutaneous	**8** Irrigating Substance	**X** Diagnostic **Z** No Qualifier
M Peritoneal Cavity ⦸	**3** Percutaneous	**8** Irrigating Substance	**X** Diagnostic **Z** No Qualifier
M Peritoneal Cavity ⦸	**3** Percutaneous	**9** Dialysate	**Z** No Qualifier

♂ 3E1N38X 3E1N38Z 3E1N78X 3E1N78Z 3E1N88X 3E1N88Z

♀ 3E1P38X 3E1P38Z 3E1P78X 3E1P78Z 3E1P88X 3E1P88Z

⦸ 3E1038X 3E1038Z 3E10X8X 3E10X8Z 3E1938X 3E1938Z 3E1978X 3E1978Z 3E1988X 3E1988Z 3E1B38X 3E1B38Z 3E1B78X
3E1B78Z 3E1B88X 3E1B88Z 3E1C38X 3E1C38Z 3E1CX8X 3E1CX8Z 3E1F38X 3E1F38Z 3E1F78X 3E1F78Z 3E1F88X 3E1F88Z
3E1G38X 3E1G38Z 3E1G78X 3E1G78Z 3E1G88X 3E1G88Z 3E1H38X 3E1H38Z 3E1H78X 3E1H78Z 3E1H88X 3E1H88Z 3E1J38X
3E1J38Z 3E1J78X 3E1J78Z 3E1J88X 3E1J88Z 3E1K38X 3E1K38Z 3E1K78X 3E1K78Z 3E1K88X 3E1K88Z 3E1L38X 3E1L38Z
3E1M38X 3E1M38Z 3E1M39Z 3E1P38X 3E1P38Z 3E1P78X 3E1P78Z 3E1P88X 3E1P88Z 3E1Q38X 3E1Q38Z 3E1R38X 3E1R38Z
3E1S38X 3E1S38Z 3E1U38X 3E1U38Z 3E1Y38X 3E1Y38Z

Measurement and Monitoring 4A0-4B0

4 Measurement and Monitoring
A Physiological Systems
0 Measurement: Determining the level of a physiological or physical function at a point in time

Body System Character 4	Approach Character 5	Function/Device Character 6	Qualifier Character 7
0 Central Nervous ⦸	**0** Open	**2** Conductivity **4** Electrical Activity **B** Pressure	**Z** No Qualifier
0 Central Nervous ⦸	**3** Percutaneous	**4** Electrical Activity	**Z** No Qualifier
0 Central Nervous ⦸	**3** Percutaneous	**B** Pressure **K** Temperature **R** Saturation	**D** Intracranial
0 Central Nervous ⦸	**7** Via Natural or Artificial Opening	**B** Pressure **K** Temperature **R** Saturation	**D** Intracranial
0 Central Nervous ⦸	**X** External	**2** Conductivity **4** Electrical Activity	**Z** No Qualifier
1 Peripheral Nervous ⦸	**0** Open **3** Percutaneous **X** External	**2** Conductivity	**9** Sensory **B** Motor
1 Peripheral Nervous ⦸	**0** Open **3** Percutaneous **X** External	**4** Electrical Activity	**Z** No Qualifier
2 Cardiac ⦸ DRG	**0** Open **3** Percutaneous	**4** Electrical Activity **9** Output **C** Rate **F** Rhythm **H** Sound **P** Action Currents	**Z** No Qualifier
2 Cardiac DRG	**0** Open **3** Percutaneous	**N** Sampling and Pressure	**6** Right Heart **7** Left Heart **8** Bilateral
2 Cardiac ⦸ CC DRG	**X** External	**4** Electrical Activity	**A** Guidance **Z** No Qualifier
2 Cardiac ⦸ DRG	**X** External	**9** Output **C** Rate **F** Rhythm **H** Sound **P** Action Currents	**Z** No Qualifier
2 Cardiac ⦸ DRG	**X** External	**M** Total Activity	**4** Stress
3 Arterial ⦸	**0** Open **3** Percutaneous	**5** Flow **J** Pulse	**1** Peripheral **3** Pulmonary **C** Coronary
3 Arterial ⦸	**0** Open **3** Percutaneous	**B** Pressure	**1** Peripheral **3** Pulmonary **C** Coronary **F** Other Thoracic
3 Arterial ⦸	**0** Open **3** Percutaneous	**H** Sound **R** Saturation	**1** Peripheral
3 Arterial ⦸	**X** External	**5** Flow **B** Pressure **H** Sound **J** Pulse **R** Saturation	**1** Peripheral

4A0 continued on next page

4A0 continued from previous page

4 Measurement and Monitoring
A Physiological Systems
0 Measurement: Determining the level of a physiological or physical function at a point in time

Body System Character 4	Approach Character 5	Function/Device Character 6	Qualifier Character 7
4 Venous ⃠	**0** Open **3** Percutaneous	**5** Flow **B** Pressure **J** Pulse	**0** Central **1** Peripheral **2** Portal **3** Pulmonary
4 Venous ⃠	**0** Open **3** Percutaneous	**R** Saturation	**1** Peripheral
4 Venous ⃠	**X** External	**5** Flow **B** Pressure **J** Pulse **R** Saturation	**1** Peripheral
5 Circulatory ⃠	**X** External	**L** Volume	**Z** No Qualifier
6 Lymphatic	**0** Open **3** Percutaneous	**5** Flow **B** Pressure	**Z** No Qualifier
7 Visual ⃠	**X** External	**0** Acuity **7** Mobility **B** Pressure	**Z** No Qualifier
8 Olfactory ⃠	**X** External	**0** Acuity	**Z** No Qualifier
9 Respiratory ⃠	**7** Via Natural or Artificial Opening **8** Via Natural or Artificial Opening Endoscopic **X** External	**1** Capacity **5** Flow **C** Rate **D** Resistance **L** Volume **M** Total Activity	**Z** No Qualifier
B Gastrointestinal ⃠	**7** Via Natural or Artificial Opening **8** Via Natural or Artificial Opening Endoscopic	**8** Motility **B** Pressure **G** Secretion	**Z** No Qualifier
C Biliary ⃠	**3** Percutaneous **4** Percutaneous Endoscopic **7** Via Natural or Artificial Opening **8** Via Natural or Artificial Opening Endoscopic	**5** Flow **B** Pressure	**Z** No Qualifier
D Urinary ⃠	**7** Via Natural or Artificial Opening	**3** Contractility **5** Flow **B** Pressure **D** Resistance **L** Volume	**Z** No Qualifier
F Musculoskeletal ⃠	**3** Percutaneous **X** External	**3** Contractility	**Z** No Qualifier
H Products of Conception, Cardiac ⃠ ♀	**7** Via Natural or Artificial Opening **8** Via Natural or Artificial Opening Endoscopic **X** External	**4** Electrical Activity **C** Rate **F** Rhythm **H** Sound	**Z** No Qualifier
J Products of Conception, Nervous ⃠ ♀	**7** Via Natural or Artificial Opening **8** Via Natural or Artificial Opening Endoscopic **X** External	**2** Conductivity **4** Electrical Activity **B** Pressure	**Z** No Qualifier
Z None ⃠	**7** Via Natural or Artificial Opening	**6** Metabolism **K** Temperature	**Z** No Qualifier
Z None ⃠	**X** External	**6** Metabolism **K** Temperature **Q** Sleep	**Z** No Qualifier

♀ 4A0H74Z 4A0H7CZ 4A0H7FZ 4A0H7HZ 4A0H84Z 4A0H8CZ 4A0H8FZ 4A0H8HZ 4A0HX4Z 4A0HXCZ 4A0HXFZ 4A0HXHZ 4A0J72Z 4A0J74Z 4A0J7BZ 4A0J82Z 4A0J84Z 4A0J8BZ 4A0JX2Z 4A0JX4Z 4A0JXBZ
⃠ 4A0002Z 4A0004Z 4A000BZ 4A0034Z 4A003BD 4A003KD 4A003RD 4A007BD 4A007KD 4A007RD 4A00X2Z 4A00X4Z 4A01029

4A0 continued on next page

4A0 continued from previous page

4A0102B 4A0104Z 4A01329 4A0132B 4A0134Z 4A01X29 4A01X2B 4A01X4Z 4A0204Z 4A0209Z 4A020CZ 4A020FZ 4A020HZ
4A020PZ 4A0234Z 4A0239Z 4A023CZ 4A023HZ 4A023PZ 4A02X4Z 4A02X9Z 4A02XCZ 4A02XFZ 4A02XHZ 4A02XM4 4A02XPZ
4A03051 4A03053 4A0305C 4A030B1 4A030B3 4A030BC 4A030BF 4A030H1 4A030J1 4A030J3 4A030JC 4A030R1 4A03351
4A03353 4A0335C 4A033B1 4A033B3 4A033BC 4A033BF 4A033H1 4A033J1 4A033J3 4A033JC 4A033R1 4A03X51 4A03XB1
4A03XH1 4A03XJ1 4A03XR1 4A04050 4A04051 4A04052 4A04053 4A040B0 4A040B1 4A040B2 4A040B3 4A040J0 4A040J1
4A040J2 4A040J3 4A040R1 4A04350 4A04351 4A04352 4A04353 4A043B0 4A043B1 4A043B2 4A043B3 4A043J0 4A043J1
4A043J2 4A043J3 4A043R1 4A04X51 4A04XB1 4A04XJ1 4A04XR1 4A05XLZ 4A07X0Z 4A07X7Z 4A07XBZ 4A08X0Z 4A0971Z
4A0975Z 4A097CZ 4A097DZ 4A097LZ 4A097MZ 4A0981Z 4A0985Z 4A098CZ 4A098DZ 4A098LZ 4A098MZ 4A09X1Z 4A09X5Z
4A09XCZ 4A09XDZ 4A09XLZ 4A09XMZ 4A0B78Z 4A0B7BZ 4A0B7GZ 4A0B88Z 4A0B8BZ 4A0B8GZ 4A0C8BZ 4A0D73Z 4A0D75Z
4A0D7BZ 4A0D7DZ 4A0D7LZ 4A0F33Z 4A0FX3Z 4A0H74Z 4A0H7CZ 4A0H7FZ 4A0H7HZ 4A0H84Z 4A0H8CZ 4A0H8FZ 4A0H8HZ
4A0HX4Z 4A0HXCZ 4A0HXFZ 4A0HXHZ 4A0J72Z 4A0J74Z 4A0J7BZ 4A0J82Z 4A0J84Z 4A0J8BZ 4A0JX2Z 4A0JX4Z 4A0JXBZ
4A0Z76Z 4A0Z7KZ 4A0ZX6Z 4A0ZXKZ 4A0ZXQZ

DRG 4A020N6 4A020N7 4A020N8 4A023FZ 4A023N6 4A023N7 4A023N8 4A02X4A

CC 4A02X4A

4 Measurement and Monitoring
A Physiological Systems
1 Monitoring: Determining the level of a physiological or physical function repetitively over a period of time

Body System Character 4	Approach Character 5	Function/Device Character 6	Qualifier Character 7
0 Central Nervous ⃠	**0** Open	**2** Conductivity **B** Pressure	**Z** No Qualifier
0 Central Nervous ⃠	**0** Open	**4** Electrical Activity	**G** Intraoperative **Z** No Qualifier
0 Central Nervous ⃠	**3** Percutaneous	**4** Electrical Activity	**G** Intraoperative **Z** No Qualifier
0 Central Nervous ⃠	**3** Percutaneous	**B** Pressure **K** Temperature **R** Saturation	**D** Intracranial
0 Central Nervous ⃠	**7** Via Natural or Artificial Opening	**B** Pressure **K** Temperature **R** Saturation	**D** Intracranial
0 Central Nervous ⃠	**X** External	**2** Conductivity	**Z** No Qualifier
0 Central Nervous ⃠	**X** External	**4** Electrical Activity	**G** Intraoperative **Z** No Qualifier
1 Peripheral Nervous ⃠	**0** Open **3** Percutaneous **X** External	**2** Conductivity	**9** Sensory **B** Motor
1 Peripheral Nervous ⃠	**0** Open **3** Percutaneous **X** External	**4** Electrical Activity	**G** Intraoperative **Z** No Qualifier
2 Cardiac ⃠	**0** Open **3** Percutaneous	**4** Electrical Activity **9** Output **C** Rate **F** Rhythm **H** Sound	**Z** No Qualifier
2 Cardiac ⃠	**X** External	**4** Electrical Activity	**5** Ambulatory **Z** No Qualifier
2 Cardiac ⃠	**X** External	**9** Output **C** Rate **F** Rhythm **H** Sound	**Z** No Qualifier
2 Cardiac ⃠	**X** External	**M** Total Activity	**4** Stress
2 Cardiac	**X** External	**S** Vascular Perfusion	**H** Indocyanine Green Dye
3 Arterial ⃠	**0** Open **3** Percutaneous	**5** Flow **B** Pressure **J** Pulse	**1** Peripheral **3** Pulmonary **C** Coronary
3 Arterial ⃠	**0** Open **3** Percutaneous	**H** Sound **R** Saturation	**1** Peripheral

4A1 continued on next page

4A1 continued from previous page

4 Measurement and Monitoring
A Physiological Systems
1 Monitoring: Determining the level of a physiological or physical function repetitively over a period of time

Body System Character 4	Approach Character 5	Function/Device Character 6	Qualifier Character 7
3 Arterial ⦸	**X** External	**5** Flow **B** Pressure **H** Sound **J** Pulse **R** Saturation	**1** Peripheral
4 Venous ⦸	**0** Open **3** Percutaneous	**5** Flow **B** Pressure **J** Pulse	**0** Central **1** Peripheral **2** Portal **3** Pulmonary
4 Venous ⦸	**0** Open **3** Percutaneous	**R** Saturation	**0** Central **2** Portal **3** Pulmonary
4 Venous ⦸	**X** External	**5** Flow **B** Pressure **J** Pulse	**1** Peripheral
6 Lymphatic	**0** Open **3** Percutaneous	**5** Flow **B** Pressure	**Z** No Qualifier
9 Respiratory ⦸	**7** Via Natural or Artificial Opening **X** External	**1** Capacity **5** Flow **C** Rate **D** Resistance **L** Volume	**Z** No Qualifier
B Gastrointestinal ⦸	**7** Via Natural or Artificial Opening **8** Via Natural or Artificial Opening Endoscopic	**8** Motility **B** Pressure **G** Secretion	**Z** No Qualifier
B Gastrointestinal ⦸	**X** External	**S** Vascular Perfusion	**H** Indocyanine Green Dye
D Urinary ⦸	**7** Via Natural or Artificial Opening	**3** Contractility **5** Flow **B** Pressure **D** Resistance **L** Volume	**Z** No Qualifier
G Skin and Breast ⦸	**X** External	**S** Vascular Perfusion	**H** Indocyanine Green Dye
H Products of Conception, Cardiac ⦸ ♀	**7** Via Natural or Artificial Opening **8** Via Natural or Artificial Opening Endoscopic **X** External	**4** Electrical Activity **C** Rate **F** Rhythm **H** Sound	**Z** No Qualifier
J Products of Conception, Nervous ⦸ ♀	**7** Via Natural or Artificial Opening **8** Via Natural or Artificial Opening Endoscopic **X** External	**2** Conductivity **4** Electrical Activity **B** Pressure	**Z** No Qualifier
Z None ⦸	**7** Via Natural or Artificial Opening	**K** Temperature	**Z** No Qualifier
Z None ⦸	**X** External	**K** Temperature **Q** Sleep	**Z** No Qualifier

♀ 4A1H74Z 4A1H7CZ 4A1H7FZ 4A1H7HZ 4A1H84Z 4A1H8CZ 4A1H8FZ 4A1H8HZ 4A1HX4Z 4A1HXCZ 4A1HXFZ 4A1HXHZ 4A1J72Z 4A1J74Z 4A1J7BZ 4A1J82Z 4A1J84Z 4A1J8BZ 4A1JX2Z 4A1JX4Z 4A1JXBZ

⦸ 4A1002Z 4A1004G 4A1004Z 4A100BZ 4A1034G 4A1034Z 4A103BD 4A103KD 4A103RD 4A107BD 4A107KD 4A107RD 4A10X2Z 4A10X4G 4A10X4Z 4A11029 4A1102B 4A1104G 4A1104Z 4A11329 4A1132B 4A1134G 4A1134Z 4A11X29 4A11X2B 4A11X4G 4A11X4Z 4A1204Z 4A1209Z 4A120CZ 4A120FZ 4A120HZ 4A1234Z 4A1239Z 4A123CZ 4A123FZ 4A123HZ 4A12X45 4A12X4Z 4A12X9Z 4A12XCZ 4A12XFZ 4A12XHZ 4A12XM4 4A12XSH 4A13051 4A13053 4A1305C 4A130B1 4A130B3 4A130BC 4A130H1 4A130J1 4A130J3 4A130JC 4A130R1 4A13351 4A13353 4A1335C 4A133B1 4A133B3 4A133BC 4A133H1 4A133J1 4A133J3 4A133JC 4A133R1 4A13X51 4A13XB1 4A13XH1 4A13XJ1 4A13XR1 4A14050 4A14051 4A14052 4A14053 4A140B0 4A140B1 4A140B2 4A140B3 4A140J0 4A140J1 4A140J2 4A140J3 4A140R0 4A140R2 4A140R3 4A14350 4A14351 4A14352 4A14353 4A143B0 4A143B1 4A143B2 4A143B3 4A143J0 4A143J1 4A143J2 4A143J3 4A143R0 4A143R2 4A143R3 4A14X51 4A14XB1 4A14XJ1 4A1971Z 4A1975Z 4A197CZ 4A197DZ 4A197LZ 4A19X1Z 4A19X5Z 4A19XCZ 4A19XDZ 4A19XLZ 4A1B78Z 4A1B7BZ 4A1B7GZ 4A1B88Z 4A1B8BZ 4A1B8GZ 4A1BXSH 4A1D73Z 4A1D75Z 4A1D7BZ 4A1D7DZ 4A1D7LZ 4A1GXSH 4A1H74Z 4A1H7CZ 4A1H7FZ 4A1H7HZ 4A1H84Z 4A1H8CZ 4A1H8FZ 4A1H8HZ 4A1HX4Z 4A1HXCZ 4A1HXFZ 4A1HXHZ 4A1J72Z 4A1J74Z 4A1J7BZ 4A1J82Z 4A1J84Z 4A1J8BZ 4A1JX2Z 4A1JX4Z 4A1JXBZ 4A1Z7KZ 4A1ZXKZ 4A1ZXQZ

4 Measurement and Monitoring
B Physiological Devices
0 Measurement: Determining the level of a physiological or physical function at a point in time

Body System Character 4	Approach Character 5	Function/Device Character 6	Qualifier Character 7
0 Central Nervous ⃠ **1** Peripheral Nervous ⃠ **F** Musculoskeletal ⃠	**X** External	**V** Stimulator	**Z** No Qualifier
2 Cardiac ⃠	**X** External	**S** Pacemaker **T** Defibrillator	**Z** No Qualifier
9 Respiratory ⃠	**X** External	**S** Pacemaker	**Z** No Qualifier

⃠ 4B00XVZ 4B01XVZ 4B02XSZ 4B02XTZ 4B09XSZ 4B0FXVZ

Extracorporeal Assistance and Performance 5A0-5A2

5 Extracorporeal Assistance and Performance
A Physiological Systems
0 Assistance: Taking over a portion of a physiological function by extracorporeal means

Body System Character 4	Duration Character 5	Function Character 6	Qualifier Character 7
2 Cardiac ⃠	1 Intermittent 2 Continuous	1 Output	0 Balloon Pump 5 Pulsatile Compression 6 Other Pump D Impeller Pump
5 Circulatory ⃠	1 Intermittent 2 Continuous	2 Oxygenation	1 Hyperbaric C Supersaturated
9 Respiratory ⃠	3 Less than 24 Consecutive Hours 4 24-96 Consecutive Hours 5 Greater than 96 Consecutive Hours	5 Ventilation	7 Continuous Positive Airway Pressure 8 Intermittent Positive Airway Pressure 9 Continuous Negative Airway Pressure B Intermittent Negative Airway Pressure Z No Qualifier

⃠ 5A02115 5A02215 5A05121 5A0512C 5A05221 5A0522C 5A09357 5A09358 5A09359 5A0935B 5A0935Z 5A09457 5A09458 5A09459 5A0945B 5A0945Z 5A09557 5A09558 5A09559 5A0955B 5A0955Z

5 Extracorporeal Assistance and Performance
A Physiological Systems
1 Performance: Completely taking over a physiological function by extracorporeal means

Body System Character 4	Duration Character 5	Function Character 6	Qualifier Character 7
2 Cardiac ⃠	0 Single	1 Output	2 Manual
2 Cardiac ⃠	1 Intermittent	3 Pacing	Z No Qualifier
2 Cardiac ⃠	2 Continuous	1 Output 3 Pacing	Z No Qualifier
5 Circulatory	2 Continuous	2 Oxygenation	3 Membrane
9 Respiratory ⃠ DRG	0 Single	5 Ventilation	4 Nonmechanical
9 Respiratory DRG	3 Less than 24 Consecutive Hours 4 24-96 Consecutive Hours 5 Greater than 96 Consecutive Hours	5 Ventilation	Z No Qualifier
C Biliary ⃠ D Urinary ⃠	0 Single 6 Multiple	0 Filtration	Z No Qualifier

⃠ 5A12012 5A1213Z 5A1221Z 5A1223Z 5A19054 5A1C00Z 5A1C60Z 5A1D00Z 5A1D60Z
DRG 5A1935Z 5A1945Z 5A1955Z

5 Extracorporeal Assistance and Performance
A Physiological Systems
2 Restoration: Returning, or attempting to return, a physiological function to its original state by extracorporeal means.

Body System Character 4	Duration Character 5	Function Character 6	Qualifier Character 7
2 Cardiac ⃠	0 Single	4 Rhythm	Z No Qualifier

⃠ 5A2204Z

Extracorporeal Therapies 6A0-6AB

6 Extracorporeal Therapies
A Physiological Systems
0 Atmospheric Control: Extracorporeal control of atmospheric pressure and composition

Body System Character 4	Duration Character 5	Qualifier Character 6	Qualifier Character 7
Z None ⦸	0 Single 1 Multiple	Z No Qualifier	Z No Qualifier

⦸ 6A0Z0ZZ 6A0Z1ZZ

6 Extracorporeal Therapies
A Physiological Systems
1 Decompression: Extracorporeal elimination of undissolved gas from body fluids

Body System Character 4	Duration Character 5	Qualifier Character 6	Qualifier Character 7
5 Circulatory ⦸	0 Single 1 Multiple	Z No Qualifier	Z No Qualifier

⦸ 6A150ZZ 6A151ZZ

6 Extracorporeal Therapies
A Physiological Systems
2 Electromagnetic Therapy: Extracorporeal treatment by electromagnetic rays

Body System Character 4	Duration Character 5	Qualifier Character 6	Qualifier Character 7
1 Urinary ⦸ 2 Central Nervous ⦸	0 Single 1 Multiple	Z No Qualifier	Z No Qualifier

⦸ 6A210ZZ 6A211ZZ 6A220ZZ 6A221ZZ

6 Extracorporeal Therapies
A Physiological Systems
3 Hyperthermia: Extracorporeal raising of body temperature

Body System Character 4	Duration Character 5	Qualifier Character 6	Qualifier Character 7
Z None ⦸	0 Single 1 Multiple	Z No Qualifier	Z No Qualifier

⦸ 6A3Z0ZZ 6A3Z1ZZ

6 Extracorporeal Therapies
A Physiological Systems
4 Hypothermia: Extracorporeal lowering of body temperature

Body System Character 4	Duration Character 5	Qualifier Character 6	Qualifier Character 7
Z None ⦸	0 Single 1 Multiple	Z No Qualifier	Z No Qualifier

⦸ 6A4Z0ZZ 6A4Z1ZZ

6 Extracorporeal Therapies
A Physiological Systems
5 Pheresis: Extracorporeal separation of blood products

Body System Character 4	Duration Character 5	Qualifier Character 6	Qualifier Character 7
5 Circulatory ⦸	0 Single 1 Multiple	Z No Qualifier	0 Erythrocytes 1 Leukocytes 2 Platelets 3 Plasma T Stem Cells, Cord Blood V Stem Cells, Hematopoietic

⦸ 6A550Z0 6A550Z1 6A550Z2 6A550Z3 6A550ZT 6A550ZV 6A551Z0 6A551Z1 6A551Z2 6A551Z3 6A551ZT 6A551ZV

6 Extracorporeal Therapies
A Physiological Systems
6 Phototherapy: Extracorporeal treatment by light rays

Body System Character 4	Duration Character 5	Qualifier Character 6	Qualifier Character 7
0 Skin ⃠ **5** Circulatory ⃠	**0** Single **1** Multiple	**Z** No Qualifier	**Z** No Qualifier

⃠ 6A600ZZ 6A601ZZ 6A650ZZ 6A651ZZ

6 Extracorporeal Therapies
A Physiological Systems
7 Ultrasound Therapy: Extracorporeal treatment by ultrasound

Body System Character 4	Duration Character 5	Qualifier Character 6	Qualifier Character 7
5 Circulatory ⃠	**0** Single **1** Multiple	**Z** No Qualifier	**4** Head and Neck Vessels **5** Heart **6** Peripheral Vessels **7** Other Vessels **Z** No Qualifier

⃠ 6A750Z4 6A750Z5 6A750Z6 6A750Z7 6A750ZZ 6A751Z4 6A751Z5 6A751Z6 6A751Z7 6A751ZZ

6 Extracorporeal Therapies
A Physiological Systems
8 Ultraviolet Light Therapy: Extracorporeal treatment by ultraviolet light

Body System Character 4	Duration Character 5	Qualifier Character 6	Qualifier Character 7
0 Skin ⃠	**0** Single **1** Multiple	**Z** No Qualifier	**Z** No Qualifier

⃠ 6A800ZZ 6A801ZZ

6 Extracorporeal Therapies
A Physiological Systems
9 Shock Wave Therapy: Extracorporeal treatment by shock waves

Body System Character 4	Duration Character 5	Qualifier Character 6	Qualifier Character 7
3 Musculoskeletal ⃠	**0** Single **1** Multiple	**Z** No Qualifier	**Z** No Qualifier

⃠ 6A930ZZ 6A931ZZ

6 Extracorporeal Therapies
A Physiological Systems
B Perfusion: Extracorporeal treatment by diffusion of therapeutic fluid

Body System Character 4	Duration Character 5	Qualifier Character 6	Qualifier Character 7
5 Circulatory ⃠ **B** Respiratory System ⃠ **F** Hepatobiliary System and Pancreas ⃠ **T** Urinary System ⃠	**0** Single	**B** Donor Organ	**Z** No Qualifier

⃠ 6AB50BZ 6ABB0BZ 6ABF0BZ 6ABT0BZ

Osteopathic 7W0

7 Osteopathic
W Anatomical Regions
0 Treatment: Manual treatment to eliminate or alleviate somatic dysfunction and related disorders

Body Region Character 4	Approach Character 5	Method Character 6	Qualifier Character 7
0 Head ⃠ **1** Cervical ⃠ **2** Thoracic ⃠ **3** Lumbar ⃠ **4** Sacrum ⃠ **5** Pelvis ⃠ **6** Lower Extremities ⃠ **7** Upper Extremities ⃠ **8** Rib Cage ⃠ **9** Abdomen ⃠	**X** External	**0** Articulatory-Raising **1** Fascial Release **2** General Mobilization **3** High Velocity-Low Amplitude **4** Indirect **5** Low Velocity-High Amplitude **6** Lymphatic Pump **7** Muscle Energy-Isometric **8** Muscle Energy-Isotonic **9** Other Method	**Z** None

⃠ 7W00X0Z 7W00X1Z 7W00X2Z 7W00X3Z 7W00X4Z 7W00X5Z 7W00X6Z 7W00X7Z 7W00X8Z 7W00X9Z 7W01X0Z 7W01X1Z 7W01X2Z 7W01X3Z 7W01X4Z 7W01X5Z 7W01X6Z 7W01X7Z 7W01X8Z 7W01X9Z 7W02X0Z 7W02X1Z 7W02X2Z 7W02X3Z 7W02X4Z 7W02X5Z 7W02X6Z 7W02X7Z 7W02X8Z 7W02X9Z 7W03X0Z 7W03X1Z 7W03X2Z 7W03X3Z 7W03X4Z 7W03X5Z 7W03X6Z 7W03X7Z 7W03X8Z 7W03X9Z 7W04X0Z 7W04X1Z 7W04X2Z 7W04X3Z 7W04X4Z 7W04X5Z 7W04X6Z 7W04X7Z 7W04X8Z 7W04X9Z 7W05X0Z 7W05X1Z 7W05X2Z 7W05X3Z 7W05X4Z 7W05X5Z 7W05X6Z 7W05X7Z 7W05X8Z 7W05X9Z 7W06X0Z 7W06X1Z 7W06X2Z 7W06X3Z 7W06X4Z 7W06X5Z 7W06X6Z 7W06X7Z 7W06X8Z 7W06X9Z 7W07X0Z 7W07X1Z 7W07X2Z 7W07X3Z 7W07X4Z 7W07X5Z 7W07X6Z 7W07X7Z 7W07X8Z 7W07X9Z 7W08X0Z 7W08X1Z 7W08X2Z 7W08X3Z 7W08X4Z 7W08X5Z 7W08X6Z 7W08X7Z 7W08X8Z 7W08X9Z 7W09X0Z 7W09X1Z 7W09X2Z 7W09X3Z 7W09X4Z 7W09X5Z 7W09X6Z 7W09X7Z 7W09X8Z 7W09X9Z

Other Procedures 8C0-8E0

8 Other Procedures
C Indwelling Device
0 Other Procedures: Methodologies which attempt to remediate or cure a disorder or disease

Body Region Character 4	Approach Character 5	Method Character 6	Qualifier Character 7
1 Nervous System ⦸	X External	6 Collection	J Cerebrospinal Fluid L Other Fluid
2 Circulatory System ⦸	X External	6 Collection	K Blood L Other Fluid

⦸ 8C01X6J 8C01X6L 8C02X6K 8C02X6L

8 Other Procedures
E Physiological Systems and Anatomical Regions
0 Other Procedures: Methodologies which attempt to remediate or cure a disorder or disease

Body Region Character 4	Approach Character 5	Method Character 6	Qualifier Character 7
1 Nervous System ⦸ U Female Reproductive System ⦸ ♂	X External	Y Other Method	7 Examination
2 Circulatory System ⦸	3 Percutaneous	D Near Infrared Spectroscopy	Z No Qualifier
9 Head and Neck Region ⦸ W Trunk Region ⦸	0 Open 3 Percutaneous 4 Percutaneous Endoscopic 7 Via Natural or Artificial Opening 8 Via Natural or Artificial Opening Endoscopic	C Robotic Assisted Procedure	Z No Qualifier
9 Head and Neck Region ⦸ W Trunk Region ⦸	X External	B Computer Assisted Procedure	F With Fluoroscopy G With Computerized Tomography H With Magnetic Resonance Imaging Z No Qualifier
9 Head and Neck Region ⦸ W Trunk Region ⦸	X External	C Robotic Assisted Procedure	Z No Qualifier
9 Head and Neck Region ⦸ W Trunk Region ⦸	X External	Y Other Method	8 Suture Removal
H Integumentary System and Breast ⦸	3 Percutaneous	0 Acupuncture	0 Anesthesia Z No Qualifier
H Integumentary System and Breast ⦸ ♀	X External	6 Collection	2 Breast Milk
H Integumentary System and Breast ⦸	X External	Y Other Method	9 Piercing
K Musculoskeletal System ⦸	X External	1 Therapeutic Massage	Z No Qualifier
K Musculoskeletal System ⦸	X External	Y Other Method	7 Examination
V Male Reproductive System ⦸ ♂	X External	1 Therapeutic Massage	C Prostate D Rectum
V Male Reproductive System ⦸ ♂	X External	6 Collection	3 Sperm
X Upper Extremity ⦸ Y Lower Extremity ⦸	0 Open 3 Percutaneous 4 Percutaneous Endoscopic	C Robotic Assisted Procedure	Z No Qualifier
X Upper Extremity ⦸ Y Lower Extremity ⦸	X External	B Computer Assisted Procedure	F With Fluoroscopy G With Computerized Tomography H With Magnetic Resonance Imaging Z No Qualifier

8E0 continued on next page

8E0 continued from previous page

8 Other Procedures
E Physiological Systems and Anatomical Regions
0 Other Procedures: Methodologies which attempt to remediate or cure a disorder or disease

Body Region Character 4	Approach Character 5	Method Character 6	Qualifier Character 7
X Upper Extremity ⦸ **Y** Lower Extremity ⦸	**X** External	**C** Robotic Assisted Procedure	**Z** No Qualifier
X Upper Extremity ⦸ **Y** Lower Extremity ⦸	**X** External	**Y** Other Method	**8** Suture Removal
Z None ⦸	**X** External	**Y** Other Method	**1** In Vitro Fertilization **4** Yoga Therapy **5** Meditation **6** Isolation

♂ 8E0VX1C 8E0VX63
♀ 8E0HX62 8E0UXY7
⦸ 8E01XY7 8E023DZ 8E090CZ 8E093CZ 8E094CZ 8E097CZ 8E098CZ 8E09XBF 8E09XBG 8E09XBH 8E09XBZ 8E09XCZ 8E09XY8 8E0H300 8E0H30Z 8E0HX62 8E0HXY9 8E0KX1Z 8E0KXY7 8E0UXY7 8E0VX1C 8E0VX1D 8E0VX63 8E0W0CZ 8E0W3CZ 8E0W4CZ 8E0W7CZ 8E0W8CZ 8E0WXBF 8E0WXBG 8E0WXBH 8E0WXBZ 8E0WXCZ 8E0WXY8 8E0X0CZ 8E0X3CZ 8E0X4CZ 8E0XXBF 8E0XXBG 8E0XXBH 8E0XXBZ 8E0XXCZ 8E0XXY8 8E0Y0CZ 8E0Y3CZ 8E0Y4CZ 8E0YXBF 8E0YXBG 8E0YXBH 8E0YXBZ 8E0YXCZ 8E0YXY8 8E0ZXY1 8E0ZXY4 8E0ZXY5 8E0ZXY6

Chiropractic 9WB

9 Chiropractic
W Anatomical Regions
B Manipulation: Manual procedure that involves a directed thrust to move a joint past the physiological range of motion, without exceeding the anatomical limit

Body Region Character 4	Approach Character 5	Method Character 6	Qualifier Character 7
0 Head ⦸	**X** External	**B** Non-Manual	**Z** None
1 Cervical ⦸		**C** Indirect Visceral	
2 Thoracic ⦸		**D** Extra-Articular	
3 Lumbar ⦸		**F** Direct Visceral	
4 Sacrum ⦸		**G** Long Lever Specific Contact	
5 Pelvis ⦸		**H** Short Lever Specific Contact	
6 Lower Extremities ⦸		**J** Long and Short Lever Specific Contact	
7 Upper Extremities ⦸		**K** Mechanically Assisted	
8 Rib Cage ⦸		**L** Other Method	
9 Abdomen ⦸			

⦸ 9WB0XBZ 9WB0XCZ 9WB0XDZ 9WB0XFZ 9WB0XGZ 9WB0XHZ 9WB0XJZ 9WB0XKZ 9WB0XLZ 9WB1XBZ 9WB1XCZ 9WB1XDZ 9WB1XFZ 9WB1XGZ 9WB1XHZ 9WB1XJZ 9WB1XKZ 9WB1XLZ 9WB2XBZ 9WB2XCZ 9WB2XDZ 9WB2XFZ 9WB2XGZ 9WB2XHZ 9WB2XJZ 9WB2XKZ 9WB2XLZ 9WB3XBZ 9WB3XCZ 9WB3XDZ 9WB3XFZ 9WB3XGZ 9WB3XHZ 9WB3XJZ 9WB3XKZ 9WB3XLZ 9WB4XBZ 9WB4XCZ 9WB4XDZ 9WB4XFZ 9WB4XGZ 9WB4XHZ 9WB4XJZ 9WB4XKZ 9WB4XLZ 9WB5XBZ 9WB5XCZ 9WB5XDZ 9WB5XFZ 9WB5XGZ 9WB5XHZ 9WB5XJZ 9WB5XKZ 9WB5XLZ 9WB6XBZ 9WB6XCZ 9WB6XDZ 9WB6XFZ 9WB6XGZ 9WB6XHZ 9WB6XJZ 9WB6XKZ 9WB6XLZ 9WB7XBZ 9WB7XCZ 9WB7XDZ 9WB7XFZ 9WB7XGZ 9WB7XHZ 9WB7XJZ 9WB7XKZ 9WB7XLZ 9WB8XBZ 9WB8XCZ 9WB8XDZ 9WB8XFZ 9WB8XGZ 9WB8XHZ 9WB8XJZ 9WB8XKZ 9WB8XLZ 9WB9XBZ 9WB9XCZ 9WB9XDZ 9WB9XFZ 9WB9XGZ 9WB9XHZ 9WB9XJZ 9WB9XKZ 9WB9XLZ

LC Limited Coverage NC Noncovered HAC HAC Associated Procedure CC Combination Cluster - See Appendix G for code lists
DRG Non-OR-Affecting MS-DRG Assignment ⦸ Non-OR-Not Affecting MS-DRG Assignment New/Revised Text in **Orange** ♂ Male ♀ Female

Imaging B00-BY4

B Imaging
0 Central Nervous System
0 Plain Radiography: Planar display of an image developed from the capture of external ionizing radiation on photographic or photoconductive plate

Body Part Character 4	Contrast Character 5	Qualifier Character 6	Qualifier Character 7
B Spinal Cord ⊘	**0** High Osmolar **1** Low Osmolar **Y** Other Contrast **Z** None	**Z** None	**Z** None

⊘ B00B0ZZ B00B1ZZ B00BYZZ B00BZZZ

B Imaging
0 Central Nervous System
1 Fluoroscopy: Single plane or bi-plane real time display of an image developed from the capture of external ionizing radiation on a fluorescent screen. The image may also be stored by either digital or analog means

Body Part Character 4	Contrast Character 5	Qualifier Character 6	Qualifier Character 7
B Spinal Cord ⊘	**0** High Osmolar **1** Low Osmolar **Y** Other Contrast **Z** None	**Z** None	**Z** None

⊘ B01B0ZZ B01B1ZZ B01BYZZ B01BZZZ

B Imaging
0 Central Nervous System
2 Computerized Tomography (CT Scan): Computer reformatted digital display of multiplanar images developed from the capture of multiple exposures of external ionizing radiation

Body Part Character 4	Contrast Character 5	Qualifier Character 6	Qualifier Character 7
0 Brain ⊘ **7** Cisterna ⊘ **8** Cerebral Ventricle(s) ⊘ **9** Sella Turcica/Pituitary Gland ⊘ **B** Spinal Cord ⊘	**0** High Osmolar **1** Low Osmolar **Y** Other Contrast	**0** Unenhanced and Enhanced **Z** None	**Z** None
0 Brain ⊘ **7** Cisterna ⊘ **8** Cerebral Ventricle(s) ⊘ **9** Sella Turcica/Pituitary Gland ⊘ **B** Spinal Cord ⊘	**Z** None	**Z** None	**Z** None

⊘ B02000Z B0200ZZ B02010Z B0201ZZ B020Y0Z B020YZZ B020ZZZ B02700Z B0270ZZ B02710Z B0271ZZ B027Y0Z B027YZZ B027ZZZ B02800Z B0280ZZ B02810Z B0281ZZ B028Y0Z B028YZZ B028ZZZ B02900Z B0290ZZ B02910Z B0291ZZ B029Y0Z B029YZZ B029ZZZ B02B00Z B02B0ZZ B02B10Z B02B1ZZ B02BY0Z B02BYZZ B02BZZZ

B Imaging
0 Central Nervous System
3 Magnetic Resonance Imaging (MRI): Computer reformatted digital display of multiplanar images developed from the capture of radiofrequency signals emitted by nuclei in a body site excited within a magnetic field

Body Part Character 4	Contrast Character 5	Qualifier Character 6	Qualifier Character 7
0 Brain ⊘ **9** Sella Turcica/Pituitary Gland ⊘ **B** Spinal Cord ⊘ **C** Acoustic Nerves ⊘	**Y** Other Contrast	**0** Unenhanced and Enhanced **Z** None	**Z** None
0 Brain ⊘ **9** Sella Turcica/Pituitary Gland ⊘ **B** Spinal Cord ⊘ **C** Acoustic Nerves ⊘	**Z** None	**Z** None	**Z** None

⊘ B030Y0Z B030YZZ B030ZZZ B039Y0Z B039YZZ B039ZZZ B03BY0Z B03BYZZ B03BZZZ B03CY0Z B03CYZZ B03CZZZ

B Imaging
0 Central Nervous System
4 Ultrasonography: Real time display of images of anatomy or flow information developed from the capture of reflected and attenuated high frequency sound waves

Body Part Character 4	Contrast Character 5	Qualifier Character 6	Qualifier Character 7
0 Brain ⦸ **B** Spinal Cord ⦸	**Z** None	**Z** None	**Z** None

⦸ B040ZZZ B04BZZZ

B Imaging
2 Heart
0 Plain Radiography: Planar display of an image developed from the capture of external ionizing radiation on photographic or photoconductive plate

Body Part Character 4	Contrast Character 5	Qualifier Character 6	Qualifier Character 7
0 Coronary Artery, Single DRG **1** Coronary Arteries, Multiple DRG **2** Coronary Artery Bypass Graft, Single DRG **3** Coronary Artery Bypass Grafts, Multiple DRG **4** Heart, Right DRG **5** Heart, Left DRG **6** Heart, Right and Left DRG **7** Internal Mammary Bypass Graft, Right DRG **8** Internal Mammary Bypass Graft, Left DRG **F** Bypass Graft, Other DRG	**0** High Osmolar **1** Low Osmolar **Y** Other Contrast	**Z** None	**Z** None

DRG B2000ZZ B2001ZZ B200YZZ B2010ZZ B2011ZZ B201YZZ B2020ZZ B2021ZZ B202YZZ B2030ZZ B2031ZZ B203YZZ B2040ZZ B2041ZZ B204YZZ B2050ZZ B2051ZZ B205YZZ B2060ZZ B2061ZZ B206YZZ B2070ZZ B2071ZZ B207YZZ B2080ZZ B2081ZZ B208YZZ B20F0ZZ B20F1ZZ B20FYZZ

B Imaging
2 Heart
1 Fluoroscopy: Single plane or bi-plane real time display of an image developed from the capture of external ionizing radiation on a fluorescent screen. The image may also be stored by either digital or analog means

Body Part Character 4	Contrast Character 5	Qualifier Character 6	Qualifier Character 7
0 Coronary Artery, Single ⦸ DRG **1** Coronary Arteries, Multiple ⦸ DRG **2** Coronary Artery Bypass Graft, Single ⦸ DRG **3** Coronary Artery Bypass Grafts, Multiple ⦸ DRG	**0** High Osmolar **1** Low Osmolar **Y** Other Contrast	**1** Laser	**0** Intraoperative
0 Coronary Artery, Single DRG **1** Coronary Arteries, Multiple DRG **2** Coronary Artery Bypass Graft, Single DRG **3** Coronary Artery Bypass Grafts, Multiple DRG	**0** High Osmolar **1** Low Osmolar **Y** Other Contrast	**Z** None	**Z** None
4 Heart, Right DRG **5** Heart, Left DRG **6** Heart, Right and Left DRG **7** Internal Mammary Bypass Graft, Right DRG **8** Internal Mammary Bypass Graft, Left DRG **F** Bypass Graft, Other DRG	**0** High Osmolar **1** Low Osmolar **Y** Other Contrast	**Z** None	**Z** None

⦸ B210010 B210110 B210Y10 B211010 B211110 B211Y10 B212010 B212110 B212Y10 B213010 B213110 B213Y10
DRG B2100ZZ B2101ZZ B210YZZ B2110ZZ B2111ZZ B211YZZ B2120ZZ B2121ZZ B212YZZ B2130ZZ B2131ZZ B213YZZ B2140ZZ B2141ZZ B214YZZ B2150ZZ B2151ZZ B215YZZ B2160ZZ B2161ZZ B216YZZ B2170ZZ B2171ZZ B217YZZ B2180ZZ B2181ZZ B218YZZ B21F0ZZ B21F1ZZ B21FYZZ

LC Limited Coverage NC Noncovered HAC HAC Associated Procedure CC Combination Cluster - See Appendix G for code lists
DRG Non-OR-Affecting MS-DRG Assignment ⦸ Non-OR-Not Affecting MS-DRG Assignment New/Revised Text in **Orange** ♂ Male ♀ Female

B Imaging
2 Heart
2 Computerized Tomography (CT Scan): Computer reformatted digital display of multiplanar images developed from the capture of multiple exposures of external ionizing radiation

Body Part Character 4	Contrast Character 5	Qualifier Character 6	Qualifier Character 7
1 Coronary Arteries, Multiple ⦸ 3 Coronary Artery Bypass Grafts, Multiple ⦸ 6 Heart, Right and Left ⦸	0 High Osmolar 1 Low Osmolar Y Other Contrast	0 Unenhanced and Enhanced Z None	Z None
1 Coronary Arteries, Multiple ⦸ 3 Coronary Artery Bypass Grafts, Multiple ⦸ 6 Heart, Right and Left ⦸	Z None	2 Intravascular Optical Coherence Z None	Z None

⦸ B22100Z B2210ZZ B22110Z B2211ZZ B221Y0Z B221YZZ B221Z2Z B221ZZZ B22300Z B2230ZZ B22310Z B2231ZZ B223Y0Z B223YZZ B223Z2Z B223ZZZ B22600Z B2260ZZ B22610Z B2261ZZ B226Y0Z B226YZZ B226Z2Z B226ZZZ

B Imaging
2 Heart
3 Magnetic Resonance Imaging (MRI): Computer reformatted digital display of multiplanar images developed from the capture of radiofrequency signals emitted by nuclei in a body site excited within a magnetic field

Body Part Character 4	Contrast Character 5	Qualifier Character 6	Qualifier Character 7
1 Coronary Arteries, Multiple ⦸ 3 Coronary Artery Bypass Grafts, Multiple ⦸ 6 Heart, Right and Left ⦸	Y Other Contrast	0 Unenhanced and Enhanced Z None	Z None
1 Coronary Arteries, Multiple ⦸ 3 Coronary Artery Bypass Grafts, Multiple ⦸ 6 Heart, Right and Left ⦸	Z None	Z None	Z None

⦸ B231Y0Z B231YZZ B231ZZZ B233Y0Z B233YZZ B233ZZZ B236Y0Z B236YZZ B236ZZZ

B Imaging
2 Heart
4 Ultrasonography: Real time display of images of anatomy or flow information developed from the capture of reflected and attenuated high frequency sound waves

Body Part Character 4	Contrast Character 5	Qualifier Character 6	Qualifier Character 7
0 Coronary Artery, Single ⦸ 1 Coronary Arteries, Multiple ⦸ 4 Heart, Right ⦸ 5 Heart, Left ⦸ 6 Heart, Right and Left ⦸ B Heart with Aorta ⦸ C Pericardium ⦸ D Pediatric Heart ⦸	Y Other Contrast	Z None	Z None
0 Coronary Artery, Single ⦸ 1 Coronary Arteries, Multiple ⦸ 4 Heart, Right ⦸ 5 Heart, Left ⦸ 6 Heart, Right and Left ⦸ B Heart with Aorta ⦸ C Pericardium ⦸ D Pediatric Heart ⦸	Z None	Z None	3 Intravascular 4 Transesophageal Z None

⦸ B240YZZ B240ZZ3 B240ZZ4 B240ZZZ B241YZZ B241ZZ3 B241ZZ4 B241ZZZ B244YZZ B244ZZ3 B244ZZ4 B244ZZZ B245YZZ B245ZZ3 B245ZZ4 B245ZZZ B246YZZ B246ZZ3 B246ZZ4 B246ZZZ B24BYZZ B24BZZ3 B24BZZ4 B24BZZZ B24CYZZ B24CZZ3 B24CZZ4 B24CZZZ B24DYZZ B24DZZ3 B24DZZ4 B24DZZZ

B Imaging
3 Upper Arteries
0 Plain Radiography: Planar display of an image developed from the capture of external ionizing radiation on photographic or photoconductive plate

Body Part Character 4	Contrast Character 5	Qualifier Character 6	Qualifier Character 7
0 Thoracic Aorta ⃠ **1** Brachiocephalic-Subclavian Artery, Right ⃠ **2** Subclavian Artery, Left ⃠ **3** Common Carotid Artery, Right ⃠ **4** Common Carotid Artery, Left ⃠ **5** Common Carotid Arteries, Bilateral ⃠ **6** Internal Carotid Artery, Right ⃠ **7** Internal Carotid Artery, Left ⃠ **8** Internal Carotid Arteries, Bilateral ⃠ **9** External Carotid Artery, Right ⃠ **B** External Carotid Artery, Left ⃠ **C** External Carotid Arteries, Bilateral ⃠ **D** Vertebral Artery, Right ⃠ **F** Vertebral Artery, Left ⃠ **G** Vertebral Arteries, Bilateral ⃠ **H** Upper Extremity Arteries, Right ⃠ **J** Upper Extremity Arteries, Left ⃠ **K** Upper Extremity Arteries, Bilateral ⃠ **L** Intercostal and Bronchial Arteries ⃠ **M** Spinal Arteries ⃠ **N** Upper Arteries, Other ⃠ **P** Thoraco-Abdominal Aorta ⃠ **Q** Cervico-Cerebral Arch ⃠ **R** Intracranial Arteries ⃠ **S** Pulmonary Artery, Right ⃠ **T** Pulmonary Artery, Left ⃠	**0** High Osmolar **1** Low Osmolar **Y** Other Contrast **Z** None	**Z** None	**Z** None

⃠ B3000ZZ B3001ZZ B300YZZ B300ZZZ B3010ZZ B3011ZZ B301YZZ B301ZZZ B3020ZZ B3021ZZ B302YZZ B302ZZZ B3030ZZ
B3031ZZ B303YZZ B303ZZZ B3040ZZ B3041ZZ B304YZZ B304ZZZ B3050ZZ B3051ZZ B305YZZ B305ZZZ B3060ZZ B3061ZZ
B306YZZ B306ZZZ B3070ZZ B3071ZZ B307YZZ B307ZZZ B3080ZZ B3081ZZ B308YZZ B308ZZZ B3090ZZ B3091ZZ B309YZZ
B309ZZZ B30B0ZZ B30B1ZZ B30BYZZ B30BZZZ B30C0ZZ B30C1ZZ B30CYZZ B30CZZZ B30D0ZZ B30D1ZZ B30DYZZ B30DZZZ
B30F0ZZ B30F1ZZ B30FYZZ B30FZZZ B30G0ZZ B30G1ZZ B30GYZZ B30GZZZ B30H0ZZ B30H1ZZ B30HYZZ B30HZZZ B30J0ZZ
B30J1ZZ B30JYZZ B30JZZZ B30K0ZZ B30K1ZZ B30KYZZ B30KZZZ B30L0ZZ B30L1ZZ B30LYZZ B30LZZZ B30M0ZZ B30M1ZZ
B30MYZZ B30MZZZ B30N0ZZ B30N1ZZ B30NYZZ B30NZZZ B30P0ZZ B30P1ZZ B30PYZZ B30PZZZ B30Q0ZZ B30Q1ZZ B30QYZZ
B30QZZZ B30R0ZZ B30R1ZZ B30RYZZ B30RZZZ B30S0ZZ B30S1ZZ B30SYZZ B30SZZZ B30T0ZZ B30T1ZZ B30TYZZ B30TZZZ

B Imaging
3 Upper Arteries
1 Fluoroscopy: Single plane or bi-plane real time display of an image developed from the capture of external ionizing radiation on a fluorescent screen. The image may also be stored by either digital or analog means

Body Part Character 4	Contrast Character 5	Qualifier Character 6	Qualifier Character 7
0 Thoracic Aorta ⃠ **1** Brachiocephalic-Subclavian Artery, Right ⃠ **2** Subclavian Artery, Left ⃠ **3** Common Carotid Artery, Right ⃠ **4** Common Carotid Artery, Left ⃠ **5** Common Carotid Arteries, Bilateral ⃠ **6** Internal Carotid Artery, Right ⃠ **7** Internal Carotid Artery, Left ⃠ **8** Internal Carotid Arteries, Bilateral ⃠ **9** External Carotid Artery, Right ⃠ **B** External Carotid Artery, Left ⃠ **C** External Carotid Arteries, Bilateral ⃠ **D** Vertebral Artery, Right ⃠ **F** Vertebral Artery, Left ⃠ **G** Vertebral Arteries, Bilateral ⃠ **H** Upper Extremity Arteries, Right ⃠ **J** Upper Extremity Arteries, Left ⃠ **K** Upper Extremity Arteries, Bilateral ⃠ **L** Intercostal and Bronchial Arteries ⃠ **M** Spinal Arteries ⃠ **N** Upper Arteries, Other ⃠ **P** Thoraco-Abdominal Aorta ⃠ **Q** Cervico-Cerebral Arch ⃠ **R** Intracranial Arteries ⃠ **S** Pulmonary Artery, Right ⃠ **T** Pulmonary Artery, Left ⃠	**0** High Osmolar **1** Low Osmolar **Y** Other Contrast	**1** Laser	**0** Intraoperative

B31 continued on next page

B Imaging
B31 continued from previous page
3 Upper Arteries
1 Fluoroscopy: Single plane or bi-plane real time display of an image developed from the capture of external ionizing radiation on a fluorescent screen. The image may also be stored by either digital or analog means

Body Part Character 4	Contrast Character 5	Qualifier Character 6	Qualifier Character 7
0 Thoracic Aorta ⃠ **1** Brachiocephalic-Subclavian Artery, Right ⃠ **2** Subclavian Artery, Left ⃠ **3** Common Carotid Artery, Right ⃠ **4** Common Carotid Artery, Left ⃠ **5** Common Carotid Arteries, Bilateral ⃠ **6** Internal Carotid Artery, Right ⃠ **7** Internal Carotid Artery, Left ⃠ **8** Internal Carotid Arteries, Bilateral ⃠ **9** External Carotid Artery, Right ⃠ **B** External Carotid Artery, Left ⃠ **C** External Carotid Arteries, Bilateral ⃠ **D** Vertebral Artery, Right ⃠ **F** Vertebral Artery, Left ⃠ **G** Vertebral Arteries, Bilateral ⃠ **H** Upper Extremity Arteries, Right ⃠ **J** Upper Extremity Arteries, Left ⃠ **K** Upper Extremity Arteries, Bilateral ⃠ **L** Intercostal and Bronchial Arteries ⃠ **M** Spinal Arteries ⃠ **N** Upper Arteries, Other ⃠ **P** Thoraco-Abdominal Aorta ⃠ **Q** Cervico-Cerebral Arch ⃠ **R** Intracranial Arteries ⃠ **S** Pulmonary Artery, Right ⃠ **T** Pulmonary Artery, Left ⃠	**0** High Osmolar **1** Low Osmolar **Y** Other Contrast	**Z** None	**Z** None

B31 continued on next page

B Imaging
3 Upper Arteries
1 Fluoroscopy: Single plane or bi-plane real time display of an image developed from the capture of external ionizing radiation on a fluorescent screen. The image may also be stored by either digital or analog means

B31 continued from previous page

Body Part Character 4	Contrast Character 5	Qualifier Character 6	Qualifier Character 7
0 Thoracic Aorta ⃠ **1** Brachiocephalic-Subclavian Artery, Right ⃠ **2** Subclavian Artery, Left ⃠ **3** Common Carotid Artery, Right ⃠ **4** Common Carotid Artery, Left ⃠ **5** Common Carotid Arteries, Bilateral ⃠ **6** Internal Carotid Artery, Right ⃠ **7** Internal Carotid Artery, Left ⃠ **8** Internal Carotid Arteries, Bilateral ⃠ **9** External Carotid Artery, Right ⃠ **B** External Carotid Artery, Left ⃠ **C** External Carotid Arteries, Bilateral ⃠ **D** Vertebral Artery, Right ⃠ **F** Vertebral Artery, Left ⃠ **G** Vertebral Arteries, Bilateral ⃠ **H** Upper Extremity Arteries, Right ⃠ **J** Upper Extremity Arteries, Left ⃠ **K** Upper Extremity Arteries, Bilateral ⃠ **L** Intercostal and Bronchial Arteries ⃠ **M** Spinal Arteries ⃠ **N** Upper Arteries, Other ⃠ **P** Thoraco-Abdominal Aorta ⃠ **Q** Cervico-Cerebral Arch ⃠ **R** Intracranial Arteries ⃠ **S** Pulmonary Artery, Right ⃠ **T** Pulmonary Artery, Left ⃠	**Z** None	**Z** None	**Z** None

⃠	B310010	B3100ZZ	B310110	B3101ZZ	B310Y10	B310YZZ	B310ZZZ	B311010	B3110ZZ	B311110	B3111ZZ	B311Y10	B311YZZ
	B311ZZZ	B312010	B3120ZZ	B312110	B3121ZZ	B312Y10	B312YZZ	B312ZZZ	B313010	B3130ZZ	B313110	B3131ZZ	B313Y10
	B313YZZ	B313ZZZ	B314010	B3140ZZ	B314110	B3141ZZ	B314Y10	B314YZZ	B314ZZZ	B315010	B3150ZZ	B315110	B3151ZZ
	B315Y10	B315YZZ	B315ZZZ	B316010	B3160ZZ	B316110	B3161ZZ	B316Y10	B316YZZ	B316ZZZ	B317010	B3170ZZ	B317110
	B3171ZZ	B317Y10	B317YZZ	B317ZZZ	B318010	B3180ZZ	B318110	B3181ZZ	B318Y10	B318YZZ	B318ZZZ	B319010	B3190ZZ
	B319110	B3191ZZ	B319Y10	B319YZZ	B319ZZZ	B31B010	B31B0ZZ	B31B110	B31B1ZZ	B31BY10	B31BYZZ	B31BZZZ	B31C010
	B31C0ZZ	B31C110	B31C1ZZ	B31CY10	B31CYZZ	B31CZZZ	B31D010	B31D0ZZ	B31D110	B31D1ZZ	B31DY10	B31DYZZ	B31DZZZ
	B31F010	B31F0ZZ	B31F110	B31F1ZZ	B31FY10	B31FYZZ	B31FZZZ	B31G010	B31G0ZZ	B31G110	B31G1ZZ	B31GY10	B31GYZZ
	B31GZZZ	B31H010	B31H0ZZ	B31H110	B31H1ZZ	B31HY10	B31HYZZ	B31HZZZ	B31J010	B31J0ZZ	B31J110	B31J1ZZ	B31JY10
	B31JYZZ	B31JZZZ	B31K010	B31K0ZZ	B31K110	B31K1ZZ	B31KY10	B31KYZZ	B31KZZZ	B31L010	B31L0ZZ	B31L110	B31L1ZZ
	B31LY10	B31LYZZ	B31LZZZ	B31M010	B31M0ZZ	B31M110	B31M1ZZ	B31MY10	B31MYZZ	B31MZZZ	B31N010	B31N0ZZ	B31N110
	B31N1ZZ	B31NY10	B31NYZZ	B31NZZZ	B31P010	B31P0ZZ	B31P110	B31P1ZZ	B31PY10	B31PYZZ	B31PZZZ	B31Q010	B31Q0ZZ
	B31Q110	B31Q1ZZ	B31QY10	B31QYZZ	B31QZZZ	B31R010	B31R0ZZ	B31R110	B31R1ZZ	B31RY10	B31RYZZ	B31RZZZ	B31S010
	B31S0ZZ	B31S110	B31S1ZZ	B31SY10	B31SYZZ	B31SZZZ	B31T010	B31T0ZZ	B31T110	B31T1ZZ	B31TY10	B31TYZZ	B31TZZZ

B Imaging
3 Upper Arteries
2 Computerized Tomography (CT Scan): Computer reformatted digital display of multiplanar images developed from the capture of multiple exposures of external ionizing radiation

Body Part Character 4	Contrast Character 5	Qualifier Character 6	Qualifier Character 7
0 Thoracic Aorta ⦸ **5** Common Carotid Arteries, Bilateral ⦸ **8** Internal Carotid Arteries, Bilateral ⦸ **G** Vertebral Arteries, Bilateral ⦸ **R** Intracranial Arteries ⦸ **S** Pulmonary Artery, Right ⦸ **T** Pulmonary Artery, Left ⦸	**0** High Osmolar **1** Low Osmolar **Y** Other Contrast	**Z** None	**Z** None
0 Thoracic Aorta ⦸ **5** Common Carotid Arteries, Bilateral ⦸ **8** Internal Carotid Arteries, Bilateral ⦸ **G** Vertebral Arteries, Bilateral ⦸ **R** Intracranial Arteries ⦸ **S** Pulmonary Artery, Right ⦸ **T** Pulmonary Artery, Left ⦸	**Z** None	**2** Intravascular Optical Coherence **Z** None	**Z** None

⦸ B3200ZZ B3201ZZ B320YZZ B320Z2Z B320ZZZ B3250ZZ B3251ZZ B325YZZ B325Z2Z B325ZZZ B3280ZZ B3281ZZ B328YZZ B328Z2Z B328ZZZ B32G0ZZ B32G1ZZ B32GYZZ B32GZ2Z B32GZZZ B32R0ZZ B32R1ZZ B32RYZZ B32RZ2Z B32RZZZ B32S0ZZ B32S1ZZ B32SYZZ B32SZ2Z B32SZZZ B32T0ZZ B32T1ZZ B32TYZZ B32TZ2Z B32TZZZ

LC Limited Coverage NC Noncovered HAC HAC Associated Procedure CC Combination Cluster - See Appendix G for code lists
DRG Non-OR-Affecting MS-DRG Assignment ⦸ Non-OR-Not Affecting MS-DRG Assignment New/Revised Text in **Orange** ♂ Male ♀ Female

B Imaging
3 Upper Arteries
3 Magnetic Resonance Imaging (MRI): Computer reformatted digital display of multiplanar images developed from the capture of radiofrequency signals emitted by nuclei in a body site excited within a magnetic field

Body Part Character 4	Contrast Character 5	Qualifier Character 6	Qualifier Character 7
0 Thoracic Aorta ⦸ **5** Common Carotid Arteries, Bilateral ⦸ **8** Internal Carotid Arteries, Bilateral ⦸ **G** Vertebral Arteries, Bilateral ⦸ **H** Upper Extremity Arteries, Right ⦸ **J** Upper Extremity Arteries, Left ⦸ **K** Upper Extremity Arteries, Bilateral ⦸ **M** Spinal Arteries ⦸ **Q** Cervico-Cerebral Arch ⦸ **R** Intracranial Arteries ⦸	**Y** Other Contrast	**0** Unenhanced and Enhanced **Z** None	**Z** None
0 Thoracic Aorta ⦸ **5** Common Carotid Arteries, Bilateral ⦸ **8** Internal Carotid Arteries, Bilateral ⦸ **G** Vertebral Arteries, Bilateral ⦸ **H** Upper Extremity Arteries, Right ⦸ **J** Upper Extremity Arteries, Left ⦸ **K** Upper Extremity Arteries, Bilateral ⦸ **M** Spinal Arteries ⦸ **Q** Cervico-Cerebral Arch ⦸ **R** Intracranial Arteries ⦸	**Z** None	**Z** None	**Z** None

⦸ B330Y0Z B330YZZ B330ZZZ B335Y0Z B335YZZ B335ZZZ B338Y0Z B338YZZ B338ZZZ B33GY0Z B33GYZZ B33GZZZ B33HY0Z B33HYZZ B33HZZZ B33JY0Z B33JYZZ B33JZZZ B33KY0Z B33KYZZ B33KZZZ B33MY0Z B33MYZZ B33MZZZ B33QY0Z B33QYZZ B33QZZZ B33RY0Z B33RYZZ B33RZZZ

B Imaging
3 Upper Arteries
4 Ultrasonography: Real time display of images of anatomy or flow information developed from the capture of reflected and attenuated high frequency sound waves

Body Part Character 4	Contrast Character 5	Qualifier Character 6	Qualifier Character 7
0 Thoracic Aorta ⦸ **1** Brachiocephalic-Subclavian Artery, Right ⦸ **2** Subclavian Artery, Left ⦸ **3** Common Carotid Artery, Right ⦸ **4** Common Carotid Artery, Left ⦸ **5** Common Carotid Arteries, Bilateral ⦸ **6** Internal Carotid Artery, Right ⦸ **7** Internal Carotid Artery, Left ⦸ **8** Internal Carotid Arteries, Bilateral ⦸ **H** Upper Extremity Arteries, Right ⦸ **J** Upper Extremity Arteries, Left ⦸ **K** Upper Extremity Arteries, Bilateral ⦸ **R** Intracranial Arteries ⦸ **S** Pulmonary Artery, Right ⦸ **T** Pulmonary Artery, Left ⦸ **V** Ophthalmic Arteries ⦸	**Z** None	**Z** None	**3** Intravascular **Z** None

B34 continued on next page

B34 continued from previous page

⃠ B340ZZ3 B340ZZZ B341ZZ3 B341ZZZ B342ZZ3 B342ZZZ B343ZZ3 B343ZZZ B344ZZ3 B344ZZZ B345ZZ3 B345ZZZ B346ZZ3 B346ZZZ B347ZZ3 B347ZZZ B348ZZ3 B348ZZZ B34HZZ3 B34HZZZ B34JZZ3 B34JZZZ B34KZZ3 B34KZZZ B34RZZ3 B34RZZZ B34SZZ3 B34SZZZ B34TZZ3 B34TZZZ B34VZZ3 B34VZZZ

B Imaging
4 Lower Arteries
0 Plain Radiography: Planar display of an image developed from the capture of external ionizing radiation on photographic or photoconductive plate

Body Part Character 4	Contrast Character 5	Qualifier Character 6	Qualifier Character 7
0 Abdominal Aorta ⃠ **2** Hepatic Artery ⃠ **3** Splenic Arteries ⃠ **4** Superior Mesenteric Artery ⃠ **5** Inferior Mesenteric Artery ⃠ **6** Renal Artery, Right ⃠ **7** Renal Artery, Left ⃠ **8** Renal Arteries, Bilateral ⃠ **9** Lumbar Arteries ⃠ **B** Intra-Abdominal Arteries, Other ⃠ **C** Pelvic Arteries ⃠ **D** Aorta and Bilateral Lower Extremity Arteries ⃠ **F** Lower Extremity Arteries, Right ⃠ **G** Lower Extremity Arteries, Left ⃠ **J** Lower Arteries, Other ⃠ **M** Renal Artery Transplant ⃠	**0** High Osmolar **1** Low Osmolar **Y** Other Contrast	**Z** None	**Z** None

⃠ B4000ZZ B4001ZZ B400YZZ B4020ZZ B4021ZZ B402YZZ B4030ZZ B4031ZZ B403YZZ B4040ZZ B4041ZZ B404YZZ B4050ZZ B4051ZZ B405YZZ B4060ZZ B4061ZZ B406YZZ B4070ZZ B4071ZZ B407YZZ B4080ZZ B4081ZZ B408YZZ B4090ZZ B4091ZZ B409YZZ B40B0ZZ B40B1ZZ B40BYZZ B40C0ZZ B40C1ZZ B40CYZZ B40D0ZZ B40D1ZZ B40DYZZ B40F0ZZ B40F1ZZ B40FYZZ B40G0ZZ B40G1ZZ B40GYZZ B40J0ZZ B40J1ZZ B40JYZZ B40M0ZZ B40M1ZZ B40MYZZ

B Imaging
4 Lower Arteries
1 Fluoroscopy: Single plane or bi-plane real time display of an image developed from the capture of external ionizing radiation on a fluorescent screen. The image may also be stored by either digital or analog means

Body Part Character 4	Contrast Character 5	Qualifier Character 6	Qualifier Character 7
0 Abdominal Aorta ⊘ **2** Hepatic Artery ⊘ **3** Splenic Arteries ⊘ **4** Superior Mesenteric Artery ⊘ **5** Inferior Mesenteric Artery ⊘ **6** Renal Artery, Right ⊘ **7** Renal Artery, Left ⊘ **8** Renal Arteries, Bilateral ⊘ **9** Lumbar Arteries ⊘ **B** Intra-Abdominal Arteries, Other ⊘ **C** Pelvic Arteries ⊘ **D** Aorta and Bilateral Lower Extremity Arteries ⊘ **F** Lower Extremity Arteries, Right ⊘ **G** Lower Extremity Arteries, Left ⊘ **J** Lower Arteries, Other ⊘	**0** High Osmolar **1** Low Osmolar **Y** Other Contrast	**1** Laser	**0** Intraoperative
0 Abdominal Aorta ⊘ **2** Hepatic Artery ⊘ **3** Splenic Arteries ⊘ **4** Superior Mesenteric Artery ⊘ **5** Inferior Mesenteric Artery ⊘ **6** Renal Artery, Right ⊘ **7** Renal Artery, Left ⊘ **8** Renal Arteries, Bilateral ⊘ **9** Lumbar Arteries ⊘ **B** Intra-Abdominal Arteries, Other ⊘ **C** Pelvic Arteries ⊘ **D** Aorta and Bilateral Lower Extremity Arteries ⊘ **F** Lower Extremity Arteries, Right ⊘ **G** Lower Extremity Arteries, Left ⊘ **J** Lower Arteries, Other ⊘	**0** High Osmolar **1** Low Osmolar **Y** Other Contrast	**Z** None	**Z** None
0 Abdominal Aorta ⊘ **2** Hepatic Artery ⊘ **3** Splenic Arteries ⊘ **4** Superior Mesenteric Artery ⊘ **5** Inferior Mesenteric Artery ⊘ **6** Renal Artery, Right ⊘ **7** Renal Artery, Left ⊘ **8** Renal Arteries, Bilateral ⊘ **9** Lumbar Arteries ⊘ **B** Intra-Abdominal Arteries, Other ⊘ **C** Pelvic Arteries ⊘ **D** Aorta and Bilateral Lower Extremity Arteries ⊘ **F** Lower Extremity Arteries, Right ⊘ **G** Lower Extremity Arteries, Left ⊘ **J** Lower Arteries, Other ⊘	**Z** None	**Z** None	**Z** None

⊘ B410010 B4100ZZ B410110 B4101ZZ B410Y10 B410YZZ B410ZZZ B412010 B4120ZZ B412110 B4121ZZ B412Y10 B412YZZ B412ZZZ B413010 B4130ZZ B413110 B4131ZZ B413Y10 B413YZZ B413ZZZ B414010 B4140ZZ B414110 B4141ZZ B414Y10 B414YZZ B414ZZZ B415010 B4150ZZ B415110 B4151ZZ B415Y10 B415YZZ B415ZZZ B416010 B4160ZZ B416110 B4161ZZ B416Y10 B416YZZ B416ZZZ B417010 B4170ZZ B417110 B4171ZZ B417Y10 B417YZZ B417ZZZ B418010 B4180ZZ B418110 B4181ZZ B418Y10 B418YZZ B418ZZZ B419010 B4190ZZ B419110 B4191ZZ B419Y10 B419YZZ B419ZZZ B41B010 B41B0ZZ B41B110 B41B1ZZ B41BY10 B41BYZZ B41BZZZ B41C010 B41C0ZZ B41C110 B41C1ZZ B41CY10 B41CYZZ B41CZZZ B41D010 B41D0ZZ B41D110 B41D1ZZ B41DY10 B41DYZZ B41DZZZ B41F010 B41F0ZZ B41F110 B41F1ZZ B41FY10 B41FYZZ B41FZZZ B41G010 B41G0ZZ B41G110 B41G1ZZ B41GY10 B41GYZZ B41GZZZ B41J010 B41J0ZZ B41J110 B41J1ZZ B41JY10 B41JYZZ B41JZZZ

B Imaging
4 Lower Arteries
2 Computerized Tomography (CT Scan): Computer reformatted digital display of multiplanar images developed from the capture of multiple exposures of external ionizing radiation

Body Part Character 4	Contrast Character 5	Qualifier Character 6	Qualifier Character 7
0 Abdominal Aorta ⊘ **1** Celiac Artery ⊘ **4** Superior Mesenteric Artery ⊘ **8** Renal Arteries, Bilateral ⊘ **C** Pelvic Arteries ⊘ **F** Lower Extremity Arteries, Right ⊘ **G** Lower Extremity Arteries, Left ⊘ **H** Lower Extremity Arteries, Bilateral ⊘ **M** Renal Artery Transplant ⊘	**0** High Osmolar **1** Low Osmolar **Y** Other Contrast	**Z** None	**Z** None
0 Abdominal Aorta ⊘ **1** Celiac Artery ⊘ **4** Superior Mesenteric Artery ⊘ **8** Renal Arteries, Bilateral ⊘ **C** Pelvic Arteries ⊘ **F** Lower Extremity Arteries, Right ⊘ **G** Lower Extremity Arteries, Left ⊘ **H** Lower Extremity Arteries, Bilateral ⊘ **M** Renal Artery Transplant ⊘	**Z** None	**2** Intravascular Optical Coherence **Z** None	**Z** None

⊘ B4200ZZ B4201ZZ B420YZZ B420Z2Z B420ZZZ B4210ZZ B4211ZZ B421YZZ B421Z2Z B421ZZZ B4240ZZ B4241ZZ B424YZZ B424Z2Z B424ZZZ B4280ZZ B4281ZZ B428YZZ B428Z2Z B428ZZZ B42C0ZZ B42C1ZZ B42CYZZ B42CZ2Z B42CZZZ B42F0ZZ B42F1ZZ B42FYZZ B42FZ2Z B42FZZZ B42G0ZZ B42G1ZZ B42GYZZ B42GZ2Z B42GZZZ B42H0ZZ B42H1ZZ B42HYZZ B42HZ2Z B42HZZZ B42M0ZZ B42M1ZZ B42MYZZ B42MZ2Z B42MZZZ

B Imaging
4 Lower Arteries
3 Magnetic Resonance Imaging (MRI): Computer reformatted digital display of multiplanar images developed from the capture of radiofrequency signals emitted by nuclei in a body site excited within a magnetic field

Body Part Character 4	Contrast Character 5	Qualifier Character 6	Qualifier Character 7
0 Abdominal Aorta ⊘ **1** Celiac Artery ⊘ **4** Superior Mesenteric Artery ⊘ **8** Renal Arteries, Bilateral ⊘ **C** Pelvic Arteries ⊘ **F** Lower Extremity Arteries, Right ⊘ **G** Lower Extremity Arteries, Left ⊘ **H** Lower Extremity Arteries, Bilateral ⊘	**Y** Other Contrast	**0** Unenhanced and Enhanced **Z** None	**Z** None
0 Abdominal Aorta ⊘ **1** Celiac Artery ⊘ **4** Superior Mesenteric Artery ⊘ **8** Renal Arteries, Bilateral ⊘ **C** Pelvic Arteries ⊘ **F** Lower Extremity Arteries, Right ⊘ **G** Lower Extremity Arteries, Left ⊘ **H** Lower Extremity Arteries, Bilateral ⊘	**Z** None	**Z** None	**Z** None

⊘ B430Y0Z B430YZZ B430ZZZ B431Y0Z B431YZZ B431ZZZ B434Y0Z B434YZZ B434ZZZ B438Y0Z B438YZZ B438ZZZ B43CY0Z B43CYZZ B43CZZZ B43FY0Z B43FYZZ B43FZZZ B43GY0Z B43GYZZ B43GZZZ B43HY0Z B43HYZZ B43HZZZ

B Imaging
4 Lower Arteries
4 Ultrasonography: Real time display of images of anatomy or flow information developed from the capture of reflected and attenuated high frequency sound waves

Body Part Character 4	Contrast Character 5	Qualifier Character 6	Qualifier Character 7
0 Abdominal Aorta ⊘ **4** Superior Mesenteric Artery ⊘ **5** Inferior Mesenteric Artery ⊘ **6** Renal Artery, Right ⊘ **7** Renal Artery, Left ⊘ **8** Renal Arteries, Bilateral ⊘ **B** Intra-Abdominal Arteries, Other ⊘ **F** Lower Extremity Arteries, Right ⊘ **G** Lower Extremity Arteries, Left ⊘ **H** Lower Extremity Arteries, Bilateral ⊘ **K** Celiac and Mesenteric Arteries ⊘ **L** Femoral Artery ⊘ **N** Penile Arteries ⊘	**Z** None	**Z** None	**3** Intravascular **Z** None

⊘ B440ZZ3 B440ZZZ B444ZZ3 B444ZZZ B445ZZ3 B445ZZZ B446ZZ3 B446ZZZ B447ZZ3 B447ZZZ B448ZZ3 B448ZZZ B44BZZ3 B44BZZZ B44FZZ3 B44FZZZ B44GZZ3 B44GZZZ B44HZZ3 B44HZZZ B44KZZ3 B44KZZZ B44LZZ3 B44LZZZ B44NZZ3 B44NZZZ

B Imaging
5 Veins
0 Plain Radiography: Planar display of an image developed from the capture of external ionizing radiation on photographic or photoconductive plate

Body Part Character 4	Contrast Character 5	Qualifier Character 6	Qualifier Character 7
0 Epidural Veins ⊘ **1** Cerebral and Cerebellar Veins ⊘ **2** Intracranial Sinuses ⊘ **3** Jugular Veins, Right ⊘ **4** Jugular Veins, Left ⊘ **5** Jugular Veins, Bilateral ⊘ **6** Subclavian Vein, Right ⊘ **7** Subclavian Vein, Left ⊘ **8** Superior Vena Cava ⊘ **9** Inferior Vena Cava ⊘ **B** Lower Extremity Veins, Right ⊘ **C** Lower Extremity Veins, Left ⊘ **D** Lower Extremity Veins, Bilateral ⊘ **F** Pelvic (Iliac) Veins, Right ⊘ **G** Pelvic (Iliac) Veins, Left ⊘ **H** Pelvic (Iliac) Veins, Bilateral ⊘ **J** Renal Vein, Right ⊘ **K** Renal Vein, Left ⊘ **L** Renal Veins, Bilateral ⊘ **M** Upper Extremity Veins, Right ⊘ **N** Upper Extremity Veins, Left ⊘ **P** Upper Extremity Veins, Bilateral ⊘ **Q** Pulmonary Vein, Right ⊘ **R** Pulmonary Vein, Left ⊘ **S** Pulmonary Veins, Bilateral ⊘ **T** Portal and Splanchnic Veins ⊘ **V** Veins, Other ⊘ **W** Dialysis Shunt/Fistula ⊘	**0** High Osmolar **1** Low Osmolar **Y** Other Contrast	**Z** None	**Z** None

⊘ B5000ZZ B5001ZZ B500YZZ B5010ZZ B5011ZZ B501YZZ B5020ZZ B5021ZZ B502YZZ B5030ZZ B5031ZZ B503YZZ B5040ZZ B5041ZZ B504YZZ B5050ZZ B5051ZZ B505YZZ B5060ZZ B5061ZZ B506YZZ B5070ZZ B5071ZZ B507YZZ B5080ZZ B5081ZZ B508YZZ B5090ZZ B5091ZZ B509YZZ B50B0ZZ B50B1ZZ B50BYZZ B50C0ZZ B50C1ZZ B50CYZZ B50D0ZZ B50D1ZZ B50DYZZ B50F0ZZ B50F1ZZ B50FYZZ B50G0ZZ B50G1ZZ B50GYZZ B50H0ZZ B50H1ZZ B50HYZZ B50J0ZZ B50J1ZZ B50JYZZ B50K0ZZ B50K1ZZ B50KYZZ B50L0ZZ B50L1ZZ B50LYZZ B50M0ZZ B50M1ZZ B50MYZZ B50N0ZZ B50N1ZZ B50NYZZ B50P0ZZ B50P1ZZ B50PYZZ B50Q0ZZ B50Q1ZZ B50QYZZ B50R0ZZ B50R1ZZ B50RYZZ B50S0ZZ B50S1ZZ B50SYZZ B50T0ZZ B50T1ZZ B50TYZZ B50V0ZZ B50V1ZZ B50VYZZ B50W0ZZ B50W1ZZ B50WYZZ

B Imaging
5 Veins
1 Fluoroscopy: Single plane or bi-plane real time display of an image developed from the capture of external ionizing radiation on a fluorescent screen. The image may also be stored by either digital or analog means

Body Part Character 4	Contrast Character 5	Qualifier Character 6	Qualifier Character 7
0 Epidural Veins ⦸ **1** Cerebral and Cerebellar Veins ⦸ **2** Intracranial Sinuses ⦸ **3** Jugular Veins, Right ⦸ CC DRG **4** Jugular Veins, Left ⦸ CC DRG **5** Jugular Veins, Bilateral ⦸ CC DRG **6** Subclavian Vein, Right ⦸ CC DRG **7** Subclavian Vein, Left ⦸ CC DRG **8** Superior Vena Cava ⦸ **9** Inferior Vena Cava ⦸ **B** Lower Extremity Veins, Right ⦸ CC DRG **C** Lower Extremity Veins, Left ⦸ CC DRG **D** Lower Extremity Veins, Bilateral ⦸ CC DRG **F** Pelvic (Iliac) Veins, Right ⦸ **G** Pelvic (Iliac) Veins, Left ⦸ **H** Pelvic (Iliac) Veins, Bilateral ⦸ **J** Renal Vein, Right ⦸ **K** Renal Vein, Left ⦸ **L** Renal Veins, Bilateral ⦸ **M** Upper Extremity Veins, Right ⦸ **N** Upper Extremity Veins, Left ⦸ **P** Upper Extremity Veins, Bilateral ⦸ **Q** Pulmonary Vein, Right ⦸ **R** Pulmonary Vein, Left ⦸ **S** Pulmonary Veins, Bilateral ⦸ **T** Portal and Splanchnic Veins ⦸ **V** Veins, Other ⦸ **W** Dialysis Shunt/Fistula ⦸	**0** High Osmolar **1** Low Osmolar **Y** Other Contrast **Z** None	**Z** None	**A** Guidance **Z** None

⦸ B5100ZA B5100ZZ B5101ZA B5101ZZ B510YZA B510YZZ B510ZZA B510ZZZ B5110ZA B5110ZZ B5111ZA B5111ZZ B511YZA B511YZZ B511ZZA B511ZZZ B5120ZA B5120ZZ B5121ZA B5121ZZ B512YZA B512YZZ B512ZZA B512ZZZ B5130ZZ B5131ZZ B513YZZ B513ZZZ B5140ZZ B5141ZZ B514YZZ B514ZZZ B5150ZZ B5151ZZ B515YZZ B515ZZZ B5160ZZ B5161ZZ B516YZZ B516ZZZ B5170ZZ B5171ZZ B517YZZ B517ZZZ B5180ZA B5180ZZ B5181ZA B5181ZZ B518YZA B518YZZ B518ZZA B518ZZZ B5190ZA B5190ZZ B5191ZA B5191ZZ B519YZA B519YZZ B519ZZA B519ZZZ B51B0ZZ B51B1ZZ B51BYZZ B51BZZZ B51C0ZZ B51C1ZZ B51CYZZ B51CZZZ B51D0ZZ B51D1ZZ B51DYZZ B51DZZZ B51F0ZA B51F0ZZ B51F1ZA B51F1ZZ B51FYZA B51FYZZ B51FZZA B51FZZZ B51G0ZA B51G0ZZ B51G1ZA B51G1ZZ B51GYZA B51GYZZ B51GZZA B51GZZZ B51H0ZA B51H0ZZ B51H1ZA B51H1ZZ B51HYZA B51HYZZ B51HZZA B51HZZZ B51J0ZA B51J0ZZ B51J1ZA B51J1ZZ B51JYZA B51JYZZ B51JZZA B51JZZZ B51K0ZA B51K0ZZ B51K1ZA B51K1ZZ B51KYZA B51KYZZ B51KZZA B51KZZZ B51L0ZA B51L0ZZ B51L1ZA B51L1ZZ B51LYZA B51LYZZ B51LZZA B51LZZZ B51M0ZA B51M0ZZ B51M1ZA B51M1ZZ B51MYZA B51MYZZ B51MZZA B51MZZZ B51N0ZA B51N0ZZ B51N1ZA B51N1ZZ B51NYZA B51NYZZ B51NZZA B51NZZZ B51P0ZA B51P0ZZ B51P1ZA B51P1ZZ B51PYZA B51PYZZ B51PZZA B51PZZZ B51Q0ZA B51Q0ZZ B51Q1ZA B51Q1ZZ B51QYZA B51QYZZ B51QZZA B51QZZZ B51R0ZA B51R0ZZ B51R1ZA B51R1ZZ B51RYZA B51RYZZ B51RZZA B51RZZZ B51S0ZA B51S0ZZ B51S1ZA B51S1ZZ B51SYZA B51SYZZ B51SZZA B51SZZZ B51T0ZA B51T0ZZ B51T1ZA B51T1ZZ B51TYZA B51TYZZ B51TZZA B51TZZZ B51V0ZA B51V0ZZ B51V1ZA B51V1ZZ B51VYZA B51VYZZ B51VZZA B51VZZZ B51W0ZA B51W0ZZ B51W1ZA B51W1ZZ B51WYZA B51WYZZ B51WZZA B51WZZZ

DRG B5130ZA B5131ZA B513YZA B513ZZA B5140ZA B5141ZA B514YZA B514ZZA B5150ZA B5151ZA B515YZA B515ZZA B5160ZA B5161ZA B516YZA B516ZZA B5170ZA B5171ZA B517YZA B517ZZA B51B0ZA B51B1ZA B51BYZA B51BZZA B51C0ZA B51C1ZA B51CYZA B51CZZA B51D0ZA B51D1ZA B51DYZA B51DZZA

CC B5130ZA B5131ZA B513YZA B513ZZA B5140ZA B5141ZA B514YZA B514ZZA B5150ZA B5151ZA B515YZA B515ZZA B5160ZA B5161ZA B516YZA B516ZZA B5170ZA B5171ZA B517YZA B517ZZA B51B0ZA B51B1ZA B51BYZA B51BZZA B51C0ZA B51C1ZA B51CYZA B51CZZA B51D0ZA B51D1ZA B51DYZA B51DZZA

B Imaging
5 Veins
2 Computerized Tomography (CT Scan): Computer reformatted digital display of multiplanar images developed from the capture of multiple exposures of external ionizing radiation

Body Part Character 4	Contrast Character 5	Qualifier Character 6	Qualifier Character 7
2 Intracranial Sinuses ⊘ **8** Superior Vena Cava ⊘ **9** Inferior Vena Cava ⊘ **F** Pelvic (Iliac) Veins, Right ⊘ **G** Pelvic (Iliac) Veins, Left ⊘ **H** Pelvic (Iliac) Veins, Bilateral ⊘ **J** Renal Vein, Right ⊘ **K** Renal Vein, Left ⊘ **L** Renal Veins, Bilateral ⊘ **Q** Pulmonary Vein, Right ⊘ **R** Pulmonary Vein, Left ⊘ **S** Pulmonary Veins, Bilateral ⊘ **T** Portal and Splanchnic Veins ⊘	**0** High Osmolar **1** Low Osmolar **Y** Other Contrast	**0** Unenhanced and Enhanced **Z** None	**Z** None
2 Intracranial Sinuses ⊘ **8** Superior Vena Cava ⊘ **9** Inferior Vena Cava ⊘ **F** Pelvic (Iliac) Veins, Right ⊘ **G** Pelvic (Iliac) Veins, Left ⊘ **H** Pelvic (Iliac) Veins, Bilateral ⊘ **J** Renal Vein, Right ⊘ **K** Renal Vein, Left ⊘ **L** Renal Veins, Bilateral ⊘ **Q** Pulmonary Vein, Right ⊘ **R** Pulmonary Vein, Left ⊘ **S** Pulmonary Veins, Bilateral ⊘ **T** Portal and Splanchnic Veins ⊘	**Z** None	**2** Intravascular Optical Coherence **Z** None	**Z** None

⊘ B52200Z B5220ZZ B52210Z B5221ZZ B522Y0Z B522YZZ B522Z2Z B522ZZZ B52800Z B5280ZZ B52810Z B5281ZZ B528Y0Z B528YZZ B528Z2Z B528ZZZ B52900Z B5290ZZ B52910Z B5291ZZ B529Y0Z B529YZZ B529Z2Z B529ZZZ B52F00Z B52F0ZZ B52F10Z B52F1ZZ B52FY0Z B52FYZZ B52FZ2Z B52FZZZ B52G00Z B52G0ZZ B52G10Z B52G1ZZ B52GY0Z B52GYZZ B52GZ2Z B52GZZZ B52H00Z B52H0ZZ B52H10Z B52H1ZZ B52HY0Z B52HYZZ B52HZ2Z B52HZZZ B52J00Z B52J0ZZ B52J10Z B52J1ZZ B52JY0Z B52JYZZ B52JZ2Z B52JZZZ B52K00Z B52K0ZZ B52K10Z B52K1ZZ B52KY0Z B52KYZZ B52KZ2Z B52KZZZ B52L00Z B52L0ZZ B52L10Z B52L1ZZ B52LY0Z B52LYZZ B52LZ2Z B52LZZZ B52Q00Z B52Q0ZZ B52Q10Z B52Q1ZZ B52QY0Z B52QYZZ B52QZ2Z B52QZZZ B52R00Z B52R0ZZ B52R10Z B52R1ZZ B52RY0Z B52RYZZ B52RZ2Z B52RZZZ B52S00Z B52S0ZZ B52S10Z B52S1ZZ B52SY0Z B52SYZZ B52SZ2Z B52SZZZ B52T00Z B52T0ZZ B52T10Z B52T1ZZ B52TY0Z B52TYZZ B52TZ2Z B52TZZZ

B Imaging
5 Veins
3 Magnetic Resonance Imaging (MRI): Computer reformatted digital display of multiplanar images developed from the capture of radiofrequency signals emitted by nuclei in a body site excited within a magnetic field

Body Part Character 4	Contrast Character 5	Qualifier Character 6	Qualifier Character 7
1 Cerebral and Cerebellar Veins ⊘ **2** Intracranial Sinuses ⊘ **5** Jugular Veins, Bilateral ⊘ **8** Superior Vena Cava ⊘ **9** Inferior Vena Cava ⊘ **B** Lower Extremity Veins, Right ⊘ **C** Lower Extremity Veins, Left ⊘ **D** Lower Extremity Veins, Bilateral ⊘ **H** Pelvic (Iliac) Veins, Bilateral ⊘ **L** Renal Veins, Bilateral ⊘ **M** Upper Extremity Veins, Right ⊘ **N** Upper Extremity Veins, Left ⊘ **P** Upper Extremity Veins, Bilateral ⊘ **S** Pulmonary Veins, Bilateral ⊘ **T** Portal and Splanchnic Veins ⊘ **V** Veins, Other ⊘	**Y** Other Contrast	**0** Unenhanced and Enhanced **Z** None	**Z** None
1 Cerebral and Cerebellar Veins ⊘ **2** Intracranial Sinuses ⊘ **5** Jugular Veins, Bilateral ⊘ **8** Superior Vena Cava ⊘ **9** Inferior Vena Cava ⊘ **B** Lower Extremity Veins, Right ⊘ **C** Lower Extremity Veins, Left ⊘ **D** Lower Extremity Veins, Bilateral ⊘ **H** Pelvic (Iliac) Veins, Bilateral ⊘ **L** Renal Veins, Bilateral ⊘ **M** Upper Extremity Veins, Right ⊘ **N** Upper Extremity Veins, Left ⊘ **P** Upper Extremity Veins, Bilateral ⊘ **S** Pulmonary Veins, Bilateral ⊘ **T** Portal and Splanchnic Veins ⊘ **V** Veins, Other ⊘	**Z** None	**Z** None	**Z** None

⊘ B531Y0Z B531YZZ B531ZZZ B532Y0Z B532YZZ B532ZZZ B535Y0Z B535YZZ B535ZZZ B538Y0Z B538YZZ B538ZZZ B539Y0Z B539YZZ B539ZZZ B53BY0Z B53BYZZ B53BZZZ B53CY0Z B53CYZZ B53CZZZ B53DY0Z B53DYZZ B53DZZZ B53HY0Z B53HYZZ B53HZZZ B53LY0Z B53LYZZ B53LZZZ B53MY0Z B53MYZZ B53MZZZ B53NY0Z B53NYZZ B53NZZZ B53PY0Z B53PYZZ B53PZZZ B53SY0Z B53SYZZ B53SZZZ B53TY0Z B53TYZZ B53TZZZ B53VY0Z B53VYZZ B53VZZZ

B Imaging
5 Veins
4 Ultrasonography: Real time display of images of anatomy or flow information developed from the capture of reflected and attenuated high frequency sound waves

Body Part Character 4	Contrast Character 5	Qualifier Character 6	Qualifier Character 7
3 Jugular Veins, Right ⊘ CC DRG **4** Jugular Veins, Left ⊘ CC DRG **6** Subclavian Vein, Right ⊘ CC DRG **7** Subclavian Vein, Left ⊘ CC DRG **8** Superior Vena Cava ⊘ **9** Inferior Vena Cava ⊘ **B** Lower Extremity Veins, Right ⊘ CC DRG **C** Lower Extremity Veins, Left ⊘ CC DRG **D** Lower Extremity Veins, Bilateral ⊘ CC DRG **J** Renal Vein, Right ⊘ **K** Renal Vein, Left ⊘ **L** Renal Veins, Bilateral ⊘ **M** Upper Extremity Veins, Right ⊘ **N** Upper Extremity Veins, Left ⊘ **P** Upper Extremity Veins, Bilateral ⊘ **T** Portal and Splanchnic Veins ⊘	**Z** None	**Z** None	**3** Intravascular **A** Guidance **Z** None

⊘ B543ZZ3 B543ZZZ B544ZZ3 B544ZZZ B546ZZ3 B546ZZZ B547ZZ3 B547ZZZ B548ZZ3 B548ZZA B548ZZZ B549ZZ3 B549ZZA B549ZZZ B54BZZ3 B54BZZZ B54CZZ3 B54CZZZ B54DZZ3 B54DZZZ B54JZZ3 B54JZZA B54JZZZ B54KZZ3 B54KZZA B54KZZZ B54LZZ3 B54LZZA B54LZZZ B54MZZ3 B54MZZA B54MZZZ B54NZZ3 B54NZZA B54NZZZ B54PZZ3 B54PZZA B54PZZZ B54TZZ3 B54TZZA B54TZZZ

DRG B543ZZA B544ZZA B546ZZA B547ZZA B54BZZA B54CZZA B54DZZA

CC B543ZZA B544ZZA B546ZZA B547ZZA B54BZZA B54CZZA B54DZZA

B Imaging
7 Lymphatic System
0 Plain Radiography: Planar display of an image developed from the capture of external ionizing radiation on photographic or photoconductive plate

Body Part Character 4	Contrast Character 5	Qualifier Character 6	Qualifier Character 7
0 Abdominal/Retroperitoneal Lymphatics, Unilateral ⊘ **1** Abdominal/Retroperitoneal Lymphatics, Bilateral ⊘ **4** Lymphatics, Head and Neck ⊘ **5** Upper Extremity Lymphatics, Right ⊘ **6** Upper Extremity Lymphatics, Left ⊘ **7** Upper Extremity Lymphatics, Bilateral ⊘ **8** Lower Extremity Lymphatics, Right ⊘ **9** Lower Extremity Lymphatics, Left ⊘ **B** Lower Extremity Lymphatics, Bilateral ⊘ **C** Lymphatics, Pelvic ⊘	**0** High Osmolar **1** Low Osmolar **Y** Other Contrast	**Z** None	**Z** None

⊘ B7000ZZ B7001ZZ B700YZZ B7010ZZ B7011ZZ B701YZZ B7040ZZ B7041ZZ B704YZZ B7050ZZ B7051ZZ B705YZZ B7060ZZ B7061ZZ B706YZZ B7070ZZ B7071ZZ B707YZZ B7080ZZ B7081ZZ B708YZZ B7090ZZ B7091ZZ B709YZZ B70B0ZZ B70B1ZZ B70BYZZ B70C0ZZ B70C1ZZ B70CYZZ

B Imaging
8 Eye
0 Plain Radiography: Planar display of an image developed from the capture of external ionizing radiation on photographic or photoconductive plate

Body Part Character 4	Contrast Character 5	Qualifier Character 6	Qualifier Character 7
0 Lacrimal Duct, Right ⦸ **1** Lacrimal Duct, Left ⦸ **2** Lacrimal Ducts, Bilateral ⦸	**0** High Osmolar **1** Low Osmolar **Y** Other Contrast	**Z** None	**Z** None
3 Optic Foramina, Right ⦸ **4** Optic Foramina, Left ⦸ **5** Eye, Right ⦸ **6** Eye, Left ⦸ **7** Eyes, Bilateral ⦸	**Z** None	**Z** None	**Z** None

⦸ B8000ZZ B8001ZZ B800YZZ B8010ZZ B8011ZZ B801YZZ B8020ZZ B8021ZZ B802YZZ B803ZZZ B804ZZZ B805ZZZ B806ZZZ B807ZZZ

B Imaging
8 Eye
2 Computerized Tomography (CT Scan): Computer reformatted digital display of multiplanar images developed from the capture of multiple exposures of external ionizing radiation

Body Part Character 4	Contrast Character 5	Qualifier Character 6	Qualifier Character 7
5 Eye, Right ⦸ **6** Eye, Left ⦸ **7** Eyes, Bilateral ⦸	**0** High Osmolar **1** Low Osmolar **Y** Other Contrast	**0** Unenhanced and Enhanced **Z** None	**Z** None
5 Eye, Right ⦸ **6** Eye, Left ⦸ **7** Eyes, Bilateral ⦸	**Z** None	**Z** None	**Z** None

⦸ B82500Z B8250ZZ B82510Z B8251ZZ B825Y0Z B825YZZ B825ZZZ B82600Z B8260ZZ B82610Z B8261ZZ B826Y0Z B826YZZ B826ZZZ B82700Z B8270ZZ B82710Z B8271ZZ B827Y0Z B827YZZ B827ZZZ

B Imaging
8 Eye
3 Magnetic Resonance Imaging (MRI): Computer reformatted digital display of multiplanar images developed from the capture of radiofrequency signals emitted by nuclei in a body site excited within a magnetic field

Body Part Character 4	Contrast Character 5	Qualifier Character 6	Qualifier Character 7
5 Eye, Right ⦸ **6** Eye, Left ⦸ **7** Eyes, Bilateral ⦸	**Y** Other Contrast	**0** Unenhanced and Enhanced **Z** None	**Z** None
5 Eye, Right ⦸ **6** Eye, Left ⦸ **7** Eyes, Bilateral ⦸	**Z** None	**Z** None	**Z** None

⦸ B835Y0Z B835YZZ B835ZZZ B836Y0Z B836YZZ B836ZZZ B837Y0Z B837YZZ B837ZZZ

B Imaging
8 Eye
4 Ultrasonography: Real time display of images of anatomy or flow information developed from the capture of reflected and attenuated high frequency sound waves

Body Part Character 4	Contrast Character 5	Qualifier Character 6	Qualifier Character 7
5 Eye, Right ⦸ **6** Eye, Left ⦸ **7** Eyes, Bilateral ⦸	**Z** None	**Z** None	**Z** None

⦸ B845ZZZ B846ZZZ B847ZZZ

B Imaging
9 Ear, Nose, Mouth and Throat
0 Plain Radiography: Planar display of an image developed from the capture of external ionizing radiation on photographic or photoconductive plate

Body Part Character 4	Contrast Character 5	Qualifier Character 6	Qualifier Character 7
2 Paranasal Sinuses ⦸ **F** Nasopharynx/Oropharynx ⦸ **H** Mastoids ⦸	**Z** None	**Z** None	**Z** None
4 Parotid Gland, Right ⦸ **5** Parotid Gland, Left ⦸ **6** Parotid Glands, Bilateral ⦸ **7** Submandibular Gland, Right ⦸ **8** Submandibular Gland, Left ⦸ **9** Submandibular Glands, Bilateral ⦸ **B** Salivary Gland, Right ⦸ **C** Salivary Gland, Left ⦸ **D** Salivary Glands, Bilateral ⦸	**0** High Osmolar **1** Low Osmolar **Y** Other Contrast	**Z** None	**Z** None

⦸ B902ZZZ B9040ZZ B9041ZZ B904YZZ B9050ZZ B9051ZZ B905YZZ B9060ZZ B9061ZZ B906YZZ B9070ZZ B9071ZZ B907YZZ B9080ZZ B9081ZZ B908YZZ B9090ZZ B9091ZZ B909YZZ B90B0ZZ B90B1ZZ B90BYZZ B90C0ZZ B90C1ZZ B90CYZZ B90D0ZZ B90D1ZZ B90DYZZ B90FZZZ B90HZZZ

B Imaging
9 Ear, Nose, Mouth and Throat
1 Fluoroscopy: Single plane or bi-plane real time display of an image developed from the capture of external ionizing radiation on a fluorescent screen. The image may also be stored by either digital or analog means

Body Part Character 4	Contrast Character 5	Qualifier Character 6	Qualifier Character 7
G Pharynx and Epiglottis ⦸ **J** Larynx ⦸	**Y** Other Contrast **Z** None	**Z** None	**Z** None

⦸ B91GYZZ B91GZZZ B91JYZZ B91JZZZ

B Imaging
9 Ear, Nose, Mouth and Throat
2 Computerized Tomography (CT Scan): Computer reformatted digital display of multiplanar images developed from the capture of multiple exposures of external ionizing radiation

Body Part Character 4	Contrast Character 5	Qualifier Character 6	Qualifier Character 7
0 Ear ⦸ **2** Paranasal Sinuses ⦸ **6** Parotid Glands, Bilateral ⦸ **9** Submandibular Glands, Bilateral ⦸ **D** Salivary Glands, Bilateral ⦸ **F** Nasopharynx/Oropharynx ⦸ **J** Larynx ⦸	**0** High Osmolar **1** Low Osmolar **Y** Other Contrast	**0** Unenhanced and Enhanced **Z** None	**Z** None
0 Ear ⦸ **2** Paranasal Sinuses ⦸ **6** Parotid Glands, Bilateral ⦸ **9** Submandibular Glands, Bilateral ⦸ **D** Salivary Glands, Bilateral ⦸ **F** Nasopharynx/Oropharynx ⦸ **J** Larynx ⦸	**Z** None	**Z** None	**Z** None

⦸ B92000Z B9200ZZ B92010Z B9201ZZ B920Y0Z B920YZZ B920ZZZ B92200Z B9220ZZ B92210Z B9221ZZ B922Y0Z B922YZZ B922ZZZ B92600Z B9260ZZ B92610Z B9261ZZ B926Y0Z B926YZZ B926ZZZ B92900Z B9290ZZ B92910Z B9291ZZ B929Y0Z B929YZZ B929ZZZ B92D00Z B92D0ZZ B92D10Z B92D1ZZ B92DY0Z B92DYZZ B92DZZZ B92F00Z B92F0ZZ B92F10Z B92F1ZZ B92FY0Z B92FYZZ B92FZZZ B92J00Z B92J0ZZ B92J10Z B92J1ZZ B92JY0Z B92JYZZ B92JZZZ

B Imaging
9 Ear, Nose, Mouth and Throat
3 Magnetic Resonance Imaging (MRI): Computer reformatted digital display of multiplanar images developed from the capture of radiofrequency signals emitted by nuclei in a body site excited within a magnetic field

Body Part Character 4	Contrast Character 5	Qualifier Character 6	Qualifier Character 7
0 Ear ⃠ 2 Paranasal Sinuses ⃠ 6 Parotid Glands, Bilateral ⃠ 9 Submandibular Glands, Bilateral ⃠ D Salivary Glands, Bilateral ⃠ F Nasopharynx/Oropharynx ⃠ J Larynx ⃠	Y Other Contrast	0 Unenhanced and Enhanced Z None	Z None
0 Ear ⃠ 2 Paranasal Sinuses ⃠ 6 Parotid Glands, Bilateral ⃠ 9 Submandibular Glands, Bilateral ⃠ D Salivary Glands, Bilateral ⃠ F Nasopharynx/Oropharynx ⃠ J Larynx ⃠	Z None	Z None	Z None

⃠ B930Y0Z B930YZZ B930ZZZ B932Y0Z B932YZZ B932ZZZ B936Y0Z B936YZZ B936ZZZ B939Y0Z B939YZZ B939ZZZ B93DY0Z B93DYZZ B93DZZZ B93FY0Z B93FYZZ B93FZZZ B93JY0Z B93JYZZ B93JZZZ

B Imaging
B Respiratory System
0 Plain Radiography: Planar display of an image developed from the capture of external ionizing radiation on photographic or photoconductive plate

Body Part Character 4	Contrast Character 5	Qualifier Character 6	Qualifier Character 7
7 Tracheobronchial Tree, Right ⃠ 8 Tracheobronchial Tree, Left ⃠ 9 Tracheobronchial Trees, Bilateral ⃠	Y Other Contrast	Z None	Z None
D Upper Airways ⃠	Z None	Z None	Z None

⃠ BB07YZZ BB08YZZ BB09YZZ BB0DZZZ

B Imaging
B Respiratory System
1 Fluoroscopy: Single plane or bi-plane real time display of an image developed from the capture of external ionizing radiation on a fluorescent screen. The image may also be stored by either digital or analog means

Body Part Character 4	Contrast Character 5	Qualifier Character 6	Qualifier Character 7
2 Lung, Right ⃠ 3 Lung, Left ⃠ 4 Lungs, Bilateral ⃠ 6 Diaphragm ⃠ C Mediastinum ⃠ D Upper Airways ⃠	Z None	Z None	Z None
7 Tracheobronchial Tree, Right ⃠ 8 Tracheobronchial Tree, Left ⃠ 9 Tracheobronchial Trees, Bilateral ⃠	Y Other Contrast	Z None	Z None

⃠ BB12ZZZ BB13ZZZ BB14ZZZ BB16ZZZ BB17YZZ BB18YZZ BB19YZZ BB1CZZZ BB1DZZZ

B Imaging
B Respiratory System
2 Computerized Tomography (CT Scan): Computer reformatted digital display of multiplanar images developed from the capture of multiple exposures of external ionizing radiation

Body Part Character 4	Contrast Character 5	Qualifier Character 6	Qualifier Character 7
4 Lungs, Bilateral ⦸ 7 Tracheobronchial Tree, Right ⦸ 8 Tracheobronchial Tree, Left ⦸ 9 Tracheobronchial Trees, Bilateral ⦸ F Trachea/Airways ⦸	0 High Osmolar 1 Low Osmolar Y Other Contrast	0 Unenhanced and Enhanced Z None	Z None
4 Lungs, Bilateral ⦸ 7 Tracheobronchial Tree, Right ⦸ 8 Tracheobronchial Tree, Left ⦸ 9 Tracheobronchial Trees, Bilateral ⦸ F Trachea/Airways ⦸	Z None	Z None	Z None

⦸ BB2400Z BB240ZZ BB2410Z BB241ZZ BB24Y0Z BB24YZZ BB24ZZZ BB2700Z BB270ZZ BB2710Z BB271ZZ BB27Y0Z BB27YZZ BB27ZZZ BB2800Z BB280ZZ BB2810Z BB281ZZ BB28Y0Z BB28YZZ BB28ZZZ BB2900Z BB290ZZ BB2910Z BB291ZZ BB29Y0Z BB29YZZ BB29ZZZ BB2F00Z BB2F0ZZ BB2F10Z BB2F1ZZ BB2FY0Z BB2FYZZ BB2FZZZ

B Imaging
B Respiratory System
3 Magnetic Resonance Imaging (MRI): Computer reformatted digital display of multiplanar images developed from the capture of radiofrequency signals emitted by nuclei in a body site excited within a magnetic field

Body Part Character 4	Contrast Character 5	Qualifier Character 6	Qualifier Character 7
G Lung Apices ⦸	Y Other Contrast	0 Unenhanced and Enhanced Z None	Z None
G Lung Apices ⦸	Z None	Z None	Z None

⦸ BB3GY0Z BB3GYZZ BB3GZZZ

B Imaging
B Respiratory System
4 Ultrasonography: Real time display of images of anatomy or flow information developed from the capture of reflected and attenuated high frequency sound waves

Body Part Character 4	Contrast Character 5	Qualifier Character 6	Qualifier Character 7
B Pleura ⦸ C Mediastinum ⦸	Z None	Z None	Z None

⦸ BB4BZZZ BB4CZZZ

B Imaging
D Gastrointestinal System
1 Fluoroscopy: Single plane or bi-plane real time display of an image developed from the capture of external ionizing radiation on a fluorescent screen. The image may also be stored by either digital or analog means

Body Part Character 4	Contrast Character 5	Qualifier Character 6	Qualifier Character 7
1 Esophagus ⦸ 2 Stomach ⦸ 3 Small Bowel ⦸ 4 Colon ⦸ 5 Upper GI ⦸ 6 Upper GI and Small Bowel ⦸ 9 Duodenum ⦸ B Mouth/Oropharynx ⦸	Y Other Contrast Z None	Z None	Z None

⦸ BD11YZZ BD11ZZZ BD12YZZ BD12ZZZ BD13YZZ BD13ZZZ BD14YZZ BD14ZZZ BD15YZZ BD15ZZZ BD16YZZ BD16ZZZ BD19YZZ BD19ZZZ BD1BYZZ BD1BZZZ

B Imaging
D Gastrointestinal System
2 Computerized Tomography (CT Scan): Computer reformatted digital display of multiplanar images developed from the capture of multiple exposures of external ionizing radiation

Body Part Character 4	Contrast Character 5	Qualifier Character 6	Qualifier Character 7
4 Colon ⦸	0 High Osmolar 1 Low Osmolar Y Other Contrast	0 Unenhanced and Enhanced Z None	Z None
4 Colon ⦸	Z None	Z None	Z None

⦸ BD2400Z BD240ZZ BD2410Z BD241ZZ BD24Y0Z BD24YZZ BD24ZZZ

B Imaging
D Gastrointestinal System
4 Ultrasonography: Real time display of images of anatomy or flow information developed from the capture of reflected and attenuated high frequency sound waves

Body Part Character 4	Contrast Character 5	Qualifier Character 6	Qualifier Character 7
1 Esophagus ⦸ 2 Stomach ⦸ 7 Gastrointestinal Tract ⦸ 8 Appendix ⦸ 9 Duodenum ⦸ C Rectum ⦸	Z None	Z None	Z None

⦸ BD41ZZZ BD42ZZZ BD47ZZZ BD48ZZZ BD49ZZZ BD4CZZZ

B Imaging
F Hepatobiliary System and Pancreas
0 Plain Radiography: Planar display of an image developed from the capture of external ionizing radiation on photographic or photoconductive plate

Body Part Character 4	Contrast Character 5	Qualifier Character 6	Qualifier Character 7
0 Bile Ducts ⦸ 3 Gallbladder and Bile Ducts C Hepatobiliary System, All	0 High Osmolar 1 Low Osmolar Y Other Contrast	Z None	Z None

⦸ BF000ZZ BF001ZZ BF00YZZ

B Imaging
F Hepatobiliary System and Pancreas
1 Fluoroscopy: Single plane or bi-plane real time display of an image developed from the capture of external ionizing radiation on a fluorescent screen. The image may also be stored by either digital or analog means

Body Part Character 4	Contrast Character 5	Qualifier Character 6	Qualifier Character 7
0 Bile Ducts ⦸ 1 Biliary and Pancreatic Ducts ⦸ 2 Gallbladder ⦸ 3 Gallbladder and Bile Ducts ⦸ 4 Gallbladder, Bile Ducts and Pancreatic Ducts ⦸ 8 Pancreatic Ducts ⦸	0 High Osmolar 1 Low Osmolar Y Other Contrast	Z None	Z None

⦸ BF100ZZ BF101ZZ BF10YZZ BF110ZZ BF111ZZ BF11YZZ BF120ZZ BF121ZZ BF12YZZ BF130ZZ BF131ZZ BF13YZZ BF140ZZ BF141ZZ BF14YZZ BF180ZZ BF181ZZ BF18YZZ

B Imaging
F Hepatobiliary System and Pancreas
2 Computerized Tomography (CT Scan): Computer reformatted digital display of multiplanar images developed from the capture of multiple exposures of external ionizing radiation

Body Part Character 4	Contrast Character 5	Qualifier Character 6	Qualifier Character 7
5 Liver ⃠ 6 Liver and Spleen ⃠ 7 Pancreas ⃠ C Hepatobiliary System, All ⃠	0 High Osmolar 1 Low Osmolar Y Other Contrast	0 Unenhanced and Enhanced Z None	Z None
5 Liver ⃠ 6 Liver and Spleen ⃠ 7 Pancreas ⃠ C Hepatobiliary System, All ⃠	Z None	Z None	Z None

⃠ BF2500Z BF250ZZ BF2510Z BF251ZZ BF25Y0Z BF25YZZ BF25ZZZ BF2600Z BF260ZZ BF2610Z BF261ZZ BF26Y0Z BF26YZZ BF26ZZZ BF2700Z BF270ZZ BF2710Z BF271ZZ BF27Y0Z BF27YZZ BF27ZZZ BF2C00Z BF2C0ZZ BF2C10Z BF2C1ZZ BF2CY0Z BF2CYZZ BF2CZZZ

B Imaging
F Hepatobiliary System and Pancreas
3 Magnetic Resonance Imaging (MRI): Computer reformatted digital display of multiplanar images developed from the capture of radiofrequency signals emitted by nuclei in a body site excited within a magnetic field

Body Part Character 4	Contrast Character 5	Qualifier Character 6	Qualifier Character 7
5 Liver ⃠ 6 Liver and Spleen ⃠ 7 Pancreas ⃠	Y Other Contrast	0 Unenhanced and Enhanced Z None	Z None
5 Liver ⃠ 6 Liver and Spleen ⃠ 7 Pancreas ⃠	Z None	Z None	Z None

⃠ BF35Y0Z BF35YZZ BF35ZZZ BF36Y0Z BF36YZZ BF36ZZZ BF37Y0Z BF37YZZ BF37ZZZ

B Imaging
F Hepatobiliary System and Pancreas
4 Ultrasonography: Real time display of images of anatomy or flow information developed from the capture of reflected and attenuated high frequency sound waves

Body Part Character 4	Contrast Character 5	Qualifier Character 6	Qualifier Character 7
0 Bile Ducts ⃠ 2 Gallbladder ⃠ 3 Gallbladder and Bile Ducts ⃠ 5 Liver ⃠ 6 Liver and Spleen ⃠ 7 Pancreas ⃠ C Hepatobiliary System, All ⃠	Z None	Z None	Z None

⃠ BF40ZZZ BF42ZZZ BF43ZZZ BF45ZZZ BF46ZZZ BF47ZZZ BF4CZZZ

B Imaging
G Endocrine System
2 Computerized Tomography (CT Scan): Computer reformatted digital display of multiplanar images developed from the capture of multiple exposures of external ionizing radiation

Body Part Character 4	Contrast Character 5	Qualifier Character 6	Qualifier Character 7
2 Adrenal Glands, Bilateral ⃠ 3 Parathyroid Glands ⃠ 4 Thyroid Gland ⃠	0 High Osmolar 1 Low Osmolar Y Other Contrast	0 Unenhanced and Enhanced Z None	Z None
2 Adrenal Glands, Bilateral ⃠ 3 Parathyroid Glands ⃠ 4 Thyroid Gland ⃠	Z None	Z None	Z None

⃠ BG2200Z BG220ZZ BG2210Z BG221ZZ BG22Y0Z BG22YZZ BG22ZZZ BG2300Z BG230ZZ BG2310Z BG231ZZ BG23Y0Z BG23YZZ BG23ZZZ BG2400Z BG240ZZ BG2410Z BG241ZZ BG24Y0Z BG24YZZ BG24ZZZ

B Imaging
G Endocrine System
3 Magnetic Resonance Imaging (MRI): Computer reformatted digital display of multiplanar images developed from the capture of radiofrequency signals emitted by nuclei in a body site excited within a magnetic field

Body Part Character 4	Contrast Character 5	Qualifier Character 6	Qualifier Character 7
2 Adrenal Glands, Bilateral ⦸ **3** Parathyroid Glands ⦸ **4** Thyroid Gland ⦸	**Y** Other Contrast	**0** Unenhanced and Enhanced **Z** None	**Z** None
2 Adrenal Glands, Bilateral ⦸ **3** Parathyroid Glands ⦸ **4** Thyroid Gland ⦸	**Z** None	**Z** None	**Z** None

⦸ BG32Y0Z BG32YZZ BG32ZZZ BG33Y0Z BG33YZZ BG33ZZZ BG34Y0Z BG34YZZ BG34ZZZ

B Imaging
G Endocrine System
4 Ultrasonography: Real time display of images of anatomy or flow information developed from the capture of reflected and attenuated high frequency sound waves

Body Part Character 4	Contrast Character 5	Qualifier Character 6	Qualifier Character 7
0 Adrenal Gland, Right ⦸ **1** Adrenal Gland, Left ⦸ **2** Adrenal Glands, Bilateral ⦸ **3** Parathyroid Glands ⦸ **4** Thyroid Gland ⦸	**Z** None	**Z** None	**Z** None

⦸ BG40ZZZ BG41ZZZ BG42ZZZ BG43ZZZ BG44ZZZ

B Imaging
H Skin, Subcutaneous Tissue and Breast
0 Plain Radiography: Planar display of an image developed from the capture of external ionizing radiation on photographic or photoconductive plate

Body Part Character 4	Contrast Character 5	Qualifier Character 6	Qualifier Character 7
0 Breast, Right ⦸ **1** Breast, Left ⦸ **2** Breasts, Bilateral ⦸	**Z** None	**Z** None	**Z** None
3 Single Mammary Duct, Right ⦸ **4** Single Mammary Duct, Left ⦸ **5** Multiple Mammary Ducts, Right ⦸ **6** Multiple Mammary Ducts, Left ⦸	**0** High Osmolar **1** Low Osmolar **Y** Other Contrast **Z** None	**Z** None	**Z** None

⦸ BH00ZZZ BH01ZZZ BH02ZZZ BH030ZZ BH031ZZ BH03YZZ BH03ZZZ BH040ZZ BH041ZZ BH04YZZ BH04ZZZ BH050ZZ BH051ZZ BH05YZZ BH05ZZZ BH060ZZ BH061ZZ BH06YZZ BH06ZZZ

B Imaging
H Skin, Subcutaneous Tissue and Breast
3 Magnetic Resonance Imaging (MRI): Computer reformatted digital display of multiplanar images developed from the capture of radiofrequency signals emitted by nuclei in a body site excited within a magnetic field

Body Part Character 4	Contrast Character 5	Qualifier Character 6	Qualifier Character 7
0 Breast, Right ⃠ 1 Breast, Left ⃠ 2 Breasts, Bilateral ⃠ D Subcutaneous Tissue, Head/Neck ⃠ F Subcutaneous Tissue, Upper Extremity ⃠ G Subcutaneous Tissue, Thorax ⃠ H Subcutaneous Tissue, Abdomen and Pelvis ⃠ J Subcutaneous Tissue, Lower Extremity ⃠	Y Other Contrast	0 Unenhanced and Enhanced Z None	Z None
0 Breast, Right ⃠ 1 Breast, Left ⃠ 2 Breasts, Bilateral ⃠ D Subcutaneous Tissue, Head/Neck ⃠ F Subcutaneous Tissue, Upper Extremity ⃠ G Subcutaneous Tissue, Thorax ⃠ H Subcutaneous Tissue, Abdomen and Pelvis ⃠ J Subcutaneous Tissue, Lower Extremity ⃠	Z None	Z None	Z None

⃠ BH30Y0Z BH30YZZ BH30ZZZ BH31Y0Z BH31YZZ BH31ZZZ BH32Y0Z BH32YZZ BH32ZZZ BH3DY0Z BH3DYZZ BH3DZZZ BH3FY0Z BH3FYZZ BH3FZZZ BH3GY0Z BH3GYZZ BH3GZZZ BH3HY0Z BH3HYZZ BH3HZZZ BH3JY0Z BH3JYZZ BH3JZZZ

B Imaging
H Skin, Subcutaneous Tissue and Breast
4 Ultrasonography: Real time display of images of anatomy or flow information developed from the capture of reflected and attenuated high frequency sound waves

Body Part Character 4	Contrast Character 5	Qualifier Character 6	Qualifier Character 7
0 Breast, Right ⃠ 1 Breast, Left ⃠ 2 Breasts, Bilateral ⃠ 7 Extremity, Upper ⃠ 8 Extremity, Lower ⃠ 9 Abdominal Wall ⃠ B Chest Wall ⃠ C Head and Neck ⃠	Z None	Z None	Z None

⃠ BH40ZZZ BH41ZZZ BH42ZZZ BH47ZZZ BH48ZZZ BH49ZZZ BH4BZZZ BH4CZZZ

B Imaging
L Connective Tissue
3 Magnetic Resonance Imaging (MRI): Computer reformatted digital display of multiplanar images developed from the capture of radiofrequency signals emitted by nuclei in a body site excited within a magnetic field

Body Part Character 4	Contrast Character 5	Qualifier Character 6	Qualifier Character 7
0 Connective Tissue, Upper Extremity ⦸ **1** Connective Tissue, Lower Extremity ⦸ **2** Tendons, Upper Extremity ⦸ **3** Tendons, Lower Extremity ⦸	**Y** Other Contrast	**0** Unenhanced and Enhanced **Z** None	**Z** None
0 Connective Tissue, Upper Extremity ⦸ **1** Connective Tissue, Lower Extremity ⦸ **2** Tendons, Upper Extremity ⦸ **3** Tendons, Lower Extremity ⦸	**Z** None	**Z** None	**Z** None

⦸ BL30Y0Z BL30YZZ BL30ZZZ BL31Y0Z BL31YZZ BL31ZZZ BL32Y0Z BL32YZZ BL32ZZZ BL33Y0Z BL33YZZ BL33ZZZ

B Imaging
L Connective Tissue
4 Ultrasonography: Real time display of images of anatomy or flow information developed from the capture of reflected and attenuated high frequency sound waves

Body Part Character 4	Contrast Character 5	Qualifier Character 6	Qualifier Character 7
0 Connective Tissue, Upper Extremity ⦸ **1** Connective Tissue, Lower Extremity ⦸ **2** Tendons, Upper Extremity ⦸ **3** Tendons, Lower Extremity ⦸	**Z** None	**Z** None	**Z** None

⦸ BL40ZZZ BL41ZZZ BL42ZZZ BL43ZZZ

B Imaging
N Skull and Facial Bones
0 Plain Radiography: Planar display of an image developed from the capture of external ionizing radiation on photographic or photoconductive plate

Body Part Character 4	Contrast Character 5	Qualifier Character 6	Qualifier Character 7
0 Skull ⦸ **1** Orbit, Right ⦸ **2** Orbit, Left ⦸ **3** Orbits, Bilateral ⦸ **4** Nasal Bones ⦸ **5** Facial Bones ⦸ **6** Mandible ⦸ **B** Zygomatic Arch, Right ⦸ **C** Zygomatic Arch, Left ⦸ **D** Zygomatic Arches, Bilateral ⦸ **G** Tooth, Single ⦸ **H** Teeth, Multiple ⦸ **J** Teeth, All ⦸	**Z** None	**Z** None	**Z** None
7 Temporomandibular Joint, Right ⦸ **8** Temporomandibular Joint, Left ⦸ **9** Temporomandibular Joints, Bilateral ⦸	**0** High Osmolar **1** Low Osmolar **Y** Other Contrast **Z** None	**Z** None	**Z** None

⦸ BN00ZZZ BN01ZZZ BN02ZZZ BN03ZZZ BN04ZZZ BN05ZZZ BN06ZZZ BN070ZZ BN071ZZ BN07YZZ BN07ZZZ BN080ZZ BN081ZZ BN08YZZ BN08ZZZ BN090ZZ BN091ZZ BN09YZZ BN09ZZZ BN0BZZZ BN0CZZZ BN0DZZZ BN0GZZZ BN0HZZZ BN0JZZZ

B Imaging
N Skull and Facial Bones
1 Fluoroscopy: Single plane or bi-plane real time display of an image developed from the capture of external ionizing radiation on a fluorescent screen. The image may also be stored by either digital or analog means

Body Part Character 4	Contrast Character 5	Qualifier Character 6	Qualifier Character 7
7 Temporomandibular Joint, Right ⦸ **8** Temporomandibular Joint, Left ⦸ **9** Temporomandibular Joints, Bilateral ⦸	**0** High Osmolar **1** Low Osmolar **Y** Other Contrast **Z** None	**Z** None	**Z** None

⦸ BN170ZZ BN171ZZ BN17YZZ BN17ZZZ BN180ZZ BN181ZZ BN18YZZ BN18ZZZ BN190ZZ BN191ZZ BN19YZZ BN19ZZZ

B Imaging
N Skull and Facial Bones
2 Computerized Tomography (CT Scan): Computer reformatted digital display of multiplanar images developed from the capture of multiple exposures of external ionizing radiation

Body Part Character 4	Contrast Character 5	Qualifier Character 6	Qualifier Character 7
0 Skull ⦸ **3** Orbits, Bilateral ⦸ **5** Facial Bones ⦸ **6** Mandible ⦸ **9** Temporomandibular Joints, Bilateral ⦸ **F** Temporal Bones ⦸	**0** High Osmolar **1** Low Osmolar **Y** Other Contrast **Z** None	**Z** None	**Z** None

⦸ BN200ZZ BN201ZZ BN20YZZ BN20ZZZ BN230ZZ BN231ZZ BN23YZZ BN23ZZZ BN250ZZ BN251ZZ BN25YZZ BN25ZZZ BN260ZZ BN261ZZ BN26YZZ BN26ZZZ BN290ZZ BN291ZZ BN29YZZ BN29ZZZ BN2F0ZZ BN2F1ZZ BN2FYZZ BN2FZZZ

B Imaging
N Skull and Facial Bones
3 Magnetic Resonance Imaging (MRI): Computer reformatted digital display of multiplanar images developed from the capture of radiofrequency signals emitted by nuclei in a body site excited within a magnetic field

Body Part Character 4	Contrast Character 5	Qualifier Character 6	Qualifier Character 7
9 Temporomandibular Joints, Bilateral ⦸	**Y** Other Contrast **Z** None	**Z** None	**Z** None

⦸ BN39YZZ BN39ZZZ

B Imaging
P Non-Axial Upper Bones
0 Plain Radiography: Planar display of an image developed from the capture of external ionizing radiation on photographic or photoconductive plate

Body Part Character 4	Contrast Character 5	Qualifier Character 6	Qualifier Character 7
0 Sternoclavicular Joint, Right ⃠ **1** Sternoclavicular Joint, Left ⃠ **2** Sternoclavicular Joints, Bilateral ⃠ **3** Acromioclavicular Joints, Bilateral ⃠ **4** Clavicle, Right ⃠ **5** Clavicle, Left ⃠ **6** Scapula, Right ⃠ **7** Scapula, Left ⃠ **A** Humerus, Right ⃠ **B** Humerus, Left ⃠ **E** Upper Arm, Right ⃠ **F** Upper Arm, Left ⃠ **J** Forearm, Right ⃠ **K** Forearm, Left ⃠ **N** Hand, Right ⃠ **P** Hand, Left ⃠ **R** Finger(s), Right ⃠ **S** Finger(s), Left ⃠ **X** Ribs, Right ⃠ **Y** Ribs, Left ⃠	**Z** None	**Z** None	**Z** None
8 Shoulder, Right ⃠ **9** Shoulder, Left ⃠ **C** Hand/Finger Joint, Right ⃠ **D** Hand/Finger Joint, Left ⃠ **G** Elbow, Right ⃠ **H** Elbow, Left ⃠ **L** Wrist, Right ⃠ **M** Wrist, Left ⃠	**0** High Osmolar **1** Low Osmolar **Y** Other Contrast **Z** None	**Z** None	**Z** None

⃠ BP00ZZZ BP01ZZZ BP02ZZZ BP03ZZZ BP04ZZZ BP05ZZZ BP06ZZZ BP07ZZZ BP080ZZ BP081ZZ BP08YZZ BP08ZZZ BP090ZZ BP091ZZ BP09YZZ BP09ZZZ BP0AZZZ BP0BZZZ BP0C0ZZ BP0C1ZZ BP0CYZZ BP0CZZZ BP0D0ZZ BP0D1ZZ BP0DYZZ BP0DZZZ BP0EZZZ BP0FZZZ BP0G0ZZ BP0G1ZZ BP0GYZZ BP0GZZZ BP0H0ZZ BP0H1ZZ BP0HYZZ BP0HZZZ BP0JZZZ BP0KZZZ BP0L0ZZ BP0L1ZZ BP0LYZZ BP0LZZZ BP0M0ZZ BP0M1ZZ BP0MYZZ BP0MZZZ BP0NZZZ BP0PZZZ BP0RZZZ BP0SZZZ BP0XZZZ BP0YZZZ

B Imaging
P Non-Axial Upper Bones
1 Fluoroscopy: Single plane or bi-plane real time display of an image developed from the capture of external ionizing radiation on a fluorescent screen. The image may also be stored by either digital or analog means

Body Part Character 4	Contrast Character 5	Qualifier Character 6	Qualifier Character 7
0 Sternoclavicular Joint, Right ⦸ 1 Sternoclavicular Joint, Left ⦸ 2 Sternoclavicular Joints, Bilateral ⦸ 3 Acromioclavicular Joints, Bilateral ⦸ 4 Clavicle, Right ⦸ 5 Clavicle, Left ⦸ 6 Scapula, Right ⦸ 7 Scapula, Left ⦸ A Humerus, Right ⦸ B Humerus, Left ⦸ E Upper Arm, Right ⦸ F Upper Arm, Left ⦸ J Forearm, Right ⦸ K Forearm, Left ⦸ N Hand, Right ⦸ P Hand, Left ⦸ R Finger(s), Right ⦸ S Finger(s), Left ⦸ X Ribs, Right ⦸ Y Ribs, Left ⦸	Z None	Z None	Z None
8 Shoulder, Right ⦸ 9 Shoulder, Left ⦸ L Wrist, Right ⦸ M Wrist, Left ⦸	0 High Osmolar 1 Low Osmolar Y Other Contrast Z None	Z None	Z None
C Hand/Finger Joint, Right ⦸ D Hand/Finger Joint, Left ⦸ G Elbow, Right ⦸ H Elbow, Left ⦸	0 High Osmolar 1 Low Osmolar Y Other Contrast	Z None	Z None

⦸ BP10ZZZ BP11ZZZ BP12ZZZ BP13ZZZ BP14ZZZ BP15ZZZ BP16ZZZ BP17ZZZ BP180ZZ BP181ZZ BP18YZZ BP18ZZZ BP190ZZ BP191ZZ BP19YZZ BP19ZZZ BP1AZZZ BP1BZZZ BP1C0ZZ BP1C1ZZ BP1CYZZ BP1D0ZZ BP1D1ZZ BP1DYZZ BP1EZZZ BP1FZZZ BP1G0ZZ BP1G1ZZ BP1GYZZ BP1H0ZZ BP1H1ZZ BP1HYZZ BP1JZZZ BP1KZZZ BP1L0ZZ BP1L1ZZ BP1LYZZ BP1LZZZ BP1M0ZZ BP1M1ZZ BP1MYZZ BP1MZZZ BP1NZZZ BP1PZZZ BP1RZZZ BP1SZZZ BP1XZZZ BP1YZZZ

B Imaging
P Non-Axial Upper Bones
2 Computerized Tomography (CT Scan): Computer reformatted digital display of multiplanar images developed from the capture of multiple exposures of external ionizing radiation

Body Part Character 4	Contrast Character 5	Qualifier Character 6	Qualifier Character 7
0 Sternoclavicular Joint, Right ⦸ **1** Sternoclavicular Joint, Left ⦸ **W** Thorax ⦸	**0** High Osmolar **1** Low Osmolar **Y** Other Contrast	**Z** None	**Z** None
2 Sternoclavicular Joints, Bilateral ⦸ **3** Acromioclavicular Joints, Bilateral ⦸ **4** Clavicle, Right ⦸ **5** Clavicle, Left ⦸ **6** Scapula, Right ⦸ **7** Scapula, Left ⦸ **8** Shoulder, Right ⦸ **9** Shoulder, Left ⦸ **A** Humerus, Right ⦸ **B** Humerus, Left ⦸ **E** Upper Arm, Right ⦸ **F** Upper Arm, Left ⦸ **G** Elbow, Right ⦸ **H** Elbow, Left ⦸ **J** Forearm, Right ⦸ **K** Forearm, Left ⦸ **L** Wrist, Right ⦸ **M** Wrist, Left ⦸ **N** Hand, Right ⦸ **P** Hand, Left ⦸ **Q** Hands and Wrists, Bilateral ⦸ **R** Finger(s), Right ⦸ **S** Finger(s), Left ⦸ **T** Upper Extremity, Right ⦸ **U** Upper Extremity, Left ⦸ **V** Upper Extremities, Bilateral ⦸ **X** Ribs, Right ⦸ **Y** Ribs, Left ⦸	**0** High Osmolar **1** Low Osmolar **Y** Other Contrast **Z** None	**Z** None	**Z** None
C Hand/Finger Joint, Right ⦸ **D** Hand/Finger Joint, Left ⦸	**Z** None	**Z** None	**Z** None

⦸	BP200ZZ	BP201ZZ	BP20YZZ	BP210ZZ	BP211ZZ	BP21YZZ	BP220ZZ	BP221ZZ	BP22YZZ	BP22ZZZ	BP230ZZ	BP231ZZ	BP23YZZ
	BP23ZZZ	BP240ZZ	BP241ZZ	BP24YZZ	BP24ZZZ	BP250ZZ	BP251ZZ	BP25YZZ	BP25ZZZ	BP260ZZ	BP261ZZ	BP26YZZ	BP26ZZZ
	BP270ZZ	BP271ZZ	BP27YZZ	BP27ZZZ	BP280ZZ	BP281ZZ	BP28YZZ	BP28ZZZ	BP290ZZ	BP291ZZ	BP29YZZ	BP29ZZZ	BP2A0ZZ
	BP2A1ZZ	BP2AYZZ	BP2AZZZ	BP2B0ZZ	BP2B1ZZ	BP2BYZZ	BP2BZZZ	BP2CZZZ	BP2DZZZ	BP2E0ZZ	BP2E1ZZ	BP2EYZZ	BP2EZZZ
	BP2F0ZZ	BP2F1ZZ	BP2FYZZ	BP2FZZZ	BP2G0ZZ	BP2G1ZZ	BP2GYZZ	BP2GZZZ	BP2H0ZZ	BP2H1ZZ	BP2HYZZ	BP2HZZZ	BP2J0ZZ
	BP2J1ZZ	BP2JYZZ	BP2JZZZ	BP2K0ZZ	BP2K1ZZ	BP2KYZZ	BP2KZZZ	BP2L0ZZ	BP2L1ZZ	BP2LYZZ	BP2LZZZ	BP2M0ZZ	BP2M1ZZ
	BP2MYZZ	BP2MZZZ	BP2N0ZZ	BP2N1ZZ	BP2NYZZ	BP2NZZZ	BP2P0ZZ	BP2P1ZZ	BP2PYZZ	BP2PZZZ	BP2Q0ZZ	BP2Q1ZZ	BP2QYZZ
	BP2QZZZ	BP2R0ZZ	BP2R1ZZ	BP2RYZZ	BP2RZZZ	BP2S0ZZ	BP2S1ZZ	BP2SYZZ	BP2SZZZ	BP2T0ZZ	BP2T1ZZ	BP2TYZZ	BP2TZZZ
	BP2U0ZZ	BP2U1ZZ	BP2UYZZ	BP2UZZZ	BP2V0ZZ	BP2V1ZZ	BP2VYZZ	BP2VZZZ	BP2W0ZZ	BP2W1ZZ	BP2WYZZ	BP2X0ZZ	BP2X1ZZ
	BP2XYZZ	BP2XZZZ	BP2Y0ZZ	BP2Y1ZZ	BP2YYZZ	BP2YZZZ							

B Imaging
P Non-Axial Upper Bones
3 Magnetic Resonance Imaging (MRI): Computer reformatted digital display of multiplanar images developed from the capture of radiofrequency signals emitted by nuclei in a body site excited within a magnetic field

Body Part Character 4	Contrast Character 5	Qualifier Character 6	Qualifier Character 7
8 Shoulder, Right ⊘ **9** Shoulder, Left ⊘ **C** Hand/Finger Joint, Right ⊘ **D** Hand/Finger Joint, Left ⊘ **E** Upper Arm, Right ⊘ **F** Upper Arm, Left ⊘ **G** Elbow, Right ⊘ **H** Elbow, Left ⊘ **J** Forearm, Right ⊘ **K** Forearm, Left ⊘ **L** Wrist, Right ⊘ **M** Wrist, Left ⊘	**Y** Other Contrast	**0** Unenhanced and Enhanced **Z** None	**Z** None
8 Shoulder, Right ⊘ **9** Shoulder, Left ⊘ **C** Hand/Finger Joint, Right ⊘ **D** Hand/Finger Joint, Left ⊘ **E** Upper Arm, Right ⊘ **F** Upper Arm, Left ⊘ **G** Elbow, Right ⊘ **H** Elbow, Left ⊘ **J** Forearm, Right ⊘ **K** Forearm, Left ⊘ **L** Wrist, Right ⊘ **M** Wrist, Left ⊘	**Z** None	**Z** None	**Z** None

⊘ BP38Y0Z BP38YZZ BP38ZZZ BP39Y0Z BP39YZZ BP39ZZZ BP3CY0Z BP3CYZZ BP3CZZZ BP3DY0Z BP3DYZZ BP3DZZZ BP3EY0Z BP3EYZZ BP3EZZZ BP3FY0Z BP3FYZZ BP3FZZZ BP3GY0Z BP3GYZZ BP3GZZZ BP3HY0Z BP3HYZZ BP3HZZZ BP3JY0Z BP3JYZZ BP3JZZZ BP3KY0Z BP3KYZZ BP3KZZZ BP3LY0Z BP3LYZZ BP3LZZZ BP3MY0Z BP3MYZZ BP3MZZZ

B Imaging
P Non-Axial Upper Bones
4 Ultrasonography: Real time display of images of anatomy or flow information developed from the capture of reflected and attenuated high frequency sound waves

Body Part Character 4	Contrast Character 5	Qualifier Character 6	Qualifier Character 7
8 Shoulder, Right ⊘ **9** Shoulder, Left ⊘ **G** Elbow, Right ⊘ **H** Elbow, Left ⊘ **L** Wrist, Right ⊘ **M** Wrist, Left ⊘ **N** Hand, Right ⊘ **P** Hand, Left ⊘	**Z** None	**Z** None	**1** Densitometry **Z** None

⊘ BP48ZZ1 BP48ZZZ BP49ZZ1 BP49ZZZ BP4GZZ1 BP4GZZZ BP4HZZ1 BP4HZZZ BP4LZZ1 BP4LZZZ BP4MZZ1 BP4MZZZ BP4NZZ1 BP4NZZZ BP4PZZ1 BP4PZZZ

B Imaging
Q Non-Axial Lower Bones
0 Plain Radiography: Planar display of an image developed from the capture of external ionizing radiation on photographic or photoconductive plate

Body Part Character 4	Contrast Character 5	Qualifier Character 6	Qualifier Character 7
0 Hip, Right ⦸ **1** Hip, Left ⦸	**0** High Osmolar **1** Low Osmolar **Y** Other Contrast	**Z** None	**Z** None
0 Hip, Right ⦸ **1** Hip, Left ⦸	**Z** None	**Z** None	**1** Densitometry **Z** None
3 Femur, Right ⦸ **4** Femur, Left ⦸	**Z** None	**Z** None	**1** Densitometry **Z** None
7 Knee, Right ⦸ **8** Knee, Left ⦸ **G** Ankle, Right ⦸ **H** Ankle, Left ⦸	**0** High Osmolar **1** Low Osmolar **Y** Other Contrast **Z** None	**Z** None	**Z** None
D Lower Leg, Right ⦸ **F** Lower Leg, Left ⦸ **J** Calcaneus, Right ⦸ **K** Calcaneus, Left ⦸ **L** Foot, Right ⦸ **M** Foot, Left ⦸ **P** Toe(s), Right ⦸ **Q** Toe(s), Left ⦸ **V** Patella, Right ⦸ **W** Patella, Left ⦸	**Z** None	**Z** None	**Z** None
X Foot/Toe Joint, Right ⦸ **Y** Foot/Toe Joint, Left ⦸	**0** High Osmolar **1** Low Osmolar **Y** Other Contrast	**Z** None	**Z** None

⦸ BQ000ZZ BQ001ZZ BQ00YZZ BQ00ZZ1 BQ00ZZZ BQ010ZZ BQ011ZZ BQ01YZZ BQ01ZZ1 BQ01ZZZ BQ03ZZ1 BQ03ZZZ BQ04ZZ1 BQ04ZZZ BQ070ZZ BQ071ZZ BQ07YZZ BQ07ZZZ BQ080ZZ BQ081ZZ BQ08YZZ BQ08ZZZ BQ0DZZZ BQ0FZZZ BQ0G0ZZ BQ0G1ZZ BQ0GYZZ BQ0GZZZ BQ0H0ZZ BQ0H1ZZ BQ0HYZZ BQ0HZZZ BQ0JZZZ BQ0KZZZ BQ0LZZZ BQ0MZZZ BQ0PZZZ BQ0QZZZ BQ0VZZZ BQ0WZZZ BQ0X0ZZ BQ0X1ZZ BQ0XYZZ BQ0Y0ZZ BQ0Y1ZZ BQ0YYZZ

B Imaging
Q Non-Axial Lower Bones
1 Fluoroscopy: Single plane or bi-plane real time display of an image developed from the capture of external ionizing radiation on a fluorescent screen. The image may also be stored by either digital or analog means

Body Part Character 4	Contrast Character 5	Qualifier Character 6	Qualifier Character 7
0 Hip, Right ⦸ **1** Hip, Left ⦸ **7** Knee, Right ⦸ **8** Knee, Left ⦸ **G** Ankle, Right ⦸ **H** Ankle, Left ⦸ **X** Foot/Toe Joint, Right ⦸ **Y** Foot/Toe Joint, Left ⦸	**0** High Osmolar **1** Low Osmolar **Y** Other Contrast **Z** None	**Z** None	**Z** None
3 Femur, Right ⦸ **4** Femur, Left ⦸ **D** Lower Leg, Right ⦸ **F** Lower Leg, Left ⦸ **J** Calcaneus, Right ⦸ **K** Calcaneus, Left ⦸ **L** Foot, Right ⦸ **M** Foot, Left ⦸ **P** Toe(s), Right ⦸ **Q** Toe(s), Left ⦸ **V** Patella, Right ⦸ **W** Patella, Left ⦸	**Z** None	**Z** None	**Z** None

⦸ BQ100ZZ BQ101ZZ BQ10YZZ BQ10ZZZ BQ110ZZ BQ111ZZ BQ11YZZ BQ11ZZZ BQ13ZZZ BQ14ZZZ BQ170ZZ BQ171ZZ BQ17YZZ BQ17ZZZ BQ180ZZ BQ181ZZ BQ18YZZ BQ18ZZZ BQ1DZZZ BQ1FZZZ BQ1G0ZZ BQ1G1ZZ BQ1GYZZ BQ1GZZZ BQ1H0ZZ BQ1H1ZZ BQ1HYZZ BQ1HZZZ BQ1JZZZ BQ1KZZZ BQ1LZZZ BQ1MZZZ BQ1PZZZ BQ1QZZZ BQ1VZZZ BQ1WZZZ BQ1X0ZZ BQ1X1ZZ BQ1XYZZ BQ1XZZZ BQ1Y0ZZ BQ1Y1ZZ BQ1YYZZ BQ1YZZZ

B Imaging
Q Non-Axial Lower Bones
2 Computerized Tomography (CT Scan): Computer reformatted digital display of multiplanar images developed from the capture of multiple exposures of external ionizing radiation

Body Part Character 4	Contrast Character 5	Qualifier Character 6	Qualifier Character 7
0 Hip, Right ⊘ **1** Hip, Left ⊘ **3** Femur, Right ⊘ **4** Femur, Left ⊘ **7** Knee, Right ⊘ **8** Knee, Left ⊘ **D** Lower Leg, Right ⊘ **F** Lower Leg, Left ⊘ **G** Ankle, Right ⊘ **H** Ankle, Left ⊘ **J** Calcaneus, Right ⊘ **K** Calcaneus, Left ⊘ **L** Foot, Right ⊘ **M** Foot, Left ⊘ **P** Toe(s), Right ⊘ **Q** Toe(s), Left ⊘ **R** Lower Extremity, Right ⊘ **S** Lower Extremity, Left ⊘ **V** Patella, Right ⊘ **W** Patella, Left ⊘ **X** Foot/Toe Joint, Right ⊘ **Y** Foot/Toe Joint, Left ⊘	**0** High Osmolar **1** Low Osmolar **Y** Other Contrast **Z** None	**Z** None	**Z** None
B Tibia/Fibula, Right ⊘ **C** Tibia/Fibula, Left ⊘	**0** High Osmolar **1** Low Osmolar **Y** Other Contrast	**Z** None	**Z** None

⊘ BQ200ZZ BQ201ZZ BQ20YZZ BQ20ZZZ BQ210ZZ BQ211ZZ BQ21YZZ BQ21ZZZ BQ230ZZ BQ231ZZ BQ23YZZ BQ23ZZZ BQ240ZZ BQ241ZZ BQ24YZZ BQ24ZZZ BQ270ZZ BQ271ZZ BQ27YZZ BQ27ZZZ BQ280ZZ BQ281ZZ BQ28YZZ BQ28ZZZ BQ2B0ZZ BQ2B1ZZ BQ2BYZZ BQ2C0ZZ BQ2C1ZZ BQ2CYZZ BQ2D0ZZ BQ2D1ZZ BQ2DYZZ BQ2DZZZ BQ2F0ZZ BQ2F1ZZ BQ2FYZZ BQ2FZZZ BQ2G0ZZ BQ2G1ZZ BQ2GYZZ BQ2GZZZ BQ2H0ZZ BQ2H1ZZ BQ2HYZZ BQ2HZZZ BQ2J0ZZ BQ2J1ZZ BQ2JYZZ BQ2JZZZ BQ2K0ZZ BQ2K1ZZ BQ2KYZZ BQ2KZZZ BQ2L0ZZ BQ2L1ZZ BQ2LYZZ BQ2LZZZ BQ2M0ZZ BQ2M1ZZ BQ2MYZZ BQ2MZZZ BQ2P0ZZ BQ2P1ZZ BQ2PYZZ BQ2PZZZ BQ2Q0ZZ BQ2Q1ZZ BQ2QYZZ BQ2QZZZ BQ2R0ZZ BQ2R1ZZ BQ2RYZZ BQ2RZZZ BQ2S0ZZ BQ2S1ZZ BQ2SYZZ BQ2SZZZ BQ2V0ZZ BQ2V1ZZ BQ2VYZZ BQ2VZZZ BQ2W0ZZ BQ2W1ZZ BQ2WYZZ BQ2WZZZ BQ2X0ZZ BQ2X1ZZ BQ2XYZZ BQ2XZZZ BQ2Y0ZZ BQ2Y1ZZ BQ2YYZZ BQ2YZZZ

B Imaging
Q Non-Axial Lower Bones
3 Magnetic Resonance Imaging (MRI): Computer reformatted digital display of multiplanar images developed from the capture of radiofrequency signals emitted by nuclei in a body site excited within a magnetic field

Body Part Character 4	Contrast Character 5	Qualifier Character 6	Qualifier Character 7
0 Hip, Right ⦸ **1** Hip, Left ⦸ **3** Femur, Right ⦸ **4** Femur, Left ⦸ **7** Knee, Right ⦸ **8** Knee, Left ⦸ **D** Lower Leg, Right ⦸ **F** Lower Leg, Left ⦸ **G** Ankle, Right ⦸ **H** Ankle, Left ⦸ **J** Calcaneus, Right ⦸ **K** Calcaneus, Left ⦸ **L** Foot, Right ⦸ **M** Foot, Left ⦸ **P** Toe(s), Right ⦸ **Q** Toe(s), Left ⦸ **V** Patella, Right ⦸ **W** Patella, Left ⦸	**Y** Other Contrast	**0** Unenhanced and Enhanced **Z** None	**Z** None
0 Hip, Right ⦸ **1** Hip, Left ⦸ **3** Femur, Right ⦸ **4** Femur, Left ⦸ **7** Knee, Right ⦸ **8** Knee, Left ⦸ **D** Lower Leg, Right ⦸ **F** Lower Leg, Left ⦸ **G** Ankle, Right ⦸ **H** Ankle, Left ⦸ **J** Calcaneus, Right ⦸ **K** Calcaneus, Left ⦸ **L** Foot, Right ⦸ **M** Foot, Left ⦸ **P** Toe(s), Right ⦸ **Q** Toe(s), Left ⦸ **V** Patella, Right ⦸ **W** Patella, Left ⦸	**Z** None	**Z** None	**Z** None

⦸ BQ30Y0Z BQ30YZZ BQ30ZZZ BQ31Y0Z BQ31YZZ BQ31ZZZ BQ33Y0Z BQ33YZZ BQ33ZZZ BQ34Y0Z BQ34YZZ BQ34ZZZ BQ37Y0Z BQ37YZZ BQ37ZZZ BQ38Y0Z BQ38YZZ BQ38ZZZ BQ3DY0Z BQ3DYZZ BQ3DZZZ BQ3FY0Z BQ3FYZZ BQ3FZZZ BQ3GY0Z BQ3GYZZ BQ3GZZZ BQ3HY0Z BQ3HYZZ BQ3HZZZ BQ3JY0Z BQ3JYZZ BQ3JZZZ BQ3KY0Z BQ3KYZZ BQ3KZZZ BQ3LY0Z BQ3LYZZ BQ3LZZZ BQ3MY0Z BQ3MYZZ BQ3MZZZ BQ3PY0Z BQ3PYZZ BQ3PZZZ BQ3QY0Z BQ3QYZZ BQ3QZZZ BQ3VY0Z BQ3VYZZ BQ3VZZZ BQ3WY0Z BQ3WYZZ BQ3WZZZ

B Imaging
Q Non-Axial Lower Bones
4 Ultrasonography: Real time display of images of anatomy or flow information developed from the capture of reflected and attenuated high frequency sound waves

Body Part Character 4	Contrast Character 5	Qualifier Character 6	Qualifier Character 7
0 Hip, Right ⦸ **1** Hip, Left ⦸ **2** Hips, Bilateral ⦸ **7** Knee, Right ⦸ **8** Knee, Left ⦸ **9** Knees, Bilateral ⦸	**Z** None	**Z** None	**Z** None

⦸ BQ40ZZZ BQ41ZZZ BQ42ZZZ BQ47ZZZ BQ48ZZZ BQ49ZZZ

B Imaging
R Axial Skeleton, Except Skull and Facial Bones
0 Plain Radiography: Planar display of an image developed from the capture of external ionizing radiation on photographic or photoconductive plate

Body Part Character 4	Contrast Character 5	Qualifier Character 6	Qualifier Character 7
0 Cervical Spine ⃠ **7** Thoracic Spine ⃠ **9** Lumbar Spine ⃠ **G** Whole Spine ⃠	**Z** None	**Z** None	**1** Densitometry **Z** None
1 Cervical Disc(s) ⃠ **2** Thoracic Disc(s) ⃠ **3** Lumbar Disc(s) ⃠ **4** Cervical Facet Joint(s) ⃠ **5** Thoracic Facet Joint(s) ⃠ **6** Lumbar Facet Joint(s) ⃠ **D** Sacroiliac Joints ⃠	**0** High Osmolar **1** Low Osmolar **Y** Other Contrast **Z** None	**Z** None	**Z** None
8 Thoracolumbar Joint ⃠ **B** Lumbosacral Joint ⃠ **C** Pelvis ⃠ **F** Sacrum and Coccyx ⃠ **H** Sternum ⃠	**Z** None	**Z** None	**Z** None

⃠ BR00ZZ1 BR00ZZZ BR010ZZ BR011ZZ BR01YZZ BR01ZZZ BR020ZZ BR021ZZ BR02YZZ BR02ZZZ BR030ZZ BR031ZZ BR03YZZ BR03ZZZ BR040ZZ BR041ZZ BR04YZZ BR04ZZZ BR050ZZ BR051ZZ BR05YZZ BR05ZZZ BR060ZZ BR061ZZ BR06YZZ BR06ZZZ BR07ZZ1 BR07ZZZ BR08ZZZ BR09ZZ1 BR09ZZZ BR0BZZZ BR0CZZZ BR0D0ZZ BR0D1ZZ BR0DYZZ BR0DZZZ BR0FZZZ BR0GZZ1 BR0GZZZ BR0HZZZ

B Imaging
R Axial Skeleton, Except Skull and Facial Bones
1 Fluoroscopy: Single plane or bi-plane real time display of an image developed from the capture of external ionizing radiation on a fluorescent screen. The image may also be stored by either digital or analog means

Body Part Character 4	Contrast Character 5	Qualifier Character 6	Qualifier Character 7
0 Cervical Spine ⃠ **1** Cervical Disc(s) ⃠ **2** Thoracic Disc(s) ⃠ **3** Lumbar Disc(s) ⃠ **4** Cervical Facet Joint(s) ⃠ **5** Thoracic Facet Joint(s) ⃠ **6** Lumbar Facet Joint(s) ⃠ **7** Thoracic Spine ⃠ **8** Thoracolumbar Joint ⃠ **9** Lumbar Spine ⃠ **B** Lumbosacral Joint ⃠ **C** Pelvis ⃠ **D** Sacroiliac Joints ⃠ **F** Sacrum and Coccyx ⃠ **G** Whole Spine ⃠ **H** Sternum ⃠	**0** High Osmolar **1** Low Osmolar **Y** Other Contrast **Z** None	**Z** None	**Z** None

⃠ BR100ZZ BR101ZZ BR10YZZ BR10ZZZ BR110ZZ BR111ZZ BR11YZZ BR11ZZZ BR120ZZ BR121ZZ BR12YZZ BR12ZZZ BR130ZZ BR131ZZ BR13YZZ BR13ZZZ BR140ZZ BR141ZZ BR14YZZ BR14ZZZ BR150ZZ BR151ZZ BR15YZZ BR15ZZZ BR160ZZ BR161ZZ BR16YZZ BR16ZZZ BR170ZZ BR171ZZ BR17YZZ BR17ZZZ BR180ZZ BR181ZZ BR18YZZ BR18ZZZ BR190ZZ BR191ZZ BR19YZZ BR19ZZZ BR1B0ZZ BR1B1ZZ BR1BYZZ BR1BZZZ BR1C0ZZ BR1C1ZZ BR1CYZZ BR1CZZZ BR1D0ZZ BR1D1ZZ BR1DYZZ BR1DZZZ BR1F0ZZ BR1F1ZZ BR1FYZZ BR1FZZZ BR1G0ZZ BR1G1ZZ BR1GYZZ BR1GZZZ BR1H0ZZ BR1H1ZZ BR1HYZZ BR1HZZZ

B Imaging
R Axial Skeleton, Except Skull and Facial Bones
2 Computerized Tomography (CT Scan): Computer reformatted digital display of multiplanar images developed from the capture of multiple exposures of external ionizing radiation

Body Part Character 4	Contrast Character 5	Qualifier Character 6	Qualifier Character 7
0 Cervical Spine ⦸ **7** Thoracic Spine ⦸ **9** Lumbar Spine ⦸ **C** Pelvis ⦸ **D** Sacroiliac Joints ⦸ **F** Sacrum and Coccyx ⦸	**0** High Osmolar **1** Low Osmolar **Y** Other Contrast **Z** None	**Z** None	**Z** None

⦸ BR200ZZ BR201ZZ BR20YZZ BR20ZZZ BR270ZZ BR271ZZ BR27YZZ BR27ZZZ BR290ZZ BR291ZZ BR29YZZ BR29ZZZ BR2C0ZZ BR2C1ZZ BR2CYZZ BR2CZZZ BR2D0ZZ BR2D1ZZ BR2DYZZ BR2DZZZ BR2F0ZZ BR2F1ZZ BR2FYZZ BR2FZZZ

B Imaging
R Axial Skeleton, Except Skull and Facial Bones
3 Magnetic Resonance Imaging (MRI): Computer reformatted digital display of multiplanar images developed from the capture of radiofrequency signals emitted by nuclei in a body site excited within a magnetic field

Body Part Character 4	Contrast Character 5	Qualifier Character 6	Qualifier Character 7
0 Cervical Spine ⦸ **1** Cervical Disc(s) ⦸ **2** Thoracic Disc(s) ⦸ **3** Lumbar Disc(s) ⦸ **7** Thoracic Spine ⦸ **9** Lumbar Spine ⦸ **C** Pelvis ⦸ **F** Sacrum and Coccyx ⦸	**Y** Other Contrast	**0** Unenhanced and Enhanced **Z** None	**Z** None
0 Cervical Spine ⦸ **1** Cervical Disc(s) ⦸ **2** Thoracic Disc(s) ⦸ **3** Lumbar Disc(s) ⦸ **7** Thoracic Spine ⦸ **9** Lumbar Spine ⦸ **C** Pelvis ⦸ **F** Sacrum and Coccyx ⦸	**Z** None	**Z** None	**Z** None

⦸ BR30Y0Z BR30YZZ BR30ZZZ BR31Y0Z BR31YZZ BR31ZZZ BR32Y0Z BR32YZZ BR32ZZZ BR33Y0Z BR33YZZ BR33ZZZ BR37Y0Z BR37YZZ BR37ZZZ BR39Y0Z BR39YZZ BR39ZZZ BR3CY0Z BR3CYZZ BR3CZZZ BR3FY0Z BR3FYZZ BR3FZZZ

B Imaging
R Axial Skeleton, Except Skull and Facial Bones
4 Ultrasonography: Real time display of images of anatomy or flow information developed from the capture of reflected and attenuated high frequency sound waves

Body Part Character 4	Contrast Character 5	Qualifier Character 6	Qualifier Character 7
0 Cervical Spine ⦸ **7** Thoracic Spine ⦸ **9** Lumbar Spine ⦸ **F** Sacrum and Coccyx ⦸	**Z** None	**Z** None	**Z** None

⦸ BR40ZZZ BR47ZZZ BR49ZZZ BR4FZZZ

LC Limited Coverage NC Noncovered HAC HAC Associated Procedure CC Combination Cluster - See Appendix G for code lists
DRG Non-OR-Affecting MS-DRG Assignment ⦸ Non-OR-Not Affecting MS-DRG Assignment New/Revised Text in **Orange** ♂ Male ♀ Female

B Imaging
T Urinary System
0 Plain Radiography: Planar display of an image developed from the capture of external ionizing radiation on photographic or photoconductive plate

Body Part Character 4	Contrast Character 5	Qualifier Character 6	Qualifier Character 7
0 Bladder ⦸ **1** Kidney, Right ⦸ **2** Kidney, Left ⦸ **3** Kidneys, Bilateral ⦸ **4** Kidneys, Ureters and Bladder ⦸ **5** Urethra ⦸ **6** Ureter, Right ⦸ **7** Ureter, Left ⦸ **8** Ureters, Bilateral ⦸ **B** Bladder and Urethra ⦸ **C** Ileal Diversion Loop ⦸	**0** High Osmolar **1** Low Osmolar **Y** Other Contrast **Z** None	**Z** None	**Z** None

⦸ BT000ZZ BT001ZZ BT00YZZ BT00ZZZ BT010ZZ BT011ZZ BT01YZZ BT01ZZZ BT020ZZ BT021ZZ BT02YZZ BT02ZZZ BT030ZZ BT031ZZ BT03YZZ BT03ZZZ BT040ZZ BT041ZZ BT04YZZ BT04ZZZ BT050ZZ BT051ZZ BT05YZZ BT05ZZZ BT060ZZ BT061ZZ BT06YZZ BT06ZZZ BT070ZZ BT071ZZ BT07YZZ BT07ZZZ BT080ZZ BT081ZZ BT08YZZ BT08ZZZ BT0B0ZZ BT0B1ZZ BT0BYZZ BT0BZZZ BT0C0ZZ BT0C1ZZ BT0CYZZ BT0CZZZ

B Imaging
T Urinary System
1 Fluoroscopy: Single plane or bi-plane real time display of an image developed from the capture of external ionizing radiation on a fluorescent screen. The image may also be stored by either digital or analog means

Body Part Character 4	Contrast Character 5	Qualifier Character 6	Qualifier Character 7
0 Bladder ⦸ **1** Kidney, Right ⦸ **2** Kidney, Left ⦸ **3** Kidneys, Bilateral ⦸ **4** Kidneys, Ureters and Bladder ⦸ **5** Urethra ⦸ **6** Ureter, Right ⦸ **7** Ureter, Left ⦸ **B** Bladder and Urethra ⦸ **C** Ileal Diversion Loop ⦸ **D** Kidney, Ureter and Bladder, Right ⦸ **F** Kidney, Ureter and Bladder, Left ⦸ **G** Ileal Loop, Ureters and Kidneys ⦸	**0** High Osmolar **1** Low Osmolar **Y** Other Contrast **Z** None	**Z** None	**Z** None

⦸ BT100ZZ BT101ZZ BT10YZZ BT10ZZZ BT110ZZ BT111ZZ BT11YZZ BT11ZZZ BT120ZZ BT121ZZ BT12YZZ BT12ZZZ BT130ZZ BT131ZZ BT13YZZ BT13ZZZ BT140ZZ BT141ZZ BT14YZZ BT14ZZZ BT150ZZ BT151ZZ BT15YZZ BT15ZZZ BT160ZZ BT161ZZ BT16YZZ BT16ZZZ BT170ZZ BT171ZZ BT17YZZ BT17ZZZ BT1B0ZZ BT1B1ZZ BT1BYZZ BT1BZZZ BT1C0ZZ BT1C1ZZ BT1CYZZ BT1CZZZ BT1D0ZZ BT1D1ZZ BT1DYZZ BT1DZZZ BT1F0ZZ BT1F1ZZ BT1FYZZ BT1FZZZ BT1G0ZZ BT1G1ZZ BT1GYZZ BT1GZZZ

B Imaging
T Urinary System
2 Computerized Tomography (CT Scan): Computer reformatted digital display of multiplanar images developed from the capture of multiple exposures of external ionizing radiation

Body Part Character 4	Contrast Character 5	Qualifier Character 6	Qualifier Character 7
0 Bladder ⃠ 1 Kidney, Right ⃠ 2 Kidney, Left ⃠ 3 Kidneys, Bilateral ⃠ 9 Kidney Transplant ⃠	0 High Osmolar 1 Low Osmolar Y Other Contrast	0 Unenhanced and Enhanced Z None	Z None
0 Bladder ⃠ 1 Kidney, Right ⃠ 2 Kidney, Left ⃠ 3 Kidneys, Bilateral ⃠ 9 Kidney Transplant ⃠	Z None	Z None	Z None

⃠ BT2000Z BT200ZZ BT2010Z BT201ZZ BT20Y0Z BT20YZZ BT20ZZZ BT2100Z BT210ZZ BT2110Z BT211ZZ BT21Y0Z BT21YZZ BT21ZZZ BT2200Z BT220ZZ BT2210Z BT221ZZ BT22Y0Z BT22YZZ BT22ZZZ BT2300Z BT230ZZ BT2310Z BT231ZZ BT23Y0Z BT23YZZ BT23ZZZ BT2900Z BT290ZZ BT2910Z BT291ZZ BT29Y0Z BT29YZZ BT29ZZZ

B Imaging
T Urinary System
3 Magnetic Resonance Imaging (MRI): Computer reformatted digital display of multiplanar images developed from the capture of radiofrequency signals emitted by nuclei in a body site excited within a magnetic field

Body Part Character 4	Contrast Character 5	Qualifier Character 6	Qualifier Character 7
0 Bladder ⃠ 1 Kidney, Right ⃠ 2 Kidney, Left ⃠ 3 Kidneys, Bilateral ⃠ 9 Kidney Transplant ⃠	Y Other Contrast	0 Unenhanced and Enhanced Z None	Z None
0 Bladder ⃠ 1 Kidney, Right ⃠ 2 Kidney, Left ⃠ 3 Kidneys, Bilateral ⃠ 9 Kidney Transplant ⃠	Z None	Z None	Z None

⃠ BT30Y0Z BT30YZZ BT30ZZZ BT31Y0Z BT31YZZ BT31ZZZ BT32Y0Z BT32YZZ BT32ZZZ BT33Y0Z BT33YZZ BT33ZZZ BT39Y0Z BT39YZZ BT39ZZZ

B Imaging
T Urinary System
4 Ultrasonography: Real time display of images of anatomy or flow information developed from the capture of reflected and attenuated high frequency sound waves

Body Part Character 4	Contrast Character 5	Qualifier Character 6	Qualifier Character 7
0 Bladder ⃠ 1 Kidney, Right ⃠ 2 Kidney, Left ⃠ 3 Kidneys, Bilateral ⃠ 5 Urethra ⃠ 6 Ureter, Right ⃠ 7 Ureter, Left ⃠ 8 Ureters, Bilateral ⃠ 9 Kidney Transplant ⃠ J Kidneys and Bladder ⃠	Z None	Z None	Z None

⃠ BT40ZZZ BT41ZZZ BT42ZZZ BT43ZZZ BT45ZZZ BT46ZZZ BT47ZZZ BT48ZZZ BT49ZZZ BT4JZZZ

B Imaging
U Female Reproductive System
0 Plain Radiography: Planar display of an image developed from the capture of external ionizing radiation on photographic or photoconductive plate

Body Part Character 4	Contrast Character 5	Qualifier Character 6	Qualifier Character 7
0 Fallopian Tube, Right ⦸ ♀ **1** Fallopian Tube, Left ⦸ ♀ **2** Fallopian Tubes, Bilateral ⦸ ♀ **6** Uterus ⦸ ♀ **8** Uterus and Fallopian Tubes ⦸ ♀ **9** Vagina ⦸ ♀	**0** High Osmolar **1** Low Osmolar **Y** Other Contrast	**Z** None	**Z** None

♀ BU000ZZ BU001ZZ BU00YZZ BU010ZZ BU011ZZ BU01YZZ BU020ZZ BU021ZZ BU02YZZ BU060ZZ BU061ZZ BU06YZZ BU080ZZ BU081ZZ BU08YZZ BU090ZZ BU091ZZ BU09YZZ

⦸ BU000ZZ BU001ZZ BU00YZZ BU010ZZ BU011ZZ BU01YZZ BU020ZZ BU021ZZ BU02YZZ BU060ZZ BU061ZZ BU06YZZ BU080ZZ BU081ZZ BU08YZZ BU090ZZ BU091ZZ BU09YZZ

B Imaging
U Female Reproductive System
1 Fluoroscopy: Single plane or bi-plane real time display of an image developed from the capture of external ionizing radiation on a fluorescent screen. The image may also be stored by either digital or analog means

Body Part Character 4	Contrast Character 5	Qualifier Character 6	Qualifier Character 7
0 Fallopian Tube, Right ⦸ ♀ **1** Fallopian Tube, Left ⦸ ♀ **2** Fallopian Tubes, Bilateral ⦸ ♀ **6** Uterus ⦸ ♀ **8** Uterus and Fallopian Tubes ⦸ ♀ **9** Vagina ⦸ ♀	**0** High Osmolar **1** Low Osmolar **Y** Other Contrast **Z** None	**Z** None	**Z** None

♀ BU100ZZ BU101ZZ BU10YZZ BU10ZZZ BU110ZZ BU111ZZ BU11YZZ BU11ZZZ BU120ZZ BU121ZZ BU12YZZ BU12ZZZ BU160ZZ BU161ZZ BU16YZZ BU16ZZZ BU180ZZ BU181ZZ BU18YZZ BU18ZZZ BU190ZZ BU191ZZ BU19YZZ BU19ZZZ

⦸ BU100ZZ BU101ZZ BU10YZZ BU10ZZZ BU110ZZ BU111ZZ BU11YZZ BU11ZZZ BU120ZZ BU121ZZ BU12YZZ BU12ZZZ BU160ZZ BU161ZZ BU16YZZ BU16ZZZ BU180ZZ BU181ZZ BU18YZZ BU18ZZZ BU190ZZ BU191ZZ BU19YZZ BU19ZZZ

B Imaging
U Female Reproductive System
3 Magnetic Resonance Imaging (MRI): Computer reformatted digital display of multiplanar images developed from the capture of radiofrequency signals emitted by nuclei in a body site excited within a magnetic field

Body Part Character 4	Contrast Character 5	Qualifier Character 6	Qualifier Character 7
3 Ovary, Right ⦸ ♀ **4** Ovary, Left ⦸ ♀ **5** Ovaries, Bilateral ⦸ ♀ **6** Uterus ⦸ ♀ **9** Vagina ⦸ ♀ **B** Pregnant Uterus ⦸ ♀ **C** Uterus and Ovaries ⦸ ♀	**Y** Other Contrast	**0** Unenhanced and Enhanced **Z** None	**Z** None
3 Ovary, Right ⦸ ♀ **4** Ovary, Left ⦸ ♀ **5** Ovaries, Bilateral ⦸ ♀ **6** Uterus ⦸ ♀ **9** Vagina ⦸ ♀ **B** Pregnant Uterus ⦸ ♀ **C** Uterus and Ovaries ⦸ ♀	**Z** None	**Z** None	**Z** None

♀ BU33Y0Z BU33YZZ BU33ZZZ BU34Y0Z BU34YZZ BU34ZZZ BU35Y0Z BU35YZZ BU35ZZZ BU36Y0Z BU36YZZ BU36ZZZ BU39Y0Z BU39YZZ BU39ZZZ BU3BY0Z BU3BYZZ BU3BZZZ BU3CY0Z BU3CYZZ BU3CZZZ

⦸ BU33Y0Z BU33YZZ BU33ZZZ BU34Y0Z BU34YZZ BU34ZZZ BU35Y0Z BU35YZZ BU35ZZZ BU36Y0Z BU36YZZ BU36ZZZ BU39Y0Z BU39YZZ BU39ZZZ BU3BY0Z BU3BYZZ BU3BZZZ BU3CY0Z BU3CYZZ BU3CZZZ

B Imaging
U Female Reproductive System
4 Ultrasonography: Real time display of images of anatomy or flow information developed from the capture of reflected and attenuated high frequency sound waves

Body Part Character 4	Contrast Character 5	Qualifier Character 6	Qualifier Character 7
0 Fallopian Tube, Right ⃠ ♀ 1 Fallopian Tube, Left ⃠ ♀ 2 Fallopian Tubes, Bilateral ⃠ ♀ 3 Ovary, Right ⃠ ♀ 4 Ovary, Left ⃠ ♀ 5 Ovaries, Bilateral ⃠ ♀ 6 Uterus ⃠ ♀ C Uterus and Ovaries ⃠ ♀	Y Other Contrast Z None	Z None	Z None

♀ BU40YZZ BU40ZZZ BU41YZZ BU41ZZZ BU42YZZ BU42ZZZ BU43YZZ BU43ZZZ BU44YZZ BU44ZZZ BU45YZZ BU45ZZZ BU46YZZ BU46ZZZ BU4CYZZ BU4CZZZ
⃠ BU40YZZ BU40ZZZ BU41YZZ BU41ZZZ BU42YZZ BU42ZZZ BU43YZZ BU43ZZZ BU44YZZ BU44ZZZ BU45YZZ BU45ZZZ BU46YZZ BU46ZZZ BU4CYZZ BU4CZZZ

B Imaging
V Male Reproductive System
0 Plain Radiography: Planar display of an image developed from the capture of external ionizing radiation on photographic or photoconductive plate

Body Part Character 4	Contrast Character 5	Qualifier Character 6	Qualifier Character 7
0 Corpora Cavernosa ⃠ ♂ 1 Epididymis, Right ⃠ ♂ 2 Epididymis, Left ⃠ ♂ 3 Prostate ⃠ ♂ 5 Testicle, Right ⃠ ♂ 6 Testicle, Left ⃠ ♂ 8 Vasa Vasorum ⃠ ♂	0 High Osmolar 1 Low Osmolar Y Other Contrast	Z None	Z None

♂ BV000ZZ BV001ZZ BV00YZZ BV010ZZ BV011ZZ BV01YZZ BV020ZZ BV021ZZ BV02YZZ BV030ZZ BV031ZZ BV03YZZ BV050ZZ BV051ZZ BV05YZZ BV060ZZ BV061ZZ BV06YZZ BV080ZZ BV081ZZ BV08YZZ
⃠ BV000ZZ BV001ZZ BV00YZZ BV010ZZ BV011ZZ BV01YZZ BV020ZZ BV021ZZ BV02YZZ BV030ZZ BV031ZZ BV03YZZ BV050ZZ BV051ZZ BV05YZZ BV060ZZ BV061ZZ BV06YZZ BV080ZZ BV081ZZ BV08YZZ

B Imaging
V Male Reproductive System
1 Fluoroscopy: Single plane or bi-plane real time display of an image developed from the capture of external ionizing radiation on a fluorescent screen. The image may also be stored by either digital or analog means

Body Part Character 4	Contrast Character 5	Qualifier Character 6	Qualifier Character 7
0 Corpora Cavernosa ⃠ ♂ 8 Vasa Vasorum ⃠ ♂	0 High Osmolar 1 Low Osmolar Y Other Contrast Z None	Z None	Z None

♂ BV100ZZ BV101ZZ BV10YZZ BV10ZZZ BV180ZZ BV181ZZ BV18YZZ BV18ZZZ
⃠ BV100ZZ BV101ZZ BV10YZZ BV10ZZZ BV180ZZ BV181ZZ BV18YZZ BV18ZZZ

B Imaging
V Male Reproductive System
2 Computerized Tomography (CT Scan): Computer reformatted digital display of multiplanar images developed from the capture of multiple exposures of external ionizing radiation

Body Part Character 4	Contrast Character 5	Qualifier Character 6	Qualifier Character 7
3 Prostate ⃠ ♂	0 High Osmolar 1 Low Osmolar Y Other Contrast	0 Unenhanced and Enhanced Z None	Z None
3 Prostate ⃠ ♂	Z None	Z None	Z None

♂ BV2300Z BV230ZZ BV2310Z BV23Y0Z BV23YZZ BV23ZZZ
⃠ BV2300Z BV230ZZ BV2310Z BV231ZZ BV23Y0Z BV23YZZ BV23ZZZ

LC Limited Coverage NC Noncovered HAC HAC Associated Procedure CC Combination Cluster - See Appendix G for code lists
DRG Non-OR-Affecting MS-DRG Assignment ⃠ Non-OR-Not Affecting MS-DRG Assignment New/Revised Text in Orange ♂ Male ♀ Female

B Imaging
V Male Reproductive System
3 Magnetic Resonance Imaging (MRI): Computer reformatted digital display of multiplanar images developed from the capture of radiofrequency signals emitted by nuclei in a body site excited within a magnetic field

Body Part Character 4	Contrast Character 5	Qualifier Character 6	Qualifier Character 7
0 Corpora Cavernosa ⦸ ♂ **3** Prostate ⦸ ♂ **4** Scrotum ⦸ ♂ **5** Testicle, Right ⦸ ♂ **6** Testicle, Left ⦸ ♂ **7** Testicles, Bilateral ⦸ ♂	**Y** Other Contrast	**0** Unenhanced and Enhanced **Z** None	**Z** None
0 Corpora Cavernosa ⦸ ♂ **3** Prostate ⦸ ♂ **4** Scrotum ⦸ ♂ **5** Testicle, Right ⦸ ♂ **6** Testicle, Left ⦸ ♂ **7** Testicles, Bilateral ⦸ ♂	**Z** None	**Z** None	**Z** None

♂ BV30Y0Z BV30YZZ BV30ZZZ BV33Y0Z BV33YZZ BV33ZZZ BV34Y0Z BV34YZZ BV34ZZZ BV35Y0Z BV35YZZ BV35ZZZ BV36Y0Z BV36YZZ BV36ZZZ BV37Y0Z BV37YZZ BV37ZZZ

⦸ BV30Y0Z BV30YZZ BV30ZZZ BV33Y0Z BV33YZZ BV33ZZZ BV34Y0Z BV34YZZ BV34ZZZ BV35Y0Z BV35YZZ BV35ZZZ BV36Y0Z BV36YZZ BV36ZZZ BV37Y0Z BV37YZZ BV37ZZZ

B Imaging
V Male Reproductive System
4 Ultrasonography: Real time display of images of anatomy or flow information developed from the capture of reflected and attenuated high frequency sound waves

Body Part Character 4	Contrast Character 5	Qualifier Character 6	Qualifier Character 7
4 Scrotum ⦸ ♂ **9** Prostate and Seminal Vesicles ⦸ ♂ **B** Penis ⦸ ♂	**Z** None	**Z** None	**Z** None

♂ BV44ZZZ BV49ZZZ BV4BZZZ

⦸ BV44ZZZ BV49ZZZ BV4BZZZ

B Imaging
W Anatomical Regions
0 Plain Radiography: Planar display of an image developed from the capture of external ionizing radiation on photographic or photoconductive plate

Body Part Character 4	Contrast Character 5	Qualifier Character 6	Qualifier Character 7
0 Abdomen ⦸ **1** Abdomen and Pelvis ⦸ **3** Chest ⦸ **B** Long Bones, All ⦸ **C** Lower Extremity ⦸ **J** Upper Extremity ⦸ **K** Whole Body ⦸ **L** Whole Skeleton ⦸ **M** Whole Body, Infant ⦸	**Z** None	**Z** None	**Z** None

⦸ BW00ZZZ BW01ZZZ BW03ZZZ BW0BZZZ BW0CZZZ BW0JZZZ BW0KZZZ BW0LZZZ BW0MZZZ

B Imaging
W Anatomical Regions
1 Fluoroscopy: Single plane or bi-plane real time display of an image developed from the capture of external ionizing radiation on a fluorescent screen. The image may also be stored by either digital or analog means

Body Part Character 4	Contrast Character 5	Qualifier Character 6	Qualifier Character 7
1 Abdomen and Pelvis ⊘ 9 Head and Neck ⊘ C Lower Extremity ⊘ J Upper Extremity ⊘	0 High Osmolar 1 Low Osmolar Y Other Contrast Z None	Z None	Z None

⊘ BW110ZZ BW111ZZ BW11YZZ BW11ZZZ BW190ZZ BW191ZZ BW19YZZ BW19ZZZ BW1C0ZZ BW1C1ZZ BW1CYZZ BW1CZZZ BW1J0ZZ BW1J1ZZ BW1JYZZ BW1JZZZ

B Imaging
W Anatomical Regions
2 Computerized Tomography (CT Scan): Computer reformatted digital display of multiplanar images developed from the capture of multiple exposures of external ionizing radiation

Body Part Character 4	Contrast Character 5	Qualifier Character 6	Qualifier Character 7
0 Abdomen ⊘ 1 Abdomen and Pelvis ⊘ 4 Chest and Abdomen ⊘ 5 Chest, Abdomen and Pelvis ⊘ 8 Head ⊘ 9 Head and Neck ⊘ F Neck ⊘ G Pelvic Region ⊘	0 High Osmolar 1 Low Osmolar Y Other Contrast	0 Unenhanced and Enhanced Z None	Z None
0 Abdomen ⊘ 1 Abdomen and Pelvis ⊘ 4 Chest and Abdomen ⊘ 5 Chest, Abdomen and Pelvis ⊘ 8 Head ⊘ 9 Head and Neck ⊘ F Neck ⊘ G Pelvic Region ⊘	Z None	Z None	Z None

⊘ BW2000Z BW200ZZ BW2010Z BW201ZZ BW20Y0Z BW20YZZ BW20ZZZ BW2100Z BW210ZZ BW2110Z BW211ZZ BW21Y0Z BW21YZZ BW21ZZZ BW2400Z BW240ZZ BW2410Z BW241ZZ BW24Y0Z BW24YZZ BW24ZZZ BW2500Z BW250ZZ BW2510Z BW251ZZ BW25Y0Z BW25YZZ BW25ZZZ BW2800Z BW280ZZ BW2810Z BW281ZZ BW28Y0Z BW28YZZ BW28ZZZ BW2900Z BW290ZZ BW2910Z BW291ZZ BW29Y0Z BW29YZZ BW29ZZZ BW2F00Z BW2F0ZZ BW2F10Z BW2F1ZZ BW2FY0Z BW2FYZZ BW2FZZZ BW2G00Z BW2G0ZZ BW2G10Z BW2G1ZZ BW2GY0Z BW2GYZZ BW2GZZZ

B Imaging
W Anatomical Regions
3 Magnetic Resonance Imaging (MRI): Computer reformatted digital display of multiplanar images developed from the capture of radiofrequency signals emitted by nuclei in a body site excited within a magnetic field

Body Part Character 4	Contrast Character 5	Qualifier Character 6	Qualifier Character 7
0 Abdomen ⊘ 8 Head ⊘ F Neck ⊘ G Pelvic Region ⊘ H Retroperitoneum ⊘ P Brachial Plexus ⊘	Y Other Contrast	0 Unenhanced and Enhanced Z None	Z None
0 Abdomen ⊘ 8 Head ⊘ F Neck ⊘ G Pelvic Region ⊘ H Retroperitoneum ⊘ P Brachial Plexus ⊘	Z None	Z None	Z None
3 Chest ⊘	Y Other Contrast	0 Unenhanced and Enhanced Z None	Z None

⊘ BW30Y0Z BW30YZZ BW30ZZZ BW33Y0Z BW33YZZ BW38Y0Z BW38YZZ BW38ZZZ BW3FY0Z BW3FYZZ BW3FZZZ BW3GY0Z BW3GYZZ BW3GZZZ BW3HY0Z BW3HYZZ BW3HZZZ BW3PY0Z BW3PYZZ BW3PZZZ

LC Limited Coverage NC Noncovered HAC HAC Associated Procedure CC Combination Cluster - See Appendix G for code lists
DRG Non-OR-Affecting MS-DRG Assignment ⊘ Non-OR-Not Affecting MS-DRG Assignment New/Revised Text in **Orange** ♂ Male ♀ Female

B Imaging
W Anatomical Regions
4 Ultrasonography: Real time display of images of anatomy or flow information developed from the capture of reflected and attenuated high frequency sound waves

Body Part Character 4	Contrast Character 5	Qualifier Character 6	Qualifier Character 7
0 Abdomen ⃠ 1 Abdomen and Pelvis ⃠ F Neck ⃠ G Pelvic Region ⃠	Z None	Z None	Z None

⃠ BW40ZZZ BW41ZZZ BW4FZZZ BW4GZZZ

B Imaging
Y Fetus and Obstetrical
3 Magnetic Resonance Imaging (MRI): Computer reformatted digital display of multiplanar images developed from the capture of radiofrequency signals emitted by nuclei in a body site excited within a magnetic field

Body Part Character 4	Contrast Character 5	Qualifier Character 6	Qualifier Character 7
0 Fetal Head ⃠ ♀ 1 Fetal Heart ⃠ ♀ 2 Fetal Thorax ⃠ ♀ 3 Fetal Abdomen ⃠ ♀ 4 Fetal Spine ⃠ ♀ 5 Fetal Extremities ⃠ ♀ 6 Whole Fetus ⃠ ♀	Y Other Contrast	0 Unenhanced and Enhanced Z None	Z None
0 Fetal Head ⃠ ♀ 1 Fetal Heart ⃠ ♀ 2 Fetal Thorax ⃠ ♀ 3 Fetal Abdomen ⃠ ♀ 4 Fetal Spine ⃠ ♀ 5 Fetal Extremities ⃠ ♀ 6 Whole Fetus ⃠ ♀	Z None	Z None	Z None

♀ BY30Y0Z BY30YZZ BY30ZZZ BY31Y0Z BY31YZZ BY31ZZZ BY32Y0Z BY32YZZ BY32ZZZ BY33Y0Z BY33YZZ BY33ZZZ BY34YZZ BY34ZZZ BY35Y0Z BY35YZZ BY35ZZZ BY36Y0Z BY36YZZ BY36ZZZ

⃠ BY30Y0Z BY30YZZ BY30ZZZ BY31Y0Z BY31YZZ BY31ZZZ BY32Y0Z BY32YZZ BY32ZZZ BY33Y0Z BY33YZZ BY33ZZZ BY34Y0Z BY34YZZ BY34ZZZ BY35Y0Z BY35YZZ BY35ZZZ BY36Y0Z BY36YZZ BY36ZZZ

B Imaging
Y Fetus and Obstetrical
4 Ultrasonography: Real time display of images of anatomy or flow information developed from the capture of reflected and attenuated high frequency sound waves

Body Part Character 4	Contrast Character 5	Qualifier Character 6	Qualifier Character 7
7 Fetal Umbilical Cord ⃠ ♀ 8 Placenta ⃠ ♀ 9 First Trimester, Single Fetus ⃠ ♀ B First Trimester, Multiple Gestation ⃠ ♀ C Second Trimester, Single Fetus ⃠ ♀ D Second Trimester, Multiple Gestation ⃠ ♀ F Third Trimester, Single Fetus ⃠ ♀ G Third Trimester, Multiple Gestation ⃠ ♀	Z None	Z None	Z None

♀ BY47ZZZ BY48ZZZ BY49ZZZ BY4BZZZ BY4CZZZ BY4DZZZ BY4FZZZ BY4GZZZ

⃠ BY47ZZZ BY48ZZZ BY49ZZZ BY4BZZZ BY4CZZZ BY4DZZZ BY4FZZZ BY4GZZZ

Nuclear Medicine C01-CW7

C Nuclear Medicine
0 Central Nervous System
1 Planar Nuclear Medicine Imaging: Introduction of radioactive materials into the body for single plane display of images developed from the capture of radioactive emissions

Body Part Character 4	Radionuclide Character 5	Qualifier Character 6	Qualifier Character 7
0 Brain ⦸	**1** Technetium 99m (Tc-99m) **Y** Other Radionuclide	**Z** None	**Z** None
5 Cerebrospinal Fluid ⦸	**D** Indium 111 (In-111) **Y** Other Radionuclide	**Z** None	**Z** None
Y Central Nervous System ⦸	**Y** Other Radionuclide	**Z** None	**Z** None

⦸ C0101ZZ C010YZZ C015DZZ C015YZZ C01YYZZ

C Nuclear Medicine
0 Central Nervous System
2 Tomographic (Tomo) Nuclear Medicine Imaging: Introduction of radioactive materials into the body for three dimensional display of images developed from the capture of radioactive emissions

Body Part Character 4	Radionuclide Character 5	Qualifier Character 6	Qualifier Character 7
0 Brain ⦸	**1** Technetium 99m (Tc-99m) **F** Iodine 123 (I-123) **S** Thallium 201 (Tl-201) **Y** Other Radionuclide	**Z** None	**Z** None
5 Cerebrospinal Fluid ⦸	**D** Indium 111 (In-111) **Y** Other Radionuclide	**Z** None	**Z** None
Y Central Nervous System ⦸	**Y** Other Radionuclide	**Z** None	**Z** None

⦸ C0201ZZ C020FZZ C020SZZ C020YZZ C025DZZ C025YZZ C02YYZZ

C Nuclear Medicine
0 Central Nervous System
3 Positron Emission Tomographic (PET) Imaging: Introduction of radioactive materials into the body for three dimensional display of images developed from the simultaneous capture, 180 degrees apart, of radioactive emissions

Body Part Character 4	Radionuclide Character 5	Qualifier Character 6	Qualifier Character 7
0 Brain ⦸	**B** Carbon 11 (C-11) **K** Fluorine 18 (F-18) **M** Oxygen 15 (O-15) **Y** Other Radionuclide	**Z** None	**Z** None
Y Central Nervous System ⦸	**Y** Other Radionuclide	**Z** None	**Z** None

⦸ C030BZZ C030KZZ C030MZZ C030YZZ C03YYZZ

C Nuclear Medicine
0 Central Nervous System
5 Nonimaging Nuclear Medicine Probe: Introduction of radioactive materials into the body for the study of distribution and fate of certain substances by the detection of radioactive emissions; or, alternatively, measurement of absorption of radioactive emissions from an external source

Body Part Character 4	Radionuclide Character 5	Qualifier Character 6	Qualifier Character 7
0 Brain ⦸	**V** Xenon 133 (Xe-133) **Y** Other Radionuclide	**Z** None	**Z** None
Y Central Nervous System ⦸	**Y** Other Radionuclide	**Z** None	**Z** None

⦸ C050VZZ C050YZZ C05YYZZ

LC Limited Coverage NC Noncovered HAC HAC Associated Procedure CC Combination Cluster - See Appendix G for code lists
DRG Non-OR-Affecting MS-DRG Assignment ⦸ Non-OR-Not Affecting MS-DRG Assignment New/Revised Text in **Orange** ♂ Male ♀ Female

C Nuclear Medicine
2 Heart
1 Planar Nuclear Medicine Imaging: Introduction of radioactive materials into the body for single plane display of images developed from the capture of radioactive emissions

Body Part Character 4	Radionuclide Character 5	Qualifier Character 6	Qualifier Character 7
6 Heart, Right and Left ⃠	**1** Technetium 99m (Tc-99m) **Y** Other Radionuclide	**Z** None	**Z** None
G Myocardium ⃠	**1** Technetium 99m (Tc-99m) **D** Indium 111 (In-111) **S** Thallium 201 (Tl-201) **Y** Other Radionuclide **Z** None	**Z** None	**Z** None
Y Heart ⃠	**Y** Other Radionuclide	**Z** None	**Z** None

⃠ C2161ZZ C216YZZ C21G1ZZ C21GDZZ C21GSZZ C21GYZZ C21GZZZ C21YYZZ

C Nuclear Medicine
2 Heart
2 Tomographic (Tomo) Nuclear Medicine Imaging: Introduction of radioactive materials into the body for three dimensional display of images developed from the capture of radioactive emissions

Body Part Character 4	Radionuclide Character 5	Qualifier Character 6	Qualifier Character 7
6 Heart, Right and Left ⃠	**1** Technetium 99m (Tc-99m) **Y** Other Radionuclide	**Z** None	**Z** None
G Myocardium ⃠	**1** Technetium 99m (Tc-99m) **D** Indium 111 (In-111) **K** Fluorine 18 (F-18) **S** Thallium 201 (Tl-201) **Y** Other Radionuclide **Z** None	**Z** None	**Z** None
Y Heart ⃠	**Y** Other Radionuclide	**Z** None	**Z** None

⃠ C2261ZZ C226YZZ C22G1ZZ C22GDZZ C22GKZZ C22GSZZ C22GYZZ C22GZZZ C22YYZZ

C Nuclear Medicine
2 Heart
3 Positron Emission Tomographic (PET) Imaging: Introduction of radioactive materials into the body for three dimensional display of images developed from the simultaneous capture, 180 degrees apart, of radioactive emissions

Body Part Character 4	Radionuclide Character 5	Qualifier Character 6	Qualifier Character 7
G Myocardium ⃠	**K** Fluorine 18 (F-18) **M** Oxygen 15 (O-15) **Q** Rubidium 82 (Rb-82) **R** Nitrogen 13 (N-13) **Y** Other Radionuclide	**Z** None	**Z** None
Y Heart ⃠	**Y** Other Radionuclide	**Z** None	**Z** None

⃠ C23GKZZ C23GMZZ C23GQZZ C23GRZZ C23GYZZ C23YYZZ

C Nuclear Medicine
2 Heart
5 Nonimaging Nuclear Medicine Probe: Introduction of radioactive materials into the body for the study of distribution and fate of certain substances by the detection of radioactive emissions; or, alternatively, measurement of absorption of radioactive emissions from an external source

Body Part Character 4	Radionuclide Character 5	Qualifier Character 6	Qualifier Character 7
6 Heart, Right and Left ⃠	**1** Technetium 99m (Tc-99m) **Y** Other Radionuclide	**Z** None	**Z** None
Y Heart ⃠	**Y** Other Radionuclide	**Z** None	**Z** None

⃠ C2561ZZ C256YZZ C25YYZZ

C Nuclear Medicine
5 Veins
1 Planar Nuclear Medicine Imaging: Introduction of radioactive materials into the body for single plane display of images developed from the capture of radioactive emissions

Body Part Character 4	Radionuclide Character 5	Qualifier Character 6	Qualifier Character 7
B Lower Extremity Veins, Right ⦸ **C** Lower Extremity Veins, Left ⦸ **D** Lower Extremity Veins, Bilateral ⦸ **N** Upper Extremity Veins, Right ⦸ **P** Upper Extremity Veins, Left ⦸ **Q** Upper Extremity Veins, Bilateral ⦸ **R** Central Veins ⦸	**1** Technetium 99m (Tc-99m) **Y** Other Radionuclide	**Z** None	**Z** None
Y Veins ⦸	**Y** Other Radionuclide	**Z** None	**Z** None

⦸ C51B1ZZ C51BYZZ C51C1ZZ C51CYZZ C51D1ZZ C51DYZZ C51N1ZZ C51NYZZ C51P1ZZ C51PYZZ C51Q1ZZ C51QYZZ C51R1ZZ C51RYZZ C51YYZZ

C Nuclear Medicine
7 Lymphatic and Hematologic System
1 Planar Nuclear Medicine Imaging: Introduction of radioactive materials into the body for single plane display of images developed from the capture of radioactive emissions

Body Part Character 4	Radionuclide Character 5	Qualifier Character 6	Qualifier Character 7
0 Bone Marrow ⦸	**1** Technetium 99m (Tc-99m) **D** Indium 111 (In-111) **Y** Other Radionuclide	**Z** None	**Z** None
2 Spleen ⦸ **5** Lymphatics, Head and Neck ⦸ **D** Lymphatics, Pelvic ⦸ **J** Lymphatics, Head ⦸ **K** Lymphatics, Neck ⦸ **L** Lymphatics, Upper Chest ⦸ **M** Lymphatics, Trunk ⦸ **N** Lymphatics, Upper Extremity ⦸ **P** Lymphatics, Lower Extremity ⦸	**1** Technetium 99m (Tc-99m) **Y** Other Radionuclide	**Z** None	**Z** None
3 Blood ⦸	**D** Indium 111 (In-111) **Y** Other Radionuclide	**Z** None	**Z** None
Y Lymphatic and Hematologic System ⦸	**Y** Other Radionuclide	**Z** None	**Z** None

⦸ C7101ZZ C710DZZ C710YZZ C7121ZZ C712YZZ C713DZZ C713YZZ C7151ZZ C715YZZ C71D1ZZ C71DYZZ C71J1ZZ C71JYZZ C71K1ZZ C71KYZZ C71L1ZZ C71LYZZ C71M1ZZ C71MYZZ C71N1ZZ C71NYZZ C71P1ZZ C71PYZZ C71YYZZ

C Nuclear Medicine
7 Lymphatic and Hematologic System
2 Tomographic (Tomo) Nuclear Medicine Imaging: Introduction of radioactive materials into the body for three dimensional display of images developed from the capture of radioactive emissions

Body Part Character 4	Radionuclide Character 5	Qualifier Character 6	Qualifier Character 7
2 Spleen ⦸	**1** Technetium 99m (Tc-99m) **Y** Other Radionuclide	**Z** None	**Z** None
Y Lymphatic and Hematologic System ⦸	**Y** Other Radionuclide	**Z** None	**Z** None

⦸ C7221ZZ C722YZZ C72YYZZ

LC Limited Coverage NC Noncovered HAC HAC Associated Procedure CC Combination Cluster - See Appendix G for code lists
DRG Non-OR-Affecting MS-DRG Assignment ⦸ Non-OR-Not Affecting MS-DRG Assignment New/Revised Text in **Orange** ♂ Male ♀ Female

C Nuclear Medicine
7 Lymphatic and Hematologic System
5 Nonimaging Nuclear Medicine Probe: Introduction of radioactive materials into the body for the study of distribution and fate of certain substances by the detection of radioactive emissions; or, alternatively, measurement of absorption of radioactive emissions from an external source

Body Part Character 4	Radionuclide Character 5	Qualifier Character 6	Qualifier Character 7
5 Lymphatics, Head and Neck ⊘ D Lymphatics, Pelvic ⊘ J Lymphatics, Head ⊘ K Lymphatics, Neck ⊘ L Lymphatics, Upper Chest ⊘ M Lymphatics, Trunk ⊘ N Lymphatics, Upper Extremity ⊘ P Lymphatics, Lower Extremity ⊘	1 Technetium 99m (Tc-99m) Y Other Radionuclide	Z None	Z None
Y Lymphatic and Hematologic System ⊘	Y Other Radionuclide	Z None	Z None

⊘ C7551ZZ C755YZZ C75D1ZZ C75DYZZ C75J1ZZ C75JYZZ C75K1ZZ C75KYZZ C75L1ZZ C75LYZZ C75M1ZZ C75MYZZ C75N1ZZ C75NYZZ C75P1ZZ C75PYZZ C75YYZZ

C Nuclear Medicine
7 Lymphatic and Hematologic System
6 Nonimaging Nuclear Medicine Assay: Introduction of radioactive materials into the body for the study of body fluids and blood elements, by the detection of radioactive emissions

Body Part Character 4	Radionuclide Character 5	Qualifier Character 6	Qualifier Character 7
3 Blood ⊘	1 Technetium 99m (Tc-99m) 7 Cobalt 58 (Co-58) C Cobalt 57 (Co-57) D Indium 111 (In-111) H Iodine 125 (I-125) W Chromium (Cr-51) Y Other Radionuclide	Z None	Z None
Y Lymphatic and Hematologic System ⊘	Y Other Radionuclide	Z None	Z None

⊘ C7631ZZ C7637ZZ C763CZZ C763DZZ C763HZZ C763WZZ C763YZZ C76YYZZ

C Nuclear Medicine
8 Eye
1 Planar Nuclear Medicine Imaging: Introduction of radioactive materials into the body for single plane display of images developed from the capture of radioactive emissions

Body Part Character 4	Radionuclide Character 5	Qualifier Character 6	Qualifier Character 7
9 Lacrimal Ducts, Bilateral ⊘	1 Technetium 99m (Tc-99m) Y Other Radionuclide	Z None	Z None
Y Eye ⊘	Y Other Radionuclide	Z None	Z None

⊘ C8191ZZ C819YZZ C81YYZZ

C Nuclear Medicine
9 Ear, Nose, Mouth and Throat
1 Planar Nuclear Medicine Imaging: Introduction of radioactive materials into the body for single plane display of images developed from the capture of radioactive emissions

Body Part Character 4	Radionuclide Character 5	Qualifier Character 6	Qualifier Character 7
B Salivary Glands, Bilateral ⊘	1 Technetium 99m (Tc-99m) Y Other Radionuclide	Z None	Z None
Y Ear, Nose, Mouth and Throat ⊘	Y Other Radionuclide	Z None	Z None

⊘ C91B1ZZ C91BYZZ C91YYZZ

C Nuclear Medicine
B Respiratory System
1 Planar Nuclear Medicine Imaging: Introduction of radioactive materials into the body for single plane display of images developed from the capture of radioactive emissions

Body Part Character 4	Radionuclide Character 5	Qualifier Character 6	Qualifier Character 7
2 Lungs and Bronchi ⃠	1 Technetium 99m (Tc-99m) 9 Krypton (Kr-81m) T Xenon 127 (Xe-127) V Xenon 133 (Xe-133) Y Other Radionuclide	Z None	Z None
Y Respiratory System ⃠	Y Other Radionuclide	Z None	Z None

⃠ CB121ZZ CB129ZZ CB12TZZ CB12VZZ CB12YZZ CB1YYZZ

C Nuclear Medicine
B Respiratory System
2 Tomographic (Tomo) Nuclear Medicine Imaging: Introduction of radioactive materials into the body for three dimensional display of images developed from the capture of radioactive emissions

Body Part Character 4	Radionuclide Character 5	Qualifier Character 6	Qualifier Character 7
2 Lungs and Bronchi ⃠	1 Technetium 99m (Tc-99m) 9 Krypton (Kr-81m) Y Other Radionuclide	Z None	Z None
Y Respiratory System ⃠	Y Other Radionuclide	Z None	Z None

⃠ CB221ZZ CB229ZZ CB22YZZ CB2YYZZ

C Nuclear Medicine
B Respiratory System
3 Positron Emission Tomographic (PET) Imaging: Introduction of radioactive materials into the body for three dimensional display of images developed from the simultaneous capture, 180 degrees apart, of radioactive emissions

Body Part Character 4	Radionuclide Character 5	Qualifier Character 6	Qualifier Character 7
2 Lungs and Bronchi ⃠	K Fluorine 18 (F-18) Y Other Radionuclide	Z None	Z None
Y Respiratory System ⃠	Y Other Radionuclide	Z None	Z None

⃠ CB32KZZ CB32YZZ CB3YYZZ

C Nuclear Medicine
D Gastrointestinal System
1 Planar Nuclear Medicine Imaging: Introduction of radioactive materials into the body for single plane display of images developed from the capture of radioactive emissions

Body Part Character 4	Radionuclide Character 5	Qualifier Character 6	Qualifier Character 7
5 Upper Gastrointestinal Tract ⃠ 7 Gastrointestinal Tract ⃠	1 Technetium 99m (Tc-99m) D Indium 111 (In-111) Y Other Radionuclide	Z None	Z None
Y Digestive System ⃠	Y Other Radionuclide	Z None	Z None

⃠ CD151ZZ CD15DZZ CD15YZZ CD171ZZ CD17DZZ CD17YZZ CD1YYZZ

C Nuclear Medicine
D Gastrointestinal System
2 Tomographic (Tomo) Nuclear Medicine Imaging: Introduction of radioactive materials into the body for three dimensional display of images developed from the capture of radioactive emissions

Body Part Character 4	Radionuclide Character 5	Qualifier Character 6	Qualifier Character 7
7 Gastrointestinal Tract ⃠	1 Technetium 99m (Tc-99m) D Indium 111 (In-111) Y Other Radionuclide	Z None	Z None
Y Digestive System ⃠	Y Other Radionuclide	Z None	Z None

⃠ CD271ZZ CD27DZZ CD27YZZ CD2YYZZ

C Nuclear Medicine
F Hepatobiliary System and Pancreas
1 Planar Nuclear Medicine Imaging: Introduction of radioactive materials into the body for single plane display of images developed from the capture of radioactive emissions

Body Part Character 4	Radionuclide Character 5	Qualifier Character 6	Qualifier Character 7
4 Gallbladder ⃠ 5 Liver ⃠ 6 Liver and Spleen ⃠ C Hepatobiliary System, All ⃠	1 Technetium 99m (Tc-99m) Y Other Radionuclide	Z None	Z None
Y Hepatobiliary System and Pancreas ⃠	Y Other Radionuclide	Z None	Z None

⃠ CF141ZZ CF14YZZ CF151ZZ CF15YZZ CF161ZZ CF16YZZ CF1C1ZZ CF1CYZZ CF1YYZZ

C Nuclear Medicine
F Hepatobiliary System and Pancreas
2 Tomographic (Tomo) Nuclear Medicine Imaging: Introduction of radioactive materials into the body for three dimensional display of images developed from the capture of radioactive emissions

Body Part Character 4	Radionuclide Character 5	Qualifier Character 6	Qualifier Character 7
4 Gallbladder ⃠ 5 Liver ⃠ 6 Liver and Spleen ⃠	1 Technetium 99m (Tc-99m) Y Other Radionuclide	Z None	Z None
Y Hepatobiliary System and Pancreas ⃠	Y Other Radionuclide	Z None	Z None

⃠ CF241ZZ CF24YZZ CF251ZZ CF25YZZ CF261ZZ CF26YZZ CF2YYZZ

C Nuclear Medicine
G Endocrine System
1 Planar Nuclear Medicine Imaging: Introduction of radioactive materials into the body for single plane display of images developed from the capture of radioactive emissions

Body Part Character 4	Radionuclide Character 5	Qualifier Character 6	Qualifier Character 7
1 Parathyroid Glands ⃠	1 Technetium 99m (Tc-99m) S Thallium 201 (Tl-201) Y Other Radionuclide	Z None	Z None
2 Thyroid Gland ⃠	1 Technetium 99m (Tc-99m) F Iodine 123 (I-123) G Iodine 131 (I-131) Y Other Radionuclide	Z None	Z None
4 Adrenal Glands, Bilateral ⃠	G Iodine 131 (I-131) Y Other Radionuclide	Z None	Z None
Y Endocrine System ⃠	Y Other Radionuclide	Z None	Z None

⃠ CG111ZZ CG11SZZ CG11YZZ CG121ZZ CG12FZZ CG12GZZ CG12YZZ CG14GZZ CG14YZZ CG1YYZZ

C Nuclear Medicine
G Endocrine System
2 Tomographic (Tomo) Nuclear Medicine Imaging: Introduction of radioactive materials into the body for three dimensional display of images developed from the capture of radioactive emissions

Body Part Character 4	Radionuclide Character 5	Qualifier Character 6	Qualifier Character 7
1 Parathyroid Glands ⃠	1 Technetium 99m (Tc-99m) S Thallium 201 (Tl-201) Y Other Radionuclide	Z None	Z None
Y Endocrine System ⃠	Y Other Radionuclide	Z None	Z None

⃠ CG211ZZ CG21SZZ CG21YZZ CG2YYZZ

C Nuclear Medicine
G Endocrine System
4 Nonimaging Nuclear Medicine Uptake: Introduction of radioactive materials into the body for measurements of organ function, from the detection of radioactive emissions

Body Part Character 4	Radionuclide Character 5	Qualifier Character 6	Qualifier Character 7
2 Thyroid Gland ⊘	1 Technetium 99m (Tc-99m) F Iodine 123 (I-123) G Iodine 131 (I-131) Y Other Radionuclide	Z None	Z None
Y Endocrine System ⊘	Y Other Radionuclide	Z None	Z None

⊘ CG421ZZ CG42FZZ CG42GZZ CG42YZZ CG4YYZZ

C Nuclear Medicine
H Skin, Subcutaneous Tissue and Breast
1 Planar Nuclear Medicine Imaging: Introduction of radioactive materials into the body for single plane display of images developed from the capture of radioactive emissions

Body Part Character 4	Radionuclide Character 5	Qualifier Character 6	Qualifier Character 7
0 Breast, Right ⊘ 1 Breast, Left ⊘ 2 Breasts, Bilateral ⊘	1 Technetium 99m (Tc-99m) S Thallium 201 (Tl-201) Y Other Radionuclide	Z None	Z None
Y Skin, Subcutaneous Tissue and Breast ⊘	Y Other Radionuclide	Z None	Z None

⊘ CH101ZZ CH10SZZ CH10YZZ CH111ZZ CH11SZZ CH11YZZ CH121ZZ CH12SZZ CH12YZZ CH1YYZZ

C Nuclear Medicine
H Skin, Subcutaneous Tissue and Breast
2 Tomographic (Tomo) Nuclear Medicine Imaging: Introduction of radioactive materials into the body for three dimensional display of images developed from the capture of radioactive emissions

Body Part Character 4	Radionuclide Character 5	Qualifier Character 6	Qualifier Character 7
0 Breast, Right ⊘ 1 Breast, Left ⊘ 2 Breasts, Bilateral ⊘	1 Technetium 99m (Tc-99m) S Thallium 201 (Tl-201) Y Other Radionuclide	Z None	Z None
Y Skin, Subcutaneous Tissue and Breast ⊘	Y Other Radionuclide	Z None	Z None

⊘ CH201ZZ CH20SZZ CH20YZZ CH211ZZ CH21SZZ CH21YZZ CH221ZZ CH22SZZ CH22YZZ CH2YYZZ

C Nuclear Medicine
P Musculoskeletal System
1 Planar Nuclear Medicine Imaging: Introduction of radioactive materials into the body for single plane display of images developed from the capture of radioactive emissions

Body Part Character 4	Radionuclide Character 5	Qualifier Character 6	Qualifier Character 7
1 Skull ⊘ 4 Thorax ⊘ 5 Spine ⊘ 6 Pelvis ⊘ 7 Spine and Pelvis ⊘ 8 Upper Extremity, Right ⊘ 9 Upper Extremity, Left ⊘ B Upper Extremities, Bilateral ⊘ C Lower Extremity, Right ⊘ D Lower Extremity, Left ⊘ F Lower Extremities, Bilateral ⊘ Z Musculoskeletal System, All ⊘	1 Technetium 99m (Tc-99m) Y Other Radionuclide	Z None	Z None
Y Musculoskeletal System, Other ⊘	Y Other Radionuclide	Z None	Z None

⊘ CP111ZZ CP11YZZ CP141ZZ CP14YZZ CP151ZZ CP15YZZ CP161ZZ CP16YZZ CP171ZZ CP17YZZ CP181ZZ CP18YZZ CP191ZZ CP19YZZ CP1B1ZZ CP1BYZZ CP1C1ZZ CP1CYZZ CP1D1ZZ CP1DYZZ CP1F1ZZ CP1FYZZ CP1YYZZ CP1Z1ZZ CP1ZYZZ

C Nuclear Medicine
P Musculoskeletal System
2 Tomographic (Tomo) Nuclear Medicine Imaging: Introduction of radioactive materials into the body for three dimensional display of images developed from the capture of radioactive emissions

Body Part Character 4	Radionuclide Character 5	Qualifier Character 6	Qualifier Character 7
1 Skull ⦸ **2** Cervical Spine ⦸ **3** Skull and Cervical Spine ⦸ **4** Thorax ⦸ **6** Pelvis ⦸ **7** Spine and Pelvis ⦸ **8** Upper Extremity, Right ⦸ **9** Upper Extremity, Left ⦸ **B** Upper Extremities, Bilateral ⦸ **C** Lower Extremity, Right ⦸ **D** Lower Extremity, Left ⦸ **F** Lower Extremities, Bilateral ⦸ **G** Thoracic Spine ⦸ **H** Lumbar Spine ⦸ **J** Thoracolumbar Spine ⦸	**1** Technetium 99m (Tc-99m) **Y** Other Radionuclide	**Z** None	**Z** None
Y Musculoskeletal System, Other ⦸	**Y** Other Radionuclide	**Z** None	**Z** None

⦸ CP211ZZ CP21YZZ CP221ZZ CP22YZZ CP231ZZ CP23YZZ CP241ZZ CP24YZZ CP261ZZ CP26YZZ CP271ZZ CP27YZZ CP281ZZ CP28YZZ CP291ZZ CP29YZZ CP2B1ZZ CP2BYZZ CP2C1ZZ CP2CYZZ CP2D1ZZ CP2DYZZ CP2F1ZZ CP2FYZZ CP2G1ZZ CP2GYZZ CP2H1ZZ CP2HYZZ CP2J1ZZ CP2JYZZ CP2YYZZ

C Nuclear Medicine
P Musculoskeletal System
5 Nonimaging Nuclear Medicine Probe: Introduction of radioactive materials into the body for the study of distribution and fate of certain substances by the detection of radioactive emissions; or, alternatively, measurement of absorption of radioactive emissions from an external source

Body Part Character 4	Radionuclide Character 5	Qualifier Character 6	Qualifier Character 7
5 Spine ⦸ **N** Upper Extremities ⦸ **P** Lower Extremities ⦸	**Z** None	**Z** None	**Z** None
Y Musculoskeletal System, Other ⦸	**Y** Other Radionuclide	**Z** None	**Z** None

⦸ CP55ZZZ CP5NZZZ CP5PZZZ CP5YYZZ

C Nuclear Medicine
T Urinary System
1 Planar Nuclear Medicine Imaging: Introduction of radioactive materials into the body for single plane display of images developed from the capture of radioactive emissions

Body Part Character 4	Radionuclide Character 5	Qualifier Character 6	Qualifier Character 7
3 Kidneys, Ureters and Bladder ⦸	**1** Technetium 99m (Tc-99m) **F** Iodine 123 (I-123) **G** Iodine 131 (I-131) **Y** Other Radionuclide	**Z** None	**Z** None
H Bladder and Ureters ⦸	**1** Technetium 99m (Tc-99m) **Y** Other Radionuclide	**Z** None	**Z** None
Y Urinary System ⦸	**Y** Other Radionuclide	**Z** None	**Z** None

⦸ CT131ZZ CT13FZZ CT13GZZ CT13YZZ CT1H1ZZ CT1HYZZ CT1YYZZ

C Nuclear Medicine
T Urinary System
2 Tomographic (Tomo) Nuclear Medicine Imaging: Introduction of radioactive materials into the body for three dimensional display of images developed from the capture of radioactive emissions

Body Part Character 4	Radionuclide Character 5	Qualifier Character 6	Qualifier Character 7
3 Kidneys, Ureters and Bladder ⦸	**1** Technetium 99m (Tc-99m) **Y** Other Radionuclide	**Z** None	**Z** None
Y Urinary System ⦸	**Y** Other Radionuclide	**Z** None	**Z** None

⦸ CT231ZZ CT23YZZ CT2YYZZ

C Nuclear Medicine
T Urinary System
6 Nonimaging Nuclear Medicine Assay: Introduction of radioactive materials into the body for the study of body fluids and blood elements, by the detection of radioactive emissions

Body Part Character 4	Radionuclide Character 5	Qualifier Character 6	Qualifier Character 7
3 Kidneys, Ureters and Bladder ⃠	**1** Technetium 99m (Tc-99m) **F** Iodine 123 (I-123) **G** Iodine 131 (I-131) **H** Iodine 125 (I-125) **Y** Other Radionuclide	**Z** None	**Z** None
Y Urinary System ⃠	**Y** Other Radionuclide	**Z** None	**Z** None

⃠ CT631ZZ CT63FZZ CT63GZZ CT63HZZ CT63YZZ CT6YYZZ

C Nuclear Medicine
V Male Reproductive System
1 Planar Nuclear Medicine Imaging: Introduction of radioactive materials into the body for single plane display of images developed from the capture of radioactive emissions

Body Part Character 4	Radionuclide Character 5	Qualifier Character 6	Qualifier Character 7
9 Testicles, Bilateral ⃠ ♂	**1** Technetium 99m (Tc-99m) **Y** Other Radionuclide	**Z** None	**Z** None
Y Male Reproductive System ⃠ ♂	**Y** Other Radionuclide	**Z** None	**Z** None

♂ CV191ZZ CV19YZZ CV1YYZZ
⃠ CV191ZZ CV19YZZ CV1YYZZ

C Nuclear Medicine
W Anatomical Regions
1 Planar Nuclear Medicine Imaging: Introduction of radioactive materials into the body for single plane display of images developed from the capture of radioactive emissions

Body Part Character 4	Radionuclide Character 5	Qualifier Character 6	Qualifier Character 7
0 Abdomen ⃠ **1** Abdomen and Pelvis ⃠ **4** Chest and Abdomen ⃠ **6** Chest and Neck ⃠ **B** Head and Neck ⃠ **D** Lower Extremity ⃠ **J** Pelvic Region ⃠ **M** Upper Extremity ⃠ **N** Whole Body ⃠	**1** Technetium 99m (Tc-99m) **D** Indium 111 (In-111) **F** Iodine 123 (I-123) **G** Iodine 131 (I-131) **L** Gallium 67 (Ga-67) **S** Thallium 201 (Tl-201) **Y** Other Radionuclide	**Z** None	**Z** None
3 Chest ⃠	**1** Technetium 99m (Tc-99m) **D** Indium 111 (In-111) **F** Iodine 123 (I-123) **G** Iodine 131 (I-131) **K** Fluorine 18 (F-18) **L** Gallium 67 (Ga-67) **S** Thallium 201 (Tl-201) **Y** Other Radionuclide	**Z** None	**Z** None
Y Anatomical Regions, Multiple ⃠	**Y** Other Radionuclide	**Z** None	**Z** None
Z Anatomical Region, Other ⃠	**Z** None	**Z** None	**Z** None

⃠ CW101ZZ CW10DZZ CW10FZZ CW10GZZ CW10LZZ CW10SZZ CW10YZZ CW111ZZ CW11DZZ CW11FZZ CW11GZZ CW11LZZ CW11SZZ CW11YZZ CW131ZZ CW13DZZ CW13FZZ CW13GZZ CW13KZZ CW13LZZ CW13SZZ CW13YZZ CW141ZZ CW14DZZ CW14FZZ CW14GZZ CW14LZZ CW14SZZ CW14YZZ CW161ZZ CW16DZZ CW16FZZ CW16GZZ CW16LZZ CW16SZZ CW16YZZ CW1B1ZZ CW1BDZZ CW1BFZZ CW1BGZZ CW1BLZZ CW1BSZZ CW1BYZZ CW1D1ZZ CW1DDZZ CW1DFZZ CW1DGZZ CW1DLZZ CW1DSZZ CW1DYZZ CW1J1ZZ CW1JDZZ CW1JFZZ CW1JGZZ CW1JLZZ CW1JSZZ CW1JYZZ CW1M1ZZ CW1MDZZ CW1MFZZ CW1MGZZ CW1MLZZ CW1MSZZ CW1MYZZ CW1N1ZZ CW1NDZZ CW1NFZZ CW1NGZZ CW1NLZZ CW1NSZZ CW1NYZZ CW1YYZZ CW1ZZZZ

C Nuclear Medicine
W Anatomical Regions
2 Tomographic (Tomo) Nuclear Medicine Imaging: Introduction of radioactive materials into the body for three dimensional display of images developed from the capture of radioactive emissions

Body Part Character 4	Radionuclide Character 5	Qualifier Character 6	Qualifier Character 7
0 Abdomen ⊘ **1** Abdomen and Pelvis ⊘ **3** Chest ⊘ **4** Chest and Abdomen ⊘ **6** Chest and Neck ⊘ **B** Head and Neck ⊘ **D** Lower Extremity ⊘ **J** Pelvic Region ⊘ **M** Upper Extremity ⊘	**1** Technetium 99m (Tc-99m) **D** Indium 111 (In-111) **F** Iodine 123 (I-123) **G** Iodine 131 (I-131) **K** Fluorine 18 (F-18) **L** Gallium 67 (Ga-67) **S** Thallium 201 (Tl-201) **Y** Other Radionuclide	**Z** None	**Z** None
Y Anatomical Regions, Multiple ⊘	**Y** Other Radionuclide	**Z** None	**Z** None

⊘ CW201ZZ CW20DZZ CW20FZZ CW20GZZ CW20KZZ CW20LZZ CW20SZZ CW20YZZ CW211ZZ CW21DZZ CW21FZZ CW21GZZ CW21KZZ CW21LZZ CW21SZZ CW21YZZ CW231ZZ CW23DZZ CW23FZZ CW23GZZ CW23KZZ CW23LZZ CW23SZZ CW23YZZ CW241ZZ CW24DZZ CW24FZZ CW24GZZ CW24KZZ CW24LZZ CW24SZZ CW24YZZ CW261ZZ CW26DZZ CW26FZZ CW26GZZ CW26KZZ CW26LZZ CW26SZZ CW26YZZ CW2B1ZZ CW2BDZZ CW2BFZZ CW2BGZZ CW2BKZZ CW2BLZZ CW2BSZZ CW2BYZZ CW2D1ZZ CW2DDZZ CW2DFZZ CW2DGZZ CW2DKZZ CW2DLZZ CW2DSZZ CW2DYZZ CW2J1ZZ CW2JDZZ CW2JFZZ CW2JGZZ CW2JKZZ CW2JLZZ CW2JSZZ CW2JYZZ CW2M1ZZ CW2MDZZ CW2MFZZ CW2MGZZ CW2MKZZ CW2MLZZ CW2MSZZ CW2MYZZ CW2YYZZ

C Nuclear Medicine
W Anatomical Regions
3 Positron Emission Tomographic (PET) Imaging: Introduction of radioactive materials into the body for three dimensional display of images developed from the simultaneous capture, 180 degrees apart, of radioactive emissions

Body Part Character 4	Radionuclide Character 5	Qualifier Character 6	Qualifier Character 7
N Whole Body ⊘	**Y** Other Radionuclide	**Z** None	**Z** None

⊘ CW3NYZZ

C Nuclear Medicine
W Anatomical Regions
5 Nonimaging Nuclear Medicine Probe: Introduction of radioactive materials into the body for the study of distribution and fate of certain substances by the detection of radioactive emissions; or, alternatively, measurement of absorption of radioactive emissions from an external source

Body Part Character 4	Radionuclide Character 5	Qualifier Character 6	Qualifier Character 7
0 Abdomen ⊘ **1** Abdomen and Pelvis ⊘ **3** Chest ⊘ **4** Chest and Abdomen ⊘ **6** Chest and Neck ⊘ **B** Head and Neck ⊘ **D** Lower Extremity ⊘ **J** Pelvic Region ⊘ **M** Upper Extremity ⊘	**1** Technetium 99m (Tc-99m) **D** Indium 111 (In-111) **Y** Other Radionuclide	**Z** None	**Z** None

⊘ CW501ZZ CW50DZZ CW50YZZ CW511ZZ CW51DZZ CW51YZZ CW531ZZ CW53DZZ CW53YZZ CW541ZZ CW54DZZ CW54YZZ CW561ZZ CW56DZZ CW56YZZ CW5B1ZZ CW5BDZZ CW5BYZZ CW5D1ZZ CW5DDZZ CW5DYZZ CW5J1ZZ CW5JDZZ CW5JYZZ CW5M1ZZ CW5MDZZ CW5MYZZ

C Nuclear Medicine
W Anatomical Regions
7 Systemic Nuclear Medicine Therapy: Introduction of unsealed radioactive materials into the body for treatment

Body Part Character 4	Radionuclide Character 5	Qualifier Character 6	Qualifier Character 7
0 Abdomen ⊘ **3** Chest ⊘	**N** Phosphorus 32 (P-32) **Y** Other Radionuclide	**Z** None	**Z** None
G Thyroid ⊘	**G** Iodine 131 (I-131) **Y** Other Radionuclide	**Z** None	**Z** None
N Whole Body ⊘	**8** Samarium 153 (Sm-153) **G** Iodine 131 (I-131) **N** Phosphorus 32 (P-32) **P** Strontium 89 (Sr-89) **Y** Other Radionuclide	**Z** None	**Z** None
Y Anatomical Regions, Multiple ⊘	**Y** Other Radionuclide	**Z** None	**Z** None

⊘ CW70NZZ CW70YZZ CW73NZZ CW73YZZ CW7GGZZ CW7GYZZ CW7N8ZZ CW7NGZZ CW7NNZZ CW7NPZZ CW7NYZZ CW7YYZZ

Radiation Therapy D00-DWY

D Radiation Therapy
0 Central and Peripheral Nervous System
0 Beam Radiation

Treatment Site Character 4	Modality Qualifier Character 5	Isotope Character 6	Qualifier Character 7
0 Brain ⊘ 1 Brain Stem ⊘ 6 Spinal Cord ⊘ 7 Peripheral Nerve ⊘	0 Photons <1 MeV 1 Photons 1 - 10 MeV 2 Photons >10 MeV 4 Heavy Particles (Protons, Ions) 5 Neutrons 6 Neutron Capture	Z None	Z None
0 Brain ⊘ 1 Brain Stem ⊘ 6 Spinal Cord ⊘ 7 Peripheral Nerve ⊘	3 Electrons	Z None	0 Intraoperative Z None

⊘ D0000ZZ D0001ZZ D0002ZZ D0003Z0 D0003ZZ D0004ZZ D0005ZZ D0006ZZ D0010ZZ D0011ZZ D0012ZZ D0013Z0 D0013ZZ D0014ZZ D0015ZZ D0016ZZ D0060ZZ D0061ZZ D0062ZZ D0063Z0 D0063ZZ D0064ZZ D0065ZZ D0066ZZ D0070ZZ D0071ZZ D0072ZZ D0073Z0 D0073ZZ D0074ZZ D0075ZZ D0076ZZ

D Radiation Therapy
0 Central and Peripheral Nervous System
1 Brachytherapy

Treatment Site Character 4	Modality Qualifier Character 5	Isotope Character 6	Qualifier Character 7
0 Brain ⊘ 1 Brain Stem ⊘ 6 Spinal Cord ⊘ 7 Peripheral Nerve ⊘	9 High Dose Rate (HDR) B Low Dose Rate (LDR)	7 Cesium 137 (Cs-137) 8 Iridium 192 (Ir-192) 9 Iodine 125 (I-125) B Palladium 103 (Pd-103) C Californium 252 (Cf-252) Y Other Isotope	Z None

⊘ D01097Z D01098Z D01099Z D0109BZ D0109CZ D0109YZ D010B7Z D010B8Z D010B9Z D010BBZ D010BCZ D010BYZ D01197Z D01198Z D01199Z D0119BZ D0119CZ D0119YZ D011B7Z D011B8Z D011B9Z D011BBZ D011BCZ D011BYZ D01697Z D01698Z D01699Z D0169BZ D0169CZ D0169YZ D016B7Z D016B8Z D016B9Z D016BBZ D016BCZ D016BYZ D01797Z D01798Z D01799Z D0179BZ D0179CZ D0179YZ D017B7Z D017B8Z D017B9Z D017BBZ D017BCZ D017BYZ

D Radiation Therapy
0 Central and Peripheral Nervous System
2 Stereotactic Radiosurgery

Treatment Site Character 4	Modality Qualifier Character 5	Isotope Character 6	Qualifier Character 7
0 Brain DRG 1 Brain Stem DRG 6 Spinal Cord DRG 7 Peripheral Nerve DRG	D Stereotactic Other Photon Radiosurgery H Stereotactic Particulate Radiosurgery J Stereotactic Gamma Beam Radiosurgery	Z None	Z None

DRG D020DZZ D020HZZ D020JZZ D021DZZ D021HZZ D021JZZ D026DZZ D026HZZ D026JZZ D027DZZ D027HZZ D027JZZ

D Radiation Therapy
0 Central and Peripheral Nervous System
Y Other Radiation

Treatment Site Character 4	Modality Qualifier Character 5	Isotope Character 6	Qualifier Character 7
0 Brain ⊘ 1 Brain Stem ⊘ 6 Spinal Cord ⊘ 7 Peripheral Nerve ⊘	7 Contact Radiation 8 Hyperthermia F Plaque Radiation K Laser Interstitial Thermal Therapy	Z None	Z None

⊘ D0Y07ZZ D0Y08ZZ D0Y0FZZ D0Y17ZZ D0Y18ZZ D0Y1FZZ D0Y67ZZ D0Y68ZZ D0Y6FZZ D0Y77ZZ D0Y78ZZ D0Y7FZZ

LC Limited Coverage NC Noncovered HAC HAC Associated Procedure CC Combination Cluster - See Appendix G for code lists
DRG Non-OR-Affecting MS-DRG Assignment ⊘ Non-OR-Not Affecting MS-DRG Assignment New/Revised Text in **Orange** ♂ Male ♀ Female

D Radiation Therapy
7 Lymphatic and Hematologic System
0 Beam Radiation

Treatment Site Character 4	Modality Qualifier Character 5	Isotope Character 6	Qualifier Character 7
0 Bone Marrow ⃠ **1** Thymus ⃠ **2** Spleen ⃠ **3** Lymphatics, Neck ⃠ **4** Lymphatics, Axillary ⃠ **5** Lymphatics, Thorax ⃠ **6** Lymphatics, Abdomen ⃠ **7** Lymphatics, Pelvis ⃠ **8** Lymphatics, Inguinal ⃠	**0** Photons <1 MeV **1** Photons 1 - 10 MeV **2** Photons >10 MeV **4** Heavy Particles (Protons, Ions) **5** Neutrons **6** Neutron Capture	**Z** None	**Z** None
0 Bone Marrow ⃠ **1** Thymus ⃠ **2** Spleen ⃠ **3** Lymphatics, Neck ⃠ **4** Lymphatics, Axillary ⃠ **5** Lymphatics, Thorax ⃠ **6** Lymphatics, Abdomen ⃠ **7** Lymphatics, Pelvis ⃠ **8** Lymphatics, Inguinal ⃠	**3** Electrons	**Z** None	**0** Intraoperative **Z** None

⃠ D7000ZZ D7001ZZ D7002ZZ D7003Z0 D7003ZZ D7004ZZ D7005ZZ D7006ZZ D7010ZZ D7011ZZ D7012ZZ D7013Z0 D7013ZZ D7014ZZ D7015ZZ D7016ZZ D7020ZZ D7021ZZ D7022ZZ D7023Z0 D7023ZZ D7024ZZ D7025ZZ D7026ZZ D7030ZZ D7031ZZ D7032ZZ D7033Z0 D7033ZZ D7034ZZ D7035ZZ D7036ZZ D7040ZZ D7041ZZ D7042ZZ D7043Z0 D7043ZZ D7044ZZ D7045ZZ D7046ZZ D7050ZZ D7051ZZ D7052ZZ D7053Z0 D7053ZZ D7054ZZ D7055ZZ D7056ZZ D7060ZZ D7061ZZ D7062ZZ D7063Z0 D7063ZZ D7064ZZ D7065ZZ D7066ZZ D7070ZZ D7071ZZ D7072ZZ D7073Z0 D7073ZZ D7074ZZ D7075ZZ D7076ZZ D7080ZZ D7081ZZ D7082ZZ D7083Z0 D7083ZZ D7084ZZ D7085ZZ D7086ZZ

D Radiation Therapy
7 Lymphatic and Hematologic System
1 Brachytherapy

Treatment Site Character 4	Modality Qualifier Character 5	Isotope Character 6	Qualifier Character 7
0 Bone Marrow ⃠ **1** Thymus ⃠ **2** Spleen ⃠ **3** Lymphatics, Neck ⃠ **4** Lymphatics, Axillary ⃠ **5** Lymphatics, Thorax ⃠ **6** Lymphatics, Abdomen ⃠ **7** Lymphatics, Pelvis ⃠ **8** Lymphatics, Inguinal ⃠	**9** High Dose Rate (HDR) **B** Low Dose Rate (LDR)	**7** Cesium 137 (Cs-137) **8** Iridium 192 (Ir-192) **9** Iodine 125 (I-125) **B** Palladium 103 (Pd-103) **C** Californium 252 (Cf-252) **Y** Other Isotope	**Z** None

⃠ D71097Z D71098Z D71099Z D7109BZ D7109CZ D7109YZ D710B7Z D710B8Z D710B9Z D710BBZ D710BCZ D710BYZ D71197Z D71198Z D71199Z D7119BZ D7119CZ D7119YZ D711B7Z D711B8Z D711B9Z D711BBZ D711BCZ D711BYZ D71297Z D71298Z D71299Z D7129BZ D7129CZ D7129YZ D712B7Z D712B8Z D712B9Z D712BBZ D712BCZ D712BYZ D71397Z D71398Z D71399Z D7139BZ D7139CZ D7139YZ D713B7Z D713B8Z D713B9Z D713BBZ D713BCZ D713BYZ D71497Z D71498Z D71499Z D7149BZ D7149CZ D7149YZ D714B7Z D714B8Z D714B9Z D714BBZ D714BCZ D714BYZ D71597Z D71598Z D71599Z D7159BZ D7159CZ D7159YZ D715B7Z D715B8Z D715B9Z D715BBZ D715BCZ D715BYZ D71697Z D71698Z D71699Z D7169BZ D7169CZ D7169YZ D716B7Z D716B8Z D716B9Z D716BBZ D716BCZ D716BYZ D71797Z D71798Z D71799Z D7179BZ D7179CZ D7179YZ D717B7Z D717B8Z D717B9Z D717BBZ D717BCZ D717BYZ D71897Z D71898Z D71899Z D7189BZ D7189CZ D7189YZ D718B7Z D718B8Z D718B9Z D718BBZ D718BCZ D718BYZ

D Radiation Therapy
7 Lymphatic and Hematologic System
2 Stereotactic Radiosurgery

Treatment Site Character 4	Modality Qualifier Character 5	Isotope Character 6	Qualifier Character 7
0 Bone Marrow DRG 1 Thymus DRG 2 Spleen DRG 3 Lymphatics, Neck DRG 4 Lymphatics, Axillary DRG 5 Lymphatics, Thorax DRG 6 Lymphatics, Abdomen DRG 7 Lymphatics, Pelvis DRG 8 Lymphatics, Inguinal DRG	D Stereotactic Other Photon Radiosurgery H Stereotactic Particulate Radiosurgery J Stereotactic Gamma Beam Radiosurgery	Z None	Z None

DRG D720DZZ D720HZZ D720JZZ D721DZZ D721HZZ D721JZZ D722DZZ D722HZZ D722JZZ D723DZZ D723HZZ D723JZZ D724DZZ D724HZZ D724JZZ D725DZZ D725HZZ D725JZZ D726DZZ D726HZZ D726JZZ D727DZZ D727HZZ D727JZZ D728DZZ D728HZZ D728JZZ

D Radiation Therapy
7 Lymphatic and Hematologic System
Y Other Radiation

Treatment Site Character 4	Modality Qualifier Character 5	Isotope Character 6	Qualifier Character 7
0 Bone Marrow ⦸ 1 Thymus ⦸ 2 Spleen ⦸ 3 Lymphatics, Neck ⦸ 4 Lymphatics, Axillary ⦸ 5 Lymphatics, Thorax ⦸ 6 Lymphatics, Abdomen ⦸ 7 Lymphatics, Pelvis ⦸ 8 Lymphatics, Inguinal ⦸	8 Hyperthermia F Plaque Radiation	Z None	Z None

⦸ D7Y08ZZ D7Y0FZZ D7Y18ZZ D7Y1FZZ D7Y28ZZ D7Y2FZZ D7Y38ZZ D7Y3FZZ D7Y48ZZ D7Y4FZZ D7Y58ZZ D7Y5FZZ D7Y68ZZ D7Y6FZZ D7Y78ZZ D7Y7FZZ D7Y88ZZ D7Y8FZZ

D Radiation Therapy
8 Eye
0 Beam Radiation

Treatment Site Character 4	Modality Qualifier Character 5	Isotope Character 6	Qualifier Character 7
0 Eye ⦸	0 Photons <1 MeV 1 Photons 1 - 10 MeV 2 Photons >10 MeV 4 Heavy Particles (Protons, Ions) 5 Neutrons 6 Neutron Capture	Z None	Z None
0 Eye ⦸	3 Electrons	Z None	0 Intraoperative Z None

⦸ D8000ZZ D8001ZZ D8002ZZ D8003Z0 D8003ZZ D8004ZZ D8005ZZ D8006ZZ

D Radiation Therapy
8 Eye
1 Brachytherapy

Treatment Site Character 4	Modality Qualifier Character 5	Isotope Character 6	Qualifier Character 7
0 Eye ⦸	9 High Dose Rate (HDR) B Low Dose Rate (LDR)	7 Cesium 137 (Cs-137) 8 Iridium 192 (Ir-192) 9 Iodine 125 (I-125) B Palladium 103 (Pd-103) C Californium 252 (Cf-252) Y Other Isotope	Z None

⦸ D81097Z D81098Z D81099Z D8109BZ D8109CZ D8109YZ D810B7Z D810B8Z D810B9Z D810BBZ D810BCZ D810BYZ

LC Limited Coverage NC Noncovered HAC HAC Associated Procedure CC Combination Cluster - See Appendix G for code lists
DRG Non-OR-Affecting MS-DRG Assignment ⦸ Non-OR-Not Affecting MS-DRG Assignment New/Revised Text in **Orange** ♂ Male ♀ Female

D Radiation Therapy
8 Eye
2 Stereotactic Radiosurgery

Treatment Site Character 4	Modality Qualifier Character 5	Isotope Character 6	Qualifier Character 7
0 Eye DRG	D Stereotactic Other Photon Radiosurgery H Stereotactic Particulate Radiosurgery J Stereotactic Gamma Beam Radiosurgery	Z None	Z None

DRG D820DZZ D820HZZ D820JZZ

D Radiation Therapy
8 Eye
Y Other Radiation

Treatment Site Character 4	Modality Qualifier Character 5	Isotope Character 6	Qualifier Character 7
0 Eye ⊘	7 Contact Radiation 8 Hyperthermia F Plaque Radiation	Z None	Z None

⊘ D8Y07ZZ D8Y08ZZ D8Y0FZZ

D Radiation Therapy
9 Ear, Nose, Mouth and Throat
0 Beam Radiation

Treatment Site Character 4	Modality Qualifier Character 5	Isotope Character 6	Qualifier Character 7
0 Ear ⊘ 1 Nose ⊘ 3 Hypopharynx ⊘ 4 Mouth ⊘ 5 Tongue ⊘ 6 Salivary Glands ⊘ 7 Sinuses ⊘ 8 Hard Palate ⊘ 9 Soft Palate ⊘ B Larynx ⊘ D Nasopharynx ⊘ F Oropharynx ⊘	0 Photons <1 MeV 1 Photons 1 - 10 MeV 2 Photons >10 MeV 4 Heavy Particles (Protons, Ions) 5 Neutrons 6 Neutron Capture	Z None	Z None
0 Ear ⊘ 1 Nose ⊘ 3 Hypopharynx ⊘ 4 Mouth ⊘ 5 Tongue ⊘ 6 Salivary Glands ⊘ 7 Sinuses ⊘ 8 Hard Palate ⊘ 9 Soft Palate ⊘ B Larynx ⊘ D Nasopharynx ⊘ F Oropharynx ⊘	3 Electrons	Z None	0 Intraoperative Z None

⊘ D9000ZZ D9001ZZ D9002ZZ D9003Z0 D9003ZZ D9004ZZ D9005ZZ D9006ZZ D9010ZZ D9011ZZ D9012ZZ D9013Z0 D9013ZZ D9014ZZ D9015ZZ D9016ZZ D9030ZZ D9031ZZ D9032ZZ D9033Z0 D9033ZZ D9034ZZ D9035ZZ D9036ZZ D9040ZZ D9041ZZ D9042ZZ D9043Z0 D9043ZZ D9044ZZ D9045ZZ D9046ZZ D9050ZZ D9051ZZ D9052ZZ D9053Z0 D9053ZZ D9054ZZ D9055ZZ D9056ZZ D9060ZZ D9061ZZ D9062ZZ D9063Z0 D9063ZZ D9064ZZ D9065ZZ D9066ZZ D9070ZZ D9071ZZ D9072ZZ D9073Z0 D9073ZZ D9074ZZ D9075ZZ D9076ZZ D9080ZZ D9081ZZ D9082ZZ D9083Z0 D9083ZZ D9084ZZ D9085ZZ D9086ZZ D9090ZZ D9091ZZ D9092ZZ D9093Z0 D9093ZZ D9094ZZ D9095ZZ D9096ZZ D90B0ZZ D90B1ZZ D90B2ZZ D90B3Z0 D90B3ZZ D90B4ZZ D90B5ZZ D90B6ZZ D90D0ZZ D90D1ZZ D90D2ZZ D90D3Z0 D90D3ZZ D90D4ZZ D90D5ZZ D90D6ZZ D90F0ZZ D90F1ZZ D90F2ZZ D90F3Z0 D90F3ZZ D90F4ZZ D90F5ZZ D90F6ZZ

LC Limited Coverage NC Noncovered HAC HAC Associated Procedure CC Combination Cluster - See Appendix G for code lists
DRG Non-OR-Affecting MS-DRG Assignment ⊘ Non-OR-Not Affecting MS-DRG Assignment New/Revised Text in Orange ♂ Male ♀ Female

D Radiation Therapy
9 Ear, Nose, Mouth and Throat
1 Brachytherapy

Treatment Site Character 4	Modality Qualifier Character 5	Isotope Character 6	Qualifier Character 7
0 Ear ⃠ 1 Nose ⃠ 3 Hypopharynx ⃠ 4 Mouth ⃠ 5 Tongue ⃠ 6 Salivary Glands ⃠ 7 Sinuses ⃠ 8 Hard Palate ⃠ 9 Soft Palate ⃠ B Larynx ⃠ D Nasopharynx ⃠ F Oropharynx ⃠	9 High Dose Rate (HDR) B Low Dose Rate (LDR)	7 Cesium 137 (Cs-137) 8 Iridium 192 (Ir-192) 9 Iodine 125 (I-125) B Palladium 103 (Pd-103) C Californium 252 (Cf-252) Y Other Isotope	Z None

⃠ D91097Z D91098Z D91099Z D9109BZ D9109CZ D9109YZ D910B7Z D910B8Z D910B9Z D910BBZ D910BCZ D910BYZ D91197Z D91198Z D91199Z D9119BZ D9119CZ D9119YZ D911B7Z D911B8Z D911B9Z D911BBZ D911BCZ D911BYZ D91397Z D91398Z D91399Z D9139BZ D9139CZ D9139YZ D913B7Z D913B8Z D913B9Z D913BBZ D913BCZ D913BYZ D91497Z D91498Z D91499Z D9149BZ D9149CZ D9149YZ D914B7Z D914B8Z D914B9Z D914BBZ D914BCZ D914BYZ D91597Z D91598Z D91599Z D9159BZ D9159CZ D9159YZ D915B7Z D915B8Z D915B9Z D915BBZ D915BCZ D915BYZ D91697Z D91698Z D91699Z D9169BZ D9169CZ D9169YZ D916B7Z D916B8Z D916B9Z D916BBZ D916BCZ D916BYZ D91797Z D91798Z D91799Z D9179BZ D9179CZ D9179YZ D917B7Z D917B8Z D917B9Z D917BBZ D917BCZ D917BYZ D91897Z D91898Z D91899Z D9189BZ D9189CZ D9189YZ D918B7Z D918B8Z D918B9Z D918BBZ D918BCZ D918BYZ D91997Z D91998Z D91999Z D9199BZ D9199CZ D9199YZ D919B7Z D919B8Z D919B9Z D919BBZ D919BCZ D919BYZ D91B97Z D91B98Z D91B99Z D91B9BZ D91B9CZ D91B9YZ D91BB7Z D91BB8Z D91BB9Z D91BBBZ D91BBCZ D91BBYZ D91D97Z D91D98Z D91D99Z D91D9BZ D91D9CZ D91D9YZ D91DB7Z D91DB8Z D91DB9Z D91DBBZ D91DBCZ D91DBYZ D91F97Z D91F98Z D91F99Z D91F9BZ D91F9CZ D91F9YZ D91FB7Z D91FB8Z D91FB9Z D91FBBZ D91FBCZ D91FBYZ

D Radiation Therapy
9 Ear, Nose, Mouth and Throat
2 Stereotactic Radiosurgery

Treatment Site Character 4	Modality Qualifier Character 5	Isotope Character 6	Qualifier Character 7
0 Ear DRG 1 Nose DRG 4 Mouth DRG 5 Tongue DRG 6 Salivary Glands DRG 7 Sinuses DRG 8 Hard Palate DRG 9 Soft Palate DRG B Larynx DRG C Pharynx DRG D Nasopharynx DRG	D Stereotactic Other Photon Radiosurgery H Stereotactic Particulate Radiosurgery J Stereotactic Gamma Beam Radiosurgery	Z None	Z None

DRG D920DZZ D920HZZ D920JZZ D921DZZ D921HZZ D921JZZ D924DZZ D924HZZ D924JZZ D925DZZ D925HZZ D925JZZ D926DZZ D926HZZ D926JZZ D927DZZ D927HZZ D927JZZ D928DZZ D928HZZ D928JZZ D929DZZ D929HZZ D929JZZ D92BDZZ D92BHZZ D92BJZZ D92CDZZ D92CHZZ D92CJZZ D92DDZZ D92DHZZ D92DJZZ

D Radiation Therapy
9 Ear, Nose, Mouth and Throat
Y Other Radiation

Treatment Site Character 4	Modality Qualifier Character 5	Isotope Character 6	Qualifier Character 7
0 Ear ⦸ 1 Nose ⦸ 5 Tongue ⦸ 6 Salivary Glands ⦸ 7 Sinuses ⦸ 8 Hard Palate ⦸ 9 Soft Palate ⦸	7 Contact Radiation 8 Hyperthermia F Plaque Radiation	Z None	Z None
3 Hypopharynx ⦸ F Oropharynx ⦸	7 Contact Radiation 8 Hyperthermia	Z None	Z None
4 Mouth ⦸ B Larynx ⦸ D Nasopharynx ⦸	7 Contact Radiation 8 Hyperthermia C Intraoperative Radiation Therapy (IORT) F Plaque Radiation	Z None	Z None
C Pharynx ⦸	C Intraoperative Radiation Therapy (IORT) F Plaque Radiation	Z None	Z None

⦸ D9Y07ZZ D9Y08ZZ D9Y0FZZ D9Y17ZZ D9Y18ZZ D9Y1FZZ D9Y37ZZ D9Y38ZZ D9Y47ZZ D9Y48ZZ D9Y4CZZ D9Y4FZZ D9Y57ZZ D9Y58ZZ D9Y5FZZ D9Y67ZZ D9Y68ZZ D9Y6FZZ D9Y77ZZ D9Y78ZZ D9Y7FZZ D9Y87ZZ D9Y88ZZ D9Y8FZZ D9Y97ZZ D9Y98ZZ D9Y9FZZ D9YB7ZZ D9YB8ZZ D9YBCZZ D9YBFZZ D9YCCZZ D9YCFZZ D9YD7ZZ D9YD8ZZ D9YDCZZ D9YDFZZ D9YF7ZZ D9YF8ZZ

D Radiation Therapy
B Respiratory System
0 Beam Radiation

Treatment Site Character 4	Modality Qualifier Character 5	Isotope Character 6	Qualifier Character 7
0 Trachea ⦸ 1 Bronchus ⦸ 2 Lung ⦸ 5 Pleura ⦸ 6 Mediastinum ⦸ 7 Chest Wall ⦸ 8 Diaphragm ⦸	0 Photons <1 MeV 1 Photons 1 - 10 MeV 2 Photons >10 MeV 4 Heavy Particles (Protons, Ions) 5 Neutrons 6 Neutron Capture	Z None	Z None
0 Trachea ⦸ 1 Bronchus ⦸ 2 Lung ⦸ 5 Pleura ⦸ 6 Mediastinum ⦸ 7 Chest Wall ⦸ 8 Diaphragm ⦸	3 Electrons	Z None	0 Intraoperative Z None

⦸ DB000ZZ DB001ZZ DB002ZZ DB003Z0 DB003ZZ DB004ZZ DB005ZZ DB006ZZ DB010ZZ DB011ZZ DB012ZZ DB013Z0 DB013ZZ DB014ZZ DB015ZZ DB016ZZ DB020ZZ DB021ZZ DB022ZZ DB023Z0 DB023ZZ DB024ZZ DB025ZZ DB026ZZ DB050ZZ DB051ZZ DB052ZZ DB053Z0 DB053ZZ DB054ZZ DB055ZZ DB056ZZ DB060ZZ DB061ZZ DB062ZZ DB063Z0 DB063ZZ DB064ZZ DB065ZZ DB066ZZ DB070ZZ DB071ZZ DB072ZZ DB073Z0 DB073ZZ DB074ZZ DB075ZZ DB076ZZ DB080ZZ DB081ZZ DB082ZZ DB083Z0 DB083ZZ DB084ZZ DB085ZZ DB086ZZ

D Radiation Therapy
B Respiratory System
1 Brachytherapy

Treatment Site Character 4	Modality Qualifier Character 5	Isotope Character 6	Qualifier Character 7
0 Trachea ⦸	9 High Dose Rate (HDR)	7 Cesium 137 (Cs-137)	Z None
1 Bronchus ⦸	B Low Dose Rate (LDR)	8 Iridium 192 (Ir-192)	
2 Lung ⦸		9 Iodine 125 (I-125)	
5 Pleura ⦸		B Palladium 103 (Pd-103)	
6 Mediastinum ⦸		C Californium 252 (Cf-252)	
7 Chest Wall ⦸		Y Other Isotope	
8 Diaphragm ⦸			

⦸ DB1097Z DB1098Z DB1099Z DB109BZ DB109CZ DB109YZ DB10B7Z DB10B8Z DB10B9Z DB10BBZ DB10BCZ DB10BYZ DB1197Z DB1198Z DB1199Z DB119BZ DB119CZ DB119YZ DB11B7Z DB11B8Z DB11B9Z DB11BBZ DB11BCZ DB11BYZ DB1297Z DB1298Z DB1299Z DB129BZ DB129CZ DB129YZ DB12B7Z DB12B8Z DB12B9Z DB12BBZ DB12BCZ DB12BYZ DB1597Z DB1598Z DB1599Z DB159BZ DB159CZ DB159YZ DB15B7Z DB15B8Z DB15B9Z DB15BBZ DB15BCZ DB15BYZ DB1697Z DB1698Z DB1699Z DB169BZ DB169CZ DB169YZ DB16B7Z DB16B8Z DB16B9Z DB16BBZ DB16BCZ DB16BYZ DB1797Z DB1798Z DB1799Z DB179BZ DB179CZ DB179YZ DB17B7Z DB17B8Z DB17B9Z DB17BBZ DB17BCZ DB17BYZ DB1897Z DB1898Z DB1899Z DB189BZ DB189CZ DB189YZ DB18B7Z DB18B8Z DB18B9Z DB18BBZ DB18BCZ DB18BYZ

D Radiation Therapy
B Respiratory System
2 Stereotactic Radiosurgery

Treatment Site Character 4	Modality Qualifier Character 5	Isotope Character 6	Qualifier Character 7
0 Trachea DRG	D Stereotactic Other Photon Radiosurgery	Z None	Z None
1 Bronchus DRG	H Stereotactic Particulate Radiosurgery		
2 Lung DRG	J Stereotactic Gamma Beam Radiosurgery		
5 Pleura DRG			
6 Mediastinum DRG			
7 Chest Wall DRG			
8 Diaphragm DRG			

DRG DB20DZZ DB20HZZ DB20JZZ DB21DZZ DB21HZZ DB21JZZ DB22DZZ DB22HZZ DB22JZZ DB25DZZ DB25HZZ DB25JZZ DB26DZZ DB26HZZ DB26JZZ DB27DZZ DB27HZZ DB27JZZ DB28DZZ DB28HZZ DB28JZZ

D Radiation Therapy
B Respiratory System
Y Other Radiation

Treatment Site Character 4	Modality Qualifier Character 5	Isotope Character 6	Qualifier Character 7
0 Trachea ⦸	7 Contact Radiation	Z None	Z None
1 Bronchus ⦸	8 Hyperthermia		
2 Lung ⦸	F Plaque Radiation		
5 Pleura ⦸	K Laser Interstitial Thermal Therapy		
6 Mediastinum ⦸			
7 Chest Wall ⦸			
8 Diaphragm ⦸			

⦸ DBY07ZZ DBY08ZZ DBY0FZZ DBY17ZZ DBY18ZZ DBY1FZZ DBY27ZZ DBY28ZZ DBY2FZZ DBY57ZZ DBY58ZZ DBY5FZZ DBY67ZZ DBY68ZZ DBY6FZZ DBY77ZZ DBY78ZZ DBY7FZZ DBY87ZZ DBY88ZZ DBY8FZZ

D Radiation Therapy
D Gastrointestinal System
0 Beam Radiation

Treatment Site Character 4	Modality Qualifier Character 5	Isotope Character 6	Qualifier Character 7
0 Esophagus ⦸ **1** Stomach ⦸ **2** Duodenum ⦸ **3** Jejunum ⦸ **4** Ileum ⦸ **5** Colon ⦸ **7** Rectum ⦸	**0** Photons <1 MeV **1** Photons 1 - 10 MeV **2** Photons >10 MeV **4** Heavy Particles (Protons, Ions) **5** Neutrons **6** Neutron Capture	**Z** None	**Z** None
0 Esophagus ⦸ **1** Stomach ⦸ **2** Duodenum ⦸ **3** Jejunum ⦸ **4** Ileum ⦸ **5** Colon ⦸ **7** Rectum ⦸	**3** Electrons	**Z** None	**0** Intraoperative **Z** None

⦸ DD000ZZ DD001ZZ DD002ZZ DD003Z0 DD003ZZ DD004ZZ DD005ZZ DD006ZZ DD010ZZ DD011ZZ DD012ZZ DD013Z0 DD013ZZ DD014ZZ DD015ZZ DD016ZZ DD020ZZ DD021ZZ DD022ZZ DD023Z0 DD023ZZ DD024ZZ DD025ZZ DD026ZZ DD030ZZ DD031ZZ DD032ZZ DD033Z0 DD033ZZ DD034ZZ DD035ZZ DD036ZZ DD040ZZ DD041ZZ DD042ZZ DD043Z0 DD043ZZ DD044ZZ DD045ZZ DD046ZZ DD050ZZ DD051ZZ DD052ZZ DD053Z0 DD053ZZ DD054ZZ DD055ZZ DD056ZZ DD070ZZ DD071ZZ DD072ZZ DD073Z0 DD073ZZ DD074ZZ DD075ZZ DD076ZZ

D Radiation Therapy
D Gastrointestinal System
1 Brachytherapy

Treatment Site Character 4	Modality Qualifier Character 5	Isotope Character 6	Qualifier Character 7
0 Esophagus ⦸ **1** Stomach ⦸ **2** Duodenum ⦸ **3** Jejunum ⦸ **4** Ileum ⦸ **5** Colon ⦸ **7** Rectum ⦸	**9** High Dose Rate (HDR) **B** Low Dose Rate (LDR)	**7** Cesium 137 (Cs-137) **8** Iridium 192 (Ir-192) **9** Iodine 125 (I-125) **B** Palladium 103 (Pd-103) **C** Californium 252 (Cf-252) **Y** Other Isotope	**Z** None

⦸ DD1097Z DD1098Z DD1099Z DD109BZ DD109CZ DD109YZ DD10B7Z DD10B8Z DD10B9Z DD10BBZ DD10BCZ DD10BYZ DD1197Z DD1198Z DD1199Z DD119BZ DD119CZ DD119YZ DD11B7Z DD11B8Z DD11B9Z DD11BBZ DD11BCZ DD11BYZ DD1297Z DD1298Z DD1299Z DD129BZ DD129CZ DD129YZ DD12B7Z DD12B8Z DD12B9Z DD12BBZ DD12BCZ DD12BYZ DD1397Z DD1398Z DD1399Z DD139BZ DD139CZ DD139YZ DD13B7Z DD13B8Z DD13B9Z DD13BBZ DD13BCZ DD13BYZ DD1497Z DD1498Z DD1499Z DD149BZ DD149CZ DD149YZ DD14B7Z DD14B8Z DD14B9Z DD14BBZ DD14BCZ DD14BYZ DD1597Z DD1598Z DD1599Z DD159BZ DD159CZ DD159YZ DD15B7Z DD15B8Z DD15B9Z DD15BBZ DD15BCZ DD15BYZ DD1797Z DD1798Z DD1799Z DD179BZ DD179CZ DD179YZ DD17B7Z DD17B8Z DD17B9Z DD17BBZ DD17BCZ DD17BYZ

D Radiation Therapy
D Gastrointestinal System
2 Stereotactic Radiosurgery

Treatment Site Character 4	Modality Qualifier Character 5	Isotope Character 6	Qualifier Character 7
0 Esophagus DRG **1** Stomach DRG **2** Duodenum DRG **3** Jejunum DRG **4** Ileum DRG **5** Colon DRG **7** Rectum DRG	**D** Stereotactic Other Photon Radiosurgery **H** Stereotactic Particulate Radiosurgery **J** Stereotactic Gamma Beam Radiosurgery	**Z** None	**Z** None

DRG DD20DZZ DD20HZZ DD20JZZ DD21DZZ DD21HZZ DD21JZZ DD22DZZ DD22HZZ DD22JZZ DD23DZZ DD23HZZ DD23JZZ DD24DZZ DD24HZZ DD24JZZ DD25DZZ DD25HZZ DD25JZZ DD27DZZ DD27HZZ DD27JZZ

D Radiation Therapy
D Gastrointestinal System
Y Other Radiation

Treatment Site Character 4	Modality Qualifier Character 5	Isotope Character 6	Qualifier Character 7
0 Esophagus ⃠	**7** Contact Radiation **8** Hyperthermia **F** Plaque Radiation **K** Laser Interstitial Thermal Therapy	**Z** None	**Z** None
1 Stomach ⃠ **2** Duodenum ⃠ **3** Jejunum ⃠ **4** Ileum ⃠ **5** Colon ⃠ **7** Rectum ⃠	**7** Contact Radiation **8** Hyperthermia **C** Intraoperative Radiation Therapy (IORT) **F** Plaque Radiation **K** Laser Interstitial Thermal Therapy	**Z** None	**Z** None
8 Anus ⃠	**C** Intraoperative Radiation Therapy (IORT) **F** Plaque Radiation **K** Laser Interstitial Thermal Therapy	**Z** None	**Z** None

⃠ DDY07ZZ DDY08ZZ DDY0FZZ DDY17ZZ DDY18ZZ DDY1CZZ DDY1FZZ DDY27ZZ DDY28ZZ DDY2CZZ DDY2FZZ DDY37ZZ DDY38ZZ DDY3CZZ DDY3FZZ DDY47ZZ DDY48ZZ DDY4CZZ DDY4FZZ DDY57ZZ DDY58ZZ DDY5CZZ DDY5FZZ DDY77ZZ DDY78ZZ DDY7CZZ DDY7FZZ DDY8CZZ DDY8FZZ

D Radiation Therapy
F Hepatobiliary System and Pancreas
0 Beam Radiation

Treatment Site Character 4	Modality Qualifier Character 5	Isotope Character 6	Qualifier Character 7
0 Liver ⃠ **1** Gallbladder ⃠ **2** Bile Ducts ⃠ **3** Pancreas ⃠	**0** Photons <1 MeV **1** Photons 1 - 10 MeV **2** Photons >10 MeV **4** Heavy Particles (Protons, Ions) **5** Neutrons **6** Neutron Capture	**Z** None	**Z** None
0 Liver ⃠ **1** Gallbladder ⃠ **2** Bile Ducts ⃠ **3** Pancreas ⃠	**3** Electrons	**Z** None	**0** Intraoperative **Z** None

⃠ DF000ZZ DF001ZZ DF002ZZ DF003Z0 DF003ZZ DF004ZZ DF005ZZ DF006ZZ DF010ZZ DF011ZZ DF012ZZ DF013Z0 DF013ZZ DF014ZZ DF015ZZ DF016ZZ DF020ZZ DF021ZZ DF022ZZ DF023Z0 DF023ZZ DF024ZZ DF025ZZ DF026ZZ DF030ZZ DF031ZZ DF032ZZ DF033Z0 DF033ZZ DF034ZZ DF035ZZ DF036ZZ

D Radiation Therapy
F Hepatobiliary System and Pancreas
1 Brachytherapy

Treatment Site Character 4	Modality Qualifier Character 5	Isotope Character 6	Qualifier Character 7
0 Liver ⃠ **1** Gallbladder ⃠ **2** Bile Ducts ⃠ **3** Pancreas ⃠	**9** High Dose Rate (HDR) **B** Low Dose Rate (LDR)	**7** Cesium 137 (Cs-137) **8** Iridium 192 (Ir-192) **9** Iodine 125 (I-125) **B** Palladium 103 (Pd-103) **C** Californium 252 (Cf-252) **Y** Other Isotope	**Z** None

⃠ DF1097Z DF1098Z DF1099Z DF109BZ DF109CZ DF109YZ DF10B7Z DF10B8Z DF10B9Z DF10BBZ DF10BCZ DF10BYZ DF1197Z DF1198Z DF1199Z DF119BZ DF119CZ DF119YZ DF11B7Z DF11B8Z DF11B9Z DF11BBZ DF11BCZ DF11BYZ DF1297Z DF1298Z DF1299Z DF129BZ DF129CZ DF129YZ DF12B7Z DF12B8Z DF12B9Z DF12BBZ DF12BCZ DF12BYZ DF1397Z DF1398Z DF1399Z DF139BZ DF139CZ DF139YZ DF13B7Z DF13B8Z DF13B9Z DF13BBZ DF13BCZ DF13BYZ

D Radiation Therapy
F Hepatobiliary System and Pancreas
2 Stereotactic Radiosurgery

Treatment Site Character 4	Modality Qualifier Character 5	Isotope Character 6	Qualifier Character 7
0 Liver DRG **1** Gallbladder DRG **2** Bile Ducts DRG **3** Pancreas DRG	**D** Stereotactic Other Photon Radiosurgery **H** Stereotactic Particulate Radiosurgery **J** Stereotactic Gamma Beam Radiosurgery	**Z** None	**Z** None

DRG DF20DZZ DF20HZZ DF20JZZ DF21DZZ DF21HZZ DF21JZZ DF22DZZ DF22HZZ DF22JZZ DF23DZZ DF23HZZ DF23JZZ

D Radiation Therapy
F Hepatobiliary System and Pancreas
Y Other Radiation

Treatment Site Character 4	Modality Qualifier Character 5	Isotope Character 6	Qualifier Character 7
0 Liver ⊘ **1** Gallbladder ⊘ **2** Bile Ducts ⊘ **3** Pancreas ⊘	**7** Contact Radiation **8** Hyperthermia **C** Intraoperative Radiation Therapy (IORT) **F** Plaque Radiation **K** Laser Interstitial Thermal Therapy	**Z** None	**Z** None

⊘ DFY07ZZ DFY08ZZ DFY0CZZ DFY0FZZ DFY17ZZ DFY18ZZ DFY1CZZ DFY1FZZ DFY27ZZ DFY28ZZ DFY2CZZ DFY2FZZ DFY37ZZ DFY38ZZ DFY3CZZ DFY3FZZ

D Radiation Therapy
G Endocrine System
0 Beam Radiation

Treatment Site Character 4	Modality Qualifier Character 5	Isotope Character 6	Qualifier Character 7
0 Pituitary Gland ⊘ **1** Pineal Body ⊘ **2** Adrenal Glands ⊘ **4** Parathyroid Glands ⊘ **5** Thyroid ⊘	**0** Photons <1 MeV **1** Photons 1 - 10 MeV **2** Photons >10 MeV **5** Neutrons **6** Neutron Capture	**Z** None	**Z** None
0 Pituitary Gland ⊘ **1** Pineal Body ⊘ **2** Adrenal Glands ⊘ **4** Parathyroid Glands ⊘ **5** Thyroid ⊘	**3** Electrons	**Z** None	**0** Intraoperative **Z** None

⊘ DG000ZZ DG001ZZ DG002ZZ DG003Z0 DG003ZZ DG005ZZ DG006ZZ DG010ZZ DG011ZZ DG012ZZ DG013Z0 DG013ZZ DG015ZZ DG016ZZ DG020ZZ DG021ZZ DG022ZZ DG023Z0 DG023ZZ DG025ZZ DG026ZZ DG040ZZ DG041ZZ DG042ZZ DG043Z0 DG043ZZ DG045ZZ DG046ZZ DG050ZZ DG051ZZ DG052ZZ DG053Z0 DG053ZZ DG055ZZ DG056ZZ

D Radiation Therapy
G Endocrine System
1 Brachytherapy

Treatment Site Character 4	Modality Qualifier Character 5	Isotope Character 6	Qualifier Character 7
0 Pituitary Gland ⊘ **1** Pineal Body ⊘ **2** Adrenal Glands ⊘ **4** Parathyroid Glands ⊘ **5** Thyroid ⊘	**9** High Dose Rate (HDR) **B** Low Dose Rate (LDR)	**7** Cesium 137 (Cs-137) **8** Iridium 192 (Ir-192) **9** Iodine 125 (I-125) **B** Palladium 103 (Pd-103) **C** Californium 252 (Cf-252) **Y** Other Isotope	**Z** None

⊘ DG1097Z DG1098Z DG1099Z DG109BZ DG109CZ DG109YZ DG10B7Z DG10B8Z DG10B9Z DG10BBZ DG10BCZ DG10BYZ DG1197Z DG1198Z DG1199Z DG119BZ DG119CZ DG119YZ DG11B7Z DG11B8Z DG11B9Z DG11BBZ DG11BCZ DG11BYZ DG1297Z DG1298Z DG1299Z DG129BZ DG129CZ DG129YZ DG12B7Z DG12B8Z DG12B9Z DG12BBZ DG12BCZ DG12BYZ DG1497Z DG1498Z DG1499Z DG149BZ DG149CZ DG149YZ DG14B7Z DG14B8Z DG14B9Z DG14BBZ DG14BCZ DG14BYZ DG1597Z DG1598Z DG1599Z DG159BZ DG159CZ DG159YZ DG15B7Z DG15B8Z DG15B9Z DG15BBZ DG15BCZ DG15BYZ

LC Limited Coverage NC Noncovered HAC HAC Associated Procedure CC Combination Cluster - See Appendix G for code lists
DRG Non-OR-Affecting MS-DRG Assignment ⊘ Non-OR-Not Affecting MS-DRG Assignment New/Revised Text in **Orange** ♂ Male ♀ Female

D Radiation Therapy
G Endocrine System
2 Stereotactic Radiosurgery

Treatment Site Character 4	Modality Qualifier Character 5	Isotope Character 6	Qualifier Character 7
0 Pituitary Gland DRG 1 Pineal Body DRG 2 Adrenal Glands DRG 4 Parathyroid Glands DRG 5 Thyroid DRG	D Stereotactic Other Photon Radiosurgery H Stereotactic Particulate Radiosurgery J Stereotactic Gamma Beam Radiosurgery	Z None	Z None

DRG DG20DZZ DG20HZZ DG20JZZ DG21DZZ DG21HZZ DG21JZZ DG22DZZ DG22HZZ DG22JZZ DG24DZZ DG24HZZ DG24JZZ DG25DZZ DG25HZZ DG25JZZ

D Radiation Therapy
G Endocrine System
Y Other Radiation

Treatment Site Character 4	Modality Qualifier Character 5	Isotope Character 6	Qualifier Character 7
0 Pituitary Gland ⊘ 1 Pineal Body ⊘ 2 Adrenal Glands ⊘ 4 Parathyroid Glands ⊘ 5 Thyroid ⊘	7 Contact Radiation 8 Hyperthermia F Plaque Radiation K Laser Interstitial Thermal Therapy	Z None	Z None

⊘ DGY07ZZ DGY08ZZ DGY0FZZ DGY17ZZ DGY18ZZ DGY1FZZ DGY27ZZ DGY28ZZ DGY2FZZ DGY47ZZ DGY48ZZ DGY4FZZ DGY57ZZ DGY58ZZ DGY5FZZ

D Radiation Therapy
H Skin
0 Beam Radiation

Treatment Site Character 4	Modality Qualifier Character 5	Isotope Character 6	Qualifier Character 7
2 Skin, Face ⊘ 3 Skin, Neck ⊘ 4 Skin, Arm ⊘ 6 Skin, Chest ⊘ 7 Skin, Back ⊘ 8 Skin, Abdomen ⊘ 9 Skin, Buttock ⊘ B Skin, Leg ⊘	0 Photons <1 MeV 1 Photons 1 - 10 MeV 2 Photons >10 MeV 4 Heavy Particles (Protons, Ions) 5 Neutrons 6 Neutron Capture	Z None	Z None
2 Skin, Face ⊘ 3 Skin, Neck ⊘ 4 Skin, Arm ⊘ 6 Skin, Chest ⊘ 7 Skin, Back ⊘ 8 Skin, Abdomen ⊘ 9 Skin, Buttock ⊘ B Skin, Leg ⊘	3 Electrons	Z None	0 Intraoperative Z None

⊘ DH020ZZ DH021ZZ DH022ZZ DH023Z0 DH023ZZ DH024ZZ DH025ZZ DH026ZZ DH030ZZ DH031ZZ DH032ZZ DH033Z0 DH033ZZ DH034ZZ DH035ZZ DH036ZZ DH040ZZ DH041ZZ DH042ZZ DH043Z0 DH043ZZ DH044ZZ DH045ZZ DH046ZZ DH060ZZ DH061ZZ DH062ZZ DH063Z0 DH063ZZ DH064ZZ DH065ZZ DH066ZZ DH070ZZ DH071ZZ DH072ZZ DH073Z0 DH073ZZ DH074ZZ DH075ZZ DH076ZZ DH080ZZ DH081ZZ DH082ZZ DH083Z0 DH083ZZ DH084ZZ DH085ZZ DH086ZZ DH090ZZ DH091ZZ DH092ZZ DH093Z0 DH093ZZ DH094ZZ DH095ZZ DH096ZZ DH0B0ZZ DH0B1ZZ DH0B2ZZ DH0B3Z0 DH0B3ZZ DH0B4ZZ DH0B5ZZ DH0B6ZZ

LC Limited Coverage NC Noncovered HAC HAC Associated Procedure CC Combination Cluster - See Appendix G for code lists
DRG Non-OR-Affecting MS-DRG Assignment ⊘ Non-OR-Not Affecting MS-DRG Assignment New/Revised Text in **Orange** ♂ Male ♀ Female

D Radiation Therapy
H Skin
Y Other Radiation

Treatment Site Character 4	Modality Qualifier Character 5	Isotope Character 6	Qualifier Character 7
2 Skin, Face ⊘ **3** Skin, Neck ⊘ **4** Skin, Arm ⊘ **6** Skin, Chest ⊘ **7** Skin, Back ⊘ **8** Skin, Abdomen ⊘ **9** Skin, Buttock ⊘ **B** Skin, Leg ⊘	**7** Contact Radiation **8** Hyperthermia **F** Plaque Radiation	**Z** None	**Z** None
5 Skin, Hand ⊘ **C** Skin, Foot ⊘	**F** Plaque Radiation	**Z** None	**Z** None

⊘ DHY27ZZ DHY28ZZ DHY2FZZ DHY37ZZ DHY38ZZ DHY3FZZ DHY47ZZ DHY48ZZ DHY4FZZ DHY5FZZ DHY67ZZ DHY68ZZ DHY6FZZ DHY77ZZ DHY78ZZ DHY7FZZ DHY87ZZ DHY88ZZ DHY8FZZ DHY97ZZ DHY98ZZ DHY9FZZ DHYB7ZZ DHYB8ZZ DHYBFZZ DHYCFZZ

D Radiation Therapy
M Breast
0 Beam Radiation

Treatment Site Character 4	Modality Qualifier Character 5	Isotope Character 6	Qualifier Character 7
0 Breast, Left ⊘ **1** Breast, Right ⊘	**0** Photons <1 MeV **1** Photons 1 - 10 MeV **2** Photons >10 MeV **4** Heavy Particles (Protons, Ions) **5** Neutrons **6** Neutron Capture	**Z** None	**Z** None
0 Breast, Left ⊘ **1** Breast, Right ⊘	**3** Electrons	**Z** None	**0** Intraoperative **Z** None

⊘ DM000ZZ DM001ZZ DM002ZZ DM003Z0 DM003ZZ DM004ZZ DM005ZZ DM006ZZ DM010ZZ DM011ZZ DM012ZZ DM013Z0 DM013ZZ DM014ZZ DM015ZZ DM016ZZ

D Radiation Therapy
M Breast
1 Brachytherapy

Treatment Site Character 4	Modality Qualifier Character 5	Isotope Character 6	Qualifier Character 7
0 Breast, Left ⊘ **1** Breast, Right ⊘	**9** High Dose Rate (HDR) **B** Low Dose Rate (LDR)	**7** Cesium 137 (Cs-137) **8** Iridium 192 (Ir-192) **9** Iodine 125 (I-125) **B** Palladium 103 (Pd-103) **C** Californium 252 (Cf-252) **Y** Other Isotope	**Z** None

⊘ DM1097Z DM1098Z DM1099Z DM109BZ DM109CZ DM109YZ DM10B7Z DM10B8Z DM10B9Z DM10BBZ DM10BCZ DM10BYZ DM1197Z DM1198Z DM1199Z DM119BZ DM119CZ DM119YZ DM11B7Z DM11B8Z DM11B9Z DM11BBZ DM11BCZ DM11BYZ

D Radiation Therapy
M Breast
2 Stereotactic Radiosurgery

Treatment Site Character 4	Modality Qualifier Character 5	Isotope Character 6	Qualifier Character 7
0 Breast, Left DRG **1** Breast, Right DRG	**D** Stereotactic Other Photon Radiosurgery **H** Stereotactic Particulate Radiosurgery **J** Stereotactic Gamma Beam Radiosurgery	**Z** None	**Z** None

DRG DM20DZZ DM20HZZ DM20JZZ DM21DZZ DM21HZZ DM21JZZ

D Radiation Therapy
M Breast
Y Other Radiation

Treatment Site Character 4	Modality Qualifier Character 5	Isotope Character 6	Qualifier Character 7
0 Breast, Left ⦸ **1** Breast, Right ⦸	**7** Contact Radiation **8** Hyperthermia **F** Plaque Radiation **K** Laser Interstitial Thermal Therapy	**Z** None	**Z** None

⦸ DMY07ZZ DMY08ZZ DMY0FZZ DMY17ZZ DMY18ZZ DMY1FZZ

D Radiation Therapy
P Musculoskeletal System
0 Beam Radiation

Treatment Site Character 4	Modality Qualifier Character 5	Isotope Character 6	Qualifier Character 7
0 Skull ⦸ **2** Maxilla ⦸ **3** Mandible ⦸ **4** Sternum ⦸ **5** Rib(s) ⦸ **6** Humerus ⦸ **7** Radius/Ulna ⦸ **8** Pelvic Bones ⦸ **9** Femur ⦸ **B** Tibia/Fibula ⦸ **C** Other Bone ⦸	**0** Photons <1 MeV **1** Photons 1 - 10 MeV **2** Photons >10 MeV **4** Heavy Particles (Protons, Ions) **5** Neutrons **6** Neutron Capture	**Z** None	**Z** None
0 Skull ⦸ **2** Maxilla ⦸ **3** Mandible ⦸ **4** Sternum ⦸ **5** Rib(s) ⦸ **6** Humerus ⦸ **7** Radius/Ulna ⦸ **8** Pelvic Bones ⦸ **9** Femur ⦸ **B** Tibia/Fibula ⦸ **C** Other Bone ⦸	**3** Electrons	**Z** None	**0** Intraoperative **Z** None

⦸ DP000ZZ DP001ZZ DP002ZZ DP003Z0 DP003ZZ DP004ZZ DP005ZZ DP006ZZ DP020ZZ DP021ZZ DP022ZZ DP023Z0 DP023ZZ
DP024ZZ DP025ZZ DP026ZZ DP030ZZ DP031ZZ DP032ZZ DP033Z0 DP033ZZ DP034ZZ DP035ZZ DP036ZZ DP040ZZ DP041ZZ
DP042ZZ DP043Z0 DP043ZZ DP044ZZ DP045ZZ DP046ZZ DP050ZZ DP051ZZ DP052ZZ DP053Z0 DP053ZZ DP054ZZ DP055ZZ
DP056ZZ DP060ZZ DP061ZZ DP062ZZ DP063Z0 DP063ZZ DP064ZZ DP065ZZ DP066ZZ DP070ZZ DP071ZZ DP072ZZ DP073Z0
DP073ZZ DP074ZZ DP075ZZ DP076ZZ DP080ZZ DP081ZZ DP082ZZ DP083Z0 DP083ZZ DP084ZZ DP085ZZ DP086ZZ DP090ZZ
DP091ZZ DP092ZZ DP093Z0 DP093ZZ DP094ZZ DP095ZZ DP096ZZ DP0B0ZZ DP0B1ZZ DP0B2ZZ DP0B3Z0 DP0B3ZZ DP0B4ZZ
DP0B5ZZ DP0B6ZZ DP0C0ZZ DP0C1ZZ DP0C2ZZ DP0C3Z0 DP0C3ZZ DP0C4ZZ DP0C5ZZ DP0C6ZZ

D Radiation Therapy
P Musculoskeletal System
Y Other Radiation

Treatment Site Character 4	Modality Qualifier Character 5	Isotope Character 6	Qualifier Character 7
0 Skull ⦸ 2 Maxilla ⦸ 3 Mandible ⦸ 4 Sternum ⦸ 5 Rib(s) ⦸ 6 Humerus ⦸ 7 Radius/Ulna ⦸ 8 Pelvic Bones ⦸ 9 Femur ⦸ B Tibia/Fibula ⦸ C Other Bone ⦸	7 Contact Radiation 8 Hyperthermia F Plaque Radiation	Z None	Z None

⦸ DPY07ZZ DPY08ZZ DPY0FZZ DPY27ZZ DPY28ZZ DPY2FZZ DPY37ZZ DPY38ZZ DPY3FZZ DPY47ZZ DPY48ZZ DPY4FZZ DPY57ZZ DPY58ZZ DPY5FZZ DPY67ZZ DPY68ZZ DPY6FZZ DPY77ZZ DPY78ZZ DPY7FZZ DPY87ZZ DPY88ZZ DPY8FZZ DPY97ZZ DPY98ZZ DPY9FZZ DPYB7ZZ DPYB8ZZ DPYBFZZ DPYC7ZZ DPYC8ZZ DPYCFZZ

D Radiation Therapy
T Urinary System
0 Beam Radiation

Treatment Site Character 4	Modality Qualifier Character 5	Isotope Character 6	Qualifier Character 7
0 Kidney ⦸ 1 Ureter ⦸ 2 Bladder ⦸ 3 Urethra ⦸	0 Photons <1 MeV 1 Photons 1 - 10 MeV 2 Photons >10 MeV 4 Heavy Particles (Protons, Ions) 5 Neutrons 6 Neutron Capture	Z None	Z None
0 Kidney ⦸ 1 Ureter ⦸ 2 Bladder ⦸ 3 Urethra ⦸	3 Electrons	Z None	0 Intraoperative Z None

⦸ DT000ZZ DT001ZZ DT002ZZ DT003Z0 DT003ZZ DT004ZZ DT005ZZ DT006ZZ DT010ZZ DT011ZZ DT012ZZ DT013Z0 DT013ZZ DT014ZZ DT015ZZ DT016ZZ DT020ZZ DT021ZZ DT022ZZ DT023Z0 DT023ZZ DT024ZZ DT025ZZ DT026ZZ DT030ZZ DT031ZZ DT032ZZ DT033Z0 DT033ZZ DT034ZZ DT035ZZ DT036ZZ

D Radiation Therapy
T Urinary System
1 Brachytherapy

Treatment Site Character 4	Modality Qualifier Character 5	Isotope Character 6	Qualifier Character 7
0 Kidney ⦸ 1 Ureter ⦸ 2 Bladder ⦸ 3 Urethra ⦸	9 High Dose Rate (HDR) B Low Dose Rate (LDR)	7 Cesium 137 (Cs-137) 8 Iridium 192 (Ir-192) 9 Iodine 125 (I-125) B Palladium 103 (Pd-103) C Californium 252 (Cf-252) Y Other Isotope	Z None

⦸ DT1097Z DT1098Z DT1099Z DT109BZ DT109CZ DT109YZ DT10B7Z DT10B8Z DT10B9Z DT10BBZ DT10BCZ DT10BYZ DT1197Z DT1198Z DT1199Z DT119BZ DT119CZ DT119YZ DT11B7Z DT11B8Z DT11B9Z DT11BBZ DT11BCZ DT11BYZ DT1297Z DT1298Z DT1299Z DT129BZ DT129CZ DT129YZ DT12B7Z DT12B8Z DT12B9Z DT12BBZ DT12BCZ DT12BYZ DT1397Z DT1398Z DT1399Z DT139BZ DT139CZ DT139YZ DT13B7Z DT13B8Z DT13B9Z DT13BBZ DT13BCZ DT13BYZ

D Radiation Therapy
T Urinary System
2 Stereotactic Radiosurgery

Treatment Site Character 4	Modality Qualifier Character 5	Isotope Character 6	Qualifier Character 7
0 Kidney DRG **1** Ureter DRG **2** Bladder DRG **3** Urethra DRG	**D** Stereotactic Other Photon Radiosurgery **H** Stereotactic Particulate Radiosurgery **J** Stereotactic Gamma Beam Radiosurgery	**Z** None	**Z** None

DRG DT20DZZ DT20HZZ DT20JZZ DT21DZZ DT21HZZ DT21JZZ DT22DZZ DT22HZZ DT22JZZ DT23DZZ DT23HZZ DT23JZZ

D Radiation Therapy
T Urinary System
Y Other Radiation

Treatment Site Character 4	Modality Qualifier Character 5	Isotope Character 6	Qualifier Character 7
0 Kidney ⊘ **1** Ureter ⊘ **2** Bladder ⊘ **3** Urethra ⊘	**7** Contact Radiation **8** Hyperthermia **C** Intraoperative Radiation Therapy (IORT) **F** Plaque Radiation	**Z** None	**Z** None

⊘ DTY07ZZ DTY08ZZ DTY0CZZ DTY0FZZ DTY17ZZ DTY18ZZ DTY1CZZ DTY1FZZ DTY27ZZ DTY28ZZ DTY2CZZ DTY2FZZ DTY37ZZ DTY38ZZ DTY3CZZ DTY3FZZ

D Radiation Therapy
U Female Reproductive System
0 Beam Radiation

Treatment Site Character 4	Modality Qualifier Character 5	Isotope Character 6	Qualifier Character 7
0 Ovary ⊘ ♀ **1** Cervix ⊘ ♀ **2** Uterus ⊘ ♀	**0** Photons <1 MeV **1** Photons 1 - 10 MeV **2** Photons >10 MeV **4** Heavy Particles (Protons, Ions) **5** Neutrons **6** Neutron Capture	**Z** None	**Z** None
0 Ovary ⊘ ♀ **1** Cervix ⊘ ♀ **2** Uterus ⊘ ♀	**3** Electrons	**Z** None	**0** Intraoperative **Z** None

♀ DU000ZZ DU001ZZ DU002ZZ DU003Z0 DU003ZZ DU004ZZ DU005ZZ DU006ZZ DU010ZZ DU011ZZ DU012ZZ DU013Z0 DU013ZZ DU014ZZ DU015ZZ DU016ZZ DU020ZZ DU021ZZ DU022ZZ DU023Z0 DU023ZZ DU024ZZ DU025ZZ DU026ZZ

⊘ DU000ZZ DU001ZZ DU002ZZ DU003Z0 DU003ZZ DU004ZZ DU005ZZ DU006ZZ DU010ZZ DU011ZZ DU012ZZ DU013Z0 DU013ZZ DU014ZZ DU015ZZ DU016ZZ DU020ZZ DU021ZZ DU022ZZ DU023Z0 DU023ZZ DU024ZZ DU025ZZ DU026ZZ

LC Limited Coverage NC Noncovered HAC HAC Associated Procedure CC Combination Cluster - See Appendix G for code lists
DRG Non-OR-Affecting MS-DRG Assignment ⊘ Non-OR-Not Affecting MS-DRG Assignment New/Revised Text in **Orange** ♂ Male ♀ Female

D Radiation Therapy
U Female Reproductive System
1 Brachytherapy

Treatment Site Character 4	Modality Qualifier Character 5	Isotope Character 6	Qualifier Character 7
0 Ovary ⊘ ♀ **1** Cervix ⊘ ♀ **2** Uterus ⊘ ♀	**9** High Dose Rate (HDR) **B** Low Dose Rate (LDR)	**7** Cesium 137 (Cs-137) **8** Iridium 192 (Ir-192) **9** Iodine 125 (I-125) **B** Palladium 103 (Pd-103) **C** Californium 252 (Cf-252) **Y** Other Isotope	**Z** None

♀ DU1097Z DU1098Z DU1099Z DU109BZ DU109CZ DU109YZ DU10B7Z DU10B8Z DU10B9Z DU10BBZ DU10BCZ DU10BYZ DU1197Z DU1198Z DU1199Z DU119BZ DU119CZ DU119YZ DU11B7Z DU11B8Z DU11B9Z DU11BBZ DU11BCZ DU11BYZ DU1297Z DU1298Z DU1299Z DU129BZ DU129CZ DU129YZ DU12B7Z DU12B8Z DU12B9Z DU12BBZ DU12BCZ DU12BYZ

⊘ DU1097Z DU1098Z DU1099Z DU109BZ DU109CZ DU109YZ DU10B7Z DU10B8Z DU10B9Z DU10BBZ DU10BCZ DU10BYZ DU1197Z DU1198Z DU1199Z DU119BZ DU119CZ DU119YZ DU11B7Z DU11B8Z DU11B9Z DU11BBZ DU11BCZ DU11BYZ DU1297Z DU1298Z DU1299Z DU129BZ DU129CZ DU129YZ DU12B7Z DU12B8Z DU12B9Z DU12BBZ DU12BCZ DU12BYZ

D Radiation Therapy
U Female Reproductive System
2 Stereotactic Radiosurgery

Treatment Site Character 4	Modality Qualifier Character 5	Isotope Character 6	Qualifier Character 7
0 Ovary ♀ DRG **1** Cervix ♀ DRG **2** Uterus ♀ DRG	**D** Stereotactic Other Photon Radiosurgery **H** Stereotactic Particulate Radiosurgery **J** Stereotactic Gamma Beam Radiosurgery	**Z** None	**Z** None

♀ DU20DZZ DU20HZZ DU20JZZ DU21DZZ DU21HZZ DU21JZZ DU22DZZ DU22HZZ DU22JZZ

DRG DU20DZZ DU20HZZ DU20JZZ DU21DZZ DU21HZZ DU21JZZ DU22DZZ DU22HZZ DU22JZZ

D Radiation Therapy
U Female Reproductive System
Y Other Radiation

Treatment Site Character 4	Modality Qualifier Character 5	Isotope Character 6	Qualifier Character 7
0 Ovary ⊘ ♀ **1** Cervix ⊘ ♀ **2** Uterus ⊘ ♀	**7** Contact Radiation **8** Hyperthermia **C** Intraoperative Radiation Therapy (IORT) **F** Plaque Radiation	**Z** None	**Z** None

♀ DUY07ZZ DUY08ZZ DUY0CZZ DUY0FZZ DUY17ZZ DUY18ZZ DUY1CZZ DUY1FZZ DUY27ZZ DUY28ZZ DUY2CZZ DUY2FZZ

⊘ DUY07ZZ DUY08ZZ DUY0CZZ DUY0FZZ DUY17ZZ DUY18ZZ DUY1CZZ DUY1FZZ DUY27ZZ DUY28ZZ DUY2CZZ DUY2FZZ

D Radiation Therapy
V Male Reproductive System
0 Beam Radiation

Treatment Site Character 4	Modality Qualifier Character 5	Isotope Character 6	Qualifier Character 7
0 Prostate ⊘ ♂ **1** Testis ⊘ ♂	**0** Photons <1 MeV **1** Photons 1 - 10 MeV **2** Photons >10 MeV **4** Heavy Particles (Protons, Ions) **5** Neutrons **6** Neutron Capture	**Z** None	**Z** None
0 Prostate ⊘ ♂ **1** Testis ⊘ ♂	**3** Electrons	**Z** None	**0** Intraoperative **Z** None

♂ DV000ZZ DV001ZZ DV002ZZ DV003Z0 DV003ZZ DV004ZZ DV005ZZ DV006ZZ DV010ZZ DV011ZZ DV012ZZ DV013Z0 DV013ZZ DV014ZZ DV015ZZ DV016ZZ

⊘ DV000ZZ DV001ZZ DV002ZZ DV003Z0 DV003ZZ DV004ZZ DV005ZZ DV006ZZ DV010ZZ DV011ZZ DV012ZZ DV013Z0 DV013ZZ DV014ZZ DV015ZZ DV016ZZ

LC Limited Coverage NC Noncovered HAC HAC Associated Procedure CC Combination Cluster - See Appendix G for code lists
DRG Non-OR-Affecting MS-DRG Assignment ⊘ Non-OR-Not Affecting MS-DRG Assignment New/Revised Text in **Orange** ♂ Male ♀ Female

D Radiation Therapy
V Male Reproductive System
1 Brachytherapy

Treatment Site Character 4	Modality Qualifier Character 5	Isotope Character 6	Qualifier Character 7
0 Prostate ⃠ ♂ **1** Testis ⃠ ♂	**9** High Dose Rate (HDR) **B** Low Dose Rate (LDR)	**7** Cesium 137 (Cs-137) **8** Iridium 192 (Ir-192) **9** Iodine 125 (I-125) **B** Palladium 103 (Pd-103) **C** Californium 252 (Cf-252) **Y** Other Isotope	**Z** None

♂ DV1097Z DV1098Z DV1099Z DV109BZ DV109CZ DV109YZ DV10B7Z DV10B8Z DV10B9Z DV10BBZ DV10BCZ DV10BYZ DV1197Z DV1198Z DV1199Z DV119BZ DV119CZ DV119YZ DV11B7Z DV11B8Z DV11B9Z DV11BBZ DV11BCZ DV11BYZ

⃠ DV1097Z DV1098Z DV1099Z DV109BZ DV109CZ DV109YZ DV10B7Z DV10B8Z DV10B9Z DV10BBZ DV10BCZ DV10BYZ DV1197Z DV1198Z DV1199Z DV119BZ DV119CZ DV119YZ DV11B7Z DV11B8Z DV11B9Z DV11BBZ DV11BCZ DV11BYZ

D Radiation Therapy
V Male Reproductive System
2 Stereotactic Radiosurgery

Treatment Site Character 4	Modality Qualifier Character 5	Isotope Character 6	Qualifier Character 7
0 Prostate ♂ DRG **1** Testis ♂ DRG	**D** Stereotactic Other Photon Radiosurgery **H** Stereotactic Particulate Radiosurgery **J** Stereotactic Gamma Beam Radiosurgery	**Z** None	**Z** None

♂ DV20DZZ DV20HZZ DV20JZZ DV21DZZ DV21HZZ DV21JZZ

DRG DV20DZZ DV20HZZ DV20JZZ DV21DZZ DV21HZZ DV21JZZ

D Radiation Therapy
V Male Reproductive System
Y Other Radiation

Treatment Site Character 4	Modality Qualifier Character 5	Isotope Character 6	Qualifier Character 7
0 Prostate ⃠ ♂	**7** Contact Radiation **8** Hyperthermia **C** Intraoperative Radiation Therapy (IORT) **F** Plaque Radiation **K** Laser Interstitial Thermal Therapy	**Z** None	**Z** None
1 Testis ⃠ ♂	**7** Contact Radiation **8** Hyperthermia **F** Plaque Radiation	**Z** None	**Z** None

♂ DVY07ZZ DVY08ZZ DVY0CZZ DVY0FZZ DVY0KZZ DVY17ZZ DVY18ZZ DVY1FZZ

⃠ DVY07ZZ DVY08ZZ DVY0CZZ DVY0FZZ DVY17ZZ DVY18ZZ DVY1FZZ

D Radiation Therapy
W Anatomical Regions
0 Beam Radiation

Treatment Site Character 4	Modality Qualifier Character 5	Isotope Character 6	Qualifier Character 7
1 Head and Neck ⃠ 2 Chest ⃠ 3 Abdomen ⃠ 4 Hemibody ⃠ 5 Whole Body ⃠ 6 Pelvic Region ⃠	0 Photons <1 MeV 1 Photons 1 - 10 MeV 2 Photons >10 MeV 4 Heavy Particles (Protons, Ions) 5 Neutrons 6 Neutron Capture	Z None	Z None
1 Head and Neck ⃠ 2 Chest ⃠ 3 Abdomen ⃠ 4 Hemibody ⃠ 5 Whole Body ⃠ 6 Pelvic Region ⃠	3 Electrons	Z None	0 Intraoperative Z None

⃠ DW010ZZ DW011ZZ DW012ZZ DW013Z0 DW013ZZ DW014ZZ DW015ZZ DW016ZZ DW020ZZ DW021ZZ DW022ZZ DW023Z0 DW023ZZ DW024ZZ DW025ZZ DW026ZZ DW030ZZ DW031ZZ DW032ZZ DW033Z0 DW033ZZ DW034ZZ DW035ZZ DW036ZZ DW040ZZ DW041ZZ DW042ZZ DW043Z0 DW043ZZ DW044ZZ DW045ZZ DW046ZZ DW050ZZ DW051ZZ DW052ZZ DW053Z0 DW053ZZ DW054ZZ DW055ZZ DW056ZZ DW060ZZ DW061ZZ DW062ZZ DW063Z0 DW063ZZ DW064ZZ DW065ZZ DW066ZZ

D Radiation Therapy
W Anatomical Regions
1 Brachytherapy

Treatment Site Character 4	Modality Qualifier Character 5	Isotope Character 6	Qualifier Character 7
1 Head and Neck ⃠ 2 Chest ⃠ 3 Abdomen ⃠ 6 Pelvic Region ⃠	9 High Dose Rate (HDR) B Low Dose Rate (LDR)	7 Cesium 137 (Cs-137) 8 Iridium 192 (Ir-192) 9 Iodine 125 (I-125) B Palladium 103 (Pd-103) C Californium 252 (Cf-252) Y Other Isotope	Z None

⃠ DW1197Z DW1198Z DW1199Z DW119BZ DW119CZ DW119YZ DW11B7Z DW11B8Z DW11B9Z DW11BBZ DW11BCZ DW11BYZ DW1297Z DW1298Z DW1299Z DW129BZ DW129CZ DW129YZ DW12B7Z DW12B8Z DW12B9Z DW12BBZ DW12BCZ DW12BYZ DW1397Z DW1398Z DW1399Z DW139BZ DW139CZ DW139YZ DW13B7Z DW13B8Z DW13B9Z DW13BBZ DW13BCZ DW13BYZ DW1697Z DW1698Z DW1699Z DW169BZ DW169CZ DW169YZ DW16B7Z DW16B8Z DW16B9Z DW16BBZ DW16BCZ DW16BYZ

D Radiation Therapy
W Anatomical Regions
2 Stereotactic Radiosurgery

Treatment Site Character 4	Modality Qualifier Character 5	Isotope Character 6	Qualifier Character 7
1 Head and Neck DRG 2 Chest DRG 3 Abdomen DRG 6 Pelvic Region DRG	D Stereotactic Other Photon Radiosurgery H Stereotactic Particulate Radiosurgery J Stereotactic Gamma Beam Radiosurgery	Z None	Z None

DRG DW21DZZ DW21HZZ DW21JZZ DW22DZZ DW22HZZ DW22JZZ DW23DZZ DW23HZZ DW23JZZ DW26DZZ DW26HZZ DW26JZZ

D Radiation Therapy
W Anatomical Regions
Y Other Radiation

Treatment Site Character 4	Modality Qualifier Character 5	Isotope Character 6	Qualifier Character 7
1 Head and Neck ⃠ 2 Chest ⃠ 3 Abdomen ⃠ 4 Hemibody ⃠ 6 Pelvic Region ⃠	7 Contact Radiation 8 Hyperthermia F Plaque Radiation	Z None	Z None
5 Whole Body ⃠	7 Contact Radiation 8 Hyperthermia F Plaque Radiation	Z None	Z None
5 Whole Body ⃠	G Isotope Administration	D Iodine 131 (I-131) F Phosphorus 32 (P-32) G Strontium 89 (Sr-89) H Strontium 90 (Sr-90) Y Other Isotope	Z None

⃠ DWY17ZZ DWY18ZZ DWY1FZZ DWY27ZZ DWY28ZZ DWY2FZZ DWY37ZZ DWY38ZZ DWY3FZZ DWY47ZZ DWY48ZZ DWY4FZZ DWY57ZZ DWY58ZZ DWY5FZZ DWY5GDZ DWY5GFZ DWY5GGZ DWY5GHZ DWY5GYZ DWY67ZZ DWY68ZZ DWY6FZZ

Physical Rehabilitation and Diagnostic Audiology F00-F15

F Physical Rehabilitation and Diagnostic Audiology
0 Rehabilitation
0 Speech Assessment: Measurement of speech and related functions

Body system/ Region Character 4	Type Qualifier Character 5	Equipment Character 6	Qualifier Character 7
3 Neurological System - Whole Body DRG	**G** Communicative/Cognitive Integration Skills	**K** Audiovisual **M** Augmentative / Alternative Communication **P** Computer **Y** Other Equipment **Z** None	**Z** None
Z None DRG	**0** Filtered Speech **3** Staggered Spondaic Word **Q** Performance Intensity Phonetically Balanced Speech Discrimination **R** Brief Tone Stimuli **S** Distorted Speech **T** Dichotic Stimuli **V** Temporal Ordering of Stimuli **W** Masking Patterns	**1** Audiometer **2** Sound Field / Booth **K** Audiovisual **Z** None	**Z** None
Z None DRG	**1** Speech Threshold **2** Speech/Word Recognition	**1** Audiometer **2** Sound Field / Booth **9** Cochlear Implant **K** Audiovisual **Z** None	**Z** None
Z None DRG	**4** Sensorineural Acuity Level	**1** Audiometer **2** Sound Field / Booth **Z** None	**Z** None
Z None DRG	**5** Synthetic Sentence Identification	**1** Audiometer **2** Sound Field / Booth **9** Cochlear Implant **K** Audiovisual	**Z** None
Z None DRG	**6** Speech and/or Language Screening **7** Nonspoken Language **8** Receptive/Expressive Language **C** Aphasia **G** Communicative/Cognitive Integration Skills **L** Augmentative/Alternative Communication System	**K** Audiovisual **M** Augmentative / Alternative Communication **P** Computer **Y** Other Equipment **Z** None	**Z** None
Z None DRG	**9** Articulation/Phonology	**K** Audiovisual **P** Computer **Q** Speech Analysis **Y** Other Equipment **Z** None	**Z** None
Z None DRG	**B** Motor Speech	**K** Audiovisual **N** Biosensory Feedback **P** Computer **Q** Speech Analysis **T** Aerodynamic Function **Y** Other Equipment **Z** None	**Z** None

F00 continued on next page

F Physical Rehabilitation and Diagnostic Audiology
0 Rehabilitation
0 Speech Assessment: Measurement of speech and related functions

F00 continued from previous page

Body system/ Region Character 4	Type Qualifier Character 5	Equipment Character 6	Qualifier Character 7
Z None DRG	**D** Fluency	**K** Audiovisual **N** Biosensory Feedback **P** Computer **Q** Speech Analysis **S** Voice Analysis **T** Aerodynamic Function **Y** Other Equipment **Z** None	**Z** None
Z None DRG	**F** Voice	**K** Audiovisual **N** Biosensory Feedback **P** Computer **S** Voice Analysis **T** Aerodynamic Function **Y** Other Equipment **Z** None	**Z** None
Z None DRG	**H** Bedside Swallowing and Oral Function **P** Oral Peripheral Mechanism	**Y** Other Equipment **Z** None	**Z** None
Z None DRG	**J** Instrumental Swallowing and Oral Function	**T** Aerodynamic Function **W** Swallowing **Y** Other Equipment	**Z** None
Z None DRG	**K** Orofacial Myofunctional	**K** Audiovisual **P** Computer **Y** Other Equipment **Z** None	**Z** None
Z None DRG	**M** Voice Prosthetic	**K** Audiovisual **P** Computer **S** Voice Analysis **V** Speech Prosthesis **Y** Other Equipment **Z** None	**Z** None
Z None DRG	**N** Non-invasive Instrumental Status	**N** Biosensory Feedback **P** Computer **Q** Speech Analysis **S** Voice Analysis **T** Aerodynamic Function **Y** Other Equipment	**Z** None
Z None DRG	**X** Other Specified Central Auditory Processing	**Z** None	**Z** None

DRG F003GKZ F003GMZ F003GPZ F003GYZ F003GZZ F00Z01Z F00Z02Z F00Z0KZ F00Z0ZZ F00Z11Z F00Z12Z F00Z19Z F00Z1KZ F00Z1ZZ F00Z21Z F00Z22Z F00Z29Z F00Z2KZ F00Z2ZZ F00Z31Z F00Z32Z F00Z3KZ F00Z3ZZ F00Z41Z F00Z42Z F00Z4ZZ F00Z51Z F00Z52Z F00Z59Z F00Z5KZ F00Z6KZ F00Z6MZ F00Z6PZ F00Z6YZ F00Z6ZZ F00Z7KZ F00Z7MZ F00Z7PZ F00Z7YZ F00Z7ZZ F00Z8KZ F00Z8MZ F00Z8PZ F00Z8YZ F00Z8ZZ F00Z9KZ F00Z9PZ F00Z9QZ F00Z9YZ F00Z9ZZ F00ZBKZ F00ZBNZ F00ZBPZ F00ZBQZ F00ZBTZ F00ZBYZ F00ZBZZ F00ZCKZ F00ZCMZ F00ZCPZ F00ZCYZ F00ZCZZ F00ZDKZ F00ZDNZ F00ZDPZ F00ZDQZ F00ZDSZ F00ZDTZ F00ZDYZ F00ZDZZ F00ZFKZ F00ZFNZ F00ZFPZ F00ZFSZ F00ZFTZ F00ZFYZ F00ZFZZ F00ZGKZ F00ZGMZ F00ZGPZ F00ZGYZ F00ZGZZ F00ZHYZ F00ZHZZ F00ZJTZ F00ZJWZ F00ZJYZ F00ZKKZ F00ZKPZ F00ZKYZ F00ZKZZ F00ZLKZ F00ZLMZ F00ZLPZ F00ZLYZ F00ZLZZ F00ZMKZ F00ZMPZ F00ZMSZ F00ZMVZ F00ZMYZ F00ZMZZ F00ZNNZ F00ZNPZ F00ZNQZ F00ZNSZ F00ZNTZ F00ZNYZ F00ZPYZ F00ZPZZ F00ZQ1Z F00ZQ2Z F00ZQKZ F00ZQZZ F00ZR1Z F00ZR2Z F00ZRKZ F00ZRZZ F00ZS1Z F00ZS2Z F00ZSKZ F00ZSZZ F00ZT1Z F00ZT2Z F00ZTKZ F00ZTZZ F00ZV1Z F00ZV2Z F00ZVKZ F00ZVZZ F00ZW1Z F00ZW2Z F00ZWKZ F00ZWZZ F00ZXZZ

F Physical Rehabilitation and Diagnostic Audiology
0 Rehabilitation
1 Motor and/or Nerve Function Assessment: Measurement of motor, nerve, and related functions

Body system/ Region Character 4	Type Qualifier Character 5	Equipment Character 6	Qualifier Character 7
0 Neurological System - Head and Neck DRG **1** Neurological System - Upper Back / Upper Extremity DRG **2** Neurological System - Lower Back / Lower Extremity DRG **3** Neurological System - Whole Body DRG	**0** Muscle Performance	**E** Orthosis **F** Assistive, Adaptive, Supportive or Protective **U** Prosthesis **Y** Other Equipment **Z** None	**Z** None
0 Neurological System - Head and Neck DRG **1** Neurological System - Upper Back / Upper Extremity DRG **2** Neurological System - Lower Back / Lower Extremity DRG **3** Neurological System - Whole Body DRG	**1** Integumentary Integrity **3** Coordination/Dexterity **4** Motor Function **G** Reflex Integrity	**Z** None	**Z** None
0 Neurological System - Head and Neck DRG **1** Neurological System - Upper Back / Upper Extremity DRG **2** Neurological System - Lower Back / Lower Extremity DRG **3** Neurological System - Whole Body DRG	**5** Range of Motion and Joint Integrity **6** Sensory Awareness/Processing/ Integrity	**Y** Other Equipment **Z** None	**Z** None
D Integumentary System - Head and Neck DRG **F** Integumentary System - Upper Back / Upper Extremity DRG **G** Integumentary System - Lower Back / Lower Extremity DRG **H** Integumentary System - Whole Body DRG **J** Musculoskeletal System - Head and Neck DRG **K** Musculoskeletal System - Upper Back / Upper Extremity DRG **L** Musculoskeletal System - Lower Back / Lower Extremity DRG **M** Musculoskeletal System - Whole Body DRG	**0** Muscle Performance	**E** Orthosis **F** Assistive, Adaptive, Supportive or Protective **U** Prosthesis **Y** Other Equipment **Z** None	**Z** None
D Integumentary System - Head and Neck DRG **F** Integumentary System - Upper Back / Upper Extremity DRG **G** Integumentary System - Lower Back / Lower Extremity DRG **H** Integumentary System - Whole Body DRG **J** Musculoskeletal System - Head and Neck DRG **K** Musculoskeletal System - Upper Back / Upper Extremity DRG **L** Musculoskeletal System - Lower Back / Lower Extremity DRG **M** Musculoskeletal System - Whole Body DRG	**1** Integumentary Integrity	**Z** None	**Z** None

F01 continued on next page

F01 continued from previous page

F Physical Rehabilitation and Diagnostic Audiology
0 Rehabilitation
1 Motor and/or Nerve Function Assessment: Measurement of motor, nerve, and related functions

Body system/ Region Character 4	Type Qualifier Character 5	Equipment Character 6	Qualifier Character 7
D Integumentary System - Head and Neck DRG **F** Integumentary System - Upper Back / Upper Extremity DRG **G** Integumentary System - Lower Back / Lower Extremity DRG **H** Integumentary System - Whole Body DRG **J** Musculoskeletal System - Head and Neck DRG **K** Musculoskeletal System - Upper Back / Upper Extremity DRG **L** Musculoskeletal System - Lower Back / Lower Extremity DRG **M** Musculoskeletal System - Whole Body DRG	**5** Range of Motion and Joint Integrity **6** Sensory Awareness/Processing/ Integrity	**Y** Other Equipment **Z** None	**Z** None
N Genitourinary System DRG	**0** Muscle Performance	**E** Orthosis **F** Assistive, Adaptive, Supportive or Protective **U** Prosthesis **Y** Other Equipment **Z** None	**Z** None
Z None DRG	**2** Visual Motor Integration	**K** Audiovisual **M** Augmentative / Alternative Communication **N** Biosensory Feedback **P** Computer **Q** Speech Analysis **S** Voice Analysis **Y** Other Equipment **Z** None	**Z** None
Z None DRG	**7** Facial Nerve Function	**7** Electrophysiologic	**Z** None
Z None DRG	**9** Somatosensory Evoked Potentials	**J** Somatosensory	**Z** None
Z None DRG	**B** Bed Mobility **C** Transfer **F** Wheelchair Mobility	**E** Orthosis **F** Assistive, Adaptive, Supportive or Protective **U** Prosthesis **Z** None	**Z** None
Z None DRG	**D** Gait and/or Balance	**E** Orthosis **F** Assistive, Adaptive, Supportive or Protective **U** Prosthesis **Y** Other Equipment **Z** None	**Z** None

DRG F0100EZ F0100FZ F0100UZ F0100YZ F0100ZZ F0101ZZ F0103ZZ F0104ZZ F0105YZ F0105ZZ F0106YZ F0106ZZ F010GZZ
F0110EZ F0110FZ F0110UZ F0110YZ F0110ZZ F0111ZZ F0113ZZ F0114ZZ F0115YZ F0115ZZ F0116YZ F0116ZZ F011GZZ
F0120EZ F0120FZ F0120UZ F0120YZ F0120ZZ F0121ZZ F0123ZZ F0124ZZ F0125YZ F0125ZZ F0126YZ F0126ZZ F012GZZ
F0130EZ F0130FZ F0130UZ F0130YZ F0130ZZ F0131ZZ F0133ZZ F0134ZZ F0135YZ F0135ZZ F0136YZ F0136ZZ F013GZZ
F01D0EZ F01D0FZ F01D0UZ F01D0YZ F01D0ZZ F01D1ZZ F01D5YZ F01D5ZZ F01D6YZ F01D6ZZ F01F0EZ F01F0FZ F01F0UZ
F01F0YZ F01F0ZZ F01F1ZZ F01F5YZ F01F5ZZ F01F6YZ F01F6ZZ F01G0EZ F01G0FZ F01G0UZ F01G0YZ F01G0ZZ F01G1ZZ
F01G5YZ F01G5ZZ F01G6YZ F01G6ZZ F01H0EZ F01H0FZ F01H0UZ F01H0YZ F01H0ZZ F01H1ZZ F01H5YZ F01H5ZZ F01H6YZ
F01H6ZZ F01J0EZ F01J0FZ F01J0UZ F01J0YZ F01J0ZZ F01J1ZZ F01J5YZ F01J5ZZ F01J6YZ F01J6ZZ F01K0EZ F01K0FZ
F01K0UZ F01K0YZ F01K0ZZ F01K1ZZ F01K5YZ F01K5ZZ F01K6YZ F01K6ZZ F01L0EZ F01L0FZ F01L0UZ F01L0YZ F01L0ZZ
F01L1ZZ F01L5YZ F01L5ZZ F01L6YZ F01L6ZZ F01M0EZ F01M0FZ F01M0UZ F01M0YZ F01M0ZZ F01M1ZZ F01M5YZ F01M5ZZ
F01M6YZ F01M6ZZ F01N0EZ F01N0FZ F01N0UZ F01N0YZ F01N0ZZ F01Z2KZ F01Z2MZ F01Z2NZ F01Z2PZ F01Z2QZ F01Z2SZ
F01Z2YZ F01Z2ZZ F01Z77Z F01Z9JZ F01ZBEZ F01ZBFZ F01ZBUZ F01ZBZZ F01ZCEZ F01ZCFZ F01ZCUZ F01ZCZZ F01ZDEZ
F01ZDFZ F01ZDUZ F01ZDYZ F01ZDZZ F01ZFEZ F01ZFFZ F01ZFUZ F01ZFZZ

LC Limited Coverage NC Noncovered HAC HAC Associated Procedure CC Combination Cluster - See Appendix G for code lists
DRG Non-OR-Affecting MS-DRG Assignment ⃠ Non-OR-Not Affecting MS-DRG Assignment New/Revised Text in **Orange** ♂ Male ♀ Female

F Physical Rehabilitation and Diagnostic Audiology
0 Rehabilitation
2 Activities of Daily Living Assessment: Measurement of functional level for activities of daily living

Body system/ Region Character 4	Type Qualifier Character 5	Equipment Character 6	Qualifier Character 7
0 Neurological System - Head and Neck DRG	**9** Cranial Nerve Integrity **D** Neuromotor Development	**Y** Other Equipment **Z** None	**Z** None
1 Neurological System - Upper Back / Upper Extremity DRG **2** Neurological System - Lower Back / Lower Extremity DRG **3** Neurological System - Whole Body DRG	**D** Neuromotor Development	**Y** Other Equipment **Z** None	**Z** None
4 Circulatory System - Head and Neck DRG **5** Circulatory System - Upper Back / Upper Extremity DRG **6** Circulatory System - Lower Back / Lower Extremity DRG **8** Respiratory System - Head and Neck DRG **9** Respiratory System - Upper Back / Upper Extremity DRG **B** Respiratory System - Lower Back / Lower Extremity DRG	**G** Ventilation, Respiration and Circulation	**C** Mechanical **G** Aerobic Endurance and Conditioning **Y** Other Equipment **Z** None	**Z** None
7 Circulatory System - Whole Body DRG **C** Respiratory System - Whole Body DRG	**7** Aerobic Capacity and Endurance	**E** Orthosis **G** Aerobic Endurance and Conditioning **U** Prosthesis **Y** Other Equipment **Z** None	**Z** None
7 Circulatory System - Whole Body DRG **C** Respiratory System - Whole Body DRG	**G** Ventilation, Respiration and Circulation	**C** Mechanical **G** Aerobic Endurance and Conditioning **Y** Other Equipment **Z** None	**Z** None
Z None DRG	**0** Bathing/Showering **1** Dressing **3** Grooming/Personal Hygiene **4** Home Management	**E** Orthosis **F** Assistive, Adaptive, Supportive or Protective **U** Prosthesis **Z** None	**Z** None
Z None DRG	**2** Feeding/Eating **8** Anthropometric Characteristics **F** Pain	**Y** Other Equipment **Z** None	**Z** None
Z None DRG	**5** Perceptual Processing	**K** Audiovisual **M** Augmentative / Alternative Communication **N** Biosensory Feedback **P** Computer **Q** Speech Analysis **S** Voice Analysis **Y** Other Equipment **Z** None	**Z** None
Z None DRG	**6** Psychosocial Skills	**Z** None	**Z** None
Z None DRG	**B** Environmental, Home and Work Barriers **C** Ergonomics and Body Mechanics	**E** Orthosis **F** Assistive, Adaptive, Supportive or Protective **U** Prosthesis **Y** Other Equipment **Z** None	**Z** None

F02 continued on next page

F02 continued from previous page

F Physical Rehabilitation and Diagnostic Audiology
0 Rehabilitation
2 Activities of Daily Living Assessment: Measurement of functional level for activities of daily living

Body system/ Region Character 4	Type Qualifier Character 5	Equipment Character 6	Qualifier Character 7
Z None DRG	**H** Vocational Activities and Functional Community or Work Reintegration Skills	**E** Orthosis **F** Assistive, Adaptive, Supportive or Protective **G** Aerobic Endurance and Conditioning **U** Prosthesis **Y** Other Equipment **Z** None	**Z** None

DRG F0209YZ F0209ZZ F020DYZ F020DZZ F021DYZ F021DZZ F022DYZ F022DZZ F023DYZ F023DZZ F024GCZ F024GGZ F024GYZ F024GZZ F025GCZ F025GGZ F025GYZ F025GZZ F026GCZ F026GGZ F026GYZ F026GZZ F0277EZ F0277GZ F0277UZ F0277YZ F0277ZZ F027GCZ F027GGZ F027GYZ F027GZZ F028GCZ F028GGZ F028GYZ F028GZZ F029GCZ F029GGZ F029GYZ F029GZZ F02BGCZ F02BGGZ F02BGYZ F02BGZZ F02C7EZ F02C7GZ F02C7UZ F02C7YZ F02C7ZZ F02CGCZ F02CGGZ F02CGYZ F02CGZZ F02Z0EZ F02Z0FZ F02Z0UZ F02Z0ZZ F02Z1EZ F02Z1FZ F02Z1UZ F02Z1ZZ F02Z2YZ F02Z2ZZ F02Z3EZ F02Z3FZ F02Z3UZ F02Z3ZZ F02Z4EZ F02Z4FZ F02Z4UZ F02Z4ZZ F02Z5KZ F02Z5MZ F02Z5NZ F02Z5PZ F02Z5QZ F02Z5SZ F02Z5YZ F02Z5ZZ F02Z6ZZ F02Z8YZ F02Z8ZZ F02ZBEZ F02ZBFZ F02ZBUZ F02ZBYZ F02ZBZZ F02ZCEZ F02ZCFZ F02ZCUZ F02ZCYZ F02ZCZZ F02ZFYZ F02ZFZZ F02ZHEZ F02ZHFZ F02ZHGZ F02ZHUZ F02ZHYZ F02ZHZZ

F Physical Rehabilitation and Diagnostic Audiology
0 Rehabilitation
6 Speech Treatment: Application of techniques to improve, augment, or compensate for speech and related functional impairment

Body system/ Region Character 4	Type Qualifier Character 5	Equipment Character 6	Qualifier Character 7
3 Neurological System - Whole Body DRG	**6** Communicative/Cognitive Integration Skills	**K** Audiovisual **M** Augmentative / Alternative Communication **P** Computer **Y** Other Equipment **Z** None	**Z** None
Z None DRG	**0** Nonspoken Language **3** Aphasia **6** Communicative/Cognitive Integration Skills	**K** Audiovisual **M** Augmentative / Alternative Communication **P** Computer **Y** Other Equipment **Z** None	**Z** None
Z None DRG	**1** Speech-Language Pathology and Related Disorders Counseling **2** Speech-Language Pathology and Related Disorders Prevention	**K** Audiovisual **Z** None	**Z** None
Z None DRG	**4** Articulation/Phonology	**K** Audiovisual **P** Computer **Q** Speech Analysis **T** Aerodynamic Function **Y** Other Equipment **Z** None	**Z** None
Z None DRG	**5** Aural Rehabilitation	**K** Audiovisual **L** Assistive Listening **M** Augmentative / Alternative Communication **N** Biosensory Feedback **P** Computer **Q** Speech Analysis **S** Voice Analysis **Y** Other Equipment **Z** None	**Z** None

F06 continued on next page

LC Limited Coverage NC Noncovered HAC HAC Associated Procedure CC Combination Cluster - See Appendix G for code lists
DRG Non-OR-Affecting MS-DRG Assignment ⊘ Non-OR-Not Affecting MS-DRG Assignment New/Revised Text in **Orange** ♂ Male ♀ Female

F06 continued from previous page

F Physical Rehabilitation and Diagnostic Audiology
0 Rehabilitation
6 Speech Treatment: Application of techniques to improve, augment, or compensate for speech and related functional impairment

Body system/ Region Character 4	Type Qualifier Character 5	Equipment Character 6	Qualifier Character 7
Z None DRG	**7** Fluency	**4** Electroacoustic Immittance / Acoustic Reflex **K** Audiovisual **N** Biosensory Feedback **Q** Speech Analysis **S** Voice Analysis **T** Aerodynamic Function **Y** Other Equipment **Z** None	**Z** None
Z None DRG	**8** Motor Speech	**K** Audiovisual **N** Biosensory Feedback **P** Computer **Q** Speech Analysis **S** Voice Analysis **T** Aerodynamic Function **Y** Other Equipment **Z** None	**Z** None
Z None DRG	**9** Orofacial Myofunctional	**K** Audiovisual **P** Computer **Y** Other Equipment **Z** None	**Z** None
Z None DRG	**B** Receptive/Expressive Language	**K** Audiovisual **L** Assistive Listening **M** Augmentative / Alternative Communication **P** Computer **Y** Other Equipment **Z** None	**Z** None
Z None DRG	**C** Voice	**K** Audiovisual **N** Biosensory Feedback **P** Computer **S** Voice Analysis **T** Aerodynamic Function **V** Speech Prosthesis **Y** Other Equipment **Z** None	**Z** None
Z None DRG	**D** Swallowing Dysfunction	**M** Augmentative / Alternative Communication **T** Aerodynamic Function **V** Speech Prosthesis **Y** Other Equipment **Z** None	**Z** None

DRG F0636KZ F0636MZ F0636PZ F0636YZ F0636ZZ F06Z0KZ F06Z0MZ F06Z0PZ F06Z0YZ F06Z0ZZ F06Z1KZ F06Z1ZZ F06Z2KZ F06Z2ZZ F06Z3KZ F06Z3MZ F06Z3PZ F06Z3YZ F06Z3ZZ F06Z4KZ F06Z4PZ F06Z4QZ F06Z4TZ F06Z4YZ F06Z4ZZ F06Z5KZ F06Z5LZ F06Z5MZ F06Z5NZ F06Z5PZ F06Z5QZ F06Z5SZ F06Z5YZ F06Z5ZZ F06Z6KZ F06Z6MZ F06Z6PZ F06Z6YZ F06Z6ZZ F06Z74Z F06Z7KZ F06Z7NZ F06Z7QZ F06Z7SZ F06Z7TZ F06Z7YZ F06Z7ZZ F06Z8KZ F06Z8NZ F06Z8PZ F06Z8QZ F06Z8SZ F06Z8TZ F06Z8YZ F06Z8ZZ F06Z9KZ F06Z9PZ F06Z9YZ F06Z9ZZ F06ZBKZ F06ZBLZ F06ZBMZ F06ZBPZ F06ZBYZ F06ZBZZ F06ZCKZ F06ZCNZ F06ZCPZ F06ZCSZ F06ZCTZ F06ZCVZ F06ZCYZ F06ZCZZ F06ZDMZ F06ZDTZ F06ZDVZ F06ZDYZ F06ZDZZ

LC Limited Coverage NC Noncovered HAC HAC Associated Procedure CC Combination Cluster - See Appendix G for code lists
DRG Non-OR-Affecting MS-DRG Assignment ⊘ Non-OR-Not Affecting MS-DRG Assignment New/Revised Text in **Orange** ♂ Male ♀ Female

F Physical Rehabilitation and Diagnostic Audiology
0 Rehabilitation
7 Motor Treatment: Exercise or activities to increase or facilitate motor function

Body system/ Region Character 4	Type Qualifier Character 5	Equipment Character 6	Qualifier Character 7
0 Neurological System - Head and Neck DRG **1** Neurological System - Upper Back / Upper Extremity DRG **2** Neurological System - Lower Back / Lower Extremity DRG **3** Neurological System - Whole Body DRG **D** Integumentary System - Head and Neck DRG **F** Integumentary System - Upper Back / Upper Extremity DRG **G** Integumentary System - Lower Back / Lower Extremity DRG **H** Integumentary System - Whole Body DRG **J** Musculoskeletal System - Head and Neck DRG **K** Musculoskeletal System - Upper Back / Upper Extremity DRG **L** Musculoskeletal System - Lower Back / Lower Extremity DRG **M** Musculoskeletal System - Whole Body DRG	**0** Range of Motion and Joint Mobility **1** Muscle Performance **2** Coordination/Dexterity **3** Motor Function	**E** Orthosis **F** Assistive, Adaptive, Supportive or Protective **U** Prosthesis **Y** Other Equipment **Z** None	**Z** None
0 Neurological System - Head and Neck DRG **1** Neurological System - Upper Back / Upper Extremity DRG **2** Neurological System - Lower Back / Lower Extremity DRG **3** Neurological System - Whole Body DRG **D** Integumentary System - Head and Neck DRG **F** Integumentary System - Upper Back / Upper Extremity DRG **G** Integumentary System - Lower Back / Lower Extremity DRG **H** Integumentary System - Whole Body DRG **J** Musculoskeletal System - Head and Neck DRG **K** Musculoskeletal System - Upper Back / Upper Extremity DRG **L** Musculoskeletal System - Lower Back / Lower Extremity DRG **M** Musculoskeletal System - Whole Body DRG	**6** Therapeutic Exercise	**B** Physical Agents **C** Mechanical **D** Electrotherapeutic **E** Orthosis **F** Assistive, Adaptive, Supportive or Protective **G** Aerobic Endurance and Conditioning **H** Mechanical or Electromechanical **U** Prosthesis **Y** Other Equipment **Z** None	**Z** None

F07 continued on next page

F Physical Rehabilitation and Diagnostic Audiology
0 Rehabilitation
7 Motor Treatment: Exercise or activities to increase or facilitate motor function

F07 continued from previous page

Body system/ Region Character 4	Type Qualifier Character 5	Equipment Character 6	Qualifier Character 7
0 Neurological System - Head and Neck DRG **1** Neurological System - Upper Back / Upper Extremity DRG **2** Neurological System - Lower Back / Lower Extremity DRG **3** Neurological System - Whole Body DRG **D** Integumentary System - Head and Neck DRG **F** Integumentary System - Upper Back / Upper Extremity DRG **G** Integumentary System - Lower Back / Lower Extremity DRG **H** Integumentary System - Whole Body DRG **J** Musculoskeletal System - Head and Neck DRG **K** Musculoskeletal System - Upper Back / Upper Extremity DRG **L** Musculoskeletal System - Lower Back / Lower Extremity DRG **M** Musculoskeletal System - Whole Body DRG	**7** Manual Therapy Techniques	**Z** None	**Z** None
4 Circulatory System - Head and Neck DRG **5** Circulatory System - Upper Back / Upper Extremity DRG **6** Circulatory System - Lower Back / Lower Extremity DRG **7** Circulatory System - Whole Body DRG **8** Respiratory System - Head and Neck DRG **9** Respiratory System - Upper Back / Upper Extremity DRG **B** Respiratory System - Lower Back / Lower Extremity DRG **C** Respiratory System - Whole Body DRG	**6** Therapeutic Exercise	**B** Physical Agents **C** Mechanical **D** Electrotherapeutic **E** Orthosis **F** Assistive, Adaptive, Supportive or Protective **G** Aerobic Endurance and Conditioning **H** Mechanical or Electromechanical **U** Prosthesis **Y** Other Equipment **Z** None	**Z** None
N Genitourinary System DRG	**1** Muscle Performance	**E** Orthosis **F** Assistive, Adaptive, Supportive or Protective **U** Prosthesis **Y** Other Equipment **Z** None	**Z** None
N Genitourinary System DRG	**6** Therapeutic Exercise	**B** Physical Agents **C** Mechanical **D** Electrotherapeutic **E** Orthosis **F** Assistive, Adaptive, Supportive or Protective **G** Aerobic Endurance and Conditioning **H** Mechanical or Electromechanical **U** Prosthesis **Y** Other Equipment **Z** None	**Z** None

F07 continued on next page

F Physical Rehabilitation and Diagnostic Audiology
0 Rehabilitation
7 Motor Treatment: Exercise or activities to increase or facilitate motor function

F07 continued from previous page

Body system/ Region Character 4	Type Qualifier Character 5	Equipment Character 6	Qualifier Character 7
Z None DRG	**4** Wheelchair Mobility	**D** Electrotherapeutic **E** Orthosis **F** Assistive, Adaptive, Supportive or Protective **U** Prosthesis **Y** Other Equipment **Z** None	**Z** None
Z None DRG	**5** Bed Mobility	**C** Mechanical **E** Orthosis **F** Assistive, Adaptive, Supportive or Protective **U** Prosthesis **Y** Other Equipment **Z** None	**Z** None
Z None DRG	**8** Transfer Training	**C** Mechanical **D** Electrotherapeutic **E** Orthosis **F** Assistive, Adaptive, Supportive or Protective **U** Prosthesis **Y** Other Equipment **Z** None	**Z** None
Z None DRG	**9** Gait Training/Functional Ambulation	**C** Mechanical **D** Electrotherapeutic **E** Orthosis **F** Assistive, Adaptive, Supportive or Protective **G** Aerobic Endurance and Conditioning **U** Prosthesis **Y** Other Equipment **Z** None	**Z** None

DRG F0700EZ F0700FZ F0700UZ F0700YZ F0700ZZ F0701EZ F0701FZ F0701UZ F0701YZ F0701ZZ F0702EZ F0702FZ F0702UZ
F0702YZ F0702ZZ F0703EZ F0703FZ F0703UZ F0703YZ F0703ZZ F0706BZ F0706CZ F0706DZ F0706EZ F0706FZ F0706GZ
F0706HZ F0706UZ F0706YZ F0706ZZ F0707ZZ F0710EZ F0710FZ F0710UZ F0710YZ F0710ZZ F0711EZ F0711FZ F0711UZ
F0711YZ F0711ZZ F0712EZ F0712FZ F0712UZ F0712YZ F0712ZZ F0713EZ F0713FZ F0713UZ F0713YZ F0713ZZ F0716BZ
F0716CZ F0716DZ F0716EZ F0716FZ F0716GZ F0716HZ F0716UZ F0716YZ F0716ZZ F0717ZZ F0720EZ F0720FZ F0720UZ
F0720YZ F0720ZZ F0721EZ F0721FZ F0721UZ F0721YZ F0721ZZ F0722EZ F0722FZ F0722UZ F0722YZ F0722ZZ F0723EZ
F0723FZ F0723UZ F0723YZ F0723ZZ F0726BZ F0726CZ F0726DZ F0726EZ F0726FZ F0726GZ F0726HZ F0726UZ F0726YZ
F0726ZZ F0727ZZ F0730EZ F0730FZ F0730UZ F0730YZ F0730ZZ F0731EZ F0731FZ F0731UZ F0731YZ F0731ZZ F0732EZ
F0732FZ F0732UZ F0732YZ F0732ZZ F0733EZ F0733FZ F0733UZ F0733YZ F0733ZZ F0736BZ F0736CZ F0736DZ F0736EZ
F0736FZ F0736GZ F0736HZ F0736UZ F0736YZ F0736ZZ F0737ZZ F0746BZ F0746CZ F0746DZ F0746EZ F0746FZ F0746GZ
F0746HZ F0746UZ F0746YZ F0746ZZ F0756BZ F0756CZ F0756DZ F0756EZ F0756FZ F0756GZ F0756HZ F0756UZ F0756YZ
F0756ZZ F0766BZ F0766CZ F0766DZ F0766EZ F0766FZ F0766GZ F0766HZ F0766UZ F0766YZ F0766ZZ F0776BZ F0776CZ
F0776DZ F0776EZ F0776FZ F0776GZ F0776HZ F0776UZ F0776YZ F0776ZZ F0786BZ F0786CZ F0786DZ F0786EZ F0786FZ
F0786GZ F0786HZ F0786UZ F0786YZ F0786ZZ F0796BZ F0796CZ F0796DZ F0796EZ F0796FZ F0796GZ F0796HZ F0796UZ
F0796YZ F0796ZZ F07B6BZ F07B6CZ F07B6DZ F07B6EZ F07B6FZ F07B6GZ F07B6HZ F07B6UZ F07B6YZ F07B6ZZ F07C6BZ
F07C6CZ F07C6DZ F07C6EZ F07C6FZ F07C6GZ F07C6HZ F07C6UZ F07C6YZ F07C6ZZ F07D0EZ F07D0FZ F07D0UZ F07D0YZ
F07D0ZZ F07D1EZ F07D1FZ F07D1UZ F07D1YZ F07D1ZZ F07D2EZ F07D2FZ F07D2UZ F07D2YZ F07D2ZZ F07D3EZ F07D3FZ
F07D3UZ F07D3YZ F07D3ZZ F07D6BZ F07D6CZ F07D6DZ F07D6EZ F07D6FZ F07D6GZ F07D6HZ F07D6UZ F07D6YZ F07D6ZZ
F07D7ZZ F07F0EZ F07F0FZ F07F0UZ F07F0YZ F07F0ZZ F07F1EZ F07F1FZ F07F1UZ F07F1YZ F07F1ZZ F07F2EZ F07F2FZ
F07F2UZ F07F2YZ F07F2ZZ F07F3EZ F07F3FZ F07F3UZ F07F3YZ F07F3ZZ F07F6BZ F07F6CZ F07F6DZ F07F6EZ F07F6FZ
F07F6GZ F07F6HZ F07F6UZ F07F6YZ F07F6ZZ F07F7ZZ F07G0EZ F07G0FZ F07G0UZ F07G0YZ F07G0ZZ F07G1EZ F07G1FZ
F07G1UZ F07G1YZ F07G1ZZ F07G2EZ F07G2FZ F07G2UZ F07G2YZ F07G2ZZ F07G3EZ F07G3FZ F07G3UZ F07G3YZ F07G3ZZ
F07G6BZ F07G6CZ F07G6DZ F07G6EZ F07G6FZ F07G6GZ F07G6HZ F07G6UZ F07G6YZ F07G6ZZ F07G7ZZ F07H0EZ F07H0FZ
F07H0UZ F07H0YZ F07H0ZZ F07H1EZ F07H1FZ F07H1UZ F07H1YZ F07H1ZZ F07H2EZ F07H2FZ F07H2UZ F07H2YZ F07H2ZZ
F07H3EZ F07H3FZ F07H3UZ F07H3YZ F07H3ZZ F07H6BZ F07H6CZ F07H6DZ F07H6EZ F07H6FZ F07H6GZ F07H6HZ F07H6UZ
F07H6YZ F07H6ZZ F07H7ZZ F07J0EZ F07J0FZ F07J0UZ F07J0YZ F07J0ZZ F07J1EZ F07J1FZ F07J1UZ F07J1YZ F07J1ZZ
F07J2EZ F07J2FZ F07J2UZ F07J2YZ F07J2ZZ F07J3EZ F07J3FZ F07J3UZ F07J3YZ F07J3ZZ F07J6BZ F07J6CZ F07J6DZ
F07J6EZ F07J6FZ F07J6GZ F07J6HZ F07J6UZ F07J6YZ F07J6ZZ F07J7ZZ F07K0EZ F07K0FZ F07K0UZ F07K0YZ F07K0ZZ
F07K1EZ F07K1FZ F07K1UZ F07K1YZ F07K1ZZ F07K2EZ F07K2FZ F07K2UZ F07K2YZ F07K2ZZ F07K3EZ F07K3FZ F07K3UZ
F07K3YZ F07K3ZZ F07K6BZ F07K6CZ F07K6DZ F07K6EZ F07K6FZ F07K6GZ F07K6HZ F07K6UZ F07K6YZ F07K6ZZ F07K7ZZ

F07 continued on next page

F07 continued from previous page

F07L0EZ	F07L0FZ	F07L0UZ	F07L0YZ	F07L0ZZ	F07L1EZ	F07L1FZ	F07L1UZ	F07L1YZ	F07L1ZZ	F07L2EZ	F07L2FZ	F07L2UZ
F07L2YZ	F07L2ZZ	F07L3EZ	F07L3FZ	F07L3UZ	F07L3YZ	F07L3ZZ	F07L6BZ	F07L6CZ	F07L6DZ	F07L6EZ	F07L6FZ	F07L6GZ
F07L6HZ	F07L6UZ	F07L6YZ	F07L6ZZ	F07L7ZZ	F07M0EZ	F07M0FZ	F07M0UZ	F07M0YZ	F07M0ZZ	F07M1EZ	F07M1FZ	F07M1UZ
F07M1YZ	F07M1ZZ	F07M2EZ	F07M2FZ	F07M2UZ	F07M2YZ	F07M2ZZ	F07M3EZ	F07M3FZ	F07M3UZ	F07M3YZ	F07M3ZZ	F07M6BZ
F07M6CZ	F07M6DZ	F07M6EZ	F07M6FZ	F07M6GZ	F07M6HZ	F07M6UZ	F07M6YZ	F07M6ZZ	F07M7ZZ	F07N1EZ	F07N1FZ	F07N1UZ
F07N1YZ	F07N1ZZ	F07N6BZ	F07N6CZ	F07N6DZ	F07N6EZ	F07N6FZ	F07N6GZ	F07N6HZ	F07N6UZ	F07N6YZ	F07N6ZZ	F07Z4DZ
F07Z4EZ	F07Z4FZ	F07Z4UZ	F07Z4YZ	F07Z4ZZ	F07Z5CZ	F07Z5EZ	F07Z5FZ	F07Z5UZ	F07Z5YZ	F07Z5ZZ	F07Z8CZ	F07Z8DZ
F07Z8EZ	F07Z8FZ	F07Z8UZ	F07Z8YZ	F07Z8ZZ	F07Z9CZ	F07Z9DZ	F07Z9EZ	F07Z9FZ	F07Z9GZ	F07Z9UZ	F07Z9YZ	F07Z9ZZ

F Physical Rehabilitation and Diagnostic Audiology
0 Rehabilitation
8 Activities of Daily Living Treatment: Exercise or activities to facilitate functional competence for activities of daily living

Body system/ Region Character 4	Type Qualifier Character 5	Equipment Character 6	Qualifier Character 7
D Integumentary System - Head and Neck DRG **F** Integumentary System - Upper Back / Upper Extremity DRG **G** Integumentary System - Lower Back / Lower Extremity DRG **H** Integumentary System - Whole Body DRG **J** Musculoskeletal System - Head and Neck DRG **K** Musculoskeletal System - Upper Back / Upper Extremity DRG **L** Musculoskeletal System - Lower Back / Lower Extremity DRG **M** Musculoskeletal System - Whole Body DRG	**5** Wound Management	**B** Physical Agents **C** Mechanical **D** Electrotherapeutic **E** Orthosis **F** Assistive, Adaptive, Supportive or Protective **U** Prosthesis **Y** Other Equipment **Z** None	**Z** None
Z None DRG	**0** Bathing/Showering Techniques **1** Dressing Techniques **2** Grooming/Personal Hygiene	**E** Orthosis **F** Assistive, Adaptive, Supportive or Protective **U** Prosthesis **Y** Other Equipment **Z** None	**Z** None
Z None DRG	**3** Feeding/Eating	**C** Mechanical **D** Electrotherapeutic **E** Orthosis **F** Assistive, Adaptive, Supportive or Protective **U** Prosthesis **Y** Other Equipment **Z** None	**Z** None
Z None DRG	**4** Home Management	**D** Electrotherapeutic **E** Orthosis **F** Assistive, Adaptive, Supportive or Protective **U** Prosthesis **Y** Other Equipment **Z** None	**Z** None
Z None DRG	**6** Psychosocial Skills	**Z** None	**Z** None
Z None DRG	**7** Vocational Activities and Functional Community or Work Reintegration Skills	**B** Physical Agents **C** Mechanical **D** Electrotherapeutic **E** Orthosis **F** Assistive, Adaptive, Supportive or Protective **G** Aerobic Endurance and Conditioning **U** Prosthesis **Y** Other Equipment **Z** None	**Z** None

DRG F08D5BZ F08D5CZ F08D5DZ F08D5EZ F08D5FZ F08D5UZ F08D5YZ F08D5ZZ F08F5BZ F08F5CZ F08F5DZ F08F5EZ F08F5FZ F08F5UZ F08F5YZ F08F5ZZ F08G5BZ F08G5CZ F08G5DZ F08G5EZ F08G5FZ F08G5UZ F08G5YZ F08G5ZZ F08H5BZ F08H5CZ

F08 continued on next page

F08 continued from previous page

F08H5DZ F08H5EZ F08H5FZ F08H5UZ F08H5YZ F08H5ZZ F08J5BZ F08J5CZ F08J5DZ F08J5EZ F08J5FZ F08J5UZ F08J5YZ
F08J5ZZ F08K5BZ F08K5CZ F08K5DZ F08K5EZ F08K5FZ F08K5UZ F08K5YZ F08K5ZZ F08L5BZ F08L5CZ F08L5DZ F08L5EZ
F08L5FZ F08L5UZ F08L5YZ F08L5ZZ F08M5BZ F08M5CZ F08M5DZ F08M5EZ F08M5FZ F08M5UZ F08M5YZ F08M5ZZ F08Z0EZ
F08Z0FZ F08Z0UZ F08Z0YZ F08Z0ZZ F08Z1EZ F08Z1FZ F08Z1UZ F08Z1YZ F08Z1ZZ F08Z2EZ F08Z2FZ F08Z2UZ F08Z2YZ
F08Z2ZZ F08Z3CZ F08Z3DZ F08Z3EZ F08Z3FZ F08Z3UZ F08Z3YZ F08Z3ZZ F08Z4DZ F08Z4EZ F08Z4FZ F08Z4UZ F08Z4YZ
F08Z4ZZ F08Z6ZZ F08Z7BZ F08Z7CZ F08Z7DZ F08Z7EZ F08Z7FZ F08Z7GZ F08Z7UZ F08Z7YZ F08Z7ZZ

F Physical Rehabilitation and Diagnostic Audiology
0 Rehabilitation
9 Hearing Treatment: Application of techniques to improve, augment, or compensate for hearing and related functional impairment

Body system/ Region Character 4	Type Qualifier Character 5	Equipment Character 6	Qualifier Character 7
Z None DRG	0 Hearing and Related Disorders Counseling 1 Hearing and Related Disorders Prevention	K Audiovisual Z None	Z None
Z None DRG	2 Auditory Processing	K Audiovisual L Assistive Listening P Computer Y Other Equipment Z None	Z None
Z None DRG	3 Cerumen Management	X Cerumen Management Z None	Z None

DRG F09Z0KZ F09Z0ZZ F09Z1KZ F09Z1ZZ F09Z2KZ F09Z2LZ F09Z2PZ F09Z2YZ F09Z2ZZ F09Z3XZ F09Z3ZZ

F Physical Rehabilitation and Diagnostic Audiology
0 Rehabilitation
B Cochlear Implant Treatment: Application of techniques to improve the communication abilities of individuals with cochlear implant

Body system/ Region Character 4	Type Qualifier Character 5	Equipment Character 6	Qualifier Character 7
Z None DRG	0 Cochlear Implant Rehabilitation	1 Audiometer 2 Sound Field / Booth 9 Cochlear Implant K Audiovisual P Computer Y Other Equipment	Z None

DRG F0BZ01Z F0BZ02Z F0BZ09Z F0BZ0KZ F0BZ0PZ F0BZ0YZ

F Physical Rehabilitation and Diagnostic Audiology
0 Rehabilitation
C Vestibular Treatment: Application of techniques to improve, augment, or compensate for vestibular and related functional impairment

Body system/ Region Character 4	Type Qualifier Character 5	Equipment Character 6	Qualifier Character 7
3 Neurological System - Whole Body DRG H Integumentary System - Whole Body DRG M Musculoskeletal System - Whole Body DRG	3 Postural Control	E Orthosis F Assistive, Adaptive, Supportive or Protective U Prosthesis Y Other Equipment Z None	Z None
Z None DRG	0 Vestibular	8 Vestibular / Balance Z None	Z None
Z None DRG	1 Perceptual Processing 2 Visual Motor Integration	K Audiovisual L Assistive Listening N Biosensory Feedback P Computer Q Speech Analysis S Voice Analysis T Aerodynamic Function Y Other Equipment Z None	Z None

DRG F0C33EZ F0C33FZ F0C33UZ F0C33YZ F0C33ZZ F0CH3EZ F0CH3FZ F0CH3UZ F0CH3YZ F0CH3ZZ F0CM3EZ F0CM3FZ F0CM3UZ
F0CM3YZ F0CM3ZZ F0CZ08Z F0CZ0ZZ F0CZ1KZ F0CZ1LZ F0CZ1NZ F0CZ1PZ F0CZ1QZ F0CZ1SZ F0CZ1TZ F0CZ1YZ F0CZ1ZZ
F0CZ2KZ F0CZ2LZ F0CZ2NZ F0CZ2PZ F0CZ2QZ F0CZ2SZ F0CZ2TZ F0CZ2YZ F0CZ2ZZ

LC Limited Coverage NC Noncovered HAC HAC Associated Procedure CC Combination Cluster - See Appendix G for code lists
DRG Non-OR-Affecting MS-DRG Assignment ⊘ Non-OR-Not Affecting MS-DRG Assignment New/Revised Text in **Orange** ♂ Male ♀ Female

F Physical Rehabilitation and Diagnostic Audiology
0 Rehabilitation
D Device Fitting: Fitting of a device designed to facilitate or support achievement of a higher level of function

Body system/ Region Character 4	Type Qualifier Character 5	Equipment Character 6	Qualifier Character 7
Z None DRG	**0** Tinnitus Masker	**5** Hearing Aid Selection / Fitting / Test **Z** None	**Z** None
Z None DRG	**1** Monaural Hearing Aid **2** Binaural Hearing Aid **5** Assistive Listening Device	**1** Audiometer **2** Sound Field / Booth **5** Hearing Aid Selection / Fitting / Test **K** Audiovisual **L** Assistive Listening **Z** None	**Z** None
Z None DRG	**3** Augmentative/Alternative Communication System	**M** Augmentative / Alternative Communication	**Z** None
Z None DRG	**4** Voice Prosthetic	**S** Voice Analysis **V** Speech Prosthesis	**Z** None
Z None DRG	**6** Dynamic Orthosis **7** Static Orthosis **8** Prosthesis **9** Assistive, Adaptive, Supportive or Protective Devices	**E** Orthosis **F** Assistive, Adaptive, Supportive or Protective **U** Prosthesis **Z** None	**Z** None

DRG F0DZ05Z F0DZ0ZZ F0DZ11Z F0DZ12Z F0DZ15Z F0DZ1KZ F0DZ1LZ F0DZ1ZZ F0DZ21Z F0DZ22Z F0DZ25Z F0DZ2KZ F0DZ2LZ
F0DZ2ZZ F0DZ3MZ F0DZ4SZ F0DZ4VZ F0DZ51Z F0DZ52Z F0DZ55Z F0DZ5KZ F0DZ5LZ F0DZ5ZZ F0DZ6EZ F0DZ6FZ F0DZ6UZ
F0DZ6ZZ F0DZ7EZ F0DZ7FZ F0DZ7UZ F0DZ7ZZ F0DZ8EZ F0DZ8FZ F0DZ8UZ

F Physical Rehabilitation and Diagnostic Audiology
0 Rehabilitation
F Caregiver Training: Training in activities to support patient's optimal level of function

Body system/ Region Character 4	Type Qualifier Character 5	Equipment Character 6	Qualifier Character 7
Z None DRG	**0** Bathing/Showering Technique **1** Dressing **2** Feeding and Eating **3** Grooming/Personal Hygiene **4** Bed Mobility **5** Transfer **6** Wheelchair Mobility **7** Therapeutic Exercise **8** Airway Clearance Techniques **9** Wound Management **B** Vocational Activities and Functional Community or Work Reintegration Skills **C** Gait Training/Functional Ambulation **D** Application, Proper Use and Care of Devices **F** Application, Proper Use and Care of Orthoses **G** Application, Proper Use and Care of Prosthesis **H** Home Management	**E** Orthosis **F** Assistive, Adaptive, Supportive or Protective **U** Prosthesis **Z** None	**Z** None
Z None DRG	**J** Communication Skills	**K** Audiovisual **L** Assistive Listening **M** Augmentative / Alternative Communication **P** Computer **Z** None	**Z** None

DRG F0FZ0EZ F0FZ0FZ F0FZ0UZ F0FZ0ZZ F0FZ1EZ F0FZ1FZ F0FZ1UZ F0FZ1ZZ F0FZ2EZ F0FZ2FZ F0FZ2UZ F0FZ2ZZ F0FZ3EZ
F0FZ3FZ F0FZ3UZ F0FZ3ZZ F0FZ4EZ F0FZ4FZ F0FZ4UZ F0FZ4ZZ F0FZ5EZ F0FZ5FZ F0FZ5UZ F0FZ5ZZ F0FZ6EZ F0FZ6FZ
F0FZ6UZ F0FZ6ZZ F0FZ7EZ F0FZ7FZ F0FZ7UZ F0FZ7ZZ F0FZ8EZ F0FZ8FZ F0FZ8UZ F0FZ8ZZ F0FZ9EZ F0FZ9FZ F0FZ9UZ
F0FZ9ZZ F0FZBEZ F0FZBFZ F0FZBUZ F0FZBZZ F0FZCEZ F0FZCFZ F0FZCUZ F0FZCZZ F0FZDEZ F0FZDFZ F0FZDUZ F0FZDZZ
F0FZFEZ F0FZFFZ F0FZFUZ F0FZFZZ F0FZGEZ F0FZGFZ F0FZGUZ F0FZGZZ F0FZHEZ F0FZHFZ F0FZHUZ F0FZHZZ F0FZJKZ
F0FZJLZ F0FZJMZ F0FZJPZ F0FZJZZ

F Physical Rehabilitation and Diagnostic Audiology
1 Diagnostic Audiology
3 Hearing Assessment: Measurement of hearing and related functions

Body system/ Region Character 4	Type Qualifier Character 5	Equipment Character 6	Qualifier Character 7
Z None ⦸	**0** Hearing Screening	**0** Occupational Hearing **1** Audiometer **2** Sound Field / Booth **3** Tympanometer **8** Vestibular / Balance **9** Cochlear Implant **Z** None	**Z** None
Z None ⦸	**1** Pure Tone Audiometry, Air **2** Pure Tone Audiometry, Air and Bone	**0** Occupational Hearing **1** Audiometer **2** Sound Field / Booth **Z** None	**Z** None
Z None ⦸	**3** Bekesy Audiometry **6** Visual Reinforcement Audiometry **9** Short Increment Sensitivity Index **B** Stenger **C** Pure Tone Stenger	**1** Audiometer **2** Sound Field / Booth **Z** None	**Z** None
Z None ⦸	**4** Conditioned Play Audiometry **5** Select Picture Audiometry	**1** Audiometer **2** Sound Field / Booth **K** Audiovisual **Z** None	**Z** None
Z None ⦸	**7** Alternate Binaural or Monaural Loudness Balance	**1** Audiometer **K** Audiovisual **Z** None	**Z** None
Z None ⦸	**8** Tone Decay **D** Tympanometry **F** Eustachian Tube Function **G** Acoustic Reflex Patterns **H** Acoustic Reflex Threshold **J** Acoustic Reflex Decay	**3** Tympanometer **4** Electroacoustic Immittance / Acoustic Reflex **Z** None	**Z** None
Z None ⦸	**K** Electrocochleography **L** Auditory Evoked Potentials	**7** Electrophysiologic **Z** None	**Z** None
Z None ⦸	**M** Evoked Otoacoustic Emissions, Screening **N** Evoked Otoacoustic Emissions, Diagnostic	**6** Otoacoustic Emission (OAE) **Z** None	**Z** None
Z None ⦸	**P** Aural Rehabilitation Status	**1** Audiometer **2** Sound Field / Booth **4** Electroacoustic Immittance / Acoustic Reflex **9** Cochlear Implant **K** Audiovisual **L** Assistive Listening **P** Computer **Z** None	**Z** None
Z None ⦸	**Q** Auditory Processing	**K** Audiovisual **P** Computer **Y** Other Equipment **Z** None	**Z** None

⦸ F13Z00Z F13Z01Z F13Z02Z F13Z03Z F13Z08Z F13Z09Z F13Z0ZZ F13Z10Z F13Z11Z F13Z12Z F13Z1ZZ F13Z20Z F13Z21Z F13Z22Z F13Z2ZZ F13Z31Z F13Z32Z F13Z3ZZ F13Z41Z F13Z42Z F13Z4KZ F13Z4ZZ F13Z51Z F13Z52Z F13Z5KZ F13Z5ZZ F13Z61Z F13Z62Z F13Z6ZZ F13Z71Z F13Z7KZ F13Z7ZZ F13Z83Z F13Z84Z F13Z8ZZ F13Z91Z F13Z92Z F13Z9ZZ F13ZB1Z F13ZB2Z F13ZBZZ F13ZC1Z F13ZC2Z F13ZCZZ F13ZD3Z F13ZD4Z F13ZDZZ F13ZF3Z F13ZF4Z F13ZFZZ F13ZG3Z F13ZG4Z F13ZGZZ F13ZH3Z F13ZH4Z F13ZHZZ F13ZJ3Z F13ZJ4Z F13ZJZZ F13ZK7Z F13ZKZZ F13ZL7Z F13ZLZZ F13ZM6Z F13ZMZZ F13ZN6Z F13ZNZZ F13ZP1Z F13ZP2Z F13ZP4Z F13ZP9Z F13ZPKZ F13ZPLZ F13ZPPZ F13ZPZZ F13ZQKZ F13ZQPZ F13ZQYZ F13ZQZZ

F Physical Rehabilitation and Diagnostic Audiology
1 Diagnostic Audiology
4 Hearing Aid Assessment: Measurement of the appropriateness and/or effectiveness of a hearing device

Body system/ Region Character 4	Type Qualifier Character 5	Equipment Character 6	Qualifier Character 7
Z None ⃠	**0** Cochlear Implant	**1** Audiometer **2** Sound Field / Booth **3** Tympanometer **4** Electroacoustic Immittance / Acoustic Reflex **5** Hearing Aid Selection / Fitting / Test **7** Electrophysiologic **9** Cochlear Implant **K** Audiovisual **L** Assistive Listening **P** Computer **Y** Other Equipment **Z** None	**Z** None
Z None ⃠	**1** Ear Canal Probe Microphone **6** Binaural Electroacoustic Hearing Aid Check **8** Monaural Electroacoustic Hearing Aid Check	**5** Hearing Aid Selection / Fitting / Test **Z** None	**Z** None
Z None ⃠	**2** Monaural Hearing Aid **3** Binaural Hearing Aid	**1** Audiometer **2** Sound Field / Booth **3** Tympanometer **4** Electroacoustic Immittance / Acoustic Reflex **5** Hearing Aid Selection / Fitting / Test **K** Audiovisual **L** Assistive Listening **P** Computer **Z** None	**Z** None
Z None ⃠	**4** Assistive Listening System/ Device Selection	**1** Audiometer **2** Sound Field / Booth **3** Tympanometer **4** Electroacoustic Immittance / Acoustic Reflex **K** Audiovisual **L** Assistive Listening **Z** None	**Z** None
Z None ⃠	**5** Sensory Aids	**1** Audiometer **2** Sound Field / Booth **3** Tympanometer **4** Electroacoustic Immittance / Acoustic Reflex **5** Hearing Aid Selection / Fitting / Test **K** Audiovisual **L** Assistive Listening **Z** None	**Z** None
Z None ⃠	**7** Ear Protector Attenuation	**0** Occupational Hearing **Z** None	**Z** None

⃠ F14Z01Z F14Z02Z F14Z03Z F14Z04Z F14Z05Z F14Z07Z F14Z09Z F14Z0KZ F14Z0LZ F14Z0PZ F14Z0YZ F14Z0ZZ F14Z15Z F14Z1ZZ F14Z21Z F14Z22Z F14Z23Z F14Z24Z F14Z25Z F14Z2KZ F14Z2LZ F14Z2PZ F14Z2ZZ F14Z31Z F14Z32Z F14Z33Z F14Z34Z F14Z35Z F14Z3KZ F14Z3LZ F14Z3PZ F14Z3ZZ F14Z41Z F14Z42Z F14Z43Z F14Z44Z F14Z4KZ F14Z4LZ F14Z4ZZ F14Z51Z F14Z52Z F14Z53Z F14Z54Z F14Z55Z F14Z5KZ F14Z5LZ F14Z5ZZ F14Z65Z F14Z6ZZ F14Z70Z F14Z7ZZ F14Z85Z F14Z8ZZ

F Physical Rehabilitation and Diagnostic Audiology
1 Diagnostic Audiology
5 Vestibular Assessment: Measurement of the vestibular system and related functions

Body system/ Region Character 4	Type Qualifier Character 5	Equipment Character 6	Qualifier Character 7
Z None ⃠	**0** Bithermal, Binaural Caloric Irrigation **1** Bithermal, Monaural Caloric Irrigation **2** Unithermal Binaural Screen **3** Oscillating Tracking **4** Sinusoidal Vertical Axis Rotational **5** Dix-Hallpike Dynamic **6** Computerized Dynamic Posturography	**8** Vestibular / Balance **Z** None	**Z** None
Z None ⃠	**7** Tinnitus Masker	**5** Hearing Aid Selection / Fitting / Test **Z** None	**Z** None

⃠ F15Z08Z F15Z0ZZ F15Z18Z F15Z1ZZ F15Z28Z F15Z2ZZ F15Z38Z F15Z3ZZ F15Z48Z F15Z4ZZ F15Z58Z F15Z5ZZ F15Z68Z F15Z6ZZ F15Z75Z F15Z7ZZ

Mental Health GZ1-GZJ

G Mental Health
Z None
1 Psychological Tests: The administration and interpretation of standardized psychological tests and measurement instruments for the assessment of psychological function

Qualifier Character 4	Qualifier Character 5	Qualifier Character 6	Qualifier Character 7
0 Developmental ⦸ 1 Personality and Behavioral ⦸ 2 Intellectual and Psychoeducational ⦸ 3 Neuropsychological ⦸ 4 Neurobehavioral and Cognitive Status ⦸	Z None	Z None	Z None

⦸ GZ10ZZZ GZ11ZZZ GZ12ZZZ GZ13ZZZ GZ14ZZZ

G Mental Health
Z None
2 Crisis Intervention: Treatment of a traumatized, acutely disturbed or distressed individual for the purpose of short-term stabilization

Qualifier Character 4	Qualifier Character 5	Qualifier Character 6	Qualifier Character 7
Z None ⦸	Z None	Z None	Z None

⦸ GZ2ZZZZ

G Mental Health
Z None
3 Medication Management: Monitoring and adjusting the use of medications for the treatment of a mental health disorder

Qualifier Character 4	Qualifier Character 5	Qualifier Character 6	Qualifier Character 7
Z None ⦸	Z None	Z None	Z None

⦸ GZ3ZZZZ

G Mental Health
Z None
5 Individual Psychotherapy: Treatment of an individual with a mental health disorder by behavioral, cognitive, psychoanalytic, psychodynamic or psychophysiological means to improve functioning or well-being

Qualifier Character 4	Qualifier Character 5	Qualifier Character 6	Qualifier Character 7
0 Interactive ⦸ 1 Behavioral ⦸ 2 Cognitive ⦸ 3 Interpersonal ⦸ 4 Psychoanalysis ⦸ 5 Psychodynamic ⦸ 6 Supportive ⦸ 8 Cognitive-Behavioral ⦸ 9 Psychophysiological ⦸	Z None	Z None	Z None

⦸ GZ50ZZZ GZ51ZZZ GZ52ZZZ GZ53ZZZ GZ54ZZZ GZ55ZZZ GZ56ZZZ GZ58ZZZ GZ59ZZZ

G Mental Health
Z None
6 Counseling: The application of psychological methods to treat an individual with normal developmental issues and psychological problems in order to increase function, improve well-being, alleviate distress, maladjustment or resolve crises

Qualifier Character 4	Qualifier Character 5	Qualifier Character 6	Qualifier Character 7
0 Educational ⦸ 1 Vocational ⦸ 3 Other Counseling ⦸	Z None	Z None	Z None

⦸ GZ60ZZZ GZ61ZZZ GZ63ZZZ

G Mental Health
Z None
7 Family Psychotherapy: Treatment that includes one or more family members of an individual with a mental health disorder by behavioral, cognitive, psychoanalytic, psychodynamic or psychophysiological means to improve functioning or well-being

Qualifier Character 4	Qualifier Character 5	Qualifier Character 6	Qualifier Character 7
2 Other Family Psychotherapy ⃠	Z None	Z None	Z None

⃠ GZ72ZZZ

G Mental Health
Z None
B Electroconvulsive Therapy: The application of controlled electrical voltages to treat a mental health disorder

Qualifier Character 4	Qualifier Character 5	Qualifier Character 6	Qualifier Character 7
0 Unilateral-Single Seizure ⃠ 1 Unilateral-Multiple Seizure ⃠ 2 Bilateral-Single Seizure ⃠ 3 Bilateral-Multiple Seizure ⃠ 4 Other Electroconvulsive Therapy ⃠	Z None	Z None	Z None

⃠ GZB0ZZZ GZB1ZZZ GZB2ZZZ GZB3ZZZ GZB4ZZZ

G Mental Health
Z None
C Biofeedback: Provision of information from the monitoring and regulating of physiological processes in conjunction with cognitive-behavioral techniques to improve patient functioning or well-being

Qualifier Character 4	Qualifier Character 5	Qualifier Character 6	Qualifier Character 7
9 Other Biofeedback ⃠	Z None	Z None	Z None

⃠ GZC9ZZZ

G Mental Health
Z None
F Hypnosis: Induction of a state of heightened suggestibility by auditory, visual and tactile techniques to elicit an emotional or behavioral response

Qualifier Character 4	Qualifier Character 5	Qualifier Character 6	Qualifier Character 7
Z None ⃠	Z None	Z None	Z None

⃠ GZFZZZZ

G Mental Health
Z None
G Narcosynthesis: Administration of intravenous barbiturates in order to release suppressed or repressed thoughts

Qualifier Character 4	Qualifier Character 5	Qualifier Character 6	Qualifier Character 7
Z None ⃠	Z None	Z None	Z None

⃠ GZGZZZZ

G Mental Health
Z None
H Group Psychotherapy: Treatment of two or more individuals with a mental health disorder by behavioral, cognitive, psychoanalytic, psychodynamic or psychophysiological means to improve functioning or well-being

Qualifier Character 4	Qualifier Character 5	Qualifier Character 6	Qualifier Character 7
Z None ⃠	Z None	Z None	Z None

⃠ GZHZZZZ

G Mental Health
Z None
J Light Therapy: Application of specialized light treatments to improve functioning or well-being

Qualifier Character 4	Qualifier Character 5	Qualifier Character 6	Qualifier Character 7
Z None ⃠	**Z** None	**Z** None	**Z** None

⃠ GZJZZZZ

Substance Abuse Treatment HZ2-HZ9

H Substance Abuse Treatment
Z None
2 Detoxification Services: Detoxification from alcohol and/or drugs

Qualifier Character 4	Qualifier Character 5	Qualifier Character 6	Qualifier Character 7
Z None ⦸	Z None	Z None	Z None

⦸ HZ2ZZZZ

H Substance Abuse Treatment
Z None
3 Individual Counseling: The application of psychological methods to treat an individual with addictive behavior

Qualifier Character 4	Qualifier Character 5	Qualifier Character 6	Qualifier Character 7
0 Cognitive DRG 1 Behavioral DRG 2 Cognitive-Behavioral DRG 3 12-Step DRG 4 Interpersonal DRG 5 Vocational DRG 6 Psychoeducation DRG 7 Motivational Enhancement DRG 8 Confrontational DRG 9 Continuing Care DRG B Spiritual DRG C Pre/Post-Test Infectious Disease ⦸	Z None	Z None	Z None

DRG HZ30ZZZ HZ31ZZZ HZ32ZZZ HZ33ZZZ HZ34ZZZ HZ35ZZZ HZ36ZZZ HZ37ZZZ HZ38ZZZ HZ39ZZZ HZ3BZZZ
⦸ HZ3CZZZ

H Substance Abuse Treatment
Z None
4 Group Counseling: The application of psychological methods to treat two or more individuals with addictive behavior

Qualifier Character 4	Qualifier Character 5	Qualifier Character 6	Qualifier Character 7
0 Cognitive DRG 1 Behavioral DRG 2 Cognitive-Behavioral DRG 3 12-Step DRG 4 Interpersonal DRG 5 Vocational DRG 6 Psychoeducation DRG 7 Motivational Enhancement DRG 8 Confrontational DRG 9 Continuing Care DRG B Spiritual DRG C Pre/Post-Test Infectious Disease ⦸	Z None	Z None	Z None

DRG HZ40ZZZ HZ41ZZZ HZ42ZZZ HZ43ZZZ HZ44ZZZ HZ45ZZZ HZ46ZZZ HZ47ZZZ HZ48ZZZ HZ49ZZZ HZ4BZZZ
⦸ HZ4CZZZ

H Substance Abuse Treatment
Z None
5 Individual Psychotherapy: Treatment of an individual with addictive behavior by behavioral, cognitive, psychoanalytic, psychodynamic or psychophysiological means

Qualifier Character 4	Qualifier Character 5	Qualifier Character 6	Qualifier Character 7
0 Cognitive DRG 1 Behavioral DRG 2 Cognitive-Behavioral DRG 3 12-Step DRG 4 Interpersonal DRG 5 Interactive DRG 6 Psychoeducation DRG 7 Motivational Enhancement DRG 8 Confrontational DRG 9 Supportive DRG B Psychoanalysis DRG C Psychodynamic DRG D Psychophysiological DRG	Z None	Z None	Z None

DRG HZ50ZZZ HZ51ZZZ HZ52ZZZ HZ53ZZZ HZ54ZZZ HZ55ZZZ HZ56ZZZ HZ57ZZZ HZ58ZZZ HZ59ZZZ HZ5BZZZ HZ5CZZZ HZ5DZZZ

H Substance Abuse Treatment
Z None
6 Family Counseling: The application of psychological methods that includes one or more family members to treat an individual with addictive behavior

Qualifier Character 4	Qualifier Character 5	Qualifier Character 6	Qualifier Character 7
3 Other Family Counseling ⦸	Z None	Z None	Z None

⦸ HZ63ZZZ

H Substance Abuse Treatment
Z None
8 Medication Management: Monitoring and adjusting the use of replacement medications for the treatment of addiction

Qualifier Character 4	Qualifier Character 5	Qualifier Character 6	Qualifier Character 7
0 Nicotine Replacement ⦸ 1 Methadone Maintenance ⦸ 2 Levo-alpha-acetyl-methadol (LAAM) ⦸ 3 Antabuse ⦸ 4 Naltrexone ⦸ 5 Naloxone ⦸ 6 Clonidine ⦸ 7 Bupropion ⦸ 8 Psychiatric Medication ⦸ 9 Other Replacement Medication ⦸	Z None	Z None	Z None

⦸ HZ80ZZZ HZ81ZZZ HZ82ZZZ HZ83ZZZ HZ84ZZZ HZ85ZZZ HZ86ZZZ HZ87ZZZ HZ88ZZZ HZ89ZZZ

H Substance Abuse Treatment
Z None
9 Pharmacotherapy: The use of replacement medications for the treatment of addiction

Qualifier Character 4	Qualifier Character 5	Qualifier Character 6	Qualifier Character 7
0 Nicotine Replacement ⃠ **1** Methadone Maintenance ⃠ **2** Levo-alpha-acetyl-methadol (LAAM) ⃠ **3** Antabuse ⃠ **4** Naltrexone ⃠ **5** Naloxone ⃠ **6** Clonidine ⃠ **7** Bupropion ⃠ **8** Psychiatric Medication ⃠ **9** Other Replacement Medication ⃠	**Z** None	**Z** None	**Z** None

⃠ HZ90ZZZ HZ91ZZZ HZ92ZZZ HZ93ZZZ HZ94ZZZ HZ95ZZZ HZ96ZZZ HZ97ZZZ HZ98ZZZ HZ99ZZZ

New Technology, Cardiovascular System X2A -X2R

X New Technology
2 Cardiovascular System
A Extirpation: Taking over a portion of a physiological function by extracorporeal means

Body Part Character 4	Approach Character 5	Device/Substance/Technology Character 6	Qualifier Character 7
5 Innominate Artery and Left Common Carotid Artery ⦸	3 Percutaneous	1 Cerebral Embolic Filtration, Dual Filter	2 New Technology Group 2

⦸ X2A5312

X New Technology
2 Cardiovascular System
C Extirpation: Taking or cutting out solid matter from a body part

Body Part Character 4	Approach Character 5	Device/Substance/Technology Character 6	Qualifier Character 7
0 Coronary Artery, One Artery 1 Coronary Artery, Two Arteries 2 Coronary Artery, Three Arteries 3 Coronary Artery, Four or More Arteries	3 Percutaneous	6 Orbital Atherectomy Technology	1 New Technology Group 1

X New Technology
2 Cardiovascular System
R Replacement: Putting in or on biological or synthetic material that physically takes the place and/or function of all or a portion of a body part

Body Part Character 4	Approach Character 5	Device/Substance/Technology Character 6	Qualifier Character 7
F Aortic Valve ⦸	0 Open 3 Percutaneous 4 Percutaneous Endoscopic	3 Zooplastic Tissue, Rapid Deployment Technique	2 New Technology Group 2

⦸ X2RF032 X2RF332 X2RF432

New Technology, Skin, Subcutaneous Tissue, Fascia and Breast XHR

X New Technology
H Skin, Subcutaneous Tissue, Fascia and Breast
R Replacement: Putting in or on biological or synthetic material that physically takes the place and/or function of all or a portion of a body part

Body Part Character 4	Approach Character 5	Device/Substance/Technology Character 6	Qualifier Character 7
P Skin ⃠	X External	L Skin Substitute, Porcine Liver Derived	2 New Technology Group 2

⃠ XHRPXL2

New Technology, Bones XNS

X New Technology
N Bones
S Reposition: Moving to its normal location, or other suitable location, all or a portion of a body part

Body Part Character 4	Approach Character 5	Device/Substance/Technology Character 6	Qualifier Character 7
0 Lumbar Vertebra ⊘ 3 Cervical Vertebra ⊘ 4 Thoracic Vertebra ⊘	0 Open 4 Percutaneous Endoscopic	3 Magnetically Controlled Growth Rod(s)	2 New Technology Group 2

⊘ XNS0032 XNS0432 XNS3032 XNS3432 XNS4032 XNS4432

New Technology, Joints XR2 - XRG

X New Technology
R Joints
2 Monitoring: Determining the level of a physiological or physical function repetitively over a period of time

Body Part Character 4	Approach Character 5	Device/Substance/Technology Character 6	Qualifier Character 7
G Knee Joint, Right **H** Knee Joint, Left ⊘	**0** Open	**2** Intraoperative Knee Replacement Sensor	**1** New Technology Group 1

⊘ XR2H021

X New Technology
R Joints
G Fusion: Joining together portions of an articular body part rendering the articular body part immobile

Body Part Character 4	Approach Character 5	Device/Substance/Technology Character 6	Qualifier Character 7
0 Occipital-cervical Joint ⊘ **1** Cervical Vertebral Joint ⊘ **2** Cervical Vertebral Joints, 2 or more ⊘ **4** Cervicothoracic Vertebral Joint ⊘ **6** Thoracic Vertebral Joint ⊘ **7** Thoracic Vertebral Joints, 2 to 7 ⊘ **8** Thoracic Vertebral Joints, 8 or more ⊘ **A** Thoracolumbar Vertebral Joint ⊘ **B** Lumbar Vertebral Joint ⊘ **C** Lumbar Vertebral Joints, 2 or more ⊘ **D** Lumbosacral Joint ⊘	**0** Open	**9** Interbody Fusion Device, Nanotextured Surface	**2** New Technology Group 2

⊘ XRG0092 XRG1092 XRG2092 XRG4092 XRG6092 XRG7092 XRG8092 XRGA092 XRGB092 XRGC092 XRGD092

New Technology, Anatomical Regions XW0

X New Technology
W Anatomical Regions
0 Introduction: Putting in or on a therapeutic, diagnostic, nutritional, physiological, or prophylactic substance except blood or blood products

Body Part Character 4	Approach Character 5	Device/Substance/Technology Character 6	Qualifier Character 7
3 Peripheral Vein ⦸	**3** Percutaneous	**2** Ceftazidime-Avibactam Anti-infective **3** Idarucizumab, Dabigatran Reversal Agent **4** Isavuconazole Anti-infective **5** Blinatumomab Antineoplastic Immunotherapy	**1** New Technology Group 1
3 Peripheral Vein ⦸	**3** Percutaneous	**7** Andexanet Alfa, Factor Xa Inhibitor Reversal Agent **9** Defibrotide Sodium Anticoagulant	**2** New Technology Group 2
4 Central Vein ⦸	**3** Percutaneous	**2** Ceftazidime-Avibactam Anti-infective **3** Idarucizumab, Dabigatran Reversal Agent **4** Isavuconazole Antiinfective **5** Blinatumomab Antineoplastic Immunotherapy	**1** New Technology Group 1
4 Central Vein ⦸	**3** Percutaneous	**7** Andexanet Alfa, Factor Xa Inhibitor Reversal Agent **9** Defibrotide Sodium Anticoagulant	**2** New Technology Group 2
D Mouth and Pharynx ⦸	**X** External	**8** Uridine Triacetate	**2** New Technology Group 2

⦸ XW03321 XW03331 XW03341 XW03351 XW03372 XW03392 XW04321 XW04331 XW04341 XW04351 XW04372 XW04392 XW0DX82

This page intentionally left blank

Appendix A: Root Operations Definitions

0 - Medical and Surgical		
Value	**Root Operation**	**Definition/Explanation**
0	Alteration	**Definition:** Modifying the anatomic structure of a body part without affecting the function of the body part **Explanation:** Principal purpose is to improve appearance **Includes/Examples:** Face lift, breast augmentation
1	Bypass	**Definition:** Altering the route of passage of the contents of a tubular body part **Explanation:** Rerouting contents of a body part to a downstream area of the normal route, to a similar route and body part, or to an abnormal route and dissimilar body part. Includes one or more anastomoses, with or without the use of a device **Includes/Examples:** Coronary artery bypass, colostomy formation
2	Change	**Definition:** Taking out or off a device from a body part and putting back an identical or similar device in or on the same body part without cutting or puncturing the skin or a mucous membrane **Explanation:** All CHANGE procedures are coded using the approach EXTERNAL **Includes/Examples:** Urinary catheter change, gastrostomy tube change
3	Control	**Definition:** Stopping, or attempting to stop, postprocedural or other acute bleeding **Explanation:** The site of the bleeding is coded as an anatomical region and not to a specific body part **Includes/Examples:** Control of post-prostatectomy hemorrhage, control of intracranial subdural hemorrhage, control of bleeding duodenal ulcer, control of retroperitoneal hemorrhage
4	Creation	**Definition:** Putting in or on biological or synthetic material to form a new body part that to the extent possible replicates the anatomic structure or function of an absent body part **Explanation:** Used for gender reassignment surgery and corrective procedures in individuals with congenital anomalies **Includes/Examples:** Creation of vagina in a male, creation of right and left atrioventricular valve from common atrioventricular valve
5	Destruction	**Definition:** Physical eradication of all or a portion of a body part by the direct use of energy, force, or a destructive agent **Explanation:** None of the body part is physically taken out **Includes/Examples:** Fulguration of rectal polyp, cautery of skin lesion
6	Detachment	**Definition:** Cutting off all or a portion of the upper or lower extremities **Explanation:** The body part value is the site of the detachment, with a qualifier if applicable to further specify the level where the extremity was detached **Includes/Examples:** Below knee amputation, disarticulation of shoulder
7	Dilation	**Definition:** Expanding an orifice or the lumen of a tubular body part **Explanation:** The orifice can be a natural orifice or an artificially created orifice. Accomplished by stretching a tubular body part using intraluminal pressure or by cutting part of the orifice or wall of the tubular body part **Includes/Examples:** Percutaneous transluminal angioplasty, pyloromyotomy
8	Division	**Definition:** Cutting into a body part, without draining fluids and/or gases from the body part, in order to separate or transect a body part **Explanation:** All or a portion of the body part is separated into two or more portions **Includes/Examples:** Spinal cordotomy, osteotomy
9	Drainage	**Definition:** Taking or letting out fluids and/or gases from a body part **Explanation:** The qualifier DIAGNOSTIC is used to identify drainage procedures that are biopsies **Includes/Examples:** Thoracentesis, incision and drainage
B	Excision	**Definition:** Cutting out or off, without replacement, a portion of a body part **Explanation:** The qualifier DIAGNOSTIC is used to identify excision procedures that are biopsies **Includes/Examples:** Partial nephrectomy, liver biopsy

0 - Medical and Surgical		
Value	**Root Operation**	**Definition/Explanation**
C	Extirpation	**Definition:** Taking or cutting out solid matter from a body part **Explanation:** The solid matter may be an abnormal byproduct of a biological function or a foreign body; it may be imbedded in a body part or in the lumen of a tubular body part. The solid matter may or may not have been previously broken into pieces **Includes/Examples:** Thrombectomy, choledocholithotomy
D	Extraction	**Definition:** Pulling or stripping out or off all or a portion of a body part by the use of force **Explanation:** The qualifier DIAGNOSTIC is used to identify extraction procedures that are biopsies **Includes/Examples:** Dilation and curettage, vein stripping
F	Fragmentation	**Definition:** Breaking solid matter in a body part into pieces **Explanation:** Physical force (e.g., manual, ultrasonic) applied directly or indirectly is used to break the solid matter into pieces. The solid matter may be an abnormal byproduct of a biological function or a foreign body. The pieces of solid matter are not taken out **Includes/Examples:** Extracorporeal shockwave lithotripsy, transurethral lithotripsy
G	Fusion	**Definition:** Joining together portions of an articular body part rendering the articular body part immobile **Explanation:** The body part is joined together by fixation device, bone graft, or other means **Includes/Examples:** Spinal fusion, ankle arthrodesis
H	Insertion	**Definition:** Putting in a nonbiological appliance that monitors, assists, performs, or prevents a physiological function but does not physically take the place of a body part **Explanation:** None **Includes/Examples:** Insertion of radioactive implant, insertion of central venous catheter
J	Inspection	**Definition:** Visually and/or manually exploring a body part **Explanation:** Visual exploration may be performed with or without optical instrumentation. Manual exploration may be performed directly or through intervening body layers **Includes/Examples:** Diagnostic arthroscopy, exploratory laparotomy
K	Map	**Definition:** Locating the route of passage of electrical impulses and/or locating functional areas in a body part **Explanation:** Applicable only to the cardiac conduction mechanism and the central nervous system **Includes/Examples:** Cardiac mapping, cortical mapping
L	Occlusion	**Definition:** Completely closing an orifice or the lumen of a tubular body part **Explanation:** The orifice can be a natural orifice or an artificially created orifice **Includes/Examples:** Fallopian tube ligation, ligation of inferior vena cava
M	Reattachment	**Definition:** Putting back in or on all or a portion of a separated body part to its normal location or other suitable location **Explanation:** Vascular circulation and nervous pathways may or may not be reestablished **Includes/Examples:** Reattachment of hand, reattachment of avulsed kidney
N	Release	**Definition:** Freeing a body part from an abnormal physical constraint by cutting or by the use of force **Explanation:** Some of the restraining tissue may be taken out but none of the body part is taken out **Includes/Examples:** Adhesiolysis, carpal tunnel release
P	Removal	**Definition:** Taking out or off a device from a body part **Explanation:** If a device is taken out and a similar device put in without cutting or puncturing the skin or mucous membrane, the procedure is coded to the root operation CHANGE. Otherwise, the procedure for taking out a device is coded to the root operation REMOVAL **Includes/Examples:** Drainage tube removal, cardiac pacemaker removal
Q	Repair	**Definition:** Restoring, to the extent possible, a body part to its normal anatomic structure and function **Explanation:** Used only when the method to accomplish the repair is not one of the other root operations **Includes/Examples:** Colostomy takedown, suture of laceration

0 - Medical and Surgical		
Value	**Root Operation**	**Definition/Explanation**
R	Replacement	**Definition:** Putting in or on biological or synthetic material that physically takes the place and/or function of all or a portion of a body part **Explanation:** The body part may have been taken out or replaced, or may be taken out, physically eradicated, or rendered nonfunctional during the Replacement procedure. A Removal procedure is coded for taking out the device used in a previous replacement procedure **Includes/Examples:** Total hip replacement, bone graft, free skin graft
S	Reposition	**Definition:** Moving to its normal location, or other suitable location, all or a portion of a body part **Explanation:** The body part is moved to a new location from an abnormal location, or from a normal location where it is not functioning correctly. The body part may or may not be cut out or off to be moved to the new location **Includes/Examples:** Reposition of undescended testicle, fracture reduction
T	Resection	**Definition:** Cutting out or off, without replacement, all of a body part **Explanation:** None **Includes/Examples:** Total nephrectomy, total lobectomy of lung
V	Restriction	**Definition:** Partially closing an orifice or the lumen of a tubular body part **Explanation:** The orifice can be a natural orifice or an artificially created orifice **Includes/Examples:** Esophagogastric fundoplication, cervical cerclage
W	Revision	**Definition:** Correcting, to the extent possible, a portion of a malfunctioning device or the position of a displaced device **Explanation:** Revision can include correcting a malfunctioning or displaced device by taking out or putting in components of the device such as a screw or pin **Includes/Examples:** Adjustment of position of pacemaker lead, recementing of hip prosthesis
U	Supplement	**Definition:** Putting in or on biological or synthetic material that physically reinforces and/or augments the function of a portion of a body part **Explanation:** The biological material is non-living, or is living and from the same individual. The body part may have been previously replaced, and the Supplement procedure is performed to physically reinforce and/or augment the function of the replaced body part **Includes/Examples:** Herniorrhaphy using mesh, free nerve graft, mitral valve ring annuloplasty, put a new acetabular liner in a previous hip replacement
X	Transfer	**Definition:** Moving, without taking out, all or a portion of a body part to another location to take over the function of all or a portion of a body part **Explanation:** The body part transferred remains connected to its vascular and nervous supply **Includes/Examples:** Tendon transfer, skin pedicle flap transfer
Y	Transplantation	**Definition:** Putting in or on all or a portion of a living body part taken from another individual or animal to physically take the place and/or function of all or a portion of a similar body part **Explanation:** The native body part may or may not be taken out, and the transplanted body part may take over all or a portion of its function **Includes/Examples:** Kidney transplant, heart transplant

1 - Obstetrics		
Value	**Root Operation**	**Definition/Explanation**
A	Abortion	**Definition:** Artificially terminating a pregnancy
2	Change	**Definition:** Taking out or off a device from a body part and putting back an identical or similar device in or on the same body part without cutting or puncturing the skin or a mucous membrane **Explanation:** All CHANGE procedures are coded using the approach EXTERNAL
E	Delivery	**Definition:** Assisting the passage of the products of conception from the genital canal
9	Drainage	**Definition:** Taking or letting out fluids and/or gases from a body part **Explanation:** The qualifier DIAGNOSTIC is used to identify drainage procedures that are biopsies

1 - Obstetrics		
Value	**Root Operation**	**Definition/Explanation**
D	Extraction	**Definition:** Pulling or stripping out or off all or a portion of a body part by the use of force **Explanation:** The qualifier DIAGNOSTIC is used to identify extraction procedures that are biopsies
H	Insertion	**Definition:** Putting in a nonbiological appliance that monitors, assists, performs, or prevents a physiological function but does not physically take the place of a body part
J	Inspection	**Definition:** Visually and/or manually exploring a body part **Explanation:** Visual exploration may be performed with or without optical instrumentation. Manual exploration may be performed directly or through intervening body layers
P	Removal	**Definition:** Taking out or off a device from a body part, region or orifice **Explanation:** If a device is taken out and a similar device put in without cutting or puncturing the skin or mucous membrane, the procedure is coded to the root operation CHANGE. Otherwise, the procedure for taking out a device is coded to the root operation REMOVAL
Q	Repair	**Definition:** Restoring, to the extent possible, a body part to its normal anatomic structure and function **Explanation:** Used only when the method to accomplish the repair is not one of the other root operations
S	Reposition	**Definition:** Moving to its normal location, or other suitable location, all or a portion of a body part **Explanation:** The body part is moved to a new location from an abnormal location, or from a normal location where it is not functioning correctly. The body part may or may not be cut out or off to be moved to the new location
T	Resection	**Definition:** Cutting out or off, without replacement, all of a body part
Y	Transplantation	**Definition:** Putting in or on all or a portion of a living body part taken from another individual or animal to physically take the place and/or function of all or a portion of a similar body part **Explanation:** The native body part may or may not be taken out, and the transplanted body part may take over all or a portion of its function

2 - Placement		
Value	**Root Operation**	**Definition/Explanation**
0	Change	**Definition:** Taking out or off a device from a body part and putting back an identical or similar device in or on the same body part without cutting or puncturing the skin or a mucous membrane
1	Compression	**Definition:** Putting pressure on a body region
2	Dressing	**Definition:** Putting material on a body region for protection
3	Immobilization	**Definition:** Limiting or preventing motion of a body region
4	Packing	**Definition:** Putting material in a body region or orifice
5	Removal	**Definition:** Taking out or off a device from a body part
6	Traction	**Definition:** Exerting a pulling force on a body region in a distal direction

3 - Administration		
Value	**Root Operation**	**Definition/Explanation**
0	Introduction	**Definition:** Putting in or on a therapeutic, diagnostic, nutritional, physiological, or prophylactic substance except blood or blood products
1	Irrigation	**Definition:** Putting in or on a cleansing substance
2	Transfusion	**Definition:** Putting in blood or blood products

4 - Measurement and Monitoring		
Value	**Root Operation**	**Definition/Explanation**
0	Measurement	**Definition:** Determining the level of a physiological or physical function at a point in time
1	Monitoring	**Definition:** Determining the level of a physiological or physical function repetitively over a period of time

5 - Extracorporeal Assistance and Performance		
Value	**Root Operation**	**Definition/Explanation**
0	Assistance	**Definition:** Taking over a portion of a physiological function by extracorporeal means
1	Performance	**Definition:** Completely taking over a physiological function by extracorporeal means
2	Restoration	**Definition:** Returning, or attempting to return, a physiological function to its original state by extracorporeal means.

6 - Extracorporeal Therapies		
Value	**Root Operation**	**Definition/Explanation**
0	Atmospheric Control	**Definition:** Extracorporeal control of atmospheric pressure and composition
1	Decompression	**Definition:** Extracorporeal elimination of undissolved gas from body fluids
2	Electromagnetic Therapy	**Definition:** Extracorporeal treatment by electromagnetic rays
3	Hyperthermia	**Definition:** Extracorporeal raising of body temperature
4	Hypothermia	**Definition:** Extracorporeal lowering of body temperature
B	Perfusion	**Definition:** Extracorporeal treatment by diffusion of therapeutic fluid
5	Pheresis	**Definition:** Extracorporeal separation of blood products
6	Phototherapy	**Definition:** Extracorporeal treatment by light rays
9	Shock Wave Therapy	**Definition:** Extracorporeal treatment by shock waves
7	Ultrasound Therapy	**Definition:** Extracorporeal treatment by ultrasound
8	Ultraviolet Light Therapy	**Definition:** Extracorporeal treatment by ultraviolet light

7 - Osteopathic		
Value	**Root Operation**	**Definition/Explanation**
0	Treatment	**Definition:** Manual treatment to eliminate or alleviate somatic dysfunction and related disorders

8 - Other Procedures		
Value	**Root Operation**	**Definition/Explanation**
0	Other Procedures	**Definition:** Methodologies which attempt to remediate or cure a disorder or disease

9 - Chiropractic		
Value	**Root Operation**	**Definition/Explanation**
B	Manipulation	**Definition:** Manual procedure that involves a directed thrust to move a joint past the physiological range of motion, without exceeding the anatomical limit

X - New Technology		
Value	**Root Operation**	**Definition/Explanation**
A	Assistance	**Definition:** Taking over a portion of a physiological function by extracorporeal means
C	Extirpation	**Definition:** Taking or cutting out solid matter from a body part **Explanation:** The solid matter may be an abnormal byproduct of a biological function or a foreign body; it may be imbedded in a body part or in the lumen of a tubular body part. The solid matter may or may not have been previously broken into pieces **Includes/Examples:** Thrombectomy, choledocholithotomy
G	Fusion	**Definition:** Joining together portions of an articular body part rendering the articular body part immobile **Explanation:** The body part is joined together by fixation device, bone graft, or other means **Includes/Examples:** Spinal fusion, ankle arthrodesis
NA	Insertion	**Definition:** Putting in a nonbiological appliance that monitors, assists, performs, or prevents a physiological function but does not physically take the place of a body part **Includes/Examples:** Insertion of radioactive implant, insertion of central venous catheter
0	Introduction	**Definition:** Putting in or on a therapeutic, diagnostic, nutritional, physiological, or prophylactic substance except blood or blood products
2	Monitoring	**Definition:** Determining the level of a physiological or physical function repetitively over a period of time
NA	Removal	**Definition:** Taking out or off a device from a body part **Explanation:** If a device is taken out and a similar device put in without cutting or puncturing the skin or mucous membrane, the procedure is coded to the root operation CHANGE. Otherwise, the procedure for taking out a device is coded to the root operation REMOVAL **Includes/Examples:** Drainage tube removal, cardiac pacemaker removal
R	Replacement	**Definition:** Putting in or on biological or synthetic material that physically takes the place and/or function of all or a portion of a body part **Explanation:** The body part may have been taken out or replaced, or may be taken out, physically eradicated, or rendered nonfunctional during the Replacement procedure. A Removal procedure is coded for taking out the device used in a previous replacement procedure **Includes/Examples:** Total hip replacement, bone graft, free skin graft
S	Reposition	**Definition:** Moving to its normal location, or other suitable location, all or a portion of a body part **Explanation:** The body part is moved to a new location from an abnormal location, or from a normal location where it is not functioning correctly. The body part may or may not be cut out or off to be moved to the new location **Includes/Examples:** Reposition of undescended testicle, fracture reduction
NA	Revision	**Definition:** Correcting, to the extent possible, a portion of a malfunctioning device or the position of a displaced device **Explanation:** Revision can include correcting a malfunctioning or displaced device by taking out or putting in components of the device such as a screw or pin **Includes/Examples:** Adjustment of position of pacemaker lead, recementing of hip prosthesis

NA = Not yet assigned

Appendix B: Body Part Key

Anatomical Term	ICD-10-PCS Value
Abdominal aortic plexus	Abdominal Sympathetic Nerve
Abdominal esophagus	Esophagus, Lower
Abductor hallucis muscle	Foot Muscle, Right
	Foot Muscle, Left
Accessory cephalic vein	Cephalic Vein, Right
	Cephalic Vein, Left
Accessory obturator nerve	Lumbar Plexus
Accessory phrenic nerve	Phrenic Nerve
Accessory spleen	Spleen
Acetabulofemoral joint	Hip Joint, Right
	Hip Joint, Left
Achilles tendon	Lower Leg Tendon, Right
	Lower Leg Tendon, Left
Acromioclavicular ligament	Shoulder Bursa and Ligament, Right
	Shoulder Bursa and Ligament, Left
Acromion (process)	Scapula, Right
	Scapula, Left
Adductor brevis muscle	Upper Leg Muscle, Right
	Upper Leg Muscle, Left
Adductor hallucis muscle	Foot Muscle, Right
	Foot Muscle, Left
Adductor longus muscle	Upper Leg Muscle, Right
	Upper Leg Muscle, Left
Adductor magnus muscle	Upper Leg Muscle, Right
	Upper Leg Muscle, Left
Adenohypophysis	Pituitary Gland
Alar ligament of axis	Head and Neck Bursa and Ligament
Alveolar process of mandible	Mandible, Right
	Mandible, Left
Alveolar process of maxilla	Maxilla, Right
	Maxilla, Left
Anal orifice	Anus
Anatomical snuffbox	Lower Arm and Wrist Muscle, Right
	Lower Arm and Wrist Muscle, Left
Angular artery	Face Artery
Angular vein	Face Vein, Right
	Face Vein, Left
Annular ligament	Elbow Bursa and Ligament, Right
	Elbow Bursa and Ligament, Left
Anorectal junction	Rectum
Ansa cervicalis	Cervical Plexus
Antebrachial fascia	Subcutaneous Tissue and Fascia, Right Lower Arm
	Subcutaneous Tissue and Fascia, Left Lower Arm
Anterior (pectoral) lymph node	Lymphatic, Right Axillary
	Lymphatic, Left Axillary
Anterior cerebral artery	Intracranial Artery
Anterior cerebral vein	Intracranial Vein
Anterior choroidal artery	Intracranial Artery
Anterior circumflex humeral artery	Axillary Artery, Right
	Axillary Artery, Left

Anatomical Term	ICD-10-PCS Value
Anterior communicating artery	Intracranial Artery
Anterior cruciate ligament (ACL)	Knee Bursa and Ligament, Right
	Knee Bursa and Ligament, Left
Anterior crural nerve	Femoral Nerve
Anterior facial vein	Face Vein, Right
	Face Vein, Left
Anterior intercostal artery	Internal Mammary Artery, Right
	Internal Mammary Artery, Left
Anterior interosseous nerve	Median Nerve
Anterior lateral malleolar artery	Anterior Tibial Artery, Right
	Anterior Tibial Artery, Left
Anterior lingual gland	Minor Salivary Gland
Anterior medial malleolar artery	Anterior Tibial Artery, Right
	Anterior Tibial Artery, Left
Anterior spinal artery	Vertebral Artery, Right
	Vertebral Artery, Left
Anterior tibial recurrent artery	Anterior Tibial Artery, Right
	Anterior Tibial Artery, Left
Anterior ulnar recurrent artery	Ulnar Artery, Right
	Ulnar Artery, Left
Anterior vagal trunk	Vagus Nerve
Anterior vertebral muscle	Neck Muscle, Right
	Neck Muscle, Left
Antihelix	External Ear, Right
	External Ear, Left
	External Ear, Bilateral
Antitragus	External Ear, Right
	External Ear, Left
	External Ear, Bilateral
Antrum of Highmore	Maxillary Sinus, Right
	Maxillary Sinus, Left
Aortic annulus	Aortic Valve
Aortic arch	Thoracic Aorta, Ascending/Arch
Aortic intercostal artery	Upper Artery
Apical (subclavicular) lymph node	Lymphatic, Right Axillary
	Lymphatic, Left Axillary
Apneustic center	Pons
Aqueduct of Sylvius	Cerebral Ventricle
Aqueous humor	Anterior Chamber, Right
	Anterior Chamber, Left
Arachnoid mater, intracranial	Cerebral Meninges
Arachnoid mater, spinal	Spinal Meninges
Arcuate artery	Foot Artery, Right
	Foot Artery, Left
Areola	Nipple, Right
	Nipple, Left
Arterial canal (duct)	Pulmonary Artery, Left
Aryepiglottic fold	Larynx
Arytenoid cartilage	Larynx
Arytenoid muscle	Neck Muscle, Right
	Neck Muscle, Left

Anatomical Term	ICD-10-PCS Value
Ascending aorta	Thoracic Aorta, Ascending/Arch
Ascending palatine artery	Face Artery
Ascending pharyngeal artery	External Carotid Artery, Right
	External Carotid Artery, Left
Atlantoaxial joint	Cervical Vertebral Joint
Atrioventricular node	Conduction Mechanism
Atrium dextrum cordis	Atrium, Right
Atrium pulmonale	Atrium, Left
Auditory tube	Eustachian Tube, Right
	Eustachian Tube, Left
Auerbach's (myenteric) plexus	Abdominal Sympathetic Nerve
Auricle	External Ear, Right
	External Ear, Left
	External Ear, Bilateral
Auricularis muscle	Head Muscle
Axillary fascia	Subcutaneous Tissue and Fascia, Right Upper Arm
	Subcutaneous Tissue and Fascia, Left Upper Arm
Axillary nerve	Brachial Plexus
Bartholin's (greater vestibular) gland	Vestibular Gland
Basal (internal) cerebral vein	Intracranial Vein
Basal nuclei	Basal Ganglia
Base of Tongue	Pharynx
Basilar artery	Intracranial Artery
Basis pontis	Pons
Biceps brachii muscle	Upper Arm Muscle, Right
	Upper Arm Muscle, Left
Biceps femoris muscle	Upper Leg Muscle, Right
	Upper Leg Muscle, Left
Bicipital aponeurosis	Subcutaneous Tissue and Fascia, Right Lower Arm
	Subcutaneous Tissue and Fascia, Left Lower Arm
Bicuspid valve	Mitral Valve
Body of femur	Femoral Shaft, Right
	Femoral Shaft, Left
Body of fibula	Fibula, Right
	Fibula, Left
Bony labyrinth	Inner Ear, Right
	Inner Ear, Left
Bony orbit	Orbit, Right
	Orbit, Left
Bony vestibule	Inner Ear, Right
	Inner Ear, Left
Botallo's duct	Pulmonary Artery, Left
Brachial (lateral) lymph node	Lymphatic, Right Axillary
	Lymphatic, Left Axillary
Brachialis muscle	Upper Arm Muscle, Right
	Upper Arm Muscle, Left
Brachiocephalic artery	Innominate Artery
Brachiocephalic trunk	Innominate Artery
Brachiocephalic vein	Innominate Vein, Right
	Innominate Vein, Left
Brachioradialis muscle	Lower Arm and Wrist Muscle, Right
	Lower Arm and Wrist Muscle, Left
Broad ligament	Uterine Supporting Structure
Bronchial artery	Upper Artery
Bronchus Intermedius	Main Bronchus, Right
Buccal gland	Buccal Mucosa
Buccinator lymph node	Lymphatic, Head
Buccinator muscle	Facial Muscle
Bulbospongiosus muscle	Perineum Muscle
Bulbourethral (Cowper's) gland	Urethra
Bundle of His	Conduction Mechanism
Bundle of Kent	Conduction Mechanism
Calcaneocuboid joint	Tarsal Joint, Right
	Tarsal Joint, Left
Calcaneocuboid ligament	Foot Bursa and Ligament, Right
	Foot Bursa and Ligament, Left
Calcaneofibular ligament	Ankle Bursa and Ligament, Right
	Ankle Bursa and Ligament, Left
Calcaneus	Tarsal, Right
	Tarsal, Left
Capitate bone	Carpal, Right
	Carpal, Left
Cardia	Esophagogastric Junction
Cardiac plexus	Thoracic Sympathetic Nerve
Cardioesophageal junction	Esophagogastric Junction
Caroticotympanic artery	Internal Carotid Artery, Right
	Internal Carotid Artery, Left
Carotid glomus	Carotid Body, Left
	Carotid Body, Right
	Carotid Bodies, Bilateral
Carotid sinus	Internal Carotid Artery, Right
	Internal Carotid Artery, Left
Carotid sinus nerve	Glossopharyngeal Nerve
Carpometacarpal (CMC) joint	Metacarpocarpal Joint, Right
	Metacarpocarpal Joint, Left
Carpometacarpal ligament	Hand Bursa and Ligament, Right
	Hand Bursa and Ligament, Left
Cauda equina	Lumbar Spinal Cord
Cavernous plexus	Head and Neck Sympathetic Nerve
Celiac (solar) plexus	Abdominal Sympathetic Nerve
Celiac ganglion	Abdominal Sympathetic Nerve
Celiac lymph node	Lymphatic, Aortic
Celiac trunk	Celiac Artery
Central axillary lymph node	Lymphatic, Right Axillary
	Lymphatic, Left Axillary
Cerebral aqueduct (Sylvius)	Cerebral Ventricle
Cerebrum	Brain
Cervical esophagus	Esophagus, Upper
Cervical facet joint	Cervical Vertebral Joint
	Cervical Vertebral Joints, 2 or more
Cervical ganglion	Head and Neck Sympathetic Nerve

Anatomical Term	ICD-10-PCS Value
Cervical interspinous ligament	Head and Neck Bursa and Ligament
Cervical intertransverse ligament	Head and Neck Bursa and Ligament
Cervical ligamentum flavum	Head and Neck Bursa and Ligament
Cervical lymph node	Lymphatic, Right Neck
	Lymphatic, Left Neck
Cervicothoracic facet joint	Cervicothoracic Vertebral Joint
Choana	Nasopharynx
Chondroglossus muscle	Tongue, Palate, Pharynx Muscle
Chorda tympani	Facial Nerve
Choroid plexus	Cerebral Ventricle
Ciliary body	Eye, Right
	Eye, Left
Ciliary ganglion	Head and Neck Sympathetic Nerve
Circle of Willis	Intracranial Artery
Circumflex iliac artery	Femoral Artery, Right
	Femoral Artery, Left
Claustrum	Basal Ganglia
Coccygeal body	Coccygeal Glomus
Coccygeus muscle	Trunk Muscle, Right
	Trunk Muscle, Left
Cochlea	Inner Ear, Right
	Inner Ear, Left
Cochlear nerve	Acoustic Nerve
Columella	Nose
Common digital vein	Foot Vein, Right
	Foot Vein, Left
Common facial vein	Face Vein, Right
	Face Vein, Left
Common fibular nerve	Peroneal Nerve
Common hepatic artery	Hepatic Artery
Common iliac (subaortic) lymph node	Lymphatic, Pelvis
Common interosseous artery	Ulnar Artery, Right
	Ulnar Artery, Left
Common peroneal nerve	Peroneal Nerve
Condyloid process	Mandible, Right
	Mandible, Left
Conus arteriosus	Ventricle, Right
Conus medullaris	Lumbar Spinal Cord
Coracoacromial ligament	Shoulder Bursa and Ligament, Right
	Shoulder Bursa and Ligament, Left
Coracobrachialis muscle	Upper Arm Muscle, Right
	Upper Arm Muscle, Left
Coracoclavicular ligament	Shoulder Bursa and Ligament, Right
	Shoulder Bursa and Ligament, Left
Coracohumeral ligament	Shoulder Bursa and Ligament, Right
	Shoulder Bursa and Ligament, Left
Coracoid process	Scapula, Right
	Scapula, Left
Corniculate cartilage	Larynx
Corpus callosum	Brain
Corpus cavernosum	Penis
Corpus spongiosum	Penis

Anatomical Term	ICD-10-PCS Value
Corpus striatum	Basal Ganglia
Corrugator supercilii muscle	Facial Muscle
Costocervical trunk	Subclavian Artery, Right
	Subclavian Artery, Left
Costoclavicular ligament	Shoulder Bursa and Ligament, Right
	Shoulder Bursa and Ligament, Left
Costotransverse joint	Thoracic Vertebral Joint
Costotransverse ligament	Thorax Bursa and Ligament, Right
	Thorax Bursa and Ligament, Left
Costovertebral joint	Thoracic Vertebral Joint
Costoxiphoid ligament	Thorax Bursa and Ligament, Right
	Thorax Bursa and Ligament, Left
Cowper's (bulbourethral) gland	Urethra
Cremaster muscle	Perineum Muscle
Cribriform plate	Ethmoid Bone, Right
	Ethmoid Bone, Left
Cricoid cartilage	Trachea
Cricothyroid artery	Thyroid Artery, Right
	Thyroid Artery, Left
Cricothyroid muscle	Neck Muscle, Right
	Neck Muscle, Left
Crural fascia	Subcutaneous Tissue and Fascia, Right Upper Leg
	Subcutaneous Tissue and Fascia, Left Upper Leg
Cubital lymph node	Lymphatic, Right Upper Extremity
	Lymphatic, Left Upper Extremity
Cubital nerve	Ulnar Nerve
Cuboid bone	Tarsal, Right
	Tarsal, Left
Cuboideonavicular joint	Tarsal Joint, Right
	Tarsal Joint, Left
Culmen	Cerebellum
Cuneiform cartilage	Larynx
Cuneonavicular joint	Tarsal Joint, Right
	Tarsal Joint, Left
Cuneonavicular ligament	Foot Bursa and Ligament, Right
	Foot Bursa and Ligament, Left
Cutaneous (transverse) cervical nerve	Cervical Plexus
Deep cervical fascia	Subcutaneous Tissue and Fascia, Anterior Neck
Deep cervical vein	Vertebral Vein, Right
	Vertebral Vein, Left
Deep circumflex iliac artery	External Iliac Artery, Right
	External Iliac Artery, Left
Deep facial vein	Face Vein, Right
	Face Vein, Left
Deep femoral (profunda femoris) vein	Femoral Vein, Right
	Femoral Vein, Left
Deep femoral artery	Femoral Artery, Right
	Femoral Artery, Left
Deep palmar arch	Hand Artery, Right
	Hand Artery, Left

Anatomical Term	ICD-10-PCS Value
Deep transverse perineal muscle	Perineum Muscle
Deferential artery	Internal Iliac Artery, Right
	Internal Iliac Artery, Left
Deltoid fascia	Subcutaneous Tissue and Fascia, Right Upper Arm
	Subcutaneous Tissue and Fascia, Left Upper Arm
Deltoid ligament	Ankle Bursa and Ligament, Right
	Ankle Bursa and Ligament, Left
Deltoid muscle	Shoulder Muscle, Right
	Shoulder Muscle, Left
Deltopectoral (infraclavicular) lymph node	Lymphatic, Right Upper Extremity
	Lymphatic, Left Upper Extremity
Denticulate (dentate) ligament	Spinal Meninges
Depressor anguli oris muscle	Facial Muscle
Depressor labii inferioris muscle	Facial Muscle
Depressor septi nasi muscle	Facial Muscle
Depressor supercilii muscle	Facial Muscle
Dermis	Skin
Descending genicular artery	Femoral Artery, Right
	Femoral Artery, Left
Diaphragma sellae	Dura Mater
Distal humerus	Humeral Shaft, Right
	Humeral Shaft, Left
Distal humerus, involving joint	Elbow Joint, Right
	Elbow Joint, Left
Distal radioulnar joint	Wrist Joint, Right
	Wrist Joint, Left
Dorsal digital nerve	Radial Nerve
Dorsal metacarpal vein	Hand Vein, Right
	Hand Vein, Left
Dorsal metatarsal artery	Foot Artery, Right
	Foot Artery, Left
Dorsal metatarsal vein	Foot Vein, Right
	Foot Vein, Left
Dorsal scapular artery	Subclavian Artery, Right
	Subclavian Artery, Left
Dorsal scapular nerve	Brachial Plexus
Dorsal venous arch	Foot Vein, Right
	Foot Vein, Left
Dorsalis pedis artery	Anterior Tibial Artery, Right
	Anterior Tibial Artery, Left
Duct of Santorini	Pancreatic Duct, Accessory
Duct of Wirsung	Pancreatic Duct
Ductus deferens	Vas Deferens, Right
	Vas Deferens, Left
	Vas Deferens, Bilateral
	Vas Deferens
Duodenal ampulla	Ampulla of Vater
Duodenojejunal flexure	Jejunum
Dura mater, intracranial	Dura Mater
Dura mater, spinal	Spinal Meninges
Dural venous sinus	Intracranial Vein
Earlobe	External Ear, Right
	External Ear, Left
	External Ear, Bilateral
Eighth cranial nerve	Acoustic Nerve
Ejaculatory duct	Vas Deferens, Right
	Vas Deferens, Left
	Vas Deferens, Bilateral
	Vas Deferens
Eleventh cranial nerve	Accessory Nerve
Encephalon	Brain
Ependyma	Cerebral Ventricle
Epidermis	Skin
Epidural space, intracranial	Epidural Space
Epidural space, spinal	Spinal Canal
Epiploic foramen	Peritoneum
Epithalamus	Thalamus
Epitrochlear lymph node	Lymphatic, Right Upper Extremity
	Lymphatic, Left Upper Extremity
Erector spinae muscle	Trunk Muscle, Right
	Trunk Muscle, Left
Esophageal artery	Upper Artery
Esophageal plexus	Thoracic Sympathetic Nerve
Ethmoidal air cell	Ethmoid Sinus, Right
	Ethmoid Sinus, Left
Extensor carpi radialis muscle	Lower Arm and Wrist Muscle, Right
	Lower Arm and Wrist Muscle, Left
Extensor carpi ulnaris muscle	Lower Arm and Wrist Muscle, Right
	Lower Arm and Wrist Muscle, Left
Extensor digitorum brevis muscle	Foot Muscle, Right
	Foot Muscle, Left
Extensor digitorum longus muscle	Lower Leg Muscle, Right
	Lower Leg Muscle, Left
Extensor hallucis brevis muscle	Foot Muscle, Right
	Foot Muscle, Left
Extensor hallucis longus muscle	Lower Leg Muscle, Right
	Lower Leg Muscle, Left
External anal sphincter	Anal Sphincter
External auditory meatus	External Auditory Canal, Right
	External Auditory Canal, Left
External maxillary artery	Face Artery
External naris	Nose
External oblique aponeurosis	Subcutaneous Tissue and Fascia, Trunk
External oblique muscle	Abdomen Muscle, Right
	Abdomen Muscle, Left
External popliteal nerve	Peroneal Nerve
External pudendal artery	Femoral Artery, Right
	Femoral Artery, Left
External pudendal vein	Greater Saphenous Vein, Right
	Greater Saphenous Vein, Left
External urethral sphincter	Urethra
Extradural space, intracranial	Epidural Space
Extradural space, spinal	Spinal Canal

APPENDIX B: BODY PART KEY

Anatomical Term	ICD-10-PCS Value
Facial artery	Face Artery
False vocal cord	Larynx
Falx cerebri	Dura Mater
Fascia lata	Subcutaneous Tissue and Fascia, Right Upper Leg
	Subcutaneous Tissue and Fascia, Left Upper Leg
Femoral head	Upper Femur, Right
	Upper Femur, Left
Femoral lymph node	Lymphatic, Right Lower Extremity
	Lymphatic, Left Lower Extremity
Femoropatellar joint	Knee Joint, Right
	Knee Joint, Left
	Knee Joint, Femoral Surface, Right
	Knee Joint, Femoral Surface, Left
Femorotibial joint	Knee Joint, Right
	Knee Joint, Left
	Knee Joint, Tibial Surface, Right
	Knee Joint, Tibial Surface, Left
Fibular artery	Peroneal Artery, Right
	Peroneal Artery, Left
Fibularis brevis muscle	Lower Leg Muscle, Right
	Lower Leg Muscle, Left
Fibularis longus muscle	Lower Leg Muscle, Right
	Lower Leg Muscle, Left
Fifth cranial nerve	Trigeminal Nerve
Filum terminale	Spinal Meninges
First cranial nerve	Olfactory Nerve
First intercostal nerve	Brachial Plexus
Flexor carpi radialis muscle	Lower Arm and Wrist Muscle, Right
	Lower Arm and Wrist Muscle, Left
Flexor carpi ulnaris muscle	Lower Arm and Wrist Muscle, Right
	Lower Arm and Wrist Muscle, Left
Flexor digitorum brevis muscle	Foot Muscle, Right
	Foot Muscle, Left
Flexor digitorum longus muscle	Lower Leg Muscle, Right
	Lower Leg Muscle, Left
Flexor hallucis brevis muscle	Foot Muscle, Right
	Foot Muscle, Left
Flexor hallucis longus muscle	Lower Leg Muscle, Right
	Lower Leg Muscle, Left
Flexor pollicis longus muscle	Lower Arm and Wrist Muscle, Right
	Lower Arm and Wrist Muscle, Left
Foramen magnum	Occipital Bone, Right
	Occipital Bone, Left
Foramen of Monro (intraventricular)	Cerebral Ventricle
Foreskin	Prepuce
Fossa of Rosenmuller	Nasopharynx
Fourth cranial nerve	Trochlear Nerve
Fourth ventricle	Cerebral Ventricle
Fovea	Retina, Right
	Retina, Left
Frenulum labii inferioris	Lower Lip
Frenulum labii superioris	Upper Lip
Frenulum linguae	Tongue
Frontal lobe	Cerebral Hemisphere
Frontal vein	Face Vein, Right
	Face Vein, Left
Fundus uteri	Uterus
Galea aponeurotica	Subcutaneous Tissue and Fascia, Scalp
Ganglion impar (ganglion of Walther)	Sacral Sympathetic Nerve
Gasserian ganglion	Trigeminal Nerve
Gastric lymph node	Lymphatic, Aortic
Gastric plexus	Abdominal Sympathetic Nerve
Gastrocnemius muscle	Lower Leg Muscle, Right
	Lower Leg Muscle, Left
Gastrocolic ligament	Greater Omentum
Gastrocolic omentum	Greater Omentum
Gastroduodenal artery	Hepatic Artery
Gastroesophageal (GE) junction	Esophagogastric Junction
Gastrohepatic omentum	Lesser Omentum
Gastrophrenic ligament	Greater Omentum
Gastrosplenic ligament	Greater Omentum
Gemellus muscle	Hip Muscle, Right
	Hip Muscle, Left
Geniculate ganglion	Facial Nerve
Geniculate nucleus	Thalamus
Genioglossus muscle	Tongue, Palate, Pharynx Muscle
Genitofemoral nerve	Lumbar Plexus
Glans penis	Prepuce
Glenohumeral joint	Shoulder Joint, Right
	Shoulder Joint, Left
Glenohumeral ligament	Shoulder Bursa and Ligament, Right
	Shoulder Bursa and Ligament, Left
Glenoid fossa (of scapula)	Glenoid Cavity, Right
	Glenoid Cavity, Left
Glenoid ligament (labrum)	Shoulder Joint, Right
	Shoulder Joint, Left
Globus pallidus	Basal Ganglia
Glossoepiglottic fold	Epiglottis
Glottis	Larynx
Gluteal lymph node	Lymphatic, Pelvis
Gluteal vein	Hypogastric Vein, Right
	Hypogastric Vein, Left
Gluteus maximus muscle	Hip Muscle, Right
	Hip Muscle, Left
Gluteus medius muscle	Hip Muscle, Right
	Hip Muscle, Left
Gluteus minimus muscle	Hip Muscle, Right
	Hip Muscle, Left
Gracilis muscle	Upper Leg Muscle, Right
	Upper Leg Muscle, Left
Great auricular nerve	Cervical Plexus
Great cerebral vein	Intracranial Vein
Great saphenous vein	Greater Saphenous Vein, Right
	Greater Saphenous Vein, Left

Anatomical Term	ICD-10-PCS Value
Greater alar cartilage	Nose
Greater occipital nerve	Cervical Nerve
Greater splanchnic nerve	Thoracic Sympathetic Nerve
Greater superficial petrosal nerve	Facial Nerve
Greater trochanter	Upper Femur, Right
	Upper Femur, Left
Greater tuberosity	Humeral Head, Right
	Humeral Head, Left
Greater vestibular (Bartholin's) gland	Vestibular Gland
Greater wing	Sphenoid Bone, Right
	Sphenoid Bone, Left
Hallux	1st Toe, Right
	1st Toe, Left
Hamate bone	Carpal, Right
	Carpal, Left
Head of fibula	Fibula, Right
	Fibula, Left
Helix	External Ear, Right
	External Ear, Left
	External Ear, Bilateral
Hepatic artery proper	Hepatic Artery
Hepatic flexure	Ascending Colon
Hepatic lymph node	Lymphatic, Aortic
Hepatic plexus	Abdominal Sympathetic Nerve
Hepatic portal vein	Portal Vein
Hepatogastric ligament	Lesser Omentum
Hepatopancreatic ampulla	Ampulla of Vater
Humeroradial joint	Elbow Joint, Right
	Elbow Joint, Left
Humeroulnar joint	Elbow Joint, Right
	Elbow Joint, Left
Humerus, distal	Humeral Shaft, Right
	Humeral Shaft, Left
Hyoglossus muscle	Tongue, Palate, Pharynx Muscle
Hyoid artery	Thyroid Artery, Right
	Thyroid Artery, Left
Hypogastric artery	Internal Iliac Artery, Right
	Internal Iliac Artery, Left
Hypopharynx	Pharynx
Hypophysis	Pituitary Gland
Hypothenar muscle	Hand Muscle, Right
	Hand Muscle, Left
Ileal artery	Superior Mesenteric Artery
Ileocolic artery	Superior Mesenteric Artery
Ileocolic vein	Colic Vein
Iliac crest	Pelvic Bone, Right
	Pelvic Bone, Left
Iliac fascia	Subcutaneous Tissue and Fascia, Right Upper Leg
	Subcutaneous Tissue and Fascia, Left Upper Leg
Iliac lymph node	Lymphatic, Pelvis

Anatomical Term	ICD-10-PCS Value
Iliacus muscle	Hip Muscle, Right
	Hip Muscle, Left
Iliofemoral ligament	Hip Bursa and Ligament, Right
	Hip Bursa and Ligament, Left
Iliohypogastric nerve	Lumbar Plexus
Ilioinguinal nerve	Lumbar Plexus
Iliolumbar artery	Internal Iliac Artery, Right
	Internal Iliac Artery, Left
Iliolumbar ligament	Trunk Bursa and Ligament, Right
	Trunk Bursa and Ligament, Left
Iliotibial tract (band)	Subcutaneous Tissue and Fascia, Right Upper Leg
	Subcutaneous Tissue and Fascia, Left Upper Leg
Ilium	Pelvic Bone, Right
	Pelvic Bone, Left
Incus	Auditory Ossicle, Right
	Auditory Ossicle, Left
Inferior cardiac nerve	Thoracic Sympathetic Nerve
Inferior cerebellar vein	Intracranial Vein
Inferior cerebral vein	Intracranial Vein
Inferior epigastric artery	External Iliac Artery, Right
	External Iliac Artery, Left
Inferior epigastric lymph node	Lymphatic, Pelvis
Inferior genicular artery	Popliteal Artery, Right
	Popliteal Artery, Left
Inferior gluteal artery	Internal Iliac Artery, Right
	Internal Iliac Artery, Left
Inferior gluteal nerve	Sacral Plexus
Inferior hypogastric plexus	Abdominal Sympathetic Nerve
Inferior labial artery	Face Artery
Inferior longitudinal muscle	Tongue, Palate, Pharynx Muscle
Inferior mesenteric ganglion	Abdominal Sympathetic Nerve
Inferior mesenteric lymph node	Lymphatic, Mesenteric
Inferior mesenteric plexus	Abdominal Sympathetic Nerve
Inferior oblique muscle	Extraocular Muscle, Right
	Extraocular Muscle, Left
Inferior pancreaticoduodenal artery	Superior Mesenteric Artery
Inferior phrenic artery	Abdominal Aorta
Inferior rectus muscle	Extraocular Muscle, Right
	Extraocular Muscle, Left
Inferior suprarenal artery	Renal Artery, Right
	Renal Artery, Left
Inferior tarsal plate	Lower Eyelid, Right
	Lower Eyelid, Left
Inferior thyroid vein	Innominate Vein, Right
	Innominate Vein, Left
Inferior tibiofibular joint	Ankle Joint, Right
	Ankle Joint, Left
Inferior turbinate	Nasal Turbinate
Inferior ulnar collateral artery	Brachial Artery, Right
	Brachial Artery, Left

Anatomical Term	ICD-10-PCS Value
Inferior vesical artery	Internal Iliac Artery, Right
	Internal Iliac Artery, Left
Infraauricular lymph node	Lymphatic, Head
Infraclavicular (deltopectoral) lymph node	Lymphatic, Right Upper Extremity
	Lymphatic, Left Upper Extremity
Infrahyoid muscle	Neck Muscle, Right
	Neck Muscle, Left
Infraparotid lymph node	Lymphatic, Head
Infraspinatus fascia	Subcutaneous Tissue and Fascia, Right Upper Arm
	Subcutaneous Tissue and Fascia, Left Upper Arm
Infraspinatus muscle	Shoulder Muscle, Right
	Shoulder Muscle, Left
Infundibulopelvic ligament	Uterine Supporting Structure
Inguinal canal	Inguinal Region, Right
	Inguinal Region, Left
	Inguinal Region, Bilateral
Inguinal triangle	Inguinal Region, Right
	Inguinal Region, Left
	Inguinal Region, Bilateral
Interatrial septum	Atrial Septum
Intercarpal joint	Carpal Joint, Right
	Carpal Joint, Left
Intercarpal ligament	Hand Bursa and Ligament, Right
	Hand Bursa and Ligament, Left
Interclavicular ligament	Shoulder Bursa and Ligament, Right
	Shoulder Bursa and Ligament, Left
Intercostal lymph node	Lymphatic, Thorax
Intercostal muscle	Thorax Muscle, Right
	Thorax Muscle, Left
Intercostal nerve	Thoracic Nerve
Intercostobrachial nerve	Thoracic Nerve
Intercuneiform joint	Tarsal Joint, Right
	Tarsal Joint, Left
Intercuneiform ligament	Foot Bursa and Ligament, Right
	Foot Bursa and Ligament, Left
Intermediate bronchus	Main Bronchus, Right
Intermediate cuneiform bone	Tarsal, Right
	Tarsal, Left
Internal (basal) cerebral vein	Intracranial Vein
Internal anal sphincter	Anal Sphincter
Internal carotid artery, intracranial portion	Intracranial Artery
Internal carotid plexus	Head and Neck Sympathetic Nerve
Internal iliac vein	Hypogastric Vein, Right
	Hypogastric Vein, Left
Internal maxillary artery	External Carotid Artery, Right
	External Carotid Artery, Left
Internal naris	Nose
Internal oblique muscle	Abdomen Muscle, Right
	Abdomen Muscle, Left
Internal pudendal artery	Internal Iliac Artery, Right
	Internal Iliac Artery, Left

Anatomical Term	ICD-10-PCS Value
Internal pudendal vein	Hypogastric Vein, Right
	Hypogastric Vein, Left
Internal thoracic artery	Internal Mammary Artery, Right
	Internal Mammary Artery, Left
	Subclavian Artery, Right
	Subclavian Artery, Left
Internal urethral sphincter	Urethra
Interphalangeal (IP) joint	Finger Phalangeal Joint, Right
	Finger Phalangeal Joint, Left
	Toe Phalangeal Joint, Right
	Toe Phalangeal Joint, Left
Interphalangeal ligament	Hand Bursa and Ligament, Right
	Hand Bursa and Ligament, Left
	Foot Bursa and Ligament, Right
	Foot Bursa and Ligament, Left
Interspinalis muscle	Trunk Muscle, Right
	Trunk Muscle, Left
Interspinous ligament	Head and Neck Bursa and Ligament
	Trunk Bursa and Ligament, Right
	Trunk Bursa and Ligament, Left
Intertransversarius muscle	Trunk Muscle, Right
	Trunk Muscle, Left
Intertransverse ligament	Trunk Bursa and Ligament, Right
	Trunk Bursa and Ligament, Left
Interventricular foramen (Monro)	Cerebral Ventricle
Interventricular septum	Ventricular Septum
Intestinal lymphatic trunk	Cisterna Chyli
Ischiatic nerve	Sciatic Nerve
Ischiocavernosus muscle	Perineum Muscle
Ischiofemoral ligament	Hip Bursa and Ligament, Right
	Hip Bursa and Ligament, Left
Ischium	Pelvic Bone, Right
	Pelvic Bone, Left
Jejunal artery	Superior Mesenteric Artery
Jugular body	Glomus Jugulare
Jugular lymph node	Lymphatic, Right Neck
	Lymphatic, Left Neck
Labia majora	Vulva
Labia minora	Vulva
Labial gland	Upper Lip
	Lower Lip
Lacrimal canaliculus	Lacrimal Duct, Right
	Lacrimal Duct, Left
Lacrimal punctum	Lacrimal Duct, Right
	Lacrimal Duct, Left
Lacrimal sac	Lacrimal Duct, Right
	Lacrimal Duct, Left
Laryngopharynx	Pharynx
Lateral (brachial) lymph node	Lymphatic, Right Axillary
	Lymphatic, Left Axillary
Lateral canthus	Upper Eyelid, Right
	Upper Eyelid, Left

Anatomical Term	ICD-10-PCS Value
Lateral collateral ligament (LCL)	Knee Bursa and Ligament, Right
	Knee Bursa and Ligament, Left
Lateral condyle of femur	Lower Femur, Right
	Lower Femur, Left
Lateral condyle of tibia	Tibia, Right
	Tibia, Left
Lateral cuneiform bone	Tarsal, Right
	Tarsal, Left
Lateral epicondyle of femur	Lower Femur, Right
	Lower Femur, Left
Lateral epicondyle of humerus	Humeral Shaft, Right
	Humeral Shaft, Left
Lateral femoral cutaneous nerve	Lumbar Plexus
Lateral malleolus	Fibula, Right
	Fibula, Left
Lateral meniscus	Knee Joint, Right
	Knee Joint, Left
Lateral nasal cartilage	Nose
Lateral plantar artery	Foot Artery, Right
	Foot Artery, Left
Lateral plantar nerve	Tibial Nerve
Lateral rectus muscle	Extraocular Muscle, Right
	Extraocular Muscle, Left
Lateral sacral artery	Internal Iliac Artery, Right
	Internal Iliac Artery, Left
Lateral sacral vein	Hypogastric Vein, Right
	Hypogastric Vein, Left
Lateral sural cutaneous nerve	Peroneal Nerve
Lateral tarsal artery	Foot Artery, Right
	Foot Artery, Left
Lateral temporomandibular ligament	Head and Neck Bursa and Ligament
Lateral thoracic artery	Axillary Artery, Right
	Axillary Artery, Left
Latissimus dorsi muscle	Trunk Muscle, Right
	Trunk Muscle, Left
Least splanchnic nerve	Thoracic Sympathetic Nerve
Left ascending lumbar vein	Hemiazygos Vein
Left atrioventricular valve	Mitral Valve
Left auricular appendix	Atrium, Left
Left colic vein	Colic Vein
Left coronary sulcus	Heart, Left
Left gastric artery	Gastric Artery
Left gastroepiploic artery	Splenic Artery
Left gastroepiploic vein	Splenic Vein
Left inferior phrenic vein	Renal Vein, Left
Left inferior pulmonary vein	Pulmonary Vein, Left
Left jugular trunk	Thoracic Duct
Left lateral ventricle	Cerebral Ventricle
Left ovarian vein	Renal Vein, Left
Left second lumbar vein	Renal Vein, Left
Left subclavian trunk	Thoracic Duct
Left subcostal vein	Hemiazygos Vein

Anatomical Term	ICD-10-PCS Value
Left superior pulmonary vein	Pulmonary Vein, Left
Left suprarenal vein	Renal Vein, Left
Left testicular vein	Renal Vein, Left
Leptomeninges, intracranial	Cerebral Meninges
Leptomeninges, spinal	Spinal Meninges
Lesser alar cartilage	Nose
Lesser occipital nerve	Cervical Plexus
Lesser splanchnic nerve	Thoracic Sympathetic Nerve
Lesser trochanter	Upper Femur, Right
	Upper Femur, Left
Lesser tuberosity	Humeral Head, Right
	Humeral Head, Left
Lesser wing	Sphenoid Bone, Right
	Sphenoid Bone, Left
Levator anguli oris muscle	Facial Muscle
Levator ani muscle	Perineum Muscle
Levator labii superioris alaeque nasi muscle	Facial Muscle
Levator labii superioris muscle	Facial Muscle
Levator palpebrae superioris muscle	Upper Eyelid, Right
	Upper Eyelid, Left
Levator scapulae muscle	Neck Muscle, Right
	Neck Muscle, Left
Levator veli palatini muscle	Tongue, Palate, Pharynx Muscle
Levatores costarum muscle	Thorax Muscle, Right
	Thorax Muscle, Left
Ligament of head of fibula	Knee Bursa and Ligament, Right
	Knee Bursa and Ligament, Left
Ligament of the lateral malleolus	Ankle Bursa and Ligament, Right
	Ankle Bursa and Ligament, Left
Ligamentum flavum	Trunk Bursa and Ligament, Right
	Trunk Bursa and Ligament, Left
Lingual artery	External Carotid Artery, Right
	External Carotid Artery, Left
Lingual tonsil	Tongue
Locus ceruleus	Pons
Long thoracic nerve	Brachial Plexus
Lumbar artery	Abdominal Aorta
Lumbar facet joint	Lumbar Vertebral Joint
Lumbar ganglion	Lumbar Sympathetic Nerve
Lumbar lymph node	Lymphatic, Aortic
Lumbar lymphatic trunk	Cisterna Chyli
Lumbar splanchnic nerve	Lumbar Sympathetic Nerve
Lumbosacral facet joint	Lumbosacral Joint
Lumbosacral trunk	Lumbar Nerve
Lunate bone	Carpal, Right
	Carpal, Left
Lunotriquetral ligament	Hand Bursa and Ligament, Right
	Hand Bursa and Ligament, Left
Macula	Retina, Right
	Retina, Left
Malleus	Auditory Ossicle, Right
	Auditory Ossicle, Left

Anatomical Term	ICD-10-PCS Value
Mammary duct	Breast, Right
	Breast, Left
	Breast, Bilateral
Mammary gland	Breast, Right
	Breast, Left
	Breast, Bilateral
Mammillary body	Hypothalamus
Mandibular nerve	Trigeminal Nerve
Mandibular notch	Mandible, Right
	Mandible, Left
Manubrium	Sternum
Masseter muscle	Head Muscle
Masseteric fascia	Subcutaneous Tissue and Fascia, Face
Mastoid (postauricular) lymph node	Lymphatic, Right Neck
	Lymphatic, Left Neck
Mastoid air cells	Mastoid Sinus, Right
	Mastoid Sinus, Left
Mastoid process	Temporal Bone, Right
	Temporal Bone, Left
Maxillary artery	External Carotid Artery, Right
	External Carotid Artery, Left
Maxillary nerve	Trigeminal Nerve
Medial canthus	Lower Eyelid, Right
	Lower Eyelid, Left
Medial collateral ligament (MCL)	Knee Bursa and Ligament, Right
	Knee Bursa and Ligament, Left
Medial condyle of femur	Lower Femur, Right
	Lower Femur, Left
Medial condyle of tibia	Tibia, Right
	Tibia, Left
Medial cuneiform bone	Tarsal, Right
	Tarsal, Left
Medial epicondyle of femur	Lower Femur, Right
	Lower Femur, Left
Medial epicondyle of humerus	Humeral Shaft, Right
	Humeral Shaft, Left
Medial malleolus	Tibia, Right
	Tibia, Left
Medial meniscus	Knee Joint, Right
	Knee Joint, Left
Medial plantar artery	Foot Artery, Right
	Foot Artery, Left
Medial plantar nerve	Tibial Nerve
Medial popliteal nerve	Tibial Nerve
Medial rectus muscle	Extraocular Muscle, Right
	Extraocular Muscle, Left
Medial sural cutaneous nerve	Tibial Nerve
Median antebrachial vein	Basilic Vein, Right
	Basilic Vein, Left
Median cubital vein	Basilic Vein, Right
	Basilic Vein, Left
Median sacral artery	Abdominal Aorta
Mediastinal lymph node	Lymphatic, Thorax

Anatomical Term	ICD-10-PCS Value
Meissner's (submucous) plexus	Abdominal Sympathetic Nerve
Membranous urethra	Urethra
Mental foramen	Mandible, Right
	Mandible, Left
Mentalis muscle	Facial Muscle
Mesoappendix	Mesentery
Mesocolon	Mesentery
Metacarpal ligament	Hand Bursa and Ligament, Right
	Hand Bursa and Ligament, Left
Metacarpophalangeal ligament	Hand Bursa and Ligament, Right
	Hand Bursa and Ligament, Left
Metatarsal ligament	Foot Bursa and Ligament, Right
	Foot Bursa and Ligament, Left
Metatarsophalangeal (MTP) joint	Metatarsal-Phalangeal Joint, Right
	Metatarsal-Phalangeal Joint, Left
Metatarsophalangeal ligament	Foot Bursa and Ligament, Right
	Foot Bursa and Ligament, Left
Metathalamus	Thalamus
Midcarpal joint	Carpal Joint, Right
	Carpal Joint, Left
Middle cardiac nerve	Thoracic Sympathetic Nerve
Middle cerebral artery	Intracranial Artery
Middle cerebral vein	Intracranial Vein
Middle colic vein	Colic Vein
Middle genicular artery	Popliteal Artery, Right
	Popliteal Artery, Left
Middle hemorrhoidal vein	Hypogastric Vein, Right
	Hypogastric Vein, Left
Middle rectal artery	Internal Iliac Artery, Right
	Internal Iliac Artery, Left
Middle suprarenal artery	Abdominal Aorta
Middle temporal artery	Temporal Artery, Right
	Temporal Artery, Left
Middle turbinate	Nasal Turbinate
Mitral annulus	Mitral Valve
Molar gland	Buccal Mucosa
Musculocutaneous nerve	Brachial Plexus
Musculophrenic artery	Internal Mammary Artery, Right
	Internal Mammary Artery, Left
Musculospiral nerve	Radial Nerve
Myelencephalon	Medulla Oblongata
Myenteric (Auerbach's) plexus	Abdominal Sympathetic Nerve
Myometrium	Uterus
Nail bed	Finger Nail
	Toe Nail
Nail plate	Finger Nail
	Toe Nail
Nasal cavity	Nose
Nasal concha	Nasal Turbinate
Nasalis muscle	Facial Muscle
Nasolacrimal duct	Lacrimal Duct, Right
	Lacrimal Duct, Left

Anatomical Term	ICD-10-PCS Value
Navicular bone	Tarsal, Right
	Tarsal, Left
Neck of femur	Upper Femur, Right
	Upper Femur, Left
Neck of humerus (anatomical)(surgical)	Humeral Head, Right
	Humeral Head, Left
Nerve to the stapedius	Facial Nerve
Neurohypophysis	Pituitary Gland
Ninth cranial nerve	Glossopharyngeal Nerve
Nostril	Nose
Obturator artery	Internal Iliac Artery, Right
	Internal Iliac Artery, Left
Obturator lymph node	Lymphatic, Pelvis
Obturator muscle	Hip Muscle, Right
	Hip Muscle, Left
Obturator nerve	Lumbar Plexus
Obturator vein	Hypogastric Vein, Right
	Hypogastric Vein, Left
Obtuse margin	Heart, Left
Occipital artery	External Carotid Artery, Right
	External Carotid Artery, Left
Occipital lobe	Cerebral Hemisphere
Occipital lymph node	Lymphatic, Right Neck
	Lymphatic, Left Neck
Occipitofrontalis muscle	Facial Muscle
Olecranon bursa	Elbow Bursa and Ligament, Right
	Elbow Bursa and Ligament, Left
Olecranon process	Ulna, Right
	Ulna, Left
Olfactory bulb	Olfactory Nerve
Ophthalmic artery	Intracranial Artery
Ophthalmic nerve	Trigeminal Nerve
Ophthalmic vein	Intracranial Vein
Optic chiasma	Optic Nerve
Optic disc	Retina, Right
	Retina, Left
Optic foramen	Sphenoid Bone, Right
	Sphenoid Bone, Left
Orbicularis oculi muscle	Upper Eyelid, Right
	Upper Eyelid, Left
Orbicularis oris muscle	Facial Muscle
Orbital fascia	Subcutaneous Tissue and Fascia, Face
Orbital portion of ethmoid bone	Orbit, Right
	Orbit, Left
Orbital portion of frontal bone	Orbit, Right
	Orbit, Left
Orbital portion of lacrimal bone	Orbit, Right
	Orbit, Left
Orbital portion of maxilla	Orbit, Right
	Orbit, Left
Orbital portion of palatine bone	Orbit, Right
	Orbit, Left

Anatomical Term	ICD-10-PCS Value
Orbital portion of sphenoid bone	Orbit, Right
	Orbit, Left
Orbital portion of zygomatic bone	Orbit, Right
	Orbit, Left
Oropharynx	Pharynx
Otic ganglion	Head and Neck Sympathetic Nerve
Oval window	Middle Ear, Right
	Middle Ear, Left
Ovarian artery	Abdominal Aorta
Ovarian ligament	Uterine Supporting Structure
Oviduct	Fallopian Tube, Right
	Fallopian Tube, Left
Palatine gland	Buccal Mucosa
Palatine tonsil	Tonsils
Palatine uvula	Uvula
Palatoglossal muscle	Tongue, Palate, Pharynx Muscle
Palatopharyngeal muscle	Tongue, Palate, Pharynx Muscle
Palmar (volar) digital vein	Hand Vein, Right
	Hand Vein, Left
Palmar (volar) metacarpal vein	Hand Vein, Right
	Hand Vein, Left
Palmar cutaneous nerve	Median Nerve
	Radial Nerve
Palmar fascia (aponeurosis)	Subcutaneous Tissue and Fascia, Right Hand
	Subcutaneous Tissue and Fascia, Left Hand
Palmar interosseous muscle	Hand Muscle, Right
	Hand Muscle, Left
Palmar ulnocarpal ligament	Wrist Bursa and Ligament, Right
	Wrist Bursa and Ligament, Left
Palmaris longus muscle	Lower Arm and Wrist Muscle, Right
	Lower Arm and Wrist Muscle, Left
Pancreatic artery	Splenic Artery
Pancreatic plexus	Abdominal Sympathetic Nerve
Pancreatic vein	Splenic Vein
Pancreaticosplenic lymph node	Lymphatic, Aortic
Paraaortic lymph node	Lymphatic, Aortic
Pararectal lymph node	Lymphatic, Mesenteric
Parasternal lymph node	Lymphatic, Thorax
Paratracheal lymph node	Lymphatic, Thorax
Paraurethral (Skene's) gland	Vestibular Gland
Parietal lobe	Cerebral Hemisphere
Parotid lymph node	Lymphatic, Head
Parotid plexus	Facial Nerve
Pars flaccida	Tympanic Membrane, Right
	Tympanic Membrane, Left
Patellar ligament	Knee Bursa and Ligament, Right
	Knee Bursa and Ligament, Left
Patellar tendon	Knee Tendon, Right
	Knee Tendon, Left

Anatomical Term	ICD-10-PCS Value
Patellofemoral joint	Knee Joint, Right
	Knee Joint, Left
	Knee Joint, Femoral Surface, Right
	Knee Joint, Femoral Surface, Left
Pectineus muscle	Upper Leg Muscle, Right
	Upper Leg Muscle, Left
Pectoral (anterior) lymph node	Lymphatic, Right Axillary
	Lymphatic, Left Axillary
Pectoral fascia	Subcutaneous Tissue and Fascia, Chest
Pectoralis major muscle	Thorax Muscle, Right
	Thorax Muscle, Left
Pectoralis minor muscle	Thorax Muscle, Right
	Thorax Muscle, Left
Pelvic splanchnic nerve	Abdominal Sympathetic Nerve
	Sacral Sympathetic Nerve
Penile urethra	Urethra
Pericardiophrenic artery	Internal Mammary Artery, Right
	Internal Mammary Artery, Left
Perimetrium	Uterus
Peroneus brevis muscle	Lower Leg Muscle, Right
	Lower Leg Muscle, Left
Peroneus longus muscle	Lower Leg Muscle, Right
	Lower Leg Muscle, Left
Petrous part of temporal bone	Temporal Bone, Right
	Temporal Bone, Left
Pharyngeal constrictor muscle	Tongue, Palate, Pharynx Muscle
Pharyngeal plexus	Vagus Nerve
Pharyngeal recess	Nasopharynx
Pharyngeal tonsil	Adenoids
Pharyngotympanic tube	Eustachian Tube, Right
	Eustachian Tube, Left
Pia mater, intracranial	Cerebral Meninges
Pia mater, spinal	Spinal Meninges
Pinna	External Ear, Right
	External Ear, Left
	External Ear, Bilateral
Piriform recess (sinus)	Pharynx
Piriformis muscle	Hip Muscle, Right
	Hip Muscle, Left
Pisiform bone	Carpal, Right
	Carpal, Left
Pisohamate ligament	Hand Bursa and Ligament, Right
	Hand Bursa and Ligament, Left
Pisometacarpal ligament	Hand Bursa and Ligament, Right
	Hand Bursa and Ligament, Left
Plantar digital vein	Foot Vein, Right
	Foot Vein, Left
Plantar fascia (aponeurosis)	Subcutaneous Tissue and Fascia, Right Foot
	Subcutaneous Tissue and Fascia, Left Foot
Plantar metatarsal vein	Foot Vein, Right
	Foot Vein, Left

Anatomical Term	ICD-10-PCS Value
Plantar venous arch	Foot Vein, Right
	Foot Vein, Left
Platysma muscle	Neck Muscle, Right
	Neck Muscle, Left
Plica semilunaris	Conjunctiva, Right
	Conjunctiva, Left
Pneumogastric nerve	Vagus Nerve
Pneumotaxic center	Pons
Pontine tegmentum	Pons
Popliteal ligament	Knee Bursa and Ligament, Right
	Knee Bursa and Ligament, Left
Popliteal lymph node	Lymphatic, Right Lower Extremity
	Lymphatic, Left Lower Extremity
Popliteal vein	Femoral Vein, Right
	Femoral Vein, Left
Popliteus muscle	Lower Leg Muscle, Right
	Lower Leg Muscle, Left
Postauricular (mastoid) lymph node	Lymphatic, Right Neck
	Lymphatic, Left Neck
Postcava	Inferior Vena Cava
Posterior (subscapular) lymph node	Lymphatic, Right Axillary
	Lymphatic, Left Axillary
Posterior auricular artery	External Carotid Artery, Right
	External Carotid Artery, Left
Posterior auricular nerve	Facial Nerve
Posterior auricular vein	External Jugular Vein, Right
	External Jugular Vein, Left
Posterior cerebral artery	Intracranial Artery
Posterior chamber	Eye, Right
	Eye, Left
Posterior circumflex humeral artery	Axillary Artery, Right
	Axillary Artery, Left
Posterior communicating artery	Intracranial Artery
Posterior cruciate ligament (PCL)	Knee Bursa and Ligament, Right
	Knee Bursa and Ligament, Left
Posterior facial (retromandibular) vein	Face Vein, Right
	Face Vein, Left
Posterior femoral cutaneous nerve	Sacral Plexus
Posterior inferior cerebellar artery(PICA)	Intracranial Artery
Posterior interosseous nerve	Radial Nerve
Posterior labial nerve	Pudendal Nerve
Posterior scrotal nerve	Pudendal Nerve
Posterior spinal artery	Vertebral Artery, Right
	Vertebral Artery, Left
Posterior tibial recurrent artery	Anterior Tibial Artery, Right
	Anterior Tibial Artery, Left
Posterior ulnar recurrent artery	Ulnar Artery, Right
	Ulnar Artery, Left
Posterior vagal trunk	Vagus Nerve
Preauricular lymph node	Lymphatic, Head
Precava	Superior Vena Cava

Anatomical Term	ICD-10-PCS Value
Prepatellar bursa	Knee Bursa and Ligament, Right
	Knee Bursa and Ligament, Left
Pretracheal fascia	Subcutaneous Tissue and Fascia, Anterior Neck
Prevertebral fascia	Subcutaneous Tissue and Fascia, Posterior Neck
Princeps pollicis artery	Hand Artery, Right
	Hand Artery, Left
Procerus muscle	Facial Muscle
Profunda brachii	Brachial Artery, Right
	Brachial Artery, Left
Profunda femoris (deep femoral) vein	Femoral Vein, Right
	Femoral Vein, Left
Pronator quadratus muscle	Lower Arm and Wrist Muscle, Right
	Lower Arm and Wrist Muscle, Left
Pronator teres muscle	Lower Arm and Wrist Muscle, Right
	Lower Arm and Wrist Muscle, Left
Prostatic urethra	Urethra
Proximal radioulnar joint	Elbow Joint, Right
	Elbow Joint, Left
Psoas muscle	Hip Muscle, Right
	Hip Muscle, Left
Pterygoid muscle	Head Muscle
Pterygoid process	Sphenoid Bone, Right
	Sphenoid Bone, Left
Pterygopalatine (sphenopalatine)ganglion	Head and Neck Sympathetic Nerve
Pubic ligament	Trunk Bursa and Ligament, Right
	Trunk Bursa and Ligament, Left
Pubis	Pelvic Bone, Right
	Pelvic Bone, Left
Pubofemoral ligament	Hip Bursa and Ligament, Right
	Hip Bursa and Ligament, Left
Pudendal nerve	Sacral Plexus
Pulmoaortic canal	Pulmonary Artery, Left
Pulmonary annulus	Pulmonary Valve
Pulmonary plexus	Vagus Nerve
	Thoracic Sympathetic Nerve
Pulmonic valve	Pulmonary Valve
Pulvinar	Thalamus
Pyloric antrum	Stomach, Pylorus
Pyloric canal	Stomach, Pylorus
Pyloric sphincter	Stomach, Pylorus
Pyramidalis muscle	Abdomen Muscle, Right
	Abdomen Muscle, Left
Quadrangular cartilage	Nasal Septum
Quadrate lobe	Liver
Quadratus femoris muscle	Hip Muscle, Right
	Hip Muscle, Left
Quadratus lumborum muscle	Trunk Muscle, Right
	Trunk Muscle, Left
Quadratus plantae muscle	Foot Muscle, Right
	Foot Muscle, Left
Quadriceps (femoris)	Upper Leg Muscle, Right
	Upper Leg Muscle, Left

Anatomical Term	ICD-10-PCS Value
Radial collateral carpal ligament	Wrist Bursa and Ligament, Right
	Wrist Bursa and Ligament, Left
Radial collateral ligament	Elbow Bursa and Ligament, Right
	Elbow Bursa and Ligament, Left
Radial notch	Ulna, Right
	Ulna, Left
Radial recurrent artery	Radial Artery, Right
	Radial Artery, Left
Radial vein	Brachial Vein, Right
	Brachial Vein, Left
Radialis indicis	Hand Artery, Right
	Hand Artery, Left
Radiocarpal joint	Wrist Joint, Right
	Wrist Joint, Left
Radiocarpal ligament	Wrist Bursa and Ligament, Right
	Wrist Bursa and Ligament, Left
Radioulnar ligament	Wrist Bursa and Ligament, Right
	Wrist Bursa and Ligament, Left
Rectosigmoid junction	Sigmoid Colon
Rectus abdominis muscle	Abdomen Muscle, Right
	Abdomen Muscle, Left
Rectus femoris muscle	Upper Leg Muscle, Right
	Upper Leg Muscle, Left
Recurrent laryngeal nerve	Vagus Nerve
Renal calyx	Kidney, Right
	Kidney, Left
	Kidneys, Bilateral
	Kidney
Renal capsule	Vagus Nerve
	Kidney, Right
	Kidney, Left
	Kidneys, Bilateral
	Kidney
Renal cortex	Vagus Nerve
	Kidney, Right
	Kidney, Left
	Kidneys, Bilateral
	Kidney
Renal plexus	Abdominal Sympathetic Nerve
Renal segment	Kidney, Right
	Kidney, Left
	Kidneys, Bilateral
	Kidney
Renal segmental artery	Renal Artery, Right
	Renal Artery, Left
Retroperitoneal lymph node	Lymphatic, Aortic
Retroperitoneal space	Retroperitoneum
Retropharyngeal lymph node	Lymphatic, Right Neck
	Lymphatic, Left Neck
Retropubic space	Pelvic Cavity
Rhinopharynx	Nasopharynx
Rhomboid major muscle	Trunk Muscle, Right
	Trunk Muscle, Left

Anatomical Term	ICD-10-PCS Value
Rhomboid minor muscle	Trunk Muscle, Right
	Trunk Muscle, Left
Right ascending lumbar vein	Azygos Vein
Right atrioventricular valve	Tricuspid Valve
Right auricular appendix	Atrium, Right
Right colic vein	Colic Vein
Right coronary sulcus	Heart, Right
Right gastric artery	Gastric Artery
Right gastroepiploic vein	Superior Mesenteric Vein
Right inferior phrenic vein	Inferior Vena Cava
Right inferior pulmonary vein	Pulmonary Vein, Right
Right jugular trunk	Lymphatic, Right Neck
Right lateral ventricle	Cerebral Ventricle
Right lymphatic duct	Lymphatic, Right Neck
Right ovarian vein	Inferior Vena Cava
Right second lumbar vein	Inferior Vena Cava
Right subclavian trunk	Lymphatic, Right Neck
Right subcostal vein	Azygos Vein
Right superior pulmonary vein	Pulmonary Vein, Right
Right suprarenal vein	Inferior Vena Cava
Right testicular vein	Inferior Vena Cava
Rima glottidis	Larynx
Risorius muscle	Facial Muscle
Round ligament of uterus	Uterine Supporting Structure
Round window	Inner Ear, Right
	Inner Ear, Left
Sacral ganglion	Sacral Sympathetic Nerve
Sacral lymph node	Lymphatic, Pelvis
Sacral splanchnic nerve	Sacral Sympathetic Nerve
Sacrococcygeal ligament	Trunk Bursa and Ligament, Right
	Trunk Bursa and Ligament, Left
Sacrococcygeal symphysis	Sacrococcygeal Joint
Sacroiliac ligament	Trunk Bursa and Ligament, Right
	Trunk Bursa and Ligament, Left
Sacrospinous ligament	Trunk Bursa and Ligament, Right
	Trunk Bursa and Ligament, Left
Sacrotuberous ligament	Trunk Bursa and Ligament, Right
	Trunk Bursa and Ligament, Left
Salpingopharyngeus muscle	Tongue, Palate, Pharynx Muscle
Salpinx	Fallopian Tube, Right
	Fallopian Tube, Left
Saphenous nerve	Femoral Nerve
Sartorius muscle	Upper Leg Muscle, Right
	Upper Leg Muscle, Left
Scalene muscle	Neck Muscle, Right
	Neck Muscle, Left
Scaphoid bone	Carpal, Right
	Carpal, Left
Scapholunate ligament	Hand Bursa and Ligament, Right
	Hand Bursa and Ligament, Left
Scaphotrapezium ligament	Hand Bursa and Ligament, Right
	Hand Bursa and Ligament, Left
Scarpa's (vestibular) ganglion	Acoustic Nerve

Anatomical Term	ICD-10-PCS Value
Sebaceous gland	Skin
Second cranial nerve	Optic Nerve
Sella turcica	Sphenoid Bone, Right
	Sphenoid Bone, Left
Semicircular canal	Inner Ear, Right
	Inner Ear, Left
Semimembranosus muscle	Upper Leg Muscle, Right
	Upper Leg Muscle, Left
Semitendinosus muscle	Upper Leg Muscle, Right
	Upper Leg Muscle, Left
Septal cartilage	Nasal Septum
Serratus anterior muscle	Thorax Muscle, Right
	Thorax Muscle, Left
Serratus posterior muscle	Trunk Muscle, Right
	Trunk Muscle, Left
Seventh cranial nerve	Facial Nerve
Short gastric artery	Splenic Artery
Sigmoid artery	Inferior Mesenteric Artery
Sigmoid flexure	Sigmoid Colon
Sigmoid vein	Inferior Mesenteric Vein
Sinoatrial node	Conduction Mechanism
Sinus venosus	Atrium, Right
Sixth cranial nerve	Abducens Nerve
Skene's (paraurethral) gland	Vestibular Gland
Small saphenous vein	Lesser Saphenous Vein, Right
	Lesser Saphenous Vein, Left
Solar (celiac) plexus	Abdominal Sympathetic Nerve
Soleus muscle	Lower Leg Muscle, Right
	Lower Leg Muscle, Left
Sphenomandibular ligament	Head and Neck Bursa and Ligament
Sphenopalatine (pterygopalatine)ganglion	Head and Neck Sympathetic Nerve
Spinal nerve, cervical	Cervical Nerve
Spinal nerve, lumbar	Lumbar Nerve
Spinal nerve, sacral	Sacral Nerve
Spinal nerve, thoracic	Thoracic Nerve
Spinous process	Cervical Vertebra
	Thoracic Vertebra
	Lumbar Vertebra
Spiral ganglion	Acoustic Nerve
Splenic flexure	Transverse Colon
Splenic plexus	Abdominal Sympathetic Nerve
Splenius capitis muscle	Head Muscle
Splenius cervicis muscle	Neck Muscle, Right
	Neck Muscle, Left
Stapes	Auditory Ossicle, Right
	Auditory Ossicle, Left
Stellate ganglion	Head and Neck Sympathetic Nerve
Stensen's duct	Parotid Duct, Right
	Parotid Duct, Left
Sternoclavicular ligament	Shoulder Bursa and Ligament, Right
	Shoulder Bursa and Ligament, Left
Sternocleidomastoid artery	Thyroid Artery, Right
	Thyroid Artery, Left

Anatomical Term	ICD-10-PCS Value
Sternocleidomastoid muscle	Neck Muscle, Right
	Neck Muscle, Left
Sternocostal ligament	Thorax Bursa and Ligament, Right
	Thorax Bursa and Ligament, Left
Styloglossus muscle	Tongue, Palate, Pharynx Muscle
Stylomandibular ligament	Head and Neck Bursa and Ligament
Stylopharyngeus muscle	Tongue, Palate, Pharynx Muscle
Subacromial bursa	Shoulder Bursa and Ligament, Right
	Shoulder Bursa and Ligament, Left
Subaortic (common iliac) lymph node	Lymphatic, Pelvis
Subarachnoid space, intracranial	Subarachnoid Space
Subarachnoid space, spinal	Spinal Canal
Subclavicular (apical) lymph node	Lymphatic, Right Axillary
	Lymphatic, Left Axillary
Subclavius muscle	Thorax Muscle, Right
	Thorax Muscle, Left
Subclavius nerve	Brachial Plexus
Subcostal artery	Upper Artery
Subcostal muscle	Thorax Muscle, Right
	Thorax Muscle, Left
Subcostal nerve	Thoracic Nerve
Subdural space, intracranial	Subdural Space
Subdural space, spinal	Spinal Canal
Submandibular ganglion	Facial Nerve
	Head and Neck Sympathetic Nerve
Submandibular gland	Submaxillary Gland, Right
	Submaxillary Gland, Left
Submandibular lymph node	Lymphatic, Head
Submaxillary ganglion	Head and Neck Sympathetic Nerve
Submaxillary lymph node	Lymphatic, Head
Submental artery	Face Artery
Submental lymph node	Lymphatic, Head
Submucous (Meissner's) plexus	Abdominal Sympathetic Nerve
Suboccipital nerve	Cervical Nerve
Suboccipital venous plexus	Vertebral Vein, Right
	Vertebral Vein, Left
Subparotid lymph node	Lymphatic, Head
Subscapular (posterior) lymph node	Lymphatic, Right Axillary
	Lymphatic, Left Axillary
Subscapular aponeurosis	Subcutaneous Tissue and Fascia, Right Upper Arm
	Subcutaneous Tissue and Fascia, Left Upper Arm
Subscapular artery	Axillary Artery, Right
	Axillary Artery, Left
Subscapularis muscle	Shoulder Muscle, Right
	Shoulder Muscle, Left
Substantia nigra	Basal Ganglia
Subtalar (talocalcaneal) joint	Tarsal Joint, Right
	Tarsal Joint, Left
Subtalar ligament	Foot Bursa and Ligament, Right
	Foot Bursa and Ligament, Left

Anatomical Term	ICD-10-PCS Value
Subthalamic nucleus	Basal Ganglia
Superficial circumflex iliac vein	Greater Saphenous Vein, Right
	Greater Saphenous Vein, Left
Superficial epigastric artery	Femoral Artery, Right
	Femoral Artery, Left
Superficial epigastric vein	Greater Saphenous Vein, Right
	Greater Saphenous Vein, Left
Superficial palmar arch	Hand Artery, Right
	Hand Artery, Left
Superficial palmar venous arch	Hand Vein, Right
	Hand Vein, Left
Superficial temporal artery	Temporal Artery, Right
	Temporal Artery, Left
Superficial transverse perineal muscle	Perineum Muscle
Superior cardiac nerve	Thoracic Sympathetic Nerve
Superior cerebellar vein	Intracranial Vein
Superior cerebral vein	Intracranial Vein
Superior clunic (cluneal) nerve	Lumbar Nerve
Superior epigastric artery	Internal Mammary Artery, Right
	Internal Mammary Artery, Left
Superior genicular artery	Popliteal Artery, Right
	Popliteal Artery, Left
Superior gluteal artery	Internal Iliac Artery, Right
	Internal Iliac Artery, Left
Superior gluteal nerve	Lumbar Plexus
Superior hypogastric plexus	Abdominal Sympathetic Nerve
Superior labial artery	Face Artery
Superior laryngeal artery	Thyroid Artery, Right
	Thyroid Artery, Left
Superior laryngeal nerve	Vagus Nerve
Superior longitudinal muscle	Tongue, Palate, Pharynx Muscle
Superior mesenteric ganglion	Abdominal Sympathetic Nerve
Superior mesenteric lymph node	Lymphatic, Mesenteric
Superior mesenteric plexus	Abdominal Sympathetic Nerve
Superior oblique muscle	Extraocular Muscle, Right
	Extraocular Muscle, Left
Superior olivary nucleus	Pons
Superior rectal artery	Inferior Mesenteric Artery
Superior rectal vein	Inferior Mesenteric Vein
Superior rectus muscle	Extraocular Muscle, Right
	Extraocular Muscle, Left
Superior tarsal plate	Upper Eyelid, Right
	Upper Eyelid, Left
Superior thoracic artery	Axillary Artery, Right
	Axillary Artery, Left
Superior thyroid artery	External Carotid Artery, Right
	External Carotid Artery, Left
	Thyroid Artery, Right
	Thyroid Artery, Left
Superior turbinate	Nasal Turbinate
Superior ulnar collateral artery	Brachial Artery, Right
	Brachial Artery, Left

Anatomical Term	ICD-10-PCS Value
Supraclavicular (Virchow's) lymph node	Lymphatic, Right Neck
	Lymphatic, Left Neck
Supraclavicular nerve	Cervical Plexus
Suprahyoid lymph node	Lymphatic, Head
Suprahyoid muscle	Neck Muscle, Right
	Neck Muscle, Left
Suprainguinal lymph node	Lymphatic, Pelvis
Supraorbital vein	Face Vein, Right
	Face Vein, Left
Suprarenal gland	Adrenal Gland, Left
	Adrenal Gland, Right
	Adrenal Glands, Bilateral
	Adrenal Gland
Suprarenal plexus	Abdominal Sympathetic Nerve
Suprascapular nerve	Brachial Plexus
Supraspinatus fascia	Subcutaneous Tissue and Fascia, Right Upper Arm
	Subcutaneous Tissue and Fascia, Left Upper Arm
Supraspinatus muscle	Shoulder Muscle, Right
	Shoulder Muscle, Left
Supraspinous ligament	Trunk Bursa and Ligament, Right
	Trunk Bursa and Ligament, Left
Suprasternal notch	Sternum
Supratrochlear lymph node	Lymphatic, Right Upper Extremity
	Lymphatic, Left Upper Extremity
Sural artery	Popliteal Artery, Right
	Popliteal Artery, Left
Sweat gland	Skin
Talocalcaneal (subtalar) joint	Tarsal Joint, Right
	Tarsal Joint, Left
Talocalcaneal ligament	Foot Bursa and Ligament, Right
	Foot Bursa and Ligament, Left
Talocalcaneonavicular joint	Tarsal Joint, Right
	Tarsal Joint, Left
Talocalcaneonavicular ligament	Foot Bursa and Ligament, Right
	Foot Bursa and Ligament, Left
Talocrural joint	Ankle Joint, Right
	Ankle Joint, Left
Talofibular ligament	Ankle Bursa and Ligament, Right
	Ankle Bursa and Ligament, Left
Talus bone	Tarsal, Right
	Tarsal, Left
Tarsometatarsal joint	Metatarsal-Tarsal Joint, Right
	Metatarsal-Tarsal Joint, Left
Tarsometatarsal ligament	Foot Bursa and Ligament, Right
	Foot Bursa and Ligament, Left
Temporal lobe	Cerebral Hemisphere
Temporalis muscle	Head Muscle
Temporoparietalis muscle	Head Muscle
Tensor fasciae latae muscle	Hip Muscle, Right
	Hip Muscle, Left
Tensor veli palatini muscle	Tongue, Palate, Pharynx Muscle
Tenth cranial nerve	Vagus Nerve
Tentorium cerebelli	Dura Mater

Anatomical Term	ICD-10-PCS Value
Teres major muscle	Shoulder Muscle, Right
	Shoulder Muscle, Left
Teres minor muscle	Shoulder Muscle, Right
	Shoulder Muscle, Left
Testicular artery	Abdominal Aorta
Thenar muscle	Hand Muscle, Right
	Hand Muscle, Left
Third cranial nerve	Oculomotor Nerve
Third occipital nerve	Cervical Nerve
Third ventricle	Cerebral Ventricle
Thoracic aortic plexus	Thoracic Sympathetic Nerve
Thoracic esophagus	Esophagus, Middle
Thoracic facet joint	Thoracic Vertebral Joint
Thoracic ganglion	Thoracic Sympathetic Nerve
Thoracoacromial artery	Axillary Artery, Right
	Axillary Artery, Left
Thoracolumbar facet joint	Thoracolumbar Vertebral Joint
Thymus gland	Thymus
Thyroarytenoid muscle	Neck Muscle, Right
	Neck Muscle, Left
Thyrocervical trunk	Thyroid Artery, Right
	Thyroid Artery, Left
Thyroid cartilage	Larynx
Tibialis anterior muscle	Lower Leg Muscle, Right
	Lower Leg Muscle, Left
Tibialis posterior muscle	Lower Leg Muscle, Right
	Lower Leg Muscle, Left
Tibiofemoral joint	Knee Joint, Right
	Knee Joint, Left
	Knee Joint, Tibial Surface, Right
	Knee Joint, Tibial Surface, Left
Tongue, base of	Pharynx
Tracheobronchial lymph node	Lymphatic, Thorax
Tragus	External Ear, Right
	External Ear, Left
	External Ear, Bilateral
Transversalis fascia	Subcutaneous Tissue and Fascia, Trunk
Transverse (cutaneous) cervical nerve	Cervical Plexus
Transverse acetabular ligament	Hip Bursa and Ligament, Right
	Hip Bursa and Ligament, Left
Transverse facial artery	Temporal Artery, Right
	Temporal Artery, Left
Transverse humeral ligament	Shoulder Bursa and Ligament, Right
	Shoulder Bursa and Ligament, Left
Transverse ligament of atlas	Head and Neck Bursa and Ligament
Transverse scapular ligament	Shoulder Bursa and Ligament, Right
	Shoulder Bursa and Ligament, Left
Transverse thoracis muscle	Thorax Muscle, Right
	Thorax Muscle, Left
Transversospinalis muscle	Trunk Muscle, Right
	Trunk Muscle, Left

Anatomical Term	ICD-10-PCS Value
Transversus abdominis muscle	Abdomen Muscle, Right
	Abdomen Muscle, Left
Trapezium bone	Carpal, Right
	Carpal, Left
Trapezius muscle	Trunk Muscle, Right
	Trunk Muscle, Left
Trapezoid bone	Carpal, Right
	Carpal, Left
Triceps brachii muscle	Upper Arm Muscle, Right
	Upper Arm Muscle, Left
Tricuspid annulus	Tricuspid Valve
Trifacial nerve	Trigeminal Nerve
Trigone of bladder	Bladder
Triquetral bone	Carpal, Right
	Carpal, Left
Trochanteric bursa	Hip Bursa and Ligament, Right
	Hip Bursa and Ligament, Left
Twelfth cranial nerve	Hypoglossal Nerve
Tympanic cavity	Middle Ear, Right
	Middle Ear, Left
Tympanic nerve	Glossopharyngeal Nerve
Tympanic part of temporal bone	Temporal Bone, Right
	Temporal Bone, Left
Ulnar collateral carpal ligament	Wrist Bursa and Ligament, Right
	Wrist Bursa and Ligament, Left
Ulnar collateral ligament	Elbow Bursa and Ligament, Right
	Elbow Bursa and Ligament, Left
Ulnar notch	Radius, Right
	Radius, Left
Ulnar vein	Brachial Vein, Right
	Brachial Vein, Left
Umbilical artery	Internal Iliac Artery, Right
	Internal Iliac Artery, Left
Ureteral orifice	Ureter, Right
	Ureter, Left
	Ureters, Bilateral
	Ureter
Ureteropelvic junction (UPJ)	Kidney Pelvis, Right
	Kidney Pelvis, Left
Ureterovesical orifice	Ureter, Right
	Ureter, Left
	Ureters, Bilateral
	Ureter
Uterine Artery	Internal Iliac Artery, Right
	Internal Iliac Artery, Left
Uterine cornu	Uterus
Uterine tube	Fallopian Tube, Right
	Fallopian Tube, Left
Uterine vein	Hypogastric Vein, Right
	Hypogastric Vein, Left
Vaginal artery	Internal Iliac Artery, Right
	Internal Iliac Artery, Left
Vaginal vein	Hypogastric Vein, Right
	Hypogastric Vein, Left

Anatomical Term	ICD-10-PCS Value
Vastus intermedius muscle	Upper Leg Muscle, Right
	Upper Leg Muscle, Left
Vastus lateralis muscle	Upper Leg Muscle, Right
	Upper Leg Muscle, Left
Vastus medialis muscle	Upper Leg Muscle, Right
	Upper Leg Muscle, Left
Ventricular fold	Larynx
Vermiform appendix	Appendix
Vermilion border	Upper Lip
	Lower Lip
Vertebral arch	Cervical Vertebra
	Thoracic Vertebra
	Lumbar Vertebra
Vertebral canal	Spinal Canal
Vertebral foramen	Cervical Vertebra
	Thoracic Vertebra
	Lumbar Vertebra
Vertebral lamina	Cervical Vertebra
	Thoracic Vertebra
	Lumbar Vertebra
Vertebral pedicle	Cervical Vertebra
	Thoracic Vertebra
	Lumbar Vertebra
Vesical vein	Hypogastric Vein, Right
	Hypogastric Vein, Left
Vestibular (Scarpa's) ganglion	Acoustic Nerve
Vestibular nerve	Acoustic Nerve
Vestibulocochlear nerve	Acoustic Nerve
Virchow's (supraclavicular) lymph node	Lymphatic, Right Neck
	Lymphatic, Left Neck
Vitreous body	Vitreous, Right
	Vitreous, Left
Vocal fold	Vocal Cord, Right
	Vocal Cord, Left
Volar (palmar) digital vein	Hand Vein, Right
	Hand Vein, Left
Volar (palmar) metacarpal vein	Hand Vein, Right
	Hand Vein, Left
Vomer bone	Nasal Septum
Vomer of nasal septum	Nasal Bone
Xiphoid process	Sternum
Zonule of Zinn	Lens, Right
	Lens, Left
Zygomatic process of frontal bone	Frontal Bone, Right
	Frontal Bone, Left
Zygomatic process of temporal bone	Temporal Bone, Right
	Temporal Bone, Left
Zygomaticus muscle	Facial Muscle

Appendix C: Device Key

Device Term	ICD-10-PCS Value
3f® (Aortic) Bioprosthesis valve	Zooplastic Tissue in Heart and Great Vessels
AbioCor® Total Replacement Heart	Synthetic Substitute
Absolute Pro® Vascular (OTW) Self-Expanding Stent System	Intraluminal Device
Acculink™ (RX) Carotid Stent System	Intraluminal Device
Acellular Hydrated Dermis	Nonautologous Tissue Substitute
Acetabular cup	Liner in Lower Joints
Activa PC® neurostimulator	Stimulator Generator, Multiple Array for Insertion in Subcutaneous Tissue and Fascia
Activa RC® neurostimulator	Stimulator Generator, Multiple Array Rechargeable for Insertion in Subcutaneous Tissue and Fascia
Activa SC® neurostimulator	Stimulator Generator, Single Array for Insertion in Subcutaneous Tissue and Fascia
ACUITY™ Steerable Lead	Cardiac Lead, Pacemaker for Insertion in Heart and Great Vessels
	Cardiac Lead, Defibrillator for Insertion in Heart and Great Vessels
Advisa MRI™	Pacemaker, Dual Chamber for Insertion in Subcutaneous Tissue and Fascia
AFX® Endovascular AAA System	Intraluminal Device
AMPLATZER® Muscular VSD Occluder	Synthetic Substitute
AMS 800® Urinary Control System	Artificial Sphincter in Urinary System
AneuRx® AAA Advantage®	Intraluminal Device
Annuloplasty ring	Synthetic Substitute
Artificial anal sphincter (AAS)	Artificial Sphincter in Gastrointestinal System
Artificial bowel sphincter (neosphincter)	Artificial Sphincter in Gastrointestinal System
Artificial urinary sphincter (AUS)	Artificial Sphincter in Urinary System
Ascenda Intrathecal Catheter	Infusion Device
Assurant Cobalt® stent	Intraluminal Device
Attain Ability® lead	Cardiac Lead, Pacemaker for Insertion in Heart and Great Vessels
	Cardiac Lead, Defibrillator for Insertion in Heart and Great Vessels
Attain StarFix® (OTW) lead	Cardiac Lead, Pacemaker for Insertion in Heart and Great Vessels
	Cardiac Lead, Defibrillator for Insertion in Heart and Great Vessels
Autograft	Autologous Tissue Substitute
Autologous artery graft	Autologous Arterial Tissue in Heart and Great Vessels
	Autologous Arterial Tissue in Upper Arteries
	Autologous Arterial Tissue in Lower Arteries
	Autologous Arterial Tissue in Upper Veins
	Autologous Arterial Tissue in Lower Veins
Autologous vein graft	Autologous Venous Tissue in Heart and Great Vessels
	Autologous Venous Tissue in Upper Arteries
	Autologous Venous Tissue in Lower Arteries
	Autologous Venous Tissue in Upper Veins
	Autologous Venous Tissue in Lower Veins
Axial Lumbar Interbody Fusion System	Interbody Fusion Device in Lower Joints
AxiaLIF® System	Interbody Fusion Device in Lower Joints
BAK/C® Interbody Cervical Fusion System	Interbody Fusion Device in Upper Joints
Bard® Composix® (E/X)(LP) mesh	Synthetic Substitute
Bard® Composix® Kugel® patch	Synthetic Substitute
Bard® Dulex™ mesh	Synthetic Substitute
Bard® Ventralex™ hernia patch	Synthetic Substitute
Baroreflex Activation Therapy® (BAT®)	Stimulator Lead in Upper Arteries
	Stimulator Generator in Subcutaneous Tissue and Fascia
Berlin Heart Ventricular Assist Device	Implantable Heart Assist System in Heart and Great Vessels
Bioactive embolization coil(s)	Intraluminal Device, Bioactive in Upper Arteries
Biventricular external heart assist system	External Heart Assist System in Heart and Great Vessels
Blood glucose monitoring system	Monitoring Device
Bone anchored hearing device	Hearing Device, Bone Conduction for Insertion in Ear, Nose, Sinus
	Hearing Device in Head and Facial Bones
Bone bank bone graft	Nonautologous Tissue Substitute

Device Term	ICD-10-PCS Value
Bone screw (interlocking)(lag)(pedicle)(recessed)	Internal Fixation Device in Head and Facial Bones
	Internal Fixation Device in Upper Bones
	Internal Fixation Device in Lower Bones
Bovine pericardial valve	Zooplastic Tissue in Heart and Great Vessels
Bovine pericardium graft	Zooplastic Tissue in Heart and Great Vessels
Brachytherapy seeds	Radioactive Element
BRYAN® Cervical Disc System	Synthetic Substitute
BVS 5000 Ventricular Assist Device	External Heart Assist System in Heart and Great Vessels
Cardiac contractility modulation lead	Cardiac Lead in Heart and Great Vessels
Cardiac event recorder	Monitoring Device
Cardiac resynchronization therapy (CRT) lead	Cardiac Lead, Pacemaker for Insertion in Heart and Great Vessels
	Cardiac Lead, Defibrillator for Insertion in Heart and Great Vessels
CardioMEMS® pressure sensor	Monitoring Device, Pressure Sensor for Insertion in Heart and Great Vessels
Carotid (artery) sinus (baroreceptor) lead	Stimulator Lead in Upper Arteries
Carotid WALLSTENT® Monorail® Endoprosthesis	Intraluminal Device
Centrimag® Blood Pump	External Heart Assist System in Heart and Great Vessels
Ceramic on ceramic bearing surface	Synthetic Substitute, Ceramic for Replacement in Lower Joints
Clamp and rod internal fixation system (CRIF)	Internal Fixation Device in Upper Bones
	Internal Fixation Device in Lower Bones
CoAxia NeuroFlo catheter	Intraluminal Device
Cobalt/chromium head and polyethylene socket	Synthetic Substitute, Metal on Polyethylene for Replacement in Lower Joints
Cobalt/chromium head and socket	Synthetic Substitute, Metal for Replacement in Lower Joints
Cochlear implant (CI), multiple channel (electrode)	Hearing Device, Multiple Channel Cochlear Prosthesis for Insertion in Ear, Nose, Sinus
Cochlear implant (CI), single channel (electrode)	Hearing Device, Single Channel Cochlear Prosthesis for Insertion in Ear, Nose, Sinus
COGNIS® CRT-D	Cardiac Resynchronization Defibrillator Pulse Generator for Insertion in Subcutaneous Tissue and Fascia
Colonic Z-Stent®	Intraluminal Device

Device Term	ICD-10-PCS Value
Complete® (SE) stent	Intraluminal Device
Concerto® II CRT-D	Cardiac Resynchronization Defibrillator Pulse Generator for Insertion in Subcutaneous Tissue and Fascia
CONSERVE® PLUS Total Resurfacing Hip System	Resurfacing Device in Lower Joints
Consulta® CRT-D	Cardiac Resynchronization Defibrillator Pulse Generator for Insertion in Subcutaneous Tissue and Fascia
Consulta® CRT-P	Cardiac Resynchronization Pacemaker Pulse Generator for Insertion in Subcutaneous Tissue and Fascia
CONTAK RENEWAL® 3 RF (HE) CRT-D	Cardiac Resynchronization Defibrillator Pulse Generator for Insertion in Subcutaneous Tissue and Fascia
Contegra® Pulmonary Valved Conduit	Zooplastic Tissue in Heart and Great Vessels
Continuous Glucose Monitoring (CGM) device	Monitoring Device
Cook Biodesign® Fistula Plug(s)	Nonautologous Tissue Substitute
Cook Biodesign® Hernia Graft(s)	Nonautologous Tissue Substitute
Cook Biodesign® Layered Graft(s)	Nonautologous Tissue Substitute
Cook Zenapro™ Layered Graft(s)	Nonautologous Tissue Substitute
Cook Zenith AAA Endovascular Graft	Intraluminal Device, Branched or Fenestrated, One or Two Arteries for Restriction in Lower Arteries
	Intraluminal Device, Branched or Fenestrated, Three or More Arteries for Restriction in Lower Arteries
	Intraluminal Device
CoreValve™ transcatheter aortic valve	Zooplastic Tissue in Heart and Great Vessels
Cormet™ Hip Resurfacing System	Resurfacing Device in Lower Joints
CoRoent® XL	Interbody Fusion Device in Lower Joints
Corox® (OTW) Bipolar Lead	Cardiac Lead, Pacemaker for Insertion in Heart and Great Vessels
	Cardiac Lead, Defibrillator for Insertion in Heart and Great Vessels
Cortical strip neurostimulator lead	Neurostimulator Lead in Central Nervous System
Cultured epidermal cell autograft	Autologous Tissue Substitute
CYPHER® Stent	Intraluminal Device, Drug-eluting in Heart and Great Vessels
Cystostomy tube	Drainage Device
DBS lead	Neurostimulator Lead in Central Nervous System
DeBakey Left Ventricular Assist Device	Implantable Heart Assist System in Heart and Great Vessels

Device Term	ICD-10-PCS Value
Deep brain neurostimulator lead	Neurostimulator Lead in Central Nervous System
Delta frame external fixator	External Fixation Device, Hybrid for Insertion in Upper Bones
	External Fixation Device, Hybrid for Reposition in Upper Bones
	External Fixation Device, Hybrid for Insertion in Lower Bones
	External Fixation Device, Hybrid for Reposition in Lower Bones
Delta III™ Reverse shoulder prosthesis	Synthetic Substitute, Reverse Ball and Socket for Replacement in Upper Joints
Diaphragmatic pacemaker generator	Stimulator Generator in Subcutaneous Tissue and Fascia
Direct Lateral Interbody Fusion (DLIF) device	Interbody Fusion Device in Lower Joints
Driver stent (RX) (OTW)	Intraluminal Device
DuraHeart® Left Ventricular Assist System	Implantable Heart Assist System in Heart and Great Vessels
Durata® Defibrillation Lead	Cardiac Lead, Defibrillator for Insertion in Heart and Great Vessels
Dynesys® Dynamic Stabilization System	Spinal Stabilization Device, Pedicle-Based for Insertion in Upper Joints
	Spinal Stabilization Device, Pedicle-Based for Insertion in Lower Joints
E-Luminexx™ (Biliary)(Vascular) Stent	Intraluminal Device
EDWARDS INTUITY Elite™ valve system	Zooplastic Tissue, Rapid Deployment Technique in New Technology
Electrical bone growth stimulator (EBGS)	Bone Growth Stimulator in Head and Facial Bones
	Bone Growth Stimulator in Upper Bones
	Bone Growth Stimulator in Lower Bones
Electrical muscle stimulation (EMS) lead	Stimulator Lead in Muscles
Electronic muscle stimulator lead	Stimulator Lead in Muscles
Embolization coil(s)	Intraluminal Device
Endeavor® (III)(IV) (Sprint) Zotarolimus-eluting Coronary Stent System	Intraluminal Device, Drug-eluting in Heart and Great Vessels
Endologix AFX® Endovascular AAA System	Intraluminal Device
EndoSure® sensor	Monitoring Device, Pressure Sensor for Insertion in Heart and Great Vessels
ENDOTAK RELIANCE® (G) Defibrillation Lead	Cardiac Lead, Defibrillator for Insertion in Heart and Great Vessels
Endotracheal tube (cuffed)(double-lumen)	Intraluminal Device, Endotracheal Airway in Respiratory System
Endurant® Endovascular Stent Graft	Intraluminal Device
Endurant® II AAA stent graft system	Intraluminal Device
EnRhythm®	Pacemaker, Dual Chamber for Insertion in Subcutaneous Tissue and Fascia
Enterra® gastric neurostimulator	Stimulator Generator, Multiple Array for Insertion in Subcutaneous Tissue and Fascia
Epic™ Stented Tissue Valve (aortic)	Zooplastic Tissue in Heart and Great Vessels
Epicel® cultured epidermal autograft	Autologous Tissue Substitute
Esophageal obturator airway (EOA)	Intraluminal Device, Airway in Gastrointestinal System
Esteem® implantable hearing system	Hearing Device in Ear, Nose, Sinus
Evera™ (XT)(S)(DR/VR)	Defibrillator Generator for Insertion in Subcutaneous Tissue and Fascia
Everolimus-eluting coronary stent	Intraluminal Device, Drug-eluting in Heart and Great Vessels
Ex-PRESS™ mini glaucoma shunt	Synthetic Substitute
EXCLUDER® AAA Endoprosthesis	Intraluminal Device, Branched or Fenestrated, One or Two Arteries for Restriction in Lower Arteries
EXCLUDER® AAA Endoprosthesis	Intraluminal Device, Branched or Fenestrated, Three or More Arteries for Restriction in Lower Arteries
EXCLUDER® AAA Endoprosthesis	Intraluminal Device
EXCLUDER® IBE Endoprosthesis	Intraluminal Device, Branched or Fenestrated, One or Two Arteries for Restriction in Lower Arteries
Express® (LD) Premounted Stent System	Intraluminal Device
Express® Biliary SD Monorail® Premounted Stent System	Intraluminal Device
Express® SD Renal Monorail® Premounted Stent System	Intraluminal Device
External fixator	External Fixation Device in Head and Facial Bones
	External Fixation Device in Upper Bones
	External Fixation Device in Lower Bones
	External Fixation Device in Upper Joints
	External Fixation Device in Lower Joints
EXtreme Lateral Interbody Fusion (XLIF) device	Interbody Fusion Device in Lower Joints

Device Term	ICD-10-PCS Value
Facet replacement spinal stabilization device	Spinal Stabilization Device, Facet Replacement for Insertion in Upper Joints
	Spinal Stabilization Device, Facet Replacement for Insertion in Lower Joints
FLAIR® Endovascular Stent Graft	Intraluminal Device
Flexible Composite Mesh	Synthetic Substitute
Foley catheter	Drainage Device
Formula™ Balloon-Expandable Renal Stent System	Intraluminal Device
Freestyle (Stentless) Aortic Root Bioprosthesis	Zooplastic Tissue in Heart and Great Vessels
Fusion screw (compression)(lag)(locking)	Internal Fixation Device in Upper Joints
	Internal Fixation Device in Lower Joints
Gastric electrical stimulation (GES) lead	Stimulator Lead in Gastrointestinal System
Gastric pacemaker lead	Stimulator Lead in Gastrointestinal System
GORE EXCLUDER® AAA Endoprosthesis	Intraluminal Device, Branched or Fenestrated, One or Two Arteries for Restriction in Lower Arteries
	Intraluminal Device, Branched or Fenestrated, Three or More Arteries for Restriction in Lower Arteries
	Intraluminal Device
GORE EXCLUDER® IBE Endoprosthesis	Intraluminal Device, Branched or Fenestrated, One or Two Arteries for Restriction in Lower Arteries
GORE TAG® Thoracic Endoprosthesis	Intraluminal Device
GORE® DUALMESH®	Synthetic Substitute
Guedel airway	Intraluminal Device, Airway in Mouth and Throat
Hancock® Bioprosthesis (aortic)(mitral) valve	Zooplastic Tissue in Heart and Great Vessels
Hancock® Bioprosthetic Valved Conduit	Zooplastic Tissue in Heart and Great Vessels
HeartMate II® Left Ventricular Assist Device (LVAD)	Implantable Heart Assist System in Heart and Great Vessels
HeartMate XVE® Left Ventricular Assist Device (LVAD)	Implantable Heart Assist System in Heart and Great Vessels
Herculink® (RX) Elite Renal Stent System	Intraluminal Device
Hip (joint) liner	Liner in Lower Joints
Holter valve ventricular shunt	Synthetic Substitute

Device Term	ICD-10-PCS Value
Ilizarov external fixator	External Fixation Device, Ring for Insertion in Upper Bones
	External Fixation Device, Ring for Reposition in Upper Bones
	External Fixation Device, Ring for Insertion in Lower Bones
	External Fixation Device, Ring for Reposition in Lower Bones
Ilizarov-Vecklich device	External Fixation Device, Limb Lengthening for Insertion in Upper Bones
	External Fixation Device, Limb Lengthening for Insertion in Lower Bones
Implantable cardioverter-defibrillator (ICD)	Defibrillator Generator for Insertion in Subcutaneous Tissue and Fascia
Implantable drug infusion pump (antispasmodic)(chemotherapy)(pain)	Infusion Device, Pump in Subcutaneous Tissue and Fascia
Implantable glucose monitoring device	Monitoring Device
Implantable hemodynamic monitor (IHM)	Monitoring Device, Hemodynamic for Insertion in Subcutaneous Tissue and Fascia
Implantable hemodynamic monitoring system (IHMS)	Monitoring Device, Hemodynamic for Insertion in Subcutaneous Tissue and Fascia
Implantable Miniature Telescope™ (IMT)	Synthetic Substitute, Intraocular Telescope for Replacement in Eye
Implanted (venous)(access) port	Vascular Access Device, Reservoir in Subcutaneous Tissue and Fascia
InDura® intrathecal catheter (1P) (spinal)	Infusion Device
Injection reservoir, port	Vascular Access Device, Reservoir in Subcutaneous Tissue and Fascia
Injection reservoir, pump	Infusion Device, Pump in Subcutaneous Tissue and Fascia
Interbody fusion (spine) cage	Interbody Fusion Device in Upper Joints
	Interbody Fusion Device in Lower Joints
Interspinous process spinal stabilization device	Spinal Stabilization Device, Interspinous Process for Insertion in Upper Joints
	Spinal Stabilization Device, Interspinous Process for Insertion in Lower Joints
InterStim® Therapy lead	Neurostimulator Lead in Peripheral Nervous System
InterStim® Therapy neurostimulator	Stimulator Generator, Single Array for Insertion in Subcutaneous Tissue and Fascia

Device Term	ICD-10-PCS Value
Intramedullary (IM) rod (nail)	Internal Fixation Device, Intramedullary in Upper Bones
	Internal Fixation Device, Intramedullary in Lower Bones
Intramedullary skeletal kinetic distractor (ISKD)	Internal Fixation Device, Intramedullary in Upper Bones
	Internal Fixation Device, Intramedullary in Lower Bones
Intrauterine device (IUD)	Contraceptive Device in Female Reproductive System
INTUITY Elite® valve system, EDWARDS	Zooplastic Tissue, Rapid Deployment Technique in New Technology
Itrel® (3)(4) neurostimulator	Stimulator Generator, Single Array for Insertion in Subcutaneous Tissue and Fascia
Joint fixation plate	Internal Fixation Device in Upper Joints
	Internal Fixation Device in Lower Joints
Joint liner (insert)	Liner in Lower Joints
Joint spacer (antibiotic)	Spacer in Upper Joints
	Spacer in Lower Joints
Kappa®	Pacemaker, Dual Chamber for Insertion in Subcutaneous Tissue and Fascia
Kirschner wire (K-wire)	Internal Fixation Device in Head and Facial Bones
	Internal Fixation Device in Upper Bones
	Internal Fixation Device in Lower Bones
	Internal Fixation Device in Upper Joints
	Internal Fixation Device in Lower Joints
Knee (implant) insert	Liner in Lower Joints
Kuntscher nail	Internal Fixation Device, Intramedullary in Upper Bones
	Internal Fixation Device, Intramedullary in Lower Bones
LAP-BAND® adjustable gastric banding system	Extraluminal Device
LifeStent® (Flexstar)(XL) Vascular Stent System	Intraluminal Device
LIVIAN™ CRT-D	Cardiac Resynchronization Defibrillator Pulse Generator for Insertion in Subcutaneous Tissue and Fascia
Loop recorder, implantable	Monitoring Device
MAGEC® Spinal Bracing and Distraction System	Magnetically Controlled Growth Rod(s) in New Technology

Device Term	ICD-10-PCS Value
Mark IV™ Breathing Pacemaker System	Stimulator Generator in Subcutaneous Tissue and Fascia
Maximo® II DR (VR)	Defibrillator Generator for Insertion in Subcutaneous Tissue and Fascia
Maximo® II DR CRT-D	Cardiac Resynchronization Defibrillator Pulse Generator for Insertion in Subcutaneous Tissue and Fascia
Medtronic Endurant® II AAA stent graft system	Intraluminal Device
Melody® transcatheter pulmonary valve	Zooplastic Tissue in Heart and Great Vessels
Metal on metal bearing surface	Synthetic Substitute, Metal for Replacement in Lower Joints
Micro-Driver® stent (RX) (OTW)	Intraluminal Device
MicroMed HeartAssist™	Implantable Heart Assist System in Heart and Great Vessels
Micrus CERECYTE® microcoil	Intraluminal Device, Bioactive in Upper Arteries
MIRODERM™ Biologic Wound Matrix	Skin Substitute, Porcine Liver Derived in New Technology
MitraClip® valve repair system	Synthetic Substitute
Mitroflow® Aortic Pericardial Heart Valve	Zooplastic Tissue in Heart and Great Vessels
Mosaic® Bioprosthesis (aortic) (mitral) valve	Zooplastic Tissue in Heart and Great Vessels
MULTI-LINK (VISION®)(MINI-VISION®)(ULTRA™) Coronary Stent System	Intraluminal Device
nanoLOCK™ interbody fusion device	Interbody Fusion Device, Nanotextured Surface in New Technology
Nasopharyngeal airway (NPA)	Intraluminal Device, Airway in Ear, Nose, Sinus
Neuromuscular electrical stimulation (NEMS) lead	Stimulator Lead in Muscles
Neurostimulator generator, multiple channel	Stimulator Generator, Multiple Array for Insertion in Subcutaneous Tissue and Fascia
Neurostimulator generator, multiple channel rechargeable	Stimulator Generator, Multiple Array Rechargeable for Insertion in Subcutaneous Tissue and Fascia
Neurostimulator generator, single channel	Stimulator Generator, Single Array for Insertion in Subcutaneous Tissue and Fascia
Neurostimulator generator, single channel rechargeable	Stimulator Generator, Single Array Rechargeable for Insertion in Subcutaneous Tissue and Fascia
Neutralization plate	Internal Fixation Device in Head and Facial Bones
	Internal Fixation Device in Upper Bones
	Internal Fixation Device in Lower Bones
Nitinol framed polymer mesh	Synthetic Substitute

Device Term	ICD-10-PCS Value
Non-tunneled central venous catheter	Infusion Device
Novacor® Left Ventricular Assist Device	Implantable Heart Assist System in Heart and Great Vessels
Novation® Ceramic AHS® (Articulation Hip System)	Synthetic Substitute, Ceramic for Replacement in Lower Joints
Omnilink Elite® Vascular Balloon Expandable Stent System	Intraluminal Device
Open Pivot™ (mechanical) valve	Synthetic Substitute
Open Pivot™ Aortic Valve Graft (AVG)	Synthetic Substitute
Optimizer™ III implantable pulse generator	Contractility Modulation Device for Insertion in Subcutaneous Tissue and Fascia
Oropharyngeal airway (OPA)	Intraluminal Device, Airway in Mouth and Throat
Ovatio™ CRT-D	Cardiac Resynchronization Defibrillator Pulse Generator for Insertion in Subcutaneous Tissue and Fascia
Oxidized zirconium ceramic hip bearing surface	Synthetic Substitute, Ceramic on Polyethylene for Replacement in Lower Joints
Paclitaxel-eluting coronary stent	Intraluminal Device, Drug-eluting in Heart and Great Vessels
Paclitaxel-eluting peripheral stent	Intraluminal Device, Drug-eluting in Upper Arteries
	Intraluminal Device, Drug-eluting in Lower Arteries
Partially absorbable mesh	Synthetic Substitute
Pedicle-based dynamic stabilization device	Spinal Stabilization Device, Pedicle-Based for Insertion in Upper Joints
	Spinal Stabilization Device, Pedicle-Based for Insertion in Lower Joints
Perceval sutureless valve	Zooplastic Tissue, Rapid Deployment Technique in New Technology
Percutaneous endoscopic gastrojejunostomy (PEG/J) tube	Feeding Device in Gastrointestinal System
Percutaneous endoscopic gastrostomy (PEG) tube	Feeding Device in Gastrointestinal System
Percutaneous nephrostomy catheter	Drainage Device
Peripherally inserted central catheter (PICC)	Infusion Device
Pessary ring	Intraluminal Device, Pessary in Female Reproductive System
Phrenic nerve stimulator generator	Stimulator Generator in Subcutaneous Tissue and Fascia
Phrenic nerve stimulator lead	Diaphragmatic Pacemaker Lead in Respiratory System
PHYSIOMESH™ Flexible Composite Mesh	Synthetic Substitute
Pipeline™ Embolization device (PED)	Intraluminal Device

Device Term	ICD-10-PCS Value
Polyethylene socket	Synthetic Substitute, Polyethylene for Replacement in Lower Joints
Polymethylmethacrylate (PMMA)	Synthetic Substitute
Polypropylene mesh	Synthetic Substitute
Porcine (bioprosthetic) valve	Zooplastic Tissue in Heart and Great Vessels
PRESTIGE® Cervical Disc	Synthetic Substitute
PrimeAdvanced® neurostimulator (SureScan®)(MRI Safe)	Stimulator Generator, Multiple Array for Insertion in Subcutaneous Tissue and Fascia
PROCEED™ Ventral Patch	Synthetic Substitute
Prodisc-C™	Synthetic Substitute
Prodisc-L™	Synthetic Substitute
PROLENE® Polypropylene Hernia System (PHS)	Synthetic Substitute
Protecta™ XT CRT-D	Cardiac Resynchronization Defibrillator Pulse Generator for Insertion in Subcutaneous Tissue and Fascia
Protecta™ XT DR (XT VR)	Defibrillator Generator for Insertion in Subcutaneous Tissue and Fascia
Protege® RX Carotid Stent System	Intraluminal Device
Pump reservoir	Infusion Device, Pump in Subcutaneous Tissue and Fascia
REALIZE® Adjustable Gastric Band	Extraluminal Device
Rebound HRD® (Hernia Repair Device)	Synthetic Substitute
RestoreAdvanced® neurostimulator (SureScan®)(MRI Safe)	Stimulator Generator, Multiple Array Rechargeable for Insertion in Subcutaneous Tissue and Fascia
RestoreSensor® neurostimulator (SureScan®)(MRI Safe)	Stimulator Generator, Multiple Array Rechargeable for Insertion in Subcutaneous Tissue and Fascia
RestoreUltra® neurostimulator (SureScan®)(MRI Safe)	Stimulator Generator, Multiple Array Rechargeable for Insertion in Subcutaneous Tissue and Fascia
Reveal® (DX)(XT)	Monitoring Device
Reverse® Shoulder Prosthesis	Synthetic Substitute, Reverse Ball and Socket for Replacement in Upper Joints
Revo MRI™ SureScan® pacemaker	Pacemaker, Dual Chamber for Insertion in Subcutaneous Tissue and Fascia
Rheos® System device	Stimulator Generator in Subcutaneous Tissue and Fascia
Rheos® System lead	Stimulator Lead in Upper Arteries
RNS® System lead	Neurostimulator Lead in Central Nervous System
RNS® system neurostimulator generator	Neurostimulator Generator in Head and Facial Bones
Sacral nerve modulation (SNM) lead	Stimulator Lead in Urinary System
Sacral neuromodulation lead	Stimulator Lead in Urinary System

Device Term	ICD-10-PCS Value
SAPIEN® transcatheter aortic valve	Zooplastic Tissue in Heart and Great Vessels
Secura™ (DR) (VR)	Defibrillator Generator for Insertion in Subcutaneous Tissue and Fascia
Sheffield hybrid external fixator	External Fixation Device, Hybrid for Insertion in Upper Bones
	External Fixation Device, Hybrid for Reposition in Upper Bones
	External Fixation Device, Hybrid for Insertion in Lower Bones
	External Fixation Device, Hybrid for Reposition in Lower Bones
Sheffield ring external fixator	External Fixation Device, Ring for Insertion in Upper Bones
	External Fixation Device, Ring for Reposition in Upper Bones
	External Fixation Device, Ring for Insertion in Lower Bones
	External Fixation Device, Ring for Reposition in Lower Bones
Single lead pacemaker (atrium) (ventricle)	Pacemaker, Single Chamber for Insertion in Subcutaneous Tissue and Fascia
Single lead rate responsive pacemaker (atrium)(ventricle)	Pacemaker, Single Chamber Rate Responsive for Insertion in Subcutaneous Tissue and Fascia
Sirolimus-eluting coronary stent	Intraluminal Device, Drug-eluting in Heart and Great Vessels
SJM Biocor® Stented Valve System	Zooplastic Tissue in Heart and Great Vessels
Spinal cord neurostimulator lead	Neurostimulator Lead in Central Nervous System
Spinal growth rods, magnetically controlled	Magnetically Controlled Growth Rod(s) in New Technology
Spiration IBV™ Valve System	Intraluminal Device, Endobronchial Valve in Respiratory System
Stent, intraluminal (cardiovascular) (gastrointestinal)(hepatobiliary) (urinary)	Intraluminal Device
Stented tissue valve	Zooplastic Tissue in Heart and Great Vessels
Stratos LV®	Cardiac Resynchronization Pacemaker Pulse Generator for Insertion in Subcutaneous Tissue and Fascia
Subcutaneous injection reservoir, port	Vascular Access Device, Reservoir in Subcutaneous Tissue and Fascia
Subcutaneous injection reservoir, pump	Infusion Device, Pump in Subcutaneous Tissue and Fascia
Subdermal progesterone implant	Contraceptive Device in Subcutaneous Tissue and Fascia
Sutureless valve, Perceval™	Zooplastic Tissue, Rapid Deployment Technique in New Technology

Device Term	ICD-10-PCS Value
SynCardia™ Total Artificial Heart	Synthetic Substitute
Synchra™ CRT-P	Cardiac Resynchronization Pacemaker Pulse Generator for Insertion in Subcutaneous Tissue and Fascia
SynchroMed® pump	Infusion Device, Pump in Subcutaneous Tissue and Fascia
Talent® Converter	Intraluminal Device
Talent® Occluder	Intraluminal Device
Talent® Stent Graft (abdominal) (thoracic)	Intraluminal Device
TandemHeart® System	External Heart Assist System in Heart and Great Vessels
TAXUS® Liberte® Paclitaxel-eluting Coronary Stent System	Intraluminal Device, Drug-eluting in Heart and Great Vessels
Therapeutic occlusion coil(s)	Intraluminal Device
Thoracostomy tube	Drainage Device
Thoratec® IVAD (Implantable Ventricular Assist Device)	Implantable Heart Assist System in Heart and Great Vessels
Thoratec Paracorporeal Ventricular Assist Device	External Heart Assist System in Heart and Great Vessels
Tibial insert	Liner in Lower Joints
TigerPaw® system for closure of left atrial appendage	Extraluminal Device
Tissue bank graft	Nonautologous Tissue Substitute
Tissue expander (inflatable) (injectable)	Tissue Expander in Skin and Breast
	Tissue Expander in Subcutaneous Tissue and Fascia
Titanium Sternal Fixation System (TSFS)	Internal Fixation Device, Rigid Plate for Insertion in Upper Bones
	Internal Fixation Device, Rigid Plate for Reposition in Upper Bones
Total artificial (replacement) heart	Synthetic Substitute
Tracheostomy tube	Tracheostomy Device in Respiratory System
Trifecta™ Valve (aortic)	Zooplastic Tissue in Heart and Great Vessels
Tunneled central venous catheter	Vascular Access Device in Subcutaneous Tissue and Fascia
Tunneled spinal (intrathecal) catheter	Infusion Device
Two lead pacemaker	Pacemaker, Dual Chamber for Insertion in Subcutaneous Tissue and Fascia
Ultraflex™ Precision Colonic Stent System	Intraluminal Device
ULTRAPRO® Hernia System (UHS)	Synthetic Substitute
ULTRAPRO® Partially Absorbable Lightweight Mesh	Synthetic Substitute
ULTRAPRO® Plug	Synthetic Substitute

Device Term	ICD-10-PCS Value
Ultrasonic osteogenic stimulator	Bone Growth Stimulator in Head and Facial Bones
	Bone Growth Stimulator in Upper Bones
	Bone Growth Stimulator in Lower Bones
Ultrasound bone healing system	Bone Growth Stimulator in Head and Facial Bones
	Bone Growth Stimulator in Upper Bones
	Bone Growth Stimulator in Lower Bones
Uniplanar external fixator	External Fixation Device, Monoplanar for Insertion in Upper Bones
	External Fixation Device, Monoplanar for Reposition in Upper Bones
	External Fixation Device, Monoplanar for Insertion in Lower Bones
	External Fixation Device, Monoplanar for Reposition in Lower Bones
Urinary incontinence stimulator lead	Stimulator Lead in Urinary System
Vaginal pessary	Intraluminal Device, Pessary in Female Reproductive System
Valiant® Thoracic Stent Graft	Intraluminal Device
Vectra® Vascular Access Graft	Vascular Access Device in Subcutaneous Tissue and Fascia
Ventrio™ Hernia Patch	Synthetic Substitute
Versa®	Pacemaker, Dual Chamber for Insertion in Subcutaneous Tissue and Fascia
Virtuoso® (II) (DR) (VR)	Defibrillator Generator for Insertion in Subcutaneous Tissue and Fascia
Viva™ (XT)(S)	Cardiac Resynchronization Defibrillator Pulse Generator for Insertion in Subcutaneous Tissue and Fascia
WALLSTENT® Endoprosthesis	Intraluminal Device
X-STOP® Spacer	Spinal Stabilization Device, Interspinous Process for Insertion in Upper Joints
	Spinal Stabilization Device, Interspinous Process for Insertion in Lower Joints
XACT® Carotid Stent System	Intraluminal Device
Xenograft	Zooplastic Tissue in Heart and Great Vessels
XIENCE™ Everolimus Eluting Coronary Stent System	Intraluminal Device, Drug-eluting in Heart and Great Vessels

Device Term	ICD-10-PCS Value
XLIF® System	Interbody Fusion Device in Lower Joints
Zenith® AAA Endovascular Graft	Intraluminal Device, Branched or Fenestrated, One or Two Arteries for Restriction in Lower Arteries
	Intraluminal Device, Branched or Fenestrated, Three or More Arteries for Restriction in Lower Arteries
	Intraluminal Device
Zenith Flex® AAA Endovascular Graft	Intraluminal Device
Zenith TX2® TAA Endovascular Graft	Intraluminal Device
Zenith® Renu™ AAA Ancillary Graft	Intraluminal Device
Zilver® PTX® (paclitaxel) Drug-Eluting Peripheral Stent	Intraluminal Device, Drug-eluting in Upper Arteries
	Intraluminal Device, Drug-eluting in Lower Arteries
Zimmer® NexGen® LPS Mobile Bearing Knee	Synthetic Substitute
Zimmer® NexGen® LPS-Flex Mobile Knee	Synthetic Substitute
Zotarolimus-eluting coronary stent	Intraluminal Device, Drug-eluting in Heart and Great Vessels

Appendix D: Device Aggregation Table

Specific Device	For Operation	In Body System	General Device
Autologous Arterial Tissue	All applicable	Heart and Great Vessels	**7** Autologous Tissue Substitute
		Lower Arteries	
		Lower Veins	
		Upper Arteries	
		Upper Veins	
Autologous Venous Tissue	All applicable	Heart and Great Vessels	**7** Autologous Tissue Substitute
		Lower Arteries	
		Lower Veins	
		Upper Arteries	
		Upper Veins	
Cardiac Lead, Defibrillator	Insertion	Heart and Great Vessels	**M** Cardiac Lead
Cardiac Lead, Pacemaker	Insertion	Heart and Great Vessels	**M** Cardiac Lead
Cardiac Resynchronization Defibrillator Pulse Generator	Insertion	Subcutaneous Tissue and Fascia	**P** Cardiac Rhythm Related Device
Cardiac Resynchronization Pacemaker Pulse Generator	Insertion	Subcutaneous Tissue and Fascia	**P** Cardiac Rhythm Related Device
Contractility Modulation Device	Insertion	Subcutaneous Tissue and Fascia	**P** Cardiac Rhythm Related Device
Defibrillator Generator	Insertion	Subcutaneous Tissue and Fascia	**P** Cardiac Rhythm Related Device
Epiretinal Visual Prosthesis	All applicable	Eye	**J** Synthetic Substitute
External Fixation Device, Hybrid	Insertion	Lower Bones	**5** External Fixation Device
		Upper Bones	
External Fixation Device, Hybrid	Reposition	Lower Bones	**5** External Fixation Device
		Upper Bones	
External Fixation Device, Limb Lengthening, Hybrid	Insertion	Lower Bones	**5** External Fixation Device
		Upper Bones	
External Fixation Device, Monoplanar	Insertion	Lower Bones	**5** External Fixation Device
		Upper Bones	
External Fixation Device, Monoplanar	Reposition	Lower Bones	**5** External Fixation Device
		Upper Bones	
External Fixation Device, Ring	Insertion	Lower Bones	**5** External Fixation Device
		Upper Bones	
External Fixation Device, Ring	Reposition	Lower Bones	**5** External Fixation Device
		Upper Bones	
Hearing Device, Bone Conduction	Insertion	Ear, Nose, Sinus	**S** Hearing Device
Hearing Device, Multiple Channel Cochlear Prosthesis	Insertion	Ear, Nose, Sinus	**S** Hearing Device
Hearing Device, Single Channel Cochlear Prosthesis	Insertion	Ear, Nose, Sinus	**S** Hearing Device
Internal Fixation Device, Intramedullary	All applicable	Lower Bones	**4** Internal Fixation Device
		Upper Bones	
Internal Fixation Device, Rigid Plate	Insertion	Lower Bones	**4** Internal Fixation Device
Internal Fixation Device, Rigid Plate	Reposition	Upper Bones	
Intraluminal Device, Airway	All applicable	Ear, Nose, Sinus Gastrointestinal System Mouth and Throat	**D** Intraluminal Device
Intraluminal Device, Bioactive	All applicable	Upper Arteries	**D** Intraluminal Device

Specific Device	For Operation	In Body System	General Device
Intraluminal Device, Branched or Fenestrated, One or Two Arteries	Restriction	Heart and Great Vessels Lower Arteries	**D** Intraluminal Device
Intraluminal Device, Branched or Fenestrated, Three or More Arteries	Restriction	Heart and Great Vessels	**D** Intraluminal Device
		Lower Arteries	
Intraluminal Device, Drug-eluting	All applicable	Heart and Great Vessels	**D** Intraluminal Device
		Lower Arteries	
		Upper Arteries	
Intraluminal Device, Drug-eluting, Four or More	All applicable	Heart and Great Vessels	**D** Intraluminal Device
		Lower Arteries	
		Upper Arteries	
Intraluminal Device, Drug-eluting, Three	All applicable	Heart and Great Vessels	**D** Intraluminal Device
		Lower Arteries	
		Upper Arteries	
Intraluminal Device, Drug-eluting, Two	All applicable	Heart and Great Vessels	**D** Intraluminal Device
		Lower Arteries	
		Upper Arteries	
Intraluminal Device, Endobronchial Valve	All applicable	Respiratory System	**D** Intraluminal Device
Intraluminal Device, Endotracheal Airway	All applicable	Respiratory System	**D** Intraluminal Device
Intraluminal Device, Four or More	All applicable	Heart and Great Vessels	**D** Intraluminal Device
		Lower Arteries	
		Upper Arteries	
Intraluminal Device, Pessary	All applicable	Female Reproductive System	**D** Intraluminal Device
Intraluminal Device, Radioactive	All applicable	Heart and Great Vessels	**D** Intraluminal Device
Intraluminal Device, Three	All applicable	Heart and Great Vessels	**D** Intraluminal Device
		Lower Arteries	
		Upper Arteries	
Intraluminal Device, Two	All applicable	Heart and Great Vessels	**D** Intraluminal Device
		Lower Arteries	
		Upper Arteries	
Monitoring Device, Hemodynamic	Insertion	Subcutaneous Tissue and Fascia	**2** Monitoring Device
Monitoring Device, Pressure Sensor	Insertion	Heart and Great Vessels	**2** Monitoring Device
Pacemaker, Dual Chamber	Insertion	Subcutaneous Tissue and Fascia	**P** Cardiac Rhythm Related Device
Pacemaker, Single Chamber	Insertion	Subcutaneous Tissue and Fascia	**P** Cardiac Rhythm Related Device
Pacemaker, Single Chamber Rate Responsive	Insertion	Subcutaneous Tissue and Fascia	**P** Cardiac Rhythm Related Device
Spinal Stabilization Device, Facet Replacement	Insertion	Lower Joints	**4** Internal Fixation Device
		Upper Joints	
Spinal Stabilization Device, Interspinous Process	Insertion	Lower Joints	**4** Internal Fixation Device
		Upper Joints	
Spinal Stabilization Device, Pedicle-Based	Insertion	Lower Joints	**4** Internal Fixation Device
		Upper Joints	
Stimulator Generator, Multiple Array	Insertion	Subcutaneous Tissue and Fascia	**M** Stimulator Generator
Stimulator Generator, Multiple Array Rechargeable	Insertion	Subcutaneous Tissue and Fascia	**M** Stimulator Generator
Stimulator Generator, Single Array	Insertion	Subcutaneous Tissue and Fascia	**M** Stimulator Generator

Specific Device	For Operation	In Body System	General Device
Stimulator Generator, Single Array Rechargeable	Insertion	Subcutaneous Tissue and Fascia	**M** Stimulator Generator
Synthetic Substitute, Ceramic	Replacement	Lower Joints	**J** Synthetic Substitute
Synthetic Substitute, Ceramic on Polyethylene	Replacement	Lower Joints	**J** Synthetic Substitute
Synthetic Substitute, Intraocular Telescope	Replacement	Eye	**J** Synthetic Substitute
Synthetic Substitute, Metal	Replacement	Lower Joints	**J** Synthetic Substitute
Synthetic Substitute, Metal on Polyethylene	Replacement	Lower Joints	**J** Synthetic Substitute
Synthetic Substitute, Polyethylene	Replacement	Lower Joints	**J** Synthetic Substitute
Synthetic Substitute, Reverse Ball and Socket	Replacement	Upper Joints	**J** Synthetic Substitute
Synthetic Substitute, Unicondylar	Replacement	Lower Joints	**J** Synthetic Substitute

This page intentionally left blank

Appendix E: Character Meaning

0: Medical and Surgical
0: Central Nervous System

Operation-Character 3	Body Part-Character 4	Approach-Character 5	Device-Character 6	Qualifier-Character 7
1 Bypass	**0** Brain	**0** Open	**0** Drainage Device	**0** Nasopharynx
2 Change	**1** Cerebral Meninges	**3** Percutaneous	**2** Monitoring Device	**1** Mastoid Sinus
5 Destruction	**2** Dura Mater	**4** Percutaneous Endoscopic	**3** Infusion Device	**2** Atrium
8 Division	**3** Epidural Space	**X** External	**7** Autologous Tissue Substitute	**3** Blood Vessel
9 Drainage	**4** Subdural Space		**J** Synthetic Substitute	**4** Pleural Cavity
B Excision	**5** Subarachnoid Space		**K** Nonautologous Tissue Substitute	**5** Intestine
C Extirpation	**6** Cerebral Ventricle		**M** Neurostimulator Lead	**6** Peritoneal Cavity
D Extraction	**7** Cerebral Hemisphere		**Y** Other Device	**7** Urinary Tract
F Fragmentation	**8** Basal Ganglia		**Z** No Device	**8** Bone Marrow
H Insertion	**9** Thalamus			**9** Fallopian Tube
J Inspection	**A** Hypothalamus			**B** Cerebral Cisterns
K Map	**B** Pons			**F** Olfactory Nerve
N Release	**C** Cerebellum			**G** Optic Nerve
P Removal	**D** Medulla Oblongata			**H** Oculomotor Nerve
Q Repair	**E** Cranial Nerve			**J** Trochlear Nerve
S Reposition	**F** Olfactory Nerve			**K** Trigeminal Nerve
T Resection	**G** Optic Nerve			**L** Abducens Nerve
U Supplement	**H** Oculomotor Nerve			**M** Facial Nerve
W Revision	**J** Trochlear Nerve			**N** Acoustic Nerve
X Transfer	**K** Trigeminal Nerve			**P** Glossopharyngeal Nerve
	L Abducens Nerve			**Q** Vagus Nerve
	M Facial Nerve			**R** Accessory Nerve
	N Acoustic Nerve			**S** Hypoglossal Nerve
	P Glossopharyngeal Nerve			**X** Diagnostic
	Q Vagus Nerve			**Z** No Qualifier
	R Accessory Nerve			
	S Hypoglossal Nerve			
	T Spinal Meninges			
	U Spinal Canal			
	V Spinal Cord			
	W Cervical Spinal Cord			
	X Thoracic Spinal Cord			
	Y Lumbar Spinal Cord			

0: Medical and Surgical
1: Peripheral Nervous System

Operation-Character 3	Body Part-Character 4	Approach-Character 5	Device-Character 6	Qualifier-Character 7
2 Change	**0** Cervical Plexus	**0** Open	**0** Drainage Device	**1** Cervical Nerve
5 Destruction	**1** Cervical Nerve	**3** Percutaneous	**2** Monitoring Device	**2** Phrenic Nerve
8 Division	**2** Phrenic Nerve	**4** Percutaneous Endoscopic	**7** Autologous Tissue Substitute	**4** Ulnar Nerve
9 Drainage	**3** Brachial Plexus	**X** External	**M** Neurostimulator Lead	**5** Median Nerve
B Excision	**4** Ulnar Nerve		**Y** Other Device	**6** Radial Nerve
C Extirpation	**5** Median Nerve		**Z** No Device	**8** Thoracic Nerve
D Extraction	**6** Radial Nerve			**B** Lumbar Nerve
H Insertion	**8** Thoracic Nerve			**C** Perineal Nerve
J Inspection	**9** Lumbar Plexus			**D** Femoral Nerve
N Release	**A** Lumbosacral Plexus			**F** Sciatic Nerve
P Removal	**B** Lumbar Nerve			**G** Tibial Nerve
Q Repair	**C** Pudendal Nerve			**H** Peroneal Nerve
S Reposition	**D** Femoral Nerve			**X** Diagnostic
U Supplement	**F** Sciatic Nerve			**Z** No Qualifier
W Revision	**G** Tibial Nerve			
X Transfer	**H** Peroneal Nerve			
	K Head and Neck Sympathetic Nerve			
	L Thoracic Sympathetic Nerve			
	M Abdominal Sympathetic Nerve			
	N Lumbar Sympathetic Nerve			
	P Sacral Sympathetic Nerve			
	Q Sacral Plexus			
	R Sacral Nerve			
	Y Peripheral Nerve			

0: Medical and Surgical
2: Heart and Great Vessels

Operation-Character 3	Body Part-Character 4	Approach-Character 5	Device-Character 6	Qualifier-Character 7
1 Bypass	**0** Coronary Artery, One Artery	**0** Open	**0** Monitoring Device, Pressure Sensor	**0** Allogeneic
4 Creation	**1** Coronary Artery, Two Arteries	**3** Percutaneous	**2** Monitoring Device	**1** Syngeneic
5 Destruction	**2** Coronary Artery, Three Arteries	**4** Percutaneous Endoscopic	**3** Infusion Device	**2** Zooplastic
7 Dilation	**3** Coronary Artery, Four or More Arteries	**X** External	**4** Intraluminal Device, Drug-eluting	**2** Common Atrioventricular Valve
8 Division	**4** Coronary Vein		**5** Intraluminal Device, Drug-Eluting, Two	**3** Coronary Artery
B Excision	**5** Atrial Septum		**6** Intraluminal Device, Drug-Eluting, Three	**4** Coronary Vein
C Extirpation	**6** Atrium, Right		**7** Intraluminal Device, Drug-Eluting, Four or More	**5** Coronary Circulation
F Fragmentation	**7** Atrium, Left		**7** Autologous Tissue Substitute	**6** Bifurcation
H Insertion	**8** Conduction Mechanism		**8** Zooplastic Tissue	**7** Atrium, Left
J Inspection	**9** Chordae Tendineae		**9** Autologous Venous Tissue	**8** Internal Mammary, Right
K Map	**A** Heart		**A** Autologous Arterial Tissue	**9** Internal Mammary, Left
L Occlusion	**B** Heart, Right		**C** Extraluminal Device	**A** Innominate Artery
N Release	**C** Heart, Left		**D** Intraluminal Device	**B** Subclavian
P Removal	**D** Papillary Muscle		**E** Intraluminal Device, Two	**C** Thoracic Artery
Q Repair	**F** Aortic Valve		**E** Intraluminal Device, Branched or Fenestrated, One or Two Arteries	**D** Carotid
R Replacement	**G** Mitral Valve		**F** Intraluminal Device, Three	**E** Atrioventricular Valve, Left
S Reposition	**H** Pulmonary Valve		**F** Intraluminal Device, Branched or Fenestrated, Three or More Arteries	**F** Abdominal Artery
T Resection	**J** Tricuspid Valve		**G** Intraluminal Device, Four or More	**G** Atrioventricular Valve, Right
U Supplement	**K** Ventricle, Right		**J** Cardiac Lead, Pacemaker	**H** Transapical
V Restriction	**L** Ventricle, Left		**J** Synthetic Substitute	**J** Truncal Valve
W Revision	**M** Ventricular Septum		**K** Cardiac Lead, Defibrillator	**K** Left Atrial Appendage
Y Transplantation	**N** Pericardium		**K** Nonautologous Tissue Substitute	**P** Pulmonary Trunk
	P Pulmonary Trunk		**M** Cardiac Lead	**Q** Pulmonary Artery, Right
	Q Pulmonary Artery, Right		**N** Intracardiac Pacemaker	**R** Pulmonary Artery, Left
	R Pulmonary Artery, Left		**Q** Implantable Heart Assist System	**S** Biventricular
	S Pulmonary Vein, Right		**R** External Heart Assist System	**S** Pulmonary Vein, Right
	T Pulmonary Vein, Left		**T** Intraluminal Device, Radioactive	**T** Pulmonary Vein, Left
	V Superior Vena Cava		**Z** No Device	**T** Ductus Arteriosus
	W Thoracic Aorta			**U** Pulmonary Vein, Confluence
	Y Great Vessel			**W** Aorta
				X Diagnostic
				Z No Qualifier

0: Medical and Surgical
3: Upper Arteries

Operation-Character 3	Body Part-Character 4	Approach-Character 5	Device-Character 6	Qualifier-Character 7
1 Bypass	**0** Internal Mammary Artery, Right	**0** Open	**0** Drainage Device	**0** Upper Arm Artery, Right
5 Destruction	**1** Internal Mammary Artery, Left	**3** Percutaneous	**2** Monitoring Device	**1** Upper Arm Artery, Left
7 Dilation	**2** Innominate Artery	**4** Percutaneous Endoscopic	**3** Infusion Device	**2** Upper Arm Artery, Bilateral
9 Drainage	**3** Subclavian Artery, Right	**X** External	**4** Intraluminal Device, Drug-eluting	**3** Lower Arm Artery, Right
B Excision	**4** Subclavian Artery, Left		**5** Intraluminal Device, Drug-eluting, Two	**4** Lower Arm Artery, Left
C Extirpation	**5** Axillary Artery, Right		**6** Intraluminal Device, Drug-eluting, , Three	**5** Lower Arm Artery, Bilateral
H Insertion	**6** Axillary Artery, Left		**7** Intraluminal Device, Drug-eluting, Four or More	**6** Upper Leg Artery, Right
J Inspection	**7** Brachial Artery, Right		**7** Autologous Tissue Substitute	**6** Bifurcation
L Occlusion	**8** Brachial Artery, Left		**9** Autologous Venous Tissue	**7** Upper Leg Artery, Left
N Release	**9** Ulnar Artery, Right		**A** Autologous Arterial Tissue	**8** Upper Leg Artery, Bilateral
P Removal	**A** Ulnar Artery, Left		**B** Intraluminal Device, Bioactive	**9** Lower Leg Artery, Right
Q Repair	**B** Radial Artery, Right		**C** Extraluminal Device	**B** Lower Leg Artery, Left
R Replacement	**C** Radial Artery, Left		**D** Intraluminal Device	**C** Lower Leg Artery, Bilateral
S Reposition	**D** Hand Artery, Right		**E** Intraluminal Device, Two	**D** Upper Arm Vein
U Supplement	**F** Hand Artery, Left		**F** Intraluminal Device, Three	**F** Lower Arm Vein
V Restriction	**G** Intracranial Artery		**G** Intraluminal Device, Four or More	**G** Intracranial Artery
W Revision	**H** Common Carotid Artery, Right		**J** Synthetic Substitute	**J** Extracranial Artery, Right
	J Common Carotid Artery, Left		**K** Nonautologous Tissue Substitute	**K** Extracranial Artery, Left
	K Internal Carotid Artery, Right		**M** Stimulator Lead	**M** Pulmonary Artery, Right
	L Internal Carotid Artery, Left		**Z** No Device	**N** Pulmonary Artery, Left
	M External Carotid Artery, Right			**X** Diagnostic
	N External Carotid Artery, Left			**Z** No Qualifier
	P Vertebral Artery, Right			
	Q Vertebral Artery, Left			
	R Face Artery			
	S Temporal Artery, Right			
	T Temporal Artery, Left			
	U Thyroid Artery, Right			
	V Thyroid Artery, Left			
	Y Upper Artery			

0: Medical and Surgical
4: Lower Arteries

Operation-Character 3	Body Part-Character 4	Approach-Character 5	Device-Character 6	Qualifier-Character 7
1 Bypass	**0** Abdominal Aorta	**0** Open	**0** Drainage Device	**0** Abdominal Aorta
5 Destruction	**1** Celiac Artery	**3** Percutaneous	**1** Radioactive Element	**1** Celiac Artery
7 Dilation	**2** Gastric Artery	**4** Percutaneous Endoscopic	**2** Monitoring Device	**1** Drug-Coated Balloon
9 Drainage	**3** Hepatic Artery	**X** External	**3** Infusion Device	**2** Mesenteric Artery
B Excision	**4** Splenic Artery		**4** Intraluminal Device, Drug-eluting	**3** Renal Artery, Right
C Extirpation	**5** Superior Mesenteric Artery		**5** Intraluminal Device, Drug-eluting, Two	**4** Renal Artery, Left
H Insertion	**6** Colic Artery, Right		**6** Intraluminal Device, Drug-eluting, , Three	**5** Renal Artery, Bilateral
J Inspection	**7** Colic Artery, Left		**7** Intraluminal Device, Drug-eluting, Four or More	**6** Bifurcation
L Occlusion	**8** Colic Artery, Middle		**7** Autologous Tissue Substitute	**6** Common Iliac Artery, Right
N Release	**9** Renal Artery, Right		**9** Autologous Venous Tissue	**7** Common Iliac Artery, Left
P Removal	**A** Renal Artery, Left		**A** Autologous Arterial Tissue	**8** Common Iliac Arteries, Bilateral
Q Repair	**B** Inferior Mesenteric Artery		**C** Extraluminal Device	**9** Internal Iliac Artery, Right
R Replacement	**C** Common Iliac Artery, Right		**D** Intraluminal Device	**B** Internal Iliac Artery, Left
S Reposition	**D** Common Iliac Artery, Left		**E** Intraluminal Device, Two	**C** Internal Iliac Arteries, Bilateral
U Supplement	**E** Internal Iliac Artery, Right		**E** Intraluminal Device, Branched or Fenestrated, One or Two Arteries	**D** External Iliac Artery, Right
V Restriction	**F** Internal Iliac Artery, Left		**F** Intraluminal Device, Three	**F** External Iliac Artery, Left
W Revision	**H** External Iliac Artery, Right		**F** Intraluminal Device, Branched or Fenestrated, Three or More Arteries	**G** External Iliac Arteries, Bilateral
	J External Iliac Artery, Left		**G** Intraluminal Device, Four or More	**H** Femoral Artery, Right
	K Femoral Artery, Right		**J** Synthetic Substitute	**J** Temporary
	L Femoral Artery, Left		**K** Nonautologous Tissue Substitute	**J** Femoral Artery, Left
	M Popliteal Artery, Right		**Z** No Device	**K** Femoral Arteries, Bilateral
	N Popliteal Artery, Left			**L** Popliteal Artery
	P Anterior Tibial Artery, Right			**M** Peroneal Artery
	Q Anterior Tibial Artery, Left			**N** Posterior Tibial Artery
	R Posterior Tibial Artery, Right			**P** Foot Artery
	S Posterior Tibial Artery, Left			**Q** Lower Extremity Artery
	T Peroneal Artery, Right			**R** Lower Artery
	U Peroneal Artery, Left			**S** Lower Extremity Vein
	V Foot Artery, Right			**T** Uterine Artery, Right
	W Foot Artery, Left			**U** Uterine Artery, Left
	Y Lower Artery			**X** Diagnostic
				Z No Qualifier

0: Medical and Surgical
5: Upper Veins

Operation-Character 3	Body Part-Character 4	Approach-Character 5	Device-Character 6	Qualifier-Character 7
1 Bypass	**0** Azygos Vein	**0** Open	**0** Drainage Device	**X** Diagnostic
5 Destruction	**1** Hemiazygos Vein	**3** Percutaneous	**2** Monitoring Device	**Y** Upper Vein
7 Dilation	**3** Innominate Vein, Right	**4** Percutaneous Endoscopic	**3** Infusion Device	**Z** No Qualifier
9 Drainage	**4** Innominate Vein, Left	**X** External	**7** Autologous Tissue Substitute	
B Excision	**5** Subclavian Vein, Right		**9** Autologous Venous Tissue	
C Extirpation	**6** Subclavian Vein, Left		**A** Autologous Arterial Tissue	
D Extraction	**7** Axillary Vein, Right		**C** Extraluminal Device	
H Insertion	**8** Axillary Vein, Left		**D** Intraluminal Device	
J Inspection	**9** Brachial Vein, Right		**J** Synthetic Substitute	
L Occlusion	**A** Brachial Vein, Left		**K** Nonautologous Tissue Substitute	
N Release	**B** Basilic Vein, Right		**M** Neurostimulator Lead	
P Removal	**C** Basilic Vein, Left		**Z** No Device	
Q Repair	**D** Cephalic Vein, Right			
R Replacement	**F** Cephalic Vein, Left			
S Reposition	**G** Hand Vein, Right			
U Supplement	**H** Hand Vein, Left			
V Restriction	**L** Intracranial Vein			
W Revision	**M** Internal Jugular Vein, Right			
	N Internal Jugular Vein, Left			
	P External Jugular Vein, Right			
	Q External Jugular Vein, Left			
	R Vertebral Vein, Right			
	S Vertebral Vein, Left			
	T Face Vein, Right			
	V Face Vein, Left			
	Y Upper Vein			

0: Medical and Surgical
6: Lower Veins

Operation-Character 3	Body Part-Character 4	Approach-Character 5	Device-Character 6	Qualifier-Character 7
1 Bypass	**0** Inferior Vena Cava	**0** Open	**0** Drainage Device	**5** Superior Mesenteric Vein
5 Destruction	**1** Splenic Vein	**3** Percutaneous	**2** Monitoring Device	**6** Inferior Mesenteric Vein
7 Dilation	**2** Gastric Vein	**4** Percutaneous Endoscopic	**3** Infusion Device	**9** Renal Vein, Right
9 Drainage	**3** Esophageal Vein	**X** External	**7** Autologous Tissue Substitute	**B** Renal Vein, Left
B Excision	**4** Hepatic Vein		**9** Autologous Venous Tissue	**C** Hemorrhoidal Plexus
C Extirpation	**5** Superior Mesenteric Vein		**A** Autologous Arterial Tissue	**T** Via Umbilical Vein
D Extraction	**6** Inferior Mesenteric Vein		**C** Extraluminal Device	**X** Diagnostic
H Insertion	**7** Colic Vein		**D** Intraluminal Device	**Y** Lower Vein
J Inspection	**8** Portal Vein		**J** Synthetic Substitute	**Z** No Qualifier
L Occlusion	**9** Renal Vein, Right		**K** Nonautologous Tissue Substitute	
N Release	**B** Renal Vein, Left		**Z** No Device	
P Removal	**C** Common Iliac Vein, Right			
Q Repair	**D** Common Iliac Vein, Left			
R Replacement	**F** External Iliac Vein, Right			
S Reposition	**G** External Iliac Vein, Left			
U Supplement	**H** Hypogastric Vein, Right			
V Restriction	**J** Hypogastric Vein, Left			
W Revision	**M** Femoral Vein, Right			
	N Femoral Vein, Left			
	P Greater Saphenous Vein, Right			
	Q Greater Saphenous Vein, Left			
	R Lesser Saphenous Vein, Right			
	S Lesser Saphenous Vein, Left			
	T Foot Vein, Right			
	V Foot Vein, Left			
	Y Lower Vein			

0: Medical and Surgical
7: Lymphatic and Hemic Systems

Operation-Character 3	Body Part-Character 4	Approach-Character 5	Device-Character 6	Qualifier-Character 7
2 Change	**0** Lymphatic, Head	**0** Open	**0** Drainage Device	**0** Allogeneic
5 Destruction	**1** Lymphatic, Right Neck	**3** Percutaneous	**3** Infusion Device	**1** Syngeneic
9 Drainage	**2** Lymphatic, Left Neck	**4** Percutaneous Endoscopic	**7** Autologous Tissue Substitute	**2** Zooplastic
B Excision	**3** Lymphatic, Right Upper Extremity	**X** External	**C** Extraluminal Device	**X** Diagnostic
C Extirpation	**4** Lymphatic, Left Upper Extremity		**D** Intraluminal Device	**Z** No Qualifier
D Extraction	**5** Lymphatic, Right Axillary		**J** Synthetic Substitute	
H Insertion	**6** Lymphatic, Left Axillary		**K** Nonautologous Tissue Substitute	
J Inspection	**7** Lymphatic, Thorax		**Y** Other Device	
L Occlusion	**8** Lymphatic, Internal Mammary, Right		**Z** No Device	
N Release	**9** Lymphatic, Internal Mammary, Left			
P Removal	**B** Lymphatic, Mesenteric			
Q Repair	**C** Lymphatic, Pelvis			
S Reposition	**D** Lymphatic, Aortic			
T Resection	**F** Lymphatic, Right Lower Extremity			
U Supplement	**G** Lymphatic, Left Lower Extremity			
V Restriction	**H** Lymphatic, Right Inguinal			
W Revision	**J** Lymphatic, Left Inguinal			
Y Transplantation	**K** Thoracic Duct			
	L Cisterna Chyli			
	M Thymus			
	N Lymphatic			
	P Spleen			
	Q Bone Marrow, Sternum			
	R Bone Marrow, Iliac			
	S Bone Marrow, Vertebral			
	T Bone Marrow			

0: Medical and Surgical
8: Eye

Operation-Character 3	Body Part-Character 4	Approach-Character 5	Device-Character 6	Qualifier-Character 7
0 Alteration	**0** Eye, Right	**0** Open	**0** Drainage Device	**3** Nasal Cavity
1 Bypass	**1** Eye, Left	**3** Percutaneous	**0** Synthetic Substitute, Intraocular Telescope	**4** Sclera
2 Change	**2** Anterior Chamber, Right	**7** Via Natural or Artificial Opening	**1** Radioactive Element	**X** Diagnostic
5 Destruction	**3** Anterior Chamber, Left	**8** Via Natural or Artificial Opening Endoscopic	**3** Infusion Device	**Z** No Qualifier
7 Dilation	**4** Vitreous, Right	**X** External	**5** Epiretinal Visual Prosthesis	
9 Drainage	**5** Vitreous, Left		**7** Autologous Tissue Substitute	
B Excision	**6** Sclera, Right		**C** Extraluminal Device	
C Extirpation	**7** Sclera, Left		**D** Intraluminal Device	
D Extraction	**8** Cornea, Right		**J** Synthetic Substitute	
F Fragmentation	**9** Cornea, Left		**K** Nonautologous Tissue Substitute	
H Insertion	**A** Choroid, Right		**Y** Other Device	
J Inspection	**B** Choroid, Left		**Z** No Device	
L Occlusion	**C** Iris, Right			
M Reattachment	**D** Iris, Left			
N Release	**E** Retina, Right			
P Removal	**F** Retina, Left			
Q Repair	**G** Retinal Vessel, Right			
R Replacement	**H** Retinal Vessel, Left			
S Reposition	**J** Lens, Right			
T Resection	**K** Lens, Left			
U Supplement	**L** Extraocular Muscle, Right			
V Restriction	**M** Extraocular Muscle, Left			
W Revision	**N** Upper Eyelid, Right			
X Transfer	**P** Upper Eyelid, Left			
	Q Lower Eyelid, Right			
	R Lower Eyelid, Left			
	S Conjunctiva, Right			
	T Conjunctiva, Left			
	V Lacrimal Gland, Right			
	W Lacrimal Gland, Left			
	X Lacrimal Duct, Right			
	Y Lacrimal Duct, Left			

0: Medical and Surgical
9: Ear, Nose, Sinus

Operation-Character 3	Body Part-Character 4	Approach-Character 5	Device-Character 6	Qualifier-Character 7
0 Alteration	**0** External Ear, Right	**0** Open	**0** Drainage Device	**0** Endolymphatic
1 Bypass	**1** External Ear, Left	**3** Percutaneous	**4** Hearing Device, Bone Conduction	**X** Diagnostic
2 Change	**2** External Ear, Bilateral	**4** Percutaneous Endoscopic	**5** Hearing Device, Single Channel Cochlear Prosthesis	**Z** No Qualifier
5 Destruction	**3** External Auditory Canal, Right	**7** Via Natural or Artificial Opening	**6** Hearing Device, Multiple Channel Cochlear Prosthesis	
7 Dilation	**4** External Auditory Canal, Left	**8** Via Natural or Artificial Opening Endoscopic	**7** Autologous Tissue Substitute	
8 Division	**5** Middle Ear, Right	**X** External	**B** Intraluminal Device, Airway	
9 Drainage	**6** Middle Ear, Left		**D** Intraluminal Device	
B Excision	**7** Tympanic Membrane, Right		**J** Synthetic Substitute	
C Extirpation	**8** Tympanic Membrane, Left		**K** Nonautologous Tissue Substitute	
D Extraction	**9** Auditory Ossicle, Right		**S** Hearing Device	
H Insertion	**A** Auditory Ossicle, Left		**Y** Other Device	
J Inspection	**B** Mastoid Sinus, Right		**Z** No Device	
M Reattachment	**C** Mastoid Sinus, Left			
N Release	**D** Inner Ear, Right			
P Removal	**E** Inner Ear, Left			
Q Repair	**F** Eustachian Tube, Right			
R Replacement	**G** Eustachian Tube, Left			
S Reposition	**H** Ear, Right			
T Resection	**J** Ear, Left			
U Supplement	**K** Nose			
W Revision	**L** Nasal Turbinate			
	M Nasal Septum			
	N Nasopharynx			
	P Accessory Sinus			
	Q Maxillary Sinus, Right			
	R Maxillary Sinus, Left			
	S Frontal Sinus, Right			
	T Frontal Sinus, Left			
	U Ethmoid Sinus, Right			
	V Ethmoid Sinus, Left			
	W Sphenoid Sinus, Right			
	X Sphenoid Sinus, Left			
	Y Sinus			

0: Medical and Surgical
B: Respiratory System

Operation-Character 3	Body Part-Character 4	Approach-Character 5	Device-Character 6	Qualifier-Character 7
1 Bypass	**0** Tracheobronchial Tree	**0** Open	**0** Drainage Device	**0** Allogeneic
2 Change	**1** Trachea	**3** Percutaneous	**1** Radioactive Element	**1** Syngeneic
5 Destruction	**2** Carina	**4** Percutaneous Endoscopic	**2** Monitoring Device	**2** Zooplastic
7 Dilation	**3** Main Bronchus, Right	**7** Via Natural or Artificial Opening	**3** Infusion Device	**4** Cutaneous
9 Drainage	**4** Upper Lobe Bronchus, Right	**8** Via Natural or Artificial Opening Endoscopic	**7** Autologous Tissue Substitute	**6** Esophagus
B Excision	**5** Middle Lobe Bronchus, Right	**X** External	**C** Extraluminal Device	**X** Diagnostic
C Extirpation	**6** Lower Lobe Bronchus, Right		**D** Intraluminal Device	**Z** No Qualifier
D Extraction	**7** Main Bronchus, Left		**E** Intraluminal Device, Endotracheal Airway	
F Fragmentation	**8** Upper Lobe Bronchus, Left		**F** Tracheostomy Device	
H Insertion	**9** Lingula Bronchus		**G** Intraluminal Device, Endobronchial Valve	
J Inspection	**B** Lower Lobe Bronchus, Left		**J** Synthetic Substitute	
L Occlusion	**C** Upper Lung Lobe, Right		**K** Nonautologous Tissue Substitute	
M Reattachment	**D** Middle Lung Lobe, Right		**M** Diaphragmatic Pacemaker Lead	
N Release	**F** Lower Lung Lobe, Right		**Y** Other Device	
P Removal	**G** Upper Lung Lobe, Left		**Z** No Device	
Q Repair	**H** Lung Lingula			
S Reposition	**J** Lower Lung Lobe, Left			
T Resection	**K** Lung, Right			
U Supplement	**L** Lung, Left			
V Restriction	**M** Lungs, Bilateral			
W Revision	**N** Pleura, Right			
Y Transplantation	**P** Pleura, Left			
	Q Pleura			
	R Diaphragm, Right			
	S Diaphragm, Left			
	T Diaphragm			

0: Medical and Surgical
C: Mouth and Throat

Operation-Character 3	Body Part-Character 4	Approach-Character 5	Device-Character 6	Qualifier-Character 7
0 Alteration	**0** Upper Lip	**0** Open	**0** Drainage Device	**0** Single
2 Change	**1** Lower Lip	**3** Percutaneous	**1** Radioactive Element	**1** Multiple
5 Destruction	**2** Hard Palate	**4** Percutaneous Endoscopic	**5** External Fixation Device	**2** All
7 Dilation	**3** Soft Palate	**7** Via Natural or Artificial Opening	**7** Autologous Tissue Substitute	**X** Diagnostic
9 Drainage	**4** Buccal Mucosa	**8** Via Natural or Artificial Opening Endoscopic	**B** Intraluminal Device, Airway	**Z** No Qualifier
B Excision	**5** Upper Gingiva	**X** External	**C** Extraluminal Device	
C Extirpation	**6** Lower Gingiva		**D** Intraluminal Device	
D Extraction	**7** Tongue		**J** Synthetic Substitute	
F Fragmentation	**8** Parotid Gland, Right		**K** Nonautologous Tissue Substitute	
H Insertion	**9** Parotid Gland, Left		**Y** Other Device	
J Inspection	**A** Salivary Gland		**Z** No Device	
L Occlusion	**B** Parotid Duct, Right			
M Reattachment	**C** Parotid Duct, Left			
N Release	**D** Sublingual Gland, Right			
P Removal	**F** Sublingual Gland, Left			
Q Repair	**G** Submaxillary Gland, Right			
R Replacement	**H** Submaxillary Gland, Left			
S Reposition	**J** Minor Salivary Gland			
T Resection	**M** Pharynx			
U Supplement	**N** Uvula			
V Restriction	**P** Tonsils			
W Revision	**Q** Adenoids			
X Transfer	**R** Epiglottis			
	S Larynx			
	T Vocal Cord, Right			
	V Vocal Cord, Left			
	W Upper Tooth			
	X Lower Tooth			
	Y Mouth and Throat			

0: Medical and Surgical
D: Gastrointestinal System

Operation-Character 3	Body Part-Character 4	Approach-Character 5	Device-Character 6	Qualifier-Character 7
1 Bypass	**0** Upper Intestinal Tract	**0** Open	**0** Drainage Device	**0** Allogeneic
2 Change	**1** Esophagus, Upper	**3** Percutaneous	**1** Radioactive Element	**1** Syngeneic
5 Destruction	**2** Esophagus, Middle	**4** Percutaneous Endoscopic	**2** Monitoring Device	**2** Zooplastic
7 Dilation	**3** Esophagus, Lower	**7** Via Natural or Artificial Opening	**3** Infusion Device	**3** Vertical
8 Division	**4** Esophagogastric Junction	**8** Via Natural or Artificial Opening Endoscopic	**7** Autologous Tissue Substitute	**4** Cutaneous
9 Drainage	**5** Esophagus	**X** External	**B** Intraluminal Device, Airway	**5** Esophagus
B Excision	**6** Stomach		**C** Extraluminal Device	**6** Stomach
C Extirpation	**7** Stomach, Pylorus		**D** Intraluminal Device	**9** Duodenum
F Fragmentation	**8** Small Intestine		**J** Synthetic Substitute	**A** Jejunum
H Insertion	**9** Duodenum		**K** Nonautologous Tissue Substitute	**B** Ileum
J Inspection	**A** Jejunum		**L** Artificial Sphincter	**H** Cecum
L Occlusion	**B** Ileum		**M** Stimulator Lead	**K** Ascending Colon
M Reattachment	**C** Ileocecal Valve		**U** Feeding Device	**L** Transverse Colon
N Release	**D** Lower Intestinal Tract		**Y** Other Device	**M** Descending Colon
P Removal	**E** Large Intestine		**Z** No Device	**N** Sigmoid Colon
Q Repair	**F** Large Intestine, Right			**P** Rectum
R Replacement	**G** Large Intestine, Left			**Q** Anus
S Reposition	**H** Cecum			**X** Diagnostic
T Resection	**J** Appendix			**Z** No Qualifier
U Supplement	**K** Ascending Colon			
V Restriction	**L** Transverse Colon			
W Revision	**M** Descending Colon			
X Transfer	**N** Sigmoid Colon			
Y Transplantation	**P** Rectum			
	Q Anus			
	R Anal Sphincter			
	S Greater Omentum			
	T Lesser Omentum			
	U Omentum			
	V Mesentery			
	W Peritoneum			

0: Medical and Surgical
F: Hepatobiliary System and Pancreas

Operation-Character 3	Body Part-Character 4	Approach-Character 5	Device-Character 6	Qualifier-Character 7
1 Bypass	**0** Liver	**0** Open	**0** Drainage Device	**0** Allogeneic
2 Change	**1** Liver, Right Lobe	**3** Percutaneous	**1** Radioactive Element	**1** Syngeneic
5 Destruction	**2** Liver, Left Lobe	**4** Percutaneous Endoscopic	**2** Monitoring Device	**2** Zooplastic
7 Dilation	**4** Gallbladder	**7** Via Natural or Artificial Opening	**3** Infusion Device	**3** Duodenum
8 Division	**5** Hepatic Duct, Right	**8** Via Natural or Artificial Opening Endoscopic	**7** Autologous Tissue Substitute	**4** Stomach
9 Drainage	**6** Hepatic Duct, Left	**X** External	**C** Extraluminal Device	**5** Hepatic Duct, Right
B Excision	**8** Cystic Duct		**D** Intraluminal Device	**6** Hepatic Duct, Left
C Extirpation	**9** Common Bile Duct		**J** Synthetic Substitute	**7** Hepatic Duct, Caudate
F Fragmentation	**B** Hepatobiliary Duct		**K** Nonautologous Tissue Substitute	**8** Cystic Duct
H Insertion	**C** Ampulla of Vater		**Y** Other Device	**9** Common Bile Duct
J Inspection	**D** Pancreatic Duct		**Z** No Device	**B** Small Intestine
L Occlusion	**F** Pancreatic Duct, Accessory			**C** Large Intestine
M Reattachment	**G** Pancreas			**X** Diagnostic
N Release				**Z** No Qualifier
P Removal				
Q Repair				
R Replacement				
S Reposition				
T Resection				
U Supplement				
V Restriction				
W Revision				
Y Transplantation				

0: Medical and Surgical
G: Endocrine System

Operation-Character 3	Body Part-Character 4	Approach-Character 5	Device-Character 6	Qualifier-Character 7
2 Change	**0** Pituitary Gland	**0** Open	**0** Drainage Device	**X** Diagnostic
5 Destruction	**1** Pineal Body	**3** Percutaneous	**2** Monitoring Device	**Z** No Qualifier
8 Division	**2** Adrenal Gland, Left	**4** Percutaneous Endoscopic	**3** Infusion Device	
9 Drainage	**3** Adrenal Gland, Right	**X** External	**Y** Other Device	
B Excision	**4** Adrenal Glands, Bilateral		**Z** No Device	
C Extirpation	**5** Adrenal Gland			
H Insertion	**6** Carotid Body, Left			
J Inspection	**7** Carotid Body, Right			
M Reattachment	**8** Carotid Bodies, Bilateral			
N Release	**9** Para-aortic Body			
P Removal	**B** Coccygeal Glomus			
Q Repair	**C** Glomus Jugulare			
S Reposition	**D** Aortic Body			
T Resection	**F** Paraganglion Extremity			
W Revision	**G** Thyroid Gland Lobe, Left			
	H Thyroid Gland Lobe, Right			
	J Thyroid Gland Isthmus			
	K Thyroid Gland			
	L Superior Parathyroid Gland, Right			
	M Superior Parathyroid Gland, Left			
	N Inferior Parathyroid Gland, Right			
	P Inferior Parathyroid Gland, Left			
	Q Parathyroid Glands, Multiple			
	R Parathyroid Gland			
	S Endocrine Gland			

0: Medical and Surgical
H: Skin and Breast

Operation-Character 3	Body Part-Character 4	Approach-Character 5	Device-Character 6	Qualifier-Character 7
0 Alteration	**0** Skin, Scalp	**0** Open	**0** Drainage Device	**3** Full Thickness
2 Change	**1** Skin, Face	**3** Percutaneous	**1** Radioactive Element	**4** Partial Thickness
5 Destruction	**2** Skin, Right Ear	**7** Via Natural or Artificial Opening	**7** Autologous Tissue Substitute	**5** Latissimus Dorsi Myocutaneous Flap
8 Division	**3** Skin, Left Ear	**8** Via Natural or Artificial Opening Endoscopic	**J** Synthetic Substitute	**6** Transverse Rectus Abdominis Myocutaneous Flap
9 Drainage	**4** Skin, Neck	**X** External	**K** Nonautologous Tissue Substitute	**7** Deep Inferior Epigastric Artery Perforator Flap
B Excision	**5** Skin, Chest		**N** Tissue Expander	**8** Superficial Inferior Epigastric Artery Flap
C Extirpation	**6** Skin, Back		**Y** Other Device	**9** Gluteal Artery Perforator Flap
D Extraction	**7** Skin, Abdomen		**Z** No Device	**D** Multiple
H Insertion	**8** Skin, Buttock			**X** Diagnostic
J Inspection	**9** Skin, Perineum			**Z** No Qualifier
M Reattachment	**A** Skin, Genitalia			
N Release	**B** Skin, Right Upper Arm			
P Removal	**C** Skin, Left Upper Arm			
Q Repair	**D** Skin, Right Lower Arm			
R Replacement	**E** Skin, Left Lower Arm			
S Reposition	**F** Skin, Right Hand			
T Resection	**G** Skin, Left Hand			
U Supplement	**H** Skin, Right Upper Leg			
W Revision	**J** Skin, Left Upper Leg			
X Transfer	**K** Skin, Right Lower Leg			
	L Skin, Left Lower Leg			
	M Skin, Right Foot			
	N Skin, Left Foot			
	P Skin			
	Q Finger Nail			
	R Toe Nail			
	S Hair			
	T Breast, Right			
	U Breast, Left			
	V Breast, Bilateral			
	W Nipple, Right			
	X Nipple, Left			
	Y Supernumerary Breast			

0: Medical and Surgical
J: Subcutaneous Tissue and Fascia

Operation-Character 3	Body Part-Character 4	Approach-Character 5	Device-Character 6	Qualifier-Character 7
0 Alteration	**0** Subcutaneous Tissue and Fascia, Scalp	**0** Open	**0** Drainage Device	**B** Skin and Subcutaneous Tissue
2 Change	**1** Subcutaneous Tissue and Fascia, Face	**3** Percutaneous	**0** Monitoring Device, Hemodynamic	**C** Skin, Subcutaneous Tissue and Fascia
5 Destruction	**4** Subcutaneous Tissue and Fascia, Anterior Neck	**X** External	**1** Radioactive Element	**X** Diagnostic
8 Division	**5** Subcutaneous Tissue and Fascia, Posterior Neck		**2** Monitoring Device	**Z** No Qualifier
9 Drainage	**6** Subcutaneous Tissue and Fascia, Chest		**3** Infusion Device	
B Excision	**7** Subcutaneous Tissue and Fascia, Back		**4** Pacemaker, Single Chamber	
C Extirpation	**8** Subcutaneous Tissue and Fascia, Abdomen		**5** Pacemaker, Single Chamber Rate Responsive	
D Extraction	**9** Subcutaneous Tissue and Fascia, Buttock		**6** Pacemaker, Dual Chamber	
H Insertion	**B** Subcutaneous Tissue and Fascia, Perineum		**7** Autologous Tissue Substitute	
J Inspection	**C** Subcutaneous Tissue and Fascia, Pelvic Region		**7** Cardiac Resynchronization Pacemaker Pulse Generator	
N Release	**D** Subcutaneous Tissue and Fascia, Right Upper Arm		**8** Defibrillator Generator	
P Removal	**F** Subcutaneous Tissue and Fascia, Left Upper Arm		**9** Cardiac Resynchronization Defibrillator Pulse Generator	
Q Repair	**G** Subcutaneous Tissue and Fascia, Right Lower Arm		**A** Contractility Modulation Device	
R Replacement	**H** Subcutaneous Tissue and Fascia, Left Lower Arm		**B** Stimulator Generator, Single Array	
U Supplement	**J** Subcutaneous Tissue and Fascia, Right Hand		**C** Stimulator Generator, Single Array Rechargeable	
W Revision	**K** Subcutaneous Tissue and Fascia, Left Hand		**D** Stimulator Generator, Multiple Array	
X Transfer	**L** Subcutaneous Tissue and Fascia, Right Upper Leg		**E** Stimulator Generator, Multiple Array Rechargeable	
	M Subcutaneous Tissue and Fascia, Left Upper Leg		**H** Contraceptive Device	
	N Subcutaneous Tissue and Fascia, Right Lower Leg		**J** Synthetic Substitute	
	P Subcutaneous Tissue and Fascia, Left Lower Leg		**K** Nonautologous Tissue Substitute	
	Q Subcutaneous Tissue and Fascia, Right Foot		**M** Stimulator Generator	
	R Subcutaneous Tissue and Fascia, Left Foot		**N** Tissue Expander	
	S Subcutaneous Tissue and Fascia, Head and Neck		**P** Cardiac Rhythm Related Device	
	T Subcutaneous Tissue and Fascia, Trunk		**V** Infusion Device, Pump	
	V Subcutaneous Tissue and Fascia, Upper Extremity		**W** Vascular Access Device, Reservoir	
	W Subcutaneous Tissue and Fascia, Lower Extremity		**X** Vascular Access Device	
			Y Other Device	
			Z No Device	

0: Medical and Surgical
K: Muscles

Operation-Character 3	Body Part-Character 4	Approach-Character 5	Device-Character 6	Qualifier-Character 7
2 Change	**0** Head Muscle	**0** Open	**0** Drainage Device	**0** Skin
5 Destruction	**1** Facial Muscle	**3** Percutaneous	**7** Autologous Tissue Substitute	**1** Subcutaneous Tissue
8 Division	**2** Neck Muscle, Right	**4** Percutaneous Endoscopic	**J** Synthetic Substitute	**2** Skin and Subcutaneous Tissue
9 Drainage	**3** Neck Muscle, Left	**X** External	**K** Nonautologous Tissue Substitute	**6** Transverse Rectus Abdominis Myocutaneous Flap
B Excision	**4** Tongue, Palate, Pharynx Muscle		**M** Stimulator Lead	**X** Diagnostic
C Extirpation	**5** Shoulder Muscle, Right		**Y** Other Device	**Z** No Qualifier
H Insertion	**6** Shoulder Muscle, Left		**Z** No Device	
J Inspection	**7** Upper Arm Muscle, Right			
M Reattachment	**8** Upper Arm Muscle, Left			
N Release	**9** Lower Arm and Wrist Muscle, Right			
P Removal	**B** Lower Arm and Wrist Muscle, Left			
Q Repair	**C** Hand Muscle, Right			
S Reposition	**D** Hand Muscle, Left			
T Resection	**F** Trunk Muscle, Right			
U Supplement	**G** Trunk Muscle, Left			
W Revision	**H** Thorax Muscle, Right			
X Transfer	**J** Thorax Muscle, Left			
	K Abdomen Muscle, Right			
	L Abdomen Muscle, Left			
	M Perineum Muscle			
	N Hip Muscle, Right			
	P Hip Muscle, Left			
	Q Upper Leg Muscle, Right			
	R Upper Leg Muscle, Left			
	S Lower Leg Muscle, Right			
	T Lower Leg Muscle, Left			
	V Foot Muscle, Right			
	W Foot Muscle, Left			
	X Upper Muscle			
	Y Lower Muscle			

0: Medical and Surgical
L: Tendons

Operation-Character 3	Body Part-Character 4	Approach-Character 5	Device-Character 6	Qualifier-Character 7
2 Change	**0** Head and Neck Tendon	**0** Open	**0** Drainage Device	**X** Diagnostic
5 Destruction	**1** Shoulder Tendon, Right	**3** Percutaneous	**7** Autologous Tissue Substitute	**Z** No Qualifier
8 Division	**2** Shoulder Tendon, Left	**4** Percutaneous Endoscopic	**J** Synthetic Substitute	
9 Drainage	**3** Upper Arm Tendon, Right	**X** External	**K** Nonautologous Tissue Substitute	
B Excision	**4** Upper Arm Tendon, Left		**Y** Other Device	
C Extirpation	**5** Lower Arm and Wrist Tendon, Right		**Z** No Device	
J Inspection	**6** Lower Arm and Wrist Tendon, Left			
M Reattachment	**7** Hand Tendon, Right			
N Release	**8** Hand Tendon, Left			
P Removal	**9** Trunk Tendon, Right			
Q Repair	**B** Trunk Tendon, Left			
R Replacement	**C** Thorax Tendon, Right			
S Reposition	**D** Thorax Tendon, Left			
T Resection	**F** Abdomen Tendon, Right			
U Supplement	**G** Abdomen Tendon, Left			
W Revision	**H** Perineum Tendon			
X Transfer	**J** Hip Tendon, Right			
	K Hip Tendon, Left			
	L Upper Leg Tendon, Right			
	M Upper Leg Tendon, Left			
	N Lower Leg Tendon, Right			
	P Lower Leg Tendon, Left			
	Q Knee Tendon, Right			
	R Knee Tendon, Left			
	S Ankle Tendon, Right			
	T Ankle Tendon, Left			
	V Foot Tendon, Right			
	W Foot Tendon, Left			
	X Upper Tendon			
	Y Lower Tendon			

0: Medical and Surgical
M: Bursae and Ligaments

Operation-Character 3	Body Part-Character 4	Approach-Character 5	Device-Character 6	Qualifier-Character 7
2 Change	**0** Head and Neck Bursa and Ligament	**0** Open	**0** Drainage Device	**X** Diagnostic
5 Destruction	**1** Shoulder Bursa and Ligament, Right	**3** Percutaneous	**7** Autologous Tissue Substitute	**Z** No Qualifier
8 Division	**2** Shoulder Bursa and Ligament, Left	**4** Percutaneous Endoscopic	**J** Synthetic Substitute	
9 Drainage	**3** Elbow Bursa and Ligament, Right	**X** External	**K** Nonautologous Tissue Substitute	
B Excision	**4** Elbow Bursa and Ligament, Left		**Y** Other Device	
C Extirpation	**5** Wrist Bursa and Ligament, Right		**Z** No Device	
D Extraction	**6** Wrist Bursa and Ligament, Left			
J Inspection	**7** Hand Bursa and Ligament, Right			
M Reattachment	**8** Hand Bursa and Ligament, Left			
N Release	**9** Upper Extremity Bursa and Ligament, Right			
P Removal	**B** Upper Extremity Bursa and Ligament, Left			
Q Repair	**C** Trunk Bursa and Ligament, Right			
S Reposition	**D** Trunk Bursa and Ligament, Left			
T Resection	**F** Thorax Bursa and Ligament, Right			
U Supplement	**G** Thorax Bursa and Ligament, Left			
W Revision	**H** Abdomen Bursa and Ligament, Right			
X Transfer	**J** Abdomen Bursa and Ligament, Left			
	K Perineum Bursa and Ligament			
	L Hip Bursa and Ligament, Right			
	M Hip Bursa and Ligament, Left			
	N Knee Bursa and Ligament, Right			
	P Knee Bursa and Ligament, Left			
	Q Ankle Bursa and Ligament, Right			
	R Ankle Bursa and Ligament, Left			
	S Foot Bursa and Ligament, Right			
	T Foot Bursa and Ligament, Left			
	V Lower Extremity Bursa and Ligament, Right			
	W Lower Extremity Bursa and Ligament, Left			
	X Upper Bursa and Ligament			
	Y Lower Bursa and Ligament			

0: Medical and Surgical
N: Head and Facial Bones

Operation-Character 3	Body Part-Character 4	Approach-Character 5	Device-Character 6	Qualifier-Character 7
2 Change	**0** Skull	**0** Open	**0** Drainage Device	**X** Diagnostic
5 Destruction	**1** Frontal Bone, Right	**3** Percutaneous	**4** Internal Fixation Device	**Z** No Qualifier
8 Division	**2** Frontal Bone, Left	**4** Percutaneous Endoscopic	**5** External Fixation Device	
9 Drainage	**3** Parietal Bone, Right	**X** External	**7** Autologous Tissue Substitute	
B Excision	**4** Parietal Bone, Left		**J** Synthetic Substitute	
C Extirpation	**5** Temporal Bone, Right		**K** Nonautologous Tissue Substitute	
H Insertion	**6** Temporal Bone, Left		**M** Bone Growth Stimulator	
J Inspection	**7** Occipital Bone, Right		**N** Neurostimulator Generator	
N Release	**8** Occipital Bone, Left		**S** Hearing Device	
P Removal	**B** Nasal Bone		**Y** Other Device	
Q Repair	**C** Sphenoid Bone, Right		**Z** No Device	
R Replacement	**D** Sphenoid Bone, Left			
S Reposition	**F** Ethmoid Bone, Right			
T Resection	**G** Ethmoid Bone, Left			
U Supplement	**H** Lacrimal Bone, Right			
W Revision	**J** Lacrimal Bone, Left			
	K Palatine Bone, Right			
	L Palatine Bone, Left			
	M Zygomatic Bone, Right			
	N Zygomatic Bone, Left			
	P Orbit, Right			
	Q Orbit, Left			
	R Maxilla, Right			
	S Maxilla, Left			
	T Mandible, Right			
	V Mandible, Left			
	W Facial Bone			
	X Hyoid Bone			

0: Medical and Surgical
P: Upper Bones

Operation-Character 3	Body Part-Character 4	Approach-Character 5	Device-Character 6	Qualifier-Character 7
2 Change	**0** Sternum	**0** Open	**0** Drainage Device	**X** Diagnostic
5 Destruction	**1** Rib, Right	**3** Percutaneous	**0** Internal Fixation Device, Rigid Plate	**Z** No Qualifier
8 Division	**2** Rib, Left	**4** Percutaneous Endoscopic	**4** Internal Fixation Device	
9 Drainage	**3** Cervical Vertebra	**X** External	**5** External Fixation Device	
B Excision	**4** Thoracic Vertebra		**6** Internal Fixation Device, Intramedullary	
C Extirpation	**5** Scapula, Right		**7** Autologous Tissue Substitute	
H Insertion	**6** Scapula, Left		**8** External Fixation Device, Limb Lengthening	
J Inspection	**7** Glenoid Cavity, Right		**B** External Fixation Device, Monoplanar	
N Release	**8** Glenoid Cavity, Left		**C** External Fixation Device, Ring	
P Removal	**9** Clavicle, Right		**D** External Fixation Device, Hybrid	
Q Repair	**B** Clavicle, Left		**J** Synthetic Substitute	
R Replacement	**C** Humeral Head, Right		**K** Nonautologous Tissue Substitute	
S Reposition	**D** Humeral Head, Left		**M** Bone Growth Stimulator	
T Resection	**F** Humeral Shaft, Right		**Y** Other Device	
U Supplement	**G** Humeral Shaft, Left		**Z** No Device	
W Revision	**H** Radius, Right			
	J Radius, Left			
	K Ulna, Right			
	L Ulna, Left			
	M Carpal, Right			
	N Carpal, Left			
	P Metacarpal, Right			
	Q Metacarpal, Left			
	R Thumb Phalanx, Right			
	S Thumb Phalanx, Left			
	T Finger Phalanx, Right			
	V Finger Phalanx, Left			
	Y Upper Bone			

0: Medical and Surgical
Q: Lower Bones

Operation-Character 3	Body Part-Character 4	Approach-Character 5	Device-Character 6	Qualifier-Character 7
2 Change	**0** Lumbar Vertebra	**0** Open	**0** Drainage Device	**X** Diagnostic
5 Destruction	**1** Sacrum	**3** Percutaneous	**4** Internal Fixation Device	**Z** No Qualifier
8 Division	**2** Pelvic Bone, Right	**4** Percutaneous Endoscopic	**5** External Fixation Device	
9 Drainage	**3** Pelvic Bone, Left	**X** External	**6** Internal Fixation Device, Intramedullary	
B Excision	**4** Acetabulum, Right		**7** Autologous Tissue Substitute	
C Extirpation	**5** Acetabulum, Left		**8** External Fixation Device, Limb Lengthening	
H Insertion	**6** Upper Femur, Right		**B** External Fixation Device, Monoplanar	
J Inspection	**7** Upper Femur, Left		**C** External Fixation Device, Ring	
N Release	**8** Femoral Shaft, Right		**D** External Fixation Device, Hybrid	
P Removal	**9** Femoral Shaft, Left		**J** Synthetic Substitute	
Q Repair	**B** Lower Femur, Right		**K** Nonautologous Tissue Substitute	
R Replacement	**C** Lower Femur, Left		**M** Bone Growth Stimulator	
S Reposition	**D** Patella, Right		**Y** Other Device	
T Resection	**F** Patella, Left		**Z** No Device	
U Supplement	**G** Tibia, Right			
W Revision	**H** Tibia, Left			
	J Fibula, Right			
	K Fibula, Left			
	L Tarsal, Right			
	M Tarsal, Left			
	N Metatarsal, Right			
	P Metatarsal, Left			
	Q Toe Phalanx, Right			
	R Toe Phalanx, Left			
	S Coccyx			
	Y Lower Bone			

0: Medical and Surgical
R: Upper Joints

Operation-Character 3	Body Part-Character 4	Approach-Character 5	Device-Character 6	Qualifier-Character 7
2 Change	**0** Occipital-cervical Joint	**0** Open	**0** Drainage Device	**0** Anterior Approach, Anterior Column
5 Destruction	**1** Cervical Vertebral Joint	**3** Percutaneous	**0** Synthetic Substitute, Reverse Ball and Socket	**1** Posterior Approach, Posterior Column
9 Drainage	**2** Cervical Vertebral Joints, 2 or more	**4** Percutaneous Endoscopic	**3** Infusion Device	**6** Humeral Surface
B Excision	**3** Cervical Vertebral Disc	**X** External	**4** Internal Fixation Device	**7** Glenoid Surface
C Extirpation	**4** Cervicothoracic Vertebral Joint		**5** External Fixation Device	**J** Posterior Approach, Anterior Column
G Fusion	**5** Cervicothoracic Vertebral Disc		**7** Autologous Tissue Substitute	**X** Diagnostic
H Insertion	**6** Thoracic Vertebral Joint		**8** Spacer	**Z** No Qualifier
J Inspection	**7** Thoracic Vertebral Joints, 2 to 7		**A** Interbody Fusion Device	
N Release	**8** Thoracic Vertebral Joints, 8 or more		**B** Spinal Stabilization Device, Interspinous Process	
P Removal	**9** Thoracic Vertebral Disc		**C** Spinal Stabilization Device, Pedicle-Based	
Q Repair	**A** Thoracolumbar Vertebral Joint		**D** Spinal Stabilization Device, Facet Replacement	
R Replacement	**B** Thoracolumbar Vertebral Disc		**J** Synthetic Substitute	
S Reposition	**C** Temporomandibular Joint, Right		**K** Nonautologous Tissue Substitute	
T Resection	**D** Temporomandibular Joint, Left		**Y** Other Device	
U Supplement	**E** Sternoclavicular Joint, Right		**Z** No Device	
W Revision	**F** Sternoclavicular Joint, Left			
	G Acromioclavicular Joint, Right			
	H Acromioclavicular Joint, Left			
	J Shoulder Joint, Right			
	K Shoulder Joint, Left			
	L Elbow Joint, Right			
	M Elbow Joint, Left			
	N Wrist Joint, Right			
	P Wrist Joint, Left			
	Q Carpal Joint, Right			
	R Carpal Joint, Left			
	S Metacarpocarpal Joint, Right			
	T Metacarpocarpal Joint, Left			
	U Metacarpophalangeal Joint, Right			
	V Metacarpophalangeal Joint, Left			
	W Finger Phalangeal Joint, Right			
	X Finger Phalangeal Joint, Left			
	Y Upper Joint			

0: Medical and Surgical
S: Lower Joints

Operation-Character 3	Body Part-Character 4	Approach-Character 5	Device-Character 6	Qualifier-Character 7
2 Change	**0** Lumbar Vertebral Joint	**0** Open	**0** Drainage Device	**0** Anterior Approach, Anterior Column
5 Destruction	**1** Lumbar Vertebral Joints, 2 or more	**3** Percutaneous	**0** Synthetic Substitute, Polyethylene	**1** Posterior Approach, Posterior Column
9 Drainage	**2** Lumbar Vertebral Disc	**4** Percutaneous Endoscopic	**1** Synthetic Substitute, Metal	**9** Cemented
B Excision	**3** Lumbosacral Joint	**X** External	**2** Synthetic Substitute, Metal on Polyethylene	**A** Uncemented
C Extirpation	**4** Lumbosacral Disc		**3** Infusion Device	**C** Patellar Surface
G Fusion	**5** Sacrococcygeal Joint		**3** Synthetic Substitute, Ceramic	**J** Posterior Approach, Anterior Column
H Insertion	**6** Coccygeal Joint		**4** Internal Fixation Device	**X** Diagnostic
J Inspection	**7** Sacroiliac Joint, Right		**4** Synthetic Substitute, Ceramic on Polyethylene	**Z** No Qualifier
N Release	**8** Sacroiliac Joint, Left		**5** External Fixation Device	
P Removal	**9** Hip Joint, Right		**7** Autologous Tissue Substitute	
Q Repair	**A** Hip Joint, Acetabular Surface, Right		**8** Spacer	
R Replacement	**B** Hip Joint, Left		**9** Liner	
S Reposition	**C** Knee Joint, Right		**A** Interbody Fusion Device	
T Resection	**D** Knee Joint, Left		**B** Resurfacing Device	
U Supplement	**E** Hip Joint, Acetabular Surface, Left		**B** Spinal Stabilization Device, Interspinous Process	
W Revision	**F** Ankle Joint, Right		**C** Spinal Stabilization Device, Pedicle-Based	
	G Ankle Joint, Left		**D** Spinal Stabilization Device, Facet Replacement	
	H Tarsal Joint, Right		**J** Synthetic Substitute	
	J Tarsal Joint, Left		**K** Nonautologous Tissue Substitute	
	K Metatarsal-Tarsal Joint, Right		**L** Synthetic Substitute, Unicondylar	
	L Metatarsal-Tarsal Joint, Left		**Y** Other Device	
	M Metatarsal-Phalangeal Joint, Right		**Z** No Device	
	N Metatarsal-Phalangeal Joint, Left			
	P Toe Phalangeal Joint, Right			
	Q Toe Phalangeal Joint, Left			
	R Hip Joint, Femoral Surface, Right			
	S Hip Joint, Femoral Surface, Left			
	T Knee Joint, Femoral Surface, Right			
	U Knee Joint, Femoral Surface, Left			
	V Knee Joint, Tibial Surface, Right			
	W Knee Joint, Tibial Surface, Left			
	Y Lower Joint			

0: Medical and Surgical
T: Urinary System

Operation-Character 3	Body Part-Character 4	Approach-Character 5	Device-Character 6	Qualifier-Character 7
1 Bypass	**0** Kidney, Right	**0** Open	**0** Drainage Device	**0** Allogeneic
2 Change	**1** Kidney, Left	**3** Percutaneous	**2** Monitoring Device	**1** Syngeneic
5 Destruction	**2** Kidneys, Bilateral	**4** Percutaneous Endoscopic	**3** Infusion Device	**2** Zooplastic
7 Dilation	**3** Kidney Pelvis, Right	**7** Via Natural or Artificial Opening	**7** Autologous Tissue Substitute	**3** Kidney Pelvis, Right
8 Division	**4** Kidney Pelvis, Left	**8** Via Natural or Artificial Opening Endoscopic	**C** Extraluminal Device	**4** Kidney Pelvis, Left
9 Drainage	**5** Kidney	**X** External	**D** Intraluminal Device	**6** Ureter, Right
B Excision	**6** Ureter, Right		**J** Synthetic Substitute	**7** Ureter, Left
C Extirpation	**7** Ureter, Left		**K** Nonautologous Tissue Substitute	**8** Colon
D Extraction	**8** Ureters, Bilateral		**L** Artificial Sphincter	**9** Colocutaneous
F Fragmentation	**9** Ureter		**M** Stimulator Lead	**A** Ileum
H Insertion	**B** Bladder		**Y** Other Device	**B** Bladder
J Inspection	**C** Bladder Neck		**Z** No Device	**C** Ileocutaneous
L Occlusion	**D** Urethra			**D** Cutaneous
M Reattachment				**X** Diagnostic
N Release				**Z** No Qualifier
P Removal				
Q Repair				
R Replacement				
S Reposition				
T Resection				
U Supplement				
V Restriction				
W Revision				
Y Transplantation				

0: Medical and Surgical
U: Female Reproductive System

Operation-Character 3	Body Part-Character 4	Approach-Character 5	Device-Character 6	Qualifier-Character 7
1 Bypass	**0** Ovary, Right	**0** Open	**0** Drainage Device	**0** Allogeneic
2 Change	**1** Ovary, Left	**3** Percutaneous	**1** Radioactive Element	**1** Syngeneic
5 Destruction	**2** Ovaries, Bilateral	**4** Percutaneous Endoscopic	**3** Infusion Device	**2** Zooplastic
7 Dilation	**3** Ovary	**7** Via Natural or Artificial Opening	**7** Autologous Tissue Substitute	**5** Fallopian Tube, Right
8 Division	**4** Uterine Supporting Structure	**8** Via Natural or Artificial Opening Endoscopic	**C** Extraluminal Device	**6** Fallopian Tube, Left
9 Drainage	**5** Fallopian Tube, Right	**F** Via Natural or Artificial Opening With Percutaneous Endoscopic Assistance	**D** Intraluminal Device	**9** Uterus
B Excision	**6** Fallopian Tube, Left	**X** External	**G** Intraluminal Device, Pessary	**X** Diagnostic
C Extirpation	**7** Fallopian Tubes, Bilateral		**H** Contraceptive Device	**Z** No Qualifier
D Extraction	**8** Fallopian Tube		**J** Synthetic Substitute	
F Fragmentation	**9** Uterus		**K** Nonautologous Tissue Substitute	
H Insertion	**B** Endometrium		**Y** Other Device	
J Inspection	**C** Cervix		**Z** No Device	
L Occlusion	**D** Uterus and Cervix			
M Reattachment	**F** Cul-de-sac			
N Release	**G** Vagina			
P Removal	**H** Vagina and Cul-de-sac			
Q Repair	**J** Clitoris			
S Reposition	**K** Hymen			
T Resection	**L** Vestibular Gland			
U Supplement	**M** Vulva			
V Restriction	**N** Ova			
W Revision				
Y Transplantation				

0: Medical and Surgical
V: Male Reproductive System

Operation-Character 3	Body Part-Character 4	Approach-Character 5	Device-Character 6	Qualifier-Character 7
1 Bypass	**0** Prostate	**0** Open	**0** Drainage Device	**J** Epididymis, Right
2 Change	**1** Seminal Vesicle, Right	**3** Percutaneous	**1** Radioactive Element	**K** Epididymis, Left
5 Destruction	**2** Seminal Vesicle, Left	**4** Percutaneous Endoscopic	**3** Infusion Device	**N** Vas Deferens, Right
7 Dilation	**3** Seminal Vesicles, Bilateral	**7** Via Natural or Artificial Opening	**7** Autologous Tissue Substitute	**P** Vas Deferens, Left
9 Drainage	**4** Prostate and Seminal Vesicles	**8** Via Natural or Artificial Opening Endoscopic	**C** Extraluminal Device	**X** Diagnostic
B Excision	**5** Scrotum	**X** External	**D** Intraluminal Device	**Z** No Qualifier
C Extirpation	**6** Tunica Vaginalis, Right		**J** Synthetic Substitute	
H Insertion	**7** Tunica Vaginalis, Left		**K** Nonautologous Tissue Substitute	
J Inspection	**8** Scrotum and Tunica Vaginalis		**Y** Other Device	
L Occlusion	**9** Testis, Right		**Z** No Device	
M Reattachment	**B** Testis, Left			
N Release	**C** Testes, Bilateral			
P Removal	**D** Testis			
Q Repair	**F** Spermatic Cord, Right			
R Replacement	**G** Spermatic Cord, Left			
S Reposition	**H** Spermatic Cords, Bilateral			
T Resection	**J** Epididymis, Right			
U Supplement	**K** Epididymis, Left			
W Revision	**L** Epididymis, Bilateral			
	M Epididymis and Spermatic Cord			
	N Vas Deferens, Right			
	P Vas Deferens, Left			
	Q Vas Deferens, Bilateral			
	R Vas Deferens			
	S Penis			
	T Prepuce			

0: Medical and Surgical
W: Anatomical Regions, General

Operation-Character 3	Body Part-Character 4	Approach-Character 5	Device-Character 6	Qualifier-Character 7
0 Alteration	**0** Head	**0** Open	**0** Drainage Device	**0** Vagina
1 Bypass	**1** Cranial Cavity	**3** Percutaneous	**1** Radioactive Element	**0** Allogeneic
2 Change	**2** Face	**4** Percutaneous Endoscopic	**3** Infusion Device	**1** Penis
3 Control	**3** Oral Cavity and Throat	**7** Via Natural or Artificial Opening	**7** Autologous Tissue Substitute	**1** Syngeneic
4 Creation	**4** Upper Jaw	**8** Via Natural or Artificial Opening Endoscopic	**J** Synthetic Substitute	**2** Stoma
8 Division	**5** Lower Jaw	**X** External	**K** Nonautologous Tissue Substitute	**4** Cutaneous
9 Drainage	**6** Neck		**Y** Other Device	**9** Pleural Cavity, Right
B Excision	**8** Chest Wall		**Z** No Device	**B** Pleural Cavity, Left
C Extirpation	**9** Pleural Cavity, Right			**G** Peritoneal Cavity
F Fragmentation	**B** Pleural Cavity, Left			**J** Pelvic Cavity
H Insertion	**C** Mediastinum			**X** Diagnostic
J Inspection	**D** Pericardial Cavity			**Y** Lower Vein
M Reattachment	**F** Abdominal Wall			**Z** No Qualifier
P Removal	**G** Peritoneal Cavity			
Q Repair	**H** Retroperitoneum			
U Supplement	**J** Pelvic Cavity			
W Revision	**K** Upper Back			
Y Transplantation	**L** Lower Back			
	M Perineum, Male			
	N Perineum, Female			
	P Gastrointestinal Tract			
	Q Respiratory Tract			
	R Genitourinary Tract			

0: Medical and Surgical
X: Anatomical Regions, Upper Extremities

Operation-Character 3	Body Part-Character 4	Approach-Character 5	Device-Character 6	Qualifier-Character 7
0 Alteration	**0** Forequarter, Right	**0** Open	**0** Drainage Device	**0** Complete
2 Change	**1** Forequarter, Left	**3** Percutaneous	**1** Radioactive Element	**0** Allogeneic
3 Control	**2** Shoulder Region, Right	**4** Percutaneous Endoscopic	**3** Infusion Device	**1** Syngeneic
6 Detachment	**3** Shoulder Region, Left	**X** External	**7** Autologous Tissue Substitute	**1** High
9 Drainage	**4** Axilla, Right		**J** Synthetic Substitute	**2** Mid
B Excision	**5** Axilla, Left		**K** Nonautologous Tissue Substitute	**3** Low
H Insertion	**6** Upper Extremity, Right		**Y** Other Device	**4** Complete 1st Ray
J Inspection	**7** Upper Extremity, Left		**Z** No Device	**5** Complete 2nd Ray
M Reattachment	**8** Upper Arm, Right			**6** Complete 3rd Ray
P Removal	**9** Upper Arm, Left			**7** Complete 4th Ray
Q Repair	**B** Elbow Region, Right			**8** Complete 5th Ray
R Replacement	**C** Elbow Region, Left			**9** Partial 1st Ray
U Supplement	**D** Lower Arm, Right			**B** Partial 2nd Ray
W Revision	**F** Lower Arm, Left			**C** Partial 3rd Ray
X Transfer	**G** Wrist Region, Right			**D** Partial 4th Ray
Y Transplantation	**H** Wrist Region, Left			**F** Partial 5th Ray
	J Hand, Right			**L** Thumb, Right
	K Hand, Left			**M** Thumb, Left
	L Thumb, Right			**N** Toe, Right
	M Thumb, Left			**P** Toe, Left
	N Index Finger, Right			**X** Diagnostic
	P Index Finger, Left			**Z** No Qualifier
	Q Middle Finger, Right			
	R Middle Finger, Left			
	S Ring Finger, Right			
	T Ring Finger, Left			
	V Little Finger, Right			
	W Little Finger, Left			

0: Medical and Surgical
Y: Anatomical Regions, Lower Extremities

Operation-Character 3	Body Part-Character 4	Approach-Character 5	Device-Character 6	Qualifier-Character 7
0 Alteration	**0** Buttock, Right	**0** Open	**0** Drainage Device	**0** Complete
2 Change	**1** Buttock, Left	**3** Percutaneous	**1** Radioactive Element	**1** High
3 Control	**2** Hindquarter, Right	**4** Percutaneous Endoscopic	**3** Infusion Device	**2** Mid
6 Detachment	**3** Hindquarter, Left	**X** External	**7** Autologous Tissue Substitute	**3** Low
9 Drainage	**4** Hindquarter, Bilateral		**J** Synthetic Substitute	**4** Complete 1st Ray
B Excision	**5** Inguinal Region, Right		**K** Nonautologous Tissue Substitute	**5** Complete 2nd Ray
H Insertion	**6** Inguinal Region, Left		**Y** Other Device	**6** Complete 3rd Ray
J Inspection	**7** Femoral Region, Right		**Z** No Device	**7** Complete 4th Ray
M Reattachment	**8** Femoral Region, Left			**8** Complete 5th Ray
P Removal	**9** Lower Extremity, Right			**9** Partial 1st Ray
Q Repair	**A** Inguinal Region, Bilateral			**B** Partial 2nd Ray
U Supplement	**B** Lower Extremity, Left			**C** Partial 3rd Ray
W Revision	**C** Upper Leg, Right			**D** Partial 4th Ray
	D Upper Leg, Left			**F** Partial 5th Ray
	E Femoral Region, Bilateral			**X** Diagnostic
	F Knee Region, Right			**Z** No Qualifier
	G Knee Region, Left			
	H Lower Leg, Right			
	J Lower Leg, Left			
	K Ankle Region, Right			
	L Ankle Region, Left			
	M Foot, Right			
	N Foot, Left			
	P 1st Toe, Right			
	Q 1st Toe, Left			
	R 2nd Toe, Right			
	S 2nd Toe, Left			
	T 3rd Toe, Right			
	U 3rd Toe, Left			
	V 4th Toe, Right			
	W 4th Toe, Left			
	X 5th Toe, Right			
	Y 5th Toe, Left			

1: Obstetrics
0: Pregnancy

Operation-Character 3	Body Part-Character 4	Approach-Character 5	Device-Character 6	Qualifier-Character 7
2 Change	**0** Products of Conception	**0** Open	**3** Monitoring Electrode	**0** Classical
9 Drainage	**1** Products of Conception, Retained	**3** Percutaneous	**Y** Other Device	**1** Low Cervical
A Abortion	**2** Products of Conception, Ectopic	**4** Percutaneous Endoscopic	**Z** No Device	**2** Extraperitoneal
D Extraction		**7** Via Natural or Artificial Opening		**3** Low Forceps
E Delivery		**8** Via Natural or Artificial Opening Endoscopic		**4** Mid Forceps
H Insertion		**X** External		**5** High Forceps
J Inspection				**6** Vacuum
P Removal				**7** Internal Version
Q Repair				**8** Other
S Reposition				**9** Fetal Blood
T Resection				**A** Fetal Cerebrospinal Fluid
Y Transplantation				**B** Fetal Fluid, Other
				C Amniotic Fluid, Therapeutic
				D Fluid, Other
				E Nervous System
				F Cardiovascular System
				G Lymphatics and Hemic
				H Eye
				J Ear, Nose and Sinus
				K Respiratory System
				L Mouth and Throat
				M Gastrointestinal System
				N Hepatobiliary and Pancreas
				P Endocrine System
				Q Skin
				R Musculoskeletal System
				S Urinary System
				T Female Reproductive System
				U Amniotic Fluid, Diagnostic
				V Male Reproductive System
				W Laminaria
				X Abortifacient
				Y Other Body System
				Z No Qualifier

2: Placement
W: Anatomical Regions

Operation-Character 3	Body Region-Character 4	Approach-Character 5	Device-Character 6	Qualifier-Character 7
0 Change	**0** Head	**X** External	**0** Traction Apparatus	**Z** No Qualifier
1 Compression	**1** Face		**1** Splint	
2 Dressing	**2** Neck		**2** Cast	
3 Immobilization	**3** Abdominal Wall		**3** Brace	
4 Packing	**4** Chest Wall		**4** Bandage	
5 Removal	**5** Back		**5** Packing Material	
6 Traction	**6** Inguinal Region, Right		**6** Pressure Dressing	
	7 Inguinal Region, Left		**7** Intermittent Pressure Device	
	8 Upper Extremity, Right		**9** Wire	
	9 Upper Extremity, Left		**Y** Other Device	
	A Upper Arm, Right		**Z** No Device	
	B Upper Arm, Left			
	C Lower Arm, Right			
	D Lower Arm, Left			
	E Hand, Right			
	F Hand, Left			
	G Thumb, Right			
	H Thumb, Left			
	J Finger, Right			
	K Finger, Left			
	L Lower Extremity, Right			
	M Lower Extremity, Left			
	N Upper Leg, Right			
	P Upper Leg, Left			
	Q Lower Leg, Right			
	R Lower Leg, Left			
	S Foot, Right			
	T Foot, Left			
	U Toe, Right			
	V Toe, Left			

2: Placement
Y: Anatomical Orifices

Operation-Character 3	Body Region-Character 4	Approach-Character 5	Device-Character 6	Qualifier-Character 7
0 Change	**0** Mouth and Pharynx	**X** External	**5** Packing Material	**Z** No Qualifier
4 Packing	**1** Nasal			
5 Removal	**2** Ear			
	3 Anorectal			
	4 Female Genital Tract			
	5 Urethra			

3: Administration
0: Circulatory

Operation-Character 3	Body System/ Region- Character 4	Approach-Character 5	Substance-Character 6	Qualifier-Character 7
2 Transfusion	**3** Peripheral Vein	**0** Open	**A** Stem Cells, Embryonic	**0** Autologous
	4 Central Vein	**3** Percutaneous	**B** 4-Factor Prothrombin Complex Concentrate	**1** Nonautologous
	5 Peripheral Artery	**7** Via Natural or Artificial Opening	**G** Bone Marrow	**2** Allogeneic, Related
	6 Central Artery		**H** Whole Blood	**3** Allogeneic, Unrelated
	7 Products of Conception, Circulatory		**J** Serum Albumin	**4** Allogeneic, Unspecified
	8 Vein		**K** Frozen Plasma	**Z** No Qualifier
			L Fresh Plasma	
			M Plasma Cryoprecipitate	
			N Red Blood Cells	
			P Frozen Red Cells	
			Q White Cells	
			R Platelets	
			S Globulin	
			T Fibrinogen	
			V Antihemophilic Factors	
			W Factor IX	
			X Stem Cells, Cord Blood	
			Y Stem Cells, Hematopoietic	

3: Administration
C: Indwelling Device

Operation-Character 3	Body System/ Region- Character 4	Approach-Character 5	Substance-Character 6	Qualifier-Character 7
1 Irrigation	**Z** None	**X** External	**8** Irrigating Substance	**Z** No Qualifier

3: Administration
E: Physiological Systems and Anatomical Regions

Operation-Character 3	Body System/ Region-Character 4	Approach-Character 5	Substance-Character 6	Qualifier-Character 7
0 Introduction	**0** Skin and Mucous Membranes	**0** Open	**0** Antineoplastic	**0** Autologous
1 Irrigation	**1** Subcutaneous Tissue	**3** Percutaneous	**1** Thrombolytic	**1** Nonautologous
	2 Muscle	**7** Via Natural or Artificial Opening	**2** Anti-infective	**2** High-dose Interleukin-2
	3 Peripheral Vein	**8** Via Natural or Artificial Opening Endoscopic	**3** Anti-inflammatory	**3** Low-dose Interleukin-2
	4 Central Vein	**X** External	**4** Serum, Toxoid and Vaccine	**4** Liquid Brachytherapy Radioisotope
	5 Peripheral Artery		**5** Adhesion Barrier	**5** Other Antineoplastic
	6 Central Artery		**6** Nutritional Substance	**6** Recombinant Human-activated Protein C
	7 Coronary Artery		**7** Electrolytic and Water Balance Substance	**7** Other Thrombolytic
	8 Heart		**8** Irrigating Substance	**8** Oxazolidinones
	9 Nose		**9** Dialysate	**9** Other Anti-infective
	A Bone Marrow		**A** Stem Cells, Embryonic	**A** Anti-Infective Envelope
	B Ear		**B** Local Anesthetic	**B** Recombinant Bone Morphogenetic Protein
	C Eye		**C** Regional Anesthetic	**C** Other Substance
	D Mouth and Pharynx		**D** Inhalation Anesthetic	**D** Nitric Oxide
	E Products of Conception		**E** Stem Cells, Somatic	**F** Other Gas
	F Respiratory Tract		**F** Intracirculatory Anesthetic	**G** Insulin
	G Upper GI		**G** Other Therapeutic Substance	**H** Human B-type Natriuretic Peptide
	H Lower GI		**H** Radioactive Substance	**J** Other Hormone
	J Biliary and Pancreatic Tract		**K** Other Diagnostic Substance	**K** Immunostimulator
	K Genitourinary Tract		**L** Sperm	**L** Immunosuppressive
	L Pleural Cavity		**M** Pigment	**M** Monoclonal Antibody
	M Peritoneal Cavity		**N** Analgesics, Hypnotics, Sedatives	**N** Blood Brain Barrier Disruption
	N Male Reproductive		**P** Platelet Inhibitor	**P** Clofarabine
	P Female Reproductive		**Q** Fertilized Ovum	**Q** Glucarpidase
	Q Cranial Cavity and Brain		**R** Antiarrhythmic	**X** Diagnostic
	R Spinal Canal		**S** Gas	**Z** No Qualifier
	S Epidural Space		**T** Destructive Agent	
	T Peripheral Nerves and Plexi		**U** Pancreatic Islet Cells	
	U Joints		**V** Hormone	
	V Bones		**W** Immunotherapeutic	
	W Lymphatics		**X** Vasopressor	
	X Cranial Nerves			
	Y Pericardial Cavity			

4: Measurement and Monitoring
A: Physiological Systems

Operation-Character 3	Body System-Character 4	Approach-Character 5	Function/ Device-Character 6	Qualifier-Character 7
0 Measurement	**0** Central Nervous	**0** Open	**0** Acuity	**0** Central
1 Monitoring	**1** Peripheral Nervous	**3** Percutaneous	**1** Capacity	**1** Peripheral
	2 Cardiac	**4** Percutaneous Endoscopic	**2** Conductivity	**2** Portal
	3 Arterial	**7** Via Natural or Artificial Opening	**3** Contractility	**3** Pulmonary
	4 Venous	**8** Via Natural or Artificial Opening Endoscopic	**4** Electrical Activity	**4** Stress
	5 Circulatory	**X** External	**5** Flow	**5** Ambulatory
	6 Lymphatic		**6** Metabolism	**6** Right Heart
	7 Visual		**7** Mobility	**7** Left Heart
	8 Olfactory		**8** Motility	**8** Bilateral
	9 Respiratory		**9** Output	**9** Sensory
	B Gastrointestinal		**B** Pressure	**A** Guidance
	C Biliary		**C** Rate	**B** Motor
	D Urinary		**D** Resistance	**C** Coronary
	F Musculoskeletal		**F** Rhythm	**D** Intracranial
	G Skin and Breast		**G** Secretion	**F** Other Thoracic
	H Products of Conception, Cardiac		**H** Sound	**G** Intraoperative
	J Products of Conception, Nervous		**J** Pulse	**H** Indocyanine Green Dye
	Z None		**K** Temperature	**Z** No Qualifier
			L Volume	
			M Total Activity	
			N Sampling and Pressure	
			P Action Currents	
			Q Sleep	
			R Saturation	
			S Vascular Perfusion	

4: Measurement and Monitoring
B: Physiological Devices

Operation-Character 3	Body System-Character 4	Approach-Character 5	Function/ Device-Character 6	Qualifier-Character 7
0 Measurement	**0** Central Nervous	**X** External	**S** Pacemaker	**Z** No Qualifier
	1 Peripheral Nervous		**T** Defibrillator	
	2 Cardiac		**V** Stimulator	
	9 Respiratory			
	F Musculoskeletal			

5: Extracorporeal Assistance and Performance
A: Physiological Systems

Operation-Character 3	Body System-Character 4	Duration-Character 5	Function-Character 6	Qualifier-Character 7
0 Assistance	**2** Cardiac	**0** Single	**0** Filtration	**0** Balloon Pump
1 Performance	**5** Circulatory	**1** Intermittent	**1** Output	**1** Hyperbaric
2 Restoration	**9** Respiratory	**2** Continuous	**2** Oxygenation	**2** Manual
	C Biliary	**3** Less than 24 Consecutive Hours	**3** Pacing	**3** Membrane
	D Urinary	**4** 24-96 Consecutive Hours	**4** Rhythm	**4** Nonmechanical
		5 Greater than 96 Consecutive Hours	**5** Ventilation	**5** Pulsatile Compression
		6 Multiple		**6** Other Pump
				7 Continuous Positive Airway Pressure
				8 Intermittent Positive Airway Pressure
				9 Continuous Negative Airway Pressure
				B Intermittent Negative Airway Pressure
				C Supersaturated
				D Impeller Pump
				Z No Qualifier

6: Extracorporeal Therapies
A: Physiological Systems

Operation-Character 3	Body System-Character 4	Duration-Character 5	Qualifier-Character 6	Qualifier-Character 7
0 Atmospheric Control	**0** Skin	**0** Single	**B** Donor Organ	**0** Erythrocytes
1 Decompression	**1** Urinary	**1** Multiple	**Z** No Qualifier	**1** Leukocytes
2 Electromagnetic Therapy	**2** Central Nervous			**2** Platelets
3 Hyperthermia	**3** Musculoskeletal			**3** Plasma
4 Hypothermia	**5** Circulatory			**4** Head and Neck Vessels
5 Pheresis	**B** Respiratory System			**5** Heart
6 Phototherapy	**F** Hepatobiliary System and Pancreas			**6** Peripheral Vessels
7 Ultrasound Therapy	**T** Urinary System			**7** Other Vessels
8 Ultraviolet Light Therapy	**Z** None			**T** Stem Cells, Cord Blood
9 Shock Wave Therapy				**V** Stem Cells, Hematopoietic
B Perfusion				**Z** No Qualifier

7: Osteopathic
W: Anatomical Regions

Operation-Character 3	Body Region-Character 4	Approach-Character 5	Method-Character 6	Qualifier-Character 7
0 Treatment	**0** Head	**X** External	**0** Articulatory-Raising	**Z** None
	1 Cervical		**1** Fascial Release	
	2 Thoracic		**2** General Mobilization	
	3 Lumbar		**3** High Velocity-Low Amplitude	
	4 Sacrum		**4** Indirect	
	5 Pelvis		**5** Low Velocity-High Amplitude	
	6 Lower Extremities		**6** Lymphatic Pump	
	7 Upper Extremities		**7** Muscle Energy-Isometric	
	8 Rib Cage		**8** Muscle Energy-Isotonic	
	9 Abdomen		**9** Other Method	

8: Other Procedures
C: Indwelling Device

Operation-Character 3	Body Region-Character 4	Approach-Character 5	Method-Character 6	Qualifier-Character 7
0 Other Procedures	**1** Nervous System	**X** External	**6** Collection	**J** Cerebrospinal Fluid
	2 Circulatory System			**K** Blood
				L Other Fluid

8: Other Procedures
E: Physiological Systems and Anatomical Regions

Operation-Character 3	Body Region-Character 4	Approach-Character 5	Method-Character 6	Qualifier-Character 7
0 Other Procedures	**1** Nervous System	**0** Open	**0** Acupuncture	**0** Anesthesia
	2 Circulatory System	**3** Percutaneous	**1** Therapeutic Massage	**1** In Vitro Fertilization
	9 Head and Neck Region	**4** Percutaneous Endoscopic	**6** Collection	**2** Breast Milk
	H Integumentary System and Breast	**7** Via Natural or Artificial Opening	**B** Computer Assisted Procedure	**3** Sperm
	K Musculoskeletal System	**8** Via Natural or Artificial Opening Endoscopic	**C** Robotic Assisted Procedure	**4** Yoga Therapy
	U Female Reproductive System	**X** External	**D** Near Infrared Spectroscopy	**5** Meditation
	V Male Reproductive System		**Y** Other Method	**6** Isolation
	W Trunk Region			**7** Examination
	X Upper Extremity			**8** Suture Removal
	Y Lower Extremity			**9** Piercing
	Z None			**C** Prostate
				D Rectum
				F With Fluoroscopy
				G With Computerized Tomography
				H With Magnetic Resonance Imaging
				Z No Qualifier

9: Chiropractic
W: Anatomical Regions

Operation-Character 3	Body Region-Character 4	Approach-Character 5	Method-Character 6	Qualifier-Character 7
B Manipulation	**0** Head	**X** External	**B** Non-Manual	**Z** None
	1 Cervical		**C** Indirect Visceral	
	2 Thoracic		**D** Extra-Articular	
	3 Lumbar		**F** Direct Visceral	
	4 Sacrum		**G** Long Lever Specific Contact	
	5 Pelvis		**H** Short Lever Specific Contact	
	6 Lower Extremities		**J** Long and Short Lever Specific Contact	
	7 Upper Extremities		**K** Mechanically Assisted	
	8 Rib Cage		**L** Other Method	
	9 Abdomen			

B: Imaging
0: Central Nervous System

Type-Character 3	Body Part-Character 4	Contrast-Character 5	Qualifier-Character 6	Qualifier-Character 7
0 Plain Radiography	**0** Brain	**0** High Osmolar	**0** Unenhanced and Enhanced	**Z** None
1 Fluoroscopy	**7** Cisterna	**1** Low Osmolar	**Z** None	
2 Computerized Tomography (CT Scan)	**8** Cerebral Ventricle(s)	**Y** Other Contrast		
3 Magnetic Resonance Imaging (MRI)	**9** Sella Turcica/Pituitary Gland	**Z** None		
4 Ultrasonography	**B** Spinal Cord			
	C Acoustic Nerves			

B: Imaging
2: Heart

Type-Character 3	Body Part-Character 4	Contrast-Character 5	Qualifier-Character 6	Qualifier-Character 7
0 Plain Radiography	**0** Coronary Artery, Single	**0** High Osmolar	**0** Unenhanced and Enhanced	**0** Intraoperative
1 Fluoroscopy	**1** Coronary Arteries, Multiple	**1** Low Osmolar	**1** Laser	**3** Intravascular
2 Computerized Tomography (CT Scan)	**2** Coronary Artery Bypass Graft, Single	**Y** Other Contrast	**2** Intravascular Optical Coherence	**4** Transesophageal
3 Magnetic Resonance Imaging (MRI)	**3** Coronary Artery Bypass Grafts, Multiple	**Z** None	**Z** None	**Z** None
4 Ultrasonography	**4** Heart, Right			
	5 Heart, Left			
	6 Heart, Right and Left			
	7 Internal Mammary Bypass Graft, Right			
	8 Internal Mammary Bypass Graft, Left			
	B Heart with Aorta			
	C Pericardium			
	D Pediatric Heart			
	F Bypass Graft, Other			

B: Imaging
3: Upper Arteries

Type-Character 3	Body Part-Character 4	Contrast-Character 5	Qualifier-Character 6	Qualifier-Character 7
0 Plain Radiography	**0** Thoracic Aorta	**0** High Osmolar	**0** Unenhanced and Enhanced	**0** Intraoperative
1 Fluoroscopy	**1** Brachiocephalic-Subclavian Artery, Right	**1** Low Osmolar	**1** Laser	**3** Intravascular
2 Computerized Tomography (CT Scan)	**2** Subclavian Artery, Left	**Y** Other Contrast	**2** Intravascular Optical Coherence	**Z** None
3 Magnetic Resonance Imaging (MRI)	**3** Common Carotid Artery, Right	**Z** None	**Z** None	
4 Ultrasonography	**4** Common Carotid Artery, Left			
	5 Common Carotid Arteries, Bilateral			
	6 Internal Carotid Artery, Right			
	7 Internal Carotid Artery, Left			
	8 Internal Carotid Arteries, Bilateral			
	9 External Carotid Artery, Right			
	B External Carotid Artery, Left			
	C External Carotid Arteries, Bilateral			
	D Vertebral Artery, Right			
	F Vertebral Artery, Left			
	G Vertebral Arteries, Bilateral			
	H Upper Extremity Arteries, Right			
	J Upper Extremity Arteries, Left			
	K Upper Extremity Arteries, Bilateral			
	L Intercostal and Bronchial Arteries			
	M Spinal Arteries			
	N Upper Arteries, Other			
	P Thoraco-Abdominal Aorta			
	Q Cervico-Cerebral Arch			
	R Intracranial Arteries			
	S Pulmonary Artery, Right			
	T Pulmonary Artery, Left			
	V Ophthalmic Arteries			

B: Imaging
4: Lower Arteries

Type-Character 3	Body Part-Character 4	Contrast-Character 5	Qualifier-Character 6	Qualifier-Character 7
0 Plain Radiography	**0** Abdominal Aorta	**0** High Osmolar	**0** Unenhanced and Enhanced	**0** Intraoperative
1 Fluoroscopy	**1** Celiac Artery	**1** Low Osmolar	**1** Laser	**3** Intravascular
2 Computerized Tomography (CT Scan)	**2** Hepatic Artery	**Y** Other Contrast	**2** Intravascular Optical Coherence	**Z** None
3 Magnetic Resonance Imaging (MRI)	**3** Splenic Arteries	**Z** None	**Z** None	
4 Ultrasonography	**4** Superior Mesenteric Artery			
	5 Inferior Mesenteric Artery			
	6 Renal Artery, Right			
	7 Renal Artery, Left			
	8 Renal Arteries, Bilateral			
	9 Lumbar Arteries			
	B Intra-Abdominal Arteries, Other			
	C Pelvic Arteries			
	D Aorta and Bilateral Lower Extremity Arteries			
	F Lower Extremity Arteries, Right			
	G Lower Extremity Arteries, Left			
	H Lower Extremity Arteries, Bilateral			
	J Lower Arteries, Other			
	K Celiac and Mesenteric Arteries			
	L Femoral Artery			
	M Renal Artery Transplant			
	N Penile Arteries			

B: Imaging
5: Veins

Type-Character 3	Body Part-Character 4	Contrast-Character 5	Qualifier-Character 6	Qualifier-Character 7
0 Plain Radiography	**0** Epidural Veins	**0** High Osmolar	**0** Unenhanced and Enhanced	**3** Intravascular
1 Fluoroscopy	**1** Cerebral and Cerebellar Veins	**1** Low Osmolar	**2** Intravascular Optical Coherence	**A** Guidance
2 Computerized Tomography (CT Scan)	**2** Intracranial Sinuses	**Y** Other Contrast	**Z** None	**Z** None
3 Magnetic Resonance Imaging (MRI)	**3** Jugular Veins, Right	**Z** None		
4 Ultrasonography	**4** Jugular Veins, Left			
	5 Jugular Veins, Bilateral			
	6 Subclavian Vein, Right			
	7 Subclavian Vein, Left			
	8 Superior Vena Cava			
	9 Inferior Vena Cava			
	B Lower Extremity Veins, Right			
	C Lower Extremity Veins, Left			
	D Lower Extremity Veins, Bilateral			
	F Pelvic (Iliac) Veins, Right			
	G Pelvic (Iliac) Veins, Left			
	H Pelvic (Iliac) Veins, Bilateral			
	J Renal Vein, Right			
	K Renal Vein, Left			
	L Renal Veins, Bilateral			
	M Upper Extremity Veins, Right			
	N Upper Extremity Veins, Left			
	P Upper Extremity Veins, Bilateral			
	Q Pulmonary Vein, Right			
	R Pulmonary Vein, Left			
	S Pulmonary Veins, Bilateral			
	T Portal and Splanchnic Veins			
	V Veins, Other			
	W Dialysis Shunt/Fistula			

B: Imaging
7: Lymphatic System

Type-Character 3	Body Part-Character 4	Contrast-Character 5	Qualifier-Character 6	Qualifier-Character 7
0 Plain Radiography	**0** Abdominal/Retroperitoneal Lymphatics, Unilateral	**0** High Osmolar	**Z** None	**Z** None
	1 Abdominal/Retroperitoneal Lymphatics, Bilateral	**1** Low Osmolar		
	4 Lymphatics, Head and Neck	**Y** Other Contrast		
	5 Upper Extremity Lymphatics, Right			
	6 Upper Extremity Lymphatics, Left			
	7 Upper Extremity Lymphatics, Bilateral			
	8 Lower Extremity Lymphatics, Right			
	9 Lower Extremity Lymphatics, Left			
	B Lower Extremity Lymphatics, Bilateral			
	C Lymphatics, Pelvic			

B: Imaging
8: Eye

Type-Character 3	Body Part-Character 4	Contrast-Character 5	Qualifier-Character 6	Qualifier-Character 7
0 Plain Radiography	**0** Lacrimal Duct, Right	**0** High Osmolar	**0** Unenhanced and Enhanced	**Z** None
2 Computerized Tomography (CT Scan)	**1** Lacrimal Duct, Left	**1** Low Osmolar	**Z** None	
3 Magnetic Resonance Imaging (MRI)	**2** Lacrimal Ducts, Bilateral	**Y** Other Contrast		
4 Ultrasonography	**3** Optic Foramina, Right	**Z** None		
	4 Optic Foramina, Left			
	5 Eye, Right			
	6 Eye, Left			
	7 Eyes, Bilateral			

B: Imaging
9: Ear, Nose, Mouth and Throat

Type-Character 3	Body Part-Character 4	Contrast-Character 5	Qualifier-Character 6	Qualifier-Character 7
0 Plain Radiography	**0** Ear	**0** High Osmolar	**0** Unenhanced and Enhanced	**Z** None
1 Fluoroscopy	**2** Paranasal Sinuses	**1** Low Osmolar	**Z** None	
2 Computerized Tomography (CT Scan)	**4** Parotid Gland, Right	**Y** Other Contrast		
3 Magnetic Resonance Imaging (MRI)	**5** Parotid Gland, Left	**Z** None		
	6 Parotid Glands, Bilateral			
	7 Submandibular Gland, Right			
	8 Submandibular Gland, Left			
	9 Submandibular Glands, Bilateral			
	B Salivary Gland, Right			
	C Salivary Gland, Left			
	D Salivary Glands, Bilateral			
	F Nasopharynx/Oropharynx			
	G Pharynx and Epiglottis			
	H Mastoids			
	J Larynx			

B: Imaging
B: Respiratory System

Type-Character 3	Body Part-Character 4	Contrast-Character 5	Qualifier-Character 6	Qualifier-Character 7
0 Plain Radiography	**2** Lung, Right	**0** High Osmolar	**0** Unenhanced and Enhanced	**Z** None
1 Fluoroscopy	**3** Lung, Left	**1** Low Osmolar	**Z** None	
2 Computerized Tomography (CT Scan)	**4** Lungs, Bilateral	**Y** Other Contrast		
3 Magnetic Resonance Imaging (MRI)	**6** Diaphragm	**Z** None		
4 Ultrasonography	**7** Tracheobronchial Tree, Right			
	8 Tracheobronchial Tree, Left			
	9 Tracheobronchial Trees, Bilateral			
	B Pleura			
	C Mediastinum			
	D Upper Airways			
	F Trachea/Airways			
	G Lung Apices			

B: Imaging
D: Gastrointestinal System

Type-Character 3	Body Part-Character 4	Contrast-Character 5	Qualifier-Character 6	Qualifier-Character 7
1 Fluoroscopy	**1** Esophagus	**0** High Osmolar	**0** Unenhanced and Enhanced	**Z** None
2 Computerized Tomography (CT Scan)	**2** Stomach	**1** Low Osmolar	**Z** None	
4 Ultrasonography	**3** Small Bowel	**Y** Other Contrast		
	4 Colon	**Z** None		
	5 Upper GI			
	6 Upper GI and Small Bowel			
	7 Gastrointestinal Tract			
	8 Appendix			
	9 Duodenum			
	B Mouth/Oropharynx			
	C Rectum			

B: Imaging
F: Hepatobiliary System and Pancreas

Type-Character 3	Body Part-Character 4	Contrast-Character 5	Qualifier-Character 6	Qualifier-Character 7
0 Plain Radiography	**0** Bile Ducts	**0** High Osmolar	**0** Unenhanced and Enhanced	**Z** None
1 Fluoroscopy	**1** Biliary and Pancreatic Ducts	**1** Low Osmolar	**Z** None	
2 Computerized Tomography (CT Scan)	**2** Gallbladder	**Y** Other Contrast		
3 Magnetic Resonance Imaging (MRI)	**3** Gallbladder and Bile Ducts	**Z** None		
4 Ultrasonography	**4** Gallbladder, Bile Ducts and Pancreatic Ducts			
	5 Liver			
	6 Liver and Spleen			
	7 Pancreas			
	8 Pancreatic Ducts			
	C Hepatobiliary System, All			

B: Imaging
G: Endocrine System

Type-Character 3	Body Part-Character 4	Contrast-Character 5	Qualifier-Character 6	Qualifier-Character 7
2 Computerized Tomography (CT Scan)	**0** Adrenal Gland, Right	**0** High Osmolar	**0** Unenhanced and Enhanced	**Z** None
3 Magnetic Resonance Imaging (MRI)	**1** Adrenal Gland, Left	**1** Low Osmolar	**Z** None	
4 Ultrasonography	**2** Adrenal Glands, Bilateral	**Y** Other Contrast		
	3 Parathyroid Glands	**Z** None		
	4 Thyroid Gland			

B: Imaging
H: Skin, Subcutaneous Tissue and Breast

Type-Character 3	Body Part-Character 4	Contrast-Character 5	Qualifier-Character 6	Qualifier-Character 7
0 Plain Radiography	**0** Breast, Right	**0** High Osmolar	**0** Unenhanced and Enhanced	**Z** None
3 Magnetic Resonance Imaging (MRI)	**1** Breast, Left	**1** Low Osmolar	**Z** None	
4 Ultrasonography	**2** Breasts, Bilateral	**Y** Other Contrast		
	3 Single Mammary Duct, Right	**Z** None		
	4 Single Mammary Duct, Left			
	5 Multiple Mammary Ducts, Right			
	6 Multiple Mammary Ducts, Left			
	7 Extremity, Upper			
	8 Extremity, Lower			
	9 Abdominal Wall			
	B Chest Wall			
	C Head and Neck			
	D Subcutaneous Tissue, Head/Neck			
	F Subcutaneous Tissue, Upper Extremity			
	G Subcutaneous Tissue, Thorax			
	H Subcutaneous Tissue, Abdomen and Pelvis			
	J Subcutaneous Tissue, Lower Extremity			

B: Imaging
L: Connective Tissue

Type-Character 3	Body Part-Character 4	Contrast-Character 5	Qualifier-Character 6	Qualifier-Character 7
3 Magnetic Resonance Imaging (MRI)	**0** Connective Tissue, Upper Extremity	**Y** Other Contrast	**0** Unenhanced and Enhanced	**Z** None
4 Ultrasonography	**1** Connective Tissue, Lower Extremity	**Z** None	**Z** None	
	2 Tendons, Upper Extremity			
	3 Tendons, Lower Extremity			

B: Imaging
N: Skull and Facial Bones

Type-Character 3	Body Part-Character 4	Contrast-Character 5	Qualifier-Character 6	Qualifier-Character 7
0 Plain Radiography	**0** Skull	**0** High Osmolar	**Z** None	**Z** None
1 Fluoroscopy	**1** Orbit, Right	**1** Low Osmolar		
2 Computerized Tomography (CT Scan)	**2** Orbit, Left	**Y** Other Contrast		
3 Magnetic Resonance Imaging (MRI)	**3** Orbits, Bilateral	**Z** None		
	4 Nasal Bones			
	5 Facial Bones			
	6 Mandible			
	7 Temporomandibular Joint, Right			
	8 Temporomandibular Joint, Left			
	9 Temporomandibular Joints, Bilateral			
	B Zygomatic Arch, Right			
	C Zygomatic Arch, Left			
	D Zygomatic Arches, Bilateral			
	F Temporal Bones			
	G Tooth, Single			
	H Teeth, Multiple			
	J Teeth, All			

B: Imaging
P: Non-Axial Upper Bones

Type-Character 3	Body Part-Character 4	Contrast-Character 5	Qualifier-Character 6	Qualifier-Character 7
0 Plain Radiography	**0** Sternoclavicular Joint, Right	**0** High Osmolar	**0** Unenhanced and Enhanced	**1** Densitometry
1 Fluoroscopy	**1** Sternoclavicular Joint, Left	**1** Low Osmolar	**Z** None	**Z** None
2 Computerized Tomography (CT Scan)	**2** Sternoclavicular Joints, Bilateral	**Y** Other Contrast		
3 Magnetic Resonance Imaging (MRI)	**3** Acromioclavicular Joints, Bilateral	**Z** None		
4 Ultrasonography	**4** Clavicle, Right			
	5 Clavicle, Left			
	6 Scapula, Right			
	7 Scapula, Left			
	8 Shoulder, Right			
	9 Shoulder, Left			
	A Humerus, Right			
	B Humerus, Left			
	C Hand/Finger Joint, Right			
	D Hand/Finger Joint, Left			
	E Upper Arm, Right			
	F Upper Arm, Left			
	G Elbow, Right			
	H Elbow, Left			
	J Forearm, Right			
	K Forearm, Left			
	L Wrist, Right			
	M Wrist, Left			
	N Hand, Right			
	P Hand, Left			
	Q Hands and Wrists, Bilateral			
	R Finger(s), Right			
	S Finger(s), Left			
	T Upper Extremity, Right			
	U Upper Extremity, Left			
	V Upper Extremities, Bilateral			
	W Thorax			
	X Ribs, Right			
	Y Ribs, Left			

B: Imaging
Q: Non-Axial Lower Bones

Type-Character 3	Body Part-Character 4	Contrast-Character 5	Qualifier-Character 6	Qualifier-Character 7
0 Plain Radiography	**0** Hip, Right	**0** High Osmolar	**0** Unenhanced and Enhanced	**1** Densitometry
1 Fluoroscopy	**1** Hip, Left	**1** Low Osmolar	**Z** None	**Z** None
2 Computerized Tomography (CT Scan)	**2** Hips, Bilateral	**Y** Other Contrast		
3 Magnetic Resonance Imaging (MRI)	**3** Femur, Right	**Z** None		
4 Ultrasonography	**4** Femur, Left			
	7 Knee, Right			
	8 Knee, Left			
	9 Knees, Bilateral			
	B Tibia/Fibula, Right			
	C Tibia/Fibula, Left			
	D Lower Leg, Right			
	F Lower Leg, Left			
	G Ankle, Right			
	H Ankle, Left			
	J Calcaneus, Right			
	K Calcaneus, Left			
	L Foot, Right			
	M Foot, Left			
	P Toe(s), Right			
	Q Toe(s), Left			
	R Lower Extremity, Right			
	S Lower Extremity, Left			
	V Patella, Right			
	W Patella, Left			
	X Foot/Toe Joint, Right			
	Y Foot/Toe Joint, Left			

B: Imaging
R: Axial Skeleton, Except Skull and Facial Bones

Type-Character 3	Body Part-Character 4	Contrast-Character 5	Qualifier-Character 6	Qualifier-Character 7
0 Plain Radiography	**0** Cervical Spine	**0** High Osmolar	**0** Unenhanced and Enhanced	**1** Densitometry
1 Fluoroscopy	**1** Cervical Disc(s)	**1** Low Osmolar	**Z** None	**Z** None
2 Computerized Tomography (CT Scan)	**2** Thoracic Disc(s)	**Y** Other Contrast		
3 Magnetic Resonance Imaging (MRI)	**3** Lumbar Disc(s)	**Z** None		
4 Ultrasonography	**4** Cervical Facet Joint(s)			
	5 Thoracic Facet Joint(s)			
	6 Lumbar Facet Joint(s)			
	7 Thoracic Spine			
	8 Thoracolumbar Joint			
	9 Lumbar Spine			
	B Lumbosacral Joint			
	C Pelvis			
	D Sacroiliac Joints			
	F Sacrum and Coccyx			
	G Whole Spine			
	H Sternum			

B: Imaging
T: Urinary System

Type-Character 3	Body Part-Character 4	Contrast-Character 5	Qualifier-Character 6	Qualifier-Character 7
0 Plain Radiography	**0** Bladder	**0** High Osmolar	**0** Unenhanced and Enhanced	**Z** None
1 Fluoroscopy	**1** Kidney, Right	**1** Low Osmolar	**Z** None	
2 Computerized Tomography (CT Scan)	**2** Kidney, Left	**Y** Other Contrast		
3 Magnetic Resonance Imaging (MRI)	**3** Kidneys, Bilateral	**Z** None		
4 Ultrasonography	**4** Kidneys, Ureters and Bladder			
	5 Urethra			
	6 Ureter, Right			
	7 Ureter, Left			
	8 Ureters, Bilateral			
	9 Kidney Transplant			
	B Bladder and Urethra			
	C Ileal Diversion Loop			
	D Kidney, Ureter and Bladder, Right			
	F Kidney, Ureter and Bladder, Left			
	G Ileal Loop, Ureters and Kidneys			
	J Kidneys and Bladder			

B: Imaging
U: Female Reproductive System

Type-Character 3	Body Part-Character 4	Contrast-Character 5	Qualifier-Character 6	Qualifier-Character 7
0 Plain Radiography	**0** Fallopian Tube, Right	**0** High Osmolar	**0** Unenhanced and Enhanced	**Z** None
1 Fluoroscopy	**1** Fallopian Tube, Left	**1** Low Osmolar	**Z** None	
3 Magnetic Resonance Imaging (MRI)	**2** Fallopian Tubes, Bilateral	**Y** Other Contrast		
4 Ultrasonography	**3** Ovary, Right	**Z** None		
	4 Ovary, Left			
	5 Ovaries, Bilateral			
	6 Uterus			
	8 Uterus and Fallopian Tubes			
	9 Vagina			
	B Pregnant Uterus			
	C Uterus and Ovaries			

B: Imaging
V: Male Reproductive System

Type-Character 3	Body Part-Character 4	Contrast-Character 5	Qualifier-Character 6	Qualifier-Character 7
0 Plain Radiography	**0** Corpora Cavernosa	**0** High Osmolar	**0** Unenhanced and Enhanced	**Z** None
1 Fluoroscopy	**1** Epididymis, Right	**1** Low Osmolar	**Z** None	
2 Computerized Tomography (CT Scan)	**2** Epididymis, Left	**Y** Other Contrast		
3 Magnetic Resonance Imaging (MRI)	**3** Prostate	**Z** None		
4 Ultrasonography	**4** Scrotum			
	5 Testicle, Right			
	6 Testicle, Left			
	7 Testicles, Bilateral			
	8 Vasa Vasorum			
	9 Prostate and Seminal Vesicles			
	B Penis			

B: Imaging
W: Anatomical Regions

Type-Character 3	Body Part-Character 4	Contrast-Character 5	Qualifier-Character 6	Qualifier-Character 7
0 Plain Radiography	**0** Abdomen	**0** High Osmolar	**0** Unenhanced and Enhanced	**Z** None
1 Fluoroscopy	**1** Abdomen and Pelvis	**1** Low Osmolar	**Z** None	
2 Computerized Tomography (CT Scan)	**3** Chest	**Y** Other Contrast		
3 Magnetic Resonance Imaging (MRI)	**4** Chest and Abdomen	**Z** None		
4 Ultrasonography	**5** Chest, Abdomen and Pelvis			
	8 Head			
	9 Head and Neck			
	B Long Bones, All			
	C Lower Extremity			
	F Neck			
	G Pelvic Region			
	H Retroperitoneum			
	J Upper Extremity			
	K Whole Body			
	L Whole Skeleton			
	M Whole Body, Infant			
	P Brachial Plexus			

B: Imaging
Y: Fetus and Obstetrical

Type-Character 3	Body Part-Character 4	Contrast-Character 5	Qualifier-Character 6	Qualifier-Character 7
3 Magnetic Resonance Imaging (MRI)	**0** Fetal Head	**Y** Other Contrast	**0** Unenhanced and Enhanced	**Z** None
4 Ultrasonography	**1** Fetal Heart	**Z** None	**Z** None	
	2 Fetal Thorax			
	3 Fetal Abdomen			
	4 Fetal Spine			
	5 Fetal Extremities			
	6 Whole Fetus			
	7 Fetal Umbilical Cord			
	8 Placenta			
	9 First Trimester, Single Fetus			
	B First Trimester, Multiple Gestation			
	C Second Trimester, Single Fetus			
	D Second Trimester, Multiple Gestation			
	F Third Trimester, Single Fetus			
	G Third Trimester, Multiple Gestation			

C: Nuclear Medicine
0: Central Nervous System

Type-Character 3	Body Part-Character 4	Radionuclide-Character 5	Qualifier-Character 6	Qualifier-Character 7
1 Planar Nuclear Medicine Imaging	**0** Brain	**1** Technetium 99m (Tc-99m)	**Z** None	**Z** None
2 Tomographic (Tomo) Nuclear Medicine Imaging	**5** Cerebrospinal Fluid	**B** Carbon 11 (C-11)		
3 Positron Emission Tomographic (PET) Imaging	**Y** Central Nervous System	**D** Indium 111 (In-111)		
5 Nonimaging Nuclear Medicine Probe		**F** Iodine 123 (I-123)		
		K Fluorine 18 (F-18)		
		M Oxygen 15 (O-15)		
		S Thallium 201 (Tl-201)		
		V Xenon 133 (Xe-133)		
		Y Other Radionuclide		

C: Nuclear Medicine
2: Heart

Type-Character 3	Body Part-Character 4	Radionuclide-Character 5	Qualifier-Character 6	Qualifier-Character 7
1 Planar Nuclear Medicine Imaging	**6** Heart, Right and Left	**1** Technetium 99m (Tc-99m)	**Z** None	**Z** None
2 Tomographic (Tomo) Nuclear Medicine Imaging	**G** Myocardium	**D** Indium 111 (In-111)		
3 Positron Emission Tomographic (PET) Imaging	**Y** Heart	**K** Fluorine 18 (F-18)		
5 Nonimaging Nuclear Medicine Probe		**M** Oxygen 15 (O-15)		
		Q Rubidium 82 (Rb-82)		
		R Nitrogen 13 (N-13)		
		S Thallium 201 (Tl-201)		
		Y Other Radionuclide		
		Z None		

C: Nuclear Medicine
5: Veins

Type-Character 3	Body Part-Character 4	Radionuclide-Character 5	Qualifier-Character 6	Qualifier-Character 7
1 Planar Nuclear Medicine Imaging	**B** Lower Extremity Veins, Right	**1** Technetium 99m (Tc-99m)	**Z** None	**Z** None
	C Lower Extremity Veins, Left	**Y** Other Radionuclide		
	D Lower Extremity Veins, Bilateral			
	N Upper Extremity Veins, Right			
	P Upper Extremity Veins, Left			
	Q Upper Extremity Veins, Bilateral			
	R Central Veins			
	Y Veins			

C: Nuclear Medicine
7: Lymphatic and Hematologic System

Type-Character 3	Body Part-Character 4	Radionuclide-Character 5	Qualifier-Character 6	Qualifier-Character 7
1 Planar Nuclear Medicine Imaging	**0** Bone Marrow	**1** Technetium 99m (Tc-99m)	**Z** None	**Z** None
2 Tomographic (Tomo) Nuclear Medicine Imaging	**2** Spleen	**7** Cobalt 58 (Co-58)		
5 Nonimaging Nuclear Medicine Probe	**3** Blood	**C** Cobalt 57 (Co-57)		
6 Nonimaging Nuclear Medicine Assay	**5** Lymphatics, Head and Neck	**D** Indium 111 (In-111)		
	D Lymphatics, Pelvic	**H** Iodine 125 (I-125)		
	J Lymphatics, Head	**W** Chromium (Cr-51)		
	K Lymphatics, Neck	**Y** Other Radionuclide		
	L Lymphatics, Upper Chest			
	M Lymphatics, Trunk			
	N Lymphatics, Upper Extremity			
	P Lymphatics, Lower Extremity			
	Y Lymphatic and Hematologic System			

C: Nuclear Medicine
8: Eye

Type-Character 3	Body Part-Character 4	Radionuclide-Character 5	Qualifier-Character 6	Qualifier-Character 7
1 Planar Nuclear Medicine Imaging	**9** Lacrimal Ducts, Bilateral	**1** Technetium 99m (Tc-99m)	**Z** None	**Z** None
	Y Eye	**Y** Other Radionuclide		

C: Nuclear Medicine
9: Ear, Nose, Mouth and Throat

Type-Character 3	Body Part-Character 4	Radionuclide-Character 5	Qualifier-Character 6	Qualifier-Character 7
1 Planar Nuclear Medicine Imaging	**B** Salivary Glands, Bilateral	**1** Technetium 99m (Tc-99m)	**Z** None	**Z** None
	Y Ear, Nose, Mouth and Throat	**Y** Other Radionuclide		

C: Nuclear Medicine
B: Respiratory System

Type-Character 3	Body Part-Character 4	Radionuclide-Character 5	Qualifier-Character 6	Qualifier-Character 7
1 Planar Nuclear Medicine Imaging	**2** Lungs and Bronchi	**1** Technetium 99m (Tc-99m)	**Z** None	**Z** None
2 Tomographic (Tomo) Nuclear Medicine Imaging	**Y** Respiratory System	**9** Krypton (Kr-81m)		
3 Positron Emission Tomographic (PET) Imaging		**K** Fluorine 18 (F-18)		
		T Xenon 127 (Xe-127)		
		V Xenon 133 (Xe-133)		
		Y Other Radionuclide		

C: Nuclear Medicine
D: Gastrointestinal System

Type-Character 3	Body Part-Character 4	Radionuclide-Character 5	Qualifier-Character 6	Qualifier-Character 7
1 Planar Nuclear Medicine Imaging	**5** Upper Gastrointestinal Tract	**1** Technetium 99m (Tc-99m)	**Z** None	**Z** None
2 Tomographic (Tomo) Nuclear Medicine Imaging	**7** Gastrointestinal Tract	**D** Indium 111 (In-111)		
	Y Digestive System	**Y** Other Radionuclide		

C: Nuclear Medicine
F: Hepatobiliary System and Pancreas

Type-Character 3	Body Part-Character 4	Radionuclide-Character 5	Qualifier-Character 6	Qualifier-Character 7
1 Planar Nuclear Medicine Imaging	**4** Gallbladder	**1** Technetium 99m (Tc-99m)	**Z** None	**Z** None
2 Tomographic (Tomo) Nuclear Medicine Imaging	**5** Liver	**Y** Other Radionuclide		
	6 Liver and Spleen			
	C Hepatobiliary System, All			
	Y Hepatobiliary System and Pancreas			

C: Nuclear Medicine
G: Endocrine System

Type-Character 3	Body Part-Character 4	Radionuclide-Character 5	Qualifier-Character 6	Qualifier-Character 7
1 Planar Nuclear Medicine Imaging	**1** Parathyroid Glands	**1** Technetium 99m (Tc-99m)	**Z** None	**Z** None
2 Tomographic (Tomo) Nuclear Medicine Imaging	**2** Thyroid Gland	**F** Iodine 123 (I-123)		
4 Nonimaging Nuclear Medicine Uptake	**4** Adrenal Glands, Bilateral	**G** Iodine 131 (I-131)		
	Y Endocrine System	**S** Thallium 201 (Tl-201)		
		Y Other Radionuclide		

C: Nuclear Medicine
H: Skin, Subcutaneous Tissue and Breast

Type-Character 3	Body Part-Character 4	Radionuclide-Character 5	Qualifier-Character 6	Qualifier-Character 7
1 Planar Nuclear Medicine Imaging	**0** Breast, Right	**1** Technetium 99m (Tc-99m)	**Z** None	**Z** None
2 Tomographic (Tomo) Nuclear Medicine Imaging	**1** Breast, Left	**S** Thallium 201 (Tl-201)		
	2 Breasts, Bilateral	**Y** Other Radionuclide		
	Y Skin, Subcutaneous Tissue and Breast			

C: Nuclear Medicine
P: Musculoskeletal System

Type-Character 3	Body Part-Character 4	Radionuclide-Character 5	Qualifier-Character 6	Qualifier-Character 7
1 Planar Nuclear Medicine Imaging	**1** Skull	**1** Technetium 99m (Tc-99m)	**Z** None	**Z** None
2 Tomographic (Tomo) Nuclear Medicine Imaging	**2** Cervical Spine	**Y** Other Radionuclide		
5 Nonimaging Nuclear Medicine Probe	**3** Skull and Cervical Spine	**Z** None		
	4 Thorax			
	5 Spine			
	6 Pelvis			
	7 Spine and Pelvis			
	8 Upper Extremity, Right			
	9 Upper Extremity, Left			
	B Upper Extremities, Bilateral			
	C Lower Extremity, Right			
	D Lower Extremity, Left			
	F Lower Extremities, Bilateral			
	G Thoracic Spine			
	H Lumbar Spine			
	J Thoracolumbar Spine			
	N Upper Extremities			
	P Lower Extremities			
	Y Musculoskeletal System, Other			
	Z Musculoskeletal System, All			

C: Nuclear Medicine
T: Urinary System

Type-Character 3	Body Part-Character 4	Radionuclide-Character 5	Qualifier-Character 6	Qualifier-Character 7
1 Planar Nuclear Medicine Imaging	**3** Kidneys, Ureters and Bladder	**1** Technetium 99m (Tc-99m)	**Z** None	**Z** None
2 Tomographic (Tomo) Nuclear Medicine Imaging	**H** Bladder and Ureters	**F** Iodine 123 (I-123)		
6 Nonimaging Nuclear Medicine Assay	**Y** Urinary System	**G** Iodine 131 (I-131)		
		H Iodine 125 (I-125)		
		Y Other Radionuclide		

C: Nuclear Medicine
V: Male Reproductive System

Type-Character 3	Body Part-Character 4	Radionuclide-Character 5	Qualifier-Character 6	Qualifier-Character 7
1 Planar Nuclear Medicine Imaging	**9** Testicles, Bilateral	**1** Technetium 99m (Tc-99m)	**Z** None	**Z** None
	Y Male Reproductive System	**Y** Other Radionuclide		

C: Nuclear Medicine
W: Anatomical Regions

Type-Character 3	Body Part-Character 4	Radionuclide-Character 5	Qualifier-Character 6	Qualifier-Character 7
1 Planar Nuclear Medicine Imaging	**0** Abdomen	**1** Technetium 99m (Tc-99m)	**Z** None	**Z** None
2 Tomographic (Tomo) Nuclear Medicine Imaging	**1** Abdomen and Pelvis	**8** Samarium 153 (Sm-153)		
3 Positron Emission Tomographic (PET) Imaging	**3** Chest	**D** Indium 111 (In-111)		
5 Nonimaging Nuclear Medicine Probe	**4** Chest and Abdomen	**F** Iodine 123 (I-123)		
7 Systemic Nuclear Medicine Therapy	**6** Chest and Neck	**G** Iodine 131 (I-131)		
	B Head and Neck	**K** Fluorine 18 (F-18)		
	D Lower Extremity	**L** Gallium 67 (Ga-67)		
	G Thyroid	**N** Phosphorus 32 (P-32)		
	J Pelvic Region	**P** Strontium 89 (Sr-89)		
	M Upper Extremity	**S** Thallium 201 (Tl-201)		
	N Whole Body	**Y** Other Radionuclide		
	Y Anatomical Regions, Multiple	**Z** None		
	Z Anatomical Region, Other			

D: Radiation Therapy
0: Central and Peripheral Nervous System

Modality-Character 3	Treatment Site -Character 4	Modality Qualifier-Character 5	Isotope -Character 6	Qualifier-Character 7
0 Beam Radiation	**0** Brain	**0** Photons <1 MeV	**7** Cesium 137 (Cs-137)	**0** Intraoperative
1 Brachytherapy	**1** Brain Stem	**1** Photons 1 - 10 MeV	**8** Iridium 192 (Ir-192)	**Z** None
2 Stereotactic Radiosurgery	**6** Spinal Cord	**2** Photons >10 MeV	**9** Iodine 125 (I-125)	
Y Other Radiation	**7** Peripheral Nerve	**3** Electrons	**B** Palladium 103 (Pd-103)	
		4 Heavy Particles (Protons, Ions)	**C** Californium 252 (Cf-252)	
		5 Neutrons	**Y** Other Isotope	
		6 Neutron Capture	**Z** None	
		7 Contact Radiation		
		8 Hyperthermia		
		9 High Dose Rate (HDR)		
		B Low Dose Rate (LDR)		
		D Stereotactic Other Photon Radiosurgery		
		F Plaque Radiation		
		H Stereotactic Particulate Radiosurgery		
		J Stereotactic Gamma Beam Radiosurgery		
		K Laser Interstitial Thermal Therapy		

D: Radiation Therapy
7: Lymphatic and Hematologic System

Modality-Character 3	Treatment Site -Character 4	Modality Qualifier-Character 5	Isotope -Character 6	Qualifier-Character 7
0 Beam Radiation	**0** Bone Marrow	**0** Photons <1 MeV	**7** Cesium 137 (Cs-137)	**0** Intraoperative
1 Brachytherapy	**1** Thymus	**1** Photons 1 - 10 MeV	**8** Iridium 192 (Ir-192)	**Z** None
2 Stereotactic Radiosurgery	**2** Spleen	**2** Photons >10 MeV	**9** Iodine 125 (I-125)	
Y Other Radiation	**3** Lymphatics, Neck	**3** Electrons	**B** Palladium 103 (Pd-103)	
	4 Lymphatics, Axillary	**4** Heavy Particles (Protons, Ions)	**C** Californium 252 (Cf-252)	
	5 Lymphatics, Thorax	**5** Neutrons	**Y** Other Isotope	
	6 Lymphatics, Abdomen	**6** Neutron Capture	**Z** None	
	7 Lymphatics, Pelvis	**8** Hyperthermia		
	8 Lymphatics, Inguinal	**9** High Dose Rate (HDR)		
		B Low Dose Rate (LDR)		
		D Stereotactic Other Photon Radiosurgery		
		F Plaque Radiation		
		H Stereotactic Particulate Radiosurgery		
		J Stereotactic Gamma Beam Radiosurgery		

D: Radiation Therapy
8: Eye

Modality-Character 3	Treatment Site -Character 4	Modality Qualifier-Character 5	Isotope -Character 6	Qualifier-Character 7
0 Beam Radiation	**0** Eye	**0** Photons <1 MeV	**7** Cesium 137 (Cs-137)	**0** Intraoperative
1 Brachytherapy		**1** Photons 1 - 10 MeV	**8** Iridium 192 (Ir-192)	**Z** None
2 Stereotactic Radiosurgery		**2** Photons >10 MeV	**9** Iodine 125 (I-125)	
Y Other Radiation		**3** Electrons	**B** Palladium 103 (Pd-103)	
		4 Heavy Particles (Protons, Ions)	**C** Californium 252 (Cf-252)	
		5 Neutrons	**Y** Other Isotope	
		6 Neutron Capture	**Z** None	
		7 Contact Radiation		
		8 Hyperthermia		
		9 High Dose Rate (HDR)		
		B Low Dose Rate (LDR)		
		D Stereotactic Other Photon Radiosurgery		
		F Plaque Radiation		
		H Stereotactic Particulate Radiosurgery		
		J Stereotactic Gamma Beam Radiosurgery		

D: Radiation Therapy
9: Ear, Nose, Mouth and Throat

Modality-Character 3	Treatment Site -Character 4	Modality Qualifier-Character 5	Isotope -Character 6	Qualifier-Character 7
0 Beam Radiation	**0** Ear	**0** Photons <1 MeV	**7** Cesium 137 (Cs-137)	**0** Intraoperative
1 Brachytherapy	**1** Nose	**1** Photons 1 - 10 MeV	**8** Iridium 192 (Ir-192)	**Z** None
2 Stereotactic Radiosurgery	**3** Hypopharynx	**2** Photons >10 MeV	**9** Iodine 125 (I-125)	
Y Other Radiation	**4** Mouth	**3** Electrons	**B** Palladium 103 (Pd-103)	
	5 Tongue	**4** Heavy Particles (Protons, Ions)	**C** Californium 252 (Cf-252)	
	6 Salivary Glands	**5** Neutrons	**Y** Other Isotope	
	7 Sinuses	**6** Neutron Capture	**Z** None	
	8 Hard Palate	**7** Contact Radiation		
	9 Soft Palate	**8** Hyperthermia		
	B Larynx	**9** High Dose Rate (HDR)		
	C Pharynx	**B** Low Dose Rate (LDR)		
	D Nasopharynx	**C** Intraoperative Radiation Therapy (IORT)		
	F Oropharynx	**D** Stereotactic Other Photon Radiosurgery		
		F Plaque Radiation		
		H Stereotactic Particulate Radiosurgery		
		J Stereotactic Gamma Beam Radiosurgery		

D: Radiation Therapy
B: Respiratory System

Modality-Character 3	Treatment Site -Character 4	Modality Qualifier-Character 5	Isotope -Character 6	Qualifier-Character 7
0 Beam Radiation	**0** Trachea	**0** Photons <1 MeV	**7** Cesium 137 (Cs-137)	**0** Intraoperative
1 Brachytherapy	**1** Bronchus	**1** Photons 1 - 10 MeV	**8** Iridium 192 (Ir-192)	**Z** None
2 Stereotactic Radiosurgery	**2** Lung	**2** Photons >10 MeV	**9** Iodine 125 (I-125)	
Y Other Radiation	**5** Pleura	**3** Electrons	**B** Palladium 103 (Pd-103)	
	6 Mediastinum	**4** Heavy Particles (Protons, Ions)	**C** Californium 252 (Cf-252)	
	7 Chest Wall	**5** Neutrons	**Y** Other Isotope	
	8 Diaphragm	**6** Neutron Capture	**Z** None	
		7 Contact Radiation		
		8 Hyperthermia		
		9 High Dose Rate (HDR)		
		B Low Dose Rate (LDR)		
		D Stereotactic Other Photon Radiosurgery		
		F Plaque Radiation		
		H Stereotactic Particulate Radiosurgery		
		J Stereotactic Gamma Beam Radiosurgery		
		K Laser Interstitial Thermal Therapy		

D: Radiation Therapy
D: Gastrointestinal System

Modality-Character 3	Treatment Site -Character 4	Modality Qualifier-Character 5	Isotope -Character 6	Qualifier-Character 7
0 Beam Radiation	**0** Esophagus	**0** Photons <1 MeV	**7** Cesium 137 (Cs-137)	**0** Intraoperative
1 Brachytherapy	**1** Stomach	**1** Photons 1 - 10 MeV	**8** Iridium 192 (Ir-192)	**Z** None
2 Stereotactic Radiosurgery	**2** Duodenum	**2** Photons >10 MeV	**9** Iodine 125 (I-125)	
Y Other Radiation	**3** Jejunum	**3** Electrons	**B** Palladium 103 (Pd-103)	
	4 Ileum	**4** Heavy Particles (Protons, Ions)	**C** Californium 252 (Cf-252)	
	5 Colon	**5** Neutrons	**Y** Other Isotope	
	7 Rectum	**6** Neutron Capture	**Z** None	
	8 Anus	**7** Contact Radiation		
		8 Hyperthermia		
		9 High Dose Rate (HDR)		
		B Low Dose Rate (LDR)		
		C Intraoperative Radiation Therapy (IORT)		
		D Stereotactic Other Photon Radiosurgery		
		F Plaque Radiation		
		H Stereotactic Particulate Radiosurgery		
		J Stereotactic Gamma Beam Radiosurgery		
		K Laser Interstitial Thermal Therapy		

D: Radiation Therapy
F: Hepatobiliary System and Pancreas

Modality-Character 3	Treatment Site -Character 4	Modality Qualifier-Character 5	Isotope -Character 6	Qualifier-Character 7
0 Beam Radiation	**0** Liver	**0** Photons <1 MeV	**7** Cesium 137 (Cs-137)	**0** Intraoperative
1 Brachytherapy	**1** Gallbladder	**1** Photons 1 - 10 MeV	**8** Iridium 192 (Ir-192)	**Z** None
2 Stereotactic Radiosurgery	**2** Bile Ducts	**2** Photons >10 MeV	**9** Iodine 125 (I-125)	
Y Other Radiation	**3** Pancreas	**3** Electrons	**B** Palladium 103 (Pd-103)	
		4 Heavy Particles (Protons, Ions)	**C** Californium 252 (Cf-252)	
		5 Neutrons	**Y** Other Isotope	
		6 Neutron Capture	**Z** None	
		7 Contact Radiation		
		8 Hyperthermia		
		9 High Dose Rate (HDR)		
		B Low Dose Rate (LDR)		
		C Intraoperative Radiation Therapy (IORT)		
		D Stereotactic Other Photon Radiosurgery		
		F Plaque Radiation		
		H Stereotactic Particulate Radiosurgery		
		J Stereotactic Gamma Beam Radiosurgery		
		K Laser Interstitial Thermal Therapy		

D: Radiation Therapy
G: Endocrine System

Modality-Character 3	Treatment Site -Character 4	Modality Qualifier-Character 5	Isotope -Character 6	Qualifier-Character 7
0 Beam Radiation	**0** Pituitary Gland	**0** Photons <1 MeV	**7** Cesium 137 (Cs-137)	**0** Intraoperative
1 Brachytherapy	**1** Pineal Body	**1** Photons 1 - 10 MeV	**8** Iridium 192 (Ir-192)	**Z** None
2 Stereotactic Radiosurgery	**2** Adrenal Glands	**2** Photons >10 MeV	**9** Iodine 125 (I-125)	
Y Other Radiation	**4** Parathyroid Glands	**3** Electrons	**B** Palladium 103 (Pd-103)	
	5 Thyroid	**5** Neutrons	**C** Californium 252 (Cf-252)	
		6 Neutron Capture	**Y** Other Isotope	
		7 Contact Radiation	**Z** None	
		8 Hyperthermia		
		9 High Dose Rate (HDR)		
		B Low Dose Rate (LDR)		
		D Stereotactic Other Photon Radiosurgery		
		F Plaque Radiation		
		H Stereotactic Particulate Radiosurgery		
		J Stereotactic Gamma Beam Radiosurgery		
		K Laser Interstitial Thermal Therapy		

D: Radiation Therapy
H: Skin

Modality-Character 3	Treatment Site -Character 4	Modality Qualifier-Character 5	Isotope -Character 6	Qualifier-Character 7
0 Beam Radiation	**2** Skin, Face	**0** Photons <1 MeV	**Z** None	**0** Intraoperative
Y Other Radiation	**3** Skin, Neck	**1** Photons 1 - 10 MeV		**Z** None
	4 Skin, Arm	**2** Photons >10 MeV		
	5 Skin, Hand	**3** Electrons		
	6 Skin, Chest	**4** Heavy Particles (Protons, Ions)		
	7 Skin, Back	**5** Neutrons		
	8 Skin, Abdomen	**6** Neutron Capture		
	9 Skin, Buttock	**7** Contact Radiation		
	B Skin, Leg	**8** Hyperthermia		
	C Skin, Foot	**F** Plaque Radiation		

D: Radiation Therapy
M: Breast

Modality-Character 3	Treatment Site -Character 4	Modality Qualifier-Character 5	Isotope -Character 6	Qualifier-Character 7
0 Beam Radiation	**0** Breast, Left	**0** Photons <1 MeV	**7** Cesium 137 (Cs-137)	**0** Intraoperative
1 Brachytherapy	**1** Breast, Right	**1** Photons 1 - 10 MeV	**8** Iridium 192 (Ir-192)	**Z** None
2 Stereotactic Radiosurgery		**2** Photons >10 MeV	**9** Iodine 125 (I-125)	
Y Other Radiation		**3** Electrons	**B** Palladium 103 (Pd-103)	
		4 Heavy Particles (Protons, Ions)	**C** Californium 252 (Cf-252)	
		5 Neutrons	**Y** Other Isotope	
		6 Neutron Capture	**Z** None	
		7 Contact Radiation		
		8 Hyperthermia		
		9 High Dose Rate (HDR)		
		B Low Dose Rate (LDR)		
		D Stereotactic Other Photon Radiosurgery		
		F Plaque Radiation		
		H Stereotactic Particulate Radiosurgery		
		J Stereotactic Gamma Beam Radiosurgery		
		K Laser Interstitial Thermal Therapy		

D: Radiation Therapy
P: Musculoskeletal System

Modality-Character 3	Treatment Site -Character 4	Modality Qualifier-Character 5	Isotope -Character 6	Qualifier-Character 7
0 Beam Radiation	**0** Skull	**0** Photons <1 MeV	**Z** None	**0** Intraoperative
Y Other Radiation	**2** Maxilla	**1** Photons 1 - 10 MeV		**Z** None
	3 Mandible	**2** Photons >10 MeV		
	4 Sternum	**3** Electrons		
	5 Rib(s)	**4** Heavy Particles (Protons, Ions)		
	6 Humerus	**5** Neutrons		
	7 Radius/Ulna	**6** Neutron Capture		
	8 Pelvic Bones	**7** Contact Radiation		
	9 Femur	**8** Hyperthermia		
	B Tibia/Fibula	**F** Plaque Radiation		
	C Other Bone			

D: Radiation Therapy
T: Urinary System

Modality-Character 3	Treatment Site -Character 4	Modality Qualifier-Character 5	Isotope -Character 6	Qualifier-Character 7
0 Beam Radiation	**0** Kidney	**0** Photons <1 MeV	**7** Cesium 137 (Cs-137)	**0** Intraoperative
1 Brachytherapy	**1** Ureter	**1** Photons 1 - 10 MeV	**8** Iridium 192 (Ir-192)	**Z** None
2 Stereotactic Radiosurgery	**2** Bladder	**2** Photons >10 MeV	**9** Iodine 125 (I-125)	
Y Other Radiation	**3** Urethra	**3** Electrons	**B** Palladium 103 (Pd-103)	
		4 Heavy Particles (Protons, Ions)	**C** Californium 252 (Cf-252)	
		5 Neutrons	**Y** Other Isotope	
		6 Neutron Capture	**Z** None	
		7 Contact Radiation		
		8 Hyperthermia		
		9 High Dose Rate (HDR)		
		B Low Dose Rate (LDR)		
		C Intraoperative Radiation Therapy (IORT)		
		D Stereotactic Other Photon Radiosurgery		
		F Plaque Radiation		
		H Stereotactic Particulate Radiosurgery		
		J Stereotactic Gamma Beam Radiosurgery		

D: Radiation Therapy
U: Female Reproductive System

Modality-Character 3	Treatment Site -Character 4	Modality Qualifier-Character 5	Isotope -Character 6	Qualifier-Character 7
0 Beam Radiation	**0** Ovary	**0** Photons <1 MeV	**7** Cesium 137 (Cs-137)	**0** Intraoperative
1 Brachytherapy	**1** Cervix	**1** Photons 1 - 10 MeV	**8** Iridium 192 (Ir-192)	**Z** None
2 Stereotactic Radiosurgery	**2** Uterus	**2** Photons >10 MeV	**9** Iodine 125 (I-125)	
Y Other Radiation		**3** Electrons	**B** Palladium 103 (Pd-103)	
		4 Heavy Particles (Protons, Ions)	**C** Californium 252 (Cf-252)	
		5 Neutrons	**Y** Other Isotope	
		6 Neutron Capture	**Z** None	
		7 Contact Radiation		
		8 Hyperthermia		
		9 High Dose Rate (HDR)		
		B Low Dose Rate (LDR)		
		C Intraoperative Radiation Therapy (IORT)		
		D Stereotactic Other Photon Radiosurgery		
		F Plaque Radiation		
		H Stereotactic Particulate Radiosurgery		
		J Stereotactic Gamma Beam Radiosurgery		

D: Radiation Therapy
V: Male Reproductive System

Modality-Character 3	Treatment Site -Character 4	Modality Qualifier-Character 5	Isotope -Character 6	Qualifier-Character 7
0 Beam Radiation	**0** Prostate	**0** Photons <1 MeV	**7** Cesium 137 (Cs-137)	**0** Intraoperative
1 Brachytherapy	**1** Testis	**1** Photons 1 - 10 MeV	**8** Iridium 192 (Ir-192)	**Z** None
2 Stereotactic Radiosurgery		**2** Photons >10 MeV	**9** Iodine 125 (I-125)	
Y Other Radiation		**3** Electrons	**B** Palladium 103 (Pd-103)	
		4 Heavy Particles (Protons, Ions)	**C** Californium 252 (Cf-252)	
		5 Neutrons	**Y** Other Isotope	
		6 Neutron Capture	**Z** None	
		7 Contact Radiation		
		8 Hyperthermia		
		9 High Dose Rate (HDR)		
		B Low Dose Rate (LDR)		
		C Intraoperative Radiation Therapy (IORT)		
		D Stereotactic Other Photon Radiosurgery		
		F Plaque Radiation		
		H Stereotactic Particulate Radiosurgery		
		J Stereotactic Gamma Beam Radiosurgery		
		K Laser Interstitial Thermal Therapy		

D: Radiation Therapy
W: Anatomical Regions

Modality-Character 3	Treatment Site -Character 4	Modality Qualifier-Character 5	Isotope -Character 6	Qualifier-Character 7
0 Beam Radiation	**1** Head and Neck	**0** Photons <1 MeV	**7** Cesium 137 (Cs-137)	**0** Intraoperative
1 Brachytherapy	**2** Chest	**1** Photons 1 - 10 MeV	**8** Iridium 192 (Ir-192)	**Z** None
2 Stereotactic Radiosurgery	**3** Abdomen	**2** Photons >10 MeV	**9** Iodine 125 (I-125)	
Y Other Radiation	**4** Hemibody	**3** Electrons	**B** Palladium 103 (Pd-103)	
	5 Whole Body	**4** Heavy Particles (Protons, Ions)	**C** Californium 252 (Cf-252)	
	6 Pelvic Region	**5** Neutrons	**D** Iodine 131 (I-131)	
		6 Neutron Capture	**F** Phosphorus 32 (P-32)	
		7 Contact Radiation	**G** Strontium 89 (Sr-89)	
		8 Hyperthermia	**H** Strontium 90 (Sr-90)	
		9 High Dose Rate (HDR)	**Y** Other Isotope	
		B Low Dose Rate (LDR)	**Z** None	
		D Stereotactic Other Photon Radiosurgery		
		F Plaque Radiation		
		G Isotope Administration		
		H Stereotactic Particulate Radiosurgery		
		J Stereotactic Gamma Beam Radiosurgery		

F: Physical Rehabilitation and Diagnostic Audiology
0: Rehabilitation

Type-Character 3	Body System / Region-Character 4	Type Qualifier-Character 5	Equipment-Character 6	Qualifier-Character 7
0 Speech Assessment	**0** Neurological System - Head and Neck	**0** Bathing/Showering	**1** Audiometer	**Z** None
1 Motor and/or Nerve Function Assessment	**1** Neurological System - Upper Back / Upper Extremity	**0** Bathing/Showering Technique	**2** Sound Field / Booth	
2 Activities of Daily Living Assessment	**2** Neurological System - Lower Back / Lower Extremity	**0** Bathing/Showering Techniques	**4** Electroacoustic Immittance / Acoustic Reflex	
6 Speech Treatment	**3** Neurological System - Whole Body	**0** Cochlear Implant Rehabilitation	**5** Hearing Aid Selection / Fitting / Test	
7 Motor Treatment	**4** Circulatory System - Head and Neck	**0** Filtered Speech	**7** Electrophysiologic	
8 Activities of Daily Living Treatment	**5** Circulatory System - Upper Back / Upper Extremity	**0** Hearing and Related Disorders Counseling	**8** Vestibular / Balance	
9 Hearing Treatment	**6** Circulatory System - Lower Back / Lower Extremity	**0** Muscle Performance	**9** Cochlear Implant	
B Cochlear Implant Treatment	**7** Circulatory System - Whole Body	**0** Nonspoken Language	**B** Physical Agents	
C Vestibular Treatment	**8** Respiratory System - Head and Neck	**0** Range of Motion and Joint Mobility	**C** Mechanical	
D Device Fitting	**9** Respiratory System - Upper Back / Upper Extremity	**0** Tinnitus Masker	**D** Electrotherapeutic	
F Caregiver Training	**B** Respiratory System - Lower Back / Lower Extremity	**0** Vestibular	**E** Orthosis	
	C Respiratory System - Whole Body	**1** Dressing	**F** Assistive, Adaptive, Supportive or Protective	
	D Integumentary System - Head and Neck	**1** Dressing Techniques	**G** Aerobic Endurance and Conditioning	
	F Integumentary System - Upper Back / Upper Extremity	**1** Hearing and Related Disorders Prevention	**H** Mechanical or Electromechanical	
	G Integumentary System - Lower Back / Lower Extremity	**1** Integumentary Integrity	**J** Somatosensory	
	H Integumentary System - Whole Body	**1** Monaural Hearing Aid	**K** Audiovisual	
	J Musculoskeletal System - Head and Neck	**1** Muscle Performance	**L** Assistive Listening	
	K Musculoskeletal System - Upper Back / Upper Extremity	**1** Perceptual Processing	**M** Augmentative / Alternative Communication	
	L Musculoskeletal System - Lower Back / Lower Extremity	**1** Speech Threshold	**N** Biosensory Feedback	
	M Musculoskeletal System - Whole Body	**1** Speech-Language Pathology and Related Disorders Counseling	**P** Computer	
	N Genitourinary System	**2** Auditory Processing	**Q** Speech Analysis	
	Z None	**2** Binaural Hearing Aid	**S** Voice Analysis	
		2 Coordination/Dexterity	**T** Aerodynamic Function	
		2 Feeding and Eating	**U** Prosthesis	
		2 Feeding/Eating	**V** Speech Prosthesis	
		2 Grooming/Personal Hygiene	**W** Swallowing	
		2 Speech-Language Pathology and Related Disorders Prevention	**X** Cerumen Management	
		2 Speech/Word Recognition	**Y** Other Equipment	
		2 Visual Motor Integration	**Z** None	
		3 Aphasia		
		3 Augmentative/Alternative Communication System		
		3 Cerumen Management		
		3 Coordination/Dexterity		

Type-Character 3	Body System / Region-Character 4	Type Qualifier-Character 5	Equipment-Character 6	Qualifier-Character 7
		3 Feeding/Eating		
		3 Grooming/Personal Hygiene		
		3 Motor Function		
		3 Postural Control		
		3 Staggered Spondaic Word		
		4 Articulation/Phonology		
		4 Bed Mobility		
		4 Home Management		
		4 Motor Function		
		4 Sensorineural Acuity Level		
		4 Voice Prosthetic		
		4 Wheelchair Mobility		
		5 Assistive Listening Device		
		5 Aural Rehabilitation		
		5 Bed Mobility		
		5 Perceptual Processing		
		5 Range of Motion and Joint Integrity		
		5 Synthetic Sentence Identification		
		5 Transfer		
		5 Wound Management		
		6 Communicative/Cognitive Integration Skills		
		6 Dynamic Orthosis		
		6 Psychosocial Skills		
		6 Sensory Awareness/Processing/Integrity		
		6 Speech and/or Language Screening		
		6 Therapeutic Exercise		
		6 Wheelchair Mobility		
		7 Aerobic Capacity and Endurance		
		7 Facial Nerve Function		
		7 Fluency		
		7 Manual Therapy Techniques		
		7 Nonspoken Language		
		7 Static Orthosis		
		7 Therapeutic Exercise		
		7 Vocational Activities and Functional Community or Work Reintegration Skills		
		8 Airway Clearance Techniques		
		8 Anthropometric Characteristics		
		8 Motor Speech		
		8 Prosthesis		
		8 Receptive/Expressive Language		
		8 Transfer Training		
		9 Articulation/Phonology		
		9 Assistive, Adaptive, Supportive or Protective Devices		
		9 Cranial Nerve Integrity		
		9 Gait Training/Functional Ambulation		
		9 Orofacial Myofunctional		
		9 Somatosensory Evoked Potentials		
		9 Wound Management		
		B Bed Mobility		

Type-Character 3	Body System / Region-Character 4	Type Qualifier-Character 5	Equipment-Character 6	Qualifier-Character 7
		B Environmental, Home and Work Barriers		
		B Motor Speech		
		B Receptive/Expressive Language		
		B Vocational Activities and Functional Community or Work Reintegration Skills		
		C Aphasia		
		C Ergonomics and Body Mechanics		
		C Gait Training/Functional Ambulation		
		C Transfer		
		C Voice		
		D Application, Proper Use and Care of Devices		
		D Fluency		
		D Gait and/or Balance		
		D Neuromotor Development		
		D Swallowing Dysfunction		
		F Application, Proper Use and Care of Orthoses		
		F Pain		
		F Voice		
		F Wheelchair Mobility		
		G Application, Proper Use and Care of Prosthesis		
		G Communicative/Cognitive Integration Skills		
		G Reflex Integrity		
		G Ventilation, Respiration and Circulation		
		H Bedside Swallowing and Oral Function		
		H Home Management		
		H Vocational Activities and Functional Community or Work Reintegration Skills		
		J Communication Skills		
		J Instrumental Swallowing and Oral Function		
		K Orofacial Myofunctional		
		L Augmentative/Alternative Communication System		
		M Voice Prosthetic		
		N Non-invasive Instrumental Status		
		P Oral Peripheral Mechanism		
		Q Performance Intensity Phonetically Balanced Speech Discrimination		
		R Brief Tone Stimuli		
		S Distorted Speech		
		T Dichotic Stimuli		
		V Temporal Ordering of Stimuli		
		W Masking Patterns		
		X Other Specified Central Auditory Processing		

F: Physical Rehabilitation and Diagnostic Audiology
1: Diagnostic Audiology

Type-Character 3	Body System / Region-Character 4	Type Qualifier-Character 5	Equipment-Character 6	Qualifier-Character 7
3 Hearing Assessment	**Z** None	**0** Bithermal, Binaural Caloric Irrigation	**0** Occupational Hearing	**Z** None
4 Hearing Aid Assessment		**0** Cochlear Implant	**1** Audiometer	
5 Vestibular Assessment		**0** Hearing Screening	**2** Sound Field / Booth	
		1 Bithermal, Monaural Caloric Irrigation	**3** Tympanometer	
		1 Ear Canal Probe Microphone	**4** Electroacoustic Immittance / Acoustic Reflex	
		1 Pure Tone Audiometry, Air	**5** Hearing Aid Selection / Fitting / Test	
		2 Monaural Hearing Aid	**6** Otoacoustic Emission (OAE)	
		2 Pure Tone Audiometry, Air and Bone	**7** Electrophysiologic	
		2 Unithermal Binaural Screen	**8** Vestibular / Balance	
		3 Bekesy Audiometry	**9** Cochlear Implant	
		3 Binaural Hearing Aid	**K** Audiovisual	
		3 Oscillating Tracking	**L** Assistive Listening	
		4 Assistive Listening System/Device Selection	**P** Computer	
		4 Conditioned Play Audiometry	**Y** Other Equipment	
		4 Sinusoidal Vertical Axis Rotational	**Z** None	
		5 Dix-Hallpike Dynamic		
		5 Select Picture Audiometry		
		5 Sensory Aids		
		6 Binaural Electroacoustic Hearing Aid Check		
		6 Computerized Dynamic Posturography		
		6 Visual Reinforcement Audiometry		
		7 Alternate Binaural or Monaural Loudness Balance		
		7 Ear Protector Attenuation		
		7 Tinnitus Masker		
		8 Monaural Electroacoustic Hearing Aid Check		
		8 Tone Decay		
		9 Short Increment Sensitivity Index		
		B Stenger		
		C Pure Tone Stenger		
		D Tympanometry		
		F Eustachian Tube Function		
		G Acoustic Reflex Patterns		
		H Acoustic Reflex Threshold		
		J Acoustic Reflex Decay		
		K Electrocochleography		
		L Auditory Evoked Potentials		
		M Evoked Otoacoustic Emissions, Screening		
		N Evoked Otoacoustic Emissions, Diagnostic		
		P Aural Rehabilitation Status		
		Q Auditory Processing		

G: Mental Health
Z: None

Type-Character 3	Qualifier-Character 4	Qualifier-Character 5	Qualifier-Character 6	Qualifier-Character 7
1 Psychological Tests	**0** Developmental	**Z** None	**Z** None	**Z** None
2 Crisis Intervention	**0** Educational			
3 Medication Management	**0** Interactive			
5 Individual Psychotherapy	**0** Unilateral-Single Seizure			
6 Counseling	**1** Behavioral			
7 Family Psychotherapy	**1** Personality and Behavioral			
B Electroconvulsive Therapy	**1** Unilateral-Multiple Seizure			
C Biofeedback	**1** Vocational			
F Hypnosis	**2** Bilateral-Single Seizure			
G Narcosynthesis	**2** Cognitive			
H Group Psychotherapy	**2** Intellectual and Psychoeducational			
J Light Therapy	**2** Other Family Psychotherapy			
	3 Bilateral-Multiple Seizure			
	3 Interpersonal			
	3 Neuropsychological			
	3 Other Counseling			
	4 Neurobehavioral and Cognitive Status			
	4 Other Electroconvulsive Therapy			
	4 Psychoanalysis			
	5 Psychodynamic			
	6 Supportive			
	8 Cognitive-Behavioral			
	9 Other Biofeedback			
	9 Psychophysiological			
	Z None			

H: Substance Abuse Treatment
Z: None

Type-Character 3	Qualifier-Character 4	Qualifier-Character 5	Qualifier-Character 6	Qualifier-Character 7
2 Detoxification Services	**0** Cognitive	**Z** None	**Z** None	**Z** None
3 Individual Counseling	**0** Nicotine Replacement			
4 Group Counseling	**1** Behavioral			
5 Individual Psychotherapy	**1** Methadone Maintenance			
6 Family Counseling	**2** Cognitive-Behavioral			
8 Medication Management	**2** Levo-alpha-acetyl-methadol (LAAM)			
9 Pharmacotherapy	**3** 12-Step			
	3 Antabuse			
	3 Other Family Counseling			
	4 Interpersonal			
	4 Naltrexone			
	5 Interactive			
	5 Naloxone			
	5 Vocational			
	6 Clonidine			
	6 Psychoeducation			
	7 Bupropion			
	7 Motivational Enhancement			
	8 Confrontational			
	8 Psychiatric Medication			
	9 Continuing Care			
	9 Other Replacement Medication			
	9 Supportive			
	B Psychoanalysis			
	B Spiritual			
	C Pre/Post-Test Infectious Disease			
	C Psychodynamic			
	D Psychophysiological			
	Z None			

X: New Technology
2: Cardiovascular System

Operation-Character 3	Body Part-Character 4	Approach-Character 5	Device-Character 6	Qualifier-Character 7
A Assistance	**0** Coronary Artery, One Artery	**0** Open	**1** Cerebral Embolic Filtration, Dual Filter	**1** New Technology Group 1
C Extirpation	**1** Coronary Artery, Two Arteries	**3** Percutaneous	**3** Zooplastic Tissue, Rapid Deployment Technique	**2** New Technology Group 2
R Replacement	**2** Coronary Artery, Three Arteries	**4** Percutaneous Endoscopic	**6** Orbital Atherectomy Technology	
	3 Coronary Artery, Four or More Arteries			

X: New Technology
2: Skin, Subcutaneous Tissue, Fascia and Breast

Operation-Character 3	Body Part-Character 4	Approach-Character 5	Device-Character 6	Qualifier-Character 7
R Replacement	**P** Skin	**X** External	**L** Skin Substitute, Porcine, Liver Derived	**2** New Technology, Group 2

X: New Technology
N: Bones

Operation-Character 3	Body Part-Character 4	Approach-Character 5	Device-Character 6	Qualifier-Character 7
S Reposition	**0** Lumbar Vertebra	**0** Open	**3** Magnetically Controlled Growth Rod(s)	**2** New Technology Group 2
	3 Cervical Vertebra	**4** Percutaneous Endoscopic		
	4 Thoracic Vertebra			

X: New Technology
R: Joints

Operation-Character 3	Body Part-Character 4	Approach-Character 5	Device-Character 6	Qualifier-Character 7
2 Monitoring	**0** Occipital-cervical Joint	**0** Open	**2** Intraoperative Knee Replacement Sensor	**1** New Technology Group 1
G Fusion	**1** Cervical Vertebral Joint		**9** Interbody Fusion Device, Nanotextured Surface	**2** New Technology Group 2
	2 Cervical Vertebral Joints, 2 or more			
	4 Cervicothoracic Vertebral Joint			
	6 Thoracic Vertebral Joint			
	7 Thoracic Vertebral Joints, 2 to 7			
	8 Thoracic Vertebral Joints, 8 or more			
	A Thoracolumbar Vertebral Joint			
	B Lumbar Vertebral Joint			
	C Lumbar Vertebral Joints, 2 or more			
	D Lumbosacral Joint			
	G Knee Joint, Right			
	H Knee Joint, Left			

X: New Technology
W: Anatomical Regions

Operation-Character 3	Body Part-Character 4	Approach-Character 5	Device-Character 6	Qualifier-Character 7
0 Introduction	**3** Peripheral Vein	**3** Percutaneous	**2** Ceftazidime-Avibactam Anti-infective	**1** New Technology Group 1
	4 Central Vein	**X** External	**3** Idarucizumab, Dabigatran Reversal Agent	**2** New Technology Group 2
	D Mouth and Pharynx		**4** Isavuconazole Anti-infective	
			5 Blinatumomab Antineoplastic Immunotherapy	
			7 Andexanet Alfa, Factor Xa Inhibitor Reversal Agent	
			8 Uridine Triacetate	
			9 Defibrotide Sodium Anticoagulant	

Appendix F: Substance Key

Substance Term	ICD-10-PCS Value
AIGISRx® Antibacterial Envelope	Anti-Infective Envelope
AIGISRx® Antimicrobial envelope	Anti-Infective Envelope
Bone morphogenetic protein 2 (BMP 2)	Recombinant Bone Morphogenetic Protein
Clolar®	Clofarabine
Defitelio®	Defibrotide Sodium Anticoagulant
Factor Xa Inhibitor Reversal Agent, Andexanet Alfa	Andexanet Alfa, Factor Xa Inhibitor Reversal Agent
Kcentra®	4-Factor Prothrombin Complex Concentrate
Nesiritide®	Human B-type Natriuretic Peptide
rhBMP-2	Recombinant Bone Morphogenetic Protein
Seprafilm®	Adhesion Barrier
Tissue Plasminogen Activator (tPA)(rtPA)	Other Thrombolytic
Vistogard®	Uridine Triacetate
Voraxaze®	Glucarpidase
Zyvox®	Oxazolidinones

This page intentionally left blank

Appendix G: Combination Clusters

Due to the nature of a specific procedure, the first code in the cluster needs to be reported with one or more of the additional codes listed for all codes to be considered valid. The example below is for insertion of a cardiac pacemaker lead into a coronary vein (highlighted code). The additional procedures describe the exact location of where the lead is inserted, which is required for correct reporting:

02H40JZ
and 02H60JZ
and 02HK0JZ
and 0JH607Z

You would need to review the first procedure in the combination/cluster to determine whether you need to report one or more of the additional codes. The CMS site also provides additional information on combinations/clusters.

02H40JZ
and 02H60JZ
and 02HK0JZ
and 0JH607Z

02H40JZ
and 02H60JZ
and 02HK0JZ
and 0JH637Z

02H40JZ
and 02H60JZ
and 02HK0JZ
and 0JH807Z

02H40JZ
and 02H60JZ
and 02HK0JZ
and 0JH837Z

02H40JZ
and 02H60JZ
and 02HK3JZ
and 0JH607Z

02H40JZ
and 02H60JZ
and 02HK3JZ
and 0JH637Z

02H40JZ
and 02H60JZ
and 02HK3JZ
and 0JH807Z

02H40JZ
and 02H60JZ
and 02HK3JZ
and 0JH837Z

02H40JZ
and 02H60JZ
and 02HK4JZ
and 0JH607Z

02H40JZ
and 02H60JZ
and 02HK4JZ
and 0JH637Z

02H40JZ
and 02H60JZ
and 02HK4JZ
and 0JH807Z

02H40JZ
and 02H60JZ
and 02HK4JZ
and 0JH837Z

02H40JZ
and 02H60JZ
and 02HL0JZ
and 0JH607Z

02H40JZ
and 02H60JZ
and 02HL0JZ
and 0JH637Z

02H40JZ
and 02H60JZ
and 02HL0JZ
and 0JH807Z

02H40JZ
and 02H60JZ
and 02HL0JZ
and 0JH837Z

02H40JZ
and 02H60JZ
and 02HL3JZ
and 0JH607Z

02H40JZ
and 02H60JZ
and 02HL3JZ
and 0JH637Z

02H40JZ
and 02H60JZ
and 02HL3JZ
and 0JH807Z

02H40JZ
and 02H60JZ
and 02HL3JZ
and 0JH837Z

02H40JZ
and 02H60JZ
and 02HL4JZ
and 0JH607Z

02H40JZ
and 02H60JZ
and 02HL4JZ
and 0JH637Z

02H40JZ
and 02H60JZ
and 02HL4JZ
and 0JH807Z

02H40JZ
and 02H60JZ
and 02HL4JZ
and 0JH837Z

02H40JZ
and 02H63JZ
and 02HK0JZ
and 0JH607Z

02H40JZ
and 02H63JZ
and 02HK0JZ
and 0JH637Z

02H40JZ
and 02H63JZ
and 02HK0JZ
and 0JH807Z

02H40JZ
and 02H63JZ
and 02HK0JZ
and 0JH837Z

02H40JZ
and 02H63JZ
and 02HK3JZ
and 0JH607Z

02H40JZ
and 02H63JZ
and 02HK3JZ
and 0JH637Z

02H40JZ
and 02H63JZ
and 02HK3JZ
and 0JH807Z

02H40JZ
and 02H63JZ
and 02HK3JZ
and 0JH837Z

02H40JZ
and 02H63JZ
and 02HK4JZ
and 0JH607Z

02H40JZ
and 02H63JZ
and 02HK4JZ
and 0JH637Z

02H40JZ
and 02H63JZ
and 02HK4JZ
and 0JH807Z

02H40JZ
and 02H63JZ
and 02HK4JZ
and 0JH837Z

02H40JZ
and 02H63JZ
and 02HL0JZ
and 0JH607Z

02H40JZ
and 02H63JZ
and 02HL0JZ
and 0JH637Z

02H40JZ
and 02H63JZ
and 02HL0JZ
and 0JH807Z

02H40JZ
and 02H63JZ
and 02HL0JZ
and 0JH837Z

02H40JZ
and 02H63JZ
and 02HL3JZ
and 0JH607Z

02H40JZ
and 02H63JZ
and 02HL3JZ
and 0JH637Z

02H40JZ
and 02H63JZ
and 02HL3JZ
and 0JH807Z

02H40JZ
and 02H63JZ
and 02HL3JZ
and 0JH837Z

02H40JZ
and 02H63JZ
and 02HL4JZ
and 0JH607Z

02H40JZ
and 02H63JZ
and 02HL4JZ
and 0JH637Z

02H40JZ
and 02H63JZ
and 02HL4JZ
and 0JH807Z

02H40JZ
and 02H63JZ
and 02HL4JZ
and 0JH837Z

02H40JZ
and 02H64JZ
and 02HK0JZ
and 0JH607Z

02H40JZ
and 02H64JZ
and 02HK0JZ
and 0JH637Z

02H40JZ
and 02H64JZ
and 02HK0JZ
and 0JH807Z

02H40JZ
and 02H64JZ
and 02HK0JZ
and 0JH837Z

02H40JZ
and 02H64JZ
and 02HK3JZ
and 0JH607Z

02H40JZ
and 02H64JZ
and 02HK3JZ
and 0JH637Z

02H40JZ
and 02H64JZ
and 02HK3JZ
and 0JH807Z

02H40JZ
and 02H64JZ
and 02HK3JZ
and 0JH837Z

02H40JZ
and 02H64JZ
and 02HK4JZ
and 0JH607Z

02H40JZ
and 02H64JZ
and 02HK4JZ
and 0JH637Z

02H40JZ
and 02H64JZ
and 02HK4JZ
and 0JH807Z

02H40JZ
and 02H64JZ
and 02HK4JZ
and 0JH837Z

02H40JZ
and 02H64JZ
and 02HL0JZ
and 0JH607Z

02H40JZ
and 02H64JZ
and 02HL0JZ
and 0JH637Z

02H40JZ
and 02H64JZ
and 02HL0JZ
and 0JH807Z

02H40JZ
and 02H64JZ
and 02HL0JZ
and 0JH837Z

02H40JZ
and 02H64JZ
and 02HL3JZ
and 0JH607Z

02H40JZ
and 02H64JZ
and 02HL3JZ
and 0JH637Z

02H40JZ
and 02H64JZ
and 02HL3JZ
and 0JH807Z

02H40JZ
and 02H64JZ
and 02HL3JZ
and 0JH837Z

02H40JZ
and 02H64JZ
and 02HL4JZ
and 0JH607Z

02H40JZ
and 02H64JZ
and 02HL4JZ
and 0JH637Z

02H40JZ
and 02H64JZ
and 02HL4JZ
and 0JH807Z

02H40JZ
and 02H64JZ
and 02HL4JZ
and 0JH837Z

02H43JZ
and 02H60JZ
and 02HK0JZ
and 0JH607Z

02H43JZ
and 02H60JZ
and 02HK0JZ
and 0JH637Z

02H43JZ
and 02H60JZ
and 02HK0JZ
and 0JH807Z

02H43JZ
and 02H60JZ
and 02HK0JZ
and 0JH837Z

02H43JZ
and 02H60JZ
and 02HK3JZ
and 0JH607Z

02H43JZ
and 02H60JZ
and 02HK3JZ
and 0JH637Z

02H43JZ
and 02H60JZ
and 02HK3JZ
and 0JH807Z

02H43JZ
and 02H60JZ
and 02HK3JZ
and 0JH837Z

02H43JZ
and 02H60JZ
and 02HK4JZ
and 0JH607Z

02H43JZ
and 02H60JZ
and 02HK4JZ
and 0JH637Z

02H43JZ
and 02H60JZ
and 02HK4JZ
and 0JH807Z

02H43JZ
and 02H60JZ
and 02HK4JZ
and 0JH837Z

02H43JZ
and 02H60JZ
and 02HL0JZ
and 0JH607Z

02H43JZ
and 02H60JZ
and 02HL0JZ
and 0JH637Z

02H43JZ
and 02H60JZ
and 02HL0JZ
and 0JH807Z

02H43JZ
and 02H60JZ
and 02HL0JZ
and 0JH837Z

02H43JZ
and 02H60JZ
and 02HL3JZ
and 0JH607Z

02H43JZ
and 02H60JZ
and 02HL3JZ
and 0JH637Z

02H43JZ
and 02H60JZ
and 02HL3JZ
and 0JH807Z

02H43JZ
and 02H60JZ
and 02HL3JZ
and 0JH837Z

02H43JZ
and 02H60JZ
and 02HL4JZ
and 0JH607Z

02H43JZ
and 02H60JZ
and 02HL4JZ
and 0JH637Z

02H43JZ
and 02H60JZ
and 02HL4JZ
and 0JH807Z

02H43JZ
and 02H60JZ
and 02HL4JZ
and 0JH837Z

02H43JZ
and 02H63JZ
and 02HK0JZ
and 0JH607Z

02H43JZ
and 02H63JZ
and 02HK0JZ
and 0JH637Z

02H43JZ
and 02H63JZ
and 02HK0JZ
and 0JH807Z

02H43JZ
and 02H63JZ
and 02HK0JZ
and 0JH837Z

02H43JZ
and 02H63JZ
and 02HK3JZ
and 0JH607Z

02H43JZ
and 02H63JZ
and 02HK3JZ
and 0JH637Z

02H43JZ
and 02H63JZ
and 02HK3JZ
and 0JH807Z

02H43JZ
and 02H63JZ
and 02HK3JZ
and 0JH837Z

02H43JZ
and 02H63JZ
and 02HK4JZ
and 0JH607Z

02H43JZ
and 02H63JZ
and 02HK4JZ
and 0JH637Z

02H43JZ
and 02H63JZ
and 02HK4JZ
and 0JH807Z

02H43JZ
and 02H63JZ
and 02HK4JZ
and 0JH837Z

02H43JZ
and 02H63JZ
and 02HL0JZ
and 0JH607Z

02H43JZ
and 02H63JZ
and 02HL0JZ
and 0JH637Z

02H43JZ
and 02H63JZ
and 02HL0JZ
and 0JH807Z

02H43JZ
and 02H63JZ
and 02HL0JZ
and 0JH837Z

02H43JZ
and 02H63JZ
and 02HL3JZ
and 0JH607Z

02H43JZ
and 02H63JZ
and 02HL3JZ
and 0JH637Z

02H43JZ
and 02H63JZ
and 02HL3JZ
and 0JH807Z

02H43JZ
and 02H63JZ
and 02HL3JZ
and 0JH837Z

02H43JZ
and 02H63JZ
and 02HL4JZ
and 0JH607Z

02H43JZ
and 02H63JZ
and 02HL4JZ
and 0JH637Z

02H43JZ
and 02H63JZ
and 02HL4JZ
and 0JH807Z

02H43JZ
and 02H63JZ
and 02HL4JZ
and 0JH837Z

02H43JZ
and 02H64JZ
and 02HK0JZ
and 0JH607Z

02H43JZ
and 02H64JZ
and 02HK0JZ
and 0JH637Z

02H43JZ
and 02H64JZ
and 02HK0JZ
and 0JH807Z

02H43JZ
and 02H64JZ
and 02HK0JZ
and 0JH837Z

02H43JZ
and 02H64JZ
and 02HK3JZ
and 0JH607Z

02H43JZ
and 02H64JZ
and 02HK3JZ
and 0JH637Z

02H43JZ
and 02H64JZ
and 02HK3JZ
and 0JH807Z

02H43JZ
and 02H64JZ
and 02HK3JZ
and 0JH837Z

02H43JZ
and 02H64JZ
and 02HK4JZ
and 0JH607Z

02H43JZ
and 02H64JZ
and 02HK4JZ
and 0JH637Z

02H43JZ
and 02H64JZ
and 02HK4JZ
and 0JH807Z

02H43JZ
and 02H64JZ
and 02HK4JZ
and 0JH837Z

02H43JZ
and 02H64JZ
and 02HL0JZ
and 0JH607Z

02H43JZ
and 02H64JZ
and 02HL0JZ
and 0JH637Z

02H43JZ
and 02H64JZ
and 02HL0JZ
and 0JH807Z

02H43JZ
and 02H64JZ
and 02HL0JZ
and 0JH837Z

02H43JZ
and 02H64JZ
and 02HL3JZ
and 0JH607Z

02H43JZ
and 02H64JZ
and 02HL3JZ
and 0JH637Z

02H43JZ
and 02H64JZ
and 02HL3JZ
and 0JH807Z

02H43JZ
and 02H64JZ
and 02HL3JZ
and 0JH837Z

02H43JZ
and 02H64JZ
and 02HL4JZ
and 0JH607Z

02H43JZ
and 02H64JZ
and 02HL4JZ
and 0JH637Z

02H43JZ
and 02H64JZ
and 02HL4JZ
and 0JH807Z

02H43JZ
and 02H64JZ
and 02HL4JZ
and 0JH837Z

02H44JZ
and 02H60JZ
and 02HK0JZ
and 0JH607Z

02H44JZ
and 02H60JZ
and 02HK0JZ
and 0JH637Z

02H44JZ
and 02H60JZ
and 02HK0JZ
and 0JH807Z

02H44JZ
and 02H60JZ
and 02HK0JZ
and 0JH837Z

02H44JZ
and 02H60JZ
and 02HK3JZ
and 0JH607Z

02H44JZ
and 02H60JZ
and 02HK3JZ
and 0JH637Z

02H44JZ
and 02H60JZ
and 02HK3JZ
and 0JH807Z

02H44JZ
and 02H60JZ
and 02HK3JZ
and 0JH837Z

02H44JZ
and 02H60JZ
and 02HK4JZ
and 0JH607Z

02H44JZ
and 02H60JZ
and 02HK4JZ
and 0JH637Z

02H44JZ
and 02H60JZ
and 02HK4JZ
and 0JH807Z

02H44JZ
and 02H60JZ
and 02HK4JZ
and 0JH837Z

02H44JZ
and 02H60JZ
and 02HL0JZ
and 0JH607Z

02H44JZ
and 02H60JZ
and 02HL0JZ
and 0JH637Z

02H44JZ
and 02H60JZ
and 02HL0JZ
and 0JH807Z

02H44JZ
and 02H60JZ
and 02HL0JZ
and 0JH837Z

02H44JZ
and 02H60JZ
and 02HL3JZ
and 0JH607Z

02H44JZ
and 02H60JZ
and 02HL3JZ
and 0JH637Z

02H44JZ
and 02H60JZ

and 02HL3JZ
and 0JH807Z

02H44JZ
and 02H60JZ
and 02HL3JZ
and 0JH837Z

02H44JZ
and 02H60JZ
and 02HL4JZ
and 0JH607Z

02H44JZ
and 02H60JZ
and 02HL4JZ
and 0JH637Z

02H44JZ
and 02H60JZ
and 02HL4JZ
and 0JH807Z

02H44JZ
and 02H60JZ
and 02HL4JZ
and 0JH837Z

02H44JZ
and 02H63JZ
and 02HK0JZ
and 0JH607Z

02H44JZ
and 02H63JZ
and 02HK0JZ
and 0JH637Z

02H44JZ
and 02H63JZ
and 02HK0JZ
and 0JH807Z

02H44JZ
and 02H63JZ
and 02HK0JZ
and 0JH837Z

02H44JZ
and 02H63JZ
and 02HK3JZ
and 0JH607Z

02H44JZ
and 02H63JZ
and 02HK3JZ
and 0JH637Z

02H44JZ
and 02H63JZ
and 02HK3JZ
and 0JH807Z

02H44JZ
and 02H63JZ
and 02HK3JZ
and 0JH837Z

02H44JZ
and 02H63JZ
and 02HK4JZ
and 0JH607Z

02H44JZ
and 02H63JZ
and 02HK4JZ
and 0JH637Z

02H44JZ
and 02H63JZ
and 02HK4JZ
and 0JH807Z

02H44JZ
and 02H63JZ
and 02HK4JZ
and 0JH837Z

02H44JZ
and 02H63JZ
and 02HL0JZ
and 0JH607Z

02H44JZ
and 02H63JZ
and 02HL0JZ
and 0JH637Z

02H44JZ
and 02H63JZ
and 02HL0JZ
and 0JH807Z

02H44JZ
and 02H63JZ
and 02HL0JZ
and 0JH837Z

02H44JZ
and 02H63JZ
and 02HL3JZ
and 0JH607Z

02H44JZ
and 02H63JZ
and 02HL3JZ
and 0JH637Z

02H44JZ
and 02H63JZ
and 02HL3JZ
and 0JH807Z

02H44JZ
and 02H63JZ
and 02HL3JZ
and 0JH837Z

02H44JZ
and 02H63JZ
and 02HL4JZ
and 0JH607Z

02H44JZ
and 02H63JZ
and 02HL4JZ
and 0JH637Z

02H44JZ
and 02H63JZ
and 02HL4JZ
and 0JH807Z

02H44JZ
and 02H63JZ
and 02HL4JZ
and 0JH837Z

02H44JZ
and 02H64JZ
and 02HK0JZ
and 0JH607Z

02H44JZ
and 02H64JZ
and 02HK0JZ
and 0JH637Z

02H44JZ
and 02H64JZ
and 02HK0JZ
and 0JH807Z

02H44JZ
and 02H64JZ
and 02HK0JZ
and 0JH837Z

02H44JZ
and 02H64JZ
and 02HK3JZ
and 0JH607Z

02H44JZ
and 02H64JZ
and 02HK3JZ
and 0JH637Z

02H44JZ
and 02H64JZ
and 02HK3JZ
and 0JH807Z

02H44JZ
and 02H64JZ
and 02HK3JZ
and 0JH837Z

02H44JZ
and 02H64JZ
and 02HK4JZ
and 0JH607Z

02H44JZ
and 02H64JZ
and 02HK4JZ
and 0JH637Z

02H44JZ
and 02H64JZ
and 02HK4JZ
and 0JH807Z

02H44JZ
and 02H64JZ
and 02HK4JZ
and 0JH837Z

02H44JZ
and 02H64JZ
and 02HL0JZ
and 0JH607Z

02H44JZ
and 02H64JZ
and 02HL0JZ
and 0JH637Z

02H44JZ
and 02H64JZ
and 02HL0JZ
and 0JH807Z

02H44JZ
and 02H64JZ
and 02HL0JZ
and 0JH837Z

02H44JZ
and 02H64JZ
and 02HL3JZ
and 0JH607Z

02H44JZ
and 02H64JZ
and 02HL3JZ
and 0JH637Z

02H44JZ
and 02H64JZ
and 02HL3JZ
and 0JH807Z

02H44JZ
and 02H64JZ
and 02HL3JZ
and 0JH837Z

02H44JZ
and 02H64JZ
and 02HL4JZ
and 0JH607Z

02H44JZ
and 02H64JZ
and 02HL4JZ
and 0JH637Z

02H44JZ
and 02H64JZ
and 02HL4JZ
and 0JH807Z

02H44JZ
and 02H64JZ
and 02HL4JZ
and 0JH837Z

02H60KZ
and 0JH608Z

02H60KZ
and 0JH638Z

02H60KZ
and 0JH808Z

02H60KZ
and 0JH838Z

02H63JZ
and 02PA0MZ

02H63JZ
and 02PA3MZ

02H63JZ
and 02PA4MZ

02H63JZ
and 02PAXMZ

02H63KZ
and 0JH608Z

02H63KZ
and 0JH638Z

02H63KZ
and 0JH808Z

02H63KZ
and 0JH838Z

02H64KZ
and 0JH608Z

02H64KZ
and 0JH638Z

02H64KZ
and 0JH808Z

02H64KZ
and 0JH838Z

02H70KZ
and 0JH608Z

02H70KZ
and 0JH638Z

02H70KZ
and 0JH808Z

02H70KZ
and 0JH838Z

02H73JZ
and 02PA0MZ

02H73JZ
and 02PA3MZ

02H73JZ
and 02PA4MZ

02H73JZ
and 02PAXMZ

02H73KZ
and 0JH608Z

02H73KZ
and 0JH638Z

02H73KZ
and 0JH808Z

02H73KZ
and 0JH838Z

02H74KZ
and 0JH608Z

02H74KZ
and 0JH638Z

02H74KZ
and 0JH808Z

02H74KZ
and 0JH838Z

02HA0RS
and 02PA0RZ

02HA0RS
and 02PA3RZ

02HA0RS
and 02PA4RZ

02HA0RZ
and 02PA0RZ

02HA0RZ
and 02PA3RZ

02HA0RZ
and 02PA4RZ

02HA3RS
and 02PA0RZ

02HA3RS
and 02PA3RZ

02HA3RS
and 02PA4RZ

02HA4RS
and 02PA0RZ

02HA4RS
and 02PA3RZ

02HA4RS
and 02PA4RZ

02HA4RZ
and 02PA0RZ

02HA4RZ
and 02PA3RZ

02HA4RZ
and 02PA4RZ

02HK00Z
and 0JH600Z

02HK00Z
and 0JH630Z

02HK00Z
and 0JH800Z

02HK00Z
and 0JH830Z

02HK02Z
and 0JH600Z

02HK02Z
and 0JH630Z

02HK02Z
and 0JH800Z

02HK02Z
and 0JH830Z

02HK0KZ
and 0JH608Z

02HK0KZ
and 0JH609Z

02HK0KZ
and 0JH638Z

02HK0KZ
and 0JH639Z

02HK0KZ
and 0JH808Z

02HK0KZ
and 0JH809Z

02HK0KZ
and 0JH838Z

02HK0KZ
and 0JH839Z

02HK30Z
and 0JH600Z

02HK30Z
and 0JH630Z

02HK30Z
and 0JH800Z

02HK30Z
and 0JH830Z

02HK32Z
and 0JH600Z

02HK32Z
and 0JH630Z

02HK32Z
and 0JH800Z

02HK32Z
and 0JH830Z

02HK3JZ
and 02PA0MZ

02HK3JZ
and 02PA3MZ

02HK3JZ
and 02PA4MZ

02HK3JZ
and 02PAXMZ

02HK3KZ
and 0JH608Z

02HK3KZ
and 0JH609Z

02HK3KZ
and 0JH638Z

02HK3KZ
and 0JH639Z

02HK3KZ
and 0JH808Z

02HK3KZ
and 0JH809Z

02HK3KZ
and 0JH838Z

02HK3KZ
and 0JH839Z

02HK40Z
and 0JH600Z

02HK40Z
and 0JH630Z

02HK40Z
and 0JH800Z

02HK40Z
and 0JH830Z

02HK42Z
and 0JH600Z

02HK42Z
and 0JH630Z

02HK42Z
and 0JH800Z

02HK42Z
and 0JH830Z

02HK4KZ
and 0JH608Z

02HK4KZ
and 0JH609Z

02HK4KZ
and 0JH638Z

02HK4KZ
and 0JH639Z

02HK4KZ
and 0JH808Z

02HK4KZ
and 0JH809Z

02HK4KZ
and 0JH838Z

02HK4KZ
and 0JH839Z

02HL0KZ
and 0JH608Z

02HL0KZ
and 0JH609Z

02HL0KZ
and 0JH638Z

02HL0KZ
and 0JH639Z

02HL0KZ
and 0JH808Z

02HL0KZ
and 0JH809Z

02HL0KZ
and 0JH838Z

02HL0KZ
and 0JH839Z

02HL0MZ
and 0JH60AZ

02HL0MZ
and 0JH63AZ

02HL0MZ
and 0JH80AZ

02HL0MZ
and 0JH83AZ

02HL3JZ
and 02PA0MZ

02HL3JZ
and 02PA3MZ

02HL3JZ
and 02PA4MZ

02HL3JZ
and 02PAXMZ

02HL3KZ
and 0JH608Z

02HL3KZ
and 0JH609Z

02HL3KZ
and 0JH638Z

02HL3KZ
and 0JH639Z

02HL3KZ
and 0JH808Z

02HL3KZ
and 0JH809Z

02HL3KZ
and 0JH838Z

02HL3KZ
and 0JH839Z

02HL3MZ
and 0JH60AZ

02HL3MZ
and 0JH63AZ

02HL3MZ
and 0JH80AZ

02HL3MZ
and 0JH83AZ

02HL4KZ
and 0JH608Z

02HL4KZ
and 0JH609Z

02HL4KZ
and 0JH638Z

02HL4KZ
and 0JH639Z

02HL4KZ
and 0JH808Z

02HL4KZ
and 0JH809Z

02HL4KZ
and 0JH838Z

02HL4KZ
and 0JH839Z

02HL4MZ
and 0JH60AZ

02HL4MZ
and 0JH63AZ

02HL4MZ
and 0JH80AZ

02HL4MZ
and 0JH83AZ

02WA0QZ
and 02PA0RZ

02WA0QZ
and 02PA3RZ

02WA0QZ
and 02PA4RZ

02WA0RZ
and 02PA0RZ

02WA0RZ
and 02PA3RZ

02WA0RZ
and 02PA4RZ

02WA3QZ
and 02PA0RZ

02WA3QZ
and 02PA3RZ

02WA3QZ
and 02PA4RZ

02WA3RZ
and 02PA0RZ

02WA3RZ
and 02PA3RZ

02WA3RZ
and 02PA4RZ

02WA4QZ
and 02PA0RZ

02WA4QZ
and 02PA3RZ

02WA4QZ
and 02PA4RZ

02WA4RZ
and 02PA0RZ

02WA4RZ
and 02PA3RZ

02WA4RZ
and 02PA4RZ

07BH0ZZ
and 0UTM0ZZ

07BH0ZZ
and 0UTMXZZ

07BH4ZZ
and 0UTM0ZZ

07BH4ZZ
and 0UTMXZZ

07BJ0ZZ
and 0UTM0ZZ

07BJ0ZZ
and 0UTMXZZ

07BJ4ZZ
and 0UTM0ZZ

07BJ4ZZ
and 0UTMXZZ

07T50ZZ
and 07T60ZZ
and 07T70ZZ
and 07T80ZZ
and 07T90ZZ
and 0HTV0ZZ
and 0KTH0ZZ
and 0KTJ0ZZ

07T50ZZ
and 07T60ZZ
and 0HTV0ZZ

07T50ZZ
and 07T60ZZ
and 0HTV0ZZ
and 0KTH0ZZ
and 0KTJ0ZZ

07T50ZZ
and 07T70ZZ
and 07T80ZZ
and 0HTT0ZZ
and 0KTH0ZZ

07T50ZZ
and 0HTT0ZZ

07T50ZZ
and 0HTT0ZZ
and 0KTH0ZZ

07T60ZZ
and 07T70ZZ
and 07T90ZZ
and 0HTU0ZZ
and 0KTJ0ZZ

07T60ZZ
and 0HTU0ZZ

07T60ZZ
and 0HTU0ZZ
and 0KTJ0ZZ

0DQ80ZZ
and 0WQFXZ2

0DQ90ZZ
and 0WQFXZ2

0DQA0ZZ
and 0WQFXZ2

0DQB0ZZ
and 0WQFXZ2

0DQE0ZZ
and 0WQFXZ2

0DQF0ZZ
and 0WQFXZ2

0DQG0ZZ
and 0WQFXZ2

0DQH0ZZ
and 0WQFXZ2

0DQK0ZZ
and 0WQFXZ2

0DQL0ZZ
and 0WQFXZ2

0DQM0ZZ
and 0WQFXZ2

0DQN0ZZ
and 0WQFXZ2

0DT90ZZ
and 0FTG0ZZ

0HRT37Z
and 0JD63ZZ

0HRT37Z
and 0JD73ZZ

0HRT37Z
and 0JD83ZZ

0HRT37Z
and 0JD93ZZ

0HRT37Z
and 0JDL3ZZ

0HRT37Z
and 0JDM3ZZ

0HRU37Z
and 0JD63ZZ

0HRU37Z
and 0JD73ZZ

0HRU37Z
and 0JD83ZZ

0HRU37Z
and 0JD93ZZ

0HRU37Z
and 0JDL3ZZ

0HRU37Z
and 0JDM3ZZ

0HRV37Z
and 0JD63ZZ

0HRV37Z
and 0JD73ZZ

0HRV37Z
and 0JD83ZZ

0HRV37Z
and 0JD93ZZ

0HRV37Z
and 0JDL3ZZ

0HRV37Z
and 0JDM3ZZ

0JH604Z
and 02H40JZ

0JH604Z
and 02H40MZ

0JH604Z
and 02H44JZ

0JH604Z
and 02H44MZ

0JH604Z
and 02H60JZ

0JH604Z
and 02H60MZ

0JH604Z
and 02H63JZ

0JH604Z
and 02H64JZ

0JH604Z
and 02H64MZ

0JH604Z
and 02H70JZ

0JH604Z
and 02H70MZ

0JH604Z
and 02H73JZ

0JH604Z
and 02H74JZ

0JH604Z
and 02H74MZ

0JH604Z
and 02HK0JZ

0JH604Z
and 02HK0MZ

0JH604Z
and 02HK3JZ

0JH604Z
and 02HK3MZ

0JH604Z
and 02HK4JZ

0JH604Z
and 02HK4MZ

0JH604Z
and 02HL0JZ

0JH604Z
and 02HL0MZ

0JH604Z
and 02HL3JZ

0JH604Z
and 02HL3MZ

0JH604Z
and 02HL4JZ

0JH604Z
and 02HL4MZ

0JH604Z
and 02HN0JZ

0JH604Z
and 02HN0MZ

0JH604Z
and 02HN3JZ

0JH604Z
and 02HN3MZ

0JH604Z
and 02HN4JZ

0JH604Z
and 02HN4MZ

0JH604Z
and 0JPT0PZ

0JH604Z
and 0JPT0PZ
and 02H40JZ

0JH604Z
and 0JPT0PZ
and 02H40MZ

0JH604Z
and 0JPT0PZ
and 02H44JZ

0JH604Z
and 0JPT0PZ
and 02H44MZ

0JH604Z
and 0JPT0PZ
and 02H60JZ

0JH604Z
and 0JPT0PZ
and 02H60MZ

0JH604Z
and 0JPT0PZ
and 02H63JZ

0JH604Z
and 0JPT0PZ
and 02H63JZ
and 02PA0MZ

0JH604Z
and 0JPT0PZ
and 02H63JZ
and 02PA3MZ

0JH604Z
and 0JPT0PZ
and 02H63JZ
and 02PA4MZ

0JH604Z
and 0JPT0PZ
and 02H63JZ
and 02PAXMZ

0JH604Z
and 0JPT0PZ
and 02H63MZ

0JH604Z
and 0JPT0PZ
and 02H64JZ

0JH604Z
and 0JPT0PZ
and 02H64MZ

0JH604Z
and 0JPT0PZ
and 02H70JZ

0JH604Z
and 0JPT0PZ
and 02H70MZ

0JH604Z
and 0JPT0PZ
and 02H73JZ

0JH604Z
and 0JPT0PZ
and 02H73JZ
and 02PA0MZ

0JH604Z
and 0JPT0PZ
and 02H73JZ
and 02PA3MZ

0JH604Z
and 0JPT0PZ
and 02H73JZ
and 02PA4MZ

0JH604Z
and 0JPT0PZ
and 02H73JZ
and 02PAXMZ

0JH604Z
and 0JPT0PZ
and 02H73MZ

0JH604Z
and 0JPT0PZ
and 02H74JZ

0JH604Z
and 0JPT0PZ
and 02H74MZ

0JH604Z
and 0JPT0PZ
and 02HK0JZ

0JH604Z
and 0JPT0PZ
and 02HK0MZ

0JH604Z
and 0JPT0PZ
and 02HK3JZ

0JH604Z
and 0JPT0PZ
and 02HK3JZ
and 02PA0MZ

0JH604Z
and 0JPT0PZ
and 02HK3JZ
and 02PA3MZ

0JH604Z
and 0JPT0PZ
and 02HK3JZ
and 02PA4MZ

0JH604Z
and 0JPT0PZ
and 02HK3JZ
and 02PAXMZ

0JH604Z
and 0JPT0PZ
and 02HK3MZ

0JH604Z
and 0JPT0PZ
and 02HK4JZ

0JH604Z
and 0JPT0PZ
and 02HK4MZ

0JH604Z
and 0JPT0PZ
and 02HL0JZ

0JH604Z
and 0JPT0PZ
and 02HL0MZ

0JH604Z
and 0JPT0PZ
and 02HL3JZ

0JH604Z
and 0JPT0PZ
and 02HL3JZ
and 02PA0MZ

0JH604Z
and 0JPT0PZ
and 02HL3JZ
and 02PA3MZ

0JH604Z
and 0JPT0PZ
and 02HL3JZ
and 02PA4MZ

0JH604Z
and 0JPT0PZ
and 02HL3JZ
and 02PAXMZ

0JH604Z
and 0JPT0PZ
and 02HL3MZ

0JH604Z
and 0JPT0PZ
and 02HL4JZ

0JH604Z
and 0JPT0PZ
and 02HL4MZ

0JH604Z
and 0JPT0PZ
and 02HN0JZ

0JH604Z
and 0JPT0PZ
and 02HN0MZ

0JH604Z
and 0JPT0PZ
and 02HN3JZ

0JH604Z
and 0JPT0PZ
and 02HN3MZ

0JH604Z
and 0JPT0PZ
and 02HN4JZ

0JH604Z
and 0JPT0PZ
and 02HN4MZ

0JH604Z
and 0JPT3PZ

0JH604Z
and 0JPT3PZ
and 02H40JZ

0JH604Z
and 0JPT3PZ
and 02H40MZ

0JH604Z
and 0JPT3PZ
and 02H44JZ

0JH604Z
and 0JPT3PZ
and 02H44MZ

0JH604Z
and 0JPT3PZ
and 02H60JZ

0JH604Z
and 0JPT3PZ
and 02H60MZ

0JH604Z
and 0JPT3PZ
and 02H63JZ

0JH604Z
and 0JPT3PZ
and 02H63JZ
and 02PA0MZ

0JH604Z
and 0JPT3PZ
and 02H63JZ
and 02PA3MZ

0JH604Z
and 0JPT3PZ
and 02H63JZ
and 02PA4MZ

0JH604Z
and 0JPT3PZ
and 02H63JZ
and 02PAXMZ

0JH604Z
and 0JPT3PZ
and 02H63MZ

0JH604Z
and 0JPT3PZ
and 02H64JZ

0JH604Z
and 0JPT3PZ
and 02H64MZ

0JH604Z
and 0JPT3PZ
and 02H70JZ

0JH604Z
and 0JPT3PZ
and 02H70MZ

0JH604Z
and 0JPT3PZ
and 02H73JZ

0JH604Z
and 0JPT3PZ
and 02H73JZ
and 02PA0MZ

0JH604Z
and 0JPT3PZ
and 02H73JZ
and 02PA3MZ

0JH604Z
and 0JPT3PZ
and 02H73JZ
and 02PA4MZ

0JH604Z
and 0JPT3PZ
and 02H73JZ
and 02PAXMZ

0JH604Z
and 0JPT3PZ
and 02H73MZ

0JH604Z
and 0JPT3PZ
and 02H74JZ

0JH604Z
and 0JPT3PZ
and 02H74MZ

0JH604Z
and 0JPT3PZ
and 02HK0JZ

0JH604Z
and 0JPT3PZ
and 02HK0MZ

0JH604Z
and 0JPT3PZ
and 02HK3JZ

0JH604Z
and 0JPT3PZ
and 02HK3JZ
and 02PA0MZ

0JH604Z
and 0JPT3PZ
and 02HK3JZ
and 02PA3MZ

0JH604Z
and 0JPT3PZ
and 02HK3JZ
and 02PA4MZ

0JH604Z
and 0JPT3PZ
and 02HK3JZ
and 02PAXMZ

0JH604Z
and 0JPT3PZ
and 02HK3MZ

0JH604Z
and 0JPT3PZ
and 02HK4JZ

0JH604Z
and 0JPT3PZ
and 02HK4MZ

0JH604Z
and 0JPT3PZ
and 02HL0JZ

0JH604Z
and 0JPT3PZ
and 02HL0MZ

0JH604Z
and 0JPT3PZ
and 02HL3JZ

0JH604Z
and 0JPT3PZ
and 02HL3JZ
and 02PA0MZ

0JH604Z
and 0JPT3PZ

and 02HL3JZ
and 02PA3MZ

0JH604Z
and 0JPT3PZ
and 02HL3JZ
and 02PA4MZ

0JH604Z
and 0JPT3PZ
and 02HL3JZ
and 02PAXMZ

0JH604Z
and 0JPT3PZ
and 02HL3MZ

0JH604Z
and 0JPT3PZ
and 02HL4JZ

0JH604Z
and 0JPT3PZ
and 02HL4MZ

0JH604Z
and 0JPT3PZ
and 02HN0JZ

0JH604Z
and 0JPT3PZ
and 02HN0MZ

0JH604Z
and 0JPT3PZ
and 02HN3JZ

0JH604Z
and 0JPT3PZ
and 02HN3MZ

0JH604Z
and 0JPT3PZ
and 02HN4JZ

0JH604Z
and 0JPT3PZ
and 02HN4MZ

0JH605Z
and 02H40JZ

0JH605Z
and 02H40MZ

0JH605Z
and 02H44JZ

0JH605Z
and 02H44MZ

0JH605Z
and 02H60JZ

0JH605Z
and 02H60MZ

0JH605Z
and 02H63JZ

0JH605Z
and 02H64JZ

0JH605Z
and 02H64MZ

0JH605Z
and 02H70JZ

0JH605Z
and 02H70MZ

0JH605Z
and 02H73JZ

0JH605Z
and 02H74JZ

0JH605Z
and 02H74MZ

0JH605Z
and 02HK0JZ

0JH605Z
and 02HK0MZ

0JH605Z
and 02HK3JZ

0JH605Z
and 02HK3MZ

0JH605Z
and 02HK4JZ

0JH605Z
and 02HK4MZ

0JH605Z
and 02HL0JZ

0JH605Z
and 02HL0MZ

0JH605Z
and 02HL3JZ

0JH605Z
and 02HL3MZ

0JH605Z
and 02HL4JZ

0JH605Z
and 02HL4MZ

0JH605Z
and 02HN0JZ

0JH605Z
and 02HN0MZ

0JH605Z
and 02HN3JZ

0JH605Z
and 02HN3MZ

0JH605Z
and 02HN4JZ

0JH605Z
and 02HN4MZ

0JH605Z
and 0JPT0PZ

0JH605Z
and 0JPT0PZ
and 02H40JZ

0JH605Z
and 0JPT0PZ
and 02H40MZ

0JH605Z
and 0JPT0PZ
and 02H44JZ

0JH605Z
and 0JPT0PZ
and 02H44MZ

0JH605Z
and 0JPT0PZ
and 02H60JZ

0JH605Z
and 0JPT0PZ
and 02H60MZ

0JH605Z
and 0JPT0PZ
and 02H63JZ

0JH605Z
and 0JPT0PZ
and 02H63JZ
and 02PA0MZ

0JH605Z
and 0JPT0PZ
and 02H63JZ
and 02PA3MZ

0JH605Z
and 0JPT0PZ
and 02H63JZ
and 02PA4MZ

0JH605Z
and 0JPT0PZ
and 02H63JZ
and 02PAXMZ

0JH605Z
and 0JPT0PZ
and 02H63MZ

0JH605Z
and 0JPT0PZ
and 02H64JZ

0JH605Z
and 0JPT0PZ
and 02H64MZ

0JH605Z
and 0JPT0PZ
and 02H70JZ

0JH605Z
and 0JPT0PZ
and 02H70MZ

0JH605Z
and 0JPT0PZ
and 02H73JZ

0JH605Z
and 0JPT0PZ
and 02H73JZ
and 02PA0MZ

0JH605Z
and 0JPT0PZ
and 02H73JZ
and 02PA3MZ

0JH605Z
and 0JPT0PZ
and 02H73JZ
and 02PA4MZ

0JH605Z
and 0JPT0PZ
and 02H73JZ
and 02PAXMZ

0JH605Z
and 0JPT0PZ
and 02H73MZ

0JH605Z
and 0JPT0PZ
and 02H74JZ

0JH605Z
and 0JPT0PZ
and 02H74MZ

0JH605Z
and 0JPT0PZ
and 02HK0JZ

0JH605Z
and 0JPT0PZ
and 02HK0MZ

0JH605Z
and 0JPT0PZ
and 02HK3JZ

0JH605Z
and 0JPT0PZ
and 02HK3JZ
and 02PA0MZ

0JH605Z
and 0JPT0PZ
and 02HK3JZ
and 02PA3MZ

0JH605Z
and 0JPT0PZ
and 02HK3JZ
and 02PA4MZ

0JH605Z
and 0JPT0PZ
and 02HK3JZ
and 02PAXMZ

0JH605Z
and 0JPT0PZ
and 02HK3MZ

0JH605Z
and 0JPT0PZ
and 02HK4JZ

0JH605Z
and 0JPT0PZ
and 02HK4MZ

0JH605Z
and 0JPT0PZ
and 02HL0JZ

0JH605Z
and 0JPT0PZ
and 02HL0MZ

0JH605Z
and 0JPT0PZ
and 02HL3JZ

0JH605Z
and 0JPT0PZ
and 02HL3JZ
and 02PA0MZ

0JH605Z
and 0JPT0PZ
and 02HL3JZ
and 02PA3MZ

0JH605Z
and 0JPT0PZ
and 02HL3JZ
and 02PA4MZ

0JH605Z
and 0JPT0PZ
and 02HL3JZ
and 02PAXMZ

0JH605Z
and 0JPT0PZ
and 02HL3MZ

0JH605Z
and 0JPT0PZ
and 02HL4JZ

0JH605Z
and 0JPT0PZ
and 02HL4MZ

0JH605Z
and 0JPT0PZ
and 02HN0JZ

0JH605Z
and 0JPT0PZ
and 02HN0MZ

0JH605Z
and 0JPT0PZ
and 02HN3JZ

0JH605Z
and 0JPT0PZ
and 02HN3MZ

0JH605Z
and 0JPT0PZ
and 02HN4JZ

0JH605Z
and 0JPT0PZ
and 02HN4MZ

0JH605Z
and 0JPT3PZ

0JH605Z
and 0JPT3PZ
and 02H40JZ

0JH605Z
and 0JPT3PZ
and 02H40MZ

0JH605Z
and 0JPT3PZ
and 02H44JZ

0JH605Z
and 0JPT3PZ
and 02H44MZ

0JH605Z
and 0JPT3PZ
and 02H60JZ

0JH605Z
and 0JPT3PZ
and 02H60MZ

0JH605Z
and 0JPT3PZ
and 02H63JZ

0JH605Z
and 0JPT3PZ
and 02H63JZ
and 02PA0MZ

0JH605Z
and 0JPT3PZ
and 02H63JZ
and 02PA3MZ

0JH605Z
and 0JPT3PZ
and 02H63JZ
and 02PA4MZ

0JH605Z
and 0JPT3PZ
and 02H63JZ
and 02PAXMZ

0JH605Z
and 0JPT3PZ
and 02H63MZ

0JH605Z
and 0JPT3PZ
and 02H64JZ

0JH605Z
and 0JPT3PZ
and 02H64MZ

0JH605Z
and 0JPT3PZ
and 02H70JZ

0JH605Z
and 0JPT3PZ
and 02H70MZ

0JH605Z
and 0JPT3PZ
and 02H73JZ

0JH605Z
and 0JPT3PZ
and 02H73JZ
and 02PA0MZ

0JH605Z
and 0JPT3PZ
and 02H73JZ
and 02PA3MZ

0JH605Z
and 0JPT3PZ
and 02H73JZ
and 02PA4MZ

0JH605Z
and 0JPT3PZ
and 02H73JZ
and 02PAXMZ

0JH605Z
and 0JPT3PZ
and 02H73MZ

0JH605Z
and 0JPT3PZ
and 02H74JZ

0JH605Z
and 0JPT3PZ
and 02H74MZ

0JH605Z
and 0JPT3PZ
and 02HK0JZ

0JH605Z
and 0JPT3PZ
and 02HK0MZ

0JH605Z
and 0JPT3PZ
and 02HK3JZ

0JH605Z
and 0JPT3PZ
and 02HK3JZ
and 02PA0MZ

0JH605Z
and 0JPT3PZ
and 02HK3JZ
and 02PA3MZ

0JH605Z
and 0JPT3PZ
and 02HK3JZ
and 02PA4MZ

0JH605Z
and 0JPT3PZ
and 02HK3JZ
and 02PAXMZ

0JH605Z
and 0JPT3PZ
and 02HK3MZ

0JH605Z
and 0JPT3PZ
and 02HK4JZ

0JH605Z
and 0JPT3PZ
and 02HK4MZ

0JH605Z
and 0JPT3PZ
and 02HL0JZ

0JH605Z
and 0JPT3PZ
and 02HL0MZ

0JH605Z
and 0JPT3PZ
and 02HL3JZ

0JH605Z
and 0JPT3PZ
and 02HL3JZ
and 02PA0MZ

0JH605Z
and 0JPT3PZ
and 02HL3JZ
and 02PA3MZ

0JH605Z
and 0JPT3PZ
and 02HL3JZ
and 02PA4MZ

0JH605Z
and 0JPT3PZ
and 02HL3JZ
and 02PAXMZ

0JH605Z
and 0JPT3PZ
and 02HL3MZ

0JH605Z
and 0JPT3PZ
and 02HL4JZ

0JH605Z
and 0JPT3PZ
and 02HL4MZ

0JH605Z
and 0JPT3PZ
and 02HN0JZ

0JH605Z
and 0JPT3PZ
and 02HN0MZ

0JH605Z
and 0JPT3PZ
and 02HN3JZ

0JH605Z
and 0JPT3PZ
and 02HN3MZ

0JH605Z
and 0JPT3PZ
and 02HN4JZ

0JH605Z
and 0JPT3PZ
and 02HN4MZ

0JH606Z
and 02HK3JZ

0JH606Z
and 02HL3JZ

0JH606Z
and 02HN0JZ

0JH606Z
and 02HN0MZ

0JH606Z
and 02HN3JZ

0JH606Z
and 02HN3MZ

0JH606Z
and 02HN4JZ

0JH606Z
and 02HN4MZ

0JH606Z
and 0JPT0PZ

0JH606Z
and 0JPT0PZ
and 02H40JZ

0JH606Z
and 0JPT0PZ
and 02H40MZ

0JH606Z
and 0JPT0PZ
and 02H44JZ

0JH606Z
and 0JPT0PZ
and 02H44MZ

0JH606Z
and 0JPT0PZ
and 02H60JZ

0JH606Z
and 0JPT0PZ
and 02H60MZ

0JH606Z
and 0JPT0PZ
and 02H63JZ

0JH606Z
and 0JPT0PZ
and 02H63JZ
and 02PA0MZ

0JH606Z
and 0JPT0PZ
and 02H63JZ
and 02PA3MZ

0JH606Z
and 0JPT0PZ
and 02H63JZ
and 02PA4MZ

0JH606Z
and 0JPT0PZ
and 02H63JZ
and 02PAXMZ

0JH606Z
and 0JPT0PZ
and 02H63MZ

0JH606Z
and 0JPT0PZ
and 02H64JZ

0JH606Z
and 0JPT0PZ
and 02H64MZ

0JH606Z
and 0JPT0PZ
and 02H70JZ

0JH606Z
and 0JPT0PZ
and 02H70MZ

0JH606Z
and 0JPT0PZ
and 02H73JZ

0JH606Z
and 0JPT0PZ
and 02H73JZ
and 02PA0MZ

0JH606Z
and 0JPT0PZ
and 02H73JZ
and 02PA3MZ

0JH606Z
and 0JPT0PZ
and 02H73JZ
and 02PA4MZ

0JH606Z
and 0JPT0PZ
and 02H73JZ
and 02PAXMZ

0JH606Z
and 0JPT0PZ
and 02H73MZ

0JH606Z
and 0JPT0PZ
and 02H74JZ

0JH606Z
and 0JPT0PZ
and 02H74MZ

0JH606Z
and 0JPT0PZ
and 02HK0JZ

0JH606Z
and 0JPT0PZ
and 02HK0MZ

0JH606Z
and 0JPT0PZ
and 02HK3JZ

0JH606Z
and 0JPT0PZ
and 02HK3JZ
and 02PA0MZ

0JH606Z
and 0JPT0PZ
and 02HK3JZ
and 02PA3MZ

0JH606Z
and 0JPT0PZ
and 02HK3JZ
and 02PA4MZ

0JH606Z
and 0JPT0PZ
and 02HK3JZ
and 02PAXMZ

0JH606Z
and 0JPT0PZ
and 02HK3MZ

0JH606Z
and 0JPT0PZ
and 02HK4JZ

0JH606Z
and 0JPT0PZ
and 02HK4MZ

0JH606Z
and 0JPT0PZ
and 02HL0JZ

0JH606Z
and 0JPT0PZ
and 02HL0MZ

0JH606Z
and 0JPT0PZ
and 02HL3JZ

0JH606Z
and 0JPT0PZ
and 02HL3JZ
and 02PA0MZ

0JH606Z
and 0JPT0PZ
and 02HL3JZ
and 02PA3MZ

0JH606Z
and 0JPT0PZ
and 02HL3JZ
and 02PA4MZ

0JH606Z
and 0JPT0PZ
and 02HL3JZ
and 02PAXMZ

0JH606Z
and 0JPT0PZ
and 02HL3MZ

0JH606Z
and 0JPT0PZ
and 02HL4JZ

0JH606Z
and 0JPT0PZ
and 02HL4MZ

0JH606Z
and 0JPT0PZ
and 02HN0JZ

0JH606Z
and 0JPT0PZ
and 02HN0MZ

0JH606Z
and 0JPT0PZ
and 02HN3JZ

0JH606Z
and 0JPT0PZ
and 02HN3MZ

0JH606Z
and 0JPT0PZ
and 02HN4JZ

0JH606Z
and 0JPT0PZ
and 02HN4MZ

0JH606Z
and 0JPT3PZ

0JH606Z
and 0JPT3PZ
and 02H40JZ

0JH606Z
and 0JPT3PZ
and 02H40MZ

0JH606Z
and 0JPT3PZ
and 02H44JZ

0JH606Z
and 0JPT3PZ
and 02H44MZ

0JH606Z
and 0JPT3PZ
and 02H60JZ

0JH606Z
and 0JPT3PZ
and 02H60MZ

0JH606Z
and 0JPT3PZ
and 02H63JZ

0JH606Z
and 0JPT3PZ
and 02H63JZ
and 02PA0MZ

0JH606Z
and 0JPT3PZ
and 02H63JZ
and 02PA3MZ

0JH606Z
and 0JPT3PZ
and 02H63JZ
and 02PA4MZ

0JH606Z
and 0JPT3PZ
and 02H63JZ
and 02PAXMZ

0JH606Z
and 0JPT3PZ
and 02H63MZ

0JH606Z
and 0JPT3PZ
and 02H64JZ

0JH606Z
and 0JPT3PZ
and 02H64MZ

0JH606Z
and 0JPT3PZ
and 02H70JZ

0JH606Z
and 0JPT3PZ
and 02H70MZ

0JH606Z
and 0JPT3PZ
and 02H73JZ

0JH606Z
and 0JPT3PZ
and 02H73JZ
and 02PA0MZ

0JH606Z
and 0JPT3PZ
and 02H73JZ
and 02PA3MZ

0JH606Z
and 0JPT3PZ
and 02H73JZ
and 02PA4MZ

0JH606Z
and 0JPT3PZ
and 02H73JZ
and 02PAXMZ

0JH606Z
and 0JPT3PZ
and 02H73MZ

0JH606Z
and 0JPT3PZ
and 02H74JZ

0JH606Z
and 0JPT3PZ
and 02H74MZ

0JH606Z
and 0JPT3PZ
and 02HK0JZ

0JH606Z
and 0JPT3PZ
and 02HK0MZ

0JH606Z
and 0JPT3PZ
and 02HK3JZ

0JH606Z
and 0JPT3PZ
and 02HK3JZ
and 02PA0MZ

0JH606Z
and 0JPT3PZ
and 02HK3JZ
and 02PA3MZ

0JH606Z
and 0JPT3PZ
and 02HK3JZ
and 02PA4MZ

0JH606Z
and 0JPT3PZ
and 02HK3JZ
and 02PAXMZ

0JH606Z
and 0JPT3PZ
and 02HK3MZ

0JH606Z
and 0JPT3PZ
and 02HK4JZ

0JH606Z
and 0JPT3PZ
and 02HK4MZ

0JH606Z
and 0JPT3PZ
and 02HL0JZ

0JH606Z
and 0JPT3PZ
and 02HL0MZ

0JH606Z
and 0JPT3PZ
and 02HL3JZ

0JH606Z
and 0JPT3PZ
and 02HL3JZ
and 02PA0MZ

0JH606Z
and 0JPT3PZ
and 02HL3JZ
and 02PA3MZ

0JH606Z
and 0JPT3PZ
and 02HL3JZ
and 02PA4MZ

0JH606Z
and 0JPT3PZ
and 02HL3JZ
and 02PAXMZ

0JH606Z
and 0JPT3PZ
and 02HL3MZ

0JH606Z
and 0JPT3PZ
and 02HL4JZ

0JH606Z
and 0JPT3PZ
and 02HL4MZ

0JH606Z
and 0JPT3PZ
and 02HN0JZ

0JH606Z
and 0JPT3PZ
and 02HN0MZ

0JH606Z
and 0JPT3PZ
and 02HN3JZ

0JH606Z
and 0JPT3PZ
and 02HN3MZ

0JH606Z
and 0JPT3PZ
and 02HN4JZ

0JH606Z
and 0JPT3PZ
and 02HN4MZ

0JH607Z
and 02H40JZ

0JH607Z
and 02H40MZ

0JH607Z
and 02H43JZ

0JH607Z
and 02H43KZ

0JH607Z
and 02H43MZ

0JH607Z
and 02H44JZ

0JH607Z
and 02H44MZ

0JH607Z
and 02H60JZ

0JH607Z
and 02H60MZ

0JH607Z
and 02H63JZ

0JH607Z
and 02H63JZ
and 02PA0MZ

0JH607Z
and 02H63JZ
and 02PA3MZ

0JH607Z
and 02H63JZ
and 02PA4MZ

0JH607Z
and 02H63JZ
and 02PAXMZ

0JH607Z
and 02H63MZ

0JH607Z
and 02H64JZ

0JH607Z
and 02H64MZ

0JH607Z
and 02H70JZ

0JH607Z
and 02H70MZ

0JH607Z
and 02H73JZ

0JH607Z
and 02H73JZ
and 02PA0MZ

0JH607Z
and 02H73JZ
and 02PA3MZ

0JH607Z
and 02H73JZ
and 02PA4MZ

0JH607Z
and 02H73JZ
and 02PAXMZ

0JH607Z
and 02H73MZ

0JH607Z
and 02H74JZ

0JH607Z
and 02H74MZ

0JH607Z
and 02HK0JZ

0JH607Z
and 02HK0MZ

0JH607Z
and 02HK3JZ

0JH607Z
and 02HK3JZ
and 02PA0MZ

0JH607Z
and 02HK3JZ
and 02PA3MZ

0JH607Z
and 02HK3JZ
and 02PA4MZ

0JH607Z
and 02HK3JZ
and 02PAXMZ

0JH607Z
and 02HK3MZ

0JH607Z
and 02HK4JZ

0JH607Z
and 02HK4MZ

0JH607Z
and 02HL0JZ

0JH607Z
and 02HL0MZ

0JH607Z
and 02HL3JZ

0JH607Z
and 02HL3JZ
and 02PA0MZ

0JH607Z
and 02HL3JZ
and 02PA3MZ

0JH607Z
and 02HL3JZ
and 02PA4MZ

0JH607Z
and 02HL3JZ
and 02PAXMZ

0JH607Z
and 02HL3MZ

0JH607Z
and 02HL4JZ

0JH607Z
and 02HL4MZ

0JH607Z
and 02HN0JZ

0JH607Z
and 02HN0MZ

0JH607Z
and 02HN3JZ

0JH607Z
and 02HN3MZ

0JH607Z
and 02HN4JZ

0JH607Z
and 02HN4MZ

0JH608Z
and 02H40KZ

0JH608Z
and 02H44KZ

0JH608Z
and 02HN0JZ

0JH608Z
and 02HN0KZ

0JH608Z
and 02HN0MZ

0JH608Z
and 02HN3JZ

0JH608Z
and 02HN3KZ

0JH608Z
and 02HN3MZ

0JH608Z
and 02HN4JZ

0JH608Z
and 02HN4KZ

0JH608Z
and 02HN4MZ

0JH609Z
and 02H40KZ

0JH609Z
and 02H43JZ

0JH609Z
and 02H43KZ

0JH609Z
and 02H43MZ

0JH609Z
and 02H44KZ

0JH609Z
and 02H60KZ

0JH609Z
and 02H63KZ

0JH609Z
and 02H64KZ

0JH609Z
and 02H70KZ

0JH609Z
and 02H73KZ

0JH609Z
and 02H74KZ

0JH609Z
and 02HN0JZ

0JH609Z
and 02HN0KZ

0JH609Z
and 02HN0MZ

0JH609Z
and 02HN3JZ

0JH609Z
and 02HN3KZ

0JH609Z
and 02HN3MZ

0JH609Z
and 02HN4JZ

0JH609Z
and 02HN4KZ

0JH609Z
and 02HN4MZ

0JH60BZ
and 00HE0MZ

0JH60BZ
and 00HE3MZ

0JH60BZ
and 00HE4MZ

0JH60BZ
and 00HU0MZ
0JH60BZ
and 00HU3MZ
0JH60BZ
and 00HU4MZ
0JH60BZ
and 00HV0MZ
0JH60BZ
and 00HV3MZ
0JH60BZ
and 00HV4MZ
0JH60BZ
and 01HY0MZ

0JH60BZ
and 01HY3MZ

0JH60BZ
and 01HY4MZ

0JH60BZ
and 0DH60MZ

0JH60BZ
and 0DH63MZ

0JH60BZ
and 0DH64MZ

0JH60CZ
and 00HE0MZ

0JH60CZ
and 00HE3MZ

0JH60CZ
and 00HE4MZ

0JH60CZ
and 00HU0MZ
0JH60CZ
and 00HU3MZ
0JH60CZ
and 00HU4MZ
0JH60CZ
and 00HV0MZ
0JH60CZ
and 00HV3MZ
0JH60CZ
and 00HV4MZ
0JH60CZ
and 01HY0MZ

0JH60CZ
and 01HY3MZ

0JH60CZ
and 01HY4MZ

0JH60CZ
and 0DH60MZ

0JH60CZ

and 0DH63MZ

0JH60CZ
and 0DH64MZ

0JH60DZ
and 00H00MZ

0JH60DZ
and 00H03MZ

0JH60DZ
and 00H04MZ

0JH60DZ
and 00H60MZ

0JH60DZ
and 00H63MZ

0JH60DZ
and 00H64MZ

0JH60DZ
and 00HE0MZ

0JH60DZ
and 00HE3MZ

0JH60DZ
and 00HE4MZ

0JH60DZ
and 00HU0MZ

0JH60DZ
and 00HU3MZ

0JH60DZ
and 00HU4MZ

0JH60DZ
and 00HV0MZ

0JH60DZ
and 00HV3MZ

0JH60DZ
and 00HV4MZ

0JH60DZ
and 01HY0MZ

0JH60DZ
and 01HY3MZ

0JH60DZ
and 01HY4MZ

0JH60DZ
and 0DH60MZ

0JH60DZ
and 0DH63MZ

0JH60DZ
and 0DH64MZ

0JH60EZ
and 00H00MZ

0JH60EZ
and 00H03MZ

0JH60EZ
and 00H04MZ

0JH60EZ
and 00H60MZ

0JH60EZ
and 00H63MZ

0JH60EZ
and 00H64MZ

0JH60EZ
and 00HE0MZ

0JH60EZ
and 00HE3MZ

0JH60EZ
and 00HE4MZ

0JH60EZ
and 00HU0MZ

0JH60EZ
and 00HU3MZ

0JH60EZ
and 00HU4MZ

0JH60EZ
and 00HV0MZ

0JH60EZ
and 00HV3MZ

0JH60EZ
and 00HV4MZ

0JH60EZ
and 01HY0MZ

0JH60EZ
and 01HY3MZ

0JH60EZ
and 01HY4MZ

0JH60EZ
and 0DH60MZ

0JH60EZ
and 0DH63MZ

0JH60EZ
and 0DH64MZ

0JH60PZ
and 02H40JZ

0JH60PZ
and 02H40MZ

0JH60PZ
and 02H44JZ

0JH60PZ
and 02H44MZ

0JH60PZ
and 02H60JZ

0JH60PZ
and 02H60MZ

0JH60PZ
and 02H63JZ

0JH60PZ
and 02H63JZ
and 02PA0MZ

0JH60PZ
and 02H63JZ
and 02PA3MZ

0JH60PZ
and 02H63JZ
and 02PA4MZ

0JH60PZ
and 02H63JZ
and 02PAXMZ

0JH60PZ
and 02H63MZ

0JH60PZ
and 02H64JZ

0JH60PZ
and 02H64MZ

0JH60PZ
and 02H70JZ

0JH60PZ
and 02H70MZ

0JH60PZ
and 02H73JZ

0JH60PZ
and 02H73JZ
and 02PA0MZ

0JH60PZ
and 02H73JZ
and 02PA3MZ

0JH60PZ
and 02H73JZ
and 02PA4MZ

0JH60PZ
and 02H73JZ
and 02PAXMZ

0JH60PZ
and 02H73MZ

0JH60PZ
and 02H74JZ

0JH60PZ
and 02H74MZ

0JH60PZ
and 02HK0JZ

0JH60PZ
and 02HK0MZ

0JH60PZ
and 02HK3JZ

0JH60PZ
and 02HK3JZ
and 02PA0MZ

0JH60PZ
and 02HK3JZ
and 02PA3MZ

0JH60PZ
and 02HK3JZ
and 02PA4MZ

0JH60PZ
and 02HK3JZ
and 02PAXMZ

0JH60PZ
and 02HK3MZ

0JH60PZ
and 02HK4JZ

0JH60PZ
and 02HK4MZ

0JH60PZ
and 02HL0JZ

0JH60PZ
and 02HL0MZ

0JH60PZ
and 02HL3JZ

0JH60PZ
and 02HL3JZ
and 02PA0MZ

0JH60PZ
and 02HL3JZ
and 02PA3MZ

0JH60PZ
and 02HL3JZ
and 02PA4MZ

0JH60PZ
and 02HL3JZ
and 02PAXMZ

0JH60PZ
and 02HL3MZ

0JH60PZ
and 02HL4JZ

0JH60PZ
and 02HL4MZ

0JH60PZ
and 02HN0JZ

0JH60PZ
and 02HN0MZ

0JH60PZ
and 02HN3JZ

0JH60PZ
and 02HN3MZ

0JH60PZ
and 02HN4JZ

0JH60PZ
and 02HN4MZ

0JH634Z
and 02H40JZ

0JH634Z
and 02H40MZ

0JH634Z
and 02H44JZ

0JH634Z
and 02H44MZ

0JH634Z
and 02H60JZ

0JH634Z
and 02H60MZ

0JH634Z
and 02H63JZ

0JH634Z
and 02H64JZ

0JH634Z
and 02H64MZ

0JH634Z
and 02H70JZ

0JH634Z
and 02H70MZ

0JH634Z
and 02H73JZ

0JH634Z
and 02H74JZ

0JH634Z
and 02H74MZ

0JH634Z
and 02HK0JZ

0JH634Z
and 02HK0MZ

0JH634Z
and 02HK3JZ

0JH634Z
and 02HK3MZ

0JH634Z
and 02HK4JZ

0JH634Z
and 02HK4MZ

0JH634Z
and 02HL0JZ

0JH634Z
and 02HL0MZ

0JH634Z
and 02HL3JZ

0JH634Z
and 02HL3MZ

0JH634Z
and 02HL4JZ

0JH634Z
and 02HL4MZ

0JH634Z
and 02HN0JZ

0JH634Z
and 02HN0MZ

0JH634Z
and 02HN3JZ

0JH634Z
and 02HN3MZ

0JH634Z
and 02HN4JZ

0JH634Z
and 02HN4MZ

0JH634Z
and 0JPT0PZ

0JH634Z
and 0JPT0PZ
and 02H40JZ

0JH634Z
and 0JPT0PZ
and 02H40MZ

0JH634Z
and 0JPT0PZ
and 02H44JZ

0JH634Z
and 0JPT0PZ
and 02H44MZ

0JH634Z
and 0JPT0PZ
and 02H60JZ

0JH634Z
and 0JPT0PZ
and 02H60MZ

0JH634Z
and 0JPT0PZ
and 02H63JZ

0JH634Z
and 0JPT0PZ
and 02H63JZ
and 02PA0MZ

0JH634Z
and 0JPT0PZ
and 02H63JZ
and 02PA3MZ

0JH634Z
and 0JPT0PZ
and 02H63JZ
and 02PA4MZ

0JH634Z
and 0JPT0PZ
and 02H63JZ
and 02PAXMZ

0JH634Z
and 0JPT0PZ
and 02H63MZ

0JH634Z
and 0JPT0PZ
and 02H64JZ

0JH634Z
and 0JPT0PZ
and 02H64MZ

0JH634Z
and 0JPT0PZ
and 02H70JZ

0JH634Z
and 0JPT0PZ
and 02H70MZ

0JH634Z
and 0JPT0PZ
and 02H73JZ

0JH634Z
and 0JPT0PZ
and 02H73JZ
and 02PA0MZ

0JH634Z

and 0JPT0PZ
and 02H73JZ
and 02PA3MZ

0JH634Z
and 0JPT0PZ
and 02H73JZ
and 02PA4MZ

0JH634Z
and 0JPT0PZ
and 02H73JZ
and 02PAXMZ

0JH634Z
and 0JPT0PZ
and 02H73MZ

0JH634Z
and 0JPT0PZ
and 02H74JZ

0JH634Z
and 0JPT0PZ
and 02H74MZ

0JH634Z
and 0JPT0PZ
and 02HK0JZ

0JH634Z
and 0JPT0PZ
and 02HK0MZ

0JH634Z
and 0JPT0PZ
and 02HK3JZ

0JH634Z
and 0JPT0PZ
and 02HK3JZ
and 02PA0MZ

0JH634Z
and 0JPT0PZ
and 02HK3JZ
and 02PA3MZ

0JH634Z
and 0JPT0PZ
and 02HK3JZ
and 02PA4MZ

0JH634Z
and 0JPT0PZ
and 02HK3JZ
and 02PAXMZ

0JH634Z
and 0JPT0PZ
and 02HK3MZ

0JH634Z
and 0JPT0PZ
and 02HK4JZ

0JH634Z
and 0JPT0PZ
and 02HK4MZ

0JH634Z
and 0JPT0PZ
and 02HL0JZ

0JH634Z
and 0JPT0PZ
and 02HL0MZ

0JH634Z
and 0JPT0PZ
and 02HL3JZ

0JH634Z
and 0JPT0PZ
and 02HL3JZ
and 02PA0MZ

0JH634Z
and 0JPT0PZ
and 02HL3JZ
and 02PA3MZ

0JH634Z
and 0JPT0PZ
and 02HL3JZ
and 02PA4MZ

0JH634Z
and 0JPT0PZ
and 02HL3JZ
and 02PAXMZ

0JH634Z
and 0JPT0PZ
and 02HL3MZ

0JH634Z
and 0JPT0PZ
and 02HL4JZ

0JH634Z
and 0JPT0PZ
and 02HL4MZ

0JH634Z
and 0JPT0PZ
and 02HN0JZ

0JH634Z
and 0JPT0PZ
and 02HN0MZ

0JH634Z
and 0JPT0PZ
and 02HN3JZ

0JH634Z
and 0JPT0PZ
and 02HN3MZ

0JH634Z
and 0JPT0PZ
and 02HN4JZ

0JH634Z
and 0JPT0PZ
and 02HN4MZ

0JH634Z
and 0JPT3PZ

0JH634Z
and 0JPT3PZ
and 02H40JZ

0JH634Z
and 0JPT3PZ
and 02H40MZ

0JH634Z
and 0JPT3PZ
and 02H44JZ

0JH634Z
and 0JPT3PZ
and 02H44MZ

0JH634Z
and 0JPT3PZ
and 02H60JZ

0JH634Z
and 0JPT3PZ
and 02H60MZ

0JH634Z
and 0JPT3PZ
and 02H63JZ

0JH634Z
and 0JPT3PZ
and 02H63JZ
and 02PA0MZ

0JH634Z
and 0JPT3PZ
and 02H63JZ
and 02PA3MZ

0JH634Z
and 0JPT3PZ
and 02H63JZ
and 02PA4MZ

0JH634Z
and 0JPT3PZ
and 02H63JZ
and 02PAXMZ

0JH634Z
and 0JPT3PZ
and 02H63MZ

0JH634Z
and 0JPT3PZ
and 02H64JZ

0JH634Z
and 0JPT3PZ
and 02H64MZ

0JH634Z
and 0JPT3PZ
and 02H70JZ

0JH634Z
and 0JPT3PZ
and 02H70MZ

0JH634Z
and 0JPT3PZ
and 02H73JZ

0JH634Z
and 0JPT3PZ
and 02H73JZ
and 02PA0MZ

0JH634Z
and 0JPT3PZ
and 02H73JZ
and 02PA3MZ

0JH634Z
and 0JPT3PZ
and 02H73JZ
and 02PA4MZ

0JH634Z
and 0JPT3PZ
and 02H73JZ
and 02PAXMZ

0JH634Z
and 0JPT3PZ
and 02H73MZ

0JH634Z
and 0JPT3PZ
and 02H74JZ

0JH634Z
and 0JPT3PZ
and 02H74MZ

0JH634Z
and 0JPT3PZ
and 02HK0JZ

0JH634Z
and 0JPT3PZ
and 02HK0MZ

0JH634Z
and 0JPT3PZ
and 02HK3JZ

0JH634Z
and 0JPT3PZ
and 02HK3JZ
and 02PA0MZ

0JH634Z
and 0JPT3PZ
and 02HK3JZ
and 02PA3MZ

0JH634Z
and 0JPT3PZ
and 02HK3JZ
and 02PA4MZ

0JH634Z
and 0JPT3PZ
and 02HK3JZ
and 02PAXMZ

0JH634Z
and 0JPT3PZ
and 02HK3MZ

0JH634Z
and 0JPT3PZ
and 02HK4JZ

0JH634Z
and 0JPT3PZ
and 02HK4MZ

0JH634Z
and 0JPT3PZ
and 02HL0JZ

0JH634Z
and 0JPT3PZ
and 02HL0MZ

0JH634Z
and 0JPT3PZ
and 02HL3JZ

0JH634Z
and 0JPT3PZ
and 02HL3JZ
and 02PA0MZ

0JH634Z
and 0JPT3PZ
and 02HL3JZ
and 02PA3MZ

0JH634Z
and 0JPT3PZ
and 02HL3JZ
and 02PA4MZ

0JH634Z
and 0JPT3PZ
and 02HL3JZ
and 02PAXMZ

0JH634Z
and 0JPT3PZ
and 02HL3MZ

0JH634Z
and 0JPT3PZ
and 02HL4JZ

0JH634Z
and 0JPT3PZ
and 02HL4MZ

0JH634Z
and 0JPT3PZ
and 02HN0JZ

0JH634Z
and 0JPT3PZ
and 02HN0MZ

0JH634Z
and 0JPT3PZ
and 02HN3JZ

0JH634Z
and 0JPT3PZ
and 02HN3MZ

0JH634Z
and 0JPT3PZ
and 02HN4JZ

0JH634Z
and 0JPT3PZ
and 02HN4MZ

0JH635Z
and 02H40JZ

0JH635Z
and 02H40MZ

0JH635Z
and 02H44JZ

0JH635Z
and 02H44MZ

0JH635Z
and 02H60JZ

0JH635Z
and 02H60MZ

0JH635Z
and 02H63JZ

0JH635Z
and 02H64JZ

0JH635Z
and 02H64MZ

0JH635Z
and 02H70JZ

0JH635Z
and 02H70MZ

0JH635Z
and 02H73JZ

0JH635Z
and 02H74JZ

0JH635Z
and 02H74MZ

0JH635Z
and 02HK0JZ

0JH635Z
and 02HK0MZ

0JH635Z
and 02HK3JZ

0JH635Z
and 02HK3MZ

0JH635Z
and 02HK4JZ

0JH635Z
and 02HK4MZ

0JH635Z
and 02HL0JZ

0JH635Z
and 02HL0MZ

0JH635Z
and 02HL3JZ

0JH635Z
and 02HL3MZ

0JH635Z
and 02HL4JZ

0JH635Z
and 02HL4MZ

0JH635Z
and 02HN0JZ

0JH635Z
and 02HN0MZ

0JH635Z
and 02HN3JZ

0JH635Z
and 02HN3MZ

0JH635Z
and 02HN4JZ

0JH635Z
and 02HN4MZ

0JH635Z
and 0JPT0PZ

0JH635Z
and 0JPT0PZ
and 02H40JZ

0JH635Z
and 0JPT0PZ

and 02H40MZ

0JH635Z
and 0JPT0PZ
and 02H44JZ

0JH635Z
and 0JPT0PZ
and 02H44MZ

0JH635Z
and 0JPT0PZ
and 02H60JZ

0JH635Z
and 0JPT0PZ
and 02H60MZ

0JH635Z
and 0JPT0PZ
and 02H63JZ

0JH635Z
and 0JPT0PZ
and 02H63JZ
and 02PA0MZ

0JH635Z
and 0JPT0PZ
and 02H63JZ
and 02PA3MZ

0JH635Z
and 0JPT0PZ
and 02H63JZ
and 02PA4MZ

0JH635Z
and 0JPT0PZ
and 02H63JZ
and 02PAXMZ

0JH635Z
and 0JPT0PZ
and 02H63MZ

0JH635Z
and 0JPT0PZ
and 02H64JZ

0JH635Z
and 0JPT0PZ
and 02H64MZ

0JH635Z
and 0JPT0PZ
and 02H70JZ

0JH635Z
and 0JPT0PZ
and 02H70MZ

0JH635Z
and 0JPT0PZ
and 02H73JZ

0JH635Z
and 0JPT0PZ
and 02H73JZ
and 02PA0MZ

0JH635Z
and 0JPT0PZ
and 02H73JZ
and 02PA3MZ

0JH635Z
and 0JPT0PZ
and 02H73JZ
and 02PA4MZ

0JH635Z
and 0JPT0PZ
and 02H73JZ
and 02PAXMZ

0JH635Z
and 0JPT0PZ
and 02H73MZ

0JH635Z
and 0JPT0PZ
and 02H74JZ

0JH635Z
and 0JPT0PZ
and 02H74MZ

0JH635Z
and 0JPT0PZ
and 02HK0JZ

0JH635Z
and 0JPT0PZ
and 02HK0MZ

0JH635Z
and 0JPT0PZ
and 02HK3JZ

0JH635Z
and 0JPT0PZ
and 02HK3JZ
and 02PA0MZ

0JH635Z
and 0JPT0PZ
and 02HK3JZ
and 02PA3MZ

0JH635Z
and 0JPT0PZ
and 02HK3JZ
and 02PA4MZ

0JH635Z
and 0JPT0PZ
and 02HK3JZ
and 02PAXMZ

0JH635Z
and 0JPT0PZ
and 02HK3MZ

0JH635Z
and 0JPT0PZ
and 02HK4JZ

0JH635Z
and 0JPT0PZ
and 02HK4MZ

0JH635Z
and 0JPT0PZ
and 02HL0JZ

0JH635Z
and 0JPT0PZ
and 02HL0MZ

0JH635Z
and 0JPT0PZ
and 02HL3JZ

0JH635Z
and 0JPT0PZ
and 02HL3JZ
and 02PA0MZ

0JH635Z
and 0JPT0PZ
and 02HL3JZ
and 02PA3MZ

0JH635Z
and 0JPT0PZ
and 02HL3JZ
and 02PA4MZ

0JH635Z
and 0JPT0PZ
and 02HL3JZ
and 02PAXMZ

0JH635Z
and 0JPT0PZ
and 02HL3MZ

0JH635Z
and 0JPT0PZ
and 02HL4JZ

0JH635Z
and 0JPT0PZ
and 02HL4MZ

0JH635Z
and 0JPT0PZ
and 02HN0JZ

0JH635Z
and 0JPT0PZ
and 02HN0MZ

0JH635Z
and 0JPT0PZ
and 02HN3JZ

0JH635Z
and 0JPT0PZ
and 02HN3MZ

0JH635Z
and 0JPT0PZ
and 02HN4JZ

0JH635Z
and 0JPT0PZ
and 02HN4MZ

0JH635Z
and 0JPT3PZ

0JH635Z
and 0JPT3PZ
and 02H40JZ

0JH635Z
and 0JPT3PZ
and 02H40MZ

0JH635Z
and 0JPT3PZ
and 02H44JZ

0JH635Z
and 0JPT3PZ
and 02H44MZ

0JH635Z
and 0JPT3PZ
and 02H60JZ

0JH635Z
and 0JPT3PZ
and 02H60MZ

0JH635Z
and 0JPT3PZ
and 02H63JZ

0JH635Z
and 0JPT3PZ
and 02H63JZ
and 02PA0MZ

0JH635Z
and 0JPT3PZ
and 02H63JZ
and 02PA3MZ

0JH635Z
and 0JPT3PZ
and 02H63JZ
and 02PA4MZ

0JH635Z
and 0JPT3PZ
and 02H63JZ
and 02PAXMZ

0JH635Z
and 0JPT3PZ
and 02H63MZ

0JH635Z
and 0JPT3PZ
and 02H64JZ

0JH635Z
and 0JPT3PZ
and 02H64MZ

0JH635Z
and 0JPT3PZ
and 02H70JZ

0JH635Z
and 0JPT3PZ
and 02H70MZ

0JH635Z
and 0JPT3PZ
and 02H73JZ

0JH635Z
and 0JPT3PZ
and 02H73JZ
and 02PA0MZ

0JH635Z
and 0JPT3PZ
and 02H73JZ
and 02PA3MZ

0JH635Z
and 0JPT3PZ
and 02H73JZ
and 02PA4MZ

0JH635Z
and 0JPT3PZ
and 02H73JZ
and 02PAXMZ

0JH635Z
and 0JPT3PZ
and 02H73MZ

0JH635Z
and 0JPT3PZ
and 02H74JZ

0JH635Z
and 0JPT3PZ
and 02H74MZ

0JH635Z
and 0JPT3PZ
and 02HK0JZ

0JH635Z
and 0JPT3PZ
and 02HK0MZ

0JH635Z
and 0JPT3PZ
and 02HK3JZ

0JH635Z
and 0JPT3PZ
and 02HK3JZ
and 02PA0MZ

0JH635Z
and 0JPT3PZ
and 02HK3JZ
and 02PA3MZ

0JH635Z
and 0JPT3PZ
and 02HK3JZ
and 02PA4MZ

0JH635Z
and 0JPT3PZ
and 02HK3JZ
and 02PAXMZ

0JH635Z
and 0JPT3PZ
and 02HK3MZ

0JH635Z
and 0JPT3PZ
and 02HK4JZ

0JH635Z
and 0JPT3PZ
and 02HK4MZ

0JH635Z
and 0JPT3PZ
and 02HL0JZ

0JH635Z
and 0JPT3PZ
and 02HL0MZ

0JH635Z
and 0JPT3PZ
and 02HL3JZ

0JH635Z
and 0JPT3PZ
and 02HL3JZ
and 02PA0MZ

0JH635Z
and 0JPT3PZ
and 02HL3JZ
and 02PA3MZ

0JH635Z
and 0JPT3PZ
and 02HL3JZ
and 02PA4MZ

0JH635Z
and 0JPT3PZ
and 02HL3JZ
and 02PAXMZ

0JH635Z
and 0JPT3PZ
and 02HL3MZ

0JH635Z
and 0JPT3PZ
and 02HL4JZ

0JH635Z
and 0JPT3PZ
and 02HL4MZ

0JH635Z
and 0JPT3PZ
and 02HN0JZ

0JH635Z
and 0JPT3PZ
and 02HN0MZ

0JH635Z
and 0JPT3PZ
and 02HN3JZ

0JH635Z
and 0JPT3PZ
and 02HN3MZ

0JH635Z
and 0JPT3PZ
and 02HN4JZ

0JH635Z
and 0JPT3PZ
and 02HN4MZ

0JH636Z
and 02HK3JZ

0JH636Z
and 02HL3JZ

0JH636Z
and 02HN0JZ

0JH636Z
and 02HN0MZ

0JH636Z
and 02HN3JZ

0JH636Z
and 02HN3MZ

0JH636Z
and 02HN4JZ

0JH636Z
and 02HN4MZ

0JH636Z
and 0JPT0PZ

0JH636Z
and 0JPT0PZ
and 02H40JZ

0JH636Z
and 0JPT0PZ

and 02H40MZ

0JH636Z and 0JPT0PZ and 02H44JZ

0JH636Z and 0JPT0PZ and 02H44MZ

0JH636Z and 0JPT0PZ and 02H60JZ

0JH636Z and 0JPT0PZ and 02H60MZ

0JH636Z and 0JPT0PZ and 02H63JZ

0JH636Z and 0JPT0PZ and 02H63JZ and 02PA0MZ

0JH636Z and 0JPT0PZ and 02H63JZ and 02PA3MZ

0JH636Z and 0JPT0PZ and 02H63JZ and 02PA4MZ

0JH636Z and 0JPT0PZ and 02H63JZ and 02PAXMZ

0JH636Z and 0JPT0PZ and 02H63MZ

0JH636Z and 0JPT0PZ and 02H64JZ

0JH636Z and 0JPT0PZ and 02H64MZ

0JH636Z and 0JPT0PZ and 02H70JZ

0JH636Z and 0JPT0PZ and 02H70MZ

0JH636Z and 0JPT0PZ and 02H73JZ

0JH636Z and 0JPT0PZ and 02H73JZ and 02PA0MZ

0JH636Z and 0JPT0PZ and 02H73JZ and 02PA3MZ

0JH636Z and 0JPT0PZ and 02H73JZ and 02PA4MZ

0JH636Z and 0JPT0PZ and 02H73JZ and 02PAXMZ

0JH636Z and 0JPT0PZ and 02H73MZ

0JH636Z and 0JPT0PZ and 02H74JZ

0JH636Z and 0JPT0PZ and 02H74MZ

0JH636Z and 0JPT0PZ and 02HK0JZ

0JH636Z and 0JPT0PZ and 02HK0MZ

0JH636Z and 0JPT0PZ and 02HK3JZ

0JH636Z and 0JPT0PZ and 02HK3JZ and 02PA0MZ

0JH636Z and 0JPT0PZ and 02HK3JZ and 02PA3MZ

0JH636Z and 0JPT0PZ and 02HK3JZ and 02PA4MZ

0JH636Z and 0JPT0PZ and 02HK3JZ and 02PAXMZ

0JH636Z and 0JPT0PZ and 02HK3MZ

0JH636Z and 0JPT0PZ and 02HK4JZ

0JH636Z and 0JPT0PZ and 02HK4MZ

0JH636Z and 0JPT0PZ and 02HL0JZ

0JH636Z and 0JPT0PZ and 02HL0MZ

0JH636Z and 0JPT0PZ and 02HL3JZ

0JH636Z and 0JPT0PZ and 02HL3JZ and 02PA0MZ

0JH636Z and 0JPT0PZ and 02HL3JZ and 02PA3MZ

0JH636Z and 0JPT0PZ and 02HL3JZ and 02PA4MZ

0JH636Z and 0JPT0PZ and 02HL3JZ and 02PAXMZ

0JH636Z and 0JPT0PZ and 02HL3MZ

0JH636Z and 0JPT0PZ and 02HL4JZ

0JH636Z and 0JPT0PZ and 02HL4MZ

0JH636Z and 0JPT0PZ and 02HN0JZ

0JH636Z and 0JPT0PZ and 02HN0MZ

0JH636Z and 0JPT0PZ and 02HN3JZ

0JH636Z and 0JPT0PZ and 02HN3MZ

0JH636Z and 0JPT0PZ and 02HN4JZ

0JH636Z and 0JPT0PZ and 02HN4MZ

0JH636Z and 0JPT3PZ

0JH636Z and 0JPT3PZ and 02H40JZ

0JH636Z and 0JPT3PZ and 02H40MZ

0JH636Z and 0JPT3PZ and 02H44JZ

0JH636Z and 0JPT3PZ and 02H44MZ

0JH636Z and 0JPT3PZ and 02H60JZ

0JH636Z and 0JPT3PZ and 02H60MZ

0JH636Z and 0JPT3PZ and 02H63JZ

0JH636Z and 0JPT3PZ and 02H63JZ and 02PA0MZ

0JH636Z and 0JPT3PZ and 02H63JZ and 02PA3MZ

0JH636Z and 0JPT3PZ and 02H63JZ and 02PA4MZ

0JH636Z and 0JPT3PZ and 02H63JZ and 02PAXMZ

0JH636Z and 0JPT3PZ and 02H63MZ

0JH636Z and 0JPT3PZ and 02H64JZ

0JH636Z and 0JPT3PZ and 02H64MZ

0JH636Z and 0JPT3PZ and 02H70JZ

0JH636Z and 0JPT3PZ and 02H70MZ

0JH636Z and 0JPT3PZ and 02H73JZ

0JH636Z and 0JPT3PZ and 02H73JZ and 02PA0MZ

0JH636Z and 0JPT3PZ and 02H73JZ and 02PA3MZ

0JH636Z and 0JPT3PZ and 02H73JZ and 02PA4MZ

0JH636Z and 0JPT3PZ and 02H73JZ and 02PAXMZ

0JH636Z and 0JPT3PZ and 02H73MZ

0JH636Z and 0JPT3PZ and 02H74JZ

0JH636Z and 0JPT3PZ and 02H74MZ

0JH636Z and 0JPT3PZ and 02HK0JZ

0JH636Z and 0JPT3PZ and 02HK0MZ

0JH636Z and 0JPT3PZ and 02HK3JZ

0JH636Z and 0JPT3PZ and 02HK3JZ and 02PA0MZ

0JH636Z and 0JPT3PZ and 02HK3JZ and 02PA3MZ

0JH636Z and 0JPT3PZ and 02HK3JZ and 02PA4MZ

0JH636Z and 0JPT3PZ and 02HK3JZ and 02PAXMZ

0JH636Z and 0JPT3PZ and 02HK3MZ

0JH636Z and 0JPT3PZ and 02HK4JZ

0JH636Z and 0JPT3PZ and 02HK4MZ

0JH636Z and 0JPT3PZ and 02HL0JZ

0JH636Z and 0JPT3PZ and 02HL0MZ

0JH636Z and 0JPT3PZ and 02HL3JZ

0JH636Z and 0JPT3PZ and 02HL3JZ and 02PA0MZ

0JH636Z and 0JPT3PZ and 02HL3JZ and 02PA3MZ

0JH636Z and 0JPT3PZ and 02HL3JZ and 02PA4MZ

0JH636Z and 0JPT3PZ and 02HL3JZ and 02PAXMZ

0JH636Z and 0JPT3PZ and 02HL3MZ

0JH636Z and 0JPT3PZ and 02HL4JZ

0JH636Z and 0JPT3PZ and 02HL4MZ

0JH636Z and 0JPT3PZ and 02HN0JZ

0JH636Z and 0JPT3PZ and 02HN0MZ

0JH636Z and 0JPT3PZ and 02HN3JZ

0JH636Z and 0JPT3PZ and 02HN3MZ

0JH636Z and 0JPT3PZ and 02HN4JZ

0JH636Z and 0JPT3PZ and 02HN4MZ

0JH637Z and 02H40JZ

0JH637Z and 02H40MZ

0JH637Z and 02H43JZ

0JH637Z and 02H43KZ

0JH637Z and 02H43MZ

0JH637Z and 02H44JZ

0JH637Z and 02H44MZ

0JH637Z and 02H60JZ

0JH637Z and 02H60MZ

0JH637Z and 02H63JZ

0JH637Z and 02H63JZ and 02PA0MZ

0JH637Z and 02H63JZ and 02PA3MZ
0JH637Z and 02H63JZ and 02PA4MZ
0JH637Z and 02H63JZ and 02PAXMZ
0JH637Z and 02H63MZ
0JH637Z and 02H64JZ
0JH637Z and 02H64MZ
0JH637Z and 02H70JZ
0JH637Z and 02H70MZ
0JH637Z and 02H73JZ
0JH637Z and 02H73JZ and 02PA0MZ
0JH637Z and 02H73JZ and 02PA3MZ
0JH637Z and 02H73JZ and 02PA4MZ
0JH637Z and 02H73JZ and 02PAXMZ
0JH637Z and 02H73MZ
0JH637Z and 02H74JZ
0JH637Z and 02H74MZ
0JH637Z and 02HK0JZ
0JH637Z and 02HK0MZ
0JH637Z and 02HK3JZ
0JH637Z and 02HK3JZ and 02PA0MZ
0JH637Z and 02HK3JZ and 02PA3MZ
0JH637Z and 02HK3JZ and 02PA4MZ
0JH637Z and 02HK3JZ and 02PAXMZ
0JH637Z and 02HK3MZ
0JH637Z and 02HK4JZ
0JH637Z and 02HK4MZ
0JH637Z and 02HL0JZ
0JH637Z and 02HL0MZ
0JH637Z and 02HL3JZ
0JH637Z and 02HL3JZ and 02PA0MZ
0JH637Z and 02HL3JZ and 02PA3MZ
0JH637Z and 02HL3JZ and 02PA4MZ
0JH637Z and 02HL3JZ and 02PAXMZ
0JH637Z and 02HL3MZ
0JH637Z and 02HL4JZ
0JH637Z and 02HL4MZ
0JH637Z and 02HN0JZ
0JH637Z and 02HN0MZ
0JH637Z and 02HN3JZ
0JH637Z and 02HN3MZ
0JH637Z and 02HN4JZ
0JH637Z and 02HN4MZ
0JH638Z and 02H40KZ
0JH638Z and 02H44KZ
0JH638Z and 02HN0JZ
0JH638Z and 02HN0KZ
0JH638Z and 02HN0MZ
0JH638Z and 02HN3JZ
0JH638Z and 02HN3KZ
0JH638Z and 02HN3MZ
0JH638Z and 02HN4JZ
0JH638Z and 02HN4KZ
0JH638Z and 02HN4MZ
0JH639Z and 02H40KZ
0JH639Z and 02H43JZ
0JH639Z and 02H43KZ
0JH639Z and 02H43MZ
0JH639Z and 02H44KZ
0JH639Z and 02H60KZ
0JH639Z and 02H63KZ
0JH639Z and 02H64KZ
0JH639Z and 02H70KZ
0JH639Z and 02H73KZ
0JH639Z and 02H74KZ
0JH639Z and 02HN0JZ
0JH639Z and 02HN0KZ
0JH639Z and 02HN0MZ
0JH639Z and 02HN3JZ
0JH639Z and 02HN3KZ
0JH639Z and 02HN3MZ
0JH639Z and 02HN4JZ
0JH639Z and 02HN4KZ
0JH639Z and 02HN4MZ
0JH63BZ and 00HE0MZ
0JH63BZ and 00HE3MZ
0JH63BZ and 00HE4MZ
0JH63BZ and 00HU0MZ
0JH63BZ and 00HU3MZ
0JH63BZ and 00HU4MZ
0JH63BZ and 00HV0MZ
0JH63BZ and 00HV3MZ
0JH63BZ and 00HV4MZ
0JH63BZ and 01HY0MZ
0JH63BZ and 01HY3MZ
0JH63BZ and 01HY4MZ
0JH63BZ and 0DH60MZ
0JH63BZ and 0DH63MZ
0JH63BZ and 0DH64MZ
0JH63CZ and 00HE0MZ
0JH63CZ and 00HE3MZ
0JH63CZ and 00HE4MZ
0JH63CZ and 00HU0MZ
0JH63CZ and 00HU3MZ
0JH63CZ and 00HU4MZ
0JH63CZ and 00HV0MZ
0JH63CZ and 00HV3MZ
0JH63CZ and 00HV4MZ
0JH63CZ and 01HY0MZ
0JH63CZ and 01HY3MZ
0JH63CZ and 01HY4MZ
0JH63CZ and 0DH60MZ
0JH63CZ and 0DH63MZ
0JH63CZ and 0DH64MZ
0JH63DZ and 00H00MZ
0JH63DZ and 00H03MZ
0JH63DZ and 00H04MZ
0JH63DZ and 00H60MZ
0JH63DZ and 00H63MZ
0JH63DZ and 00H64MZ
0JH63DZ and 00HE0MZ
0JH63DZ and 00HE3MZ
0JH63DZ and 00HE4MZ
0JH63DZ and 00HU0MZ
0JH63DZ and 00HU3MZ
0JH63DZ and 00HU4MZ
0JH63DZ and 00HV0MZ
0JH63DZ and 00HV3MZ
0JH63DZ and 00HV4MZ
0JH63DZ and 01HY0MZ
0JH63DZ and 01HY3MZ
0JH63DZ and 01HY4MZ
0JH63DZ and 0DH60MZ
0JH63DZ and 0DH63MZ
0JH63DZ and 0DH64MZ
0JH63EZ and 00H00MZ
0JH63EZ and 00H03MZ
0JH63EZ and 00H04MZ
0JH63EZ and 00H60MZ
0JH63EZ and 00H63MZ
0JH63EZ and 00H64MZ
0JH63EZ and 00HE0MZ
0JH63EZ and 00HE3MZ
0JH63EZ and 00HE4MZ
0JH63EZ and 00HU0MZ
0JH63EZ and 00HU3MZ
0JH63EZ and 00HU4MZ
0JH63EZ and 00HV0MZ
0JH63EZ and 00HV3MZ
0JH63EZ and 00HV4MZ
0JH63EZ and 01HY0MZ
0JH63EZ and 01HY3MZ
0JH63EZ and 01HY4MZ
0JH63EZ and 0DH60MZ
0JH63EZ and 0DH63MZ
0JH63EZ and 0DH64MZ
0JH63PZ and 02H40JZ
0JH63PZ and 02H40MZ
0JH63PZ and 02H44JZ
0JH63PZ and 02H44MZ
0JH63PZ and 02H60JZ
0JH63PZ and 02H60MZ
0JH63PZ and 02H63JZ
0JH63PZ and 02H63JZ and 02PA0MZ
0JH63PZ and 02H63JZ and 02PA3MZ
0JH63PZ and 02H63JZ and 02PA4MZ
0JH63PZ and 02H63JZ

and 02PAXMZ

0JH63PZ
and 02H63MZ

0JH63PZ
and 02H64JZ

0JH63PZ
and 02H64MZ

0JH63PZ
and 02H70JZ

0JH63PZ
and 02H70MZ

0JH63PZ
and 02H73JZ

0JH63PZ
and 02H73JZ
and 02PA0MZ

0JH63PZ
and 02H73JZ
and 02PA3MZ

0JH63PZ
and 02H73JZ
and 02PA4MZ

0JH63PZ
and 02H73JZ
and 02PAXMZ

0JH63PZ
and 02H73MZ

0JH63PZ
and 02H74JZ

0JH63PZ
and 02H74MZ

0JH63PZ
and 02HK0JZ

0JH63PZ
and 02HK0MZ

0JH63PZ
and 02HK3JZ

0JH63PZ
and 02HK3JZ
and 02PA0MZ

0JH63PZ
and 02HK3JZ
and 02PA3MZ

0JH63PZ
and 02HK3JZ
and 02PA4MZ

0JH63PZ
and 02HK3JZ
and 02PAXMZ

0JH63PZ
and 02HK3MZ

0JH63PZ
and 02HK4JZ

0JH63PZ
and 02HK4MZ

0JH63PZ
and 02HL0JZ

0JH63PZ
and 02HL0MZ

0JH63PZ
and 02HL3JZ

0JH63PZ
and 02HL3JZ
and 02PA0MZ

0JH63PZ
and 02HL3JZ
and 02PA3MZ

0JH63PZ
and 02HL3JZ
and 02PA4MZ

0JH63PZ
and 02HL3JZ
and 02PAXMZ

0JH63PZ
and 02HL3MZ

0JH63PZ
and 02HL4JZ

0JH63PZ
and 02HL4MZ

0JH63PZ
and 02HN0JZ

0JH63PZ
and 02HN0MZ

0JH63PZ
and 02HN3JZ

0JH63PZ
and 02HN3MZ

0JH63PZ
and 02HN4JZ

0JH63PZ
and 02HN4MZ

0JH70BZ
and 00HE0MZ

0JH70BZ
and 00HE3MZ

0JH70BZ
and 00HE4MZ

0JH70BZ
and 00HU0MZ
0JH70BZ
and 00HU3MZ
0JH70BZ
and 00HU4MZ
0JH70BZ
and 00HV0MZ
0JH70BZ
and 00HV3MZ
0JH70BZ
and 00HV4MZ
0JH70BZ
and 01HY0MZ

0JH70BZ
and 01HY3MZ

0JH70BZ
and 01HY4MZ

0JH70BZ
and 0DH60MZ

0JH70BZ
and 0DH63MZ

0JH70BZ
and 0DH64MZ

0JH70CZ
and 00HE0MZ

0JH70CZ
and 00HE3MZ

0JH70CZ
and 00HE4MZ

0JH70CZ
and 00HU0MZ
0JH70CZ
and 00HU3MZ
0JH70CZ
and 00HU4MZ
0JH70CZ
and 00HV0MZ
0JH70CZ
and 00HV3MZ
0JH70CZ
and 00HV4MZ
0JH70CZ
and 01HY0MZ

0JH70CZ
and 01HY3MZ

0JH70CZ
and 01HY4MZ

0JH70CZ
and 0DH60MZ

0JH70CZ
and 0DH63MZ

0JH70CZ
and 0DH64MZ

0JH70DZ
and 00H00MZ

0JH70DZ
and 00H03MZ

0JH70DZ
and 00H04MZ

0JH70DZ
and 00H60MZ

0JH70DZ
and 00H63MZ

0JH70DZ
and 00H64MZ

0JH70DZ
and 00HE0MZ

0JH70DZ
and 00HE3MZ

0JH70DZ
and 00HE4MZ

0JH70DZ
and 00HU0MZ
0JH70DZ
and 00HU3MZ
0JH70DZ
and 00HU4MZ
0JH70DZ
and 00HV0MZ
0JH70DZ
and 00HV3MZ
0JH70DZ
and 00HV4MZ
0JH70DZ
and 01HY0MZ

0JH70DZ
and 01HY3MZ

0JH70DZ
and 01HY4MZ

0JH70DZ
and 0DH60MZ

0JH70DZ
and 0DH63MZ

0JH70DZ
and 0DH64MZ

0JH70EZ
and 00H00MZ

0JH70EZ
and 00H03MZ

0JH70EZ
and 00H04MZ

0JH70EZ
and 00H60MZ

0JH70EZ
and 00H63MZ

0JH70EZ
and 00H64MZ

0JH70EZ
and 00HE0MZ

0JH70EZ
and 00HE3MZ

0JH70EZ
and 00HE4MZ

0JH70EZ
and 00HU0MZ
0JH70EZ
and 00HU3MZ
0JH70EZ
and 00HU4MZ
0JH70EZ
and 00HV0MZ
0JH70EZ
and 00HV3MZ
0JH70EZ
and 00HV4MZ
0JH70EZ
and 01HY0MZ

0JH70EZ
and 01HY3MZ

0JH70EZ
and 01HY4MZ

0JH70EZ
and 0DH60MZ

0JH70EZ
and 0DH63MZ

0JH70EZ
and 0DH64MZ

0JH73BZ
and 00HE0MZ

0JH73BZ
and 00HE3MZ

0JH73BZ
and 00HE4MZ

0JH73BZ
and 00HU0MZ
0JH73BZ
and 00HU3MZ
0JH73BZ
and 00HU4MZ
0JH73BZ
and 00HV0MZ
0JH73BZ
and 00HV3MZ
0JH73BZ
and 00HV4MZ
0JH73BZ
and 01HY0MZ

0JH73BZ
and 01HY3MZ

0JH73BZ
and 01HY4MZ

0JH73BZ
and 0DH60MZ

0JH73BZ
and 0DH63MZ

0JH73BZ
and 0DH64MZ

0JH73CZ
and 00HE0MZ

0JH73CZ
and 00HE3MZ

0JH73CZ
and 00HE4MZ

0JH73CZ
and 00HU0MZ
0JH73CZ
and 00HU3MZ
0JH73CZ
and 00HU4MZ
0JH73CZ
and 00HV0MZ
0JH73CZ
and 00HV3MZ
0JH73CZ
and 00HV4MZ
0JH73CZ
and 01HY0MZ

0JH73CZ
and 01HY3MZ

0JH73CZ
and 01HY4MZ

0JH73CZ
and 0DH60MZ

0JH73CZ
and 0DH63MZ

0JH73CZ
and 0DH64MZ

0JH73DZ
and 00H00MZ

0JH73DZ
and 00H03MZ

0JH73DZ
and 00H04MZ

0JH73DZ
and 00H60MZ

0JH73DZ
and 00H63MZ

0JH73DZ
and 00H64MZ

0JH73DZ
and 00HE0MZ

0JH73DZ
and 00HE3MZ

0JH73DZ
and 00HE4MZ

0JH73DZ
and 00HU0MZ
0JH73DZ
and 00HU3MZ
0JH73DZ
and 00HU4MZ
0JH73DZ
and 00HV0MZ
0JH73DZ
and 00HV3MZ
0JH73DZ
and 00HV4MZ
0JH73DZ
and 01HY0MZ

0JH73DZ
and 01HY3MZ

0JH73DZ
and 01HY4MZ

0JH73DZ
and 0DH60MZ

0JH73DZ
and 0DH63MZ

0JH73DZ
and 0DH64MZ

0JH73EZ
and 00H00MZ

0JH73EZ

and 00H03MZ

0JH73EZ
and 00H04MZ

0JH73EZ
and 00H60MZ

0JH73EZ
and 00H63MZ

0JH73EZ
and 00H64MZ

0JH73EZ
and 00HE0MZ

0JH73EZ
and 00HE3MZ

0JH73EZ
and 00HE4MZ

0JH73EZ
and 00HU0MZ

0JH73EZ
and 00HU3MZ

0JH73EZ
and 00HU4MZ

0JH73EZ
and 00HV0MZ

0JH73EZ
and 00HV3MZ

0JH73EZ
and 00HV4MZ

0JH73EZ
and 01HY0MZ

0JH73EZ
and 01HY3MZ

0JH73EZ
and 01HY4MZ

0JH73EZ
and 0DH60MZ

0JH73EZ
and 0DH63MZ

0JH73EZ
and 0DH64MZ

0JH804Z
and 02H40JZ

0JH804Z
and 02H40MZ

0JH804Z
and 02H44JZ

0JH804Z
and 02H44MZ

0JH804Z
and 02H60JZ

0JH804Z
and 02H60MZ

0JH804Z
and 02H63JZ

0JH804Z
and 02H64JZ

0JH804Z
and 02H64MZ

0JH804Z
and 02H70JZ

0JH804Z
and 02H70MZ

0JH804Z
and 02H73JZ

0JH804Z
and 02H74JZ

0JH804Z
and 02H74MZ

0JH804Z
and 02HK0JZ

0JH804Z
and 02HK0MZ

0JH804Z
and 02HK3JZ

0JH804Z
and 02HK3MZ

0JH804Z
and 02HK4JZ

0JH804Z
and 02HK4MZ

0JH804Z
and 02HL0JZ

0JH804Z
and 02HL0MZ

0JH804Z
and 02HL3JZ

0JH804Z
and 02HL3MZ

0JH804Z
and 02HL4JZ

0JH804Z
and 02HL4MZ

0JH804Z
and 02HN0JZ

0JH804Z
and 02HN0MZ

0JH804Z
and 02HN3JZ

0JH804Z
and 02HN3MZ

0JH804Z
and 02HN4JZ

0JH804Z
and 02HN4MZ

0JH804Z
and 0JPT0PZ

0JH804Z
and 0JPT0PZ
and 02H40JZ

0JH804Z
and 0JPT0PZ
and 02H40MZ

0JH804Z
and 0JPT0PZ
and 02H44JZ

0JH804Z
and 0JPT0PZ
and 02H44MZ

0JH804Z
and 0JPT0PZ
and 02H60JZ

0JH804Z
and 0JPT0PZ
and 02H60MZ

0JH804Z
and 0JPT0PZ
and 02H63JZ

0JH804Z
and 0JPT0PZ
and 02H63JZ
and 02PA0MZ

0JH804Z
and 0JPT0PZ
and 02H63JZ
and 02PA3MZ

0JH804Z
and 0JPT0PZ
and 02H63JZ
and 02PA4MZ

0JH804Z
and 0JPT0PZ
and 02H63JZ
and 02PAXMZ

0JH804Z
and 0JPT0PZ
and 02H63MZ

0JH804Z
and 0JPT0PZ
and 02H64JZ

0JH804Z
and 0JPT0PZ
and 02H64MZ

0JH804Z
and 0JPT0PZ
and 02H70JZ

0JH804Z
and 0JPT0PZ
and 02H70MZ

0JH804Z
and 0JPT0PZ
and 02H73JZ

0JH804Z
and 0JPT0PZ
and 02H73JZ
and 02PA0MZ

0JH804Z
and 0JPT0PZ
and 02H73JZ
and 02PA3MZ

0JH804Z
and 0JPT0PZ
and 02H73JZ
and 02PA4MZ

0JH804Z
and 0JPT0PZ
and 02H73JZ
and 02PAXMZ

0JH804Z
and 0JPT0PZ
and 02H73MZ

0JH804Z
and 0JPT0PZ
and 02H74JZ

0JH804Z
and 0JPT0PZ
and 02H74MZ

0JH804Z
and 0JPT0PZ
and 02HK0JZ

0JH804Z
and 0JPT0PZ
and 02HK0MZ

0JH804Z
and 0JPT0PZ
and 02HK3JZ

0JH804Z
and 0JPT0PZ
and 02HK3JZ
and 02PA0MZ

0JH804Z
and 0JPT0PZ
and 02HK3JZ
and 02PA3MZ

0JH804Z
and 0JPT0PZ
and 02HK3JZ
and 02PA4MZ

0JH804Z
and 0JPT0PZ
and 02HK3JZ
and 02PAXMZ

0JH804Z
and 0JPT0PZ
and 02HK3MZ

0JH804Z
and 0JPT0PZ
and 02HK4JZ

0JH804Z
and 0JPT0PZ
and 02HK4MZ

0JH804Z
and 0JPT0PZ
and 02HL0JZ

0JH804Z
and 0JPT0PZ
and 02HL0MZ

0JH804Z
and 0JPT0PZ
and 02HL3JZ

0JH804Z
and 0JPT0PZ
and 02HL3JZ
and 02PA0MZ

0JH804Z
and 0JPT0PZ
and 02HL3JZ
and 02PA3MZ

0JH804Z
and 0JPT0PZ
and 02HL3JZ
and 02PA4MZ

0JH804Z
and 0JPT0PZ
and 02HL3JZ
and 02PAXMZ

0JH804Z
and 0JPT0PZ
and 02HL3MZ

0JH804Z
and 0JPT0PZ
and 02HL4JZ

0JH804Z
and 0JPT0PZ
and 02HL4MZ

0JH804Z
and 0JPT0PZ
and 02HN0JZ

0JH804Z
and 0JPT0PZ
and 02HN0MZ

0JH804Z
and 0JPT0PZ
and 02HN3JZ

0JH804Z
and 0JPT0PZ
and 02HN3MZ

0JH804Z
and 0JPT0PZ
and 02HN4JZ

0JH804Z
and 0JPT0PZ
and 02HN4MZ

0JH804Z
and 0JPT3PZ

0JH804Z
and 0JPT3PZ
and 02H40JZ

0JH804Z
and 0JPT3PZ
and 02H40MZ

0JH804Z
and 0JPT3PZ
and 02H44JZ

0JH804Z
and 0JPT3PZ
and 02H44MZ

0JH804Z
and 0JPT3PZ
and 02H60JZ

0JH804Z
and 0JPT3PZ
and 02H60MZ

0JH804Z
and 0JPT3PZ
and 02H63JZ

0JH804Z
and 0JPT3PZ
and 02H63JZ
and 02PA0MZ

0JH804Z
and 0JPT3PZ
and 02H63JZ
and 02PA3MZ

0JH804Z
and 0JPT3PZ
and 02H63JZ
and 02PA4MZ

0JH804Z
and 0JPT3PZ
and 02H63JZ
and 02PAXMZ

0JH804Z
and 0JPT3PZ
and 02H63MZ

0JH804Z
and 0JPT3PZ
and 02H64JZ

0JH804Z
and 0JPT3PZ
and 02H64MZ

0JH804Z
and 0JPT3PZ
and 02H70JZ

0JH804Z
and 0JPT3PZ
and 02H70MZ

0JH804Z
and 0JPT3PZ
and 02H73JZ

0JH804Z
and 0JPT3PZ
and 02H73JZ
and 02PA0MZ

0JH804Z
and 0JPT3PZ
and 02H73JZ
and 02PA3MZ

0JH804Z
and 0JPT3PZ
and 02H73JZ
and 02PA4MZ

0JH804Z
and 0JPT3PZ
and 02H73JZ
and 02PAXMZ

0JH804Z
and 0JPT3PZ
and 02H73MZ

0JH804Z
and 0JPT3PZ
and 02H74JZ

0JH804Z
and 0JPT3PZ
and 02H74MZ

0JH804Z
and 0JPT3PZ
and 02HK0JZ

0JH804Z
and 0JPT3PZ
and 02HK0MZ

0JH804Z
and 0JPT3PZ
and 02HK3JZ

0JH804Z
and 0JPT3PZ
and 02HK3JZ
and 02PA0MZ

0JH804Z
and 0JPT3PZ
and 02HK3JZ
and 02PA3MZ

0JH804Z
and 0JPT3PZ
and 02HK3JZ
and 02PA4MZ

0JH804Z
and 0JPT3PZ
and 02HK3JZ
and 02PAXMZ

0JH804Z
and 0JPT3PZ
and 02HK3MZ

0JH804Z
and 0JPT3PZ
and 02HK4JZ

0JH804Z
and 0JPT3PZ
and 02HK4MZ

0JH804Z
and 0JPT3PZ
and 02HL0JZ

0JH804Z
and 0JPT3PZ
and 02HL0MZ

0JH804Z
and 0JPT3PZ
and 02HL3JZ

0JH804Z
and 0JPT3PZ
and 02HL3JZ
and 02PA0MZ

0JH804Z
and 0JPT3PZ
and 02HL3JZ
and 02PA3MZ

0JH804Z
and 0JPT3PZ
and 02HL3JZ
and 02PA4MZ

0JH804Z
and 0JPT3PZ
and 02HL3JZ
and 02PAXMZ

0JH804Z
and 0JPT3PZ
and 02HL3MZ

0JH804Z
and 0JPT3PZ
and 02HL4JZ

0JH804Z
and 0JPT3PZ
and 02HL4MZ

0JH804Z
and 0JPT3PZ
and 02HN0JZ

0JH804Z
and 0JPT3PZ
and 02HN0MZ

0JH804Z
and 0JPT3PZ
and 02HN3JZ

0JH804Z
and 0JPT3PZ
and 02HN3MZ

0JH804Z
and 0JPT3PZ
and 02HN4JZ

0JH804Z
and 0JPT3PZ
and 02HN4MZ

0JH805Z
and 02H40JZ

0JH805Z
and 02H40MZ

0JH805Z
and 02H44JZ

0JH805Z
and 02H44MZ

0JH805Z
and 02H60JZ

0JH805Z
and 02H60MZ

0JH805Z
and 02H63JZ

0JH805Z
and 02H64JZ

0JH805Z
and 02H64MZ

0JH805Z
and 02H70JZ

0JH805Z
and 02H70MZ

0JH805Z
and 02H73JZ

0JH805Z
and 02H74JZ

0JH805Z
and 02H74MZ

0JH805Z
and 02HK0JZ

0JH805Z
and 02HK0MZ

0JH805Z
and 02HK3JZ

0JH805Z
and 02HK3MZ

0JH805Z
and 02HK4JZ

0JH805Z
and 02HK4MZ

0JH805Z
and 02HL0JZ

0JH805Z
and 02HL0MZ

0JH805Z
and 02HL3JZ

0JH805Z
and 02HL3MZ

0JH805Z
and 02HL4JZ

0JH805Z
and 02HL4MZ

0JH805Z
and 02HN0JZ

0JH805Z
and 02HN0MZ

0JH805Z
and 02HN3JZ

0JH805Z
and 02HN3MZ

0JH805Z
and 02HN4JZ

0JH805Z
and 02HN4MZ

0JH805Z
and 0JPT0PZ

0JH805Z
and 0JPT0PZ
and 02H40JZ

0JH805Z
and 0JPT0PZ
and 02H40MZ

0JH805Z
and 0JPT0PZ
and 02H44JZ

0JH805Z
and 0JPT0PZ
and 02H44MZ

0JH805Z
and 0JPT0PZ
and 02H60JZ

0JH805Z
and 0JPT0PZ
and 02H60MZ

0JH805Z
and 0JPT0PZ
and 02H63JZ

0JH805Z
and 0JPT0PZ
and 02H63JZ
and 02PA0MZ

0JH805Z
and 0JPT0PZ
and 02H63JZ
and 02PA3MZ

0JH805Z
and 0JPT0PZ
and 02H63JZ
and 02PA4MZ

0JH805Z
and 0JPT0PZ
and 02H63JZ
and 02PAXMZ

0JH805Z
and 0JPT0PZ
and 02H63MZ

0JH805Z
and 0JPT0PZ
and 02H64JZ

0JH805Z
and 0JPT0PZ
and 02H64MZ

0JH805Z
and 0JPT0PZ
and 02H70JZ

0JH805Z
and 0JPT0PZ
and 02H70MZ

0JH805Z
and 0JPT0PZ
and 02H73JZ

0JH805Z
and 0JPT0PZ
and 02H73JZ
and 02PA0MZ

0JH805Z
and 0JPT0PZ
and 02H73JZ
and 02PA3MZ

0JH805Z
and 0JPT0PZ
and 02H73JZ
and 02PA4MZ

0JH805Z
and 0JPT0PZ
and 02H73JZ
and 02PAXMZ

0JH805Z
and 0JPT0PZ
and 02H73MZ

0JH805Z
and 0JPT0PZ
and 02H74JZ

0JH805Z
and 0JPT0PZ
and 02H74MZ

0JH805Z
and 0JPT0PZ
and 02HK0JZ

0JH805Z
and 0JPT0PZ
and 02HK0MZ

0JH805Z
and 0JPT0PZ
and 02HK3JZ

0JH805Z
and 0JPT0PZ
and 02HK3JZ
and 02PA0MZ

0JH805Z
and 0JPT0PZ
and 02HK3JZ
and 02PA3MZ

0JH805Z
and 0JPT0PZ
and 02HK3JZ
and 02PA4MZ

0JH805Z
and 0JPT0PZ
and 02HK3JZ
and 02PAXMZ

0JH805Z
and 0JPT0PZ
and 02HK3MZ

0JH805Z
and 0JPT0PZ
and 02HK4JZ

0JH805Z
and 0JPT0PZ
and 02HK4MZ

0JH805Z
and 0JPT0PZ
and 02HL0JZ

0JH805Z
and 0JPT0PZ
and 02HL0MZ

0JH805Z
and 0JPT0PZ
and 02HL3JZ

0JH805Z
and 0JPT0PZ
and 02HL3JZ
and 02PA0MZ

0JH805Z
and 0JPT0PZ
and 02HL3JZ
and 02PA3MZ

0JH805Z
and 0JPT0PZ
and 02HL3JZ
and 02PA4MZ

0JH805Z
and 0JPT0PZ
and 02HL3JZ
and 02PAXMZ

0JH805Z
and 0JPT0PZ
and 02HL3MZ

0JH805Z
and 0JPT0PZ
and 02HL4JZ

0JH805Z
and 0JPT0PZ
and 02HL4MZ

0JH805Z
and 0JPT0PZ
and 02HN0JZ

0JH805Z
and 0JPT0PZ
and 02HN0MZ

0JH805Z
and 0JPT0PZ
and 02HN3JZ

0JH805Z
and 0JPT0PZ
and 02HN3MZ

0JH805Z
and 0JPT0PZ
and 02HN4JZ

0JH805Z
and 0JPT0PZ
and 02HN4MZ

0JH805Z
and 0JPT3PZ

0JH805Z
and 0JPT3PZ
and 02H40JZ

0JH805Z
and 0JPT3PZ
and 02H40MZ

0JH805Z
and 0JPT3PZ
and 02H44JZ

0JH805Z
and 0JPT3PZ
and 02H44MZ

0JH805Z
and 0JPT3PZ
and 02H60JZ

and 02H60MZ

0JH805Z
and 0JPT3PZ
and 02H60MZ

0JH805Z
and 0JPT3PZ
and 02H63JZ

0JH805Z
and 0JPT3PZ
and 02H63JZ
and 02PA0MZ

0JH805Z
and 0JPT3PZ
and 02H63JZ
and 02PA3MZ

0JH805Z
and 0JPT3PZ
and 02H63JZ
and 02PA4MZ

0JH805Z
and 0JPT3PZ
and 02H63JZ
and 02PAXMZ

0JH805Z
and 0JPT3PZ
and 02H63MZ

0JH805Z
and 0JPT3PZ
and 02H64JZ

0JH805Z
and 0JPT3PZ
and 02H64MZ

0JH805Z
and 0JPT3PZ
and 02H70JZ

0JH805Z
and 0JPT3PZ
and 02H70MZ

0JH805Z
and 0JPT3PZ
and 02H73JZ

0JH805Z
and 0JPT3PZ
and 02H73JZ
and 02PA0MZ

0JH805Z
and 0JPT3PZ
and 02H73JZ
and 02PA3MZ

0JH805Z
and 0JPT3PZ
and 02H73JZ
and 02PA4MZ

0JH805Z
and 0JPT3PZ
and 02H73JZ
and 02PAXMZ

0JH805Z
and 0JPT3PZ
and 02H73MZ

0JH805Z
and 0JPT3PZ
and 02H74JZ

0JH805Z
and 0JPT3PZ
and 02H74MZ

0JH805Z
and 0JPT3PZ
and 02HK0JZ

0JH805Z
and 0JPT3PZ
and 02HK0MZ

0JH805Z
and 0JPT3PZ
and 02HK3JZ

0JH805Z
and 0JPT3PZ
and 02HK3JZ
and 02PA0MZ

0JH805Z
and 0JPT3PZ
and 02HK3JZ
and 02PA3MZ

0JH805Z
and 0JPT3PZ
and 02HK3JZ
and 02PA4MZ

0JH805Z
and 0JPT3PZ
and 02HK3JZ
and 02PAXMZ

0JH805Z
and 0JPT3PZ
and 02HK3MZ

0JH805Z
and 0JPT3PZ
and 02HK4JZ

0JH805Z
and 0JPT3PZ
and 02HK4MZ

0JH805Z
and 0JPT3PZ
and 02HL0JZ

0JH805Z
and 0JPT3PZ
and 02HL0MZ

0JH805Z
and 0JPT3PZ
and 02HL3JZ

0JH805Z
and 0JPT3PZ
and 02HL3JZ
and 02PA0MZ

0JH805Z
and 0JPT3PZ
and 02HL3JZ
and 02PA3MZ

0JH805Z
and 0JPT3PZ
and 02HL3JZ
and 02PA4MZ

0JH805Z
and 0JPT3PZ
and 02HL3JZ
and 02PAXMZ

0JH805Z
and 0JPT3PZ
and 02HL3MZ

0JH805Z
and 0JPT3PZ
and 02HL4JZ

0JH805Z
and 0JPT3PZ
and 02HL4MZ

0JH805Z
and 0JPT3PZ
and 02HN0JZ

0JH805Z
and 0JPT3PZ
and 02HN0MZ

0JH805Z
and 0JPT3PZ
and 02HN3JZ

0JH805Z
and 0JPT3PZ
and 02HN3MZ

0JH805Z
and 0JPT3PZ
and 02HN4JZ

0JH805Z
and 0JPT3PZ
and 02HN4MZ

0JH806Z
and 02HK3JZ

0JH806Z
and 02HL3JZ

0JH806Z
and 02HN0JZ

0JH806Z
and 02HN0MZ

0JH806Z
and 02HN3JZ

0JH806Z
and 02HN3MZ

0JH806Z
and 02HN4JZ

0JH806Z
and 02HN4MZ

0JH806Z
and 0JPT0PZ

0JH806Z
and 0JPT0PZ
and 02H40JZ

0JH806Z
and 0JPT0PZ
and 02H40MZ

0JH806Z
and 0JPT0PZ
and 02H44JZ

0JH806Z
and 0JPT0PZ
and 02H44MZ

0JH806Z
and 0JPT0PZ
and 02H60JZ

0JH806Z
and 0JPT0PZ
and 02H60MZ

0JH806Z
and 0JPT0PZ
and 02H63JZ

0JH806Z
and 0JPT0PZ
and 02H63JZ
and 02PA0MZ

0JH806Z
and 0JPT0PZ
and 02H63JZ
and 02PA3MZ

0JH806Z
and 0JPT0PZ
and 02H63JZ
and 02PA4MZ

0JH806Z
and 0JPT0PZ
and 02H63JZ
and 02PAXMZ

0JH806Z
and 0JPT0PZ
and 02H63MZ

0JH806Z
and 0JPT0PZ
and 02H64JZ

0JH806Z
and 0JPT0PZ
and 02H64MZ

0JH806Z
and 0JPT0PZ
and 02H70JZ

0JH806Z
and 0JPT0PZ
and 02H70MZ

0JH806Z
and 0JPT0PZ
and 02H73JZ

0JH806Z
and 0JPT0PZ
and 02H73JZ
and 02PA0MZ

0JH806Z
and 0JPT0PZ
and 02H73JZ
and 02PA3MZ

0JH806Z
and 0JPT0PZ
and 02H73JZ
and 02PA4MZ

0JH806Z
and 0JPT0PZ
and 02H73JZ
and 02PAXMZ

0JH806Z
and 0JPT0PZ
and 02H73MZ

0JH806Z
and 0JPT0PZ
and 02H74JZ

0JH806Z
and 0JPT0PZ
and 02H74MZ

0JH806Z
and 0JPT0PZ
and 02HK0JZ

0JH806Z
and 0JPT0PZ
and 02HK0MZ

0JH806Z
and 0JPT0PZ
and 02HK3JZ

0JH806Z
and 0JPT0PZ
and 02HK3JZ
and 02PA0MZ

0JH806Z
and 0JPT0PZ
and 02HK3JZ
and 02PA3MZ

0JH806Z
and 0JPT0PZ
and 02HK3JZ
and 02PA4MZ

0JH806Z
and 0JPT0PZ
and 02HK3JZ
and 02PAXMZ

0JH806Z
and 0JPT0PZ
and 02HK3MZ

0JH806Z
and 0JPT0PZ
and 02HK4JZ

0JH806Z
and 0JPT0PZ
and 02HK4MZ

0JH806Z
and 0JPT0PZ
and 02HL0JZ

0JH806Z
and 0JPT0PZ
and 02HL0MZ

0JH806Z
and 0JPT0PZ
and 02HL3JZ

0JH806Z
and 0JPT0PZ
and 02HL3JZ
and 02PA0MZ

0JH806Z
and 0JPT0PZ
and 02HL3JZ
and 02PA3MZ

0JH806Z
and 0JPT0PZ
and 02HL3JZ
and 02PA4MZ

0JH806Z
and 0JPT0PZ
and 02HL3JZ
and 02PAXMZ

0JH806Z
and 0JPT0PZ
and 02HL3MZ

0JH806Z
and 0JPT0PZ
and 02HL4JZ

0JH806Z
and 0JPT0PZ
and 02HL4MZ

0JH806Z
and 0JPT0PZ
and 02HN0JZ

0JH806Z
and 0JPT0PZ
and 02HN0MZ

0JH806Z
and 0JPT0PZ
and 02HN3JZ

0JH806Z
and 0JPT0PZ
and 02HN3MZ

0JH806Z
and 0JPT0PZ
and 02HN4JZ

0JH806Z
and 0JPT0PZ
and 02HN4MZ

0JH806Z
and 0JPT3PZ

0JH806Z
and 0JPT3PZ
and 02H40JZ

0JH806Z
and 0JPT3PZ
and 02H40MZ

0JH806Z
and 0JPT3PZ
and 02H44JZ

0JH806Z
and 0JPT3PZ
and 02H44MZ

0JH806Z
and 0JPT3PZ
and 02H60JZ

0JH806Z
and 0JPT3PZ
and 02H60MZ

0JH806Z
and 0JPT3PZ
and 02H63JZ

0JH806Z
and 0JPT3PZ
and 02H63JZ
and 02PA0MZ

0JH806Z
and 0JPT3PZ
and 02H63JZ
and 02PA3MZ

0JH806Z
and 0JPT3PZ
and 02H63JZ
and 02PA4MZ

0JH806Z
and 0JPT3PZ
and 02H63JZ
and 02PAXMZ

0JH806Z
and 0JPT3PZ
and 02H63MZ

0JH806Z
and 0JPT3PZ
and 02H64JZ

0JH806Z
and 0JPT3PZ
and 02H64MZ

0JH806Z
and 0JPT3PZ
and 02H70JZ

0JH806Z
and 0JPT3PZ
and 02H70MZ

0JH806Z
and 0JPT3PZ
and 02H73JZ

0JH806Z
and 0JPT3PZ
and 02H73JZ
and 02PA0MZ

0JH806Z
and 0JPT3PZ
and 02H73JZ
and 02PA3MZ

0JH806Z
and 0JPT3PZ
and 02H73JZ
and 02PA4MZ

0JH806Z
and 0JPT3PZ
and 02H73JZ
and 02PAXMZ

0JH806Z
and 0JPT3PZ
and 02H73MZ

0JH806Z
and 0JPT3PZ
and 02H74JZ

0JH806Z
and 0JPT3PZ
and 02H74MZ

0JH806Z
and 0JPT3PZ
and 02HK0JZ

0JH806Z
and 0JPT3PZ
and 02HK0MZ

0JH806Z
and 0JPT3PZ
and 02HK3JZ

0JH806Z
and 0JPT3PZ
and 02HK3JZ
and 02PA0MZ

0JH806Z
and 0JPT3PZ
and 02HK3JZ
and 02PA3MZ

0JH806Z
and 0JPT3PZ
and 02HK3JZ
and 02PA4MZ

0JH806Z
and 0JPT3PZ
and 02HK3JZ
and 02PAXMZ

0JH806Z
and 0JPT3PZ
and 02HK3MZ

0JH806Z
and 0JPT3PZ
and 02HK4JZ

0JH806Z
and 0JPT3PZ
and 02HK4MZ

0JH806Z
and 0JPT3PZ
and 02HL0JZ

0JH806Z
and 0JPT3PZ
and 02HL0MZ

0JH806Z
and 0JPT3PZ
and 02HL3JZ

0JH806Z
and 0JPT3PZ
and 02HL3JZ
and 02PA0MZ

0JH806Z
and 0JPT3PZ
and 02HL3JZ
and 02PA3MZ

0JH806Z
and 0JPT3PZ
and 02HL3JZ
and 02PA4MZ

0JH806Z
and 0JPT3PZ
and 02HL3JZ
and 02PAXMZ

0JH806Z
and 0JPT3PZ
and 02HL3MZ

0JH806Z
and 0JPT3PZ
and 02HL4JZ

0JH806Z
and 0JPT3PZ
and 02HL4MZ

0JH806Z
and 0JPT3PZ
and 02HN0JZ

0JH806Z
and 0JPT3PZ
and 02HN0MZ

0JH806Z
and 0JPT3PZ
and 02HN3JZ

0JH806Z
and 0JPT3PZ
and 02HN3MZ

0JH806Z
and 0JPT3PZ
and 02HN4JZ

0JH806Z
and 0JPT3PZ
and 02HN4MZ

0JH807Z
and 02H40JZ

0JH807Z
and 02H40MZ

0JH807Z
and 02H43JZ

0JH807Z
and 02H43KZ

0JH807Z
and 02H43MZ

0JH807Z
and 02H44JZ

0JH807Z
and 02H44MZ

0JH807Z
and 02H60JZ

0JH807Z
and 02H60MZ

0JH807Z
and 02H63JZ

0JH807Z
and 02H63JZ
and 02PA0MZ

0JH807Z
and 02H63JZ
and 02PA3MZ

0JH807Z
and 02H63JZ
and 02PA4MZ

0JH807Z
and 02H63JZ
and 02PAXMZ

0JH807Z
and 02H63MZ

0JH807Z
and 02H64JZ

0JH807Z
and 02H64MZ

0JH807Z
and 02H70JZ

0JH807Z
and 02H70MZ

0JH807Z
and 02H73JZ

0JH807Z
and 02H73JZ
and 02PA0MZ

0JH807Z
and 02H73JZ
and 02PA3MZ

0JH807Z
and 02H73JZ
and 02PA4MZ

0JH807Z
and 02H73JZ
and 02PAXMZ

0JH807Z
and 02H73MZ

0JH807Z
and 02H74JZ

0JH807Z
and 02H74MZ

0JH807Z
and 02HK0JZ

0JH807Z
and 02HK0MZ

0JH807Z
and 02HK3JZ

0JH807Z
and 02HK3JZ
and 02PA0MZ

0JH807Z
and 02HK3JZ
and 02PA3MZ

0JH807Z
and 02HK3JZ
and 02PA4MZ

0JH807Z
and 02HK3JZ
and 02PAXMZ

0JH807Z
and 02HK3MZ

0JH807Z
and 02HK4JZ

0JH807Z
and 02HK4MZ

0JH807Z
and 02HL0JZ

0JH807Z
and 02HL0MZ

0JH807Z
and 02HL3JZ

0JH807Z
and 02HL3JZ
and 02PA0MZ

0JH807Z
and 02HL3JZ
and 02PA3MZ

0JH807Z
and 02HL3JZ
and 02PA4MZ

0JH807Z
and 02HL3JZ
and 02PAXMZ

0JH807Z
and 02HL3MZ

0JH807Z
and 02HL4JZ

0JH807Z
and 02HL4MZ

0JH807Z
and 02HN0JZ

0JH807Z
and 02HN0MZ

0JH807Z
and 02HN3JZ

0JH807Z
and 02HN3MZ

0JH807Z
and 02HN4JZ

0JH807Z
and 02HN4MZ

0JH808Z
and 02H40KZ

0JH808Z
and 02H44KZ

0JH808Z
and 02HN0JZ

0JH808Z
and 02HN0KZ

0JH808Z
and 02HN0MZ

0JH808Z
and 02HN3JZ

0JH808Z
and 02HN3KZ

0JH808Z
and 02HN3MZ

0JH808Z
and 02HN4JZ

0JH808Z
and 02HN4KZ

0JH808Z
and 02HN4MZ

0JH809Z
and 02H40KZ

0JH809Z
and 02H43JZ

0JH809Z
and 02H43KZ

0JH809Z
and 02H43MZ

0JH809Z
and 02H44KZ

0JH809Z
and 02H60KZ

0JH809Z
and 02H63KZ

0JH809Z
and 02H64KZ

0JH809Z
and 02H70KZ

0JH809Z
and 02H73KZ

0JH809Z
and 02H74KZ

0JH809Z
and 02HN0JZ

0JH809Z
and 02HN0KZ

0JH809Z
and 02HN0MZ

0JH809Z
and 02HN3JZ

0JH809Z
and 02HN3KZ

0JH809Z
and 02HN3MZ

0JH809Z
and 02HN4JZ

0JH809Z
and 02HN4KZ

0JH809Z and 02HN4MZ

0JH80BZ and 00HE0MZ

0JH80BZ and 00HE3MZ

0JH80BZ and 00HE4MZ

0JH80BZ and 00HU0MZ

0JH80BZ and 00HU3MZ

0JH80BZ and 00HU4MZ

0JH80BZ and 00HV0MZ

0JH80BZ and 00HV3MZ

0JH80BZ and 00HV4MZ

0JH80BZ and 01HY0MZ

0JH80BZ and 01HY3MZ

0JH80BZ and 01HY4MZ

0JH80BZ and 0DH60MZ

0JH80BZ and 0DH63MZ

0JH80BZ and 0DH64MZ

0JH80CZ and 00HE0MZ

0JH80CZ and 00HE3MZ

0JH80CZ and 00HE4MZ

0JH80CZ and 00HU0MZ

0JH80CZ and 00HU3MZ

0JH80CZ and 00HU4MZ

0JH80CZ and 00HV0MZ

0JH80CZ and 00HV3MZ

0JH80CZ and 00HV4MZ

0JH80CZ and 01HY0MZ

0JH80CZ and 01HY3MZ

0JH80CZ and 01HY4MZ

0JH80CZ and 0DH60MZ

0JH80CZ and 0DH63MZ

0JH80CZ and 0DH64MZ

0JH80DZ and 00H00MZ

0JH80DZ and 00H03MZ

0JH80DZ and 00H04MZ

0JH80DZ and 00H60MZ

0JH80DZ and 00H63MZ

0JH80DZ and 00H64MZ

0JH80DZ and 00HE0MZ

0JH80DZ and 00HE3MZ

0JH80DZ and 00HE4MZ

0JH80DZ and 00HU0MZ

0JH80DZ and 00HU3MZ

0JH80DZ and 00HU4MZ

0JH80DZ and 00HV0MZ

0JH80DZ and 00HV3MZ

0JH80DZ and 00HV4MZ

0JH80DZ and 01HY0MZ

0JH80DZ and 01HY3MZ

0JH80DZ and 01HY4MZ

0JH80DZ and 0DH60MZ

0JH80DZ and 0DH63MZ

0JH80DZ and 0DH64MZ

0JH80EZ and 00H00MZ

0JH80EZ and 00H03MZ

0JH80EZ and 00H04MZ

0JH80EZ and 00H60MZ

0JH80EZ and 00H63MZ

0JH80EZ and 00H64MZ

0JH80EZ and 00HE0MZ

0JH80EZ and 00HE3MZ

0JH80EZ and 00HE4MZ

0JH80EZ and 00HU0MZ

0JH80EZ and 00HU3MZ

0JH80EZ and 00HU4MZ

0JH80EZ and 00HV0MZ

0JH80EZ and 00HV3MZ

0JH80EZ and 00HV4MZ

0JH80EZ and 01HY0MZ

0JH80EZ and 01HY3MZ

0JH80EZ and 01HY4MZ

0JH80EZ and 0DH60MZ

0JH80EZ and 0DH63MZ

0JH80EZ and 0DH64MZ

0JH80PZ and 02H40JZ

0JH80PZ and 02H40MZ

0JH80PZ and 02H44JZ

0JH80PZ and 02H44MZ

0JH80PZ and 02H60JZ

0JH80PZ and 02H60MZ

0JH80PZ and 02H63JZ

0JH80PZ and 02H63JZ and 02PA0MZ

0JH80PZ and 02H63JZ and 02PA3MZ

0JH80PZ and 02H63JZ and 02PA4MZ

0JH80PZ and 02H63JZ and 02PAXMZ

0JH80PZ and 02H63MZ

0JH80PZ and 02H64JZ

0JH80PZ and 02H64MZ

0JH80PZ and 02H70JZ

0JH80PZ and 02H70MZ

0JH80PZ and 02H73JZ

0JH80PZ and 02H73JZ and 02PA0MZ

0JH80PZ and 02H73JZ and 02PA3MZ

0JH80PZ and 02H73JZ and 02PA4MZ

0JH80PZ and 02H73JZ and 02PAXMZ

0JH80PZ and 02H73MZ

0JH80PZ and 02H74JZ

0JH80PZ and 02H74MZ

0JH80PZ and 02HK0JZ

0JH80PZ and 02HK0MZ

0JH80PZ and 02HK3JZ

0JH80PZ and 02HK3JZ and 02PA0MZ

0JH80PZ and 02HK3JZ and 02PA3MZ

0JH80PZ and 02HK3JZ and 02PA4MZ

0JH80PZ and 02HK3JZ and 02PAXMZ

0JH80PZ and 02HK3MZ

0JH80PZ and 02HK4JZ

0JH80PZ and 02HK4MZ

0JH80PZ and 02HL0JZ

0JH80PZ and 02HL0MZ

0JH80PZ and 02HL3JZ

0JH80PZ and 02HL3JZ and 02PA0MZ

0JH80PZ and 02HL3JZ and 02PA3MZ

0JH80PZ and 02HL3JZ and 02PA4MZ

0JH80PZ and 02HL3JZ and 02PAXMZ

0JH80PZ and 02HL3MZ

0JH80PZ and 02HL4JZ

0JH80PZ and 02HL4MZ

0JH80PZ and 02HN0JZ

0JH80PZ and 02HN0MZ

0JH80PZ and 02HN3JZ

0JH80PZ and 02HN3MZ

0JH80PZ and 02HN4JZ

0JH80PZ and 02HN4MZ

0JH834Z and 02H40JZ

0JH834Z and 02H40MZ

0JH834Z and 02H44JZ

0JH834Z and 02H44MZ

0JH834Z and 02H60JZ

0JH834Z and 02H60MZ

0JH834Z and 02H63JZ

0JH834Z and 02H64JZ

0JH834Z and 02H64MZ

0JH834Z and 02H70JZ

0JH834Z and 02H70MZ

0JH834Z and 02H73JZ

0JH834Z and 02H74JZ

0JH834Z and 02H74MZ

0JH834Z and 02HK0JZ

0JH834Z and 02HK0MZ

0JH834Z and 02HK3JZ

0JH834Z and 02HK3MZ

0JH834Z and 02HK4JZ

0JH834Z and 02HK4MZ

0JH834Z and 02HL0JZ

0JH834Z and 02HL0MZ

0JH834Z and 02HL3JZ

0JH834Z and 02HL3MZ

0JH834Z and 02HL4JZ

0JH834Z and 02HL4MZ

0JH834Z and 02HN0JZ

0JH834Z and 02HN0MZ

0JH834Z and 02HN3JZ

0JH834Z and 02HN3MZ

0JH834Z and 02HN4JZ

0JH834Z and 02HN4MZ

0JH834Z and 0JPT0PZ

0JH834Z and 0JPT0PZ

and 02H40JZ

0JH834Z
and 0JPT0PZ
and 02H40MZ

0JH834Z
and 0JPT0PZ
and 02H44JZ

0JH834Z
and 0JPT0PZ
and 02H44MZ

0JH834Z
and 0JPT0PZ
and 02H60JZ

0JH834Z
and 0JPT0PZ
and 02H60MZ

0JH834Z
and 0JPT0PZ
and 02H63JZ

0JH834Z
and 0JPT0PZ
and 02H63JZ
and 02PA0MZ

0JH834Z
and 0JPT0PZ
and 02H63JZ
and 02PA3MZ

0JH834Z
and 0JPT0PZ
and 02H63JZ
and 02PA4MZ

0JH834Z
and 0JPT0PZ
and 02H63JZ
and 02PAXMZ

0JH834Z
and 0JPT0PZ
and 02H63MZ

0JH834Z
and 0JPT0PZ
and 02H64JZ

0JH834Z
and 0JPT0PZ
and 02H64MZ

0JH834Z
and 0JPT0PZ
and 02H70JZ

0JH834Z
and 0JPT0PZ
and 02H70MZ

0JH834Z
and 0JPT0PZ
and 02H73JZ

0JH834Z
and 0JPT0PZ
and 02H73JZ
and 02PA0MZ

0JH834Z
and 0JPT0PZ
and 02H73JZ
and 02PA3MZ

0JH834Z
and 0JPT0PZ
and 02H73JZ
and 02PA4MZ

0JH834Z
and 0JPT0PZ
and 02H73JZ
and 02PAXMZ

0JH834Z
and 0JPT0PZ
and 02H73MZ

0JH834Z
and 0JPT0PZ
and 02H74JZ

0JH834Z
and 0JPT0PZ
and 02H74MZ

0JH834Z
and 0JPT0PZ
and 02HK0JZ

0JH834Z
and 0JPT0PZ
and 02HK0MZ

0JH834Z
and 0JPT0PZ
and 02HK3JZ

0JH834Z
and 0JPT0PZ
and 02HK3JZ
and 02PA0MZ

0JH834Z
and 0JPT0PZ
and 02HK3JZ
and 02PA3MZ

0JH834Z
and 0JPT0PZ
and 02HK3JZ
and 02PA4MZ

0JH834Z
and 0JPT0PZ
and 02HK3JZ
and 02PAXMZ

0JH834Z
and 0JPT0PZ
and 02HK3MZ

0JH834Z
and 0JPT0PZ
and 02HK4JZ

0JH834Z
and 0JPT0PZ
and 02HK4MZ

0JH834Z
and 0JPT0PZ
and 02HL0JZ

0JH834Z
and 0JPT0PZ
and 02HL0MZ

0JH834Z
and 0JPT0PZ
and 02HL3JZ

0JH834Z
and 0JPT0PZ
and 02HL3JZ
and 02PA0MZ

0JH834Z
and 0JPT0PZ
and 02HL3JZ
and 02PA3MZ

0JH834Z
and 0JPT0PZ
and 02HL3JZ
and 02PA4MZ

0JH834Z
and 0JPT0PZ
and 02HL3JZ
and 02PAXMZ

0JH834Z
and 0JPT0PZ
and 02HL3MZ

0JH834Z
and 0JPT0PZ
and 02HL4JZ

0JH834Z
and 0JPT0PZ
and 02HL4MZ

0JH834Z
and 0JPT0PZ
and 02HN0JZ

0JH834Z
and 0JPT0PZ
and 02HN0MZ

0JH834Z
and 0JPT0PZ
and 02HN3JZ

0JH834Z
and 0JPT0PZ
and 02HN3MZ

0JH834Z
and 0JPT0PZ
and 02HN4JZ

0JH834Z
and 0JPT0PZ
and 02HN4MZ

0JH834Z
and 0JPT3PZ

0JH834Z
and 0JPT3PZ
and 02H40JZ

0JH834Z
and 0JPT3PZ
and 02H40MZ

0JH834Z
and 0JPT3PZ
and 02H44JZ

0JH834Z
and 0JPT3PZ
and 02H44MZ

0JH834Z
and 0JPT3PZ
and 02H60JZ

0JH834Z
and 0JPT3PZ
and 02H60MZ

0JH834Z
and 0JPT3PZ
and 02H63JZ

0JH834Z
and 0JPT3PZ
and 02H63JZ
and 02PA0MZ

0JH834Z
and 0JPT3PZ
and 02H63JZ
and 02PA3MZ

0JH834Z
and 0JPT3PZ
and 02H63JZ
and 02PA4MZ

0JH834Z
and 0JPT3PZ
and 02H63JZ
and 02PAXMZ

0JH834Z
and 0JPT3PZ
and 02H63MZ

0JH834Z
and 0JPT3PZ
and 02H64JZ

0JH834Z
and 0JPT3PZ
and 02H64MZ

0JH834Z
and 0JPT3PZ
and 02H70JZ

0JH834Z
and 0JPT3PZ
and 02H70MZ

0JH834Z
and 0JPT3PZ
and 02H73JZ

0JH834Z
and 0JPT3PZ
and 02H73JZ
and 02PA0MZ

0JH834Z
and 0JPT3PZ
and 02H73JZ
and 02PA3MZ

0JH834Z
and 0JPT3PZ
and 02H73JZ
and 02PA4MZ

0JH834Z
and 0JPT3PZ
and 02H73JZ
and 02PAXMZ

0JH834Z
and 0JPT3PZ
and 02H73MZ

0JH834Z
and 0JPT3PZ
and 02H74JZ

0JH834Z
and 0JPT3PZ
and 02H74MZ

0JH834Z
and 0JPT3PZ
and 02HK0JZ

0JH834Z
and 0JPT3PZ
and 02HK0MZ

0JH834Z
and 0JPT3PZ
and 02HK3JZ

0JH834Z
and 0JPT3PZ
and 02HK3JZ
and 02PA0MZ

0JH834Z
and 0JPT3PZ
and 02HK3JZ
and 02PA3MZ

0JH834Z
and 0JPT3PZ
and 02HK3JZ
and 02PA4MZ

0JH834Z
and 0JPT3PZ
and 02HK3JZ
and 02PAXMZ

0JH834Z
and 0JPT3PZ
and 02HK3MZ

0JH834Z
and 0JPT3PZ
and 02HK4JZ

0JH834Z
and 0JPT3PZ
and 02HK4MZ

0JH834Z
and 0JPT3PZ
and 02HL0JZ

0JH834Z
and 0JPT3PZ
and 02HL0MZ

0JH834Z
and 0JPT3PZ
and 02HL3JZ

0JH834Z
and 0JPT3PZ
and 02HL3JZ
and 02PA0MZ

0JH834Z
and 0JPT3PZ
and 02HL3JZ
and 02PA3MZ

0JH834Z
and 0JPT3PZ
and 02HL3JZ
and 02PA4MZ

0JH834Z
and 0JPT3PZ
and 02HL3JZ
and 02PAXMZ

0JH834Z
and 0JPT3PZ
and 02HL3MZ

0JH834Z
and 0JPT3PZ
and 02HL4JZ

0JH834Z
and 0JPT3PZ
and 02HL4MZ

0JH834Z
and 0JPT3PZ
and 02HN0JZ

0JH834Z
and 0JPT3PZ
and 02HN0MZ

0JH834Z
and 0JPT3PZ
and 02HN3JZ

0JH834Z
and 0JPT3PZ
and 02HN3MZ

0JH834Z
and 0JPT3PZ
and 02HN4JZ

0JH834Z
and 0JPT3PZ
and 02HN4MZ

0JH835Z
and 02H40JZ

0JH835Z
and 02H40MZ

0JH835Z
and 02H44JZ

0JH835Z
and 02H44MZ

0JH835Z
and 02H60JZ

0JH835Z
and 02H60MZ

0JH835Z
and 02H63JZ

0JH835Z
and 02H64JZ

0JH835Z
and 02H64MZ

0JH835Z
and 02H70JZ

0JH835Z
and 02H70MZ

0JH835Z
and 02H73JZ

0JH835Z
and 02H74JZ

0JH835Z
and 02H74MZ

0JH835Z
and 02HK0JZ

0JH835Z
and 02HK0MZ

0JH835Z
and 02HK3JZ

0JH835Z
and 02HK3MZ

0JH835Z
and 02HK4JZ

0JH835Z
and 02HK4MZ

0JH835Z
and 02HL0JZ

0JH835Z
and 02HL0MZ

0JH835Z
and 02HL3JZ

0JH835Z
and 02HL3MZ

0JH835Z
and 02HL4JZ

0JH835Z
and 02HL4MZ

0JH835Z
and 02HN0JZ

0JH835Z
and 02HN0MZ

0JH835Z
and 02HN3JZ

0JH835Z
and 02HN3MZ

0JH835Z
and 02HN4JZ

0JH835Z
and 02HN4MZ

0JH835Z
and 0JPT0PZ

0JH835Z
and 0JPT0PZ
and 02H40JZ

0JH835Z
and 0JPT0PZ
and 02H40MZ

0JH835Z
and 0JPT0PZ
and 02H44JZ

0JH835Z
and 0JPT0PZ
and 02H44MZ

0JH835Z
and 0JPT0PZ
and 02H60JZ

0JH835Z
and 0JPT0PZ
and 02H60MZ

0JH835Z
and 0JPT0PZ
and 02H63JZ

0JH835Z
and 0JPT0PZ
and 02H63JZ
and 02PA0MZ

0JH835Z
and 0JPT0PZ
and 02H63JZ
and 02PA3MZ

0JH835Z
and 0JPT0PZ
and 02H63JZ
and 02PA4MZ

0JH835Z
and 0JPT0PZ
and 02H63JZ
and 02PAXMZ

0JH835Z
and 0JPT0PZ
and 02H63MZ

0JH835Z
and 0JPT0PZ
and 02H64JZ

0JH835Z
and 0JPT0PZ
and 02H64MZ

0JH835Z
and 0JPT0PZ
and 02H70JZ

0JH835Z
and 0JPT0PZ
and 02H70MZ

0JH835Z
and 0JPT0PZ
and 02H73JZ

0JH835Z
and 0JPT0PZ
and 02H73JZ
and 02PA0MZ

0JH835Z
and 0JPT0PZ
and 02H73JZ
and 02PA3MZ

0JH835Z
and 0JPT0PZ
and 02H73JZ
and 02PA4MZ

0JH835Z
and 0JPT0PZ
and 02H73JZ
and 02PAXMZ

0JH835Z
and 0JPT0PZ
and 02H73MZ

0JH835Z
and 0JPT0PZ
and 02H74JZ

0JH835Z
and 0JPT0PZ
and 02H74MZ

0JH835Z
and 0JPT0PZ
and 02HK0JZ

0JH835Z
and 0JPT0PZ
and 02HK0MZ

0JH835Z
and 0JPT0PZ
and 02HK3JZ

0JH835Z
and 0JPT0PZ
and 02HK3JZ
and 02PA0MZ

0JH835Z
and 0JPT0PZ
and 02HK3JZ
and 02PA3MZ

0JH835Z
and 0JPT0PZ
and 02HK3JZ
and 02PA4MZ

0JH835Z
and 0JPT0PZ
and 02HK3JZ
and 02PAXMZ

0JH835Z
and 0JPT0PZ
and 02HK3MZ

0JH835Z
and 0JPT0PZ
and 02HK4JZ

0JH835Z
and 0JPT0PZ
and 02HK4MZ

0JH835Z
and 0JPT0PZ
and 02HL0JZ

0JH835Z
and 0JPT0PZ
and 02HL0MZ

0JH835Z
and 0JPT0PZ
and 02HL3JZ

0JH835Z
and 0JPT0PZ
and 02HL3JZ
and 02PA0MZ

0JH835Z
and 0JPT0PZ
and 02HL3JZ
and 02PA3MZ

0JH835Z
and 0JPT0PZ
and 02HL3JZ
and 02PA4MZ

0JH835Z
and 0JPT0PZ
and 02HL3JZ
and 02PAXMZ

0JH835Z
and 0JPT0PZ
and 02HL3MZ

0JH835Z
and 0JPT0PZ
and 02HL4JZ

0JH835Z
and 0JPT0PZ
and 02HL4MZ

0JH835Z
and 0JPT0PZ
and 02HN0JZ

0JH835Z
and 0JPT0PZ
and 02HN0MZ

0JH835Z
and 0JPT0PZ
and 02HN3JZ

0JH835Z
and 0JPT0PZ
and 02HN3MZ

0JH835Z
and 0JPT0PZ
and 02HN4JZ

0JH835Z
and 0JPT0PZ
and 02HN4MZ

0JH835Z
and 0JPT3PZ

0JH835Z
and 0JPT3PZ
and 02H40JZ

0JH835Z
and 0JPT3PZ
and 02H40MZ

0JH835Z
and 0JPT3PZ
and 02H44JZ

0JH835Z
and 0JPT3PZ
and 02H44MZ

0JH835Z
and 0JPT3PZ
and 02H60JZ

0JH835Z
and 0JPT3PZ
and 02H60MZ

0JH835Z
and 0JPT3PZ
and 02H63JZ

0JH835Z
and 0JPT3PZ
and 02H63JZ
and 02PA0MZ

0JH835Z
and 0JPT3PZ
and 02H63JZ
and 02PA3MZ

0JH835Z
and 0JPT3PZ
and 02H63JZ
and 02PA4MZ

0JH835Z
and 0JPT3PZ
and 02H63JZ
and 02PAXMZ

0JH835Z
and 0JPT3PZ
and 02H63MZ

0JH835Z
and 0JPT3PZ
and 02H64JZ

0JH835Z
and 0JPT3PZ
and 02H64MZ

0JH835Z
and 0JPT3PZ
and 02H70JZ

0JH835Z
and 0JPT3PZ
and 02H70MZ

0JH835Z
and 0JPT3PZ
and 02H73JZ

0JH835Z
and 0JPT3PZ
and 02H73JZ
and 02PA0MZ

0JH835Z
and 0JPT3PZ
and 02H73JZ
and 02PA3MZ

0JH835Z
and 0JPT3PZ
and 02H73JZ
and 02PA4MZ

0JH835Z
and 0JPT3PZ
and 02H73JZ
and 02PAXMZ

0JH835Z
and 0JPT3PZ
and 02H73MZ

0JH835Z
and 0JPT3PZ
and 02H74JZ

0JH835Z
and 0JPT3PZ
and 02H74MZ

0JH835Z
and 0JPT3PZ
and 02HK0JZ

0JH835Z
and 0JPT3PZ
and 02HK0MZ

0JH835Z
and 0JPT3PZ
and 02HK3JZ

0JH835Z
and 0JPT3PZ
and 02HK3JZ
and 02PA0MZ

0JH835Z
and 0JPT3PZ
and 02HK3JZ
and 02PA3MZ

0JH835Z
and 0JPT3PZ
and 02HK3JZ
and 02PA4MZ

0JH835Z
and 0JPT3PZ
and 02HK3JZ
and 02PAXMZ

0JH835Z
and 0JPT3PZ
and 02HK3MZ

0JH835Z
and 0JPT3PZ
and 02HK4JZ

0JH835Z
and 0JPT3PZ
and 02HK4MZ

0JH835Z
and 0JPT3PZ
and 02HL0JZ

0JH835Z
and 0JPT3PZ
and 02HL0MZ

0JH835Z
and 0JPT3PZ
and 02HL3JZ

0JH835Z
and 0JPT3PZ
and 02HL3JZ
and 02PA0MZ

0JH835Z
and 0JPT3PZ
and 02HL3JZ
and 02PA3MZ

0JH835Z
and 0JPT3PZ
and 02HL3JZ

and 02PA4MZ

0JH835Z
and 0JPT3PZ
and 02HL3JZ
and 02PAXMZ

0JH835Z
and 0JPT3PZ
and 02HL3MZ

0JH835Z
and 0JPT3PZ
and 02HL4JZ

0JH835Z
and 0JPT3PZ
and 02HL4MZ

0JH835Z
and 0JPT3PZ
and 02HN0JZ

0JH835Z
and 0JPT3PZ
and 02HN0MZ

0JH835Z
and 0JPT3PZ
and 02HN3JZ

0JH835Z
and 0JPT3PZ
and 02HN3MZ

0JH835Z
and 0JPT3PZ
and 02HN4JZ

0JH835Z
and 0JPT3PZ
and 02HN4MZ

0JH836Z
and 02HK3JZ

0JH836Z
and 02HL3JZ

0JH836Z
and 02HN0JZ

0JH836Z
and 02HN0MZ

0JH836Z
and 02HN3JZ

0JH836Z
and 02HN3MZ

0JH836Z
and 02HN4JZ

0JH836Z
and 02HN4MZ

0JH836Z
and 0JPT0PZ

0JH836Z
and 0JPT0PZ
and 02H40JZ

0JH836Z
and 0JPT0PZ
and 02H40MZ

0JH836Z
and 0JPT0PZ
and 02H44JZ

0JH836Z
and 0JPT0PZ
and 02H44MZ

0JH836Z
and 0JPT0PZ
and 02H60JZ

0JH836Z
and 0JPT0PZ
and 02H60MZ

0JH836Z
and 0JPT0PZ
and 02H63JZ

0JH836Z
and 0JPT0PZ
and 02H63JZ
and 02PA0MZ

0JH836Z
and 0JPT0PZ
and 02H63JZ
and 02PA3MZ

0JH836Z
and 0JPT0PZ
and 02H63JZ
and 02PA4MZ

0JH836Z
and 0JPT0PZ
and 02H63JZ
and 02PAXMZ

0JH836Z
and 0JPT0PZ
and 02H63MZ

0JH836Z
and 0JPT0PZ
and 02H64JZ

0JH836Z
and 0JPT0PZ
and 02H64MZ

0JH836Z
and 0JPT0PZ
and 02H70JZ

0JH836Z
and 0JPT0PZ
and 02H70MZ

0JH836Z
and 0JPT0PZ
and 02H73JZ

0JH836Z
and 0JPT0PZ
and 02H73JZ
and 02PA0MZ

0JH836Z
and 0JPT0PZ
and 02H73JZ
and 02PA3MZ

0JH836Z
and 0JPT0PZ
and 02H73JZ
and 02PA4MZ

0JH836Z
and 0JPT0PZ
and 02H73JZ
and 02PAXMZ

0JH836Z
and 0JPT0PZ
and 02H73MZ

0JH836Z
and 0JPT0PZ
and 02H74JZ

0JH836Z
and 0JPT0PZ
and 02H74MZ

0JH836Z
and 0JPT0PZ
and 02HK0JZ

0JH836Z
and 0JPT0PZ
and 02HK0MZ

0JH836Z
and 0JPT0PZ
and 02HK3JZ

0JH836Z
and 0JPT0PZ
and 02HK3JZ
and 02PA0MZ

0JH836Z
and 0JPT0PZ
and 02HK3JZ
and 02PA3MZ

0JH836Z
and 0JPT0PZ
and 02HK3JZ
and 02PA4MZ

0JH836Z
and 0JPT0PZ
and 02HK3JZ
and 02PAXMZ

0JH836Z
and 0JPT0PZ
and 02HK3MZ

0JH836Z
and 0JPT0PZ
and 02HK4JZ

0JH836Z
and 0JPT0PZ
and 02HK4MZ

0JH836Z
and 0JPT0PZ
and 02HL0JZ

0JH836Z
and 0JPT0PZ
and 02HL0MZ

0JH836Z
and 0JPT0PZ
and 02HL3JZ

0JH836Z
and 0JPT0PZ
and 02HL3JZ
and 02PA0MZ

0JH836Z
and 0JPT0PZ
and 02HL3JZ
and 02PA3MZ

0JH836Z
and 0JPT0PZ
and 02HL3JZ
and 02PA4MZ

0JH836Z
and 0JPT0PZ
and 02HL3JZ
and 02PAXMZ

0JH836Z
and 0JPT0PZ
and 02HL3MZ

0JH836Z
and 0JPT0PZ
and 02HL4JZ

0JH836Z
and 0JPT0PZ
and 02HL4MZ

0JH836Z
and 0JPT0PZ
and 02HN0JZ

0JH836Z
and 0JPT0PZ
and 02HN0MZ

0JH836Z
and 0JPT0PZ
and 02HN3JZ

0JH836Z
and 0JPT0PZ
and 02HN3MZ

0JH836Z
and 0JPT0PZ
and 02HN4JZ

0JH836Z
and 0JPT0PZ
and 02HN4MZ

0JH836Z
and 0JPT3PZ

0JH836Z
and 0JPT3PZ
and 02H40JZ

0JH836Z
and 0JPT3PZ
and 02H40MZ

0JH836Z
and 0JPT3PZ
and 02H44JZ

0JH836Z
and 0JPT3PZ
and 02H44MZ

0JH836Z
and 0JPT3PZ
and 02H60JZ

0JH836Z
and 0JPT3PZ
and 02H60MZ

0JH836Z
and 0JPT3PZ
and 02H63JZ

0JH836Z
and 0JPT3PZ
and 02H63JZ
and 02PA0MZ

0JH836Z
and 0JPT3PZ
and 02H63JZ
and 02PA3MZ

0JH836Z
and 0JPT3PZ
and 02H63JZ
and 02PA4MZ

0JH836Z
and 0JPT3PZ
and 02H63JZ
and 02PAXMZ

0JH836Z
and 0JPT3PZ
and 02H63MZ

0JH836Z
and 0JPT3PZ
and 02H64JZ

0JH836Z
and 0JPT3PZ
and 02H64MZ

0JH836Z
and 0JPT3PZ
and 02H70JZ

0JH836Z
and 0JPT3PZ
and 02H70MZ

0JH836Z
and 0JPT3PZ
and 02H73JZ

0JH836Z
and 0JPT3PZ
and 02H73JZ
and 02PA0MZ

0JH836Z
and 0JPT3PZ
and 02H73JZ
and 02PA3MZ

0JH836Z
and 0JPT3PZ
and 02H73JZ
and 02PA4MZ

0JH836Z
and 0JPT3PZ
and 02H73JZ
and 02PAXMZ

0JH836Z
and 0JPT3PZ
and 02H73MZ

0JH836Z
and 0JPT3PZ
and 02H74JZ

0JH836Z
and 0JPT3PZ
and 02H74MZ

0JH836Z
and 0JPT3PZ
and 02HK0JZ

0JH836Z
and 0JPT3PZ
and 02HK0MZ

0JH836Z
and 0JPT3PZ
and 02HK3JZ

0JH836Z
and 0JPT3PZ
and 02HK3JZ
and 02PA0MZ

0JH836Z
and 0JPT3PZ
and 02HK3JZ
and 02PA3MZ

0JH836Z
and 0JPT3PZ
and 02HK3JZ
and 02PA4MZ

0JH836Z
and 0JPT3PZ
and 02HK3JZ
and 02PAXMZ

0JH836Z
and 0JPT3PZ
and 02HK3MZ

0JH836Z
and 0JPT3PZ
and 02HK4JZ

0JH836Z
and 0JPT3PZ
and 02HK4MZ

0JH836Z
and 0JPT3PZ
and 02HL0JZ

0JH836Z
and 0JPT3PZ
and 02HL0MZ

0JH836Z
and 0JPT3PZ
and 02HL3JZ

0JH836Z
and 0JPT3PZ
and 02HL3JZ
and 02PA0MZ

0JH836Z
and 0JPT3PZ
and 02HL3JZ
and 02PA3MZ

0JH836Z
and 0JPT3PZ
and 02HL3JZ

and 02PA4MZ

0JH836Z
and 0JPT3PZ
and 02HL3JZ
and 02PAXMZ

0JH836Z
and 0JPT3PZ
and 02HL3MZ

0JH836Z
and 0JPT3PZ
and 02HL4JZ

0JH836Z
and 0JPT3PZ
and 02HL4MZ

0JH836Z
and 0JPT3PZ
and 02HN0JZ

0JH836Z
and 0JPT3PZ
and 02HN0MZ

0JH836Z
and 0JPT3PZ
and 02HN3JZ

0JH836Z
and 0JPT3PZ
and 02HN3MZ

0JH836Z
and 0JPT3PZ
and 02HN4JZ

0JH836Z
and 0JPT3PZ
and 02HN4MZ

0JH837Z
and 02H40JZ

0JH837Z
and 02H40MZ

0JH837Z
and 02H43JZ

0JH837Z
and 02H43KZ

0JH837Z
and 02H43MZ

0JH837Z
and 02H44JZ

0JH837Z
and 02H44MZ

0JH837Z
and 02H60JZ

0JH837Z
and 02H60MZ

0JH837Z
and 02H63JZ

0JH837Z
and 02H63JZ
and 02PA0MZ

0JH837Z
and 02H63JZ
and 02PA3MZ

0JH837Z
and 02H63JZ
and 02PA4MZ

0JH837Z
and 02H63JZ
and 02PAXMZ

0JH837Z
and 02H63MZ

0JH837Z
and 02H64JZ

0JH837Z
and 02H64MZ

0JH837Z
and 02H70JZ

0JH837Z
and 02H70MZ

0JH837Z
and 02H73JZ

0JH837Z
and 02H73JZ
and 02PA0MZ

0JH837Z
and 02H73JZ
and 02PA3MZ

0JH837Z
and 02H73JZ
and 02PA4MZ

0JH837Z
and 02H73JZ
and 02PAXMZ

0JH837Z
and 02H73MZ

0JH837Z
and 02H74JZ

0JH837Z
and 02H74MZ

0JH837Z
and 02HK0JZ

0JH837Z
and 02HK0MZ

0JH837Z
and 02HK3JZ

0JH837Z
and 02HK3JZ
and 02PA0MZ

0JH837Z
and 02HK3JZ
and 02PA3MZ

0JH837Z
and 02HK3JZ
and 02PA4MZ

0JH837Z
and 02HK3JZ
and 02PAXMZ

0JH837Z
and 02HK3MZ

0JH837Z
and 02HK4JZ

0JH837Z
and 02HK4MZ

0JH837Z
and 02HL0JZ

0JH837Z
and 02HL0MZ

0JH837Z
and 02HL3JZ

0JH837Z
and 02HL3JZ
and 02PA0MZ

0JH837Z
and 02HL3JZ
and 02PA3MZ

0JH837Z
and 02HL3JZ
and 02PA4MZ

0JH837Z
and 02HL3JZ
and 02PAXMZ

0JH837Z
and 02HL3MZ

0JH837Z
and 02HL4JZ

0JH837Z
and 02HL4MZ

0JH837Z
and 02HN0JZ

0JH837Z
and 02HN0MZ

0JH837Z
and 02HN3JZ

0JH837Z
and 02HN3MZ

0JH837Z
and 02HN4JZ

0JH837Z
and 02HN4MZ

0JH838Z
and 02H40KZ

0JH838Z
and 02H44KZ

0JH838Z
and 02HN0JZ

0JH838Z
and 02HN0KZ

0JH838Z
and 02HN0MZ

0JH838Z
and 02HN3JZ

0JH838Z
and 02HN3KZ

0JH838Z
and 02HN3MZ

0JH838Z
and 02HN4JZ

0JH838Z
and 02HN4KZ

0JH838Z
and 02HN4MZ

0JH839Z
and 02H40KZ

0JH839Z
and 02H43JZ

0JH839Z
and 02H43KZ

0JH839Z
and 02H43MZ

0JH839Z
and 02H44KZ

0JH839Z
and 02H60KZ

0JH839Z
and 02H63KZ

0JH839Z
and 02H64KZ

0JH839Z
and 02H70KZ

0JH839Z
and 02H73KZ

0JH839Z
and 02H74KZ

0JH839Z
and 02HN0JZ

0JH839Z
and 02HN0KZ

0JH839Z
and 02HN0MZ

0JH839Z
and 02HN3JZ

0JH839Z
and 02HN3KZ

0JH839Z
and 02HN3MZ

0JH839Z
and 02HN4JZ

0JH839Z
and 02HN4KZ

0JH839Z
and 02HN4MZ

0JH83BZ
and 00HE0MZ

0JH83BZ
and 00HE3MZ

0JH83BZ
and 00HE4MZ

0JH83BZ
and 00HU0MZ
0JH83BZ
and 00HU3MZ
0JH83BZ
and 00HU4MZ
0JH83BZ
and 00HV0MZ
0JH83BZ
and 00HV3MZ
0JH83BZ
and 00HV4MZ
0JH83BZ
and 01HY0MZ

0JH83BZ
and 01HY3MZ

0JH83BZ
and 01HY4MZ

0JH83BZ
and 0DH60MZ

0JH83BZ
and 0DH63MZ

0JH83BZ
and 0DH64MZ

0JH83CZ
and 00HE0MZ

0JH83CZ
and 00HE3MZ

0JH83CZ
and 00HE4MZ

0JH83CZ
and 00HU0MZ
0JH83CZ
and 00HU3MZ
0JH83CZ
and 00HU4MZ
0JH83CZ
and 00HV0MZ
0JH83CZ
and 00HV3MZ
0JH83CZ
and 00HV4MZ
0JH83CZ
and 01HY0MZ

0JH83CZ
and 01HY3MZ

0JH83CZ
and 01HY4MZ

0JH83CZ
and 0DH60MZ

0JH83CZ
and 0DH63MZ

0JH83CZ
and 0DH64MZ

0JH83DZ
and 00H00MZ

0JH83DZ
and 00H03MZ

0JH83DZ
and 00H04MZ

0JH83DZ
and 00H60MZ

0JH83DZ
and 00H63MZ

0JH83DZ
and 00H64MZ

0JH83DZ
and 00HE0MZ

0JH83DZ
and 00HE3MZ

0JH83DZ
and 00HE4MZ

0JH83DZ
and 00HU0MZ
0JH83DZ
and 00HU3MZ
0JH83DZ
and 00HU4MZ
0JH83DZ
and 00HV0MZ
0JH83DZ
and 00HV3MZ
0JH83DZ
and 00HV4MZ
0JH83DZ
and 01HY0MZ

0JH83DZ
and 01HY3MZ

0JH83DZ
and 01HY4MZ

0JH83DZ
and 0DH60MZ

0JH83DZ
and 0DH63MZ

0JH83DZ
and 0DH64MZ

0JH83EZ
and 00H00MZ

0JH83EZ
and 00H03MZ

0JH83EZ
and 00H04MZ

0JH83EZ
and 00H60MZ

0JH83EZ
and 00H63MZ

0JH83EZ

and 00H64MZ

0JH83EZ and 00HE0MZ

0JH83EZ and 00HE3MZ

0JH83EZ and 00HE4MZ

0JH83EZ and 00HU0MZ

0JH83EZ and 00HU3MZ

0JH83EZ and 00HU4MZ

0JH83EZ and 00HV0MZ

0JH83EZ and 00HV3MZ

0JH83EZ and 00HV4MZ

0JH83EZ and 01HY0MZ

0JH83EZ and 01HY3MZ

0JH83EZ and 01HY4MZ

0JH83EZ and 0DH60MZ

0JH83EZ and 0DH63MZ

0JH83EZ and 0DH64MZ

0JH83PZ and 02H40JZ

0JH83PZ and 02H40MZ

0JH83PZ and 02H44JZ

0JH83PZ and 02H44MZ

0JH83PZ and 02H60JZ

0JH83PZ and 02H60MZ

0JH83PZ and 02H63JZ

0JH83PZ and 02H63JZ and 02PA0MZ

0JH83PZ and 02H63JZ and 02PA3MZ

0JH83PZ and 02H63JZ and 02PA4MZ

0JH83PZ and 02H63JZ and 02PAXMZ

0JH83PZ and 02H63MZ

0JH83PZ and 02H64JZ

0JH83PZ and 02H64MZ

0JH83PZ and 02H70JZ

0JH83PZ and 02H70MZ

0JH83PZ and 02H73JZ

0JH83PZ and 02H73JZ and 02PA0MZ

0JH83PZ and 02H73JZ and 02PA3MZ

0JH83PZ and 02H73JZ and 02PA4MZ

0JH83PZ and 02H73JZ and 02PAXMZ

0JH83PZ and 02H73MZ

0JH83PZ and 02H74JZ

0JH83PZ and 02H74MZ

0JH83PZ and 02HK0JZ

0JH83PZ and 02HK0MZ

0JH83PZ and 02HK3JZ

0JH83PZ and 02HK3JZ and 02PA0MZ

0JH83PZ and 02HK3JZ and 02PA3MZ

0JH83PZ and 02HK3JZ and 02PA4MZ

0JH83PZ and 02HK3JZ and 02PAXMZ

0JH83PZ and 02HK3MZ

0JH83PZ and 02HK4JZ

0JH83PZ and 02HK4MZ

0JH83PZ and 02HL0JZ

0JH83PZ and 02HL0MZ

0JH83PZ and 02HL3JZ

0JH83PZ and 02HL3JZ and 02PA0MZ

0JH83PZ and 02HL3JZ and 02PA3MZ

0JH83PZ and 02HL3JZ and 02PA4MZ

0JH83PZ and 02HL3JZ and 02PAXMZ

0JH83PZ and 02HL3MZ

0JH83PZ and 02HL4JZ

0JH83PZ and 02HL4MZ

0JH83PZ and 02HN0JZ

0JH83PZ and 02HN0MZ

0JH83PZ and 02HN3JZ

0JH83PZ and 02HN3MZ

0JH83PZ and 02HN4JZ

0JH83PZ and 02HN4MZ

0NH00NZ and 00H00MZ

0NH00NZ and 00H03MZ

0NH00NZ and 00H04MZ

0NH00NZ and 00H60MZ

0NH00NZ and 00H63MZ

0NH00NZ and 00H64MZ

0PS33ZZ and 0PU33JZ

0PS43ZZ and 0PU43JZ

0QS03ZZ and 0QU03JZ

0QS13ZZ and 0QU13JZ

0QSS3ZZ and 0QUS3JZ

0SP908Z and 0SR9019

0SP908Z and 0SR901A

0SP908Z and 0SR901Z

0SP908Z and 0SR9029

0SP908Z and 0SR902A

0SP908Z and 0SR902Z

0SP908Z and 0SR9039

0SP908Z and 0SR903A

0SP908Z and 0SR903Z

0SP908Z and 0SR9049

0SP908Z and 0SR904A

0SP908Z and 0SR904Z

0SP908Z and 0SR90J9

0SP908Z and 0SR90JA

0SP908Z and 0SR90JZ

0SP908Z and 0SRA009

0SP908Z and 0SRA00A

0SP908Z and 0SRA00Z

0SP908Z and 0SRA019

0SP908Z and 0SRA01A

0SP908Z and 0SRA01Z

0SP908Z and 0SRA039

0SP908Z and 0SRA03A

0SP908Z and 0SRA03Z

0SP908Z and 0SRA0J9

0SP908Z and 0SRA0JA

0SP908Z and 0SRA0JZ

0SP908Z and 0SRR019

0SP908Z and 0SRR01A

0SP908Z and 0SRR01Z

0SP908Z and 0SRR039

0SP908Z and 0SRR03A

0SP908Z and 0SRR03Z

0SP908Z and 0SRR0J9

0SP908Z and 0SRR0JA

0SP908Z and 0SRR0JZ

0SP908Z and 0SU909Z

0SP908Z and 0SUA09Z

0SP908Z and 0SUR09Z

0SP909Z and 0SR9019

0SP909Z and 0SR901A

0SP909Z and 0SR901Z

0SP909Z and 0SR9029

0SP909Z and 0SR902A

0SP909Z and 0SR902Z

0SP909Z and 0SR9039

0SP909Z and 0SR903A

0SP909Z and 0SR903Z

0SP909Z and 0SR9049

0SP909Z and 0SR904A

0SP909Z and 0SR904Z

0SP909Z and 0SR90J9

0SP909Z and 0SR90JA

0SP909Z and 0SR90JZ

0SP909Z and 0SRA009

0SP909Z and 0SRA00A

0SP909Z and 0SRA00Z

0SP909Z and 0SRA019

0SP909Z and 0SRA01A

0SP909Z and 0SRA01Z

0SP909Z and 0SRA039

0SP909Z and 0SRA03A

0SP909Z and 0SRA03Z

0SP909Z and 0SRA0J9

0SP909Z and 0SRA0JA

0SP909Z and 0SRA0JZ

0SP909Z and 0SRR019

0SP909Z and 0SRR01A

0SP909Z and 0SRR01Z

0SP909Z and 0SRR039

0SP909Z and 0SRR03A

0SP909Z and 0SRR03Z

0SP909Z and 0SRR0J9

0SP909Z and 0SRR0JA

0SP909Z and 0SRR0JZ

0SP909Z and 0SU909Z

0SP909Z and 0SUA09Z

0SP909Z and 0SUR09Z

0SP90BZ and 0SR9019

0SP90BZ and 0SR901A

0SP90BZ and 0SR901Z

0SP90BZ and 0SR9029

0SP90BZ and 0SR902A

0SP90BZ and 0SR902Z

0SP90BZ and 0SR9039

0SP90BZ and 0SR903A

0SP90BZ and 0SR903Z

0SP90BZ and 0SR9049

0SP90BZ and 0SR904A

0SP90BZ and 0SR904Z

0SP90BZ and 0SR90J9

0SP90BZ and 0SR90JA

0SP90BZ and 0SR90JZ

0SP90BZ and 0SRA009

0SP90BZ and 0SRA00A

0SP90BZ and 0SRA00Z

0SP90BZ and 0SRA019

0SP90BZ and 0SRA01A

0SP90BZ and 0SRA01Z

0SP90BZ and 0SRA039

0SP90BZ and 0SRA03A

0SP90BZ and 0SRA03Z

0SP90BZ and 0SRA0J9

0SP90BZ and 0SRA0JA

0SP90BZ and 0SRA0JZ

0SP90BZ and 0SRR019

0SP90BZ and 0SRR01A

0SP90BZ and 0SRR01Z

0SP90BZ and 0SRR039

0SP90BZ and 0SRR03A

0SP90BZ and 0SRR03Z

0SP90BZ and 0SRR0J9

0SP90BZ and 0SRR0JA

0SP90BZ and 0SRR0JZ

0SP90BZ and 0SU909Z

0SP90BZ and 0SUA09Z

0SP90BZ and 0SUR09Z

0SP90JZ and 0SR9019

0SP90JZ and 0SR901A

0SP90JZ and 0SR901Z

0SP90JZ and 0SR9029

0SP90JZ and 0SR902A

0SP90JZ and 0SR902Z

0SP90JZ and 0SR9039

0SP90JZ and 0SR903A

0SP90JZ and 0SR903Z

0SP90JZ and 0SR9049

0SP90JZ and 0SR904A

0SP90JZ and 0SR904Z

0SP90JZ and 0SR90J9

0SP90JZ and 0SR90JA

0SP90JZ and 0SR90JZ

0SP90JZ and 0SRA009

0SP90JZ and 0SRA00A

0SP90JZ and 0SRA00Z

0SP90JZ and 0SRA019

0SP90JZ and 0SRA01A

0SP90JZ and 0SRA01Z

0SP90JZ and 0SRA039

0SP90JZ and 0SRA03A

0SP90JZ and 0SRA03Z

0SP90JZ and 0SRA0J9

0SP90JZ and 0SRA0JA

0SP90JZ and 0SRA0JZ

0SP90JZ and 0SRR019

0SP90JZ and 0SRR01A

0SP90JZ and 0SRR01Z

0SP90JZ and 0SRR039

0SP90JZ and 0SRR03A

0SP90JZ and 0SRR03Z

0SP90JZ and 0SRR0J9

0SP90JZ and 0SRR0JA

0SP90JZ and 0SRR0JZ

0SP948Z and 0SR9019

0SP948Z and 0SR901A

0SP948Z and 0SR901Z

0SP948Z and 0SR9029

0SP948Z and 0SR902A

0SP948Z and 0SR902Z

0SP948Z and 0SR9039

0SP948Z and 0SR903A

0SP948Z and 0SR903Z

0SP948Z and 0SR9049

0SP948Z and 0SR904A

0SP948Z and 0SR904Z

0SP948Z and 0SR90J9

0SP948Z and 0SR90JA

0SP948Z and 0SR90JZ

0SP948Z and 0SRA009

0SP948Z and 0SRA00A

0SP948Z and 0SRA00Z

0SP948Z and 0SRA019

0SP948Z and 0SRA01A

0SP948Z and 0SRA01Z

0SP948Z and 0SRA039

0SP948Z and 0SRA03A

0SP948Z and 0SRA03Z

0SP948Z and 0SRA0J9

0SP948Z and 0SRA0JA

0SP948Z and 0SRA0JZ

0SP948Z and 0SRR019

0SP948Z and 0SRR01A

0SP948Z and 0SRR01Z

0SP948Z and 0SRR039

0SP948Z and 0SRR03A

0SP948Z and 0SRR03Z

0SP948Z and 0SRR0J9

0SP948Z and 0SRR0JA

0SP948Z and 0SRR0JZ

0SP948Z and 0SU909Z

0SP948Z and 0SUA09Z

0SP948Z and 0SUR09Z

0SP94JZ and 0SR9019

0SP94JZ and 0SR901A

0SP94JZ and 0SR901Z

0SP94JZ and 0SR9029

0SP94JZ and 0SR902A

0SP94JZ and 0SR902Z

0SP94JZ and 0SR9039

0SP94JZ and 0SR903A

0SP94JZ and 0SR903Z

0SP94JZ and 0SR9049

0SP94JZ and 0SR904A

0SP94JZ and 0SR904Z

0SP94JZ and 0SR90J9

0SP94JZ and 0SR90JA

0SP94JZ and 0SR90JZ

0SP94JZ and 0SRA009

0SP94JZ and 0SRA00A

0SP94JZ and 0SRA00Z

0SP94JZ and 0SRA019

0SP94JZ and 0SRA01A

0SP94JZ and 0SRA01Z

0SP94JZ and 0SRA039

0SP94JZ and 0SRA03A

0SP94JZ and 0SRA03Z

0SP94JZ and 0SRA0J9

0SP94JZ and 0SRA0JA

0SP94JZ and 0SRA0JZ

0SP94JZ and 0SRR019

0SP94JZ and 0SRR01A

0SP94JZ and 0SRR01Z

0SP94JZ and 0SRR039

0SP94JZ and 0SRR03A

0SP94JZ and 0SRR03Z

0SP94JZ and 0SRR0J9

0SP94JZ and 0SRR0JA

0SP94JZ and 0SRR0JZ

0SP94JZ and 0SU909Z

0SP94JZ and 0SUA09Z

0SP94JZ and 0SUR09Z

0SPB08Z and 0SRB019

0SPB08Z and 0SRB01A

0SPB08Z and 0SRB01Z

0SPB08Z and 0SRB029

0SPB08Z and 0SRB02A

0SPB08Z and 0SRB02Z

0SPB08Z and 0SRB039

0SPB08Z and 0SRB03A

0SPB08Z and 0SRB03Z

0SPB08Z and 0SRB049

0SPB08Z and 0SRB04A

0SPB08Z and 0SRB04Z

0SPB08Z and 0SRB0J9

0SPB08Z and 0SRB0JA

0SPB08Z and 0SRB0JZ

0SPB08Z and 0SRE009

0SPB08Z and 0SRE00A

0SPB08Z and 0SRE00Z

0SPB08Z and 0SRE019

0SPB08Z and 0SRE01A

0SPB08Z and 0SRE01Z

0SPB08Z and 0SRE039

0SPB08Z and 0SRE03A

0SPB08Z and 0SRE03Z

0SPB08Z and 0SRE0J9

0SPB08Z and 0SRE0JA

0SPB08Z and 0SRE0JZ

0SPB08Z and 0SRS019

0SPB08Z and 0SRS01A

0SPB08Z and 0SRS01Z

0SPB08Z and 0SRS039

0SPB08Z and 0SRS03A

0SPB08Z and 0SRS03Z

0SPB08Z and 0SRS0J9

0SPB08Z and 0SRS0JA

0SPB08Z and 0SRS0JZ

0SPB08Z and 0SUB09Z

0SPB08Z and 0SUE09Z

0SPB08Z and 0SUS09Z

0SPB09Z and 0SRB019

0SPB09Z and 0SRB01A

0SPB09Z and 0SRB01Z

0SPB09Z and 0SRB029

0SPB09Z and 0SRB02A

0SPB09Z and 0SRB02Z

0SPB09Z and 0SRB039

0SPB09Z and 0SRB03A

0SPB09Z and 0SRB03Z

0SPB09Z and 0SRB049

0SPB09Z and 0SRB04A

0SPB09Z and 0SRB04Z

0SPB09Z and 0SRB0J9

0SPB09Z and 0SRB0JA

0SPB09Z and 0SRB0JZ

0SPB09Z and 0SRE009

0SPB09Z and 0SRE00A

0SPB09Z and 0SRE00Z

0SPB09Z and 0SRE019

0SPB09Z and 0SRE01A

0SPB09Z and 0SRE01Z

0SPB09Z and 0SRE039

0SPB09Z and 0SRE03A

0SPB09Z and 0SRE03Z

0SPB09Z and 0SRE0J9

0SPB09Z and 0SRE0JA

0SPB09Z and 0SRE0JZ

0SPB09Z and 0SRS019

0SPB09Z and 0SRS01A

0SPB09Z and 0SRS01Z

0SPB09Z and 0SRS039

0SPB09Z and 0SRS03A

0SPB09Z and 0SRS03Z

0SPB09Z and 0SRS0J9

0SPB09Z and 0SRS0JA

0SPB09Z and 0SRS0JZ

0SPB09Z and 0SUB09Z

0SPB09Z and 0SUE09Z

0SPB09Z and 0SUS09Z

0SPB0BZ and 0SRB019

0SPB0BZ and 0SRB01A

0SPB0BZ and 0SRB01Z

0SPB0BZ and 0SRB029

0SPB0BZ and 0SRB02A

0SPB0BZ and 0SRB02Z

0SPB0BZ and 0SRB039

0SPB0BZ and 0SRB03A

0SPB0BZ and 0SRB03Z

0SPB0BZ and 0SRB049

0SPB0BZ and 0SRB04A

0SPB0BZ and 0SRB04Z

0SPB0BZ and 0SRB0J9

0SPB0BZ and 0SRB0JA

0SPB0BZ and 0SRB0JZ

0SPB0BZ and 0SRE009

0SPB0BZ and 0SRE00A

0SPB0BZ and 0SRE00Z

0SPB0BZ and 0SRE019

0SPB0BZ and 0SRE01A

0SPB0BZ and 0SRE01Z

0SPB0BZ and 0SRE039

0SPB0BZ and 0SRE03A

0SPB0BZ and 0SRE03Z

0SPB0BZ and 0SRE0J9

0SPB0BZ and 0SRE0JA

0SPB0BZ and 0SRE0JZ

0SPB0BZ and 0SRS019

0SPB0BZ and 0SRS01A

0SPB0BZ and 0SRS01Z

0SPB0BZ and 0SRS039

0SPB0BZ and 0SRS03A

0SPB0BZ and 0SRS03Z

0SPB0BZ and 0SRS0J9

0SPB0BZ and 0SRS0JA

0SPB0BZ and 0SRS0JZ

0SPB0BZ and 0SUB09Z

0SPB0BZ and 0SUE09Z

0SPB0BZ and 0SUS09Z

0SPB0JZ and 0SRB019

0SPB0JZ and 0SRB01A

0SPB0JZ and 0SRB01Z

0SPB0JZ and 0SRB029

0SPB0JZ and 0SRB02A

0SPB0JZ and 0SRB02Z

0SPB0JZ and 0SRB039

0SPB0JZ and 0SRB03A

0SPB0JZ and 0SRB03Z

0SPB0JZ and 0SRB049

0SPB0JZ and 0SRB04A

0SPB0JZ and 0SRB04Z

0SPB0JZ and 0SRB0J9

0SPB0JZ and 0SRB0JA

0SPB0JZ and 0SRB0JZ

0SPB0JZ and 0SRE009

0SPB0JZ and 0SRE00A

0SPB0JZ and 0SRE00Z

0SPB0JZ and 0SRE019

0SPB0JZ and 0SRE01A

0SPB0JZ and 0SRE01Z

0SPB0JZ and 0SRE039

0SPB0JZ and 0SRE03A

0SPB0JZ and 0SRE03Z

0SPB0JZ and 0SRE0J9

0SPB0JZ and 0SRE0JA

0SPB0JZ and 0SRE0JZ

0SPB0JZ and 0SRS019

0SPB0JZ and 0SRS01A

0SPB0JZ and 0SRS01Z

0SPB0JZ and 0SRS039

0SPB0JZ and 0SRS03A

0SPB0JZ and 0SRS03Z

0SPB0JZ and 0SRS0J9

0SPB0JZ and 0SRS0JA

0SPB0JZ and 0SRS0JZ

0SPB48Z and 0SRB019

0SPB48Z and 0SRB01A

0SPB48Z and 0SRB01Z

0SPB48Z and 0SRB029

0SPB48Z and 0SRB02A

0SPB48Z and 0SRB02Z

0SPB48Z and 0SRB039

0SPB48Z and 0SRB03A

0SPB48Z and 0SRB03Z

0SPB48Z and 0SRB049

0SPB48Z and 0SRB04A

0SPB48Z and 0SRB04Z

0SPB48Z and 0SRB0J9

0SPB48Z and 0SRB0JA

0SPB48Z and 0SRB0JZ

0SPB48Z and 0SRE009

0SPB48Z and 0SRE00A

0SPB48Z and 0SRE00Z

0SPB48Z and 0SRE019

0SPB48Z and 0SRE01A

0SPB48Z and 0SRE01Z

0SPB48Z and 0SRE039

0SPB48Z and 0SRE03A

0SPB48Z and 0SRE03Z

0SPB48Z and 0SRE0J9

0SPB48Z and 0SRE0JA

0SPB48Z and 0SRE0JZ

0SPB48Z and 0SRS019

0SPB48Z and 0SRS01A

0SPB48Z and 0SRS01Z

0SPB48Z and 0SRS039

0SPB48Z and 0SRS03A

0SPB48Z and 0SRS03Z

0SPB48Z and 0SRS0J9

0SPB48Z and 0SRS0JA

0SPB48Z and 0SRS0JZ

0SPB48Z and 0SUB09Z

0SPB48Z and 0SUE09Z

0SPB48Z and 0SUS09Z

0SPB4JZ and 0SRB019

0SPB4JZ and 0SRB01A

0SPB4JZ and 0SRB01Z

0SPB4JZ and 0SRB029

0SPB4JZ and 0SRB02A

0SPB4JZ and 0SRB02Z

0SPB4JZ and 0SRB039

0SPB4JZ and 0SRB03A

0SPB4JZ and 0SRB03Z

0SPB4JZ and 0SRB049

0SPB4JZ and 0SRB04A

0SPB4JZ and 0SRB04Z

0SPB4JZ and 0SRB0J9

0SPB4JZ and 0SRB0JA

0SPB4JZ and 0SRB0JZ

0SPB4JZ and 0SRE009

0SPB4JZ and 0SRE00A

0SPB4JZ and 0SRE00Z

0SPB4JZ and 0SRE019

0SPB4JZ and 0SRE01A

0SPB4JZ and 0SRE01Z

0SPB4JZ and 0SRE039

0SPB4JZ and 0SRE03A

0SPB4JZ and 0SRE03Z

0SPB4JZ and 0SRE0J9

0SPB4JZ and 0SRE0JA

0SPB4JZ and 0SRE0JZ

0SPB4JZ and 0SRS019

0SPB4JZ and 0SRS01A

0SPB4JZ and 0SRS01Z

0SPB4JZ and 0SRS039

0SPB4JZ and 0SRS03A

0SPB4JZ and 0SRS03Z

0SPB4JZ and 0SRS0J9

0SPB4JZ and 0SRS0JA

0SPB4JZ and 0SRS0JZ

0SPB4JZ and 0SUB09Z

0SPB4JZ and 0SUE09Z

0SPB4JZ and 0SUS09Z

0SPC08Z and 0SRC0J9

0SPC08Z and 0SRC0JA

0SPC08Z and 0SRC0JZ

0SPC08Z and 0SRT0J9

0SPC08Z and 0SRT0JA

0SPC08Z and 0SRT0JZ

0SPC08Z and 0SRV0J9

0SPC08Z and 0SRV0JA

0SPC08Z and 0SRV0JZ

0SPC09Z and 0SRC0J9

0SPC09Z and 0SRC0JA

0SPC09Z and 0SRC0JZ

0SPC09Z and 0SRT0J9

0SPC09Z and 0SRT0JA

0SPC09Z and 0SRT0JZ

0SPC09Z and 0SRV0J9

0SPC09Z and 0SRV0JA

0SPC09Z and 0SRV0JZ

0SPC09Z and 0SUV09Z

0SPC0JZ and 0SRC0J9

0SPC0JZ and 0SRC0JA

0SPC0JZ and 0SRC0JZ

0SPC0JZ and 0SRT0J9

0SPC0JZ and 0SRT0JA

0SPC0JZ and 0SRT0JZ

0SPC0JZ and 0SRV0J9

0SPC0JZ and 0SRV0JA

0SPC0JZ and 0SRV0JZ

0SPC38Z and 0SRC0J9

0SPC38Z and 0SRC0JA

0SPC38Z and 0SRC0JZ

0SPC38Z and 0SRT0J9

0SPC38Z and 0SRT0JA

0SPC38Z and 0SRT0JZ

0SPC38Z and 0SRV0J9

0SPC38Z and 0SRV0JA

0SPC38Z and 0SRV0JZ

0SPC48Z and 0SRC0J9

0SPC48Z and 0SRC0JA

0SPC48Z and 0SRC0JZ

0SPC48Z and 0SRT0J9

0SPC48Z and 0SRT0JA

0SPC48Z and 0SRT0JZ

0SPC48Z and 0SRV0J9

0SPC48Z and 0SRV0JA

0SPC48Z and 0SRV0JZ

0SPC4JZ and 0SRC0J9

0SPC4JZ and 0SRC0JA

0SPC4JZ and 0SRC0JZ

0SPC4JZ and 0SRT0J9

0SPC4JZ and 0SRT0JA

0SPC4JZ and 0SRT0JZ

0SPC4JZ and 0SRV0J9

0SPC4JZ and 0SRV0JA

0SPC4JZ and 0SRV0JZ

0SPD08Z and 0SRD0J9

0SPD08Z and 0SRD0JA

0SPD08Z and 0SRD0JZ

0SPD08Z and 0SRU0JA

0SPD08Z and 0SRU0JA

0SPD08Z and 0SRU0JZ

0SPD08Z and 0SRW0J9

0SPD08Z and 0SRW0JA

0SPD08Z and 0SRW0JZ

0SPD09Z and 0SRD0J9

0SPD09Z and 0SRD0JA

0SPD09Z and 0SRD0JZ

0SPD09Z and 0SRU0J9

0SPD09Z and 0SRU0JA

0SPD09Z and 0SRU0JZ

0SPD09Z and 0SRW0J9

0SPD09Z and 0SRW0JA

0SPD09Z and 0SRW0JZ

0SPD09Z and 0SUW09Z

0SPD0JZ
and 0SRD0J9

0SPD0JZ
and 0SRD0JA

0SPD0JZ
and 0SRD0JZ

0SPD0JZ
and 0SRU0J9

0SPD0JZ
and 0SRU0JA

0SPD0JZ
and 0SRU0JZ

0SPD0JZ
and 0SRW0J9

0SPD0JZ
and 0SRW0JA

0SPD0JZ
and 0SRW0JZ

0SPD38Z
and 0SRD0J9

0SPD38Z
and 0SRD0JA

0SPD38Z
and 0SRD0JZ

0SPD38Z
and 0SRU0JA

0SPD38Z
and 0SRU0JA

0SPD38Z
and 0SRU0JZ

0SPD38Z
and 0SRW0J9

0SPD38Z
and 0SRW0JA

0SPD38Z
and 0SRW0JZ

0SPD48Z
and 0SRD0J9

0SPD48Z
and 0SRD0JA

0SPD48Z
and 0SRD0JZ

0SPD48Z
and 0SRU0JA

0SPD48Z
and 0SRU0JA

0SPD48Z
and 0SRU0JZ

0SPD48Z
and 0SRW0J9

0SPD48Z
and 0SRW0JA

0SPD48Z
and 0SRW0JZ

0SPD4JZ
and 0SRD0J9

0SPD4JZ
and 0SRD0JA

0SPD4JZ
and 0SRD0JZ

0SPD4JZ
and 0SRU0J9

0SPD4JZ
and 0SRU0JA

0SPD4JZ
and 0SRU0JZ

0SPD4JZ
and 0SRW0J9

0SPD4JZ
and 0SRW0JA

0SPD4JZ
and 0SRW0JZ

0TQB0ZZ
and 0WQFXZ2

0TQB0ZZ
and 0WQFXZZ

0TQB3ZZ
and 0WQFXZ2

0TQB3ZZ
and 0WQFXZZ

0TQB4ZZ
and 0WQFXZ2

0TQB4ZZ
and 0WQFXZZ

0TTB0ZZ
and 0TTD0ZZ
and 0UT20ZZ
and 0UT70ZZ
and 0UT90ZZ
and 0UTC0ZZ
and 0UTG0ZZ

0TY00Z0
and 0FYG0Z0

0TY00Z0
and 0FYG0Z1

0TY00Z0
and 0FYG0Z2

0TY00Z1
and 0FYG0Z0

0TY00Z1
and 0FYG0Z1

0TY00Z1
and 0FYG0Z2

0TY00Z2
and 0FYG0Z0

0TY00Z2
and 0FYG0Z1

0TY00Z2
and 0FYG0Z2

0TY10Z0
and 0FYG0Z0

0TY10Z0
and 0FYG0Z1

0TY10Z0
and 0FYG0Z2

0TY10Z1
and 0FYG0Z0

0TY10Z1
and 0FYG0Z1

0TY10Z1
and 0FYG0Z2

0TY10Z2
and 0FYG0Z0

0TY10Z2
and 0FYG0Z1

0TY10Z2
and 0FYG0Z2

0UT40ZZ
and 0UT90ZZ
and 0UTC0ZZ

0UT44ZZ
and 0UT94ZZ
and 0UTC4ZZ

0UT44ZZ
and 0UT9FZZ
and 0UTC4ZZ

0UT47ZZ
and 0UT97ZZ
and 0UTC7ZZ

0UT47ZZ
and 0UT97ZZ
and 0UTC8ZZ

0UT47ZZ
and 0UT98ZZ
and 0UTC7ZZ

0UT47ZZ
and 0UT98ZZ
and 0UTC8ZZ

0UT48ZZ
and 0UT97ZZ
and 0UTC7ZZ

0UT48ZZ
and 0UT97ZZ
and 0UTC8ZZ

0UT48ZZ
and 0UT98ZZ
and 0UTC7ZZ

0UT48ZZ
and 0UT98ZZ
and 0UTC8ZZ

0VT00ZZ
and 0VT30ZZ

0VT00ZZ
and 0VT34ZZ

0VT04ZZ
and 0VT30ZZ

0VT04ZZ
and 0VT34ZZ

0VT07ZZ
and 0VT30ZZ

0VT07ZZ
and 0VT34ZZ

0VT08ZZ
and 0VT30ZZ

0VT08ZZ
and 0VT34ZZ

One of
0RG7070
0RG70A0
0RG70J0
0RG70K0
0RG70Z0
0RG7370
0RG73A0
0RG73J0
0RG73K0
0RG73Z0
0RG7470
0RG74A0
0RG74J0
0RG74K0
0RG74Z0
with one of
0SG1070
0SG10A0
0SG10J0
0SG10K0
0SG10Z0
0SG1370
0SG13A0
0SG13J0
0SG13K0
0SG13Z0
0SG1470
0SG14A0
0SG14J0
0SG14K0
0SG14Z0

One of
0RG7071
0RG707J
0RG70A1
0RG70AJ
0RG70J1
0RG70JJ
0RG70K1
0RG70KJ
0RG70Z1
0RG70ZJ
0RG7371
0RG737J
0RG73A1
0RG73AJ
0RG73J1
0RG73JJ
0RG73K1
0RG73KJ
0RG73Z1
0RG73ZJ
0RG7471
0RG747J
0RG74A1
0RG74AJ
0RG74J1
0RG74JJ
0RG74K1
0RG74KJ
0RG74Z1
0RG74ZJ
with one of
0SG1071
0SG107J
0SG10A1
0SG10AJ
0SG10J1
0SG10JJ
0SG10K1
0SG10KJ
0SG10Z1
0SG10ZJ
0SG1371
0SG137J
0SG13A1
0SG13AJ
0SG13J1
0SG13JJ
0SG13K1
0SG13KJ
0SG13Z1
0SG13ZJ
0SG1471
0SG147J
0SG14A1
0SG14AJ
0SG14J1
0SG14JJ
0SG14K1
0SG14KJ
0SG14Z1
0SG14ZJ

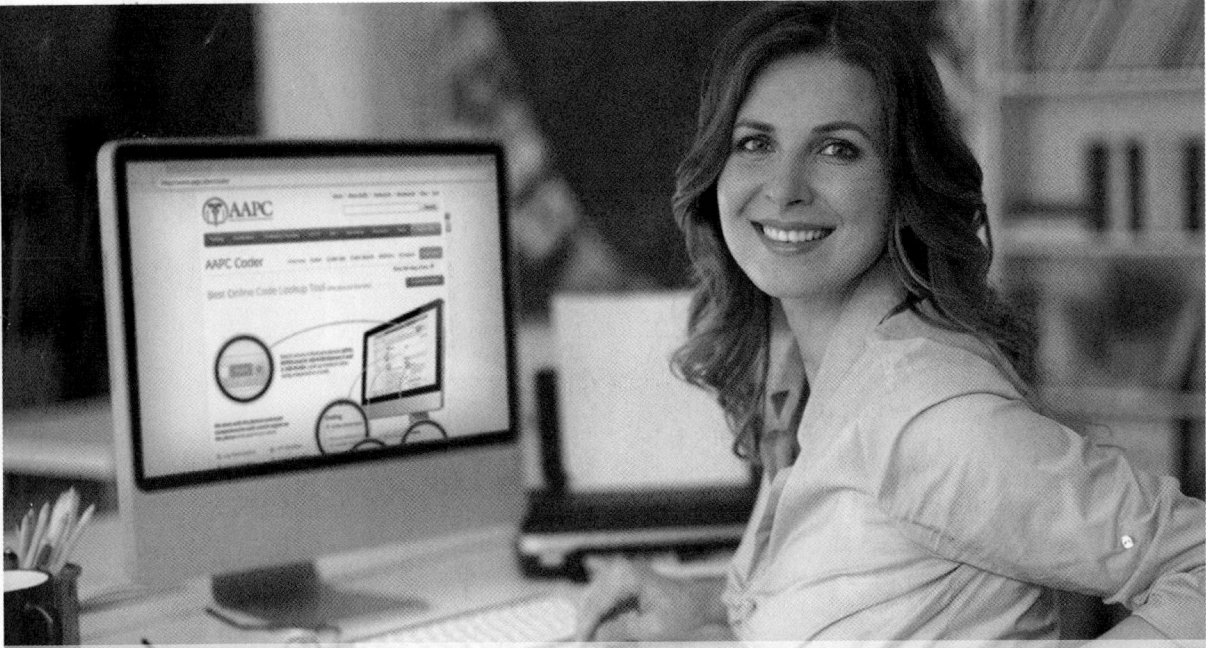

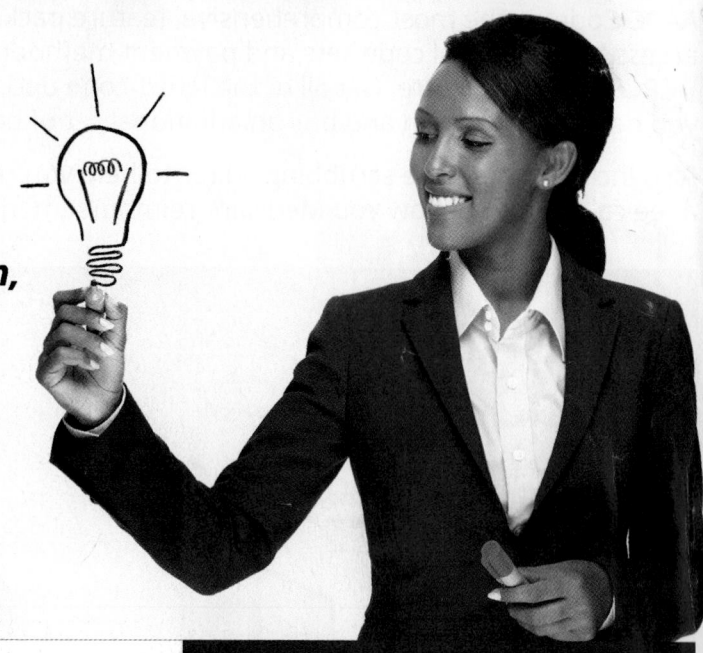